5.0 APPLY LEGAL CONCEPTS TO PRACTICE

5.1 Document Accurately

5.2 Determine Needs for Documentation and Reporting

5.3 Use Appropriate Guidelines When Releasing Records or Information

5.4 Follow Established Policy in Initiating or Terminating Medical Treatment

5.5 Dispose of Controlled Substances in Compliance With Government Regulations

5.6 Maintain Licenses and Accreditation

5.7 Monitor Legislation Related to Current Healthcare Issues and Practice

Develop* and Maintain Policy and Procedure Manuals

Establish* Risk Management Protocol for the Practice

6.0 MANAGE THE OFFICE

6.1 Maintain the Physical Plant

6.2 Operate and Maintain Facilities and Equipment Safely

6.3 Inventory Equipment and Supplies

6.4 Evaluate and Recommend Equipment and Supplies for a Practice

6.5 Maintain Liability Coverage

6.6 Exercise Efficient Time Management

Supervise* Personnel

Develop* Job Descriptions

Interview* and Recommend New Personnel

Negotiate* Leases and Prices for Equipment and Supply Contracts

7.0 PROVIDE INSTRUCTION

7.1 Orient Patients to Office Policies and Procedures

7.2 Instruct Patients With Special Needs

7.3 Teach Patients Methods of Health Promotion and Disease Prevention

7.4 Orient and Train Personnel

Provide* Health Information for Public Use

Supervise* Student Practicums

Conduct* Continuing Education Activities

Develop* Educational Materials

8.0 MANAGE PRACTICE FINANCES

8.1 Use Manual Bookkeeping Systems

8.2 Implement Current Procedural Terminology and ICD-9 Coding

8.3 Analyze and Use Current Third-Party Guidelines for Reimbursement

8.4 Manage Accounts Receivable

8.5 Manage Accounts Payable

8.6 Maintain Records for Accounting and Banking Purposes

8.7 Process Employee Payroll

Manage* Personnel Benefits and Records

*Denotes advanced-level skills.
The medical assistant should be able to perform all other skills after completing a CAHEA-accredited program and starting a first job.

DEVELOPED BY:
The American Association of Medical Assistants, Inc.

CONSULTANTS:
Mary Lee Seibert, EdD, CMA
and
Patricia A. Amos, MS

COMPREHENSIVE MEDICAL ASSISTING
Competencies for Administrative and Clinical Practice
Third Edition

Mary Ann Frew, MS, RN, CMA-C
Director, Office of Cooperative Education
Gannon University
and Former Director
Medical Assistant Program
Department of Health Sciences
Gannon University
Erie, Pennsylvania

Karen Lane, CMA-AC
Former Program Director
Medical Assisting Program
Medix School
Baltimore, Maryland
and Former Chair
Curriculum Review Board
American Association of Medical Assistants Endowment

David R. Frew, MA, DBA
Director, Health Services Administration Program
Gannon University
Erie, Pennsylvania

 F. A. DAVIS COMPANY • Philadelphia

F. A. Davis Company
1915 Arch Street
Philadelphia, PA 19103

Printed in the United States of America

Last digit indicates print number: 10 9 8 7 6 5 4 3 2

Allied Health Publisher: Jean-François Vilain
Developmental Editor: Ralph Zickgraf
Production Editor: Arofan Gregory
Cover Design: Steven R. Morrone

As new scientific information becomes available through basic and clinical research, recommended treatments and drug therapies undergo changes. The authors and publisher have done everything possible to make this book accurate, up to date, and in accord with accepted standards at the time of publication. The authors, editors, and publisher are not responsible for errors or omissions or for consequences from application of the book, and make no warranty, expressed or implied, in regard to the contents of the book. Any practice described in this book should be applied by the reader in accordance with professional standards of care used in regard to the unique circumstances that may apply in each situation. The reader is advised always to check product information (package inserts) for changes and new information regarding dose and contraindications before administering any drug. Caution is especially urged when using new or infrequently ordered drugs.

Library of Congress Cataloging in Publication Data

Frew, Mary Ann.
  Comprehensive medical assisting : competencies for administrative and clinical practice / Mary Ann Frew, Karen Lane, David R. Frew. — 3rd ed.
      p.   cm.
  Includes bibliographical references and index.
  ISBN 0-8036-3871-X (alk. paper)
    1. Medical assistants. 2. Physicians' assistants. I. Lane, Karen, 1946–   . II. Frew, David R. III. Title.
  [DNLM: 1. Physicians' Assistants. W 21.5 F892c 1995]
  R728.8.F74 1995
  610.69′53 — dc20
  DNLM/DLC
  for Library of Congress   94-13508
                                                                                  CIP

PREFACE

Since the first edition of this book was published, much has changed—in our lives, in the profession of medical assisting, and in medical assisting education. We have grown wiser, we hope, as well as older; medical assisting is a more sophisticated, respected, and demanding profession; and medical assisting education is correspondingly more rigorous. There is ever more to learn and, it seems, less time in which to teach it. Our reason for writing *Comprehensive Medical Assisting*, however, and revising it, remains the same: To help each student reach the highest level of professional knowledge and skill by focusing on the competencies required of the best prepared and most respected medical assistants working today.

In preparing a third edition, we wanted not only to update the administrative and clinical information and maintain the comprehensive coverage of a constantly evolving body of knowledge and skills, but also to make the book a more useful, more accessible, and easier one from which to learn and to teach. To reach these goals, we:

- ❏ Revised the Procedures—retaining the emphasis on Terminal Performance Objectives and underlying principles while increasing the number and quality of illustrations
- ❏ Increased the number of administrative Procedures by almost 400 percent
- ❏ Reorganized the Administrative Procedures section to make course design easier and more logical by:
  - ❏ Expanding the coverage of entry-level administrative competencies
  - ❏ Updating the chapters on communications and business machines
  - ❏ Rewriting the insurance chapter to reflect the latest changes and account, as much as possible, for the many more changes to come
- ❏ Recast the Clinical Procedures section to account for the multitude of far-reaching changes in clinical practice, particularly in regard to infection control, by:
  - ❏ Expanding one chapter on asepsis, sterilization, and office surgery to two, with complete coverage of Universal Precautions and OSHA Guidelines
  - ❏ Expanding two chapters on laboratory procedures to three, with exhaustive coverage of entry-level and advanced procedures

Throughout both the Administrative Procedures and Clinical Procedures sections, each chapter contains a discussion of patient teaching considerations relevant to and ethical and legal implications of the chapter content. And most chapters feature Highlights, which illuminate controversial topics or give glimpses of recent related developments.

In pursuit of our goal of making the third edition of *Comprehensive Medical Assisting* as useful and effective a teaching tool as possible, we carefully refined the chapter pedagogical features, which now include:

- ❏ Chapter-opening quotes that set the tone
- ❏ Outlines that map the material covered
- ❏ Learning Objectives and Performance Objectives, to help student and teacher set goals
- ❏ Listings of relevant DACUM components that identify the competencies addressed
- ❏ Glossaries that alert students to important new terms and provide definitions
- ❏ Discussion questions that relate chapter topics to the reality of medical assisting practice

In addition, extensive appendices offer easy reference to oft-needed information such as medical abbreviations, specialized vocabularies, and CDC Universal Precautions; a 24-page atlas of full-color anatomy plates helps students visualize body structures; and a vibrant, two-color page design, with many new illustrations, enhances the learning experience.

Also available is a well-conceived and well-executed Workbook, written by Anne Lilly and Mary Ann Frew. The Workbook is a package of application exercises, mastery activities, case studies, study review questions, and self-evaluation charts that will help students master the competencies and retain the knowledge presented in this book.

For instructors, May Ann Frew, Anne Lilly, and Karen Lane have prepared an Instructor's Guide that offers content overviews, tips on writing and evaluating Terminal Performance Objectives, suggested student activities, test bank, and answers to Workbook study review questions. Included in the Instructor's Guide is a demonstration diskette for the F. A. Davis Make-a-Test program, a completely interactive test-generating program that is available at no charge to instructors who adopt the text.

Throughout the lengthy and, at times, difficult process of preparing the third edition of *Comprehensive Medical Assisting*, we have had one overriding goal: to produce a textbook that will enable all the students who use it to prepare fully to succeed in all aspects of their chosen profession.

Mary Ann Frew
Karen Lane
David R. Frew

ACKNOWLEDGMENTS

Writing a textbook is a collaborative task, and we would like to thank all the participants in the process.

To the educators and clinicians who reviewed the various drafts of the manuscript of the third edition, our gratitude for their close reading, helpful comments, and encouragement: Susan A. Beamis, EdD, PT (Chatham College); Jeannie Christen, MA, CMA (Phoenix College); Patrick J. Debold (Concorde Career Colleges); Margaret R. Frazier, RN, CMA (Ivy Tech); Sue Hargrove, MA (Philips Junior College); Marilyn Mendel, MA; John Ricci, MA (Duff's Business School); Patience E. Sharp, MS, RT, ARRT (Gannon University); Cyndy Snyder, RN (Metro Health Center of Erie); Laura D. Sorg, RN, MA (Miami Jacobs Junior College); Pat Suminski, MA (Milwaukee Area Technical College); and Diane Vander Ploeg, MS, CMA (Des Moines Area Community College). David Baglia, Professor of Accounting at Gannon University, was very helpful in reviewing the bookkeeping chapters. A special thanks, and sigh of relief, to Anne Lilly, MA, RN, MA (Santa Rosa Junior College).

We remain grateful to the many whose participation in the first and second edition constitutes a valuable legacy to the third: Marcia O. Diehl, CMA-A, CMT (Grossmont College); Jean Keenon, CMA-A (University of Alabama at Birmingham); Harriet Laronge, CMA (Sarasota County Vocational-Technical Center); Marcia A. Lewis, RN, MA, EdD, CMA-AC (Olympic College); Anne Lilly, MA, RN, MA (Santa Rosa Junior College); Bonnie J. Lindsey, CMT, CMA (Riverside City College); A. Christine Payne, RN, CMA-C (Sarasota County Vocational-Technical Center); Midge Ray, MA (University of Alabama at Birmingham); Jo-Ann Rowell, BS (Anne Arundel Community College); Gretchen Spence (Cencor Career Colleges); Diane Suchman, RN (Sarasota County Vocational-Technical Center); Carol D. Tamparo, BS, PhD, CMA-A (Highline Community College); Sue Turley, RN, BS, CMT (Anne Arundel Community College); Sharon Vance, CMA-A (Crandell Junior College); Diane Vander Ploeg, MS, CMA (Des Moines Area Community College); Margaret W. Watkins, MT(ASCP), MHSA; Dianne Whalen, MT(ASCP), CMA-C (Northwestern Michigan College); and Shirley Zeitter, RN, MA, CMA (Davenport College of Business).

Hahnemann Hospital of Philadelphia graciously allowed us to take photographs for the textbook cover in the hospital Pediatric Clinic; thanks to Lisa Alpert, of Hahnemann University Publications Department, for her patience. The Hahnemann photographs were taken by Patricia Gregory.

We wish finally to express our appreciation to our co-workers, in particular the administration and faculty of Gannon University for their support, forbearance, and collegiality; and to our families, for their love and patience.

CONTENTS

TABLES

PROCEDURES

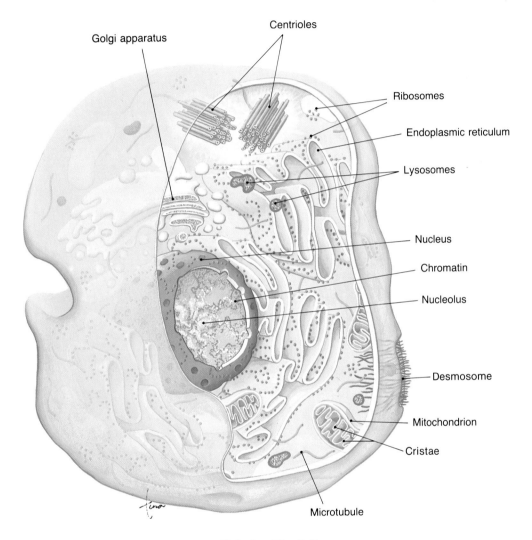

Golgi apparatus

Centrioles

Ribosomes

Endoplasmic reticulum

Lysosomes

Nucleus

Chromatin

Nucleolus

Desmosome

Mitochondrion

Cristae

Microtubule

Plate 1.   The Cell.

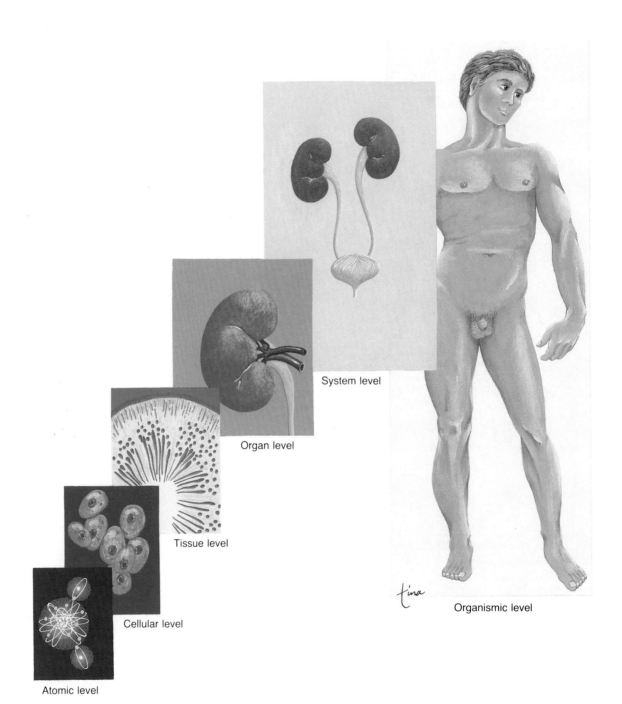

System level

Organ level

Tissue level

Cellular level

Atomic level

Organismic level

Plate 2.   Levels of Organization of the Body.

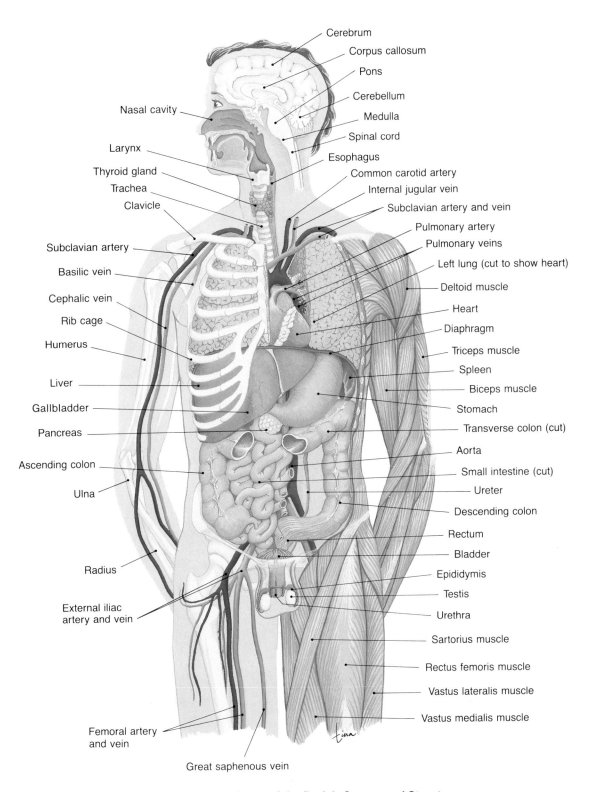

Cerebrum
Corpus callosum
Pons
Cerebellum
Medulla
Spinal cord
Esophagus
Common carotid artery
Internal jugular vein
Subclavian artery and vein
Pulmonary artery
Pulmonary veins
Left lung (cut to show heart)
Deltoid muscle
Heart
Diaphragm
Triceps muscle
Spleen
Biceps muscle
Stomach
Transverse colon (cut)
Aorta
Small intestine (cut)
Ureter
Descending colon
Rectum
Bladder
Epididymis
Testis
Urethra
Sartorius muscle
Rectus femoris muscle
Vastus lateralis muscle
Vastus medialis muscle

Nasal cavity
Larynx
Thyroid gland
Trachea
Clavicle
Subclavian artery
Basilic vein
Cephalic vein
Rib cage
Humerus
Liver
Gallbladder
Pancreas
Ascending colon
Ulna
Radius
External iliac
artery and vein
Femoral artery
and vein
Great saphenous vein

Plate 3.   Overview of Some of the Body's Organs and Structures.

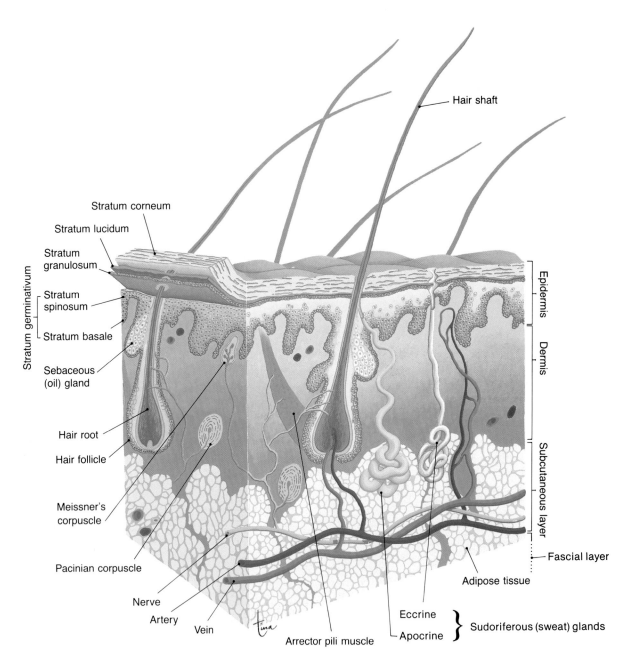

Stratum corneum

Stratum lucidum

Stratum granulosum

Stratum germinativum

Stratum spinosum

Stratum basale

Sebaceous (oil) gland

Hair root

Hair follicle

Meissner's corpuscle

Pacinian corpuscle

Nerve

Artery

Vein

Arrector pili muscle

Hair shaft

Epidermis

Dermis

Subcutaneous layer

Fascial layer

Adipose tissue

Eccrine

Apocrine

} Sudoriferous (sweat) glands

Plate 4.   Cross-Section of the Skin.

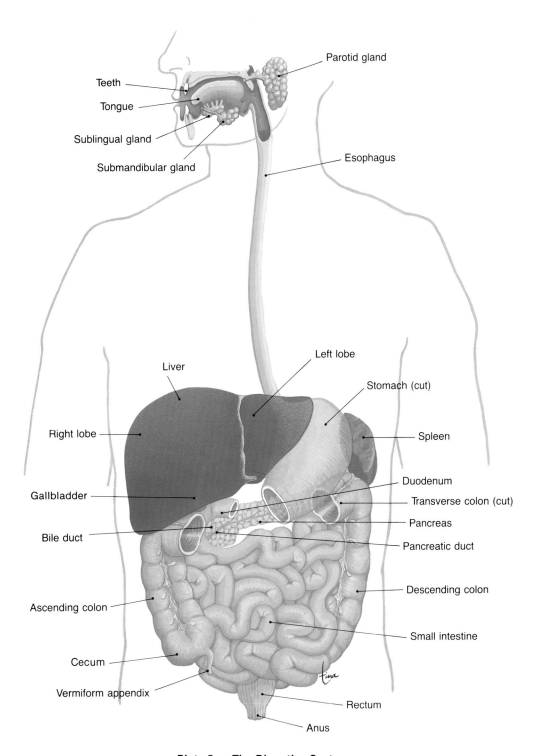

Teeth

Tongue

Sublingual gland

Submandibular gland

Parotid gland

Esophagus

Liver

Left lobe

Stomach (cut)

Right lobe

Spleen

Gallbladder

Duodenum

Transverse colon (cut)

Pancreas

Bile duct

Pancreatic duct

Descending colon

Ascending colon

Small intestine

Cecum

Vermiform appendix

Rectum

Anus

Plate 5.   The Digestive System.

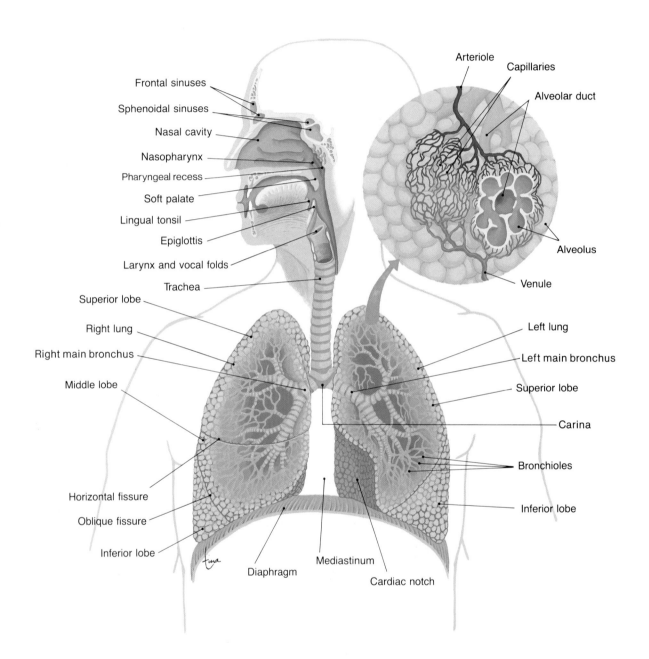

Arteriole
Capillaries
Alveolar duct
Frontal sinuses
Sphenoidal sinuses
Nasal cavity
Nasopharynx
Pharyngeal recess
Soft palate
Lingual tonsil
Epiglottis
Larynx and vocal folds
Alveolus
Trachea
Venule
Superior lobe
Right lung
Left lung
Right main bronchus
Left main bronchus
Middle lobe
Superior lobe
Carina
Bronchioles
Horizontal fissure
Oblique fissure
Inferior lobe
Inferior lobe
Diaphragm
Mediastinum
Cardiac notch

Plate 6.   The Respiratory System.

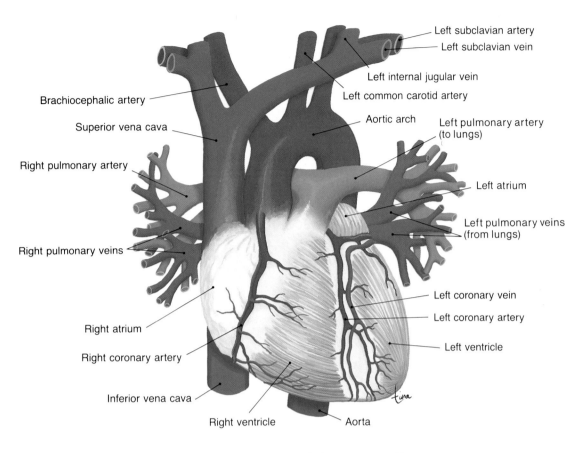

Left subclavian artery
Left subclavian vein
Left internal jugular vein
Brachiocephalic artery
Left common carotid artery
Superior vena cava
Aortic arch
Left pulmonary artery (to lungs)
Right pulmonary artery
Left atrium
Left pulmonary veins (from lungs)
Right pulmonary veins
Left coronary vein
Left coronary artery
Right atrium
Left ventricle
Right coronary artery
Inferior vena cava
Right ventricle
Aorta

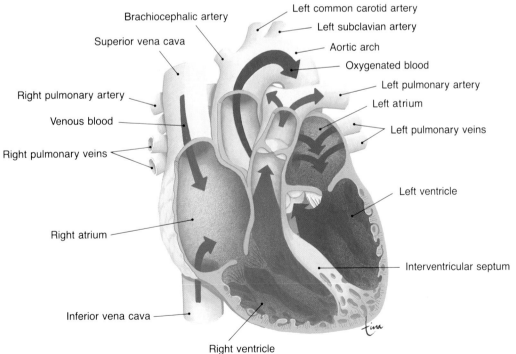

Brachiocephalic artery
Left common carotid artery
Superior vena cava
Left subclavian artery
Aortic arch
Oxygenated blood
Right pulmonary artery
Left pulmonary artery
Venous blood
Left atrium
Right pulmonary veins
Left pulmonary veins
Left ventricle
Right atrium
Interventricular septum
Inferior vena cava
Right ventricle

Plate 7.   The Exterior of the Heart, and Blood Flow Through the Heart.

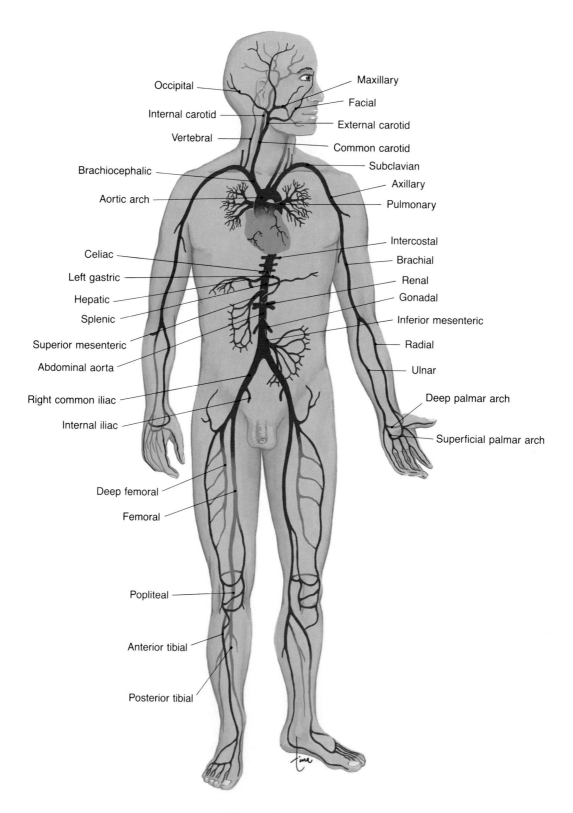

Occipital

Maxillary

Internal carotid

Facial

Vertebral

External carotid

Brachiocephalic

Common carotid

Aortic arch

Subclavian

Axillary

Pulmonary

Celiac

Intercostal

Left gastric

Brachial

Hepatic

Renal

Splenic

Gonadal

Superior mesenteric

Inferior mesenteric

Abdominal aorta

Radial

Right common iliac

Ulnar

Internal iliac

Deep palmar arch

Superficial palmar arch

Deep femoral

Femoral

Popliteal

Anterior tibial

Posterior tibial

Plate 8.   The Arteries.

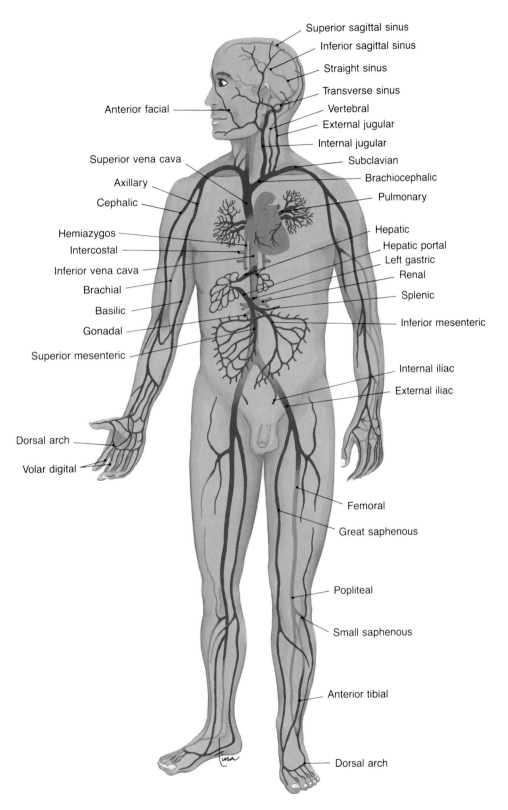

Superior sagittal sinus
Inferior sagittal sinus
Straight sinus
Transverse sinus
Anterior facial
Vertebral
External jugular
Internal jugular
Superior vena cava
Subclavian
Brachiocephalic
Axillary
Pulmonary
Cephalic
Hemiazygos
Hepatic
Intercostal
Hepatic portal
Inferior vena cava
Left gastric
Brachial
Renal
Basilic
Splenic
Gonadal
Inferior mesenteric
Superior mesenteric
Internal iliac
External iliac
Dorsal arch
Volar digital
Femoral
Great saphenous
Popliteal
Small saphenous
Anterior tibial
Dorsal arch

Plate 9.   The Veins.

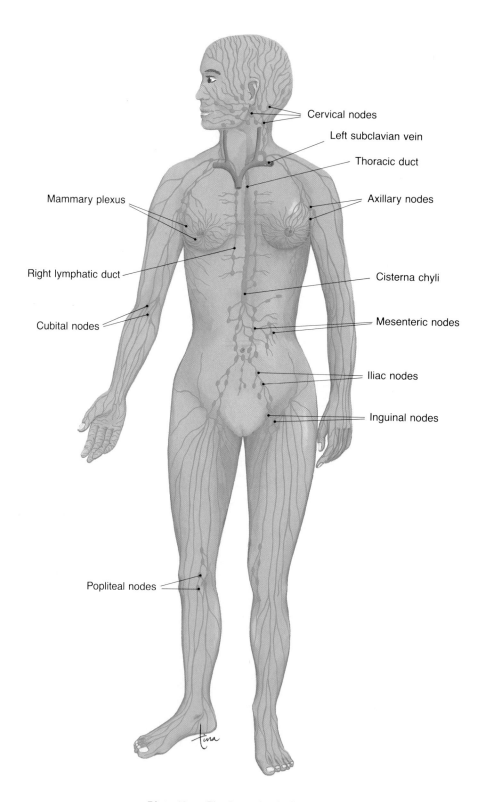

Cervical nodes

Left subclavian vein

Thoracic duct

Mammary plexus

Axillary nodes

Right lymphatic duct

Cisterna chyli

Cubital nodes

Mesenteric nodes

Iliac nodes

Inguinal nodes

Popliteal nodes

Plate 10.   The Lymphatic System.

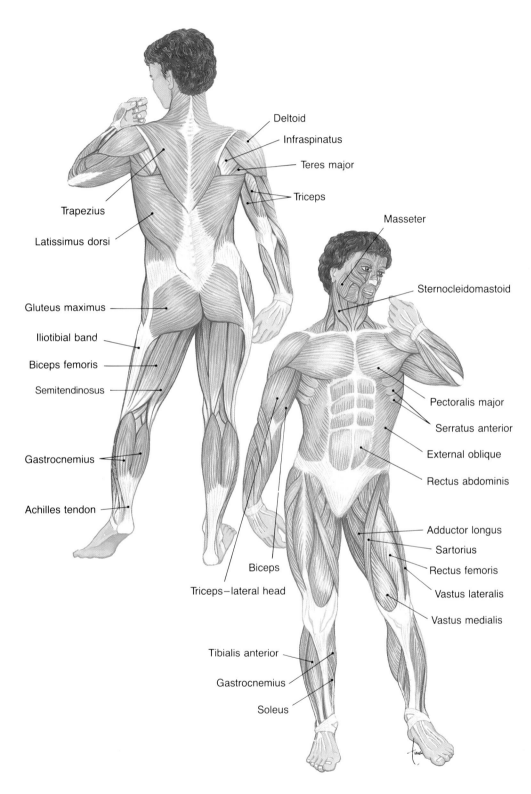

Deltoid

Infraspinatus

Teres major

Triceps

Masseter

Trapezius

Sternocleidomastoid

Latissimus dorsi

Gluteus maximus

Iliotibial band

Pectoralis major

Biceps femoris

Serratus anterior

Semitendinosus

External oblique

Rectus abdominis

Gastrocnemius

Adductor longus

Sartorius

Achilles tendon

Rectus femoris

Vastus lateralis

Vastus medialis

Biceps

Triceps–lateral head

Tibialis anterior

Gastrocnemius

Soleus

Plate 11.   Posterior and Anterior Views of the Muscles.

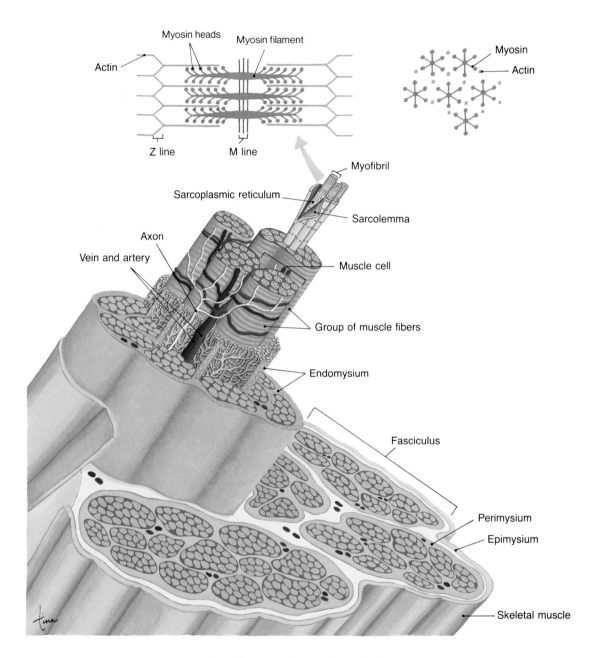

Plate 12.   Cross-Section of Skeletal Muscle.

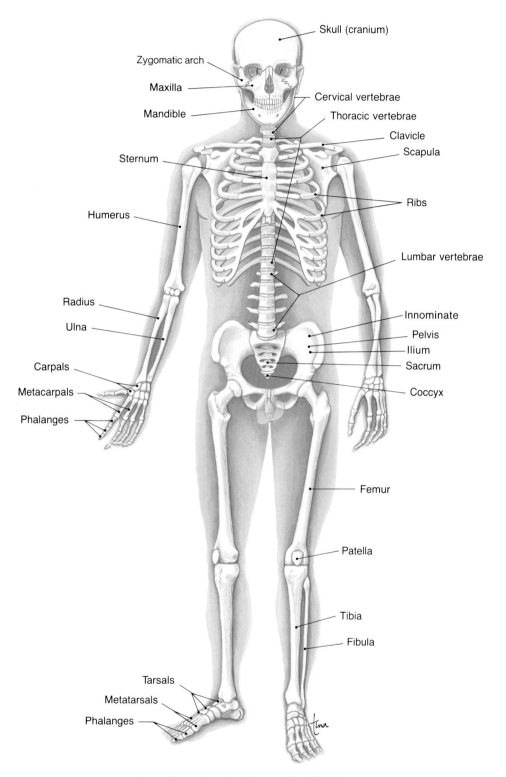

Plate 13.   Anterior View of the Skeleton.

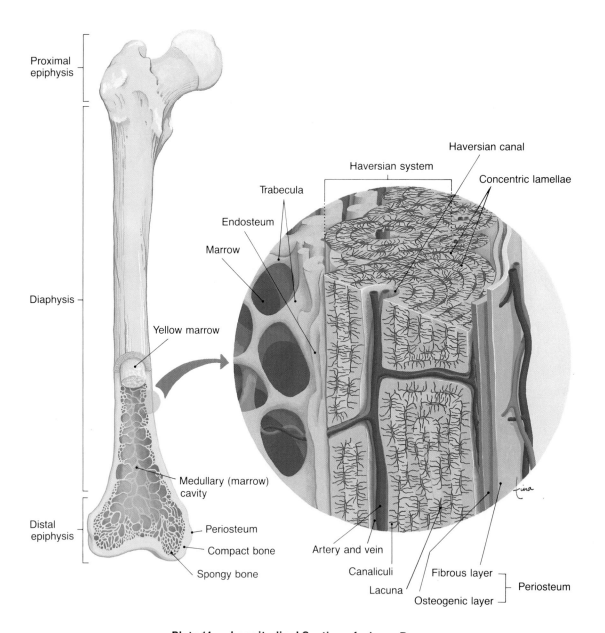

Plate 14.   Longitudinal Section of a Long Bone.

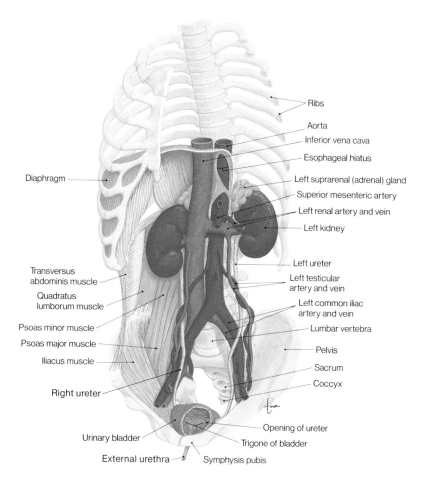

Ribs
Aorta
Inferior vena cava
Esophageal hiatus
Left suprarenal (adrenal) gland
Superior mesenteric artery
Left renal artery and vein
Left kidney
Left ureter
Left testicular artery and vein
Left common iliac artery and vein
Lumbar vertebra
Pelvis
Sacrum
Coccyx
Opening of ureter
Trigone of bladder
Symphysis pubis

Diaphragm

Transversus abdominis muscle
Quadratus lumborum muscle
Psoas minor muscle
Psoas major muscle
Iliacus muscle

Right ureter

Urinary bladder
External urethra

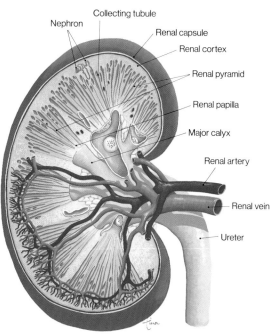

Nephron
Collecting tubule
Renal capsule
Renal cortex
Renal pyramid
Renal papilla
Major calyx
Renal artery
Renal vein
Ureter

Plate 15.   The Urinary System, and the Kidney.

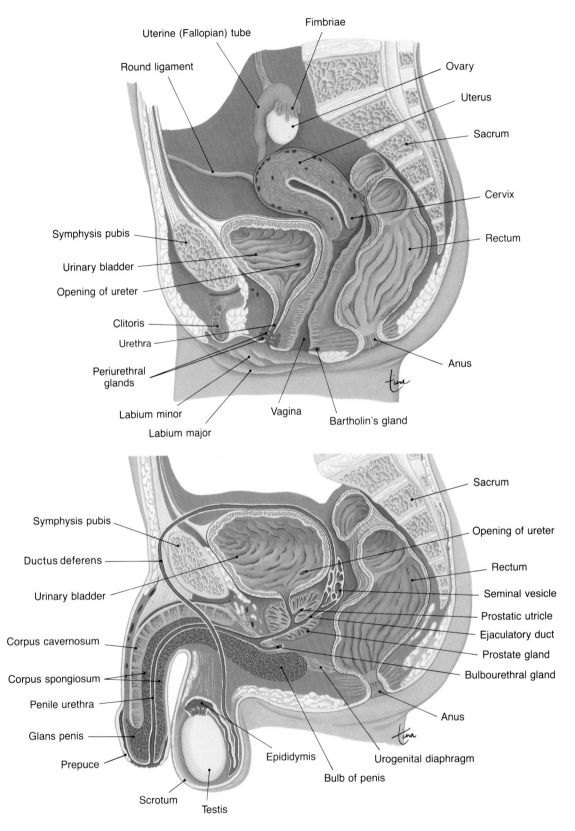

Plate 16. The Female and Male Reproductive Systems.

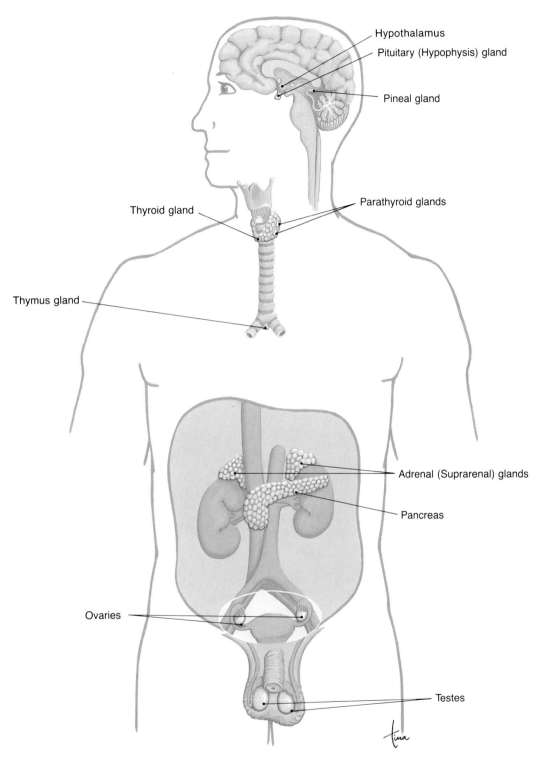

Hypothalamus

Pituitary (Hypophysis) gland

Pineal gland

Parathyroid glands

Thyroid gland

Thymus gland

Adrenal (Suprarenal) glands

Pancreas

Ovaries

Testes

Plate 17.   The Endocrine System.

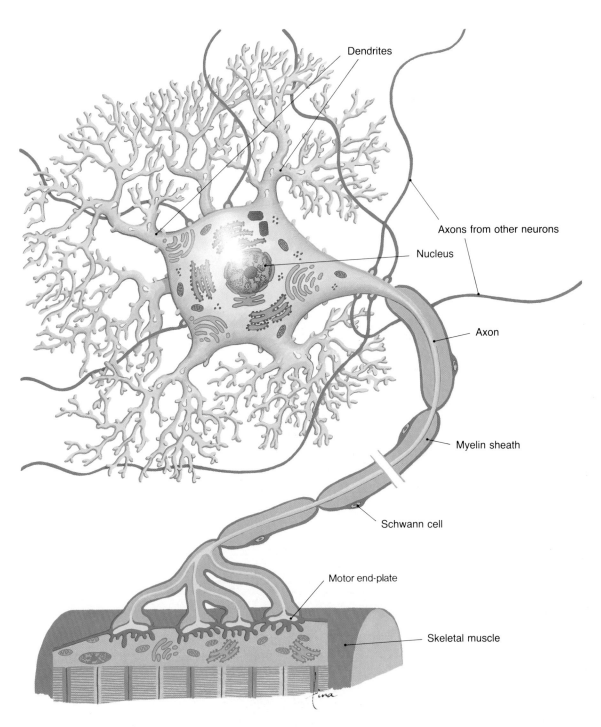

Dendrites

Axons from other neurons

Nucleus

Axon

Myelin sheath

Schwann cell

Motor end-plate

Skeletal muscle

Plate 18.   A Motor Neuron.

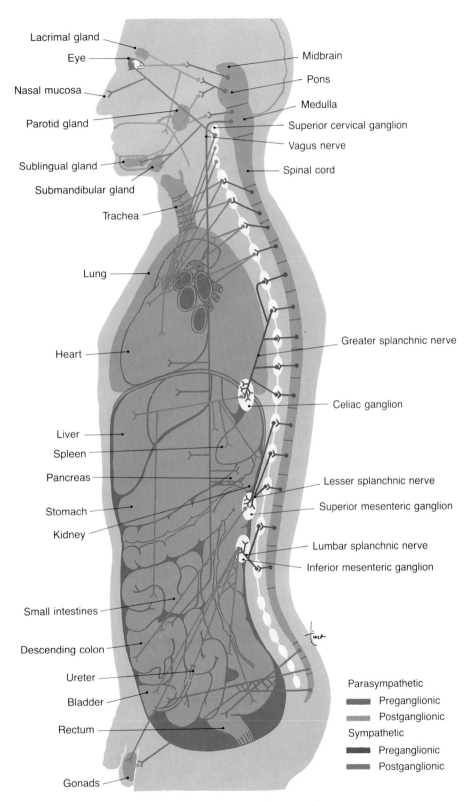

Lacrimal gland

Eye

Nasal mucosa

Parotid gland

Sublingual gland

Submandibular gland

Trachea

Lung

Heart

Liver

Spleen

Pancreas

Stomach

Kidney

Small intestines

Descending colon

Ureter

Bladder

Rectum

Gonads

Midbrain

Pons

Medulla

Superior cervical ganglion

Vagus nerve

Spinal cord

Greater splanchnic nerve

Celiac ganglion

Lesser splanchnic nerve

Superior mesenteric ganglion

Lumbar splanchnic nerve

Inferior mesenteric ganglion

Parasympathetic
  Preganglionic
  Postganglionic
Sympathetic
  Preganglionic
  Postganglionic

Plate 19.   The Autonomic Nervous System.

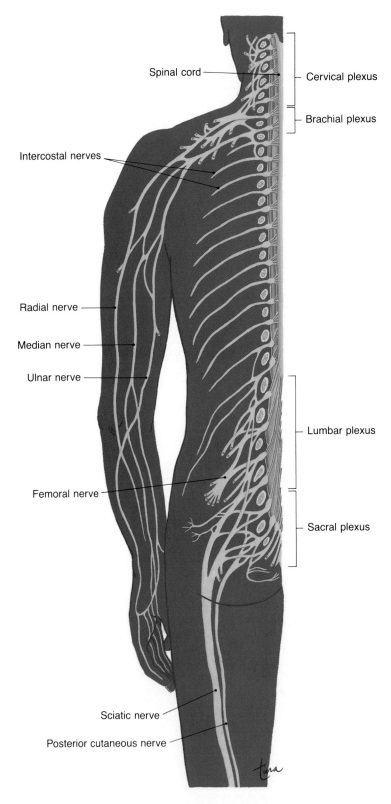

Spinal cord

Cervical plexus

Brachial plexus

Intercostal nerves

Radial nerve

Median nerve

Ulnar nerve

Lumbar plexus

Femoral nerve

Sacral plexus

Sciatic nerve

Posterior cutaneous nerve

Plate 20.   The Nervous System.

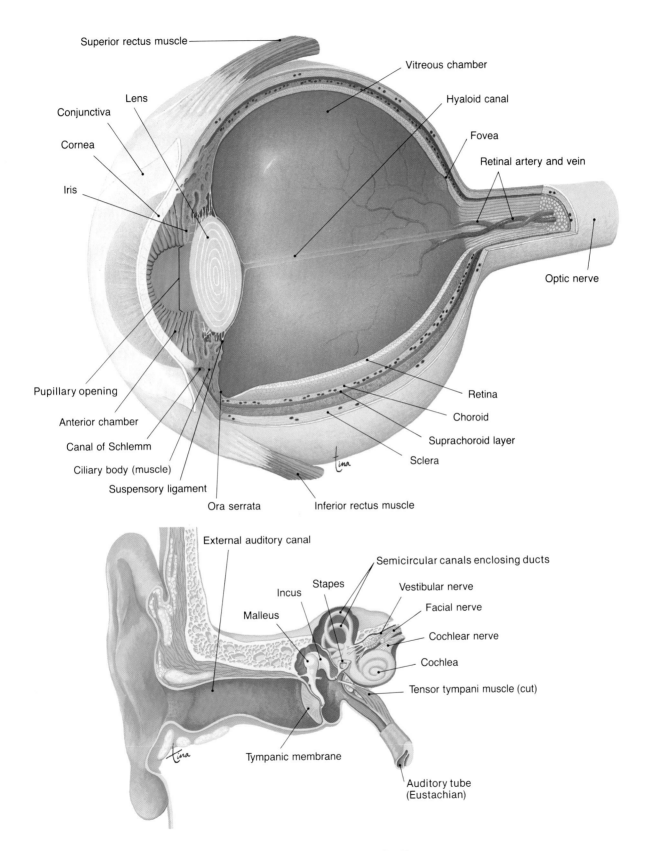

Plate 21.   The Eye, and the Ear.

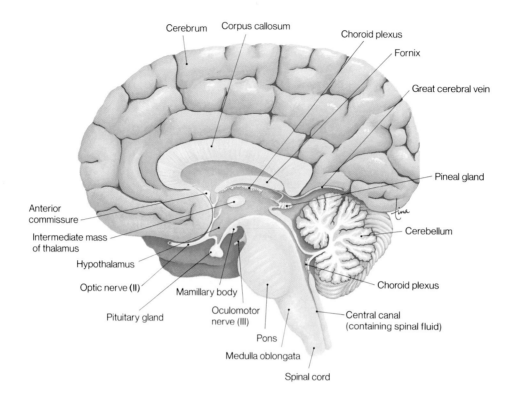

Cerebrum · Corpus callosum · Choroid plexus · Fornix · Great cerebral vein · Pineal gland · Cerebellum · Choroid plexus · Central canal (containing spinal fluid) · Anterior commissure · Intermediate mass of thalamus · Hypothalamus · Optic nerve (II) · Mamillary body · Oculomotor nerve (III) · Pituitary gland · Pons · Medulla oblongata · Spinal cord

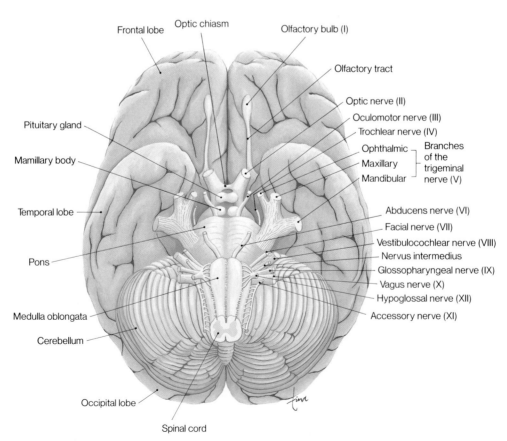

Frontal lobe · Optic chiasm · Olfactory bulb (I) · Olfactory tract · Optic nerve (II) · Oculomotor nerve (III) · Trochlear nerve (IV) · Ophthalmic · Maxillary · Mandibular · Branches of the trigeminal nerve (V) · Pituitary gland · Mamillary body · Temporal lobe · Abducens nerve (VI) · Facial nerve (VII) · Vestibulocochlear nerve (VIII) · Nervus intermedius · Glossopharyngeal nerve (IX) · Vagus nerve (X) · Hypoglossal nerve (XII) · Accessory nerve (XI) · Pons · Medulla oblongata · Cerebellum · Occipital lobe · Spinal cord

Plate 22.   Cross-Sections of the Brain, and the Cranial Nerves.

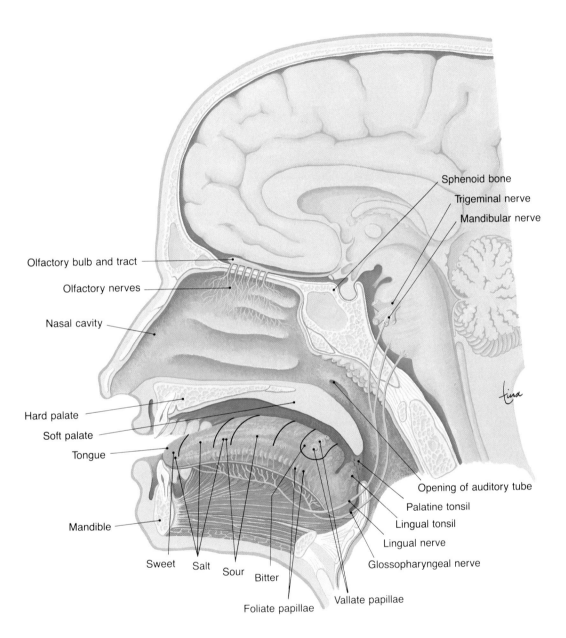

Sphenoid bone

Trigeminal nerve

Mandibular nerve

Olfactory bulb and tract

Olfactory nerves

Nasal cavity

Hard palate

Soft palate

Tongue

Mandible

Opening of auditory tube

Palatine tonsil

Lingual tonsil

Lingual nerve

Glossopharyngeal nerve

Sweet   Salt   Sour   Bitter

Foliate papillae

Vallate papillae

Plate 23.   The Centers of Smell and Taste.

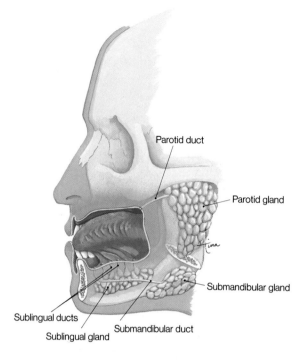

Parotid duct

Parotid gland

Submandibular gland

Sublingual ducts

Sublingual gland

Submandibular duct

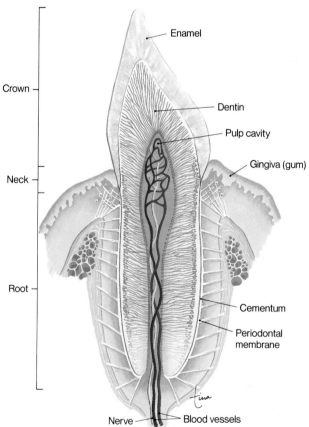

Enamel

Crown

Dentin

Pulp cavity

Gingiva (gum)

Neck

Root

Cementum

Periodontal membrane

Nerve

Blood vessels

Plate 24.   The Salivary Glands, and the Tooth.

Section I

Administrative Procedures

Unit 1

Professional Issues

The beginning chapters of this text focus on elucidating the profession of medical assisting and the complex interactions of the medical assistant with the patient and the patient's family. These chapters lay the foundation for developing an attitude appropriate to the profession. Regardless of the level of competence achieved in performing administrative and clinical skills, the medical assistant's attitude toward the profession and the patient determines his or her ability to perform the task successfully. Because of their importance, the communication skills introduced in this chapter are continually referred to throughout the text. This unit covers the basic concepts and skills that the medical assistant needs to perform all procedures correctly.

Unit Objectives

Upon completing this unit, you will be able to:

1. Define medical assisting and explain its relationship to other health professions.
2. Recognize the necessity of making a commitment to continue updating professional knowledge and skills.
3. Understand the role of ethics in medical practice and be aware of the legal responsibilities of the medical assistant.
4. Understand the transformation an individual undergoes when becoming a patient; recognize and respond appropriately to the resulting attitudes and behaviors.
5. Understand the needs of the patient's family as they relate to the concerns of family members for the patient's welfare.
6. Communicate with patients and their families in a positive manner that will help the patient become well.
7. Use specific techniques to assess the need for patient teaching.

> Developing the full potential of so large and complex an institution as medicine will require the wisdom of people in many fields and years of continuing study, theoretical formulation, clinical skill and collaboration, a common effort toward a common goal.
>
> Naomi Remen, MD

CHAPTER OUTLINE

LEARNING OBJECTIVES

Upon completing this chapter, you will be able to:

1. Define medical assisting.

Chapter **1**

*M*edical Assisting
THE VITAL LINK IN HEALTH CARE DELIVERY

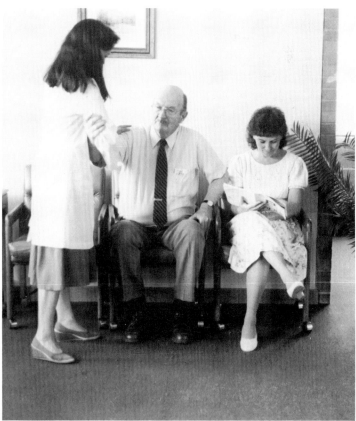

2. Describe educational programs for medical assisting.
3. Describe the method and purpose of professional certification.
4. List and describe the personal qualifications for medical assisting listed in this chapter.
5. List the duties of a medical assistant as described by the DACUM Educational Components.
6. List the work setting options available to the medical assistant.
7. List and describe the purpose and activities of the AAMA and RMA/AMT.
8. List and define the areas of responsibilities for each health profession mentioned in the chapter.

PERFORMANCE OBJECTIVE

Upon completing this chapter, you will be able to:

Describe the field of medical assisting to patients and others outside the field.

DACUM EDUCATIONAL COMPONENTS

1. Promote the profession by participating in professional meetings or seminars (1.9).
2. Use medical terminology accurately (2.1C).
3. Work as a team member by displaying an awareness of own and other team members' responsibilities (1.5A).
4. Promote the profession by acting in a professional manner (1.1E; 1.9C).
5. Serve as a liaison between the physician and others (2.5,A–B).
6. Determine the need for documentation and reporting by identifying sources of information for medicolegal documentation requirements in a given locality (5.2A,E).

Glossary

Chiropractor: A certified, licensed practitioner of chiropractic, a system of health care based on the premise that the relationship between the spinal column and nervous system is of great importance in health and disease; a chiropractor "manipulates" the spinal column to provide relief from disease attributed to dislocation and misalignment of vertebrae

Ethical: Pertaining to moral—not legal—conduct; the values and guidelines governing decisions in medical practice

Holistic medicine: A broadened concept of health care in which the spiritual, mental, emotional, and social needs of the patient are valued as much as the physical needs; holistic medicine considers each of these aspects part of an integrated whole

Legal: Concerned with, conforming to, or permitted by law

Liable: Responsible for; legally obligated

Osteopath: A physician (DO) who practices osteopathic medicine, which emphasizes the importance of normal body mechanics; osteopathic medicine uses a system of therapy that combines manipulative methods of correcting faulty structures with conventional medical and surgical procedures

Podiatrist: A physician (DPM) who diagnoses and treats conditions and diseases of the feet

Psychiatrist: A physician who specializes in the study, treatment, and prevention of mental disorders; differs from a psychologist in that a psychologist is not an MD and cannot administer drugs

---

The evolution of medical assisting, like that of so many other health professions, is intertwined with the history of physicianship. The image of the "old country doctor" is quickly fading. At the turn of the century, the country doctor was in the literal sense a general practitioner. Not only was he an internist, obstetrician, surgeon, and psychiatrist, but he also welcomed the patient, wrote receipts for payment, and made house calls. As the demands on his time multiplied, this "Marcus Welby" type was often assisted in the office by a neighbor or friend whom he trained. The population grew and the medical profession continued to change. The physician and the industry of medicine were affected by the industrial revolution and subsequently by specialization.

As specialization developed in the field of medicine, with choices of concentration, such as urology or pediatrics, becoming available, a need evolved for specialized health professionals who would work in cooperation with the physician. In 1934, a New York City physician, M. Mandl, founded a school specifically for training individuals to work in the physician's office.

The availability of specially trained personnel for the medical office provided alternatives to the hiring of individuals who had to be trained on the job, and to the training of health professionals, frequently nurses, to work in medical office settings.

The training, scope, and definition of medical assisting have changed in keeping with the pace of dramatic changes in medical practice. Today, medical assisting is a well-established profession. The medical assistant is a respected member of the health care team and possesses specific knowledge and skills most commonly obtained through completion of an educational program in a proprietary school, junior or community college, or university. Although most medical assistants are women, the profession is welcoming an increasing number of men.

EDUCATIONAL PROGRAMS FOR MEDICAL ASSISTANTS

In 1969, in cooperation with the Committee on Allied Health Education and Accreditation of the American Medical Association (AMA; the primary professional association for physicians), the American Association of Medical Assistants Endowment standardized educational programs in medical assisting and began offering accreditation to programs meeting specific standards. The minimum standards for accreditation are found in the "Essentials and Guidelines for an Accredited Educational Program for the Medical Assistant," currently published in the annual *Allied Health Education Directory*, a catalogue of accreditation requirements and guidelines for allied health education programs accredited by the AMA.

The Accrediting Bureau of Health Education Schools (ABHES), now an independent agency, first formed by the American Medical Technologists in 1974, has also established standards for accreditation of medical assisting programs. Recognized by the U.S. Department of Education, ABHES accredits medical assisting programs that meet established educational and training criteria.

DEFINITION OF THE PROFESSION

According to the 1991 AAMA *Essentials*: "Medical assisting is a multiskilled allied health profession"; practitioners work primarily in ambulatory settings such as medical offices and clinics. Medical assistants function as members of the healthcare delivery team and perform administrative and clinical procedures." Competence in the field also requires that a medical assistant display professionalism, communicate effectively, and provide instruction to patients. According to the Code of Ethics for the Registered Medical Assistant of the American Medical Technologist's Association (RMA/AMT), the medical assistant must

> always plac[e] the welfare of patients entrusted to [his/her] care above all else, with full realiza-

tion of . . . personal responsibility for the patient's best interests. . . .

The medical assistant is the medical office expert. Skilled in both administrative and clinical functions, medical assistants are often preferred to administrative secretaries or receptionists because they can contribute role and task flexibility to the physician's office. Possessing an understanding of clinical theory, the medical assistant can use this knowledge to assist the physician in front and back office areas, screening and providing information to patients and families. Unlike the nurse, whose training is oriented to bedside care, the medical assistant is specifically prepared to function in a medical office. As medical technology advances, the medical assistant's role in office practice is becoming even more diverse. Advanced training may be required in such fields as computer systems, patient education, and management.

SPECIFIC AREAS OF TRAINING

The curriculum design for accredited medical assisting programs reflects the description of the profession. In 1979, 1984, and 1990, occupational analyses for medical assisting were conducted by a group of practitioners and educators selected by the AAMA to gather information about the role and function of practicing medical assistants. The results of that study, called the DACUM (Developing a Curriculum) analysis, outline entry-level skills and skill areas that should be included in the medical assistant's role. According to the DACUM analysis, the medical assistant must develop the following general skill areas: communication, professionalism, administrative abilities, clinical abilities, management of emergency situations, management of practice finances, patient instruction, knowledge of related legal concepts, and management of facilities and personnel. The basic medical assisting program is designed to include these entry-level areas of competence. This textbook focuses on the development of the theory and skills for each area.

PERSONAL QUALIFICATIONS

In addition to the educational requirements, the medical assistant should possess certain characteristics, which would enable him or her to work successfully in the people-centered environment of medical practice.

PROFESSIONAL IMAGE

The medical assistant must not only act professional, but also look professional. A well-groomed appearance is essential for maintaining patient confidence and reducing disease transmission. Female medical assistants must take care to wear appropriate makeup and jewelry. Light day makeup, rings whose settings do not protrude excessively, earrings that are contained on the ear (not long or dangling), and necklaces that do not dangle beyond the upper chest are typically appropriate. These considerations and other employer expectations related to appearance, such as the style and color of the uniform, should be discussed before employment begins.

DEPENDABILITY

The medical assistant must be dependable and follow through on commitments such as keeping precise hours, arriving and leaving on time, completing tasks on time, accepting responsibility for one's own actions, and interacting with others in a supportive manner.

POSITIVE ATTITUDE TOWARD OTHERS

The medical assistant must have a positive regard or general liking for people and a sincere interest in helping them. By understanding the needs and behaviors of others, the medical assistant can anticipate needs, respond with positive reinforcement, and thereby contribute to the patient's care.

FLEXIBILITY

The medical assistant must be able to adapt to changing demands. For instance, plans to complete tasks may be interrupted by demands of greater priority, such as a patient emergency. The medical assistant must be able to "shift gears" without becoming disoriented and disorganized. Although this characteristic is learned with practice, being able to react flexibly to change assists an individual in becoming a medical assistant.

COMMUNICATION SKILLS

The medical assistant must develop communication skills directed at specific goals, such as helping the patient to understand and comply with treatment. However, basic verbal and writing skills are prerequisites. The aspiring medical assistant must be capable of clear and appropriate expression orally and in writing. The medical assistant must also know when not to reveal private matters according to ethical and legal principles of confidentiality.

Many other attributes are desirable for a medical assistant to possess or develop. Among these are initiative, courtesy, respect for patient rights, ethical behavior, and a realistic idea of personal abilities. The acquisition of all these characteristics enables the student to become a successful professional medical assistant.

THE CERTIFICATION EXAMINATION

Certification examinations are intended to evaluate the individual's basic competency in medical assisting. Certification examinations were instituted to ensure consistent standard of competency on which hiring physicians could rely and to which medical assistants could aspire. Although certification examinations are not legally required for practicing medical assisting, they measure and affirm the ability of individuals to function at the entry level as competent medical assistants. For medical assistants, certification is the professional credential. Ideally, every medical assistant should graduate from an accredited program and become certified.

The certification examinations consist of three primary categories: the general area of medical assisting, administrative questions, and clinical questions. Graduates of an AAMA-accredited program can take the Certified Medical Assistant (CMA) examination immediately after graduation, and are eligible for membership in the AAMA. ABHES-accredited program graduates are eligible to take the RMA/AMT certification examination and thereby become registrants (members) in the AMT Registry of its certificants. Nonaccredited program graduates must work in a medical office for a specified period before they become eligible for either examination.

Certification differs from licensure in that certification is optional and licensure is not. Licensure is administered by government agencies. Certification is administered by peer review. Although different states may have different licensure (license to practice) requirements in various other allied health professions, all states accept the passing of the medical assisting certification examinations. Passing the AAMA exam results in the awarding of the title *Certified Medical Assistant* (CMA). ABHES program graduates are required to pass the AMT certification examination to be awarded the title *Registered Medical Assistant* (RMA).

DUTIES OF THE MEDICAL ASSISTANT

Generally, the duties of the medical assistant include the physical management and maintenance of the office and the treatment and examination areas. Administrative duties include receiving patients and their families, acting as an information and education resource for patients, handling telephone and written communications, managing patient records, bookkeeping, filing, processing insurance, typing, scheduling appointments, and managing public relations. Clinical duties include preparing patients for treatment, assisting the physician with treatment, preparing and sterilizing instruments, maintaining supply inventories, obtaining laboratory specimens, performing basic laboratory tests, and educating patients. Although this list cites an array of responsibilities, it is certainly not complete. In all situations, medical assistants will find themselves attending to duties based on the particular needs of the office practice.

WORK ENVIRONMENT

Although the medical assistant was originally envisioned as assisting the physician in the medical office, medical assistants are appropriately used in several other settings. The multifaceted skills of medical assistants, along with particular regional labor market situations, have created numerous nontraditional employment opportunities. For example, many medical assistants work in clinics, hospitals, medical centers, and various other health-related settings, such as medical claims departments of insurance companies and pharmaceutical companies. An increasing number of medical assistants also work for podiatrists, psychologists, and chiropractors. Many are assuming managerial roles and patient education responsibilities, and many assist other health care practitioners. Economic trends and patient care technology may further broaden the employment scope for medical assisting and further emphasize the multicompetence, interdisciplinary approach to the education of health professionals.

PROFESSIONAL ASSOCIATIONS FOR MEDICAL ASSISTANTS

As was previously mentioned, the AAMA and its Endowment (Fig. 1–1), in collaboration with the AMA, administer the accreditation process and graduate certification examination. The association directs other professional activities as well. *The Professional Medical Assistant* journal, which includes articles of special relevance to practicing medical assistants, students, and educators, is the official bimonthly publication of the AAMA. The journal also provides articles designed to enable the reader to obtain continuing education credits.

The Continuing Education Board of the AAMA administers the continuing education of medical assistants. In 1988, the board declared revalidation of certificates mandatory for practice as a certified medical assistant (CMA). As of December 31, 1992, revalidation is required every 5 years. Two methods of revalidation are available: accumulating the required number of continuing education credits and taking the examination.

The AAMA's commitment to continuing education is also evident in the availability of official publications, such as guided study courses, and in its sponsoring of educational workshops. The AAMA has local and statewide affiliations, providing the opportunity for medical assistants to participate regularly in meetings and seminars designed to ensure the highest level of competence in the profession.

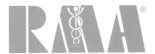

Figure 1–2. The RMA logo. (Courtesy of American Medical Technologists.)

Another nationally recognized association that addresses the needs and concerns of the medical assisting profession is the American Medical Technologists, which, in collaboration with ABHES, certifies and registers five primary designations of health personnel, one of which is the medical assistant. The publication, *Vital Signs*, published quarterly by the AMT, is directed to registered medical assistants and students of ABHES schools. AMT certified its first medical assistant in 1972; the RMA program's official inception was in 1976 (Fig. 1–2).

Similar to the AAMA, the RMA/AMT has its own bylaws, officers, state chapters, committees, conventions, awards, registrations, and revalidation processes. The RMA/AMT, like the AAMA, is dedicated to expanding the professional stature of medical assistants. The AMT, in cooperation with the AMT Institute for Education (AMTIE), offers a continuing education program for professional improvement and annual AMT Registry renewal.

THE MEDICAL ASSISTANT AS A MEMBER OF THE HEALTH CARE TEAM

The medical assistant is a significant member of the health care team, with the specific role or function of delivering patient care. Because of the complexity of medical and health care technology, various other health care professions have evolved. Each health care practitioner offers a different and necessary contribution to patient care. On the team of health care professionals, each member has a specific responsibility and yet is united to the others by the common goal of helping individuals to obtain or maintain health, or to cope with illness. As a coordinator of office tasks, a patient resource provider, and a patient educator, the medical assistant must understand the role that each health care professional plays. The medical assistant should perceive health care team members as interdependent, each relying on the others for certain areas of expertise and contributions to the patient's well-being.

In addition to understanding and respecting the various professions, the medical assistant must strive to build and maintain harmonious relationships. An office staff whose members know, respect, and like each other functions smoothly and effectively. An office staff experiencing interpersonal problems benefits neither physician nor patient. Courses in psychology are useful in assisting the development of interpersonal and communications skills.

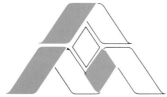

Figure 1–1. The AAMA shield and logo. (Courtesy of the America Association of Medical Assistants.)

ROLES OF HEALTH CARE PROFESSIONALS

Physicians

The term "doctor" actually signifies an academic degree awarded (usually after the attainment of a master's degree) in recognition of a person's having reached the highest academic level in a particular area. Therefore, a physician is a person who has received a doctorate in medicine. Only an individual with an earned doctorate in medicine and a license to practice can diagnose medical conditions and treat patients. The following are examples of medical degrees: Doctor of Medicine (MD), Doctor of Osteopathy (DO), Doctor of Optometry (OD), Doctor of Dentistry (DDS), and Doctor of Podiatric Medicine (DPM).

After obtaining an undergraduate degree, the aspiring physician must attend medical school, which takes 4 years. On graduation from medical school, the physician must complete an internship program (1 to 2 years) in a hospital or medical center. If the physician wants to specialize, a residency of 2 to 5 years postinternship is required. The physician must pass the licensure examination in the state in which he or she chooses to practice, and must also become certified by the US Drug Enforcement Agency to prescribe and dispense narcotics and certain other potentially dangerous medications. Board certification in specialty areas, such as pediatrics or sports medicine, is achieved by passing examinations in those disciplines. Periodic recertification is also required.

Physician Specialists

The specialist is a physician who has an expanded and detailed understanding of a single system or aspect of medicine. The specialties listed below are common work settings for medical assistants:

1. *Allergy.* Allergist. Diagnoses and treats allergic conditions (immunology is a related field).
2. *Immunology.* Immunologist. Diagnoses the causes of alterations in immunity and treats altered immune conditions.
3. *Anesthesia.* Anesthesiologist. Administers anesthesia before and during surgical procedures requiring an anesthesia-induced state of unconsciousness. Although anesthesiologists are hospital based, they may employ administrative medical assistants.
4. *Cardiology.* Cardiologist. Diagnoses and treats diseases and conditions of the heart. May perform surgery with specialized training.
5. *Dermatology.* Dermatologist. Diagnoses and treats diseases and conditions of the skin.
6. *Endocrinology.* Endocrinologist. Diagnoses and treats disorders and diseases of the glands controlling internal secretions; conditions include diabetes, obesity, menopausal conditions, and thyroid malfunctions.
7. *Family practice.* Family practitioner. Diagnoses and treats diseases and conditions within family units.
8. *Gastroenterology.* Gastroenterologist. Diagnoses and treats disorders of the stomach and the large and small intestines.
9. *Gynecology.* Gynecologist. Specializes in conditions of the female reproductive system.
10. *Internal medicine.* Internist. Diagnoses and treats diseases and conditions of the internal organs.
11. *Neurology.* Neurologist. Diagnoses and treats diseases and conditions of the central nervous system and associated systems.
12. *Obstetrics.* Obstetrician. Provides medical care during pregnancy, childbirth, and immediately after birth (postpartum).
13. *Oncology.* Oncologist. Specializes in the diagnosis and treatment of cancers.
14. *Ophthalmology.* Ophthalmologist. Cares for the eyes and related tissues and nerves.
15. *Orthopedics.* Orthopedist. Diagnoses and treats injuries and diseases of bones, tendons, and cartilage.
16. *Otorhinolaryngology.* Otorhinolaryngologist. Commonly called an "ENT physician"; specializes in treatment of *e*ars, *n*ose, and *t*hroat.
17. *Pathology.* Pathologist. Studies the nature of disease and uses laboratory methods in clinical diagnosis.
18. *Pediatrics.* Pediatrician. Specializes in a particular age group rather than a body system. Usually provides medical care to infants and young children. Some continue care through adolescence.
19. *Psychiatry.* Psychiatrist. Diagnoses and treats emotional and behavioral problems.
20. *Radiology.* Radiologist. Focuses primarily on the diagnosis and treatment of disease by radiant energy.
21. *Reconstructive and plastic surgery.* Reconstructive-plastic surgeon. Treats injuries and disease-related problems involving the skin and the functioning of body parts such as fingers and hands. May also perform elective (cosmetic) surgical procedures.
22. *Sports medicine.* Sports physician. Usually adopts an orthopedic approach and treats injuries with an emphasis on early return to athletic and other active functions.
23. *Urology.* Urologist. Diagnoses and treats diseases and conditions of the urinary systems.

Nurses

Like the physician, the nurse has responded to the increasing complexity of medicine by role differentiation and specialization. The role of the nurse is to provide health care by employing the nursing decision-making and implementation process: planning, implementing the plan, and appraising the ultimate resolution of the patient's nursing problems. These nursing interventions (simple to complex tasks) are based on self-directed judgments. For instance, helping a postoperative patient to cough is considered a basic nursing intervention and is based on the knowledge that a post-operative patient can develop pneumonia if secretions are not discharged from the lungs. The desired outcome is a complication-free postoperative recovery. The nurse's training is not designed to provide competence in administrative or laboratory functions in the medical office. Because of their specialized clinical orientation, however, nurses are commonly encountered in medical offices. Therefore, the medical assistant must understanding the nursing profession.

All nurses must pass a state licensure examination and renew their licenses periodically. With the exception of practical nurses, all nurses receive the designation of registered nurse (RN) on passing the initial licensure examination. There are specific examinations for RNs, licensed practical nurses (LPNs), and nurse practitioners. The nursing profession distinguishes among several types of nurses, including the following:

1. *Practical nurses.* Persons attend a training course, usually 1 year in length, to learn basic nursing procedures. The practical nurse must pass a state licensure examination and is awarded the designation of LPN or Licensed Vocational Nurse (LVN).
2. *Diploma school nurses.* Persons complete a 2- or 3-year training program sponsored by a hospital or medical center and receive a diploma. Diploma school training programs are decreasing in number.
3. *Associate nurses.* Persons complete a 2-year training program in a college or university. Graduates are often referred to as *nurse-technicians* and receive an associate's degree in science with a major in nursing. The nurse-technician deals with commonly occurring nursing problems and standardized, technique-oriented solutions.
4. *Baccalaureate nurses.* Individuals complete a 4-year college degree program and are awarded a Bachelor of Science (BS) degree in nursing. These nurses receive the designation of *professional nurse* and function in a wide variety of nursing careers, including the administration of health services and public health nursing.
5. *Postgraduate nurses.* BS nurses earn master's or doctoral degrees in nursing education or other nursing specialties. The term *clinical specialist* is often applied to the holder of a master's degree in nursing.
6. *Nurse practitioners.* BS or postgraduate nurses complete an additional year or more of training so that they can practice independently. The nurse practitioner is prepared to assume responsibility for the patient in a colleague relationship with the physician.

Allied Health Professionals

The list below, although not complete, gives the occupational titles of other health professionals most likely to come in contact with the medical assistant. In many cases there are two possible designations: *technician* and *technologist.* The designation *technologist* usually indicates advanced training or college credit and more expanded responsibilities than those of the technician.

1. *Electroencephalogram (EEG) technician.* Operates an electroencephalograph and obtains readings for physician interpretation.
2. *Electrocardiograph (ECG) technician.* Operates an electrocardiograph and obtains readings for physician interpretation.
3. *Medical records technician or technologist.* Maintains medical records and administers the organization of medical records in a medical center.
4. *Medical technologist.* Performs complex laboratory procedures that provide data used by physicians to determine the presence, extent, and causes of disease. Graduates of 4-year programs who pass the certification examination of the American Society of Clinical Pathologists are designated MT (ASCP).
5. *Medical laboratory technician:* Performs clinical laboratory tests. Graduates of 2-year associate degree programs who pass the certification examination of the American Society of Clinical Pathologists are designed MLT (ASCP).
6. *Medical secretary.* Performs secretarial duties; must receive specialized training in medical office procedures.
7. *Mental health counselor.* Assists patients who are experiencing emotional or psychological problems, usually in a mental health facility.
8. *Nuclear medicine technologist.* In collaboration with the physician, treats diseases and obtains diagnostic information by using radioactive nuclides.
9. *Occupational therapist.* Assists injured or handicapped patients to resume functioning at work or other activities.
10. *Physicial therapist.* Uses exercises and other types of therapy to assist in the patient's recovery.
11. *Physician's assistant.* Works under the supervision of the physician, assuming some of the physician's responsibilities in performing diagnostic and treatment procedures.
12. *Radiologic technician or technologist.* Operates x-ray and associated equipment.
13. *Registered dietitian (RD).* Prescribes dietary therapy in collaboration with the physician; instructs patients in nutrition and dietary therapy.
14. *Respiratory therapist.* Assists in the specialized therapy of persons with serious respiratory problems.

PATIENT TEACHING CONSIDERATIONS

Not all patients understand the differences among health professionals and the role of medical assistants in the health care setting. The patient may have to be educated regarding these differences. The medical assistant must allow the patient the opportunity to ask questions and should give brief, clear answers. The patient will then be encouraged to ask additional questions for further clarification. The best reference for a response to questions regarding the profession and duties of a medical assistant is the definition of a medical assistant stated earlier in this chapter.

Health professionals in any health care setting should always wear proper identification, including name and credentials. In addition, the health professional should state name and title on introduction to the patient: "Good morning, Mrs. Jones. I'm Mary Carl, a medical assistant, and I will be preparing you for examination." This introduction not only educates the patient, but also avoids confusion and saves embarrassment. Without introduction the patient may assume that the medical assistant is a different type of health professional or the physician. (Patients do not always see name pins immediately or, because of poor eyesight, cannot read the print.) In addition, medical assistants should not refer to themselves as, or imply that they are "like," nurses or other health professionals. Patients appreciate receiving the correct information and the opportunity to ask questions regarding the medical assistant's identity and function.

RELATED ETHICAL AND LEGAL IMPLICATIONS

Given its broad scope and definition, the legal practice of medical assisting warrants consideration. The medical assistant should be aware of state laws regulating the practice of medical assisting. For instance, in some states, the medical assistant may not perform a venipuncture (withdrawal of blood from a vein), and in all states, a medical assistant cannot diagnose conditions or prescribe treatment. To do so, even if the physician requests it, would be illegal and unethical. In some states, both the physician and the medical assistant could be charged with criminal action. In most employer-employee situations, however, the medical assistant is not asked to perform duties outside the scope of professional practice. The physician is ultimately responsible for all the actions of every employee under the legal doctrine of *respondeat superior,* which literally translates as "let the master answer." (This doctrine is discussed in Chapter 3.) Under the doctrine the physician-employer assumes the responsibility for hiring qualified professionals who perform tasks solely within the scope of their professional knowledge and training; the ultimate liability rests with the physician. Obviously, the medical assistant must understand and accept the areas of responsibility and the duties appropriate to the profession, and must never attempt to diagnose or suggest treatment. In addition, the medical

assistant must be careful not to permit patients to misconstrue his or her function. For example, the medical assistant may never allow the patient to think that he or she is a nurse or other type of professional. To do so is fraudulent and places the office practice, the physician, and the medical assistant in jeopardy of liability. The medical assistant's objective of functioning within the parameters of professional practice should always be safeguarded.

THE FUTURE OF MEDICAL ASSISTING

Medical assisting, in its brief history, has emerged as a well-established health profession that continues to change in definition and scope of practice. The future should bring continued advancement as the health care delivery system becomes more complex and the need for multiskilled health professionals increases.

Also emerging is a heightened sense of professionalism among medical assistants. With revalidation or certification requirements, competence-based curricula, accreditation requirements, and a well-organized professional association, medical assisting is becoming an acknowledged health profession.

The graduates of educational programs, however, will determine the future of medical assisting. Activities such as obtaining certification, becoming involved in the organization, subscribing to the journal, and committing to continuing education are essential professional responsibilities. The fulfillment of these responsibilities by each medical assistant graduate will ensure the vitality of the profession, create new career dimensions, and, perhaps most important, lead to personal satisfaction as a health professional. The common goal of developing the full potential of medicine, expressed in the quotation by Naomi Remen at the beginning of this chapter, can be achieved only if each health professional remains committed to providing the highest quality of patient care. Seeking the highest level of professional competence is, of course, a prerequisite.

SUMMARY

History has experienced the profession of medical assisting as ever growing and ever changing. The contemporary medical assistant is a highly skilled and multifaceted member of the health care team. The educational and training programs for medical assisting and the activities of the AAMA and RMA have raised the medical assistant's professional sights. Certified medical assistants have taken their place among other health professionals. All are interdependent, and each has an important role to perform, with the common objective of providing the highest quality of patient care.

DISCUSSION QUESTIONS

1. Why did you choose the profession of medical assisting?
2. After reviewing the definition and duties of a medical assistant, choose the duty least familiar to you, learn about it through library research, and then briefly describe it.
3. Review the discussions on personal qualifications. Choose two or more qualities you think particularly apply to you and explain how they do so.
4. Describe the "interdependence" team concept of health professionals in a large medical office practice.
5. Go to the library and locate a copy of *The Professional Medical Assistant*. Choose an article from a recent copy and discuss it.
6. Review the medical specialties. Which specialties sound particularly interesting to you in terms of employment possibilities? Explain why.

BIBLIOGRAPHY

Abelgas EB: The importance of professional reading for professional advancement. AMT Events 6:6, 1989.

American Medical Association: Allied Health Education Directory. American Medical Association, Chicago, 1993.

Balasa DA: The most comprehensive profile of medical assisting. The Professional Medical Assistant 24(6):23, November/December 1991.

Frew MA, Fabian D: Addressing the special needs of the nontraditional student. The Professional Medical Assistant 4(3), May/June 1991.

Institute of Medicine. Committee to Study the Role of Allied Health Personnel: Allied Health Services: Avoiding Crisis. National Academy Press, Washington DC, 1989.

Lewis M and Tamparo C: Law and Ethics in the Medical Office, ed 3. FA Davis, Philadelphia, 1993.

Thomas CL (ed): Taber's Cyclopedic Medical Directory, ed 17. FA Davis, Philadelphia, 1993.

HIGHLIGHTS

According to the US Bureau of Labor Statistics, 149,000 people were employed as medical assistants in 1988, and that number will increase 70%, to 253,000, by the year 2000. However, supply may not meet demand. During the last few years, some health care professions have experienced severe personnel shortages. How are the supply-and-demand trends shaping the future of health care delivery and what is their impact on the medical assisting profession?

Health care industry growth trends are most likely linked to increased demands for health care by an aging population that, over the next few decades, will be the largest elderly population in many years. Another factor in promoting the growth trend may be the continuing advances in medical technology.

Observable shifts in the delivery of health care services, caused by socioeconomic trends and shortages of health care personnel, are forcing changes in the professions themselves and their role expectations. Among these shifts

1. *Many changes are predicted in insurance and payment plans.* In addition to the Clinton Administration, many groups are proposing many different plans for a national health care insurance system. For medical assistants, paperwork tasks are likely to increase. The medical assistant will have to keep up with the changes in both private and government-sponsored insurance plans. Patients will most likely become more dependent on the medical assistant for instructions regarding these plans. In addition, the medical assistant will probably become a coding specialist, maintaining accuracy in assigning particular codes to specific diagnoses as mandated by government and other insurance companies. The coding of diagnoses by insurance companies for services provided in the physician's office may become standard as government efforts to contain the cost of health care increase.

   Moreover, the recent trend to managed care in the form of health maintenance organizations will probably continue. Such a fundamental change in the delivery of health care will transform the administrative procedures of many medical offices.

2. *Marketing strategies for physicians' offices will include offering services such as evening and weekend office hours.* Many physicians across the country now offer evening and weekend hours and permit walk-in office visits (as opposed to closed scheduling, in which patients are seen only by appointment). The impact of these changes on the medical assistant will include changes in the work schedule (which has previously been confined to weekdays) and increased opportunity for overtime made necessary to accommodate walk-in patients, who disrupt carefully scheduled appointments.

   Career opportunities for medical assistants also exist in public health facilities, hospitals, laboratories, medical schools, research institutions, and university medical centers. By the year 2000, some 253,000 medical assistants will be employed in such settings.

3. *Computer use in the medical office is increasing.* Medical assistants cannot afford to be computer illiterate. The future can only increase computer applications in the medical office.

4. *Patient expectations are changing and new areas of responsibility for medical assistants continue to evolve.* Today's patients are more interested in wellness, fitness, and preventive medicine than ever before. The medical assistant must respond to these expectations by becoming proficient at patient assessment and instruction, including the knowledge of and referral to community resources.

The impact of these trends on the medical assistant profession can only be estimated. However, the anticipation of change should be a stimulus for preparation. The medical assistant must be an adaptive professional, prepared for the future, informed by the past, and focused on the present. The key to success for any health care professional is to keep current—to continuously learn, observe, participate, and grow in professional stature.

Professional Growth and Personal Management

> Everyone owes some of his time to his own personal growth, and to the upbuilding of the profession to which he belongs.
>
> Theodore Roosevelt

CHAPTER OUTLINE

LEARNING OBJECTIVES

Upon completing this chapter, you will be able to:

1. Explain the conflicts that affect medical assistants in their work roles.
2. Describe the essential differences between professional and nonprofessional workers.
3. Explain the purpose of a professional membership at local, state, and national levels.
4. Describe the purpose of goal setting, goal defining (pinpointing), and time management in the medical office.

PERFORMANCE OBJECTIVES

Upon completing this chapter, you will be able to:

1. Apply problem-solving skills to goal setting, pinpointing techniques, and prioritizing needs.
2. Develop a list of pinpointed personal and professional goals.

*P*rofessional Growth and Personal Management

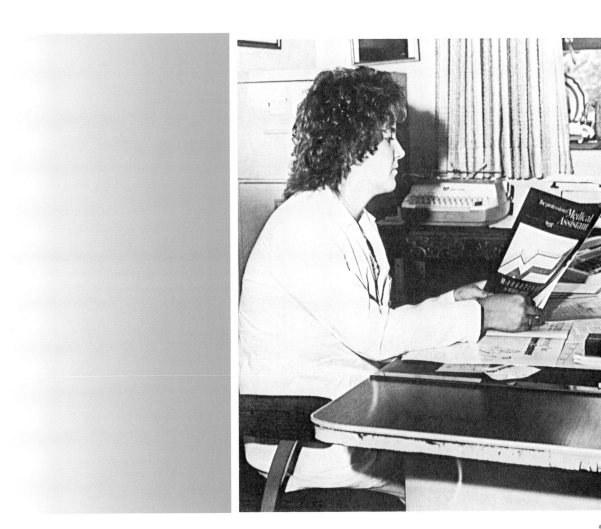

DACUM EDUCATIONAL COMPONENTS

1. Adapt to change by applying problem-solving skills to prioritize needs, adapt schedules, reassign duties, modify activities, and revise procedures (1.7C).
2. Show initiative and responsibility by recognizing work to be done, completing tasks, offering assistance, and volunteering for additional duties as time allows (1.88D,E).
3. Adapt to change by confronting the issues and people involved to assess and resolve conflicts (1.7A,B).
4. Show initiative and responsibility by designing and implementing a basic time management system (1.8A,B).

Glossary

Autonomy: Independence; self-direction; self-governance
Dynamism: A process of change responsible for development of a system
Role: Expected behavior; a part to be played

Throughout Chapter 1, we used the word "professional" many times. Perhaps, through reading and discussion, you have achieved some understanding of the meaning of the word. However, further elaboration is necessary because professionalism is more than a simply defined term. It is an attitude and a process.

PROFESSIONALISM: AN ATTITUDE AND A PROCESS

The terms *profession, job,* and *work* are sometimes used synonymously. A profession, however, differs substantially from a job. The professional medical assistant understands that other professionals function in different offices and perform similar tasks. A profession, in this instance medical assisting, binds all these persons together and allows them to communicate, share, and grow from their common experiences. Professionals can ensure a standard of practice that transcends any particular office. Similarly, they can be assured that their professionalism benefits those persons who use their services as either employers or patients.

Dr. Thomas Curtis, a professor of family medicine at Louisiana State University's School of Medicine, described the essence of being professional in the journal *The Professional Medical Assistant.* He suggests that the professional is knowledgeable in the technical area and confident of that knowledge, dedicated both to the profession and to continued understanding of it, trustworthy, self-motivated, a listener and thinker, and most important, committed. The professional must be committed to several ideals simultaneously and to the discipline of learning the profession, the quality of service delivered to clients (patients in this case), and to the employer or organization. The careful balance of the missions described by Curtis is not a simple task. It is, rather, a lofty ideal. Professionalism is an attitude be-

cause it embodies ideals and beliefs. It is a process because it is learned, experienced, and developed over time. To develop a sense of professionalism, the medical assistant must both understand his or her role in relation to other health professionals and be aware of the nature of the role itself. The purpose of this chapter, then, is to assist the student in coping with the difficulty of developing as a professional and functioning effectively.

DEVELOPING AS A PROFESSIONAL
ROLE CONFLICT

The medical assistant soon discovers that the medical office is a unique and complex setting. In ways different from other types of office stress, the pace, the critical nature of the work, and the intensity of interactions with both patients and staff members create a challenging atmosphere. The work is mentally, physically, and emotionally taxing. It also holds the potential for great personal reward and satisfaction. Medical assisting demands a professional approach because of its critical nature and service orientation. Therefore, because of the role complexity, the medical assistant must develop careful strategic approaches to achieving both high levels of office efficiency and personal job satisfaction.

Unlike the traditional factory or office, where there is a relative degree of predictability and order about work, the medical office is characterized by emergencies, sidetracks, and interruptions. It is difficult for the medical assistant to predict and plan the work systematically. Just when a report or a paperwork project is near completion, the unexpected happens, or the physician calls, and the resulting postponement causes frustration.

The medical assistant is expected to be both an assistant, whose role is to facilitate the work of the physician and the staff, and a professional person, whose role is to autonomously determine what must be accomplished and to follow though with little or no supervision. Learning to recognize and deal with these conflicting roles—those of assistant and independent professional—is essential to becoming a successful professional medical assistant.

DEVELOPING AUTONOMY

As a professional, the medical assistant must become an autonomous member of the health care delivery team. In other words, the medical assistant must be able to anticipate the needs of physician, patient, and staff, and must be self-directed and highly motivated in meeting those needs. In the medical office, the physician does not have the time or the inclination to constantly supervise and provide direction. The medical assistant who needs constant or close supervision is less valuable as an assistant. The optimally functioning assistant recognizes what is to be done and seeks to accomplish the task immediately. There is a fine line between making a decision that should not be made without the approval of the physician and other staff members, and assisting the physician by independently performing tasks perceived to be within the cope of medical assisting. The medical assistant must therefore strive to reach a delicate balance as a professional. This balance is best achieved through a thorough knowledge of the medical assisting profession and the physician's preferences.

The best safeguard against misunderstanding in this area is to maintain a continuous dialogue with the physician. It is helpful to schedule periodic meetings to discuss practical problems experienced in the office. The medical assistant will soon grow to understand the physician's expectations and will then be able to acquire more autonomy.

If the office does not have an appropriate job description for a medical assistant that would clarify areas of responsibility, the medical assistant might suggest that one be formulated. Each item within the description should be expressed in clear language. Generally, such descriptions include a list of duties and a list specifying supervisory requirements and qualifications. A well-developed job description increases both the potential for autonomy and the understanding of the role of the medical assistant.

REALITY VERSUS THEORY

The actual office procedures may be quite different from the expectations formed during the educational program. Many physicians may not fully understand the training and skills of a medical assistant. In addition, some offices have evolved systems or procedures that require the medical assistant to function in unusual ways, or that call on other staff members to carry out

tasks ordinarily performed by the medical assistant. The medical assistant may need to gradually educate both the physician and the professional staff regarding his or her training and skills. It may take months or years to finally function in all the classic roles of the professional medical assistant. It is not reasonable to expect the traditional practices of the office to immediately change when the medical assistant is employed.

A medical assistant whose skills are substantially underused should work to gain the confidence of the physician and other staff members. It is important to be clear and direct in proposing an expanded role. Communication with the physician and the staff may require patience and understanding because established systems, such as those in the physician's office, are resistant to change. For the sake of office harmony, the satisfaction of all involved, and optimum professional development, there must be general agreement about how other staff members, and medical assistants themselves, perceive the role of the professional medical assistant.

In some settings the medical assistant may be overtaxed with responsibilities (asked to do tasks beyond the medical assistant's training or experience). Professional ethics and legal considerations demand that these responsibilities be discussed with the physician or staff member involved. Although autonomy is desirable, it must be developed within the parameters of professional practice.

EXPANDING PROFESSIONAL DEVELOPMENT BEYOND THE OFFICE

One vital difference between nonprofessionals and professionals is that the highly autonomous professional is interested in work for its own sake. Whereas an employee is usually not expected to seek information about how similar jobs are conducted elsewhere, medical assistants and other professionals must constantly strive to learn about current practices in other localities, advances in the field of medical assisting, and changes in medicine itself.

There are several opportunities for staying current in one's profession. These include reading professional materials such as textbooks and journals, attending continuing education courses in medical assisting, accumulating continuing education credits, and belonging to and participating in professional associations and meetings. The American Association of Medical Assistants (AAMA) and the Registry of Medical Assistants of American Medical Technologists (RMA/AMT) have local, state, and national organizations that hold regular meetings. At these meetings the medical assistant has an opportunity to interact with other medical assistants, ask questions about current practices, learn of new developments in the field, and develop a network of professional colleagues who can be counted on for advice and support. The medical assistant should join and seek to participate in professional associations at each organizational level.

PROFESSIONAL BEHAVIOR

Chapter 3 thoroughly covers the ethical and legal issues related to professional behavior for medical assistants. The following list of desired behaviors, however, will help the beginning medical assisting student develop an awareness of the expectations for professional behavior.

1. Support the physician and the other staff members in discussions with patients. There may be disagreements between staff member and patient, between coworkers, and between staff member and physician. Differences, however, are never verbalized to patients or expressed in their company. The appropriate place for discussion is a private setting.
2. Protect patients' rights and confidentiality. Confidentiality is central to medical office practice and is the expectation and right of the patient. All health professionals understand that every patient encounter must be kept confidential, or private. Outside the medical setting, patients' names are not used, and no information is discussed that might be legally implicating. Less well understood is that every matter —not just every patient matter, but every aspect of medical office practice—should be kept confidential. The professional and personal lives of the office staff, problems that may exist in relationships with coworkers, and staff and patient evaluations of the physician are examples of matters that warrant confidentiality. The best practice is to leave what happens in the office at the office.
3. Immediately bring concerns or questions regarding patient care to the attention of the physician. It is well within the parameters of medical assisting practice to assess patient needs and concerns. The physician may not always be aware of these concerns. The medical assistant is, in fact, the patients' representative and must sometimes act as their spokesperson. Although patients should be encouraged to ask questions and discuss concerns with the physician directly, there are many reasons why they may not do so. Some patients are intimated by the physician; some are simply uncomfortable. On some occasions the medical assistant may have questions or concerns regarding patient care. It is more productive to ask, discuss, and learn the answers than to misunderstand or make wrong guesses. The physician may be unaware of the effect an aspect of patient care has on the patient. The medical assistant, having gained the patient's confidence, may provide the physician

with important data, thereby enabling the physician to provide competent, comprehensive care.
4. Become certified. Participate in association activities and continuing education within the professional association (AAMA or RMA). As was previously stated, a professional is such because of the unifying bond with others engaged in the same career. Role definition and expectation are shared by all the members who work together to safeguard and upgrade the profession. This relationship of professionals begins when a student enrolls in a medical assisting program. Students can be members of local, state, and national medical assisting organizations and can gain knowledge and support through participation.

SELF-MANAGEMENT

Because the medical assistant must become a highly motivated and autonomous contributor to the office practice, it is essential to know and apply several principles of self-management. The medical assistant cannot depend on other persons to determine and prioritize work assignments. As a self-regulating, committed professional, the medical assistant must manage and prioritize his or her own work. Of course, the medical assistant's duties are ultimately determined by the needs of the physician. However, it is the duty of the medical assistant to understand and independently fulfill those needs.

In practical terms, this requirement suggests that the medical assistant must become proficient in two skills: goal setting and time management. Goal-setting skills allow the medical assistant to clarify the nature of the tasks that must be accomplished and to develop a strategic approach to planning. Time management skills result in effective task organization and proper prioritization of responsibilities.

FULFILLING THE ROLE OF MEDICAL ASSISTANT THROUGH GOAL SETTING

Because the essence of the medical assistant's role is to assist the physician for purposes of improved efficiency and patient care (the physician uses valuable time to attend to medical rather than peripheral functions), medical assistants must guard against allowing their own professional goals to take precedence over either those of the physician or the office objectives. For instance, fast food workers who are so intent on loading napkin machines or stacking paper cups that they neglect to wait on customers, or bank tellers who do not respond to clients because they are filling out forms, are accomplishing personal goals at the expense of the mission of the business. These are examples of persons who are so intent on accomplishing a goal they have set for themselves that they neglect their essential roles.

In the medical office, the mission of the physician is to provide medical care for patients. The role of the medical assistant is to facilitate the work of the physician in accomplishing this goal. One practical method for translating principles into everyday office practice is the technique of goal setting. Most large organizations make a periodic practice of reviewing their missions and philosophies and then translating these into practical objectives. This logical practice can simplify many of the most complex issues within the medical office. The medical assistant cannot assist the physician effectively without first understanding the objectives for the office and the goals to be achieved by various staff members.

The Importance of Physician Input

The medical assistant should communicate with the physician to learn the overall objectives for the operation of the office practice and to achieve a clear understanding of the physician's goals and personal priorities. This dialogue should continue on a regular basis because, as was previously stated, objectives change over time. It is also a good practice to record and review these objectives periodically. The understanding that results can help to clarify the physician's expectations for the role of the medical assistant. Examples of goals the physician might wish to attain are: involving patients in their own treatment, making the office visit pleasant for each patient, and reducing the time patients spend in the waiting room.

Pinpointing

In setting goals it is tempting to overly generalize personal or office goals. Unless a goal is specific, it cannot be a motivator or a planning tool. Therefore, the medical assistant who is seeking direction from the physician should attempt to pinpoint goals. Pinpointing converts general missions or philosophies into clear and specific goals. A pinpointed goal is observable and measurable. For example, wanting to provide prompt service for patients is a general objective. A pinpointed goal might be to reduce the average patient waiting time to 15 minutes. Although it may be enlightening to establish the physician's philosophies and personal objectives for each office staff member, the medical assistant's ability to translate these missions into pinpointed objectives is more important.

Establishing a List of Personal Goals

After discussions with the physician, the medical assistant should create a personal list of prioritized and pinpointed goals. This exercise enhances the job description. In dynamic environments such as the medical office, job descriptions alone are rarely adequate for daily planning and priority setting. The goal list provides a periodic (annual or semiannual) check on progress, an aid to setting everyday priorities, and the basis for daily organization. Task accomplishment is best organized within the context of clear general and specific personal goals.

Two examples of specific personal goals are (1) attending at least two medical assisting conferences during the next year, and (2) spending at least 5 minutes talking with each patient in the office. Examples of general goals are (1) making more productive use of time, (2) creating an office library, and (3) improving the communication among coworkers.

THE TASK OF DAILY ORGANIZATION: TIME MANAGEMENT

Once the medical assistant understands the role of the professional and the missions and goals of the office, the concepts discussed above can be applied to the daily operation of the practice. The effective operation of a medical practice, however, also depends on a third concept: the problem of time management. Goals translated into tasks must be achieved within the framework of time constraints.

Create a Job List System

The first step in time management is to develop a system of recording tasks to be accomplished, and then to check them off as they are completed. A job list is the key organizational tool for the medical assistant. There are many ways to create such a list. A corkboard with notes attached, a blackboard, or a notebook would all suffice. Perhaps the most popular system involves either a plain form (Fig. 2–1) or a specialized design that includes the particular need categories within the office (Fig. 2–2).

The job list is both a planning guide and a reminder for tasks that are unanticipated in the daily routine, such as requests by the physician or by patients. Forms may be either attached to a clipboard or kept in a

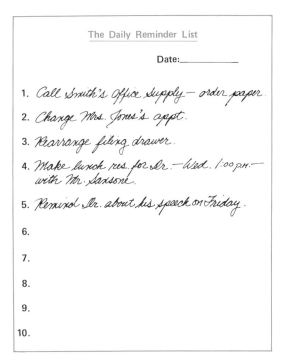

The Daily Reminder List

Date:_____

1. Call Smith's Office Supply — order paper.
2. Change Mrs. Jones's appt.
3. Rearrange filing drawer.
4. Make lunch res. for Dr. — Wed. 1:00 PM.— with Mr. Sansone.
5. Remind Dr. about his speech on Friday.
6.
7.
8.
9.
10.

Figure 2–1. A simple reminder form.

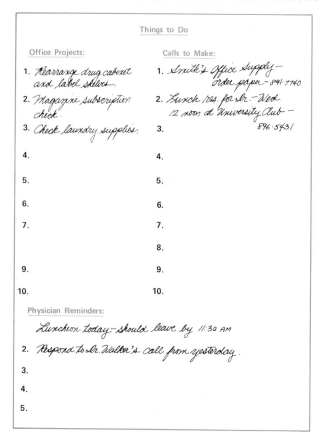

Figure 2–2. A categorized reminder form.

strategic place on the desk, so that when an assignment cannot be carried out immediately it can be recorded on the job list. The list should include any pertinent information, such as telephone numbers and due dates.

The job list is useful only if it is regularly used to organize the medical assistant's daily activities. It should always be conveniently placed, referred to often for direction and priority setting, and used for planning at the beginning and end of each work day. Regularly recording assignments on the list and using the list for planning is far more important than designing it esthetically.

Do Not Trust Memory

The most serious errors made by medical assistants and others who work in dynamic job environments are usually errors of omission rather than execution. For example, the physician may casually suggest that the medical assistant order disposable gloves because the office supply is quite low. The medical assistant is busy filing and decides to do it after lunch. However, after lunch Mrs. Jones suffers a ruptured appendix in the office, and by the time things calm down it's break time. As the day's responsibilities continue to unfold, the request is simply forgotten. Two or three days later, the physician needs the gloves and they are not available.

This vignette illustrates the most common error made by assistants in the medical office. No matter how skillful and dedicated the medical assistant may be, it is

dangerous to rely on memory for information retention. There are too many things happening to allow for reliable recall. An essential lesson for the medical assistant is to write down all messages, self-reminders, and projects. Unless it is faster to accomplish the task than write it, it should be entered on the job list. This simple habit virtually eliminates the largest single source of errors.

Use the Job List

Much of the workday will be spent in reacting to immediate concerns or emergencies. When the telephone rings, the physician calls, or a patient asks a question, the medical assistant's immediate response and full attention are required. The remainder of the workday still must be managed effectively. The purpose of the job list is to guide decisions regarding what the medical assistant should be doing with the available time. At least once and possibly twice a day, the medical assistant should review the list and identify and prioritize items with a special mark, such as a star or an underline. Most people who use a job list find that reviewing the list each morning and at the end of each day gives reasonable control over prioritization of work. Some individuals find it useful to rank the tasks on their job list either by numbering the items in descending order of priority (1, 2, 3, etc.) or by using an A-B-C system, with the letter *A* designating the most important tasks. Regardless of the system used, all tasks should be recorded and prioritized.

During the working day the list can be referred to frequently. The medical assistant must develop the discipline of concentrating on the highest-priority items. Although there may be a temptation to complete tasks that are quick or easy so they can be crossed off of the list, it is important to use the available time on high-priority items. If there is insufficient time to complete an important item, it is far more useful to begin working toward its completion than to finish a low-priority task. A list of tasks to be completed daily would probably be included in the office procedure manual, which is discussed in Chapter 7. The job list, however, is a helpful tool for ordering unanticipated daily tasks.

The procedure for designing a time management plan is described at the end of this chapter.

Avoid Double Work

As was mentioned earlier, when it would be easier and faster to complete a task rather than to enter it on the job list, it is a good practice to finish the task immediately. Not doing so often results in a duplication of effort. The medical assistant may, for example, open the mail and find that a letter requires a response that could be completed quickly. Often, instead of applying time management principles, the assistant procrastinates by making a note on the job list. In some cases this putting off of the task requires the medical assistant to think through the task again, thus wasting valuable office time.

If a project is important, it is good practice to follow through with the task at hand. This practice avoids double processing.

PATIENT TEACHING CONSIDERATIONS

With the knowledge of self-management techniques, the medical assistant can better instruct patients in lifestyle changes that may necessitate rearranging priorities and learning new ways to manage time. As later chapters illustrate, certain conditions and diseases require patients to change various aspects of their lives. For instance, a busy executive recovering from a heart attack may need to find time every day for walking. He or she may need help in learning to adjust the daily schedule to include exercise.

Self-improvement for the medical assistant automatically results in increased potential for administering to patients' holistic needs and helping patients to manage their own time.

RELATED ETHICAL AND LEGAL IMPLICATIONS

The American Association of Medical Assistants has established a code of ethics for professional medical assistants. The RMA also has a code of ethics similar in content to the AAMA code. The ethical principles are reprinted with permission of the AAMA and are included in the bylaws of the association:

> Members of AAMA dedicated to the conscientious pursuit of their profession, and thus desiring to merit the high regard of the entire medical profession and the respect of the general public which they serve, do pledge themselves to strive always to
>
> A. Render service with full respect for the dignity of humanity;
> B. Respect confidential information obtained through employment unless legally authorized or required by responsible performance of duty to divulge such information;
> C. Uphold the honor and high principles of the profession and accept its disciplines;
> D. Seek to continually improve the knowledge and skills of medical assistants for the benefit of patients and professional colleagues;
> E. Participate in additional service activities aimed toward improving the health and well-being of the community.

CREED

> I believe in the principles and purposes of the profession of medical assisting.
>
> I endeavor to be more effective.
>
> I aspire to render greater service.
>
> I protect the confidence entrusted to me.
>
> I am dedicated to the care and well-being of all patients.
>
> I am loyal to my physician-employer.
>
> I am true to the ethics of my profession.
>
> I am strengthened by compassion, courage, and faith.

SUMMARY

From the perspective of the physician, the valuable medical assistant is able to anticipate, assess, and respond to the needs of the physician, the patient, and the office staff. He or she must be able to meet all these complicated needs harmoniously without overstepping the prudent boundaries of good judgment. In addition, the medical assistant must be autonomous, but at the same time must operate within reasonable guidelines. This balance is indeed delicate and takes years of experience and effort to achieve. The constant pursuit of professional development and the effective management of personal time facilitate the accomplishment of these objectives.

DISCUSSION QUESTIONS

1. What problems related to the effective operation of the office would be created by a medical assistant who was not self-motivated?
2. What difficulties could be created by the opposite extreme, an overly aggressive medical assistant?
3. Describe the purpose of goal setting in the medical office.
4. Discuss the importance of pinpointing goals.
5. Describe the purpose of time management. Evaluate your own use of time. Discuss the problems students encounter in managing their time.

BIBLIOGRAPHY

Ash AM: Motivate before you delegate: An effective strategy. The Professional Medical Assistant 21(5):16, September/October 1988.

Curtis CT: On being a professional. The Professional Medical Assistant 13(2):24, March 1980.

Feist CM: Synergy in the medical office. The Professional Medical Assistant 23(3):6, May/June 1990.

Frew DR and Frew MA: Dimensions of professional behavior. The Professional Medical Assistant 18(6):4, November/December 1985.

Ledford J: First things first: Setting priorities. The Professional Medical Assistant 21(6):18, November/December 1988.

Liebler JG et al: Management Principles for Health Professionals, ed 2. Aspen, Gaithersburg, MD, 1992.

Purtilo R: Health Professionals and Patient Interaction, ed 4. WB Saunders, Philadelphia, 1990.

Skinner OC: Performing under pressure. AMT Events 6:6, 1989.

Upton P: The job description. The Professional Medical Assistant 19(2):20, March/April 1986.

PROCEDURE: Design a time management plan

Terminal Performance Objective: Create a strategy for managing time efficiently and setting goals for the completion of tasks.

EQUIPMENT: Office or facilities procedures manual
Typewriter and typing paper, or
Word processor and printer

PROCEDURE

1. Identify the specific goals to be achieved and the tasks to be accomplished.

2. Determine the average time required to complete each task. While you are performing the planned tasks, note the actual time used.

3. Write an action plan that lists the tasks to be achieved and the time allowed for completion. Place this plan in the procedures manual.

PRINCIPLE

1. Knowing what specific tasks must be done and why and how they are to be done, and allotting time accurately is essential to time management.

2. Although the average times may not be precise, they are useful for predicting the time needed for task completion, the essential second step in planning. Checking the time required against the time predicted helps in setting more realistic objectives the next time.

3. Writing an action plan communicates the plan to co-workers, serves as a reference for evaluation of the time-management plan, and provides a permanent record.

HIGHLIGHTS

Assertiveness, the ability to express yourself constructively in the face of disagreement, is a reflection of professional growth and personal management. Assertiveness may be an inherent trait in a few of us. Most of us, however, must consciously learn the appropriate use of assertive behaviors. Learning assertiveness can be achieved by (1) identifying areas of nonassertiveness, and (2) practicing assertive behaviors. The Book *Pulling Your Own Strings* by Wayne W. Dyer can help you identify your assertiveness strengths and weaknesses.

Everyone has areas of strength and weakness related to assertiveness. Some individuals tend to be less assertive in family relationships, whereas for others, work relationships elicit more unassertive behaviors. Knowing your strengths and weaknesses related to assertiveness is an essential beginning in developing assertiveness as a patterned response and choice of behaviors.

Practicing assertiveness rather than aggressiveness at work requires conscious effort. In the workplace, the goal in using assertiveness is to keep relationships with coworkers smooth and productive. The assertive emphasis, then, is not on sharing feelings but on acting. The assertive emphasis is not for the sake of interpersonal closeness but for that of job satisfaction, professional growth, positive interaction with coworkers, and the realization of career goals.

Verbal assertiveness on the job includes the following:

1. *Taking credit for your ideas.* "Excuse me, Dr. Smith, you were misled. I designed that brochure."
2. *Saying no to unrealistic or unreasonable demands.* "No, Mrs. Jones, I cannot stay until 7 PM every evening. When I was hired, I was assured that I would be able to leave at 5:30 each evening. It was with that understanding that I accepted this position."
3. *Making firm, reasonable requests.* "Judy, these records need to be filed. Please complete this project by Friday."
4. *Asking for what you need or want.* "Dr. Carnes, I have been here for 18 months now and my evaluations have been very good. I know I am worth more to the practice than what I am presently receiving. I would like to discuss this with you."

In expressing assertiveness, it is important to remember that face-to-face confrontation may not be the best or only alternative. Letter writing or gaining the support and cooperation of supervisors may be more appropriate, depending on the situation.

In the work environment, the ability to say no, make requests, and express constructive criticism will be determinants in career advancement. Verbal assertiveness is obviously one major component of being assertive. Assertive acts are also required in order to achieve career goals. The following is a checklist of assertive acts directed toward career advancement:

1. Be knowledgeable and competent in your performance of job responsibilities.
2. Identify the skills required for advancement.
3. Acquire the desirable skills through practice, research, or course work.
4. Ask your employer for the necessary equipment and supplies to perform your tasks well.
5. Exert an assertive image in both speaking and acting.

Being appropriately assertive is a characteristic of personal management and professional growth. Assertiveness enables you to like and respect yourself, to find satisfaction in your work, and to be respected by others.

> The first concern of medical law and ethics should be the person who seeks health rather than the professions or institutions which provide it.
>
> Ashley and O'Rourke,
> *Health Care Ethics*

CHAPTER OUTLINE

MEDICAL LAW

THE PHYSICIAN-PATIENT RELATIONSHIP

MEDICAL LICENSURE

THE LAW OF CONTRACTS
  Implications of the Contract
  Statutory Reports
  Third-Party Contracts
  Terminating a Contract

INFORMED CONSENT
  Assault and Battery
  Negligent Failure to Inform

THE AMERICAN LEGAL SYSTEM
  The Tort of Negligence
  Intentional Torts
  Damages
  Statutes of Limitations
  Criminal Offenses

THE LAW RELATING TO DRUG ADMINISTRATION
  Narcotic and Nonnarcotic Drugs
  Narcotic Inventory Control

THE LAW RELATING TO MEDICAL RECORDS
  Contents
  Ownership
  Retention and Disposal
  Documentation Guidelines
  Release

LEGAL RESPONSIBILITIES OF THE
  MEDICAL ASSISTANT

MEDICAL ETHICS
  American Medical Association Principles
  Ethical Responsibilities of Medical
    Assistants
  Contemporary Ethical Issues

SUMMARY

DISCUSSION QUESTIONS

BIBLIOGRAPHY

HIGHLIGHTS

LEARNING OBJECTIVES

Upon completing this chapter, you will be able to:

1. Describe the nature of and the criteria for the physician-patient relationship.
2. Describe the purpose of medical practice acts.
3. List the six requirements for the licensure of physicians.

Chapter 3

*M*edical Law and Ethics

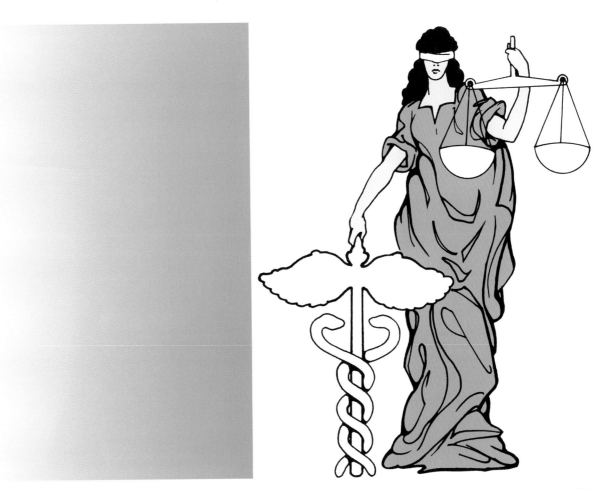

4. List two classifications of contracts, the four requirements of a valid contract, and four additional contract implications specific to the physician-patient relationship.
5. List six examples of mandatory disclosure (required by law) and give at least two examples of discretionary disclosure.
6. State the process of terminating the physician-patient relationship.
7. List the five criteria for valid and informed consent.
8. List the four elements necessary to recover damages for negligence.
9. Define *res ipsa loquitur*, the doctrine of professional discretion, the law of agency, *respondeat superior*, strict liability, and contributory negligence.
10. Define statute of limitations.
11. Describe the Drug Enforcement Agency (DEA) regulations and state regulations related to controlled substances.
12. Describe the legal ownership and retention periods of medical records.
13. Describe four aspects of the legal responsibilities of the medical assistant.
14. Define medical ethics.
15. List at least three principles of the medical assistant's and American Medical Association (AMA) codes of ethics and the Patient's Bill of Rights.
16. Describe the nature of the contents of *The Current Opinion of the Judiciary Council* of the AMA.

DACUM EDUCATIONAL COMPONENTS

1. Perform within ethical boundaries by applying ethical standards in the workplace, respecting patient rights, and recognizing practices that involve bioethical issues (1.2A–C).
2. Practice within the scope of education, training, and personal capabilities (1.3A–C).
3. Maintain confidentiality of verbal, written, and electronically generated information (1.4A).
4. Determine the needs for documenting and making correct entries in medical records and appointment books (5.1A–B; 5.2H).
5. Determine the needs for documenting and reporting to local, state, and federal agencies, and the Drug Enforcement Administration (DEA) (5.2B,C,F; 5.3B).
6. Use appropriate guidelines when releasing records or information to protect the privacy of patient health information (5.3A–D).
7. Follow established policy in initiating or terminating medical treatment (physician-patient relationship) and practice measures to prevent professional liability by identifying the significance of affirmative actions (5.4A–J).
8. Dispose of controlled substances in compliance with government regulations by complying with DEA regulations (5.5).
9. Maintain licenses and facility registration, certification, and accreditation (5.6A–C).
10. Monitor legislation related to current health care and practice (5.7A–C).

Glossary

Agent: A person acting on behalf of another
Breach: Failure to perform a legal obligation
Civil: Referring to legal rights and to proceedings between private individuals
Contract: An agreement between two or more competent individuals that obligates each to fulfill specified promises
Defendant: The individual against whom legal action is taken
Fiduciary: Based on trust and confidence
Good Samaritan law: A law that protects medical practitioners from claims of malpractice if they render care at the scene of an accident, provided that the care is competent and correct; most states have passed laws covering physicians; approximately half the laws cover nurses
Liable: Legally obligated
Libel: Defamation of character in writing
Negligence: Failure to do something that a reasonable person of ordinary prudence would do in a certain situation, or doing something that such a person would not do; negligence may be the reason for a lawsuit when the physician or medical assistant neglects to provide reasonable care to a patient and the negligence results in damage to the patient
Peer review: An evaluation by professional coworkers of equal status of the way an individual physician, nurse, or other health professional conducts practice, education, or research

Continued

Plaintiff: The individual who takes legal action
Proximate cause: An act or omission of an act directly responsible for producing an injury that would not have otherwise occurred
Release: Relinquishing of a right, claim, or title to another person
Statute: A state or federal law that commands or prohibits an act
Tort: A civil wrong caused by a breach of legal obligation

This chapter introduces the basic issues of medical law and ethics that are relevant to medical office practice. Specifically, the discussion of medical law includes the nature of legal rights and responsibilities for the patient, physician, and medical assistant. The discussion of medical ethics confronts the moral implications of situations common to medical practice.

Law and ethics are interrelated. However, *law* refers to rules of conduct that are legally binding. *Ethics* refers to rules of conduct that are not legally binding but govern the morality, or the rightness or wrongness, of behavior. Ethics, although often contained in law, may transcend legal boundaries. Laws dictate what we must do; ethics dictate what we should do. Following legal rules maintains social order and eliminates punishment. Following ethical rules not only maintains a social order but creates a challenge to achieve the highest standard of human behavior. Medical law reflects the principles of medical ethics. The following discussion of medical law focuses on legal issues related to medical office practice.

MEDICAL LAW

The contemporary physician has become a major target for lawsuits. In recent years, the number of patients initiating legal action against physicians has increased substantially. These lawsuits cover a wide spectrum of claims dealing with suspected or confirmed errors of diagnosis or treatment, and are commonly referred to as *malpractice claims.* In all cases, patients are dissatisfied with some aspect of medical care. The publicity these suits receive and the large monetary settlements awarded may contribute to the frequency with which patients seek legal counsel.

The public does not understand that the sensationalized headlines of windfall awards that get widespread attention are often decreased, reversed, or never collected. In fact, eight out of every ten malpractice cases are dismissed, withdrawn, or decided in favor of the physician. Therefore, 80% of the cases filed are *not* the result of malpractice (negligence). Studies show that the physicians sued most often are those who provide the most highly technical care in life-threatening situations, such as neurosurgeons, or obstetricians who care for "high-risk" unhealthy mothers.

The vast majority of physicians carry liability insurance that protects them against personal loss resulting from malpractice claims. However, many physicians have discounted their liability insurance or refuse to perform high-risk procedures because of the high cost of coverage. The medical assistant must understand the basics of medical law to follow current legal standards of care and help prevent lawsuits.

When physicians are sued, regardless of the outcome, their reputations are affected. For many physicians, a suit that has become public knowledge is a crushing emotional experience. If the court rules against the physician and a large settlement to the patient becomes public knowledge, the future of the physician's practice may be severely jeopardized. There is a danger that the anxiety generated by a suit will result in "defensive medicine" and dehumanized services. The sensible approach, however, is to accept the statistical probability of a lawsuit and carry on office business in a way that diminishes the likelihood of patients bringing action against the physician.

In addition to publicity, changing social values also contribute to encouraging lawsuits in medical practice. Society is increasingly sensitive to patient rights involving privacy, informed consent, confidentiality, ownership of and access to medical records, and the right to refuse treatment. Still other changes have occurred in the amount of paperwork and documentation legally required in medical practice. These latter changes, although not contributing to the number of medical malpractice suits, increase the medical assistant's legal responsibilities and require an expanded awareness of medical law related to office practice.

THE PHYSICIAN-PATIENT RELATIONSHIP

The legal relationship between the physician and the patient is defined by the law of contracts. The stated rights and obligations of physicians and patients arise from the nature of the physician-patient relationship.

The physician-patient relationship is fiduciary— based on trust and confidence. The patient trusts in the physician's knowledge and competence. The physician, in turn, is obligated by the patient's trust and confidence to put personal interests aside and act in the patient's best interests. Other examples of fiduciary relationships include those of the attorney and client, and the priest and parishioner.

Fiduciary relationships exist in contracts involving

other service provider–consumer relationships. In buyer-seller relationships, for instance, each individual is invested in his or her own best interest. An atmosphere of *caveat emptor* ("let the buyer beware") exists. No informed consent or voluntary disclosure of risks pertaining to the purchase of merchandise is required. In the physician-patient relationship, however, the physician owes the patient full disclosure. Likewise, the patient owes the physician just payment and compliance with the recommended treatment regimen. It is within the spirit of trust and confidence that the patient joins the physician in accepting certain legal rights and obligations as well as certain ethical responsibilities.

MEDICAL LICENSURE

Inherent in the physician-patient contractual agreement is the patient's right to a qualified physician. Physicians are licensed to practice medicine through state medical practice acts. These acts have regulated the practice of medicine consistently since 1899. While each state formulates its own medical practice acts, all state acts share certain characteristics:

1. They define the practice of medicine.
2. They permit the practice of medicine only to individuals who obtain a valid license.
3. They define licensing prerequisites.
4. They legitimize the authority and establishment of a medical examination board to grant licensure to individuals passing the examination.
5. They establish conditions for renewal.
6. They prescribe conditions and procedures for the suspension and revocation of licensure.

Although the process of licensure may differ from state to state, the following basic requirements may be cited. The physician must

1. Have graduated from an accredited medical school.
2. Have completed an internship approved by the state board of medical examiners.
3. Be at least 21 years of age and a United States resident.
4. Be a state resident of good moral character.
5. Satisfactorily complete the state board examination.
6. Pay a license fee.

Each practicing physician has a legal responsibility to obtain a license to practice medicine, to display it in the medical office, and to renew it periodically. Physicians who prescribe controlled substances also must obtain certificates of registration from the Drug Enforcement Agency (DEA). The registration number must appear on each prescription for a controlled substance.

Most states have a state agency on medical discipline that is empowered to suspend or revoke a physician's license to practice medicine. Physicians voluntarily serve on peer review committees to investigate complaints. If a complaint is justified, the agency can take disciplinary action. In addition, every hospital has a peer review committee that oversees the care provided by physicians. Medicare, Medicaid, and most insurance companies also require separate reviews of hospital care by independent agencies. In addition, the American Medical Association (AMA) affirms that all potentially criminal acts committed by the physician and discovered by the medical society must be reported to appropriate government officials. Most states will revoke the physician's license under the following conditions:

1. Criminal offenses
2. Unprofessional conduct
3. Fraud
4. Professional or personal incompetence

The medical practice acts of each state establish definitions and parameters for license revocation and suspension. Most complaints are received and heard by the state licensing board. If charges are made, the physician is given a hearing. The board then investigates, prosecutes, passes judgment, and sentences accordingly. Some state laws empower licensing boards to suspend a license pending investigation if a licensing board determines that a physician poses an immediate threat to the public. The Administrator of the DEA may suspend a DEA Certificate of Registration at any time for any period determined. Before a registration is revoked or suspended, the physician is issued to "show cause why such registration should not be removed or suspended," and is entitled to a hearing. DEA privileges may be revoked entirely or limited to a particular controlled substance. A physician whose DEA privileges have been suspended or revoked can still prescribe nonscheduled drugs.

THE LAW OF CONTRACTS

The physician-patient relationship begins when the physician first "lays hands" on the patient. Implied in this act is the physician's willingness to accept the responsibility for the patient's care. The patient, by first keeping a preset appointment and then permitting the physician's "laying on of hands," implies choice and consent to receive the care of the physician.

This interaction between physician and patient constitutes a contractual agreement, or implied contract. An implied contract is differentiated from an expressed contract, in which verbal or written agreement occurs. Both implied and expressed contracts are valid and binding.

A valid contract has four characteristics:

1. *Manifestation of assent.* There must be both an offer and an acceptance.
2. *Legal subject matter.* The subject of the contract may not pertain to an illegal act.

3. *Legal capacity.* Both parties must be legally capable of entering into an agreement.
4. *Consideration.* Benefits must pass between the parties.

During the patient's first visit with the physician, all four elements are present. The patient implies by his or her very presence (and often verbally) that the physician's care is desired. The actions of the patient and physician demonstrate the offer and its acceptance. The mutual exchange of promises also is implied in the behavior of these two consenting parties. Both parties have the right to refuse to make a contract. Although no formal contract is signed by patient and physician, all the components of the implied agreement are assumed within contract law.

IMPLICATIONS OF THE CONTRACT

There are several assumptions or implications in the physician-patient relationship. First is the promise that the physician (an individual licensed to practice medicine) will provide an acceptable standard of care for the patient. It is also presumed that the physician possesses a reasonable level of knowledge and skill comparable to those of other physicians practicing in the same specialty.

Regarding the standard of care, the physician is legally responsible only to provide competent care. He or she is not responsible for providing a cure. The promise of a cure becomes part of the contractual agreement only if verbalized by the physician. In this instance the physician would be held liable for failure to deliver the promised cure. This fact of law implies that *no one* in a medical office, including the medical assistant, should ever promise a cure. The medical assistant's discussions with patients should reinforce the physician's explanations relating to the diagnosis, treatment, and probable outcome. The medical assistant should never make statements such as, "Of course your broken finger can be fixed. Dr. Jones is an excellent physician, and 10 weeks from now your finger will be as good as new." Not only has a cure been promised in this statement, but a time limit has been set as well. All conversation should be directed toward helping the patient understand the physician's course of treatment and encouraging compliance without raising false expectations.

Another implication of the relationship between physician and patient is the responsibility of the physician, and consequently of the office staff, to maintain confidentiality. Information regarding the patient may not be disclosed without the patient's authorization unless disclosure is required by law. To breach the confidentiality of the physician-patient relationship is not only unethical, but unlawful.

Evidence of the seriousness of maintaining confidentiality between physicians and patients is found in several areas. The court system permits patients to sue physicians for a breach of confidence when the unauthorized disclosure is determined to be damaging to the

patient. Also, many states have enacted statutes stipulating that the betrayal of professional confidences will result in suspension or revocation of licensure.

In addition, in most states, a physician cannot testify in court regarding a patient unless the patient has authorized the disclosures or waives his or her right to confidentiality. An authorization for disclosure form (Fig. 3–1) is used to obtain written consent from the patient allowing the release of information. However, when a patient sues a physician, the physician is released from the restraints of confidentiality.

Some disclosures, however, are legally required. In cases of *mandatory* disclosure, the physician's duty to the public supersedes the patient's right to confidentiality. Disclosures can be required by (1) a subpoena or (2) a statute designed to protect the public. Disclosure is *discretionary* when a physician determines that it is necessary to protect the welfare of the patient or a third party.

A *subpoena* is a document issued by the court that orders an individual to testify and specifies the time, date, and place. When a physician is required to testify, usually the patient's medical record is also requested. In these instances, the subpoena is entitled *subpoena duces tecum*, or, "Under penalty you shall take it with you." The original record must be taken to court. A photocopy is maintained in the physician's office.

Statues or state laws requiring disclosure to protect the public welfare are related to the physician's public duties and responsibilities.

STATUTORY REPORTS

Most states require that a physician report the following:

1. Births
2. Specific infectious, communicable, or contagious diseases
3. Known or suspected incidents of drug abuse
4. Suspected child abuse
5. Injuries caused by violence
6. All deaths, including accidents or unexpected deaths

Noncompliance with state regulations may result in criminal action against the physician.

Disclosures for the protection of a patient or third party are often a matter of physician discretion. Many lawsuits against physicians occur in this area and allege inappropriate or inadequate disclosure. Our judicial system maintains that a physician has the legal obligation to instruct patients in how to notify third parties (person or persons other than patient responsible for payment to the physician, such as a parent responsible for a child, a son or daughter with power of attorney responsible for a parent, a guardian responsible for an adolescent, and so on) and refer them to health care providers. If the patient is unwilling to comply, the physician is legally bound to use confidential proce-

RELEASE AND ASSIGNMENT

Date_____

To_____
INSURANCE COMPANY

_____

Group No._____   Certificate No._____

I hereby authorize Dr._____

to release to your company or its representative, any information including the diagnosis and the records of any treatment or examination rendered to me during the period of such Medical or Surgical care.

I also authorize and request your company to pay directly to the above named doctor the amount due me in my pending claim for Medical or Surgical treatment or services, by reason of such treatment or services rendered to:

_____
PATIENT

_____   _____
WITNESS   SIGNATURE OF INSURED

_____
ADDRESS

Figure 3–1. An authorization for disclosure form.

dures to disclose information about the patient to ensure that the third party is notified. Therefore, the physician determines when such information must be disclosed. In this instance the physician's duty to society outweighs his or her duty to patient confidentiality.

Encompassed in the patient's right to confidentiality is the right to privacy. It is unlawful for the physician to engage in publicity, including journal publication, regarding a patient's medical treatment without the patient's written consent. Likewise, the physician must obtain the patient's consent before inviting other health professionals to observe the patient receiving treatment or undergoing medical procedures. Forms are available from the AMA for these situations. Figure 3–2 shows an example.

The physician-patient relationship is the basis for the court's interpretation of the contractual agreement and its four major implications: standard of care, confidentiality, mandatory and discretionary disclosure, and right to privacy. In addition to the implications discussed, the physician encounters other problems associated with the implicit contractual agreement between physician and patient. One such problem is the introduction of a third party into the agreement.

THIRD-PARTY CONTRACTS

One of the more common contractual problems for the physician is the treatment of an individual who will not be responsible for payment. Mr. Jones, who is a regular patient, brings in his next-door neighbor, Mr. Smith, and explains that Mr. Smith hurt his back help-

ing to push Mr. Jones' car out of a snowdrift. Mr. Jones offers to pay the medical bill.

On the surface this situation does not seem problematic. Sometimes, however, these matters can become complicated. For example, the physician may find that extensive treatment costing several thousand dollars is required. Meanwhile, Mr. Jones learns that Mr. Smith has had a bad back since he was injured 10 years ago playing shuffleboard. Mr. Jones now tells Mr. Smith that he will not pay; Mr. Smith tells the physician to collect the money from Mr. Jones; and the physician may find it impossible to obtain the fee.

Inherent in the implied contractual agreement between physician and patient is the assumption that the patient is legally responsible to pay for services. Difficulty in collecting fees often occurs, but promise of third-party payment causes particular problems.

The foregoing example illustrates the reason why, unless a patient asks for treatment for him- or herself or for a dependent (spouse or child), the physician must obtain a written agreement from the third party promising to pay for the services the patient receives. This agreement must be signed and witnessed. If physicians do not secure a written agreement, they will subsequently find that they may have no legal right to payment from the third party.

TERMINATING A CONTRACT

Having entered into an implied contract with a patient, the physician is legally obligated to provide continuous care. A physician who wishes to discontinue the

Consent to Operation

Saint Vincent Health Center
Erie, Pennsylvania

Patient _____ Date _____

1. I hereby authorize Dr. _____ , or a physician

    designated by him, to perform upon _____

    the following operative procedure: _____

    He is authorized to utilize in the performance of this surgical procedure the service of physicians, residents or members of the House Staff. If any unforeseen condition arises in the course of the operation calling in his judgment, for procedures in addition to or different from this now contemplated, I authorize him to do whatever he deems advisable.

2. The nature and purpose of the surgical procedure, possible alternative methods and treatment, the risks and possible consequences involved and the possibility of complication have been explained to my satisfaction. If I am a female patient, I acknowledge that any surgical procedure on my reproductive organs may REMOVE MY CAPABILITY to bear children in the future. I have discussed this with my husband and we both understand and accept this possibility. I acknowledge that no guarantee or assurance has been made as to results that may be obtained.

3. I consent to the administration of anesthesia to be administered under the direction of the Chief of the Department of Anesthesia, by one of his associates or by an individual designated by him and to the use of such anesthetics as he or she may deem advisable.

4. I consent to the administration of blood transfusions or other medications; to the disposal by authorities of Saint Vincent Health Center of any tissue or parts which may be removed; to the taking and publication of any photographs in the course of this operation and consent to the admittance of observers to the Operating Room for the purpose of advancement of medical education.

    I certify that I have read and fully understand the above consent for surgical operation and that explanations therein referred to have been made.

                        Signature of Patient_____

                        Signature of Patient's
                        Husband or Wife _____

                        Signature of person authorized
                        to consent for a minor_____

                        Relationship to Patient _____

Witness to Signature _____

Witness to Explanation _____

                                                    7117-3
                                                    T5387-38-SV19

Figure 3–2. A consent to operation form. (Courtesy of St. Vincent Health Center, Erie, Pennsylvania.)

FORM A-1

LETTER OF WITHDRAWAL FROM CASE

Dear Mr. _____

    I find it necessary to inform you that I am withdrawing from further professional attendance upon you for the reason that you have persisted in refusing to follow my medical advice and treatment. Since your condition requires medical attention, I suggest that you place yourself under the care of another physician without delay. If you so desire, I shall be available to attend you for a reasonable time after you have received this letter, but in no event for more than five days.

    This should give you ample time to select a physician of your choice from the many competent practitioners in this city. With your approval, I will make available to this physician your case history and information regarding the diagnosis and treatment which you have received from me.

Very truly yours,

_____ M.D.

Figure 3–3. A sample letter of termination. (Courtesy American Medical Association.)

relationship must write a letter of termination of services and should send it by certified mail, with a return receipt requested (Fig. 3–3). Also, a photocopy of the letter and the mail receipt should be placed in the patient record. The physician may withdraw from a case in three general instances:

1. The patient fails to uphold his or her part of the contract, either through refusal to make any payment or through not following the physician's orders. However, once treatment has been initiated, the physician cannot legally refuse to continue treatment because the patient has not paid.
2. The patient leaves the hospital without the permission of the physician or fails to keep appointments as part of follow-up care.
3. The patient requests that the physician not continue services.

Even in these instances, withdrawal is appropriate only if it involves no jeopardy for the patient. The physician who withdraws from a case must notify the patient in advance to provide opportunity for the patient to obtain alternative medical care. Failure to notify a patient of withdrawal in writing may subject the physician to liability for abandonment.

INFORMED CONSENT

Although the initial contractual agreement between physician and patient is implied, there are special treatments and procedures for which the law requires written and informed consent. In such cases the physician should secure a signed consent form, such as the one shown in Figure 3–2. The AMA suggests that this procedure be followed if a particular medical treatment either presents a recognized risk or involves hospitalization. For such a form to be binding, the patient must

be of legal age (legal age varies from state to state, but usually is 18) or be an emancipated minor (a person younger than 18 who is no longer under parental care and who has been declared of legal age by the state). Regardless of the patient's age, the contents of the form should be carefully explained. If the patient is in grave danger (a life- or limb-threatening emergency) and at the same time is unconscious or otherwise unable to respond, the physician may give emergency treatment without signed consent forms. In the instance of voluntary sterilization, the physician must obtain the signed consent of both the patient and his or her spouse. In addition, all surgical procedures and special treatments require that the patient's consent be informed and in writing.

Whenever a recognized danger or risk to the patient occurs, for instance, through a surgical procedure or the administration of a dangerous drug, informed consent is mandated by law. The fiduciary nature of the physician-patient relationship obligates physicians to disclose risks inherent in certain procedures and treatments and to obtain consent *before* beginning medical treatment. The AMA suggests that physicians follow a particular process in providing disclosures and obtaining a signed consent. Forms such as those illustrated in Figures 3–1 and 3–2 are available for such instances.

Provided that the patient is of legal age, certain other criteria must be present for consent to be informed and valid. Patients must understand the following:

1. What is going to be done, by whom, and why
2. The expected outcomes and consequences of the proposed treatment or procedure (predictable and potential)
3. The dangers or risks inherent in the proposed procedure or treatment and the likelihood of the occurrence of each
4. The severity and permanence of common side effects or complications
5. The existence of alternative procedures or treatments (including no treatment), and the probable cause of each in comparison with the proposed procedure or treatment

Obviously, the above guidelines are interpreted according to individual situations. For instance, a physician is not required by law to list every possible side effect of every drug administered. Usually, physicians assess the degree of disclosure according to the degree of risk. The physician may request the aid of the medical assistant in determining the patient's understanding of the procedure and may depend on the medical assistant to offer reinforcement. However, the physician, not the medical assistant, is legally responsible for obtaining consent. A patient who refers questions or difficulties concerning the treatment or procedure to the medical assistant should be referred to the physician.

In some instances the physician may legally withhold information. One such example is that of a patient who refuses to be informed. However, in deviating from the informed consent guidelines, a physician should seek legal counsel and protection.

There are also instances (in addition to life-threatening situations) in which consent is not required. When a state law requires certain treatment, such as vaccination, or a court order is issued to administer treatment, consent is not required.

ASSAULT AND BATTERY

A physician who treats a patient without first obtaining informed consent, in circumstances in which informed consent is appropriate, may be sued for assault and battery. *Assault* as related to medical practice refers to a deliberate attempt or threat to touch another person without consent.

Battery is forcibly touching another person against his or her will. Assault and battery claims against physicians are not frequent, but cases have been tried on those grounds and verdicts rendered in favor of the patient. The law maintains that no matter how severely ill a patient may be, a conscious, competent adult has the right to refuse treatment.

Consent at its simplest is the permission given by the patient to be touched, examined, and treated. Consent is given both by words and by action. For this reason it is extremely important for the medical assistant to introduce him- or herself to the patient and to take the time necessary to inform the patient of each procedure or treatment. Patient consent is considered given when the patient agrees to a procedure either orally or by a nonverbal action, such as a nod.

NEGLIGENT FAILURE TO INFORM

Professional negligence suits against physicians are more common than those charging assault and battery. Negligence can be alleged even if signed consent was obtained. In these instances the plaintiff (patient) charges that the physician failed or neglected to provide adequate information. The burden of proof in these cases lies in the ability of the patient or the patient's attorney's to show that the patient suffered a known risk that would routinely be disclosed by other physicians, and that if the patient knew of the risk, he or she would have declined treatment. "Professional negligence" also refers to suits alleging malpractice or physician incompetence regardless of valid consent. These situations are further explained in the following discussion of torts and criminal offenses.

THE AMERICAN LEGAL SYSTEM

The American legal system originated from several sources. As the highest law in this land, the Constitution limits the application of law in the court system and provides for civil rights, such as due process. The other sources of current law in the United States were treaties made with other governments, statutes, ordinances, administrative regulations, and executive orders.

Statutes are state laws passed by state legislatures. For example, the state can recognize the danger of radiation and enact or pass a law that prohibits or controls certain uses of radioactive material. The 51 medical practice acts are governed by individual state laws.

Administrative regulations are enacted, or passed into federal law, by Congress. The laws are then enforced by administrative agencies, such as the DEA or the Nuclear Regulatory Commission. Often state legislatures pass a state law that is already a federal law. The purpose is usually to pass down enforcement of the law to the state level, and often to make the federal law even more rigorous. States may pass their own laws based on federal laws, provided that the state law is at least as comprehensive as the federal law. One recent example of such legislation is the Occupational Safety and Health Administration Bloodborne Pathogens Protection Standard enacted by Congress in 1991. Regulated by the Departments of Labor and of Health and Human Resources, the law is designed to protect workers against occupational exposure to hepatitis B virus and human immunodeficiency virus. By 1992, 26 states had passed their own plans based on the federal standard. Other administrative laws regulating the physician's practice include the Clinical Laboratory Improvement Amendment of 1988 and the Omnibus Budget Reconciliation Act (OBRA) of 1989, which regulates the federally funded Medicare program. OBRA is enforced by the Health Care Financing Administration. All the federal laws regulating medical practice are discussed in subsequent chapters.

Arbitration is becoming increasingly popular as a method of settling disputes outside the court system. The parties in dispute select a person or persons who may or may not have been trained in law to hear and decide the dispute. Arbitration is quicker to initiate than the court system, is less formal than a trial, takes less time than a trial, and can involve an arbitrator with expertise or technical background.

In the United States, there are three types of wrongful conduct: criminal offense, tort, and breach of contract. Most lawsuits against physicians are based on tort law. A *tort* is a civil wrong or injury other than breach of contract. If a physician is sued under civil law (i.e., a malpractice suit), the basis of the litigation must be breach of contract, negligence, or intentional wrongdoing. These terms are differentiated from one another in the following discussion.

Negligence is an issue when a patient claims that a physician (or someone acting on the physician's instructions) performed an action improperly, causing harm to the patient whether or not there was intent to do harm; for example, leaving an instrument or sponge inside a patient following surgery.

Breach of contract is an issue when a patient claims that a physician did not live up to his or her part of the implied physician-patient contract. Violation of confidentiality and failure to perform prescribed services fall within this category.

Torts can be either intentional or unintentional. Unintentional torts account for a significant number of lawsuits against physicians and are based on allegations that a mistake was made, although in good faith. Intentional torts are offenses committed in the absence of good faith. Battery (unlawful touching or beating) is an intentional tort. The types of torts applicable to medical office practice are described in the following discussion.

The Tort of Negligence

Legally defined, negligence is the omission of an act that would ordinarily be done by a reasonable person, or the performance of an act that a reasonable person would not do. In lawsuits alleging professional negligence, the reasonableness of the defendant is measured against a standard of "reasonable members of the profession." For instance, the professional expectations of medical assistants would be derived from the professional definition and standards of the profession itself.

The physician is required by law to possess the same degree of knowledge or skill that other physicians possess in the same specialty or system of practice. To win a lawsuit alleging professional negligence against a physician, the patient or attorney must prove the "Four Ds": (1) that a physician-patient relationship existed (duty), (2) that the physician was negligent (dereliction of duty), (3) that the physician's negligence was the direct cause of the patient's injury (direct cause) and (4) that injury occurred to the patient (damage). *Proximate cause* refers to the cause-and-effect relationship between the negligent act and the personal injury suffered by the patient.

For the patient to be awarded a sum of money (damages or compensation), injury must have occurred. The physician is not liable for an incorrect diagnosis but is liable for failure to provide reasonable care. The physician can also be liable for death resulting from negligence by failure to provide adequate care or by noncare (abandonment). Expert testimony usually is required in negligence cases. In fact, physicians offer their services as experts in court cases. Expert testimony can be given only by a physician knowledgeable in the same specialty. The expert witness evaluates the alleged negligent act according to standards of reasonable care for the specialty. In such a case, the expert would testify that the injury might have been caused by some improper act, although the expert may not know exactly what the act was.

In some cases, injury may have been caused by any of several of possible acts. To prove a claim of contributory negligence, the patient must show that the physician's negligence was the direct cause of injury and that no intervening circumstances could have caused or contributed to the injury. If, however, the patient's failure to exercise a reasonable degree of caution and follow the physician's advice, or to otherwise exercise reasonable care, combined with the negligence of the physician in causing injury, compensation might be reduced or denied.

In some cases, the doctrine of *res ipsa loquitur* ("the thing speaks for itself") may apply. Although the patient normally has the burden of proving how and when the physician was negligent, cases that fall under this doctrine are exceptions. In this type of case, evidence of injury is apparent. The physician must then mount a defense against the evidence. An example of *res ipsa loquitur* is a postsurgery x-ray of an instrument or sponge inside a patient.

Intentional Torts

Battery, as mentioned previously, is an example of an intentional tort. Intentional torts are deliberate wrongs usually not related to medical treatment but to the interaction between physician and patient. Examples of battery include a physician slapping an uncooperative child or continuing with treatment despite the parent's or guardian's refusal.

Other intentional torts applicable to medical practice are

> *Invasion of privacy.* Unauthorized disclosure of information regarding the patient to a third party.
>
> *Defamation of character.* An untrue, unauthorized statement that damages the patient's name, reputation, or character (defamation is termed *slander* when the statement is oral and *libel* when it is written).
>
> *False imprisonment.* Restraint of a patient against his or her will.
>
> *Intentional infliction of emotional distress.* Actions designed to be so outrageous and offensive as to cause great upset.

Damages

When the court rules in favor of the injured plaintiff, the party is compensated monetarily and thereby awarded damages. Damages (monetary award) can be nominal, compensatory, special, or punitive. *Nominal* damages are for a small dollar amount and represent recognition that legal rights were violated, although no substantial injury was sustained. *Compensatory* damages are awarded on the basis of actual general or particular losses incurred. General damages represent a dollar amount awarded for pain and suffering, disability, and loss of income. *Special* damages represent payment for actual medical expenses, lost past income, and other pretrial economic losses. *Punitive* damages are awarded to impose further punishment or to deter outrageous conduct and represent a dollar amount beyond actual compensation. Punitive damages rarely are awarded. Damages are usually paid by the physician's professional liability insurance carrier.

Statutes of Limitations

A statute of limitations is a law that specifies the period in which the patient may seek legal action against a physician. This determination may be based on the time negligence occurred, the time treatment ended, or the date the injury was discovered. Statutes of limitations vary from state to state. However, in most states, taking legal action is limited to between 3 and 7 years after an injury or the discovery of an injury.

In some cases the limitation period is extended. In the case of a minor, the period of the statute may not begin until the child reaches 18, allowing the child to reach adulthood before legal action is initiated. If a pediatric injury is discovered after a child has reached 18 years of age, the usual limitation period applies. The statutes of limitations do not apply to legally insane patients until after the period of insanity has ended.

CRIMINAL OFFENSES

Criminal offenses have occasional application in medical law and warrant brief discussion. Unlike torts, which are subject to court or judicial interpretation (civil law), criminal offenses are acts defined by local, state, or federal law to be against the state or public welfare (public law). An example of a criminal offense is the practice of medicine without a license.

THE LAW RELATING TO DRUG ADMINISTRATION

Due to the growing problem of drug abuse, the Drug Enforcement Agency was established under the Controlled Substances Act of 1970. One of the primary responsibilities of the DEA is to regulate the dispensing of controlled substances, including narcotic drugs. Because of the paperwork involved in these procedures, the medical assistant usually is involved in the physician's dealings with the DEA.

Each physician prescribing controlled substances must register with the DEA. A physician supplying, administering, or dispensing controlled substances from more than one office must register each of these offices individually. Each prescription for controlled substances (nonnarcotic or narcotic drugs) requires the physician's signature and registration number. For drugs that are not controlled substances, only the physician's signature is required. Some states require that Schedule II (drugs that have a high potential for abuse and for physical or psychological dependence) narcotic prescriptions be written on specially printed, sequentially numbered duplicate or triplicate prescription blanks. If a triplicate form is required, one copy is sent to the state agency where records of all Schedule II prescriptions are kept.

NARCOTIC AND NONNARCOTIC DRUGS

Under DEA regulations, controlled substances may be divided into two distinct generic categories: narcotic and nonnarcotic. Narcotics belong to the controlled substance classification of scheduled drugs (see Chapter 23) and are potentially addictive (that is, they may cause the user to become psychologically or physically

dependent on them). Examples of narcotic drugs are morphine, meperidine (Demerol), and codeine. Although the primary concern of the agency is narcotic drugs, physicians who dispense nonnarcotic drugs on a regular basis must inventory these substances and keep an updated record of all transactions for 2 years. Agents of the DEA may ask to review these records at any time, and the physician is required by federal law to provide them.

Many pharmaceutical representatives routinely supply physicians with samples of their company's particular products so that the physician can hand them out to patients. These free samples may have a special notation on the label such as, "Sample – Not to be Sold." Many physicians accumulate drug samples and pass them along to patients. For example, if a patient requires a decongestant, the physician may simply provide a starter dose from the sample shelf. This basic approach is not considered a regular process of drug dispensing and thus does not require a record-keeping system.

NARCOTIC INVENTORY CONTROL

With substances that are defined as narcotics by the DEA, both physicians and their staffs are required to practice several routine precautionary procedures. First, and perhaps most important, all narcotics must be stored in a locked cabinet or safe, and access to keys to that container must be carefully controlled. Theft or other loss of substances from the locked area must be reported to the regional DEA office as soon as the loss is discovered. Local law enforcement agencies also should be informed.

All narcotic drugs kept in the physician's office should be ordered on DEA triplicate order forms, retaining the third part of the form (Fig. 3–4). Physicians also must maintain 2 years of inventory records for their supplies of narcotic drugs.

THE LAW RELATING TO MEDICAL RECORDS

The patient's medical record is a legal document. The importance of careful attention to the method of documenting patient care cannot be overstated. Physicians can be sued both for omission and for what is written in the medical record. The medical record should be clearly written, well organized, accurate, and complete.

CONTENTS

The medical record should contain all personal information provided by the patient and all clinically relevant information provided by the physician and authorized staff. Financial records should be kept separate from the medical record. All consent forms for office procedures, forms to authorize disclosure of information, consultation reports, and all correspondence regarding the patient should be contained in the medical record.

See Reverse of PURCHASER'S Copy for Instructions	No order form may be issued for Schedule I and II substances unless a completed application form has been received, (21 CFR 1305.04).		OMB APPROVAL No. 1117-0010

TO: *(Name of Supplier)*   ACME WHOLESALE DRUGS   STREET ADDRESS   600 NORTH AVE.

CITY and STATE   ANYTOWN, USA   DATE   TODAY'S DATE

LINE No	No. of Packages	Size of Package	Name of Item	NATIONAL DRUG CODE	No. of Packages Received	Date Received
			TO BE FILLED IN BY PURCHASER		TO BE FILLED IN BY PURCHASER	
1	3	100	Sodium pentothal Capsules, 100 mg		3	0/0/9-
2	2	100	Secobarbital Capsules, 100 mg		2	0/0/9-
3	3	100	Desoxyn Tablets, 5 mg		3	0/0/9-
4	1	30 ml	Demerol, 50mg/ml		1	0/0/9-
5	2	PINT	Robitussin A-C, 2mg/ml		2	0/0/9-
6						
7						
8						
9						
10						

5 ◀ NO. OF LINES COMPLETED   SIGNATURE OF PURCHASER OR HIS ATTORNEY OR AGENT

Date Issued	DEA Registration No.	Name and Address of Registrant
12/31/82	AD.000000	JAMES HO, M.D.
Schedules	2,2N,3,3N,4,5	1 MAIN STREET
Registered as a	No. of this Order Form	ANYWHERE, USA 55555-0000
Practitioner	PO 123456	

DEA Form -222 (Aug. 1990)

U.S. OFFICIAL ORDER FORMS - SCHEDULES I & II
DRUG ENFORCEMENT ADMINISTRATION
PURCHASER'S Copy 3

Figure 3–4. The Federal Triplicate Order Form is used to order Schedule C-II controlled substances. (From Lane, K: Medications: A Guide for the Health Profession. Philadelphia, FA Davis, 1992, p 36.)

Notations of medically significant telephone conversations and prescription refills also should be included.

OWNERSHIP

In most states, the office patient's medical record belongs to the physician. Hospital or medical facility records belong to the institution providing care. Historically, patients have not had access to their medical records unless they initiated a lawsuit. However, since 1973, as a result of the report prepared by the Commission on Medical Malpractice, the medical record has been made more available to patients who sign a consent for release of information. Several states have passed legislation permitting the patient to review the record at will.

To protect mentally or emotionally ill patients from potential harm, the courts have instituted a *doctrine of professional discretion*. This doctrine gives the physician the right to refuse access to certain portions of the medical record that the physician believes the patient could not understand or handle emotionally. If the patient challenges the physician's refusal to release the record, the physician must defend his or her position in a court of law.

RETENTION AND DISPOSAL

Individual states have laws stipulating the length of time during which a medical record should be retained. Physicians typically maintain the patient record until the statute of limitations has expired. In most instances, records are retained for 7 to 10 years from the date on which the physician or the patient terminated care. Many physicians have adopted microfilm and microfiche technology to store records.

Medical records ready for disposal should be shredded and burned to obscure the identity of the patient and ensure confidentiality.

DOCUMENTATION GUIDELINES

As is indicated in Chapter 6, the method of recording information is as important as the content. Although most of the information related to the topic is discussed in Chapter 6, it is useful to review the following points:

1. Personal option and value-laden statements should be excluded.
2. Every patient interaction, including medically significant telephone conversations, should be noted.
3. The medical assistant should initial his or her entries.
4. Entries should be made at the time of the event or shortly thereafter.
5. A medical record can be corrected but not altered. No erasures or whiteouts are permitted. Corrections are made in ink by drawing a single line through the error, placing it in parentheses, and writing the correction above or alongside the error. The correction is dated and initialed.
6. The appointment book is a legal document. If a patient fails to appear for the scheduled visit, "No show" should be entered in the appointment book and the patient record. If a patient cancels an appointment, "Canceled" should be entered in the appointment book and the patient record. Who canceled the appointment (physician or patient), and whether and when the appointment has been rescheduled, should also be noted.
7. All prescription renewals should be noted on the patient's chart.

RELEASE

Unless legally required by court order, the patient also has the right to authorize disclosure of information contained in the record. In most states, when a patient requests the release of records to another physician, a physician is not legally bound to send the record in its entirety, but is legally bound to send a written summary or photocopied excerpts from the patient's record. If the entire record is to be sent, it is photocopied and the original record is retained by the physician. A new authorization is required each time information is released.

LEGAL RESPONSIBILITIES OF THE MEDICAL ASSISTANT

Under the *law of agency*, physicians are legally responsible (liable) for the acts of their employees. Physicians who employ other physicians as associates under their supervision are responsible for their acts as well. As an employee of the physician, the medical assistant also is the agent of the physician. Therefore, when the medical assistant, acting on behalf of the physician, performs a negligent act, the physician assumes legal responsibility. The medical assistant may also be liable and can be sued.

The doctrine of *respondeat superior*, meaning "Let the master answer," is the legal term stemming from the law of agency. Although this doctrine applies to medical assistants and other employees in the medical office, it does not render any of the physician's employees immune to liability. Legal principle maintains that individuals are responsible for their own negligence. The law of agency enables the patient to seek damages from both the physician and the physician's staff. In addition, the physician-employer may sue the staff member to recover employee-caused losses.

Unfortunately, many of the lawsuits related to office practice and against physicians are the result of employee negligence. Therefore, it is essential that medical assistants understand their own legal responsibilities, not only for the sake of the physician but also for their own protection. The medical assistant must exercise extreme caution and avoid certain behaviors to prevent litigation.

Betrayal of Physician-Patient Confidence

Medical assistants are bound morally and legally as agents of the physician to protect the privacy and confidentiality of physician-patient interactions. To this end, the medical assistant must ensure the following:

1. All patient information must be obtained from the patient and exchanged with staff members in private.
2. The patient should never undergo unnecessary or inappropriate physical exposure.
3. The medical assistant should avoid discussing a particular case with anyone outside the office even when the name is withheld unless the discussion is professional. Examples include referring to a patient by another name (name is used), or classroom use of a case study (name and facts that might disclose identity are withheld).
4. Office staff members should discuss the patient or view the patient record only when it is necessary and appropriate to do so.
5. All written documents pertaining to a patient should be kept from the view of other patients or visitors to the office.

Performance of Tasks Beyond the Scope of the Medical Assisting Profession

A medical assistant is prepared to perform certain administrative and clinical tasks acceptable to the profession. Performing a task that does not fall within professional parameters increases the likelihood of litigation. Examples would include performing physical assessment (examination), giving intravenous injections, renewing prescriptions without orders, and advising the patient. For the medical assistant's own protection, the medical assistant's responsibilities in the office should be decided in agreement with the physician and should accord with acceptable standards for the profession. Ideally, the medical assistant's tasks and job description would be listed and described in the procedures manual. Obviously, the medical assistant is legally responsible for the diligent and competent performance of those tasks.

As has been stated, medical assistants who are negligent may be sued. In most cases, however, patients sue the physician because the employing physician is held liable for the actions of employees. Two of the most common areas for potential litigation involving medical assistants are (1) providing emergency care in the physician's absence and (2) misinstructing patients.

Emergency Situations

There is a reasonable chance that the medical assistant will confront a medical emergency in the physician's office when the physician and other professionals are not available. The medical assistant may provide whatever emergency care, within the limits of skill and training, is clearly indicated and consistent with routine first-aid procedures (see Chapter 27). The medical assistant should discuss this eventuality with the physician and ask for instructions regarding these situations to further avoid litigation. Emergency protocol also should be described in the procedure manual. In the event of an accidental injury in the office, an incident report should be filed (Fig. 3–5) if it is the office policy to do so. The incident report is completed by the person witnessing or associated with the incident. The physician signs the report, and a copy is usually sent to the physician's insurance company for evaluation of potential liability.

In an emergency such as an automobile accident or an injury occurring at a basketball game, physicians, nurses, or other allied health professionals may be called on to render immediate first aid. To protect such persons from later suits by the injured parties or their families, most states have passed "Good Samaritan acts." Although the exact areas of applicability vary from state to state, the general purpose of these acts is to ensure that the physician or other person who gave reasonable care in good faith is protected from civil liability under the circumstances.

Misinstructing Patients

The medical assistant must take care not to promise a cure, guarantee results from a procedure, or advise the patient regarding treatment. As an authorized agent of a physician, the medical assistant is legally presumed to be relaying the physician's instruction to the patient. The medical assistant must take extreme care in explaining treatments and other procedures, and must be sure that patients fully understand any instructions they are given.

As was previously mentioned, medical assistants also must be prudent in their choice of language with regard to appointments, diagnoses, treatments, and outcomes. If, for example, a medical assistant tells a patient that the physician will meet him or her in the emergency room in 30 minutes, the medical assistant has legally bound the physician to an agreement or contract. If the physician is an hour late due to an emergency, he or she may be subject to suit. The medical assistant should use nonspecific language.

Examples

> *Nonspecific:* "Please be at the emergency at 9 AM. The physician will see you as soon as he has completed his rounds."

> *Specific:* "Dr. Jones will meet you in the emergency room at 9 AM."
> *Nonspecific:* "Most patients find that this medication does not make them nauseated."
> *Specific:* "Don't worry. You won't get sick as a result of this drug."
> *Nonspecific:* "Several of our patients have gotten over the flu in a few days when they followed these instructions."
> *Specific:* "Take your medication, drink plenty of fluids, and you will be better by next Friday."

Although the physician is legally responsible for the actions of a representative who does not have the required professional skills or who follows physician's instructions that prove to be improper, he or she is not responsible for the patient's negligence or failure to follow instructions. Thus, it is imperative that the medical assistant, acting as agent for the physician, understands clearly and follows accurately all instructions regarding patient care.

MEDICAL ETHICS

Every profession adheres both to the legal regulations imposed on its practice and to an expected code of behavior for its practitioners. This code, based on certain defined principles, is the subject of medical ethics. The medical assistant, as a valued member of the health care team, must internalize the principles of medical ethics and acquire an understanding of the relationship between law and ethics discussed in the introduction.

The term *medical ethics* refers to the principles that reflect a code of behavior based on moral standards of medical practice. According to the AMA, medical ethics provides standards that transcend those required by law. Another dimension of medical ethics is bioethics, a new term denoting the study of moral issues as they relate to medical research and its applications. Bioethics combines the fields of medicine and philosophy in a quest for moral responsibility, judgment, and potential responses to critical questions posed by medical technology. Such questions relate to abortion, the treatment of patients with acquired immunodeficiency syndrome, artificial insemination, the cost of health care, organ transplants, the quality of life, and terminal illness.

Medical ethics is based on historic custom in general and the Hippocratic oath in particular. The oath, which Hippocrates required of his students in the fourth century BC, is still in use today (Fig. 3–6). Figure 3–7 is the *Geneva Convention Code of Medical Ethics*, adapted by the World Medical Association in 1949 and used as an alternative to the Hippocratic Oath.

AMERICAN MEDICAL ASSOCIATION PRINCIPLES

The medical profession has long subscribed to a body of ethical statements developed primarily for the benefit of the health professional. As a member of the health

CONFIDENTIAL P.E.R.T.S. REPORT
(NOT A PART OF MEDICAL RECORD)

phico INSURANCE COMPANY

"An event is any happening which is not consistent with the routine operation of the facility or the routine care of a particular patient. It may be an accident or a situation which might result in an accident. This might involve patient, visitor, volunteer."

NAME OF FACILITY, CITY & STATE: _____

PATIENT—Diagnosis and/o. procedure at time of event: _____

0501169

NAME OF ATTENDING PHYSICIAN: _____

FOR PATIENT EVENTS—Use addressograph plate or full name.
IF OTHER THAN PATIENT—Full name, address & telephone number.
OTHER THAN PATIENT—Reason in or at facility: _____

PATIENT'S ROOM NO.: _____ DATE OF EVENT: _____

DESCRIPTION OF EVENT—Facts, no opinions. Identify equipment involved by name, manufacturer, model number & serial no.: _____

PHYSICIAN'S SIGNATURE: _____ PHYSICIAN ADVISED: ☐ Yes ☐ No

WITNESS(ES)/ROOMMATE(S)—Name & address: _____

DATE OF REPORT: INDIVIDUAL PREPARING REPORT (print name): DEPARTMENT HEAD/SUPERVISOR (Indicates Review):

NAME OF FACILITY, CITY & STATE: _____

| DATE OF EVENT: | TIME (2400 clock): | SEX: ☐ 01 Male ☐ 02 Female | AGE: | STATUS: ☐01 Inpatient ☐02 Outpatient ☐03 Visitor ☐04 Volunteer ☐99 Other | DAY OF WEEK: ☐01 Sunday ☐02 Monday ☐03 Tuesday ☐04 Wednesday ☐05 Thursday ☐06 Friday ☐07 Saturday |

SELECT ONLY ONE SHADED CATEGORY (1 THRU 10) AND CHECK APPROPRIATE BOX WHICH BEST DESCRIBES THE EVENT (EXCEPT FALLS & MEDICATION):

1. TREATMENT/PROCEDURE:
☐01 Consent Problem
☐02 Change in Diagnosis
☐03 Application/Removal of Cast/Splint
☐04 Missing Specimen
☐05 Dietary Problem
☐06 Prep Problem
☐07 Reporting of Test Results
☐08 Transfer/Moving of Patient
☐09 Injection Site
☐10 Patient Refusal
☐11 Invasive Procedure/Placement
☐12 Delay
☐13 Adverse Reaction
☐14 Documenting
☐15 Identification Patient/Site
☐16 Omitted
☐17 Deviation from Established Procedure
☐18 Not Documented
☐19 Transcription Error
☐20 Monitoring
☐21 Dressing Changes
☐22 Cancellation of Procedure
☐23 Repeat Procedure
☐24 Technique
☐99 Other ___

2. EQUIPMENT:
☐01 Electrical Problem
☐02 Not Available
☐03 Improper Use
☐04 Mechanical Problem
☐05 Malfunction/Defect
☐06 Wrong Equipment
☐07 Disconnected/Dislodged
☐08 Tampered With/By Patient/Non-Patient
☐99 Other ___

3. INTRAVENOUS/BLOOD:
☐01 Infiltration
☐02 Wrong Solution/Type
☐03 Patient Identification
☐04 Rate of Flow
☐05 Mislabeled
☐06 Wrong Additive
☐07 Repeated Attempts to Start
☐08 Site Problem
☐09 Wrong Time
☐10 Omitted
☐11 Repeat Administration
☐12 Transcription Error
☐13 Incompatible Additives
☐14 Tubing Pulled Out/Broken
☐15 Tubing Not Changed
☐16 Out-of-Sequence
☐17 Not Documented
☐18 Outdated
☐19 Adverse Reaction
☐20 Crossmatch Problem
☐99 Other ___

4. MISCELLANEOUS:
☐01 Against Medical Advice
☐02 Elopement
☐03 Fire
☐04 Other Accident While Ambulating
☐05 In Bed—Other Accident
☐06 Assault
☐07 Property Missing or Damaged
☐08 Natural Disaster
☐09 Unplanned Transfer to Critical Care
☐10 Cardiac/Respiratory Arrest
☐11 Self-Inflicted Injury
☐12 Dissatisfied Patient/Family
☐13 Readmission
☐14 Excessive Length of Stay
☐15 Admission From Outpatient Unit
☐16 Aspiration
☐99 Other ___

5. ANESTHESIA:
☐01 Anesthetic Agent
☐02 Equipment
☐03 Intubation
☐04 Extubation
☐05 Aspiration
☐06 Technique
☐07 Monitoring
☐08 Position
☐99 Other ___

6. OBSTETRICS:
☐01 Contamination
☐02 Equipment
☐03 Technique
☐04 Monitoring
☐05 Complication of Augmented Labor
☐06 Complication of Forceps
☐07 Precipitous Delivery
☐08 Prolonged Labor
☐09 Unrecognized Cephalo-pelvic Disproportion
☐10 4th Degree Laceration
☐11 Apgar Score Less Than 5
☐12 Return to Delivery Room
☐13 Meconium Aspiration/Abnormal Staining
☐14 Neonatal Injury
☐15 Pregnancy Post Sterilization
☐16 Unattended Delivery
☐99 Other ___

7. EMERGENCY:
☐01 Monitoring
☐02 Delay in Treatment
☐03 Return for Same Problem
☐04 Change in Diagnosis
☐05 Discharged Without Being Seen By Physician
☐06 DOA Within 7 Days of Discharge
☐07 Held/Observed Beyond Hospital Policy
☐99 Other ___

8. SURGERY:
☐01 Contamination
☐02 Equipment
☐03 Sponge/Instrument/Needle Count
☐04 Prep
☐05 Technique
☐06 Return/Repeat Surgery
☐07 Monitoring
☐08 Identification Patient/Site
☐09 Unplanned Removal of Organ or Part of Organ
☐10 Cancelled
☐11 Delay in Starting
☐99 Other ___

9. FALL:
☐01 Bed
☐02 Chair/Stretcher/Table
☐03 While Ambulating
☐04 Bedside Commode
☐05 Fall/Slip
☐06 Scales
☐07 Found on Floor
☐08 From Toy
☐09 Recreational Activity
☐99 Other ___

CHECK ONE:
☐01 Attended
☐02 Unattended

Activity Privileges (select one per medical order):
☐01 Unlimited
☐02 Ambulate With Assistance
☐03 Ambulate With Walker
☐04 Ambulate Without Assistance
☐05 Bedrest
☐06 Up in Chair/Wheelchair
☐07 Bathroom Privileges With Assistance
☐08 Bathroom Privileges Without Assistance
☐09 Not Specified
☐99 Other ___

Siderails (indicate position at time of event, if applicable):
☐01 None
Half rails:
☐02 1 up
☐03 2 up
☐04 3 up
☐05 4 up
Full rails:
☐06 1 up
☐07 2 up
Restraints (other than side rails):
☐01 Yes
☐02 No
Medicated Past 4 Hours:
☐01 Yes (If Yes, check
☐02 No Type Medication)

10. MEDICATION:
☐01 Patient Identification
☐02 Wrong Dosage
☐03 Wrong Drug
☐04 Wrong Time
☐05 Incorrect Route
☐06 Omitted
☐07 Repeat Administration
☐08 Given Without Order
☐09 Out-of-Sequence
☐10 Transcription Error
☐11 Improper Order
☐12 Adverse Reaction
☐13 Mislabeled
☐14 Dispensing Error
☐15 Medication Given Before Culture Taken
☐16 Medication Missing
☐17 Not Documented
☐18 Patient Took Unprescribed Medication
☐99 Other ___

Type Medication (check appropriate type(s) relative to FALL or MEDICATION EVENT):
☐01 Analgesic
☐02 Antibiotic
☐03 Anticoagulant
☐04 Anticonvulsant
☐05 Antidepressant
☐06 Antiemetic
☐07 Antihistamine
☐08 Antineoplastic
☐09 Bronchodilator
☐10 Cardiovascular
☐11 Contrast Media
☐12 Diuretic
☐13 Immunizations
☐14 Insulin
☐15 Laxative
☐16 Narcotic
☐17 Oxytocics
☐18 Radionuclides
☐19 Sedative/Tranquilizer
☐20 Unmedicated IV Solution
☐21 Vasodilator
☐22 Vasopressor
☐99 Other ___

TYPE OF INJURY (select the most serious):
☐01 External Laceration
☐02 Hematoma
☐03 Abrasion
☐04 Contusion
☐05 Sprain/Strain
☐06 Fracture/Dislocation
☐07 Internal Laceration
☐08 Perforation
☐09 Infection
☐10 Electrical Shock
☐11 Retained Foreign Object
☐12 Burn
☐13 Rash/Hives
☐14 Anoxia
☐15 Neurological Deficit
☐16 Decubitus
☐17 Poisoning
☐18 Contracture
☐19 Blister
☐20 Stillborn
☐21 Deterioration in Condition
☐22 Damaged Teeth
☐23 Amputation
☐24 Excessive Blood Loss
☐25 Circulatory Impairment
☐26 Sensory Impairment
☐27 Hyperthermia
☐28 Phlebitis
☐29 Wound Disruption
☐30 Unknown
☐31 None
☐99 Other ___

SEVERITY OF INJURY:
☐01 Minor
☐02 Severe
☐03 Death
☐04 Unknown
☐05 None

DEPARTMENT, UNIT, COST CENTER (select the one where event OCCURRED):
☐01 Administration
☐02 Admitting
☐03 Ambulatory Surgery
☐04 Anesthesia
☐05 Building & Grounds
☐06 Burn Unit
☐07 Business Office
☐08 Cafeteria
☐09 Cardiopulmonary Lab
☐10 Cardiovascular Lab
☐11 Central Supply
☐12 Clinic
☐13 Coronary Care Unit
☐14 Coffee/Gift Shop
☐15 Delivery Room
☐16 Detoxification Unit
☐17 Dialysis Unit
☐18 Dietary
☐19 Emergency Services
☐20 Endoscopy Unit
☐21 Extended Care/Geriatrics
☐22 Gynecology
☐23 Heliport
☐24 Housekeeping
☐25 Intensive Care Unit
☐26 Intermediate/Progressive Care Unit
☐27 IV Therapy
☐28 Laboratory
☐29 Labor Room
☐30 Laundry/Linen
☐31 Maintenance
☐32 Medical Records
☐33 Mental Health/Mental Retardation
☐34 Neonatal Intensive Care Unit
☐35 Nuclear Medicine
☐36 Nursery
☐37 Nursing—Code #
☐38 Obstetrics/Postpartum
☐39 Occupational Therapy
☐40 Operating Room
☐41 Pediatrics
☐42 Pharmacy
☐43 Physical Therapy
☐44 Psychiatry
☐45 Radiology
☐46 Recovery Room
☐47 Rehabilitation Unit
☐48 Respiratory Therapy
☐49 Security
☐50 Social Service
☐51 Utilization Review
☐52 Home Health
☐53 Hospice
☐54 Oncology
☐55 Radiation Therapy
☐99 Other ___

LOCATION (select best description of EXACT location of event):
☐01 Patient's Room
☐02 Bathroom in Patient Room
☐03 Bathroom/Other
☐04 Driveway
☐05 Elevator/Escalator
☐06 Examining/Treatment Room
☐07 Hallway/Corridor
☐08 Medication Room
☐09 Nursing Station
☐10 Parking Lot
☐11 Recreation Area
☐12 Roof
☐13 Shower/Tub Room
☐14 Stairs
☐15 Waiting Room
☐16 Walkway/Sidewalk
☐17 Window
☐99 Other ___

0501169

ADMINISTRATION USE ONLY

| Code # | SENT TO PHICO CLAIM DEPT. ☐01 Yes ☐02 No |

Form #RM-006 (REV. 10/85) DATA COLLECTION REPORT © 1985 PHICO Insurance Company, Mechanicsburg, PA ■ ALL RIGHTS RESERVED

Figure 3–5. An incident report. (Courtesy of PHICO Insurance Company.)

professions, a physician must recognize responsibility not only to patients, but also to society, to other health professionals, and to him- or herself. The following *Principles of the American Medical Association* (adopted in 1980) are not laws, but standards of conduct that define the essentials of honorable behavior for the physician.

I. A physician shall be dedicated to providing competent medical service with compassion and respect for human dignity

II. A physician shall deal honestly with patients and colleagues, and strive to expose those physicians deficient in character or competence, or who engage in fraud or deception.

I swear by Apollo the physician, and Aesculapius, and Heth, and Allheal, and all the gods and goddesses, that, according to my ability and judgment, I will keep this oath and stipulation, to reckon him who taught me this art equally dear to me as my parents, to share my substance with him and relieve his necessities if required; to regard his offspring as on the same footing with my own brothers, and to teach them this art if they should wish to learn it, without fee or stipulation, and that by precept, lecture and every other mode of instruction, I will impart a knowledge of the art to my own sons and to those of my teachers, and to disciples bound by a stipulation and oath, according to the law of medicine, but to none other.

I will follow that method of treatment which, according to my ability and judgment, I consider for the benefit of my patients, and abstain from whatever is deleterious and mischievous. I will give no deadly medicine to anyone if asked, nor suggest any such counsel; furthermore, I will not give to a woman an instrument to produce abortion.

With purity and holiness I will pass my life and practice my art. I will not cut a person who is suffering with a stone, but will leave this to be done by practitioners of this work. Into whatever houses I enter I will go to them for the benefit of the sick and will abstain from every voluntary act of mischief and corruption; and further from the seduction of females or males, bond or free.

Whatever, in connection with my professional practice, or not in connection with it, I may see or hear in the lives of men which ought not to be spoken abroad, I will not divulge, as reckoning that all such should be kept secret.

While I continue to keep this oath unviolated, may it be granted to me to enjoy life and the practice of the art, respected by all men at all times, but should I trespass and violate this oath, may the reverse be my lot.

Figure 3-6. The Hippocratic oath.

III. A physician shall respect the law and also recognize a responsibility to seek changes in those requirements which are contrary to the best interests of the patient.

IV. A physician shall respect the rights of patients, of colleagues, and of other health professionals, and shall safeguard patient confidences within the constraints of law.

V. A physician shall continue to study, apply and advance scientific knowledge, make relevant information available to patients, colleagues, and the public, obtain consultation, and use the talents of other health professionals when indicated.

VI. A physician shall, in the provision of appropriate patient care, except in emergencies, be free to choose whom to serve, with whom to associate, and the environment in which to provide medical services.

VII. A physician shall recognize a responsibility to participate in activities contributing to an improved community.

Service to Humanity

The purpose of the medical profession is to "render service to humanity with full respect to the dignity of humanity" (AMA code of ethics). Thus, the role of each physician and supporting staff is to provide health care to the best of their combined abilities, and in so doing, to treat and regard the patient humanely. This statement rejects the notion of treating the patient as a diseased entity or body part rather than as a human being with a complex scope of sensibilities.

Physicians and their staff are thus called on to practice holistic medicine to treat the patient as a total person. Administering to the patient in this sense implies that respect for and attention to the patient's intellectual, emotional, spiritual, psychologic, and physiologic states are required to fulfill the ethical goals of the medical profession.

Continued Pursuit of Excellence

The training and education of physicians do not end with formal schooling. They are charged with the lifelong task of maintaining skills and increasing knowledge. This process applies to all professionals. However, it may be argued that because a physician practicing dated medicine imposes a more serious danger than does, say, a tax accountant who missed some recent adjustment in the tax laws, this particular ethical principle is critical for the physician. In fact, most states require continuing education units (CEUs) for continued licensure.

Physicians usually commit themselves to reading journals and current medical textbooks, to attending conferences, and to acquiring CEUs. To a great extent, the physician assumes this responsibility at the expense of interrupting the practice of medicine. Thus, the pursuit of this principle may carry a corresponding loss of income. This principle implies that the patient has the right to expect reasonably current modes of medical practice, and that the physician has the obligation to provide up-to-date, well-informed care as long as he or she intends to function as a medical practitioner.

Scientific Methods of Healing

Physicians practice the art of healing, which is based on a scientifically verifiable model of medicine. Therefore, their professional responsibilities require that they practice within the confines of their understanding of medical practices, and that they assist, if possible, in the dynamic evolution of that model by contributing their own learning experiences to the shared body of knowledge.

THE DECLARATION OF GENEVA

At the time of being admitted as a member of the medical profession:

I solemnly pledge myself to consecrate my life to the service of humanity.

I will give to my teachers the respect and gratitude which is their due;

I will practice my profession with conscience and dignity;

The health of my patient will be my first consideration;

I will respect the secrets which are confided in me;

I will maintain by all the means in my power, the honor and the noble traditions of the medical profession;

My colleagues will be my brothers;

I will not permit considerations of religion, nationality, race, party politics or social standing to intervene between my duty and my patient;

I will maintain the utmost respect for human life, from the time of conception;

Even under threat, I will not use my medical knowledge contrary to the laws of humanity.

I make these promises solemnly, freely and upon my honor.

Figure 3-7. The Declaration of Geneva. (Adopted by the Third General Assembly of the World Medical Association, at Geneva, Switzerland, September 1948.)

It would be unethical for physicians to extend their diagnoses to areas that have no basis in scientific prediction. This ethical code of behavior protects the physician, the patient, and the integrity of the medical profession.

Upholding the Profession

The physician assumes the responsibility of maintaining the "dignity and honor of the profession" (AMA code of ethics). Operationally, the ethical behavior implied is two-dimensional. On the one hand, physicians must demonstrate the utmost confidence in and respect for colleagues and must never indiscriminately criticize the approaches or methodologies of other physicians in public. On the other hand, they must do everything within their power to expose any illegal or unethical behavior by fellow physicians.

Because the practice of medicine is both technically complex and held in high esteem by the general public, physicians themselves are charged with the heavy burden of monitoring and maintaining the competent and ethical practice of their own profession. In this way the public is protected from negligent or harmful medical practice, and society's faith in the profession remains intact.

Responsibility to a Patient

Under normal circumstances, physicians are free to choose their patients. As a result of office location, specialty, or the determination of optimal practice size, physicians may effectively refuse to undertake the care of persons requesting their services. A physician may also suggest that a patient would be better served by a different physician. Withdrawal from the rendering of services requires that the patient be duly informed of the decision in writing. This responsibility is both ethical and legal. In emergencies, however, the physician should care for the patient as effectively as possible until other adequate medical care becomes available.

Physicians cannot neglect patients entrusted to their care. It is ethical to discontinue service at the completion of a treatment regimen on notifying the patient, but to delay care or abandon the patient is unethical.

Appropriate Terms and Conditions

Physicians constantly must strive to ensure that they are practicing within an environment that supports both the practice of high-quality medical care and the continuation of ethical behavior. In practical terms this principle implies that physicians should not associate with an organization (hospital or other) that pressures them to practice medicine of inferior quality or to compromise their own moral codes. Physicians should not enter into contracts with patients that would result in the same outcome. Physicians must avoid all situations that dictate that their medical procedures differ from those they would consider to be fully competent and morally acceptable.

Income for Direct Services

The physician's income should be earned in exchange for direct medical services performed either personally or by an employee under his or her supervision. Physicians should not compensate each other for referrals or consultations, thereby supplementing their income for favors bestowed or received. They should not enter the general business of supplying drugs or appliances unless dispensing these items provides a necessary service to the patient.

This principle emphasizes that the physician's fee should be compatible with the services provided and implies that fee splitting is unethical. *Fee splitting* refers to the sharing of fees when one physician refers to a patient to another and then receives a portion of the patient's fee. Fees should be reasonable and not excessive. Among the specific criteria to be considered are the complexity and quality of the service rendered, the experience of the physician, and the customary fee for the locality. Of particular interest to the medical assistant is the ethical practice of charging fees for specific ancillary services. The AMA Judicial Council states that charges should not be made for the routine processing of insurance forms. A customary fee, however, is not viewed as unethical if it pays for the processing of multiple forms or nonstandard, complex forms. The Council also directs that charging interest and setting finance charges on unpaid balances is ethical only if the patient has been made aware of this policy in writing and in advance of the services rendered.

Regarding charges for laboratory services, the Council advises the physician to state on the billing form the actual charge for any service performed by an outside laboratory and a minimal handling charge for obtaining the specimen in the office. The laboratory bills the physician at a reduced rate, rather than the patient, to reduce the cost to the patient. Thus, the total bill for laboratory fees that originate from the physician's office is less than would be incurred by the patient in direct billing from the laboratory facility.

In addition, guidelines exist for charging patients who miss an appointment or cancel an appointment with less than 24 hours' notice. The Council views reasonable charges for these situations as ethical.

The Council maintains that it is unethical for a physician to influence the patient regarding where to fill a prescription or obtain other medical services when the physician is guided by financial interests.

Consulting with Fellow Physicians

When diagnostic or treatment difficulties seem beyond the scope of the physician's experience or knowledge, or when a reasonable doubt arises and a second opinion is desired, the physician should willingly consult with colleagues or specialists known to be knowledgeable and skillful in the particular area in question.

If a patient requests a second opinion, physicians also should pursue a consulting relationship regardless of their own feelings concerning the necessity of the consultation. Physicians must never allow a patient's request for a second opinion to influence their approach. The patient retains the right to acquire a consensus in treatment or diagnostic methods. The physician who encourages patients to seek a second opinion in cases in which diagnosis or treatment poses severe consequences is generally regarded as showing integrity and high moral character.

Confidentiality

Often, information disclosed in the diagnosis or treatment of a case could be deleterious to the patient's reputation. Character flaws, personality problems, drug and alcohol addiction, and other types of potentially volatile information often are disclosed to the physician. The ethical code dictates confidentiality in all physician-patient exchanges.

Unless they are required by law to share information or believe that doing so would protect society or the patient from serious harm, physicians may not reveal the content of private conversations. When the patient's care requires that the physician discuss the case with other health care professionals, disclosures should be appropriate and made out of the hearing of the patient, other patients, and anyone else for whom the information is not intended.

Social Responsibility

The physician's ethical responsibilities to individual patients also apply to society at large. Social responsibility implies that physicians of moral character contribute to the general welfare of their communities. If physicians can benefit society by the prudent application of their professional knowledge, it is their obligation to do so. The code of ethical behavior described above contains the expectation that physicians will participate in community activities and that their involvement will reflect the ideals and ethics of the profession.

The Patient's Bill of Rights

Many hospitals and medical practices have adapted a patient's bill of rights as declared by the Joint Commission on Accreditation of Health Care Organizations. California and Minnesota have passed the rights into law, making patients' rights mandatory. Figure 3–8 is a sample declaration of patient rights.

ETHICAL RESPONSIBILITIES OF MEDICAL ASSISTANTS

The ethical responsibility of medical assistants is to uphold the moral principles established by the AMA and the American Association of Medical Assistants (AAMA). The AAMA Code of Ethics is presented in Figure 3–9.

Medical Ethics of the American Association of Medical Assistants

The similarities between the AMA and the AAMA codes of ethics are apparent. Both the physician and the medical assistant share a dedication to providing competent, comprehensive care with respect to human dignity, the law, continuing education, contributing services to the community, and the confidentiality and privacy of the patient. The medical assistant is required to make ethical decisions and therefore should continue to study and keep informed regarding ethical issues.

CONTEMPORARY ETHICAL ISSUES

Because of the dynamic nature of society and of medicine itself, problematic bioethical issues are constantly emerging. Perhaps the greatest problem in dealing with these and similar issues is that morality can be viewed from the perspective of particular religious beliefs.

It is not possible to present specific moral precepts within this chapter. Even if they could be fully presented, such precepts would offer no conclusive answers to complex moral questions occurring in medicine. However, a logical guide to preserving one's own system of personal ethics is the following:

1. Medical assistants should not be forced to violate their moral convictions because of their professional training, even if there is controversy regarding the "rightness" of an issue. An individual's right to his or her own convictions supersedes group consensus.
2. Medical assistants should not attempt to force their beliefs on other individuals, especially patients. If there is a moral controversy regarding an issue, they must allow opposing beliefs in others.
3. Medical assistants should attempt to find employment in settings that do not continually challenge their moral positions.

In issues of morality, there are no clear lines. Most controversies arise out of difficult interpretations. As a medical assistant, you will find these issues within medicine to be both dynamic and challenging. Questions of ethics in relation to the contemporary issues of medicine will never be settled. However, thought will evolve continuously regarding appropriate ethical and moral solutions to various issues. The continuing task for the medical assistant will be the active participation of a problem solver, thinker, and evaluator.

Although philosophical discussions of ethical issues are beyond the scope of this chapter, it is important for the medical assistant to have a point of reference regarding these issues.

Because the code of ethics for medical assisting is closely associated with the code of ethics for physicians, the AMA publication *Current Opinions of the Council on Ethical and Judicial Affairs* can help the medical assistant in initially examining the ethical issues from a medical perspective. Published in 1990, this text is an appendage to the latest revisions of the *Principles of Medical Ethics* previously listed. The Judicial Council of the AMA periodically reviews and revises the *Princi-*

A PATIENT'S BILL OF RIGHTS

The American Hospital Association presents Patient's Bill of Rights with the expectation that observance of these rights will contribute to more effective patient care and greater satisfaction for the patient, his physician, and the hospital organization. Further, the Association presents these rights in the expectation that they will be supported by the hospital on behalf of its patients, as an integral part of the healing process. It is recognized that a personal relationship between the physician and the patient is essential for the provision of proper medical care. The traditional physician-patient relationship takes on a new dimension when care is rendered within an organizational structure. Legal precedent has established that the institution itself also has a responsibility to the patient. It is in recognition of these factors that these rights are affirmed.

1. The patient has the right to considerate and respectful care.

2. The patient has the right to obtain from his physician complete current information concerning his diagnosis, treatment, and prognosis in terms the patient can be reasonably be expected to understand. When it is not medically advisable to give such information to the patient, the information should be made available to an appropriate person in his behalf. He has the right to know, by name, the physician responsible for coordinating his care.

3. The patient has the right to receive from his physician information necessary to give informed consent prior to the start of any procedure and/or treatment. Except in emergencies, such information for informed consent should include but not necessarily be limited to the specific procedure and/or treatment, the medically significant risks involved, and the probable duration of incapacitation. Where medically significant alternatives for care or treatment exist, or when the patient requests information concerning medical alternatives, the patient has the right to such information. The patient also has the right to know the name of the person responsible for the procedures and/or treatment.

4. The patient has the right to refuse treatment to the extent permitted by law and to be informed of the medical consequences of his action.

5. The patient has the right to every consideration of his privacy concerning his own medical care program. Case discussion, consultation, examination, and treatment are confidential and should be conducted discreetly. Those not directly involved in his care must have the permission of the patient to be present.

tion to which the patient is to be transferred must not have accepted the patient for transfer.

8. The patient has the right to obtain information as to any relationship of his hospital to other health care and educational institutions insofar as his care is concerned. The patient has the right to obtain information as to the existence of any professional relationship among individuals, by name, who are treating him.

9. The patient has the right to be advised if the hospital proposes to engage in or perform human experimentation affecting his care or treatment. The patient has the right to refuse to participate in such research projects.

10. The patient has the right to expect reasonable continuity of care. He has the right to know in advance what appointment times and physicians are available and where. The patient has the right to expect that the hospital will provide a mechanism whereby he is informed by his physician or a delegate of the physician of the patient's continuing health care requirements following discharge.

11. The patient has the right to examine and receive an explanation of his bill regardless of source of payment.

12. The patient has the right to know what hospital rules and regulations apply to his conduct as a patient.

No catalog of rights can guarantee for the patient the kind of treatment he has a right to expect. A hospital has many functions to perform, including the prevention and treatment of disease, the education of both health professionals and patients, and the conduct of clinical research. All these activities must be conducted with an overriding concern for the patient, and, above all, the recognition of his dignity as a human being. Success in achieving this recognition assures success in the defense of the rights of the patient.

Figure 3–8. A Patient's Bill of Rights. (From the American Hospital Association, with permission. Copyright 1975.)

AAMA CODE OF ETHICS

The Code of Ethics of the AAMA shall set forth principles of ethical and moral conduct as they relate to the medical profession and the particular practice of medical assisting.

Members of AAMA dedicated to the conscientious pursuit of their profession, and thus desiring to merit the high regard of the entire medical profession and the respect of the general public which they serve, do pledge themselves to strive always to:

A. Render service with full respect for the dignity of humanity
B. Respect confidential information obtained through employment unless legally authorized or required by responsible performance of duty to divulge such information
C. Uphold the honor and high principles of the profession and accept its disciplines
D. Seek to continually improve the knowledge and skills of medical assistants for the benefit of patients and professional colleagues;
E. Participate in additional service activities aimed toward improving the health and well-being of the community

Figure 3–9. The AAMA Code of Ethics.

thics and among its other functions
principles. (For further reference, a
obtained from the AMA, under the order
P632290).

edical assistant is expected to function accord-
the expectations of ethical standards set for
sicians. Adhering to the AMA and AAMA codes of
thics ensures that the medical assistant is achieving
the highest possible standard of ethical practice.

However, practical ethical considerations for medical
assistants may not be obvious in a general reading of
the *Code of Ethics* for medical assistants or the AMA
Council's *Current Opinions.* On a daily basis, the medical assistant has the opportunity to engage in ethical
practice warranted by the nature of the medical assisting profession itself. Certain areas of patient interaction
may not appear to be related to ethical practice, but are
in fact its essence.

For instance, every day medical assistants must confront their own interpersonal relationships with patients
to ascertain whether they are adversely affected by the
medical assistant's own personal judgments of the patient's behavior. Likewise, every day the medical assistant must be aware of his or her own mood so as not to
transform personal bad days into professional ones.

Achieving high ethical standards, therefore, involves
not only patient care associated with procedures, but
also patient care associated with approach.

SUMMARY

No tangible rewards or benefits result from the vigilant practice of ethically and legally correct behavior in
the medical office. However, this behavior is both expected and required. It is the cornerstone on which all
office practices are built. The medical assistant must
understand and internalize the basic principles of law
and ethics and strive to apply them to the professional
practice of medical assisting.

DISCUSSION QUESTIONS

1. What would constitute a breach of contract in the physician-patient relationship?
2. Discuss the implications that the law of agency has for the medical assistant.
3. Describe the role of the medical assistant in helping to prevent malpractice suits. Identify particular areas
   of vulnerability regarding potential claims of negligence.
4. Discuss the extent to which the medical assistant's behavior should be governed by the AAMA Code of
   Ethics and the Patient's Bill of Rights.

BIBLIOGRAPHY

American Medical Association: Current Opinions of the Council on Ethical and Judicial Affairs. American Medical Association,
Chicago, 1990.

Arras J and Rhoden J: Ethical Issues in Modern Medicine, ed 3. Mayfield, Mountain View, CA, 1989.

Flight M: Law, Liability, and Ethics for Medical Office Personnel, ed 2. Delmar, Albany, 1993.

Lewis M and Warden C: Law and Ethics in the Medical Office Including Bioethical Issues, ed 3. FA Davis, Philadelphia, 1993.

Roach, WH, Jr., et al: Medical Records and the Law, ed 2. Gaithersburg, MD, 1992.

Scott RW: Health Care Malpractice: A Primer on Legal Issues for Professionals. Slack, Thorofare, NJ, 1990.

HIGHLIGHTS

UNIFORM ANATOMIC GIFT ACT

As the successful transplantation of vital organs becomes commonplace in contemporary medicine, an increasing number of individuals are willing to donate all or some of their organs after death. These include liver, heart, kidneys, pancreas, lungs, corneas, bone, bone marrow, skin, and blood. Other individuals donate their bodies after death for use in medical research.

Before 1968, the statutes governing donations were contingent on individual state legislation regarding anatomic gifts. However, at the National Conference of Commissioners on Uniform State Laws held in 1968, the Uniform Anatomic Gift Act was drafted and approved. At present, all 50 states have either adopted this specific act or enacted similar legislation.

PROVISIONS OF THE UNIFORM ANATOMIC GIFT ACT

The Act includes the following provisions:

1. *Who may donate.* Any mentally competent adult (18 years of age or older) who is in good health may, after death, donate any or all organs for transplantation or medical research. The entire body may also be donated for medical research.
2. *Donors' rights.* The donor's rights supersede those of any family members except when state law requires an autopsy.
3. *Survivors' rights.* The decedent's survivors, in legal order of consent, may donate any part(s) of the body provided the decedent did not oppose the donation prior to death.
4. *Attending physician's role.* When part of a decedent's body is to be transplanted, the physician attending the donor may not participate in the transplantation or removal procedures. Likewise, the time of death

must be established by a physician who is not a member of the transplant team.
5. *Who may receive the gift, and for what purpose.* Specific criteria have been established that relate to, among other things, the accreditation of the hospital, the specialization and board certification of the physician, and the intent of the transplantation (e.g., in most instances, a kidney transplant solely for prophylactic purposes would not be approved).
6. *How the gift may be donated.* There are three ways in which a person may donate an anatomic gift:
   A. Through a living will, in those states in which it is valid
   B. Through an affidavit filed with the motor vehicle division of the state's department of transportation, along with a notation made on the person's driver's license
   C. Through the use of the Uniform Donor Card

UNIFORM DONOR CARDS

Uniform Donor Cards (Fig. 3–10) are legal documents and are available through the AMA and through state and national divisions of organizations associated with organ transplants. Some states allocate space for anatomic gift designation on the reverse side of the driver's license. In addition, a brightly colored "Organ Donor" sticker is attached to the license to alert emergency care providers to the donor's request.

COMMONLY ASKED QUESTIONS

The medical assistant usually is not involved in soliciting organ donors, but probably provides patient

---

LIVING DONOR CARD

OF _____
   Print or type name of donor

In the hope that I may help others, I hereby make this anatomical gift, if medically acceptable, to take effect upon my death. The words and marks below indicate my desires.

I give: (a) _____ any needed organs or parts
        (b) _____ only the following organs or parts

_____
Specify the organ(s) or part(s)
for the purpose of transplantation.

Limitations or special wishes, if any: _____
_____

Signed by the donor and the following two witnesses in the presence of each other:

_____   _____
Signature of Donor   Date of Birth of Donor

_____   _____
Date Signed   City and State

_____   _____
Witness   Witness

THIS IS A LEGAL DOCUMENT UNDER THE UNIFORM ANATOMICAL GIFT ACT OR SIMILAR LAWS.

Figure 3-10.

Continued

instruction in the form of answering patients' questions regarding organ donation. Some of the most frequently asked questions and the appropriate responses are as follows:

1. *How is the recipient of my organs chosen?* Organs available for transplantation will be tissue typed for matching purposes and then registered in a national computer bank. Also in the computer bank are the names, listed by priority, of individuals who need organ transplants. The computer matches the organ with the appropriate recipient.
2. *Will my hospital care suffer if I am an organ donor?* No. Every attempt to provide competent lifesaving care will be made.
3. *Will the recipient know that I donated the organs?* Most organ donors choose to remain anonymous. The donor is identified only if he or she wishes to be.
4. *Will my family have to pay to have my organs removed?* No.
5. *Will my family receive any money for my organs?* No. It is illegal to buy or sell organs.
6. *If I sign a donor card, can I change my mind later?* Yes. All you have to do is tear up the card and let your family know that you have changed your mind.

*U*nderstanding and Communicating with Patients and Their Families

> Communication is: How to talk so others will listen; How to listen so others will talk.
>
> A.W. Howard

CHAPTER OUTLINE

THE MEDICAL ASSISTANT AS AN ATTITUDE TRANSMITTER

THE ROLE OF EMPATHY AND IMPARTIALITY IN POSITIVE PATIENT DYNAMICS

GUIDELINES FOR EFFECTIVE PATIENT APPROACHES

UNDERSTANDING THE PATIENT
  The Experience of Loss of Self-Esteem
  The Effects of Motivational Forces
  The Effects of Cultural Background
  Common Responses to Illness

COMMUNICATING WITH THE PATIENT
  Verbal Communication
  Nonverbal Communication
  Communication Barriers

Communication Skill Development
Special Communication Problems

DEALING WITH FAMILY AND FRIENDS

PATIENT TEACHING CONSIDERATIONS

RELATED ETHICAL AND LEGAL IMPLICATIONS

SUMMARY

DISCUSSION QUESTIONS

BIBLIOGRAPHY

PROCEDURE
  Listen to and Communicate with the Patient

HIGHLIGHTS
  Understanding Terminally Ill Patients and Their Families

LEARNING OBJECTIVES

Upon completing this chapter, you will be able to:

1. Describe the medical assistant's role as an attitude transmitter.
2. Describe the role of empathy and acceptance in patient dynamics.
3. Describe the four strategies of the healing approach.
4. List and explain the losses an individual experiences in becoming a patient.
5. List three needs that motivate behavior, and describe the personality characteristics of individuals possessing those needs.
6. Explain the effects of cultural background on the patient's behavior.
7. List three common patient responses to illness.
8. List 10 defensive responses to illness and give five examples of each.
9. Explain the difference between verbal and nonverbal communication.
10. List three examples of communication barriers.
11. List and describe five ways to direct communication.
12. List the special communication problems specific to the emotionally distressed patient, the dying patient, the angry patient, the hearing- or vision-impaired patient, and the elderly patient.
13. Describe two approaches that are helpful in dealing with the patient's family and friends.
14. List three implications of communicating with patients and their families.

*U*nderstanding and Communicating with Patients and Their Families

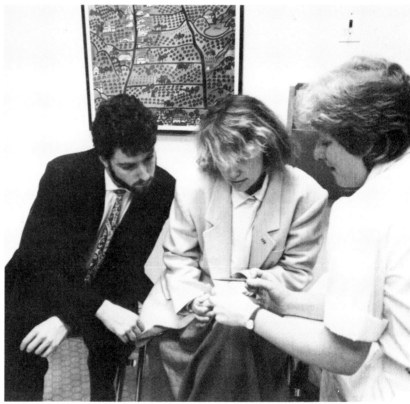

PERFORMANCE OBJECTIVES

Upon completing this chapter, you will be able to:

1. Assess patient needs through listening skills and understanding techniques.
2. Respond appropriately and effectively with empathetic and open-ended statements.

DACUM EDUCATIONAL COMPONENTS

1. Project a positive attitude (to anticipate and respond to the needs of others) (1.1A,D).
2. Conduct oneself in a courteous and diplomatic manner (by showing acceptance of patients with cultural and behavior differences) (1.6A–C).
3. Listen and observe (to identify the needs of others) (2.1A–B).
4. Treat all patients with empathy and impartiality (through verbal and nonverbal cues) (2.2A,B).
5. Adapt communications to individuals' abilities to understand (to respond effectively to patients with special needs) (2.3A,B).
6. Recognize and respond to (and evaluate) verbal and nonverbal communication (by using active listening techniques, reflection techniques, and open-ended statements) (2.4A,B; 2.6A).
7. Evaluate understanding of communication (by using positive responses to overcome communication barriers and obstacles) (1.6C; 2.4B).

Glossary

Anxiety: A state of uneasiness or apprehension that is not associated with any particular cause
Assessment: An overall evaluation or accounting
Attitude: The set of beliefs or feelings that a person has regarding a particular phenomenon
Bias: A continuing positive or negative attitude toward a person or a phenomenon that may influence objectivity in evaluation
Coping mechanism: A practiced and historical procedure for dealing with difficulties that has nothing to do with the problem at hand; a ritualistic process
Helping profession: A type of work designed to assist people
Perception: The subjective manner in which an individual interprets reality
Personality: The role that a person assumes to convey his or her conscious intentions
Stress: Psychologic or physiologic arousal due to demands from the physical or interpersonal environment

Medical assisting is a helping profession. It involves caring for patients specifically for the purpose of contributing to their wellness. By its very nature, the role of the medical assistant requires entering into a helping relationship with the patient. Through this relationship the medical assistant can understand and react to the needs, concerns, and behaviors that a person may develop in the process of becoming a patient. In addition, this relationship assumes the individuality of the patient: the differences inherent in his or her own personality and background. This relationship requires the medical assistant to develop a positive attitude toward patients and their families; acquire the ability to assess needs; prove understanding; communicate positive regard (a feeling of caring and esteem for the patient); and decide appropriate action. On the premise that self-awareness is a prerequisite to understanding others, Chapter 2 emphasized self-awareness and self-management. This chapter teaches ways to facilitate understanding of the patient, and to develop communication skills that promote positive patient interaction.

THE MEDICAL ASSISTANT AS AN ATTITUDE TRANSMITTER

The medical assistant plays a major role in shaping the patient's perception of the medical office. To a large extent, how the medical assistant relates to the patient determines the patient's general view of the office and specific reaction to the office visit. In many instances the medical assistant may spend more time with patients, particularly new patients, than the physician does. During the first visit, the administrative assistant collects information, explains office policies, and provides a general orientation to the office. The clinical assistant may also spend time with the patient when preparation for examination, treatment procedures, and patient teaching are required. The patient's perception of the medical assistant as caring and warm, empathetic, compassionate, knowledgeable, and respectful of people directly and positively affects the patient's attitude and response toward the medical assistant and the other staff members.

Attitude therefore originates with perception. Behavior, in turn, is derived from attitude. Nursing research has demonstrated that the manner in which the health professional interacts with the patient can in itself promote wellness, aggravate illness, or cause inaccurate assessment. If the interaction between the patient and the medical assistant is unpleasant, negative consequences can occur. For instance, the medical assistant could take the patient's blood pressure and obtain a higher-than-normal reading for the patient because emotion affects blood pressure. Knowledge of the abnormal reading could increase the patient's stress and adversely affect the remainder of the office visit.

Whether the patient is receiving treatment, asking to make a telephone call, requesting assistance, or expressing anger, the medical assistant must consistently transmit an attitude that communicates a clear message to the patient: "You are important. Your concerns are worthwhile. I care about you. I am willing to help you. Trust in my ability to help." Every interaction provides an opportunity to express positive regard for the patient. This transmitted attitude of caring reflects the medical assistant's ability to perceive the patient as a whole person and not just as a disease or condition.

The patient, being human, possesses a mind and spirit in addition to a body. The medical assistant must recognize that each of these interacts with the others in composing the whole person. The patient, then, is not just a person with a diseased organ, but an individual whose mental, emotional, spiritual, and social entities have been affected by illness. Therefore, the patient's needs are not limited to feeling physically well. Wellness is the state of optimal health for the whole person.

Health professionals label this perspective *holistic health*. Understanding the patient means, in addition to fostering a positive attitude, accepting the patient as a whole person and recognizing the medical assistant's role in providing holistic health care. The medical assistant must communicate with the patient in a manner that is therapeutically responsive.

THE ROLE OF EMPATHY AND IMPARTIALITY IN POSITIVE PATIENT DYNAMICS

Empathy is an attempt to view the situation through the patient's eyes and to "stand in the patient's shoes." The ability to view a situation from the individual's own frame of reference is conveyed by communicating understanding and interest. Developing an empathetic attitude and the related communication skills requires practice and experience. A way to facilitate developing such an attitude is to remember an experience similar to the patient's that may have occurred in your own life. It

may be helpful to ask self-directed questions, such as "How did I feel when this happened to me?" "How did my friend or relative feel when this happened to him?" "Is there any experience in my life that I can compare with this?" Answers to these questions may enable the medical assistant to identify with the patient's feelings and to adopt an empathetic attitude. A way to communicate empathy is to verbally acknowledge the patient's feelings and to share similar experiences and feelings. For example: "I was frightened too when I was told I had to have surgery; everyone is." A necessary caution in self-disclosure is to avoid unlimited elaboration and remember the reason for choosing a particular response. It is often more appropriate to state only that "These feelings are normal and natural." Empathy can also be communicated nonverbally by a touch or a facial expression.

Developing an attitude of empathy helps the medical assistant remain impartial (nonjudgmental and accepting). Social psychologists maintain that the more we see ourselves as similar to one another, the more accepting we are of potential differences.

The patients encountered in medical practice come from various cultural, ethnic, racial, economic, and religious backgrounds. Everyone has certain biases regarding these differences. The medical assistant must be aware of his or her own biases and of how they might interfere with objectivity and acceptance. Furthermore, acceptance is not tolerance. It is being aware of differences and respecting each individual's own uniqueness of personality and circumstance.

With empathy and impartiality, the medical assistant can relate to the patient in a way that will help the patient to achieve or sustain a sense of well-being and wholeness. This support will positively influence relationship dynamics (perceptions, communication, feelings) between the medical assistant and the patient. The guidelines that follow suggest approaches for effective communication.

GUIDELINES FOR EFFECTIVE PATIENT APPROACHES

The following strategies will help you to develop a positive approach to the patient:

1. Assume that the patient will be cooperative. When you sound confident, you appear competent. The patient feels comfortable and secure. *Example:* "Mr. Jones, please step on the scale. The doctor requires all patients to be weighed at each visit." You have made several points to the patient: (a) he does not have a choice; (b) weighing is routine; there is no cause for alarm; and (c) you expect that he will be cooperative.
2. Praise correct patient behavior when it is appropriate to do so. Positive feedback helps the patient to develop a sense of well-being. The patient feels liked and worthwhile. (*Example:* "Mrs. Kenyon, you really did a great job giving

yourself the injection." You have expressed [a] that you think she is intelligent and worthwhile; [b] that you have motivated her to continue this behavior; and [c] that you have shown approval).

3. Give opportunity for negative expression. The patient will make judgments that may be threatening. You may feel defensive. Nevertheless, allowing the patient the opportunity for negative expression without retaliation helps the patient to feel understood and accepted. (*Example: Patient:* "These appointment times are never convenient." *Medical Assistant:* "Perhaps we can do better with the next appointment." [Instead of, "Well, you made the appointment; you should have said something then."] With a positive response you have expressed [a] your acceptance of the patient's annoyance; [b] your desire to resolve the difficulty; and [c] that you will not attack or punish the patient for his or her feelings).

4. A sense of belonging is important to the patient and helps in developing a positive relationship. The medical assistant can convey this sense by (a) giving immediate attention to the patient by acknowledging his or her presence on arrival; (b) using the patient's name when talking to him or her; (c) informing the patient of delays; and (d) explaining procedures. (*Example:* "Good morning, Mrs. Rose. It's good to see you. Your appointment will be delayed about 15 minutes. Please have a seat and I will call you when the doctor is ready." You have [a] expressed a warm welcome; [b] given correct information and helped to prevent the patient's anxiety from developing; and [c] indicated what the patient can expect. Thus, you have alleviated anxiety and established positive dynamics).

An understanding of what it means to become a patient can further aid the medical assistant in developing attitudes appropriate for the profession.

UNDERSTANDING THE PATIENT

The medical assistant's purpose in attempting to understand the patient is to help the person adapt positively to the experience of being a patient. Although the office visit is not as unsettling as hospitalization for most people, assuming the role of patient usually affects the individual emotionally.

Everyone, to some degree, has basic needs related to self-worth and self-image, such as feeling good about oneself and having control over one's life. Assuming the role of patient may become problematic for some people because it interferes with their meeting basic needs.

THE EXPERIENCE OF LOSS OF SELF-ESTEEM

Health professionals do not always understand the loss of self-esteem and self-image following physical limitations imposed by injury or illness. For instance, a social worker who runs marathons and has made physical fitness his life's work suddenly contracts a lung disorder and is instructed by his physician to stop exercising. His entire lifestyle, including the way he used his work and leisure time, is changed by the constraints of the disease. The health professional would expect the patient to experience some problems maintaining a positive self-image.

Obviously, the ways in which individuals respond to disease are greatly influenced by their emotional makeup and the coping mechanisms they acquire while growing up. However, although the degrees of severity might differ, certain problems with self-esteem would be predictable in the preceding example.

Perhaps harder to recognize are feelings not specifically associated with illness, but instead related to assuming the role of patient. Some of these feelings are associated with the potential losses of self-confidence, autonomy, and privacy.

For example, on entering the office, a person may experience a sense of uneasiness. Being in unfamiliar surroundings contributes to this feeling, commonly referred to by health professionals as "culture shock." Medical practice has a culture all its own. It includes exposure to a new language (medical terminology), a new technology (diagnostic equipment), and new people and places (health professionals and medical facilities). This experience may be likened to the culture shock someone might feel visiting a foreign country where the customs, language, and surroundings are very different from those at home. In becoming a patient, the individual may respond to the culture of medical practice with feelings of insecurity and inferiority. Generally, the patient is not as self-assured as he or she might be outside the medical office.

The loss of autonomy, or the sense of not being in control, accompanies the loss of self-confidence. During the office visit, the patient gives up control over time, circumstances, and outcome. For instance, the patient may have to wait for an unanticipated amount of time to see the physician. While waiting, he or she is sitting with unfamiliar people. In addition, the circumstances (the visit itself) and outcome (what happens as a result of the visit) are outside the limits of the patient's control.

During the visit, the patient most probably discloses personal information and comes in physical contact with the physician and staff during examination and treatment procedures. This experience may cause the patient to feel uncomfortable and vulnerable and to experience the loss of privacy. The field of sociology has contributed to the health professional's understanding of these feelings. Sociologists explain that when people's personal space (psychological or physical) is invaded they become uncomfortable. Associated with physical contact, this personal space is called *social distance*. A visitor in a foreign country may have learned to be comfortable with a certain distance not respected by those native to that country. For instance, when two people from the same country are speaking to one another, they are usually both comfortable with the distance between them. However, when individuals from different countries are speaking together, one may stand closer than the distance to which the other is accustomed. Another example of social distance occurs in the interaction between individuals riding a bus. Most go to great lengths not to talk to or come in physical contact with another passenger. They look straight ahead and avoid touching the person in the next seat. Providing health care may necessarily invade the social distance acceptable to the patient.

The patient usually undresses for the examination and is touched by the medical assistant and the physician during procedures. In addition, the patient may be asked questions about personal habits, such as coping with stress, the use of leisure time, and satisfaction at work and with family relationships. Other questions may be related to an illness specifically; the patient may be asked to describe symptoms and to give a personal and a family history. Disclosing the required information may make the patient uncomfortable. He or she may be concerned with confidentiality or with the opinions of the physician and the office staff. In this instance, the patient may feel the loss of privacy because comfortable ranges of psychologic distance have been invaded.

The medical assistant's awareness of the feelings associated with becoming a patient facilitates his or her understanding of the patient. However, the medical assistant must recognize the other factors—motivation, cultural background, and personal response to illness—as being influential in shaping patient behavior.

THE EFFECTS OF MOTIVATIONAL FORCES

Personality theory suggests that it is possible to better understand and interact with someone if the needs that motivate the person's behavior can be identified. Most people are concerned with needs for achievement, dominance, and friendship. Behaviors are motivated by a desire to satisfy these needs. Achievement needs are associated with the desire to set goals and objectives and then to accomplish them. The desire to be in charge, to be the best, to be superior and in control is associated with the need to dominate. The desire to be connected with others (affiliated) and to be liked and approved of by others is the need for friendship. Psychologists explain that these needs, although part of everyone's personality, differ in degree among individuals. One person, for instance, may have a greater need to dominate than to be liked.

Certain personality characteristics are attributed to each of these needs. For instance, a patient who is goal oriented may not be as prone to being labeled a "talker"

as one who is friendship oriented. This individual may be far more interested in the task at hand than in becoming friendly with the office staff.

Individuals more concerned with dominance tend to become more frustrated with the loss of autonomy than other patients do. Persons with strong needs for approval will be more interested in conversation and personal attention.

THE EFFECTS OF CULTURAL BACKGROUND

In part, needs are conditioned by the individual's social and cultural background. Each individual is influenced by the set of beliefs, values, and accepted behaviors learned from association with a particular environment. For example, a patient may feel inclined to "keep a stiff upper lip" and show no emotion when experiencing pain due to an illness or injury because that is the expectation of the patient's particular cultural group. To do otherwise would be unacceptable, and the person would be perceived as being out of control. Another patient experiencing pain may have learned that emotional expression is acceptable or even desirable, and may look to the office staff to reinforce approval and acceptance. Knowledge of the factors affecting behavior enables the medical assistant to help the patient adapt positively to the role.

Other factors, such as gender, age, education, and income, influence an individual's response to becoming a patient. Throughout the chapter, attention is focused on these and other influences that affect patient behavior.

COMMON RESPONSES TO ILLNESS

The patient may exhibit certain predictable responses when self-worth is threatened because of illness. Anxiety and stress are two common responses. Anxiety is characterized by feelings of uneasiness, fear, worry, and nervousness. Anxiety may be mild or severe. Severe anxiety may affect overall ability to function effectively. Stress too can be mild or severe and may be physiologic (e.g., produced by running) or psychological (e.g., produced by worry).

Stress is an excessive and sometimes abrupt demand for biologic or psychological adjustment that can arise from inside or outside the individual. This demand depletes energy reserves in two stages. First is the shock stage. In this stage, signs of injury appear, heartbeat is irregular, blood pressure falls, muscle tone is lost, and body temperature drops. Second is the countershock stage. In this stage, shock reactions are reversed and the body prepares for defense: the adrenal cortex is mobilized and enlarged, and adrenalin production is stimulated. Heart rate, temperature, and blood pressure increase. Muscle tone is restored and the body is prepared for "flight or fight." Whether the stress is caused by good or bad news, the body's response is always the same. Therefore, stress management is very important because each stress-producing occurrence can cause excessive energy to be discharged through bodily organs. This discharge of energy in turn causes stress symptoms, such as headache, stomachache, or nervous tension. If stress becomes chronic and has no other outlet, chronic stress diseases, such as migraines, ulcers, or colitis, can occur.

Anxiety and stress both strain a person's sense of balance. Although everyone experiences stress daily, the degree of stress and the individual's capacity to manage it vary. These factors determine whether stress can be handled efficiently and with minimum energy expenditure and personal distress. The way in which stress is handled determines whether its effects will be positive or negative. For instance, positive stress can increase motivation to accomplish a task and to be creative and productive. Negative stress may result in disease. Cardiovascular disease, for example, is linked with prolonged stress. Thus, the medical profession has determined that, if a loss of self-esteem due to illness has caused anxiety and stress, the illness is aggravated. This effect occurs in all types of illness.

In addition to experiencing anxiety and stress, some patients may respond by behaving defensively. A defensive behavior is usually an unconscious reaction prompted by a perceived threat. It enables an individual to maintain composure and to adapt to the situation. Every person uses defensive behavior at times. Because patients may feel uneasy at becoming patients or having an illness, they often respond defensively. These defensive reactions are not necessarily unhealthy. They become harmful when they inhibit problem confrontation and resolution. Table 4–1 lists common defenses and examples of each. Understanding the needs, concerns, and common reactions of patients is essential to developing a nonjudgmental attitude appropriate for medical assisting. Coupled with self-awareness, this attitude of understanding and acceptance will help the medical assistant to communicate more effectively with patients, their families, and their friends.

COMMUNICATING WITH THE PATIENT

Communication with the patient is usually directed toward a purpose or goal. It is a necessary component of patient assessment, treatment, and education. Communication involves sending and receiving both verbal and nonverbal messages. Effective communication exists when the thoughts or ideas conveyed are mutually understood. (See procedure at the end of this chapter.)

VERBAL COMMUNICATION

Although verbal communication includes writing, this discussion focuses on the spoken word. Verbal communication, then, is the conveying of a spoken message. The sender usually uses both verbal and nonverbal techniques simultaneously. For instance, the medical assistant might say "Good morning" to the patient. The message might be accompanied by the sender's smile. For communication to have occurred, the receiver of the message must offer feedback. The patient may smile and say "Good morning" back. The greeting has been conveyed and understood by both sender and receiver. Verbal communication without feedback is ineffective. Communication with irrelevant feedback is also ineffective. For instance, the medical assistant might ask the patient, "Have you had this pain before?" The patient's reply might be a description of what was eaten for supper. Obviously, the receiver did not interpret the message correctly or was distracted from listening. Common understanding is essential in communication.

To achieve common understanding, the message itself must be clear. Language differences and different word interpretations would make the message unclear. For example, the patient may interpret the phrase "pain in my tummy" to refer to the broad area of the abdomen. Literal interpretation by the medical assistant would be "stomach." In this instance, clarification is necessary to determine the exact location of the pain. The message may need repeating or restructuring to achieve common understanding.

NONVERBAL COMMUNICATION

Messages can be sent without words. Although verbal communication is usually intentional, nonverbal communication may be unintentional; yet it is an equally important part of the message being sent and received. If "Good morning" is accompanied by a cold stare, a translation of the message will not be based solely on the words expressed. According to several factors, such as relationship, the receiver could interpret the sender to be angry, sad, or bored. The medical assistant develops the ability to understand both verbal and nonverbal messages and to differentiate between what the patient says and what he or she actually feels.

The medical assistant, aware of this process, can use nonverbal communication techniques to convey understanding. For instance, if a patient is upset, touching may be an appropriate way to convey caring. Key nonverbal communication skills include the appropriate use of space (atmosphere, face-to-face positioning at the same eye level, no physical barriers, and comfortable surroundings); time (involvement and no interruptions); posture (leaning toward the patient, avoiding rigid or defiant postures or slouching); voice inflection (warmth, concern, curiosity); and elimination of distracting body movements, such as foot shaking, pencil tapping, or looking at the clock. The most important nonverbal skill for gaining patient confidence, however, is good eye contact while talking with patients.

COMMUNICATION BARRIERS

The medical assistant must be aware of, and thus avoid, the obstacles to effective communication. Too much information given in a short time, the distraction

Table 4–1

DEFENSIVE BEHAVIORS COMMONLY ADOPTED BY PEOPLE UNDER STRESS

Defensive Responses	Example
Introjection Adopting the feelings, qualities, or values of another person or group	Mr. Carnes has been told by many of his friends to go to the physician and get the lump on his neck checked. They have said it is better to know. After several months, Mr. Carnes is convinced they are right.
Projection Imagining that another person is displaying one's own feelings.	Mr. Carnes feels irritable because he has had to wait so long in the waiting room. The medical assistant asks him a question, and he concludes that the medical assistant is irritable.
Compensation Replacing an attitude, behavior, or feeling with its opposite	Mr. Carnes is frightened that the lump on his neck may be diagnosed as cancer. However, he smiles continuously.
Sublimation Diverting unacceptable instinctual drives into acceptable channels	Mrs. Linn, feeling scared and angry at the thought of having surgery, relieves these feelings by playing tennis.
Denial Unconsciously avoiding the reality of a disturbing situation, thought, need, or feeling	Mrs. Linn has canceled her appointment to discuss and schedule surgery four times consecutively and reasons that she is just so busy—something unplanned always comes up.
Regression Returning to former behavior or aspects of personality	When Mrs. Linn was a teenager and she became worried and anxious, she would vomit deliberately. She has not engaged in this behavior for 15 years. Suddenly, she has again begun to vomit at least once a day.
Repression Putting unpleasant thoughts, feelings, or events out of one's mind	When the physician questions Mrs. Linn regarding her general state of health, she states that she occasionally has an upset stomach.
Dissociation Compartmentalizing emotions; disconnecting emotional significance from specific ideas or events	Mr. Bonan is a respiratory therapist and often instructs patients to stop smoking. Off duty, Mr. Bonan is a chain smoker.
Rationalization Justifying, sometimes illogically, thoughts, feelings, or actions to avoid truthful self-confrontation	Mr. Bonan, when asked how he could continue to smoke when he knows it is an unhealthy habit, states that he is too young to be concerned yet and that his grandfather smoked from age 14 until he died at age 94.
Displaced and Free-Floating Anger Expressing angry feelings toward objects or persons that have no significance to the emotion	Mrs. Wills leaves the office angry at the way she was treated by the medical assistant. She goes back to work and explodes when a coworker asks for assistance.

of noises, and dishonest responses are examples of communication barriers. Another common example in medical practice is the offering of false reassurance. Mrs. Jones says she is worried she might have cancer. The medical assistant replies, "Don't worry, everything will be O.K." Because the medical assistant's response minimized the patient's concerns an did not encourage her to elaborate on her feelings, further communication is most probably blocked. In addition, this comment may solicit legal problems because it promises a cure. Other errors that might inhibit communication are interrupting, prolonged silence or hesitation in responding, changing the subject abruptly, and using trite expressions to console the patient.

COMMUNICATION SKILL DEVELOPMENT

The following communication skills promote positive patient interaction and enable the medical assistant to better understand the patient's needs.

Listening

1. *Listen attentively.* To receive the message clearly, the medical assistant must examine his or her own personality for attitudes and feelings that might inhibit communication. For instance, if the medical assistant is angry or frustrated, receiving a clear message is more difficult because the barrier is within the medical assistant —the receiver—rather than in the message itself or the sender. Listening involves removing the focus on the self and giving full attention to the patient's verbal message and nonverbal cues.

2. *Check for clear interpretation.* The sender (the patient) may need to repeat the message so that the receiver (the medical assistant) can check for accuracy of interpretation. The statement may need to be rephrased to help the patient express it more clearly. *Example: Patient:* "I'm late in coming for a checkup." *Medical Assistant:* "You think you should have had the checkup before this?"

3. *Listen for feelings.* Generally, individuals with concerns tend to repeat or rephrase these concerns during conversation. Be alert for key words or themes expressed repetitively.

4. *Listen and observe.* The message conveyed is successfully interpreted when verbal messages are compatible with nonverbal expressions. *Example:* Mr. Jones' facial expression may be tense and he may be peeling the cuticle of his nails while verbally stating that he is certain the doctor will say he does not need surgery.

5. *Listen completely.* Effective listening habits include allowing the patient the opportunity to finish sentences or phrases without interruption or completion by the medical assistant.

Directing Communication

1. *Use open and closed statements purposefully.* The manner in which a question or statement is formulated helps to determine the patient's response. For instance, comments such as "Tell me more about it" and questions such as "Would you please describe it for me?" are open because they encourage the patient to elaborate freely and unpredictably. Requests such as "Tell me where you live" and questions such as "Are you married or single?" are closed because they discourage elaboration and direct the patient to make simple, brief, predictable responses. Regardless of open or closed phrasing, questions that ask "Why?" should be avoided because they tend to make the patient uncomfortable and sometimes defensive. *Example:* "Why aren't you following your diet?"

2. *Reflect the patient's statements.* Reflection is a technique used to direct conversations back to the patient by either repeating or restating the patient's words. This technique is used to direct the patient to clarify feelings, ideas, or thoughts. *Example: Patient:* "I'm so discouraged. I thought I'd be finished with those injections today." *Medical Assistant:* "Yes, I know you thought you'd be finished today." Reflection also encourages elaboration. The successful and comfortable use of this technique requires practice.

3. *Add to the patient's implied statement. Example: Patient:* "Most of the time I don't mind coming in for a checkup." *Medical Assistant:* "But today you do?" The medical assistant must use this technique with extreme caution because it may, if used repeatedly, discourage disclosure rather than encourage elaboration.

4. *Seek direct clarification when confused.* When confused, the medical assistant can use an alternative technique by confronting the confusion and stating, for example, "Mrs. Hale, I'm sorry, but I'm confused about what you are saying."

5. *Use silence when it is appropriate.* Silence is a tool that should not be forgotten in directing patient communication. Practice will enable the medical assistant to be comfortable with silence and to make good discretionary judgments concerning its use. Feelings are often conveyed in silence with a look or a touch. Silence may also give the patient needed opportunity to think before talking.

Additional techniques that are useful for directing communication are learned through exposure to other disciplines and through contact with other professionals. Communication with the patient is directed toward gaining information; learning the patient's feelings, thoughts, or ideas; providing the opportunity for talking to relieve stress; or any number of other goals. The medical assistant must first identify the goal, then choose the technique.

SPECIAL COMMUNICATION PROBLEMS

The Emotionally Distressed Patient

A common communication problem in medical settings is connected with giving distressing information and helping patients to cope. Each circumstance presents a unique problem, so a single effective solution is not possible. However, some discussion will prove helpful.

The difficulty of directing the medical assistant's response is that patients differ in what they interpret as "bad news." For some individuals a change of medication constitutes a crisis, whereas for others, impending surgery causes less distress.

The medical assistant should be vigilant for nonverbal behaviors suggesting that a patient has been overwhelmed by information. The feelings of a patient who perceives that he or she has been given bad news cannot be dismissed.

If the physician or medical assistant is aware in advance of the need to deliver unpleasant information, preparation is advisable. The medical assistant should discuss the situation with the physician, consider the personality of the patient, and plan a logical approach.

Sensitivity toward the patient and the patient's family, and complete privacy, if possible, are required. Care should be taken to ensure the physical safety of patients who may be in a high state of emotional distress. If there is any doubt regarding the patient's subsequent physical or emotional stability, the medical assistant may arrange for transportation or suggest to the patient that he or she should not attempt to drive without assistance.

Sometimes the reaction to bad news elicits withdrawal. Someone who is overwhelmed by or unable to deal with information may react by blocking out the problem. Withdrawal is evident when it is difficult to elicit conversation from the patient. When communication techniques fail to alter the patient's response, the medical assistant should notify the physician.

The Terminally Ill Patient

Terminally ill, or dying, patients present particular communication challenges to the office staff. The process of dying is not only physically but psychologically stressful for the patient and family. However, more than in other decades, society is recognizing the needs of patients and their families and the stages of grief and loss. Health care professionals are participating in innovations that address these needs, such as hospices and Living Wills. The hospice movement cares for the holistic needs of the patient, family, and friends by offering specialized inpatient and outpatient services. One such service is home visits by hospice volunteers to provide domestic help and counseling. Hospice volunteers participate in a training program specifically designed to prepare them for relating to the dying patient.

Generally, it is helpful to the medical assistant to confront his or her own concerns and fears about dying. Empathy is facilitated by a focus on similarities. Common fears of terminally ill patients are those related to dying. They include fear of pain, dependence, and death itself. The medical assistant must be willing to listen if the patient expresses the need to talk.

Because death has long been a subject met with denial, health professionals tend to "leave the patient alone." Although doing so is sometimes appropriate, the medical assistant must discern the motivation for such behavior and determine whose needs are being satisfied (the medical assistant's or the patient's). Touching, too, must be used with caution. Generally, it is best if the medical assistant does not force touching or caring on the patient if the patient does not find these behaviors natural or comfortable. Support for the patient and family are the major objectives of care in dealing with the terminally ill patient.

The Living Will and Durable Power of Attorney for Health Care

The Living Will and the Durable Power of Attorney for Health Care meet the needs of the dying patient in other ways. Through the format of the Living Will, the patient instructs health professionals and family regarding the use of life-sustaining procedures when death is imminent and the patient is unable to communicate or make meaningful decisions concerning treatment (Fig. 4–1). The patient or representative is responsible for notifying the physician of the existence of a Living Will and giving a copy of it for the medical record. New medical legislation requires hospital-admitting personnel to ask incoming patients whether a Living Will or Durable Power of Attorney for Health Care document exists, and if not, whether the patient desires to execute one or both documents.

The Living Will cannot be implemented if the patient is pregnant or younger than 18 years of age, was legally incompetent when the document was signed, or has not been determined within a reasonable degree of certainty to have a terminal illness; or if the physician believes that the patient has revoked the Living Will. In the absence of these conditions, the attending physician must specify orders for implementing the Living Will, or must make every reasonable effort to transfer the patient's care to another physician who will do so. The execution of a Living Will does not permit any deliberate act or omission to end life, other than withholding or withdrawing life-sustaining procedures.

The Durable Power of Attorney for Health Care designates another person to make decisions for the patient when at least two physicians agree that the patient cannot make decisions for himself or herself. Unlike the Living Will, this document allows another person to make decisions even if the condition is not terminal. This document is not in effect as long as the patient is able to make medical decisions. It can be cancelled any time, verbally or in writing. The document applies to health care decisions only; it does not relate to any decisions concerning money, property, or estates.

Free copies of the Living Will can be obtained from the Euthanasia Education Council, 250 West 57 Street, New York, NY 10019. In some states the Living Will is not binding at present.

The Angry Patient

Another problem that interferes with positive communication is the patient's anger or hostility, which can either be a reaction to bad news or precipitated by an unknown cause. The medical assistant must recognize that the anger may be out of character for the patient. In many cases, it is related to the medical problem being treated. The goal in dealing with anger is to help calm the patient and contain the situation.

The medical assistant must never become caught up in a cycle of escalating anger. Instead, it is imperative to remain calm and objective, yet firm and direct. The medical assistant should not give in to a patient who is making an unreasonable demand. However, it is impor-

LIVING WILL DECLARATION

I, _____ , being of sound mind, willfully and voluntarily make this declaration to be followed if I become incompetent. This declaration reflects my firm and settled commitment to refuse life-sustaining treatment under the circumstance indicated below.

I direct my attending physician to withhold or withdraw life-sustaining treatment that serves only to prolong the process of my dying, if I should be in a terminal condition or in a state of permanent unconsciousness.

I direct that treatment be limited to measures to keep me comfortable and to relieve pain, including any pain that might occur by withholding or withdrawing life-sustaining treatment.

In addition, if I am in the condition described above, I feel especially strong about the following forms of treatment:

I ❑ DO ❑ DO NOT want cardiac resuscitation.
I ❑ DO ❑ DO NOT want blood or blood products.
I ❑ DO ❑ DO NOT want tube feeding or any other artificial or invasive form of nutrition (food) or hydration (water).

I ❑ DO ❑ DO NOT want mechanical respiration.
I ❑ DO ❑ DO NOT want kidney dialysis.
I ❑ DO ❑ DO NOT want antibiotics.
I ❑ DO ❑ DO NOT want any form of surgery or invasive diagnostic tests.

I realize that if I do not specifically indicate my preference regarding any of the forms of treatment listed above, I may receive that form of treatment.

OTHER INSTRUCTIONS:
I ❑ DO ❑ DO NOT want to designate another person as my surrogate to make medical treatment decisions for me if I should be incompetent and in a terminal condition or in a state of permanent unconsciousness.

Name of surrogate (if applicable): _____

Name of substitute surrogate (if surrogate designated is unable to serve): _____

Address: _____

Address: _____

The declarant or the person on behalf of and at the direction of the declarant knowingly and voluntarily signed this writing by signature or mark in my presence.

I made this declaration on the _____ day of _____ (month, year).

Witness's signature: _____

Witness's address: _____

Declarant's signature: _____

Declarant's address: _____

Witness's signature: _____

Witness's address: _____

Figure 4-1. This example of a living will is from Pennsylvania. (Courtesy Pennsylvania State Senator Buzz Andrezeski, Harrisburg, Pennsylvania.)

tant, both for the sake of the upset person and for other patients in the office, to quickly extinguish a public display of angry behavior. If the angry person is not provoked further, the anger usually subsides.

The following is a list of suggestions for dealing with an angry person:

1. Do not allow yourself to get upset.
2. Take deep breaths and concentrate on calming yourself.
3. Do not interrupt an irrational line of verbal reasoning; just listen.
4. If the person is being loud and disruptive, use the first available opportunity to gently ask him or her to be quieter for the sake of the other patients.
5. Gently call attention to the patient's anger with a statement such as, "I realize that you are very angry, and I'm sorry, but. . . ."
6. If all else fails, isolation may work. Ask the patient to wait for a few moments alone in an

examination room. Often, time spent alone has a calming effect.

The Hearing-Impaired or Foreign-Language-Speaking Patient

In addition to communication problems of emotional origin, communication problems occur when the patient is hearing-impaired or speaks a foreign language. Although it may be desirable to learn how to communicate using sign language and other languages, this goal is somewhat unrealistic. The medical assistant should, however, know of and be able to obtain resources or to contact individuals who would be helpful in communicating with these patients.

Standing or sitting directly in front of the patient and speaking slowly and distinctly helps patients who lipread. In certain areas where a large number of the population speak a language other than English, it would be useful for the medical assistant to learn the language or key medical words in that language.

The Sight-Impaired Patient

The sight-impaired patient offers another challenge to communication and may require more touching. The patient may need to feel objects for better understanding. The medical assistant must be careful, however, to ask the patient, "How can I be of help?" rather than to take the individual's hand and place it on an object without warning. The sight-impaired person knows best what he or she needs. Again, the medical assistant's role in communicating with these patients is one of openness, flexibility, and support.

The Aging Patient

The older or aging patient also presents communication problems at times. The medical assistant may need to speak slowly and repeat information patiently. A very important caution, however, is that each older or aging adult is an individual and has communication needs, styles, and preferences based on that individuality. The medical assistant should not relate to older or aging adults in a particular manner simply because they are aging. Each patient requires and deserves individual assessment (Fig. 4–2).

The communication problems discussed above are frequently encountered in medical practice. As the medical assistant gains confidence and experience, his or her own style and preferences emerge. The preceding discussion offers general guidelines. However, all health professionals can become effective communica-tors by being uniquely themselves and being open to and aware of the needs of others.

DEALING WITH FAMILY AND FRIENDS

Patients often come to the office with one or more other persons. Usually, these friends or family members form an emotional support group for the patient. Their presence in the office suggests both their willingness to be involved and their interest in the patient. It is the medical assistant's responsibility to answer the needs and questions of the patient's friends and relatives.

In all cases, the wishes of the *patient* should be addressed. The medical assistant might, for example, ask a patient, "Mrs. Brown, would you like your husband to accompany you to the examination room?" If the patient says yes, the medical assistant can invite the husband to join his wife. The issue of privacy must be handled carefully with growing children. With very young children, it seems appropriate to have parents present at all times. But as children become young adults, it may be appropriate to allow a child privacy with the physician.

In addition, patients are concerned for their friends, and likewise their friends are concerned for them. The medical assistant must acknowledge these ancillary persons and attend to the problem of keeping them informed. For example, friends and relatives in waiting rooms can suffer needless anxiety while waiting. Thus,

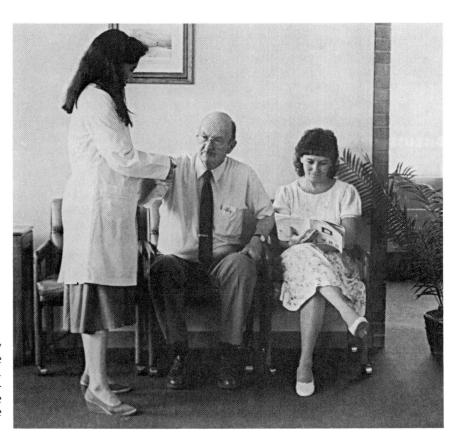

Figure 4–2. Some patients may require physical assistance to rise from a seated position or to walk. Remember, however, that patients do not automatically require such assistance simply because they are elderly.

it is courteous to update those waiting on the patient's progress and inform them of delays.

The communication problems discussed in the previous sections are as likely to occur with friends and family members as they are with patients themselves. The medical assistant must apply the same communication skills with family and friends as with the patient. Most frequently, acknowledgment is all that the patient's family and friends require of the medical assistant. These office visitors want to know that they are welcome and that their concern for the patient is valued. It is important to remember that families and friends are, in a very real sense, a significant part of the healing process for the ill patient. Their concerns are as important to successful treatment as those of the patient, but confidentiality must still be maintained.

PATIENT TEACHING CONSIDERATIONS

The medical office keeps a supply of patient teaching brochures related to disease, conditions, and health education. In addition, the medical assistant might include appropriate self-help booklets. For example, it is advisable to include brochures that suggest ways to handle stress, manage anger, and deal with emotions in general. The medical profession accepts that a cause-and-effect relationship exists between psychological factors and illness. When lifestyle changes are required, or if the patient needs help in coping with the death of a spouse, a terminal illness, or work-related stress, the physician frequently refers the patient for counseling. The medical assistant should be prepared to inform the patient of counseling services at the physician's request.

Other booklets are available for the patient's family. These publications give suggestions for coping with the patient who has a specific condition or disease, such as

diabetes. (The booklet on diabetes is published by the American Diabetes Association, 2 Park Ave, New York, NY, 10016.)

RELATED ETHICAL AND LEGAL IMPLICATIONS

The medical assistant should use caution in communicating with patients. Such statements as "Don't worry. I know you'll be absolutely fine" give false reassurance, which is unethical. From the legal perspective, this statement promises a cure for which the physician may be liable. It is important to respond honestly and to avoid well-meaning but false statements. Recording unpleasant or emotionally upsetting interactions on the patient record is the best protection against legal claims. However, the medical assistant should take care not to record value-laden, dubious statements, such as "He is unable to accept his illness." Another ethical concern is related to information disclosure: what the patient should be told and by whom. The medical assistant must never make these decisions, but may instead offer support and genuine caring to the patient.

SUMMARY

Communicating purposefully and positively with patients involves learning and practicing communication skills. However, the medical assistant must build on these skills to develop a style of communicating that is comfortable and genuine. Sincere, positive regard for patients is more important than expert use of skills. Effort and frequent practice will facilitate the medical assistant's ease in communicating with patients, their families, and their friends.

DISCUSSION QUESTIONS

Before choosing a response to the problems presented, try to think about the objectives to be achieved. Your instructor may ask that you prepare written answers to these issues.

1. *Example:* The patient comes to the desk and begins criticizing the physician.
   Objective: Refer the patient to the physician and try to prevent a disturbance at the front desk.
2. *Example:* The patient is about to have x-rays and states that she does not like x-rays.
   Objective: Reassure the patient. Accept her feelings.
   Patient: *"I don't want Dr. Jones to examine me—I want Dr. Smith."* (The two are partners and she is scheduled for Dr. Jones.)
   Patient: *"I can't understand how you would enjoy working in a doctor's office."*
   Patient's Relative: *"My nephew has been in the examining room for an hour. What could be wrong?"*
   Patient: *"I am concerned about paying for all this."*
   Patient: *"That woman waiting to see the doctor is quite ill."*
3. What is the medical assistant's role as an attitude transmitter?
4. What are the losses a person experiences in becoming a patient? Can you think of any others? How does becoming a patient affect a person's ability to understand and respond effectively?
5. How does cultural background influence patient behavior?
6. What is the definition of a defensive response? Are these responses unhealthy? Why or why not?
7. What is the purpose of listening skills? Please list them.

BIBLIOGRAPHY

Davis C: Patient Practitioner Interaction: An Experiential Manual for Developing the Art of Health Care. Slack, Thorofare, NJ, 1989.

Howard A and Howard W: Exploring the Road Less Traveled. Simon and Schuster, New York, 1985.

Kubler-Ross E: On Death and Dying. Macmillan, New York, 1974.

Lewis M and Warden CD: Law and Ethics in the Medical Office Including Bioethical Issues, ed 2. FA Davis, Philadelphia, 1988.

Purtilo R: Health Professional and Patient Interaction, ed 4. WB Saunders, Philadelphia, 1990.

PROCEDURE: Listen to and communicate with the patient

Terminal Performance Objective: Demonstrate the ability to listen to and communicate with the patient in a manner that fosters positive patient dynamics.

PROCEDURE

1. Listen attentively to the patient's verbal message.
2. Check for clear interpretation by asking the patient to repeat the message. *Example: Patient:* "I'm late in coming for a checkup." *Medical Assistant:* "You think you should have had a checkup before this?"
3. Listen for feelings.

4. Observe the patient for nonverbal expression.

5. Use open and closed statements to direct communication, and use other directing techniques (e.g., reflecting, adding to implied statements, and silence) accordingly.

PRINCIPLE

1. The listener's attention should focus on the patient.
2. The listener cannot make the correct, therapeutic response if he or she does not understand what is communicated.

3. Inflection and emphasis often convey emotional reactions to what is being said.
4. Nonverbal expression, such as facial wincing or furrowed brow, conveys emotion.
5. Different types of statements elicit different responses.

HIGHLIGHTS

Understanding Terminally Ill Patients and Their Families

It is likely that the medical assistant will at some time be involved in caring for terminally ill patients. Understanding the common characteristics of terminally ill patients helps the medical assistant provide the appropriate, supportive treatment.

RESPONSES TO THE DYING PROCESS

As a consequence of her research, Elisabeth Kubler-Ross identified "stages of dying." These stages are actually responses. It is now understood that individuals do not necessarily progress through the stages in sequential order.

On learning that they are terminally ill, many people's first reactions are shock and grief and then denial—disbelief that they will actually die. Depression, anger, hostility, bargaining, and acceptance are other responses the terminally ill patient may demonstrate.

The medical assistant must be careful to recognize that there are no right or most appropriate ways of reacting to terminal illness and the prospect of dying. Each patient has a right to his or her own unique responses. The most professional role is to provide support and the opportunity for the patient to react.

Another perspective on dying and its responses is called "dying trajectorius." Monselle Pattison (the author responsible for this theory) defined "trajectory of life" as the individual's anticipated life span and the plan for the way he or she will live out life. He theorizes that, between the time that we discover that we will die sooner than anticipated and the time we actually die, there exist "living-dying intervals." These have three phases of development. Pattison suggests that the health professional's role is to help the patient cope and live well through each phase. These phases are as follows:

1. *Acute.* The patient first discovers that the event of death has a relatively predictable cause, course, and time frame. Pattison suggests that this phase is the most emotionally wrenching.
2. *Chronic.* In this phase, the terminally ill patient begins to actually confront the concept of dying. Defense mechanisms such as denial, anger, and bargaining may be characteristic of this phase.
3. *Terminal.* In this phase, the patient may appear distant and withdrawn and may begin to accept the finality of approaching death.

THE FAMILY OF THE TERMINALLY ILL PATIENT

Family members begin the grief process (grieving for the loss of a loved one) immediately on learning of the terminal illness. Reactions of family members are not unlike those of the patient. Most family members cry frequently and suddenly, sigh often, feel depressed, and have difficulty sleeping. These same reactions continue for a long time after the patient dies. Various factors influence the nature and duration of grief. They include the specific relationship between the dying patient and family members, and the changes in the family members' own lives experienced as a result of the loss.

THE MEDICAL ASSISTANT'S ROLE

As was previously mentioned, the medical assistant's role in interacting with terminally ill patients and their families is supportive. The term "supportive" brings particular images to mind, such as displaying warmth and kindness to patients. However, being supportive also necessitates that the medical assistant realize the appropriate parameters. For instance:

1. The medical assistant should not inform the patient or family members of the terminal illness or its progression. It is the physician's responsibility to do so. The medical assistant may, however, give explanations and provide instructions.
2. It is not the medical assistant's responsibility to become the primary counselor. However, he or she may, in collaboration with the physician, refer the patient and family to specific persons, groups, and organizations that may be helpful, given the patient's particular circumstances.
3. The medical assistant must recognize that every patient is unique. Some prefer to know everything about the disease, to seek help wherever it can be found, and to express their concern verbally. Others require little information and are quiet and satisfied with limited explanation. The medical assistant cannot be judgmental. Instead, his or her own acceptance of the patient's needs is directly related to how effectively the medical assistant can provide supportive care to the terminally ill patient.

> Patient education is an active process that involves information exchange between patient and health professional; it is not something done to the patient but rather with the patient—a joint effort
>
> Donna Falvo,
> Effective Patient Education

CHAPTER OUTLINE

LEARNING OBJECTIVES

Upon completing this chapter, you will be able to:

1. State the purpose of patient teaching and the purpose of the holistic approach to patient education.
2. List eight variables that contribute to the patient's openness and readiness to learn.
3. State seven ways to create an environment that will encourage patients to ask questions.
4. Apply the legal doctrine of *respondeat superior* to the patient-teaching situation.

PERFORMANCE OBJECTIVES

Upon completing this chapter, you will be able to:

1. Use standardized instruction sheets, handouts, and verbal instructions to reinforce and clarify the physician's orders.

Chapter 5

Patient Teaching

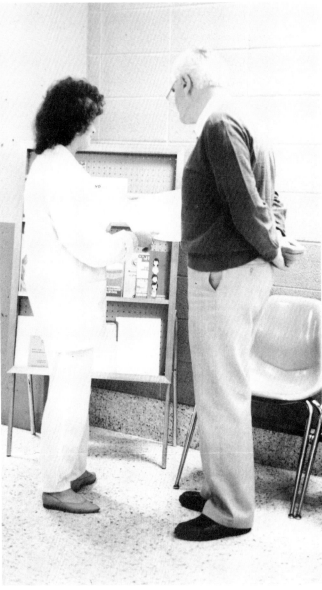

2. File informal teaching notes and formal teaching handouts in the patient's medical record.
3. Develop activities for each of the seven teaching strategies: referral, recordkeeping, journalkeeping, role playing, demonstration, family involvement, and programmed instruction.
4. Order patient instruction materials from publishing and resource agencies providing information for patients.

DACUM EDUCATIONAL COMPONENTS

1. Interview (patients and family members) effectively (by telephone and in the office (2.9A).
2. Locate resources and information for patients and employers (3.6A, B).
3. Orient patients to office policies and procedures (and to treatments by using patient education systems and literature) (7.1B).
4. Instruct patients with special needs (for self-monitoring, follow-up care, home medical equipment, and chronic disease management) (7.2A–D).
5. Teach patients methods of health promotion and disease prevention (by providing verbal and written information, demonstration, and referrals to outside resources) (7.3A–D).

Glossary

Assessment: A determination, study, or analysis
Compliance: Conforming or obeying; being in accordance with
Intervention: Interference; influential act
Journalkeeping: Writing or reporting on a regular basis
Outcome: Result
Patient education: A process that is part of total health care. It involves talking with the patient and using certain forms to help the patient clarify health issues and reach decisions compatible with his or her own needs.
Patient teaching: Actual imparting of information to the patient
Process: An ongoing system

Patient health education includes helping the patient toward some degree of competent self-care in following prescribed treatment plans. The emphasis of patient teaching, however, is directed toward helping the patient acquire and maintain high-level wellness and adopt healthy behaviors such as exercise and well-balanced nutrition. Both patients and physicians are emphasizing the need for patient teaching in medical practice.

From the patient's perspective, an accurate clinical diagnosis and satisfactory treatment are not always sufficient returns for the cost of medical care. Many patients expect to participate in their treatment and to be educated as well as treated. They are interested in learning how to improve their health, achieve optimum wellness, and prevent illness. They may, in fact, seek to become actively involved in making decisions about their own health care needs.

From the perspective of physicians and other health care professionals, well-informed patients are more likely to cooperate and to experience successful treatment. Medical scientists have acknowledged the role of patient education in the prevention of illness and disease. Illness and disease processes are known to be affected strongly by psychosocial factors, including lifestyle and personality patterns.

In light of the patient's needs for health care educa-

tion and the supportive conclusions of medical research, physicians in office practice are becoming increasingly attentive to patient education. The contemporary concept of patient education embodies a holistic view of the patient. The physician and staff who hold this view concern themselves with issues that are medically related but far exceed the diagnosis and treatment of specific illnesses. This holistic model focuses on the overall wellness of each patient by considering not only the patient's psychological and physiologic conditions, but also the intellectual and spiritual dimensions (see Highlights at the end of this chapter).

In this context, the medical assistant may prepare to assume the advanced professional skill of facilitating patient education. He or she should be aware of the role that patient education plays in holistic medicine, and should be able to develop teaching behaviors that will enable patients to participate in their own treatment and achieve their own wellness goals. For instance, the medical assistant can instruct diabetic patients on how to give themselves injections and blood tests, and other patients on how to change their own dressings or take their own blood pressure. Patients who are interested in improving their diet and exercise habits may look to the medical office staff for direction. Regardless of which behavior the patient must learn to accomplish a specific procedure or personal goal, the medical assistant's approach to teaching must be based on general principles of patient education introduced in this chapter. The medical assistant who shares patient teaching responsibilities with the physician becomes more valuable than ever in the office. The physician has more time, and thus gains greater autonomy in providing comprehensive health care.

DEFINITION AND PURPOSE OF PATIENT TEACHING

Patient education and *patient teaching*, although used synonymously throughout this chapter, have some definitive differences. Patient education is the process of teaching and learning; patient teaching is the content of these activities. Patient education is directed toward changing the patient's knowledge, attitudes, motivations, and behaviors by influencing thoughts, feelings, and actions. The holistic attitudes and teaching skills of the patient educator are used in the process. Patient education has evolved into an accepted component of comprehensive care. Its purpose is to help patients learn how to recover from and prevent diseases by changing patterns of lifestyle or personality. It is currently recognized as both the patient's right and a key to increasing the efficiency of health care.

Patient teaching, by contrast, often is limited to less comprehensive patient instruction, such as directions given in preparation for laboratory testing, special examination, specific treatments, or follow-up care. This type of instruction teaches self-care during a one-time procedure or isolated event and is not used for long-term or holistic purposes. If a handout is used to instruct, the medical assistant should discuss it with the patient, encouraging the patient to ask questions, and assessing the patient's understanding of the handout material (Fig. 5–1).

Compliance, or the following of the physician's advice, is often the purpose of patient teaching. A recent study of patients with high blood pressure found that a large percentage of the patients suffered from hypertension because they were not taking their medications properly. Similar studies, by researchers interested in learning whether patients would take the entire prescribed dose of any medication, have generally found that more than half terminated their medication prematurely.

A logical conclusion derived from such studies is that patients are likely to misunderstand or not follow even the simplest instructions. The medical assistant must be alert to the patient's potential for compliance to direct patient teaching activities appropriately.

In addition to encouraging compliance, some physicians attempt to provide articles and pamphlets for their patients suggesting behaviors for a healthy lifestyle. The purpose is to stimulate good health habits, thus preventing illness rather than treating symptoms at a later date.

Figure 5–1. Sample patient instruction sheet.

THE LEARNER

Patients possess diverse backgrounds that directly affect their desire and ability to understand information and master skills. The medical assistant must be aware of these variables and anticipate the role they play in his or her teaching relationship with the patient.

The factors listed below contribute significantly to the patient's openness and readiness to learn:

1. The patient's perception of his or her disease versus the actual state of wellness
2. The patient's need for information
3. The patient's age and level of development
4. The patient's feelings, such as anxiety, depression, or anger
5. The patient's religion, ethnicity, family experiences, and personality
6. The patient's individual learning style
7. Special problems that would affect learning, such as visual or hearing impairment
8. The medical assistant's teaching style

The medical assistant may discover these variables through conversing with and observing the patient during the regular office visit, through interviewing or formal teaching, or through the assessment process described in the following section of this chapter. Regardless of the constraints of time and resources, teaching should encourage patients to assume an active role in their own health care.

THE ROLE OF THE PATIENT EDUCATOR

The medical assistant's role as patient educator complements the physician's role and probably reflects the physician's commitment to patient education. Although the medical assistant may be responsible for formalized (scheduled and organized) patient teaching, usually he or she participates in an educational exchange with the patient during a regular office visit or telephone conversation. Regardless of the circumstance or the topic, each encounter with a patient is a potential opportunity to teach. To respond effectively, the medical assistant must be able to identify the individual needs of the patient. The information presented must be relevant, comprehensive, and directed at enabling the patient to change certain behaviors.

As a teacher, the medical assistant is usually involved with the patient continuously rather than during a single visit. This relationship is nurtured by the medical assistant's attitude of being the facilitator—the one who enables the patient to learn by creating the climate and the circumstance.

As was mentioned, much of the medical assistant's teaching is constrained by time and competing responsibilities. However, when time permits or is specifically designated for formal patient teaching, a teaching plan may be used. Regardless of the formal or informal nature of patient teaching in the medical office, the medical assistant should make every attempt to encourage questions and motivating patients to learn. The following guidelines apply:

1. Project a willingness to discuss issues and to answer the patient's questions. Asking "How do you feel about this?" or "Did you want to tell me anything before you leave the office?" is often more successful than "Do you have any questions?"
2. Post cheerful signs that convey your willingness to answer patients' questions, such as "Patients should feel free to call with questions" or "Can we help you learn more about good health?"
3. Do not react negatively or respond casually to the patient's question. Think about the importance of the question to the patient before choosing a response. To be an effective teacher, the medical assistant must be accepting, supportive, and nonjudgmental toward the learner.
4. Not all questions can be answered immediately. It is certainly acceptable to say "That's an excellent question, but I don't know the answer. I'll find out and get back to you." Tell the patient that you will ask the physician or look up the answer, and follow through as soon as possible.
5. Do not dismiss questions that may not be closely related to the matter at hand. Instead, direct the patient toward appropriate information resources.
6. Encourage patients who are leaving the office to ask any final questions and to call if any come to mind later.
7. Never assume the physician's role. Never go beyond the physician's guidelines or what he or she has revealed to the patient. Refer the patient to the physician when it would be more appropriate for the physician to answer the question.

Medical assistants must guard against setting up an alternative diagnostic or treatment center in the office and diverting patients from accepting the physician's judgments. Rather, they should provide a support system to assist patients in asking for and interpreting the physician's advice.

The medical assistant should note briefly in the patient's record the content of any teaching encounters that occur over the telephone or in person. Each entry should also be dated and initialed. Recording not only ensures consistency in direction, objectives, and content, but also provides legal protection. An example of a patient teaching notation follows:

11/6/93 Patient given verbal and written instructions during office visit re: change of dressing. (Routine instructions—Handout #24). Patient questioning the need for another office visit in 2 weeks. Referred to physician. Joyce Collins.

TEACHING STRATEGIES

Teaching strategies assist in accomplishing the goals determined by the patient and the patient educator. Those listed here are suggested for use with medical office patients and account for the time and resource limitations presented in the medical office.

REFERRAL PROGRAMS

The medical assistant may inform the patient of lectures or programs in the community that are relevant to the patient's learning needs. For example, a couple expecting their first child may be referred to prenatal classes sponsored by a community medical center, or to classes offered by independent organizations in the community, such as the Childbirth Education Association. In addition, many hospitals and medical centers have developed detailed programs to aid patients in managing chronic disorders, such as diabetes and hypertension.

RECORD AND JOURNAL KEEPING

The medical assistant may ask the patient to keep a progress record, a journal, or both. Recordkeeping permits assessment by the patient of what has been accomplished and what has not. Journal keeping, or writing feelings about the changes experienced, encourages the patient's awareness of developing new attitudes and offers reinforcement. For example, a long-time smoker who is attempting to stop smoking may find this technique helpful.

ROLE PLAYING

Depending on the type of medical office and the commitment to patient teaching, the medical assistant may use role playing to teach new behaviors and attitudes through practice. Role playing can be particularly useful for helping patients with chronic diseases to master particular skills, such as dietary management in diabetes. Using this technique, individuals are able to learn from one another and share common concerns. For children anticipating surgery or diagnostic tests, play using dolls or other toys that recreate real-life situations is often helpful.

LEARNING CONTRACT

A learning contract is a patient teaching strategy which identifies the learning goals and objectives, the responsibilities of the teacher and learner, and the method of evaluation. Figure 5–2 is an example of a learning contract.

DEMONSTRATION AND RETURN DEMONSTRATION

The medical assistant's demonstration of a procedure and the patient's return demonstration is a form of role playing that requires the participation of only the patient and the medical assistant. This technique is particularly useful for teaching specific behaviors, such as self-administration of insulin, and self-assessment procedures, such as obtaining blood pressure and performing blood and urine tests. Often, anatomic models can be used for practicing procedures such as giving injections or detecting a mass in a breast.

FAMILY INVOLVEMENT

Friends and family can offer reinforcement for the patient attempting to adopt new behaviors. Their involvement in teaching sessions can be useful only if the patient approves and is comfortable with their participation.

PROGRAMMED INSTRUCTION

Videos, self-instruction manuals, and printed handouts available from many organizations and public agencies may be useful for teaching specific behaviors or attitudes, such as child safety or wellness programs featuring diet, exercise, and stress reduction strategies. Teaching activities, of course, are selected on the basis of what information is to be learned, when, and by whom. As was mentioned earlier, the most important consideration in choosing one or several strategies is the compatibility of the strategy with the patient. The

---

Mrs. Mattis, 45-year-old female; osteoarthritis of the fingers
Goals: 1. Maintain joint motion
2. Control pain
3. Prevent deformities

Medical Assistant's Responsibilities (Joyce)

10/1/86

Instruct Mrs. Mattis concerning the physicians orders: rest, medication, other supportive techniques such as massage and heat application

Give Mrs. Mattis brochure on Osteoarthritis

Instruct Mrs. Mattis on exercise program by demonstrating each of the exercises

10/16/86

Check Mrs. Mattis's progress with self-care:
1. Medication being taken on schedule
2. Exercises properly performed
3. Use of other supportive treatments such as rest, heat application, massage

11/12/86

Meet with Mrs. Mattis during the office visit to review contract and make necessary adjustments with the physician's approval

MA Signature_____
Date_____

Patient's Responsibilities

10/1/86

Ask questions to clarify and understand instructions

Read brochure. Give verbal descriptions of self-care prescribed

Return the demonstration while Joyce supervises

10/16/86

Mrs. Mattis reports progress and reviews procedure by demonstrating exercises, massage, and describes other techniques

11/12/86

Meet with Joyce to review contract and make adjustments as necessary and approved by physician

Patient Signature_____
Date_____

Figure 5–2. An example of a learning contract.

mutual participation approach to patient teaching requires the medical assistant to be skillful not only in providing accurate information, but also in offering guidance and support based on the patient's needs.

DESIGNING AND WRITING HANDOUT MATERIALS

Although this task is rarely necessary because of the accessibility of preprinted materials, the medical assistant may elect to write handout materials to describe procedures relevant to a particular medical practice or specific to a particular patient's needs. The format depends on the type and amount of information to be included. A popular format is the question-and-answer style because it is precise and easy to read. Figure 5–3 shows a sample of this style. A question is asked as a patient would ask it and then is answered clearly and thoroughly. Another type of handout lists steps for the patient to follow in completing a procedure or mastering a technique (Fig. 5–3).

The medical assistant must recognize that whenever printed or written handouts are used, it is easy to give the handout to the patient without sufficient explanation and interaction. Communication is extremely important in using teaching aids since the patient may misinterpret information, become anxious, or be reluctant to ask questions because "it is all spelled out in the

handout." Written materials are not a substitute for learner-teacher communication and should be viewed as reinforcements, not replacements.

In addition, the medical assistant using preprinted materials should scrutinize them for readability, inclusion of essential information, and relevance to patient needs. The following example demonstrates the inappropriate and appropriate use of handouts.

Example

Diabetic Patient: I have some more questions about what to do if I start to get weak. How will I know if it's really the need to eat or I'm just feeling tired? After all, I'm 70.

Inappropriate Response: "Everything you need to know is in these booklets. Call if you have questions."

Appropriate Response: The medical assistant first answers the questions and then points out the contents of each pamphlet, asks the patient to read them, and sets up an appointment for a telephone call or follow-up office visit to discuss the information in the pamphlet and answer the patient's questions. The medical assistant may also instruct the patient to write questions while reading so as not to forget them before there has been an opportunity for discussion.

Some Answers To Common Questions About Dr. White's Office

1. What is Dr. White's Specialty?
   Answer: Dr. George White is an orthopedic specialist who has developed a sub-specialty in sports medicine. This means that he is particularly interested in the kinds of orthopedic problems that have resulted from or contribute to the inability to participate in sports.

2. Do I have to be a professional athlete to see Dr. White?
   Answer: No! Dr. White is convinced that all of us would be happier and healthier if we would maintain an active participation in lifelong sports activities. He is as interested in a grandmother who can't jog because of a sore foot as he would be in treating a professional football player.

3. Is Dr. White's service expensive?
   Answer: We will be pleased to discuss our professional fee structure with you before you begin treatment. In the long run, most persons would consider this kind of treatment to be less expensive than the surgery which might result from an undiagnosed problem.

4. How should I pay the Doctor?
   Answer: Normally, patients should pay for services at the time of the office visit. If there are extenuating circumstances, we will be happy to discuss them with you.

5. What are the office hours and how can I make an appointment?
   Answer: Except for emergency cases, all office visits are by appointment. The office is open Tuesday, Thursday, and Saturday from 10:00 A.M. to 7:00 P.M.

6. What if I have questions?
   Answer: We welcome you to call us at 412-3768 during regular office hours. We will either get an answer to your question or arrange an appointment.

7. What about emergencies or questions during non-office hours?
   Answer: If the question can wait until regular hours we would appreciate your not calling until then; but in the event that an emergency occurs, you may reach Dr. White any time by calling 412-3768 and reaching his answering service.

Figure 5–3. An example of a patient handout in the question-and-answer style.

RELATED ETHICAL AND LEGAL IMPLICATIONS

The legal issue central to patient teaching is the patient's "right to know." Whenever the patient enters into a contractual agreement with the physician and other health caretakers by presenting himself or herself for diagnosis and treatment, this right is legally guaranteed. The patient's right to know includes the right to understand the diagnosis, the suggested therapy, its rationale, the alternative treatments, and the chances for recovery. The right to know entitles the patient to education. Under the legal doctrine of *respondeat superior* ("Let the master answer."), the physician is ultimately liable for all acts, including patient teaching, performed by the medical assistant. Therefore, the physician ultimately determines the guidelines governing patient teaching and approves all written handouts and verbal instructions.

From an ethical perspective, adult patients deserve access to information regardless of the consequences. It is the patient's right to decide whether or not to comply with the advice given. In particular, the underprivileged, the poor, and members of minorities deserve special attention in patient teaching because they appear to encounter a large percentage of health care problems. In the expanded sense of ethical obligation, medical assistants share the responsibility not only to educate patients specifically, but also to respond to opportunities for educating society as a whole regarding national health care priorities.

SUMMARY

Increasingly, physicians are becoming involved in patient education with the purpose of helping patients to design a healthy life. Physicians cannot be expected to carry out patient education alone. They should be able to rely on support from a staff that is knowledgeable and aware of the holistic perspective. Medical assistants in turn should provide the catalyst for patient education. Understandably, this responsibility is reserved for advanced medical assistants with extensive experience. Entry-level medical assistants, however, can function as resource persons, anticipating questions, providing answers, intervening and interpreting when necessary, and helping to change patients' orientation from passive to active participation in their own health care.

DISCUSSION QUESTIONS

1. Discuss the importance of patient teaching to the overall objective of providing comprehensive patient care.
2. What variables may provide obstacles to learning? If a patient is resistant to learning and the variable is simply lack of interest, what would be your initial response?
3. What patient teaching opportunities can the medical assistant probably expect?
4. Using evaluative tools, the medical assistant discovers that the patient has not changed behaviors. How may the medical assistant respond? What plan of action might the medical assistant pursue?
5. Discuss the advantages and disadvantages of using printed handouts in patient teaching.

BIBLIOGRAPHY

Chatburn RL and Longh MD: Handbook of Respiratory Care, ed 2. Mosby–Year Book, St. Louis, 1990.
Falvo DR: Effective Patient Education: A Guide to Increased Compliance. Aspen, Gaithersburg, MD, 1983.
Harris RD and Ramsay AT: Health Care Counseling: A Behavioral Approach. FA Davis, Philadelphia, 1988.
Hodges P and Vickery C: Effective Counseling: Strategies for Dietary Management. Aspen, Gaithersburg, MD, 1989.
Lewis CB: Aging: The Health Care Challenge, ed 2. FA Davis, Philadelphia, 1990.
Meyers D: Client Teaching Guides for Home Health Care. Aspen, Gaithersburg, MD, 1988.
Payton OD et al: Patient Participation in Program Planning: A Manual for Therapists. FA Davis, Philadelphia, 1990.
Purtilo R: Health Professional and Patient Interaction, ed 4. WB Saunders, Philadelphia, 1990.
Reed KL and Sanderson SN: Concepts of Occupational Therapy, ed 3. Williams and Wilkins, Baltimore, 1992.
Rothstein JM et al: The Rehabilitation Specialist's Handbook. FA Davis, Philadelphia, 1991.
Swinford P: Promoting Wellness: A Nurse's Handbook. Aspen, Gaithersburg, MD, 1988.

HIGHLIGHTS
Holistic Health Planning

More than just the absence of disease, holistic health is defined as a total state of physical, mental, and social well-being. This wellness orientation depends on integrating the self with a healthy and safe environment, a healthy lifestyle (experiences based on good reasoning and healthy behavior patterns), healthy attitudes toward oneself and others, value systems that reinforce health and healing, and accessibility to medical services for health maintenance, disease prevention, treatment, and rehabilitation when necessary.

Holistic health education depends on teaching plans that integrate the individual's body, mind, spirituality, and social relationships. In addition to preventive medicine and traditional medical care, the wellness movement emphasizes a lifestyle and self-awareness that make each individual responsible for the following:

❑ Exercise
❑ Good nutrition
❑ Stress management
❑ Rest and relaxation
❑ Elimination of substance use and abuse
❑ An ecologically balanced environment

The holistic approach is a three-step process:

1. Develop a sense of responsibility.
2. Identify problem behaviors and lifestyles.
3. Modify or eliminate unhealthy behaviors and lifestyles.

Once patients begin participating in decisions about their own well-being, they can participate in developing long-term teaching plans. Extensive written plans, reference books, and pamphlets on lifestyle behaviors and modifications are especially useful if complex changes are required over long periods. Modifying lifestyles and behavior patterns can be difficult and even unpleasant. Therefore, learning contracts (discussed earlier in this chapter) may be useful to encourage patient compliance.

PHYSICAL FITNESS

A regular exercise program is important for improving cardiovascular and pulmonary functioning, carbohydrate and lipid metabolism, self-image, and mental and motor performance; controlling body weight; decreasing the risk for cardiovascular diseases; and increasing the body's ability to withstand stress.

An exercise program is designed to enhance fitness and overall conditioning by placing controlled stress on the body at regular intervals. Each exercise program must be individually planned by the physician after a complete physical examination and cardiovas-cular testing (including electrocardiography and stress testing). The patient is encouraged to select aerobic activities (walking, jogging, running, cycling, swimming, and racquet sports) that interest him or her.

Depending on the patient's age and previous exercise experience, the exercise training plan gradually increases effort and endurance until maximum benefit levels are reached. Exercise time and intensity usually increase at 2- to 3-week intervals on the basis of predicted cardiovascular endurance. When maximum levels are reached, the program is continued as a permanent routine of the patient's lifestyle.

NUTRITIONAL ADVICE

Cardiovascular disease, cancer, stroke, hypertension, diabetes, and hepatic cirrhosis are the leading causes of death in the United States. These diseases, along with obesity, are strongly linked to eating and drinking habits. Excessive intake of fat, cholesterol, sugar, salt, alcohol, and calories contribute to soaring health costs and decrease human productivity. Optimum nutritional intake is the cornerstone of holistic health.

Dietary planning varies depending on body size, gender, degree of physical activity, and metabolic rate. Eating plans and dietary information are designed to control individual dietary excesses and thus reduce the risk for cardiovascular disease and other chronic health problems. Nutritional information, such as food groups, sample menus, weight graphs, shopping lists, and food records, are used to help the patient reach the ideal weight and maintain a sound dietary program thereafter.

STRESS MANAGEMENT

When harnessed productively, stress produces innovation and vitality. When left unchecked, it can damage physical and psychologic health and personal self-esteem. When there is an excess of stressful events or when a person cannot handle them, stress becomes a problem.

External stressors include job pressures, interpersonal relationships, community or governmental pressures, and environmental stressors, such as excessive noise or pollution. Internal stressors include illness, pain, fatigue, negative emotions, and feelings of alienation. Although it is not always possible to control the external environment, medical science is showing that we can better control the internal environment by managing our reactions to stressors. A stress reduction program depends on regular exercise, improving interpersonal communications with family, friends, and coworkers, and relaxation techniques. Stress management begins with helping the individual to

Continued

clarify psychosocial and cultural values, identify the sources of stress, recognize individual manifestations of stress and tension, and then develop a personalized plan of exercise, relaxation, diet and nutrition, and social interactions to modify the effects of stress.

REST AND RELAXATION

Rest and relaxation techniques are an important adjunct to any stress modification program. Research continues to show that relaxation decreases anxiety and the arousal response to stress; improves coping abilities, self-image, and self-acceptance; improves learning ability with better retention and recall; and creates a sense of calm and a more philosophic attitude.

The relaxation response is a form of meditation—a state of concentration. Used once or twice a day and with regular practice, relaxation can reduce metabolism and decrease consumption of oxygen, blood pressure, and muscle tension. All techniques for relaxation are self-regulatory; no technique works unless the individual is motivated and chooses to practice what he or she has learned. Techniques include spiritual meditative approaches, such as Zen Buddhism, yoga, and Sufism; practical meditative approaches, such as relaxation response training, transcendental meditation, and clinically standardized meditation; visualization and hypnosis, such as guided imagery, autohypnosis, concentration, behavior modification, and autogenic training; kinesiologic or somatic approaches, such as bioenergetics, massage, progressive relaxation, acupuncture, and biofeedback; physical activity, such as a fitness program, sports, dance therapy, tai chi, and yoga; and group approaches, such as assertiveness training, psychodrama, psychosynthesis, transactional analysis groups, and various other therapy and self-formed groups.

SUBSTANCE USE AND ABUSE

All toxic substances, such as poisons, medications and other drugs, chemical additives to foods, and alcohol, nicotine, and caffeine excesses, are sources of biophysical and chemical stress. Excessive alcoholic and caffeinated beverage consumption, cigarette smoking, and the use of street drugs or prescription medications may be the first symptoms of underlying disease or may be stress related. In these situations of habit control, referral to a professional counselor or specific therapy group (for alcoholism, drug abuse, diet control, etc.) may be of the greatest value.

The following self-help references may be useful for developing patient fitness programs:

Smoking

Danaher BG and Lichtenstein E: Become an Ex-Smoker. Prentice-Hall, Englewood Cliffs, NJ, 1978.

Weight Control

Mahoney M and Mahoney K: Permanent Weight Control: A Total Solution to the Dieter's Dilemma. Norton, New York, 1976.

Nutrition

Ferguson JM and Taylor CB: A Change for Heart: Your Family and the Food You Eat. Bull, Palo Alto, 1978.

Exercise

Cooper KH: The Aerobics Way. Bantam, New York, 1978.
Benjamin BE: Sports Without Pain. Summit, New York, 1979.

Stress Control

Girdano D and Everly G: Controlling Stress and Tension: A Holistic Approach. Prentice-Hall, Englewood Cliffs, NJ, 1979.

Relaxation

Bernstein D and Borkovec T: Progressive Relaxation Training: A Manual for the Helping Professions. Research Press, Chicago, 1973.

General

Pelletier K: Mind as Healer, Mind as Slayer. Dell, New York, 1977.

Unit 2

Office Management

The chapters in this unit focus on administrative medical assisting skills. The administrative medical assistant's role is multifaceted and may include the management of any or all of the tasks described in this unit. Performing these tasks effectively and efficiently requires versatility. The medical assistant must be a competent communicator in speech and in writing, precise with details, and consistently concerned with the professional and legal ramifications of performing his or her duties. The concepts and skills discussed in the previous unit are integral to the successful performance of administrative procedures. Likewise, in many instances, skills learned throughout this unit will find expression and application in the performance of clinical tasks. Each component area of medical assisting is a building block that is essential to the construction of the profession as a whole.

Unit Objectives

Upon completing this unit, you will be able to:

1. Describe the methods of reception that help the patient to feel comfortable and welcome in the medical office setting.
2. Identify the component parts of the patient record, explain the importance of each part, and obtain and record the required information.
3. Perform medical office organizational tasks, including the filing of medical records.
4. Demonstrate letter-writing skills.
5. Distinguish between types of mailing, and list effective and efficient ways of handling incoming and outgoing mail.
6. Be proficient in dictation and transcription skills.
7. Manage telephone interactions in a manner appropriate to the medical office.
8. Assess individual needs in scheduling appointments, and use the proper scheduling method.
9. Operate business machines commonly encountered in medical office practice, and explain their functions.

> Good charting is nothing more than good communication.
>
> RN Magazine

LEARNING OBJECTIVES

Upon completing this chapter, you will be able to:

1. Explain the purpose of the patient record.
2. Describe the difference between source-oriented and problem-oriented patient records.
3. List the four steps of charting on progress notes.
4. Describe the difference between subjective and objective signs and symptoms.
5. State the usual requirements for retaining records.
6. List the circumstances under which a written release of records is not required.

PERFORMANCE OBJECTIVES

Upon completing this chapter, you will be able to:

1. Establish a source-oriented medical record for a patient in chronologic order and a problem-oriented medical record in order of patient problems.
2. Document all activity related to patient care in the medical record legibly and without omission.
3. Correct errors on a medical record.
4. Document withdrawal from care in the medical record.
5. Release information in response to written patient authorization.

DACUM EDUCATIONAL COMPONENTS

1. Prepare and maintain medical records (using both the source-oriented and problem-oriented arrangements) (3.3A–E).

Chapter 6

*E*stablishing and Maintaining the Patient Record

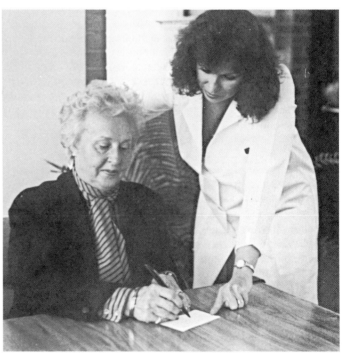

2. Interview and take a patient history (by recording the subjective and objective information obtained from the patient and during the physician's examination) (4.6).
3. Determine the needs for documenting (all activity related to patient care) (5.1A, B; 5.2H).
4. Use appropriate guidelines to maintain confidentiality when releasing records or information (5.3A–D; 1.4A).

Glossary

Diagnosis: Identification by the physician of a disease, condition, or illness
Patient record: Case history or accumulated data initiated on the first visit and terminating with the patient's discharge or withdrawal from the physician's care, or the physician's withdrawal from caring for the patient; also referred to as the *medical record*
Prognosis: Prediction by the physician of the course of a disease, or condition, or illness
Release of records: Written permission by the patient for the transfer of information from the record to a source other than the physician's office

Physicians treat thousands of patients during their professional careers. Without a system for recording each patient's medical care, valuable information contributing to the outcome of treatment would be lost. Establishing a medical record and maintaining its continuity ensures that the patient receives competent, comprehensive medical care.

Although the medical assistant does not have complete responsibility for establishing the patient record, he or she must make appropriate notations and manage the record filing system, discussed in Chapter 8. This chapter explains the purpose, content, and organization of the medical record.

The purpose of compiling the medical record is to establish a database for each patient. This database consists of pertinent facts related to the patient's health history, illness, and treatment, and is used to

1. Provide a method of communication between physician and office staff members involved in caring for the patient and managing the record
2. Serve as a document for planning patient care
3. Furnish documentary evidence regarding the type and quality of care the patient received while under the physician's supervision
4. Protect the legal interests of the physician and the patient
5. Provide clinical data for research and education.

RECORD PREPARATION AND CONTENT

The medical record is initiated at the time of the patient's first visit. The medical assistant prepares the patient record by assembling the necessary components, which include

1. File folder
2. Patient information sheet
3. Blank history form or sheet
4. Physical examination and progress notes forms

5. Other forms as appropriate for the particular specialty

Nonmedical information—address, telephone number, and occupation—are usually obtained from the patient's registration form (Fig. 6–1) and are typed in the spaces designated on the patient record. The file folder is labeled with the patient's name and is checked for completeness (inclusion of all necessary forms). The clinical medical assistant then places the folder in a designated area for use by the physician during the patient examination. The medical assistant should take care that the labeling reflects the office policy regarding filing. Typically, each file is labeled with the patient's name, and titles such as *Mr.* and *Ms.* are eliminated. Other such guidelines for filing are discussed in Chapter 7.

The record grows as correspondence, notations, diagnostic reports, and other information accumulate during the patient's subsequent visits to the office. Ultimately, the content of the record depends on the type of medical practice, the physician's preferences, and the nature of the patient's condition or illness. Generally, however, the record contains the following:

1. *Patient history.* The patient history may be recorded by either the medical assistant or the physician during the initial interview, or it may be a form given to the patient to complete. Figure 6–2 shows an example of a history to be completed by the patient. Questions are directed at identifying the patient's history regarding childhood diseases, past illnesses, past surgeries, and current health status.
2. *Physical examination findings.* At the time of the patient's first visit, the physician may perform a complete physical examination. The findings (status of each body part and system) are recorded by the physician and serve as a baseline reference for assessing the patient's health during subsequent visits.

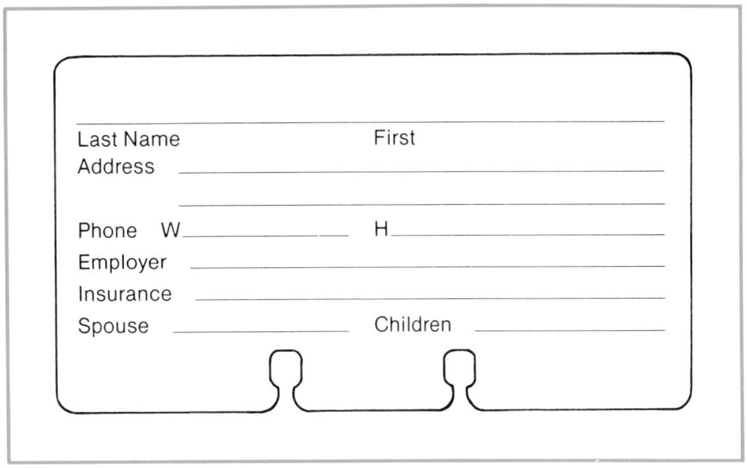

Figure 6-1. A patient registration and intake card.

3. *Diagnostic and laboratory test results.* If the physician has ordered laboratory tests during the patient's first visit, test results are reported and recorded after that visit. Test results already known during the first visit are an exception. Separate laboratory reports are usually filed with the most recent results on top.

4. *Consultation reports.* Consultation reports summarize patient evaluations performed at the request of a referring physician and with the patient's consent.

5. *Past medical records.* A summary of past records, or copies of the records themselves, may be kept in the patient's medical record if the patient has requested, in writing, the transfer of records from the office of another physician, or from a hospital or medical center that provided inpatient or outpatient care.

6. *Correspondence related to patient care.* Correspondence with or about the patient and related to diagnosis or treatment is contained in the medical record.

7. *Progress and other notes.* These notations include detailed entries by the physician, written at the first and subsequent visits, regarding impressions (health status), treatment plan, instructions to the patient, and progress notes. Comments and observations about the patient's course of illness are included.

8. *Termination summary.* If the physician has served as a consultant and has discharged the patient, or if the patient or physician terminates the relationship, the date of termination and the condition of the patient at the time of discharge are noted.

The patient record includes subjective and objective information. *Subjective information* refers to the patient's expressions of his or her feelings and opinions. *Objective information* is observable and unchanged by the patient's interpretation and is mostly supplied by the physician. For instance, the patient's symptoms are related to the description of illness and would be sub-jective information. *Patient:* "I've been nauseous and dizzy, and I have pain right here." The patient's statement contains unobservable, unmeasurable feelings. In contrast, signs of illness are examples of objective information. For instance, the physician's notes might read: "Physician's Examination Findings: On palpation of the abdomen, the patient was found to have rebound tenderness and pain in the right lower quadrant." The information obtained from examining the patient is observable, measurable, and usually acquired by scientific methods.

An important goal of organizing the patient record is to keep it precise and current. The medical assistant checks the patient record after each use to ensure that that use has been acknowledged and that each entry is clearly written for further reference. After reading a report or other section of the record that has been flagged for his or her attention, the physician initials it.

Prescription pads printed on no-smear, no-spot carbon paper facilitate the recording of prescriptions by using a timesaving, write-it-once system. The prescription blank is placed over the patient record and completed, and a copy is automatically available. Notation of unkept appointments and refusals to follow instructions should be recorded and initialed by the physician or the medical assistant. The signature must always be that of the actual recorder.

All patient contacts related to medical care, office visits, telephone conversations, and correspondence should be noted in the medical record. The patient's financial record is separated from the medical record to avoid exposing the medical record during the audit of financial records. No information that might be of subsequent use in diagnosis, prognosis, or treatment can be excluded from the medical record.

RECORD ORGANIZATION

CHRONOLOGIC-SECTIONAL METHOD

The record will be organized according to the physician's preferences and the specific needs of the staff for

CASE #

PATIENT'S NAME

ADDRESS _____ INSURANCE _____ DATE _____ NO. OF CHILDREN _____

TEL. #   REFERRED BY   OCCUPATION   AGE   SEX   SMWD

NOTE: THIS IS A CONFIDENTIAL RECORD OF YOUR MEDICAL HISTORY AND WILL BE KEPT IN THIS OFFICE. INFORMATION CONTAINED HERE WILL NOT BE RELEASED WITHOUT YOUR PERMISSION.

LIST YOUR CHIEF COMPLAINTS & SYMPTOMS

1. _____
2. _____
3. _____
4. _____
5. _____

DO YOU HAVE ANY OF THESE SYMPTOMS?

In General, do you feel Bad?	Yes	No
Your appetite is Poor?	Yes	No
Trouble with Swallowing	Yes	No
Hoarseness	Yes	No
Sore Throat	Yes	No
Chills or Fever	Yes	No
Any Eye Disease, Impaired sight	Yes	No
Any ear disease, Impaired hearing	Yes	No
Any nose, sinus, mouth trouble	Yes	No
Fainting Spells	Yes	No
Loss of Consciousness	Yes	No
Convulsions	Yes	No
Paralysis	Yes	No
Dizziness	Yes	No
Severe headache	Yes	No
Depression	Yes	No
Anxiety, Nervousness	Yes	No
Hallucinations	Yes	No
Enlarged Glands	Yes	No
Enlarged Thyroid or Goiter	Yes	No
Underactive Thyroid	Yes	No
Overactive Thyroid	Yes	No
Skin Disease	Yes	No
Chronic Cough	Yes	No
Chest Pain	Yes	No
Angina	Yes	No
Spitting up Blood	Yes	No
Night Sweats	Yex	No
Shortness of Breath	Yes	No
Palpitations or fluttering of heart	Yes	No
Swelling of hands, feet, ankles	Yes	No
Varicose Veins	Yes	No
Bladder Infection	Yes	No
Albumin, Sugar, Pus, or Blood in Urine	Yes	No
Difficulty in Urination	Yes	No
Abnormal Thirst	Yes	No
Abdominal Pain	Yes	No
Indigestion	Yes	No
Liver Enlarged	Yes	No
Fried Fatty Food Intolerance	Yes	No
Gall Bladder Disease	Yes	No
Colitis	Yes	No
Hemorrhoids	Yes	No
Rectal Bleeding	Yes	No
Constipation	Yes	No
Diarrhea	Yes	No
Change in Bowel Habits	Yes	No
Insomnia	Yes	No

PAST ILLNESSES

HAVE YOU EVER HAD?

	Yes	No
Measles	Yes	No
Duodenal Ulcer	Yes	No
Scarlet Fever, Scarletina	Yes	No
Diphtheria	Yes	No
Smallpox	Yes	No
Pneumonia	Yes	No
Tuberculosis	Yes	No
Pleurisy	Yes	No
A Murmur of the Heart	Yes	No
Heart Disease	Yes	No
Arthritis or Rheumatism	Yes	No
Bone or Joint Disease	Yes	No
Neuritis, Neuralgia	Yes	No
Bursitis, Sciatica	Yes	No
Polio, Meningitis	Yes	No
Bright's Disease	Yes	No
Kidney Stone	Yes	No
Kidney Infection	Yes	No
Recent Weight Gain	Yes	No
Recent Weight Loss	Yes	No

Weight now _____ 1 Yr. Ago _____
Maximum _____ Minimum _____

CIRCLE ALL ANSWERS

	Yes	No
Anemia	Yes	No
Jaundice	Yes	No
Easy Bleeding	Yes	No
Epilepsy	Yes	No
Migraine Headache	Yes	No
Diabetes	Yes	No
High Blood Pressure	Yes	No
Low Blood Pressure	Yes	No
Nervous Breakdown	Yes	No
Hay Fever	Yes	No
Asthma	Yes	No
Hives, Eczema	Yes	No
Boils, Frequent	Yes	No
Colds, Frequent	Yes	No.
Allergies	Yes	No
Allergies to Drugs	Yes	No
Which Ones _____		
Smoke Cigarettes	Yes	No
How many _____		
Drink Moderately	Yes	No

SURGERY

OPERATIONS	HOSPITAL	YEAR
1.		
2.		
3.		
4.		

HOSPITALIZATIONS

FOR WHAT ILLNESS
1. _____
2. _____
3. _____
4. _____

WOMEN ONLY   MENSTRUAL HISTORY

Age at Onset _____
Regular   Yes _____ No _____
Cycle _____ days (from start to start)
Usual Duration_____ Days
Heavy_____ Medium _____ Light _____
Date of Last Period_____
How Many Pregnancies _____
How Many Children _____
How Many Miscarriages _____
Complications of Pregnancy_____

FAMILY HISTORY

	IF LIVING		IF DECEASED	
	AGE	ILLNESS	AGE	CAUSE
Father				
Mother				
Sisters				
1.				
2.				
3.				
Brothers				
1.				
2.				
3.				

DID OR DOES YOUR MOTHER, FATHER, SISTER OR BROTHER HAVE

	Yes	No
Diabetes	Yes	No
Heart Trouble	Yes	No
High Blood Pressure	Yes	No
Epilepsy	Yes	No
Stroke	Yes	No
Hemophilia or Blood Diseases	Yes	No
Gout	Yes	No
Duodenal Ulcer	Yes	No
Rheumatic Fever	Yes	No

A

FORM S-41776

Figure 6-2. The portion of the patient history form that is to be completed by the patient. (Courtesy of E. Gary Lansmack, M.D.)

PHYSICAL EXAMINATION: TEMP. ____ PULSE ____ RESP. ____ B.P. ____ HT. ____ WT. ____   LABORATORY FINDINGS:

GENERAL APPEARANCE _____

SKIN _____ MUCOUS MEMBRANE _____

EYES: VISION _____ PUPIL _____ FUNDUS _____

EARS: _____

NOSE: _____   DATE

THROAT: _____ PHARYNX _____ TONSILS _____

CHEST: _____ BREASTS _____

HEART: _____

LUNGS: _____

ABDOMEN: _____

GENITALIA: _____

RECTUM: _____

PELVIC: _____

EXTREMITIES: _____ PULSES: _____

LYMPH NODES: NECK _____ AXILLA _____ INGUINAL _____ ABDOMINAL _____

NEUROLOGICAL: _____

DIAGNOSIS: _____

_____

TREATMENT: _____

PATIENT'S NAME

DATE			SUBSEQUENT VISITS AND FINDINGS	B.P.	WGT.
MO.	DAY	YR.			

B

Figure 6–2. Continued.

use and access. The *source-oriented record* is ordered according to the source of information. Sources include nurses, physicians, medical assistants, laboratory technicians, physical therapists, and any health professional who provides patient care. Generally, however, the record is arranged in chronologic order and is divided into subsections. Each subsection may be represented by a tab. The following guidelines are commonly applied:

1. Paper clips rather than staples are used to secure individual sheets to one another. Staples damage individual sheets.
2. The subsections of the record are sequenced in the following manner:
   a. *Medical history.* Data related to personal and family medical histories may be recorded on a separate form designed specifically for this purpose, or in the allotted space on the physician's notes.
   b. *Physician's notes.* As was stated above, the physician's notes may begin with the medical history. The notes detailing the initial evaluation of the patient (the physical examination) and each subsequent visit are recorded on sheets headed "Progress Notes." The file folder should open to these notes. To save time and provide the physician with easy access, progress notes are often placed in reverse chronologic order, with the most recent entry on top. Figure 6–3 shows an example of progress notes.

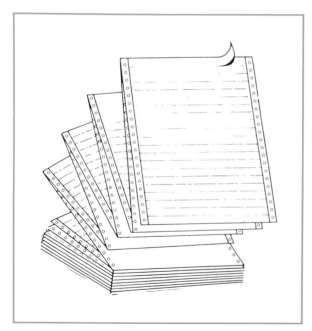

Figure 6–3. Preprinted forms for physician's progress notes. The physician may write directly on these preprinted adhesive strips, or the medical assistant may transcribe the physician's dictated notes. Once completed, the dated strip is placed in the patient's file. (Courtesy of Control-o-fax.)

c. *Diagnostic reports.* Diagnostic reports follow the physician's notes. They contain recorded results of laboratory and other diagnostic tests. They are arranged in either chronologic order or reverse chronologic order, depending on the physician's preference. Laboratory slips may also be stacked using a "shingle method," with one slip overlapping another.
   d. *Correspondence.* The correspondence section follows the diagnostic reports and contains all correspondence from other physicians (including consultations), the patient, and others. This section excludes financial matters.
   e. *Insurance forms.* Copies of insurance forms may be filed separately in either the patient's financial record or the medical record.

PROBLEM-ORIENTED MEDICAL RECORD METHOD

As an alternative to the source-oriented medical record, the *problem-oriented medical record* (POMR) organizes data according to the patient's health problem. This system was originated by Dr. Lawrence Weed and is sometimes referred to as the "Weed system."

For example, pertinent information derived from the physician's examination may be recorded on a separate sheet headed "Notes" or "Laboratory Results," which is placed in a diagnostic reports section. The POMR is, as its name implies, problem oriented. The POMR includes four basic components: (1) database, (2) problem list, (3) plans, and (4) progress notes. All pertinent information relating to diagnosis and treatment is contained under each numbered disease or condition.

The Database

The *database* includes the patient's history and profile, chief complaint, physical examination findings, and laboratory reports. A numbered and headed page is added for each medical, social, environmental, or psychological problem that requires diagnosis and treatment. For example, a patient who has visited the office at various times with chest pain, an inguinal hernia, and back pain has a separate page for each condition. All three pages are kept in one folder. Each problem page lists any other physical or psychological problems related to the condition.

The Problem List

The *problem list* is kept at the beginning of the record and indexes information by organizing it around a problem so that it does not get lost in the record. The problem list includes active and inactive problems, date of onset, and the date on which any problem is resolved. Two problem lists may be used: short term (temporary) and long term (permanent). A number is never used twice, even when a problem is resolved. The defined and numbered problem is a permanent record of a past or present problem in the database.

Example of a problem list:

Problem Number	Date Entered	Problem List	Problem Resolved	Date Resolved
1.	3/27/93	Back Pain	X	6/20/93
2.	4/28/93	Hypertension		

Plans are initial detailed descriptions of diagnostic and treatment measures and include schedules for further evaluative studies and interviews, therapeutic directions for dietary, surgical, psychologic, or physical treatments, and patient teaching plans. The plans may be modified as additional data are collected during subsequent office visits.

Example of a Numbered Problem Page with Related Problems and Initial Plan (Dated and Titled)

PROBLEM #1 3/27/93 BACK PAIN

A. Unable to work at present position as dock loader.
B. Unable to sleep through the night.

PLAN (INITIAL)

A. Refer to Physical Therapy for evaluation.
B. Tylenol with codeine on tab q.i.d. p.r.n.

Example of a Second Problem Page

PROBLEM #2 4/28/93 HYPERTENSION

PLAN (INITIAL)

A. Diet and exercise prescription for hypertension given to patient and further explained by medical assistant.
B. Aldactazine 50 mg one tablet b.i.d. for 1 week.
C. Recheck in 7 days.

Progress Notes

Progress notes are also dated, headed, and numbered for specific problems.

The approach to recording progress notes in a logical sequence is abbreviated *SOAP*:

S Subjective data (patient's symptoms, feelings, comments)
O Objective data (findings of examination and diagnostic tests)
A Assessment (diagnosis, impressions)
P Plan of action (treatment regimen: medication, consultation, surgery, further tests)

Each problem is addressed using SOAP steps.

Example:

PROBLEM #1—BACK PAIN: 5/19/93

S Patient states that pain has subsided with medication: "Feeling generally better."
O X-ray negative for fracture or displacement
A Medication offering pain relief
P Continue medication for 3 weeks. Reevaluate.

The POMR is an organizational system that allows easy review of the medical record and promotes an orderly and comprehensive approach to patient care (Figs. 6–4 and 6–5). Since its inception, other charting system designs have expanded and modified the POMR.

Figure 6–4. The problem list is attached to the front of the POMR (problem-oriented medical record) file. (Courtesy of Joseph M. DeFranco, M.D.)

Figure 6–5. Other forms commonly used with POMR files. (Courtesy of Joseph M. DeFranco, M.D.)

One such system preprints folders for age, dating, and basic information. Dividers used in the POMR are centered in the folder. Specific questionnaires (cardiovascular, gastrointestinal, gynecologic, etc.) are available for gathering a history database. Figure 6–6 shows an example of a POMR folder cover.

OTHER METHODS

As was previously stated, the physician may prefer to use the chronologic/sectional (source) method, the POMR, or both methods, selecting the most appropriate method for each situation. Alternative methods of patient recordkeeping include narrative paragraph progress notations. Regardless of the method used, the medical assistant's role in recordkeeping is to become

familiar with the method and to adhere to charting guidelines for making appropriate entries.

DOCUMENTATION GUIDELINES

Regardless of the organizational approach to establishing and maintaining the patient record, certain documentation, or charting, guidelines facilitate the precise, complete recording and provide protection against legal claims.

1. The patient's name and date should be written on each page of the record.
2. In most practices, each office visit is noted in the medical record and dated. (The medical as-

Date / /

PHONE CALL

NAME OF PATIENT:_____ **PHONE:**_____

PERSON CALLING:_____ **PHONE:**_____

PROBLEM:

ALLERGIES:
PHARMACY: PHONE:

	MEDICATION	DOSE	DISP	DIRECTIONS	REFILLS
1.					
2.					
3.					

BILLING OF HOSPITAL PATIENTS

Name of Patient	Date of Admission	Date of Discharge	Date Dr. turned into the office	Date Charged	Date Billed	Date Pmt. Rec.	Amt. Bill

PROGRESS NOTES

INITIAL H&P:_____. SEE ORANGE BOOK OR H&P SHEETS.
SEE PROBLEM LIST ON INSIDE COVER.

PROBLEM #	PLAN

B

Figure 6–5. Continued.

sistant usually stamps or writes the date on the chart before the patient is taken to the examination room).

3. Each notation (vital signs, observations, patient teaching notes) made by the medical assistant should be dated and initialed or signed.

4. Each phone call from the patient concerning medical care and prescriptions, and the staff member's response, should be recorded, dated, and initialed or signed by the receiver.

5. Failed appointments (no-shows) should be noted in the patient record.

6. The patient's refusal or failure to follow treatment plans should be recorded.

7. The patient's discharge or termination of care by the physician should be recorded.

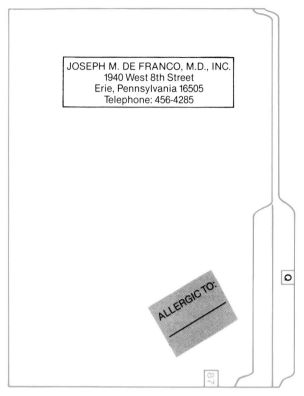

JOSEPH M. DE FRANCO, M.D., INC.
1940 West 8th Street
Erie, Pennsylvania 16505
Telephone: 456-4285

ALLERGIC TO:

Figure 6–6. A POMR folder cover. (Courtesy of Joseph M. DeFranco, M.D.)

8. Outpatient visits, hospital surgeries, consultations, and other referrals should be noted in the record and dated. *Example:* Referred to Dr. Jones for ENG* consultation 3/27/87. Appointment scheduled with Dr. Jones 4/18/87. D. Wilson.

9. Each day, the records of patients seen by the physician on that date should be checked for complete notations before refiling. Many types of alert stickers with checkoff blocks for charting sections are available.

10. The recorder should correct errors in handwritten entries by drawing a single line through the error, placing it in parentheses (optional), and writing the correction above or beside the error. The abbreviation "Corr.," the date of correction, and the recorder's signature should appear in the margin. The notation is initialed and dated. *Example:* (urine) specimen obtained. Corr. 3/29/87 D. Wilson. Typed materials with errors discovered later are corrected in the same way. If an entry is made in the wrong record, the error is identified by a single line through the entry and the following: *Example:* "Recorded by error. Information transferred to the record of Jane Brown."

11. All corrections should be written in permanent ink.

---

*Electroneurography.

THE ROLE OF THE MEDICAL ASSISTANT

The medical assistant is the agent of the physician. As such, he or she approaches the tasks of establishing and maintaining the patient record with interest in safeguarding both the physician's and the patient's rights. The medical assistant must safeguard the integrity of the patient record as a legal document, recognizing that entries are unalterable and are permissible only by authorized personnel. See the procedures at the end of this chapter for detailed descriptions of the creation and correction of patient records.

The medical assistant must scrutinize all written entries for professional appearance and content. Humorous, sarcastic, or casual remarks are never acceptable. Their inclusion invites legal claims of libel (defamation in writing). Information disclosed by the patient is best put in quotation marks rather than condensed. In addition, all typed progress notes should be signed by the physician prior to filing.

PATIENT TEACHING CONSIDERATIONS

The patient often observes the medical assistant and the physician writing in the record during an interview or conversation. To allay any anxiety about what is being charted, it is helpful for the medical assistant to explain the purpose of charting and recordkeeping to the patient. The patient should also be informed that he or she owns the information and is welcome to read the chart. If the patient requests a reading, the medical assistant notifies the physician, who usually provides supervision. Most patients do not elect to read the record and are even less inclined to do so when an explanation is provided.

RELATED ETHICAL AND LEGAL IMPLICATIONS

A major ethical and legal concern related to the patient record is confidentiality. All interactions between the physician, the office staff, and the patient are privileged communications and therefore confidential. The patient's right to privacy must be protected. The record should not be discussed with anyone, including staff members, unless this is required. Also, the record should be read only when necessary and should not be left in view of the patient. The patient should not read the record without the physician's or medical assistant's collaboration. If records must remain on the administrative assistant's or physician's desk for whatever reason, they should be placed in a locked cabinet overnight and returned to the desk the next morning.

Associated with the concern for confidentiality is the discretionary release or disclosure of confidential information. The patient owns the information; the physician owns the record. The patient has a right to a copy or a summary of the record and must make the request in writing or sign a release authorization form (Fig.

Date_____

TO WHOM IT MAY CONCERN:

This is to authorize the release of my medical records to:

Patient_____

Signature_____

Figure 6-7. A standard release-of-records form.

6-7). For release of information to other medical offices, insurance companies, attorneys, hospitals, or employers, the patient's written consent and the physician's approval are required.

A signed authorization is not required for subpoena, or in some states, for use by Medicare or county agencies that require the reporting of communicable diseases. A *subpoena duces tecum* is a court order mandating that the physician give the court any patient records pertinent to the case. When a record is subpoenaed, a copy, not the original, is released.

When a subpoena is served, the server gives the medical assistant both the subpoena and a check to cover the cost of processing the record. Some subpoena offices call in advance to check the existence of a record. If asked whether a patient is under the physician's care, the medical assistant's appropriate response is, "Please forward first the subpoena and then I will be able to check our records." This response protects the patient against a breach of confidentiality.

What information is recorded and how it is written are as important as the later handling of that information. Legally, "If it's not recorded it wasn't done." Omissions are as important as inclusions in litigation. Likewise, illegible notations and the appearance of altered records cast suspicion on the physician's compe-

tence and credibility. Although the medical assistant is not responsible for the physician's charting, he or she can help to monitor the thoroughness of the record by checking for completeness. In addition, all entries made by the medical assistant should be within the parameters of the profession. The patient record, if precise, accurate, and complete, is the physician's best defense against charges of malpractice. (Refer to Chapter 3, "Medical Law and Ethics," for further elaboration.)

In addition to the legal implications of a breach of confidentiality, several other concerns pertain to the medical record. Letters of withdrawal or discharge and warning letters regarding failure to follow treatment regimens should be sent to patients for the physician's legal protection. A copy is kept in the record with a note of the mailing date. A notation confirming that the letter was sent, the date, and the circumstances should be written in the progress notes. A copy of a letter of withdrawal (termination of care by the physician) or discharge should also be kept in the patient record. The original letter is sent by certified mail. The proof of mailing form is attached to the copy. The medical assistant should become familiar with the legal requirements regarding medical records in the state in which he or she will seek employment.

SUMMARY

The patient record provides both medical and legal documentation of the physician's diagnosis and treatment. The medical assistant does not control the format or quality of the entries made by the physician and other health professionals, but is responsible for monitoring the type and inclusion of entries. The medical assistant can be a valuable asset to the physician by combining knowledge of the recordkeeping methods with respect for their inherent medical and legal implications.

DISCUSSION QUESTIONS

1. What is the purpose of the patient record?
2. What are the components of the chronologic-sectional approach to organizing the patient record?
3. How does the POMR differ from the chronologic-sectional approach?
4. Under what circumstances is a written request for release of records not required?
5. How are charting errors corrected and why?

BIBLIOGRAPHY

American Medical Association: Medicolegal Forms with Legal Analysis. American Medical Association, Chicago, 1990.

Griff J and Ignatavicius D: The Writer's Handbook: The Complete Guide to Clinical Documentation, Professional Writing, and Research Papers. Resource Applications, Baltimore, 1986.

Huffman EK: Medical Records Management, ed. 9. Physician's Record Company, Berwyn, IL, 1990.

Kettenbach G: Writing S.O.A.P. Notes. FA Davis, Philadelphia, 1990.

Lewis MA and Warden CD: Law and Ethics in the Medical Office Including Bioethical Issues, ed 2. FA Davis, Philadelphia, 1988.

Liebler JG: Medical Records: Policies and Guidelines. Aspen, Gaithersburg, MD, 1991.

Roach WH Jr et al: Medical Records and the Law, ed. 2. Aspen, Gaithersburg, MD, 1992.

Scott RW: Health Care Malpractice: A Primer on Legal Issues for Professionals. Slack, Thorofare, NJ, 1990.

PROCEDURE: Assemble and organize the patient record

Terminal Performance Objective: Assemble and organize a patient record folder with 100 percent accuracy in the time designated.

EQUIPMENT: Patient file folder
Completed registration card
Typewriter
Medical records form
File label
Financial card

PROCEDURE

1. Assemble supplies and equipment.
2. Type the medical record label with the patient's name, or number if the facility uses the numerical system. Color code the medical record folder as appropriate to the facility. The numeric filing system requires a cross-reference card with the patient's name and an identification card.
3. Using the registration card for reference, type the patient's name and other necessary information on the patient history form.
4. Assemble other medical record components (problem- or source-oriented) in the folder. With source-oriented recordkeeping, the laboratory sheet, progress notes, and other forms are separate and organized in the order preferred by the physician. Type the patient's name on all forms to be included in the medical record.
5. Type the patient's name and other pertinent information as required on the patient's financial record.
6. Place the medical record, registration card, and financial card in the designated area.

PRINCIPLE

1. Organization and planning save time and prevent error.
2. Color coding may be used to alphabetize patient records or for other purposes. The patient uses the number on the identification card to make appointments and handle other matters that require patient identification.
3. Personal data are required for medical care.

4. Typing the patient's name on all forms in the medical record helps prevent losing or misplacing valuable information.

5. Complete information is required to process insurance forms and billing statements accurately.
6. Correct placement completes the task and prevents loss or misplacement of the patient's records.

PROCEDURE: Make corrections in the patient record

Terminal Performance Objective: Correct errors in the patient record with 100 percent accuracy in the time designated.

EQUIPMENT: Patient's medical record
Pen

PROCEDURE

1. Locate the charting error and confirm that the information is incorrect.
2. With the pen, draw a line through any errors; put parentheses at the beginning and end of the error.

3. Write the correction above or to the side of the error.

4. Write the date, your initials, and the abbreviation "Corr." next to the corrected entry.
5. Return the medical record to the designated location.

PRINCIPLE

1. Confirmation prevents further error.

2. Drawing a single line through an error is the only legally acceptable method of making corrections. Incorrect information should still be legible after it has been marked as incorrect.
3. Writing the correction near the error clarifies where the error has been made.
4. Documentation is necessary for future reference.

5. Correct placement prevents loss or misplacement of the record.

HIGHLIGHTS

Freedom of Information: The Past and the Present

Until the passing of recent legislation (Freedom of Information Act), patients have not had the right to see or obtain copies of their own medical records unless they initiated a lawsuit. In the medical office in the past, many physicians refused patients access to their medical records. Some physicians were reluctant to permit the patient to read the medical record for fear that the patient would be anxious or confused or would not know the meaning of the physician's charting notes and diagnostic findings. Still another motivation for the physician's resistance was the concern that access to records would add to the already increasing number of malpractice suits. Likewise, hospitals did not release medical records to patients without the permission of the attending physician because they believed that physicians owned the medical records and that they, the hospital staff, were merely custodians.

The rethinking of medical record ownership was brought about by changes in legislation. In 1973, the report by the Commission on Medical Malpractice recommended that the information contained in the medical record be accessible to patients without the aid of an attorney. During that same year, the 1973 US Privacy Protection Study Commission urged states to enact legislation permitting patients not only access to their own medical records, but also the right to make corrections.

Today such access is available. Legislation has given patients the right of ownership of the information in medical records. Regulations also permit fees for duplication, timing of responses, and recourse if response is denied.

At present, a physician refusing a patient access to the medical record would have to prove that he or she is exercising the Doctrine of Professional Discretion in doing so. Under this doctrine, the physician may determine that the patient's emotional health will be adversely affected if access is granted. If the patient challenged such a decision, the courts decide the validity of the physician's action. The Doctrine of Professional Discretion is usually applied by physicians treating patients who are mentally or emotionally ill.

The laws have been changed, but the debate over ownership continues. The current debate focuses on some peripheral issues of ownership: How should the information be made accessible? Should patients actually maintain their own set of records?

The Freedom of Information regulations and the related complex controversies directly affect everyone working in the health care industry. Health care professionals, recognizing this fact, should keep abreast of updated changes and opposing views to participate in formulating fair regulations that uphold both the patient's and the physician's rights.

Organizing the Office and Maintaining Records

> Each staff member contributes something different; but their efforts must be organized toward the common goal. . . .
>
> Peter Drucker

CHAPTER OUTLINE

LEARNING OBJECTIVES

Upon completing this chapter, you will be able to:

1. Explain the four primary functions of the policy and procedures manual in the physician's office.
2. Explain the basic types of records necessary for maintaining the equipment and supply inventory.
3. List the components of a color-coded patient record filing system.
4. List the five steps in the filing process.

Chapter 7

Organizing the Office and Maintaining Records

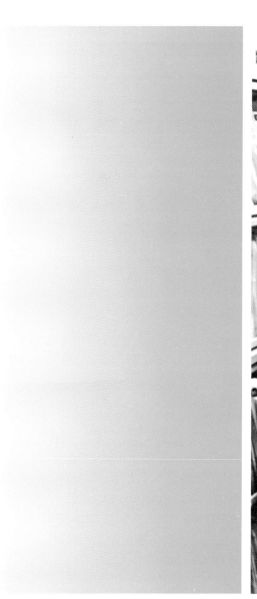
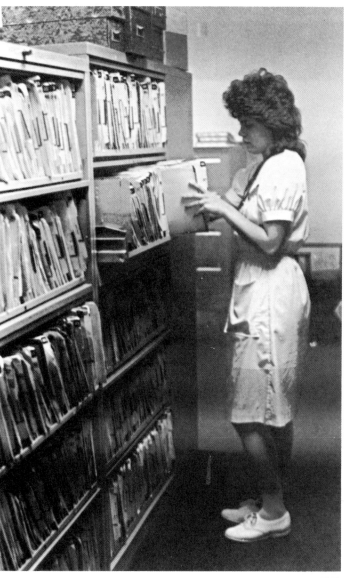

5. List the 19 basic filing rules.
6. List the 15 guidelines for efficient records management.
7. Describe the various uses of the card index system.
8. Describe the situations in which the patient and other authorized persons can have access to medical records.

PERFORMANCE OBJECTIVES

Upon completing this chapter, you will be able to:

1. Design and compose standard operating procedures.
2. Inventory and reorder supplies.
3. File patient, library, research, and personnel records.
4. Protect patient and personnel records from unauthorized access and release of information.

DACUM EDUCATIONAL COMPONENTS

1. Perform basic secretarial skills for records management (3.1B).
2. Maintain the physical plant (6.1A–B).
3. Operate and maintain facilities and equipment safely (6.2A–D).
4. Inventory equipment and supplies (6.3A–C).
5. Evaluate and recommend equipment and supplies for a practice (6.4A–D).
6. Orient patients to office policies and procedures (7.1A).
7. Orient and train personnel to office policies and procedures (7.4A).

Glossary

Color-coded files: Colors added to alphabetic order in a filing system. Color coding assists in error reduction

Critical supply items: Items such as patient receipts or checks, which are essential to the operation of the office

Cross-referencing: The use of two or more designations so that the document can be found in more than one way

Patient file: The folder that contains all the medical records of an individual patient

Procedures manual: A guide to the most common and most important operations within the office: how to order new supplies, daily duties, job descriptions, and so forth; law requires separate procedures manuals for office and laboratory quality assurance and for tasks exposing the worker to hazardous chemicals and biohazardous waste, such as blood and body fluids

Purge: To remove old and inactive files from the active storage area

Reorder quantity: The level below which a stockpile of supply items should not fall; for example, 500 patient file release forms

Surname: The last name: for John H. Smith it is "Smith"

Useful life: The length of time during which a particular item is useful and desirable

As team member or office manager, the medical assistant is expected to assist with or take responsibility for the organization and maintenance of the equipment, supplies, and filing system in the physician's office. Most physicians want to be free of daily concerns regarding office-related matters, and therefore depend on the medical assistant's expertise in this area.

The procedures described in this chapter do not always prevent frustrating office problems from occurring. However, organizing and properly designing the work environment can significantly improve the flow of office work and ensure that unanticipated problems are minimal.

Exclusive of the accounting, insurance, and banking aspects of office management (which are covered later in the text), the medical assistant is typically required to oversee the organization and maintenance of the five areas discussed in this chapter:

1. Policy and procedures manual
2. Equipment
3. Supplies
4. Patient records
5. Personnel records

As a preliminary step, however, the medical assistant

must understand the extent of his or her organizational responsibilities. Some physicians delegate complete authority for office management to the medical assistant. The medical assistant is expected to arrange furniture, purchase new equipment, and generally "manage" the office. Other physicians may prefer to be consulted about each decision. Most physicians take a position between these extremes. With gained experience and confidence, the opinion of the medical assistant becomes valued and responsibility is expanded.

THE POLICY AND PROCEDURES MANUAL

A manual that includes both policies and procedures is termed a "policy and procedures manual." Most practices, no matter how small, have overall objectives and missions that should be converted into formal policies. Many physicians include these policy statements in a section of the procedures manual. Policy statements — general statements of office purposes or objectives — often include the goals of the physician and staff. Specifically, they relate to the role of personnel, their duties, benefits, and job descriptions. "Providing the highest quality medical care," or "an excellent employment and growth opportunity" are statements that might be contained in a policy manual. In addition, policies concerning administrative functions may be included. *Example:* "It is our policy not to mail statements to patients. All office visits should be paid for in cash before the patient leaves the office."

Every practice must maintain a separate Standard Operating Procedure (SOP) manual detailing descriptions and instructions for high-risk procedures routinely performed in the workplace (see Chapter 28). A third quality assurance laboratory manual must be developed for any practice that tests human specimens.

PURPOSE OF THE PROCEDURES MANUAL

The office procedures manual is a mainstay of efficient office management. The manual has four primary functions: (1) a record of the tasks to be performed by personnel; (2) a training and monitoring device to aid in standardizing procedures; (3) a description of job titles and responsibilities for office staff members; (4) a "how to" document when temporary personnel are introduced to the office. A loose-leaf manual is preferable because it allows for additions and deletions of material with a minimum of effort and encourages frequent updating and revision.

The importance and complexity of the procedures manual grow in direct proportion to the size and scope of the office. A medical practice of any size requires the use of a manual to organize the multitude of activities and to universalize the approach to the performance of tasks. If one is nonexistent, the medical assistant should discuss the need for a manual and its ultimate design with the physician before initiating its use.

CONTENTS OF THE PROCEDURES MANUAL

The first major division within the manual consists of a checklist of tasks performed on a time schedule. These scheduled times are usually specified as daily, weekly, or monthly. Figure 7–1 provides an example of a checklist for administrative tasks. A checklist for clinical procedures schedules tasks directly related to patient care, the examination rooms, and medical records.

The following sections (many of which are discussed individually in later sections of this chapter) should also be established:

I. *Business Office Procedures*

1. The daily, weekly, and monthly task list
2. The office equipment master list
3. The equipment service list
4. The equipment preventive maintenance list
5. The critical supply list
6. The incidental supplies list
7. The periodic supplies list

II. *Quality Assurance Laboratory Program*

1. Patient preparation
2. Specimen collection
3. Labeling, preservation, and transporting of specimens
4. Corrective actions
5. Use of different testing methods
6. Inconsistent results
7. Personnel problems and corrective action
8. Complaints and subsequent investigations
9. Record keeping and control logs

III. *Occupational Safety and Health Administration Guidelines for Facility Bloodborne Pathogens Exposure Control Procedures*

1. Exposure determination listing all job classifications and the associated tasks and procedures (SOPs) performed by each employee
2. Implementation schedule and methodology
3. Compliance methods (universal precautions) regarding

   ❑ Needles
   ❑ Containers for reusable sharps
   ❑ Work area restrictions
   ❑ Specimens
   ❑ Contaminated equipment
   ❑ Personal protective equipment
   ❑ Decontamination procedures
   ❑ Regulated waste control
   ❑ Laundry procedures
   ❑ Hepatitis B vaccine

4. Postexposure evaluation and follow-up
5. Training
6. Record keeping

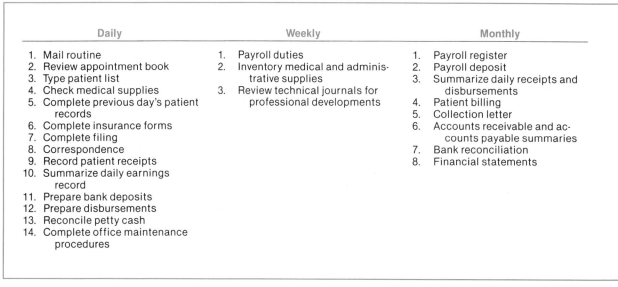

Daily	Weekly	Monthly
1. Mail routine	1. Payroll duties	1. Payroll register
2. Review appointment book	2. Inventory medical and adminis-	2. Payroll deposit
3. Type patient list	trative supplies	3. Summarize daily receipts and
4. Check medical supplies	3. Review technical journals for	disbursements
5. Complete previous day's patient	professional developments	4. Patient billing
records		5. Collection letter
6. Complete insurance forms		6. Accounts receivable and ac-
7. Complete filing		counts payable summaries
8. Correspondence		7. Bank reconciliation
9. Record patient receipts		8. Financial statements
10. Summarize daily earnings		
record		
11. Prepare bank deposits		
12. Prepare disbursements		
13. Reconcile petty cash		
14. Complete office maintenance		
procedures		

Figure 7–1. *An example of a checklist for the administrative medical assistant.*

Other major sections are as follows:

Standard Operating Procedures

The administrative and clinical procedures performed in the office are described in a detailed, stepwise approach. Examples of procedures from the administrative manual include records control and management, office maintenance, and equipment review. Examples of procedures from a clinical manual include taking the patient's temperature and taking the patient's blood pressure. In addition to a listing of clinical procedures and a stepwise approach, the SOP requires a rationale. The SOP section of the manual should include each step in the procedure and the corresponding principle, for example, the protective barriers (equipment) required, methods of disposal, sterilization procedures, and other procedures that may be necessary to guard against the possible transmission of bloodborne viruses, such as HIV. These inclusions are of particular importance for clinical tasks because SOPs are used as a training tool in assisting new employees, monitoring employees for SOP compliance, and documenting SOP accidents. All employees should have the same understanding of why a particular step is carried out. Understanding reduces the temptation to modify the procedure inappropriately. SOPs should be written for all tasks that involve a potential risk of mucous membrane or skin contact with blood, body fluid, or tissues, or a risk for spill, splash, or splatter, and therefore require protective equipment (masks, goggles, gowns, gloves). If equipment is available in case of unplanned exposure to blood and body fluids, a SOP section is again necessary. (Please refer to the clinical section of this text for an illustration of the procedure and principle format that should be included in the clinical procedure manual.)

Outside Services

A list of referral services for patients such as The Cancer Society or Women's Health Center; professional services used by the physician, such as attorneys, accountants, and insurance agents; equipment deadlines and repair services; medical supply houses; and drug and pharmaceutical concerns' contact numbers should be listed in the referral section of the office procedures manual or in the referral services manual (if available).

Patient Policies

Billing procedures for each physician, and policies related to patient ledger cards and medical histories, progress reports, laboratory reports, and correspondence, are contained in the administrative or clinical manual or the administrative or clinical section of the manual, as appropriate.

Personnel Policies

Working hours, vacations, and so forth are contained in the administrative section.

Physician

The physician data section lists resumes and a professional curriculum vitae for each physician; policies regarding office hours and hospital laboratory hours; personnel data such as addresses and call services; hospital and medical society affiliations; and a list of outside services and medical consultants who are used on a referral basis.

Record Keeping

Basic forms, such as those related to medical insurance, medical payroll, licensing, patient care, and financial records; and procedures for filling out the documents and keeping records, are described in the appropriate administrative or clinical sections or manuals.

In large offices, separate insurance and billing procedures manuals may be necessary. Important points to consider in the preparation of the procedures manual are that (1) details should be specific and inclusive; (2) extensive cross-referencing is done; and (3) the information is up-to-date and complete. Within each division and subdivision of the manual, the topic should be covered in sufficient detail to orient office personnel and to serve as a future reference source. For example, the "Basic Forms" section under the heading "Record Keeping" would contain a list of all forms used by the office and a sample of each. This section would outline procedures for filling out forms, include names and addresses for filing instructions, and outline an audit trail to the final location of each copy. A checklist of due dates would be compiled and placed at the beginning of the subsection. The entire subsection would be referenced to (1) the daily routine outline, (2) the office procedures section, (3) specific subsections within "Record Keeping" in which each form is used, and (4) the topic subsection that refers to the use of each form for medical insurance. As has been indicated, a medical office may have a separate manual for insurance processing.

Another example of cross-referencing might involve "Patient Procedures," with the subheading "Billing." A detailed schedule of each physician's fees for services would be provided and summarized in the individual patient records. The subheading would be cross-referenced to outside services with information about referral fees. The subheading "Basic Forms," would also be referenced to "Record Keeping," and would illustrate the proper billing format and procedures. This subheading would also be referenced to financial record-keeping procedures illustrating the "one-write" billing, receipt, and accounts receivable process.

USING THE PROCEDURES MANUAL

The loose-leaf procedures manual form is designed to allow for ease of modification. Ideally, the medical assistant would

1. Spend time each month reviewing the manual
2. Revise or remove outdated or unnecessary material with the physician's approval
3. Add items of current concern and interest to members of the office staff
4. Check that details are current and accurate
5. Translate sections of the manual to "tickler" (reminder) files or rotary wheel devices to provide easier and more frequent access by all members of the professional staff.

GUIDELINES FOR WRITING AND ORGANIZING THE PROCEDURES MANUAL

Initiating the use of a procedures manual may be the responsibility of the medical assistant. Therefore the medical assistant may actually have to organize and write the manual. The procedure at the end of this chapter presents a stepwise approach to the writing of individual procedure sheets.

EQUIPMENT

In addition to establishing and maintaining manuals that organize and universalize the staff's efforts, the medical assistant often must organize equipment and supplies records. Office equipment is distinguished from office supplies by its life expectancy. A typewriter is considered equipment (permanent) because the need for replacement is infrequent. Typing paper, however, is designated as a supply because it is depleted continuously. Required equipment items include telephones, typewriters, filing cabinets, examination tables and other clinical office equipment, medical instruments, and specialized medical machinery. Larger offices need various other types of equipment, such as computers.

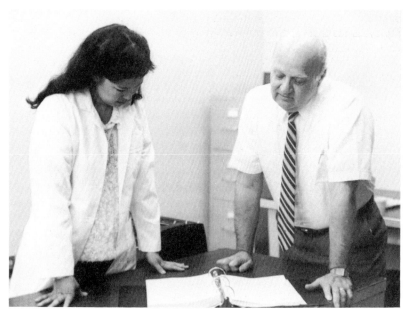

Decisions about the organization and content of the procedures manual require the input of both physician and staff.

EQUIPMENT RECORDS

The equipment used in the medical office represents a major portion of the physical assets of a physician's practice. Therefore a formal record should be maintained and updated so that at any particular time, the physician or accountant can calculate the value of these investments.

Two different types of record keeping are appropriate. First, a master list of equipment items includes description, date of purchase, purchase cost, and estimated actual life. As was stated earlier, the useful life is an estimate of how long a particular piece of equipment will be useful, serviceable, or both. The useful life may be different from the financial (depreciation) life of an item allowed in present tax codes. The latter information allows the physician to make an instant inventory of assets, to understand the depth of equipment investment, and to provide the data form from which the accountant computes depreciation information for taxation purposes (Fig. 7–2).

In addition to the master list, a separate record or file should be maintained for each major piece of equipment. The following may be included:

1. Receipts for the particular item in question, including purchase price and installation and delivery charges
2. Operating manuals, including instructions
3. Guarantees
4. Repair and preventive maintenance instructions and the dates on which maintenance checkups are due
5. List of service persons and their telephone numbers; the manufacturer's or service operator's business card can be attached to each record card or sheet
6. Any other pertinent information

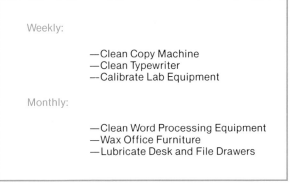

Weekly:

—Clean Copy Machine
—Clean Typewriter
—Calibrate Lab Equipment

Monthly:

—Clean Word Processing Equipment
—Wax Office Furniture
—Lubricate Desk and File Drawers

Figure 7–3. An equipment basic maintenance list.

MAINTENANCE AND REPAIRS

Most equipment requires periodic cleaning and maintenance. Complicated maintenance and repair work should be performed by qualified persons, not by the medical assistant. The medical assistant can ensure periodic preventive maintenance by keeping a master list of service personnel and contacting the appropriate maintenance person on schedule. The medical assistant or other members of the office staff may regularly perform other procedures not requiring a service specialist.

Two equipment maintenance sheets should be included in the office procedures manual: one for procedures that the medical assistant carries out, and a second for work that service personnel must perform (Figs. 7–3 and 7–4).

If equipment fails, the appropriate service person is contacted. However, the medical assistant should consult the physician before engaging the repair person and should apprise the physician of the situation as repairs progress. If, for example, a repair will be costly, the physician may wish to replace rather than repair the

No.	Item (Qty)	Total Installed Cost	Date Installed	Useful Life (Years)
	(Desks)			
1	Physician (1)	625.00	6/2/79	5
2	Medical Assistant (1)	400.00	8/2/80	10
3	Nurse (1)	400.00	10/3/82	10
4	Desk Chairs (3)	300.00	8/1/80	6
5	Telephone System (1)	1900.00	5/2/81	4
6	Typewriter (1)	2000.00	6/8/83	3
7	Word Processor (1)	1900.00	9/2/83	3
8	Copy Machine (1)	4200.00	3/1/80	4
	(File Cabinets)			
9	Acme (4)	400.00	1/12/78	10
10	Barnes (5)	1000.00	1/6/83	10
	(Reception Area)			
11	Couch (1)	600.00	1/10/80	5
12	Chairs (4)	280.00	2/16/80	5
13	Occasional Tables (4)	400.00	2/21/80	10

Figure 7–2. A typical office equipment master list.

Item	Date	Service Required	Name and Phone Of Service Person
Typewriter	June 1, Jan. 1	Cleaning and Adjusting	G. Jones 486-1212
Copy Machine	Dec. 1, Apr. 1, Aug. 1	Cleaning and Adjusting	P. Spearman 502-8306
Telephone System	July 15	Electrical Balancing and Testing	Bell Telephone 402-6868
ECG Equipment	March 1, Sept. 1	Calibration	Acme Medical Prod. 502-6161

Figure 7-4. An equipment service maintenance list.

equipment. A record of all repairs and their costs should be maintained in the equipment file.

PURCHASES

When an equipment item, such as a copier, nears the end of its useful life or becomes obsolete, the medical assistant may initiate or participate in the discussion and decision regarding its replacement. Potential vendors are usually willing to provide information and train office staff members to use the equipment. Before making a purchase decision it is important to gather as much data as possible, including the costs of service and expendable supplies, replacement costs, availability of service, training time, and the time required to operate the equipment. The physician may discuss the feasibility of a major purchase with the accountant. The medical assistant may contact several potential vendors, network with peers, and attempt to assist the physician in making the final decision.

SPACE PLANNING

The arrangement of office equipment can be critical to the attractiveness, efficiency, and safety of a medical office. Even if the most modern and efficient equipment has been purchased, it can be arranged in a way that impedes optimum traffic patterns and accessibility. Although there are no clear guidelines for optimum use, two suggestions may be helpful:

1. Ask vendors to give opinions regarding the use and placement of their products. They usually have had the opportunity to observe many different situations and can individualize the arrangement according to specific office needs.
2. Involve staff members who will be using the equipment in decisions regarding arrangement and use.

SUPPLIES

Equipment represents the fixed assets or machinery of the medical office; supplies are its "life blood." The efficient operation of an office is characterized by the steady flow of supplies, such as paper products, into and out of the office. The medical assistant must often oversee the acquisition, inventory, and flow of these supplies.

INVENTORY CONTROL

There are two competing objectives related to the management of supplies. First, the stock or inventory of a particular item should be maintained at a reasonable level. The office must store a large enough quantity of each supply item to ensure that the office does not run out. The unavailability of supplies can disrupt necessary tasks. There is, however, a second, opposing objective. Supplies should be maintained at a reasonably low level because it is an unwise business practice to spend money that could otherwise be earning interest. A large inventory also requires additional space for storage and increases the risk of loss, damage, or deterioration. Decisions pertaining to appropriate stock amounts require a formal supplies list. This list should be included in the procedures manual.

SUPPLIES LIST

A supplies list should include any item that is systematically reordered as it is used. A stapler, for example, is not a supply item. However, staples are used continuously and require replacement. Obviously, some items are more critical than others. Rubber bands, for example, may be relatively important, but running out does not precipitate a crisis. A new supply can be easily procured, and it is possible to function without them. If the office runs out of a specialized form (e.g., superbills), however, it may be impossible to replace this form in a short time and difficult to carry on efficient office practices without it.

The supplies list could therefore be broken into several categories:

1. *Critical supplies.* Items whose lack would threaten office efficiency and that are difficult to replace (long delays or special orders are required)

2. *Incidental supplies.* Paper clips, paper, rubber bands, and other items that are easily and quickly acquired
3. *Periodic supplies.* For example, calendars, appointment books, and other items that are needed at the beginning of a new year

A list of reliable discount vendors should be updated yearly and filed with the supplies list. In addition, several current supply catalogues should be kept on hand for comparison pricing and availability of desired supplies.

REORDER QUANTITIES

For critical items, such as special office forms, the medical assistant should work with the physician to determine the level of supply that is required as a safety margin and the consequent reorder point. If a particular form is used at the rate of 100 per week and it takes 3 weeks to reorder, it may be appropriate to reorder when the available supply reaches 300. To allow for a safety margin for unforeseen problems, such as late delivery or extraordinarily high use, a more prudent reorder point might be 500 or 1000. For each critical supply item, a reorder point should be established so that the medical assistant can periodically check the inventory of critical supply items and reorder those that are running low. Reorder reminder cards can be created and inserted at the supply level designated as the reorder point. Reorder reminders should be colorful or noticeable.

Figure 7–5 is an example of a critical items supply list that should be placed in a procedures manual. It might be advisable for large offices with many critical inventory items to institute a system of inventory cards, such as the one shown in Figure 7–6, or an inventory control log.

An inventory card should be maintained for each critical item or group of similar items used by the physician's office. The inventory card should be completed in detail and updated whenever supplies are reordered. The procedure for preparing the inventory and ordering supplies is included at the end of this chapter.

MANAGEMENT OF THE PATIENT RECORD

The patient record, whose contents were described in the previous chapter, must also be systematically organized to ensure against loss of important information. Therefore, the central filing activity in the physician's office is the organization of the patient record. It is the medical assistant's responsibility to manage these records precisely and efficiently and to protect both the physician's and the patient's right to privacy.

The primary purpose of the patient record filing system is to facilitate rapid and error-proof document retrieval and return. This objective requires a simplified system and careful attention to detail by all who access the filing system.

STORAGE

The patient record (file) is a historic record of personal medical data that may be critical to subsequent treatment of an illness or accident. The file should be treated with sensitivity and care. When it is removed from storage it should never be left where it could be lost, misplaced, or read by unauthorized individuals, particularly other patients. Markers or out guides should be used to indicate that the record is missing.

A well-organized system for replacing patient records includes designating a single return area for files that have been used during the day. Files are returned to that area after the physician has added notes to the record. The medical assistant refiles these documents daily.

Technically, the patient record is the property of the physician; however, the information it contains is the property of the patient. In certain situations, patients, their attorneys, or legal agencies may request information from the patient file, or the file itself. If a patient release form is signed and placed in the file, the office may release information requested by an insurance company or another physician. It is prudent to send copies and retain originals because the patient record is the physician's only proof of proper care.

No.	Description	Quantity to be Ordered	Point	To Supplies	Reorder Address
1	Checks	2000	500	First National Bank	390 Main St. Erie, PA
2	Prescription Forms	5000	1000	Ace Printing	814 Cherry Meadville, PA
3	Patient Charge Forms	2500	500	Potter Bus. Forms	114 W. 12th Erie, PA

Figure 7–5. A critical items supply list.

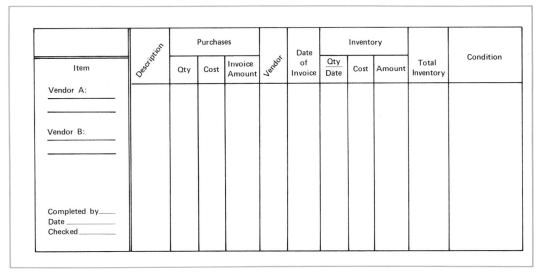

Figure 7-6. A supplies inventory card.

Although standards of file retention vary greatly depending on the geographic area and medical specialty, the conservative policy is to keep patient files indefinitely. Most physicians adopt a particular purging practice that is based on both common sense and convention and withdraw older files from the active drawers. These older records can be stored in special storage boxes in out-of-the-way areas or can be converted to microfilm as needed. Currently, the accepted standard is to periodically purge — but never destroy — patient records.

COLOR CODING

Because simplicity and speed are essential, a filing method often used in medical practices is the color-coded alphabetic system. The system of choice in most medical offices involves the following:

1. Flat or straight-edged file folders to which labels or tabs can be affixed
2. Two color-coded tabs showing the first two letters of the patient's last name
3. A white tab calling attention to the patient's full name
4. A color-coded purge tab showing the year in which the file will be purged

For a patient whose name is "Smith, John H.," for example, the file would contain a white tab for the name and three colored tabs. (The individual colors vary with the manufacturer.) A large red *S*, for instance, would be affixed in its code color. Immediately after the red S is an *M* in the code color for "M" (e.g., blue). Thus when a file drawer is opened there are several red *S*s. Some of these are followed by blue *M*s, and then green *N*s, gray *O*s, and so forth. This designation makes filing errors less frequent because the color coding immediately calls attention to misfiled records.

The file tab also contains the patient's name and a color-coded year tag (e.g., 1987, green; 1988, red; etc.).

Each time a file is used and then replaced, the medical assistant affixes the proper year tag. If adhesive tabs are used, for example, and Mr. Smith is being seen for the first time since 1986, a new color tab corresponding to this year is affixed over the old tab. In this way the medical assistant can purge old files systematically by retrieving all files of a certain color tab designation.

Some physicians prefer not to use a two-color system for last names that begin with uncommon letters. Thus patient files beginning with *Q* or *Z* can be accommodated with only one color-coded tab. Figure 7-7 illustrates a typical color-coded file drawer.

Active files may be maintained for patients or families who are seen at least every 2 years. Inactive files are maintained for up to 4 or 5 years. They may be purged and placed in storage areas.

GENERAL PRINCIPLES OF FILING SYSTEM MANAGEMENT

The medical assistant can ensure the overall integrity of the patient record and other files by understanding and following the traditional rules of records management. The four primary areas of records management are

1. *Filing management:* The design of effective filing systems with respect to methods and equipment
2. *Information retrieval:* The development of effective and rapid recall and replacement methods using the four basic approaches to filing
3. *Records protection:* The classification of documents by importance and the designation of storage methods for each classification
4. *Records retention and storage:* The determination of what, where, and for how long docu-

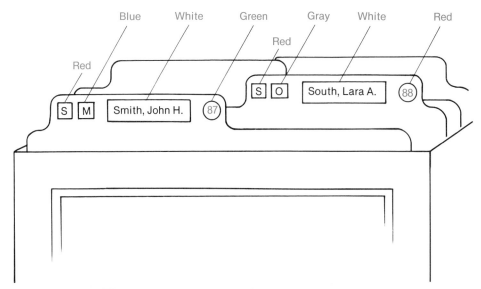

Figure 7–7. *An example of a color-coded file drawer.*

ments will be stored, and of when and how outdated documents will be purged from active files

EQUIPMENT AND SUPPLIES

Filing may be defined as a system of classifying, arranging, and storing documents in an orderly and efficient manner. Files must be systematized and kept up to date. Any deviation from the prescribed procedures results in lost documents, wasted time due to inefficient retrieval methods, outdated documents used in reference materials, and the inability of office personnel to use the records management system.

The first step in designing a records management system is to determine the most efficient records control for equipment and supplies necessary for the physician's office. Efficiency should be measured by (1) the size of the materials to be filed, (2) the number of items to be filed, (3) the physical limitations of the administrative and clinical work areas, and (4) the physical demands placed on the medical assistant. Systematization and standardization are key elements.

Standard file cabinets are available for storing documents of the two most common sizes: letter size (8½ by 11 inches) and legal size (8½ by 14 inches). Most patient files use the standard sizes. Other cabinets are available to house card files, visible records, punched cards, and computer printouts.

The typical "pull-out drawer" file cabinet (vertical file) is manufactured with multiple drawer units. False economy should be avoided: the best heavy-duty equipment should be purchased because it provides both maximum protection for patient records and financial documents and physical efficiency for the medical assistant who operates the equipment. The physical layout of the physician's office determines the number and arrangement of the file cabinets.

Because increasing numbers of patient-related and financial documents must be stored, many practices now use lateral and shelf files. Lateral cabinets look like chests of drawers and are often used for documents that must be retrieved quickly and frequently. In shelf filing, records are held upright in file folders and stacked seven or eight units high for maximum space efficiency. However, retrieval efficiency may be reduced with shelf filing unless the files are well indexed.

In addition to the standard filing equipment cited above, special equipment is available for files in various sizes. Examples of various size needs related to files are visibility where a portion of the patient record becomes a key point of the indexing system, rotary files, microfilm and microfiche, and electronic data processing records.

Filing Aids

The efficiency of the filing system is enhanced by the use of appropriate filing aids, including guides, folders, and labels.

Guides

Guides subdivide the drawer of the file cabinet for ease in referencing. They are heavy cardboard or plastic sheets the size of the file folders. A caption indicating the alphabetic range of materials filed behind the guide is printed on the top, or tab, of the guide. Primary guides indicate major divisions within the filing system. Secondary, or special, guides are subdivisions of primary guides and highlight special sections of subjects within the filing system. For an efficient system, frequent use of guides is recommended.

File Folders

Folders subdivide the drawer further as well as physically protect the documents within the drawer. They are made of heavy manila paper and are slightly larger than the documents they contain. Folders should not be overcrowded. If an individual file folder contains more than 1 inch of material, it should be subdivided and indexed as part 1, part 2, and so on.

Labels

Labels identify records within the drawer, guide units, or folders. They identify the contents of both the file cabinet and the individual folders. Captions should be consistent in terms of indexing order, capitalization, and punctuation. The medical assistant can maximize efficient retrieval by making certain that labels are current, accurate, and in good condition. Figure 7–8 represents four commonly used labeling systems. As was stated earlier, in addition to patient records the typical medical office includes records of various types of correspondence (letters from other physicians and organizations such as hospitals, medical societies, and insurance companies), business correspondence (purchase requisitions, orders, and invoices), and financial and other records.

THE FIVE-STEP FILING PROCESS

The filing process should stress the regular, orderly, and reliable collection of all retainable documents generated in-house or derived from external sources. It should designate responsibility for the flow and deposition of all materials, usually by means of a timestamp and routing index. Finally, the filing process should provide for document release, usually indicated by initials signifying that the transaction has received the required processing and that the document may be filed.

A five-step filing process is recommended for efficient and orderly document flow. This process consists of inspecting, indexing and cross-referencing, coding, sorting, and storing. The procedure for filing is included at the end of this chapter (section on related procedures); the process is described below.

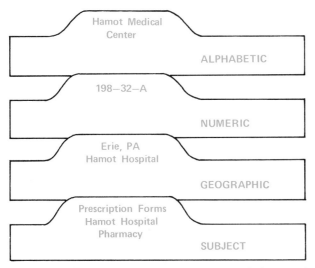

Figure 7–8. Examples of commonly used forms of labeling.

The *first* step in the filing process is to *inspect* the document for the necessary release marks.

The *second* step, *index* and *cross-reference*, determines the file folder caption under which the document will be filed. The most frequent recall pattern is determined by reference to the name on the letterhead, the name of the person to whom the letter is addressed, the signature on the letter, the subject of the document, and the name of the location. Cross-referencing by means of photocopies or a cross-reference sheet indicating the location of the original document is necessary when frequent recall for the document occurs under more than one index caption.

Coding is then necessary and is achieved by marking the index caption on the document to be filed. In a color-key system, the medical assistant either underlines the caption or indicates it in the upper right-hand corner of the record, and adds an *X* to an underlined or written index for cross-referencing to emphasize the indexing that has been completed previously.

In the *fourth* step, the documents are *sorted* in alphabetic order. The key to efficiency in these instances is to arrange the documents in small alphabetic divisions, such as A–C, D–G, H–L, M–R, and S–Z; to resort each division (A,B,C); and finally, to alphabetize the sections within each division.

In the *final* step, *storing*, the medical assistant places the documents in file folders for vertical filing. Care in this terminal step is imperative. A final document check should include agreement of the filing index, the file folder caption, and the index on the first document already contained in the folder. Documents should be filed neatly, without overcrowding the folder and with the heading to the left as a viewer faces the file. Documents should be inserted while the folder is raised and resting on the side of the file cabinet drawer to ensure correct folder section and proper document preservation.

FILING AND IDENTIFICATION SYSTEMS

Efficient information retrieval depends on the selection of an appropriate record filing system. There are four general approaches to filing: alphabetic, topical, geographic, and numeric. However, other systems may be used for other types of records. The medical assistant should be familiar with each of the four basic approaches. Figure 7–9 illustrates the basic advantages and disadvantages of each approach.

Alphabetic Filing

Alphabetic filing applies indexing rules to names of business firms, persons, or organizations. Folder captions are restricted to one correspondent or subject, and documents within the folders are arranged chronologically, with the most recent in front. File guides use alphabetic captions with a single-letter reference to indicate documents beginning behind that caption, or double-letter references to indicate the beginning and the end of the document range. Most alphabetic sys-

Methods	Advantages	Disadvantages
Alphabetic	1. Direct filing and reference 2. No index required 3. Record groupings by name 4. Record management by guides, folder colors 5. Miscellaneous files easily identified	1. Misfiling of common names 2. Related records scattered throughout the files 3. Cross-referencing may be either too simple or too extensive
Subject	1. Records grouping that establishes statistical or technical relationships 2. Unlimited expansion	1. Difficulty in classifying records for filing 2. Extensive cross-referencing necessary 3. Miscellaneous records difficult to classify 4. Frequent reference to index to determine subject heading or subdivision
Geographic	1. Direct filing and reference by location—indirect by individual 2. Records grouped by location 3. Provision for miscellaneous records	1. Location as well as name required for document retrieval 2. Triple sort—state, city, alphabet—increases error rate and raises labor costs 3. Reference to card index necessary to find document 4. Fold labels required and extensive information and maintenance
Numeric	1. Accuracy 2. Unlimited expansion 3. Cross-referencing permanent and extensive 4. Index is complete list of documents by name 5. Document retrieval by specific numeric identification with reference to name or subject (Same numeric ID can provide uniform system for all files)	1. Indirect filing and reference 2. Cumbersome index 3. Miscellaneous documents requiring separate files

Figure 7-9. Characteristics of the four basic approaches to filing.

tems use primary, special, individual, and miscellaneous captions. For facilitating retrieval, color keys correspond to the guide tabs and the folders filed behind these guides. This system is the most common approach to filing used in the medical office.

Subject Filing

Subject filing systems designate document retention and retrieval by topic rather than by alphabetic or numeric reference. These systems may be employed if (1) documents do not refer to the names of persons or organizations, (2) retrieval is more likely to be by subject than by name, (3) documents may be reasonably grouped by activities or products, or (4) too many small subdivisions would occur if records were not grouped by subject.

There are two main types of subject systems: alphabetic-subject and numeric-subject. A combination alphabetic-subject system is used when the main body of the file has an alphabetic reference and a small number of files are indexed by subject.

Alphabetic-subject systems use subject headings for main file divisions and alphabetic divisions within the subject headings. This system requires a card index or similar index to identify all heading divisions and subdivisions, and strong referencing to maximize retrieval efficiency. Such systems often look like dictionary or encyclopedia catalogues.

Numeric-subject systems use numeric captions for each subject heading, with a relative index as the key to entry into the filing system. Subject filing may be used to organize information related to disease and conditions in a particular specialty. Figure 7–10 illustrates types of alphabetic-subject and numeric-subject filings.

Geographic Filing

Geographic filing systems employ an alphabetic arrangement of the document location index. Primary guides indicate large geographic divisions, and special guides are used for subdivisions of the main geographic units. Individual folders list city and state references and are indexed in accordance with the standardized rules. A card index is used to identify the geographic location of each document and is referenced alphabetically. Cross-referencing is necessary if the index reference has more than one geographic location or if the recall reference may be made by name, subject, or location (Fig. 7–11).

Numeric Filing

Numeric filing systems use numbers as index captions on guides and folders. This system provides indirect retrieval because the user must refer to an alphabetized code to find the number assigned to the document name or subject. Numeric systems are maintained when record retention is by case history, contract, or project for an indefinite period. Although the system requires extensive cross-referencing to be effective, it preserves the anonymity of the documents, which can be a major goal of the file management system.

In a numeric system, the individual folders are assigned consecutive numeric captions and are filed in numeric sequence. Documents that have not accumulated sufficiently to warrant a numeric index are filed in miscellaneous alphabetic folders that are stored sepa-

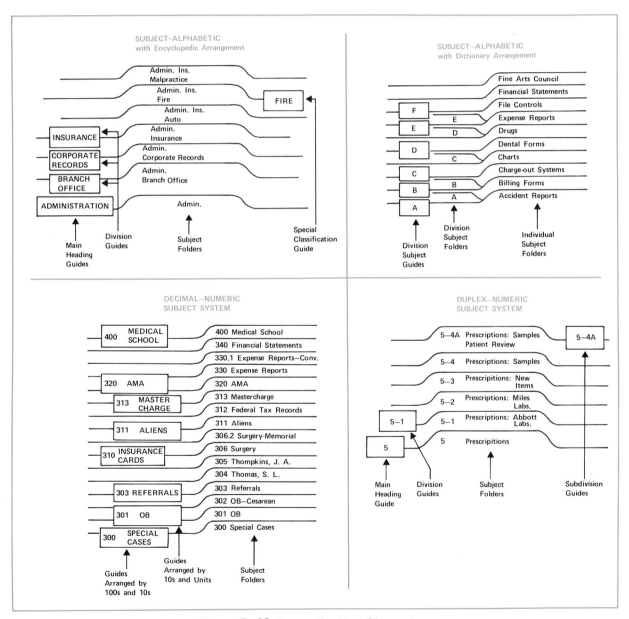

Figure 7–10. Types of subject filing systems.

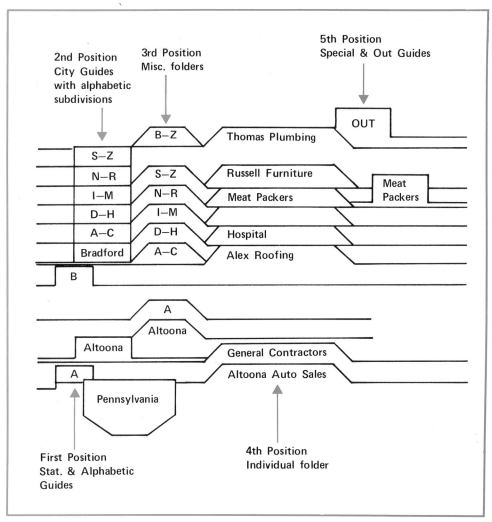

Figure 7–11. Geographic filing system.

rately. An alphabetic card index identifies the assigned numeric indexes by name and subject and accounts for all unassigned numbers. Numeric or geographic systems may be used in nonpatient filing within the medical office; examples would include the physician's personal research or professional projects.

STANDARDS FOR FILING SYSTEMS

Developing an orderly, efficient filing system requires standardized rules and procedures. The following basic rules are of use for choosing the index captions:

1. Individual names are indexed by surname, followed by given name, then middle name or initial.
2. Each unit is alphabetized by letter, starting with the order indicated above.
3. A surname used alone precedes the same surname with a first name or initial. A surname with a first initial precedes the same surname with a complete first name beginning with the same letter as the initial.
4. A surname prefix is not a separate indexing unit; for example, "McDonald" is filed under M.
5. Firm and institution names are indexed in the order written when they do not contain the complete name of an individual.
6. If a firm or institution name includes the complete name of an individual, indexing order follows rule 1 above.
7. "The" is always disregarded in indexing.
8. Hyphenated words in a firm name are indexed as separate units. Hyphenated surnames of individuals are considered as one indexing unit even when part of a firm name.
9. Abbreviations are indexed as though the words were written in full.
10. Conjunctions and prepositions (*and, for, in, of,* and *so forth*) are disregarded in indexing.
11. Names that may be written as either one or two words are indexed as one unit.

12. Parts of compound geographic names are indexed separately unless the first name is not an English word.

13. Titles and degrees are disregarded unless they indicate seniority or if the title is the initial word of the name.

14. In a possessive name, "'s" is disregarded; "s'" is indexed including the "s."

15. United States and foreign government names are indexed and subdivided by department, bureau, division, commission, and board.

16. A number in a name is considered as though spelled out and is indexed as one unit.

17. Banks are indexed by city, bank name, and state.

18. Married women are indexed as in rule 1, with husband's given and middle names noted parenthetically.

19. Cross-referencing or indexing is done if the organization is identifiable by more than the first word in the name, if the surname is not easily identifiable, if abbreviations can be readily identified, and if subject identification is possible.

Figure 7–12 illustrates the basic filing rules.

RECORDS PROTECTION

Effective and efficient retrieval methods control document flow, ensure the accountability and accessibility of all records, and designate and maintain a standard routing schedule for document movements. A charge-out system (1) initiates requests for filed materials through a requisition slip, (2) charges document materials to the individual collecting the records, and (3) institutes follow-up procedures until the documents are returned to the files.

Charge-out systems (transfer processes) use either out-guide or out-folder records to indicate who removed the individual file folder and when it was removed. Either form of charge-out record should specify the nominal index of the borrowed record, the subject of the record, the name and signature of the borrower, the date of the record, the date it was borrowed, the date when the record is to be returned, and the borrower's department or work unit. The charge-out records are removed when materials are returned or when a notation is made showing that the documents have been reclassified and filed as permanent or inactive records (Fig. 7–13).

A card index system should be used as a reminder file so that follow-up procedures are instituted when the borrowed records have been kept beyond the time stated on the charge-out record. A systematic follow-up procedure reduces the possibility of document loss, as do short, definite loan periods.

The larger the operation, the more important the records protection system. In a smaller medical office a spiral notebook may substitute for this more elaborate system.

RECORDS RETENTION AND STORAGE

Hospital records are retained for 10 years in most states (depending on the statute of limitations, or the period in which a lawsuit can be initiated). Records of medical office patients are kept indefinitely. Records of minors no longer under the physician's care are kept until the minor reaches the age of 18 or 21 (depending on the state's definition of an independent adult) and then for the number of years during which a lawsuit can be initiated according to local statutes of limitations.

File maintenance procedures are necessary to maximize efficiency and minimize the chance of error or document loss. The essential ingredients of an effective information system are fourfold: document flow, document accountability, frequent initial and replacement filing, and efficient storage.

An effective system for purging inactive files is essential. Otherwise the number of files becomes cumbersome, taking up additional office space and making document retrieval difficult. A system appropriate to the type of medical office practice and specialty should be selected as a chronologic purging system.

Frequent initial and replacement filing preserve the integrity of the documents themselves, protect the records from misplacement or loss, and provide for accurate and up-to-date information systems. Information accessibility is essential for all members of the physician's office, and the materials contained in the records management system must be current and accurate. Integrity is preserved through a rigid procedure for returning records to their respective files as quickly as possible after the physician has completed notes and any other necessary work that has been done.

Efficient storage minimizes physical strain and maximizes information retrieval methods. Design and layout of equipment and supplies should follow the procedures outlined throughout this chapter. Standardization and systematization are the key elements of effective records management.

Records retention policies determine what, where, and for how long documents are stored, and how outdated documents are to be destroyed. The physician's information requirements dictate the classification of files as active, permanent, or inactive.

Requirements imposed by federal, state, and local agencies identify specific documents that must be retained and the required retention period. Historic documents concerning the physician's practice provide valuable legal documentation as well as reference for scientific and medical research. Finally, vital patient records must be preserved and stored for case history referrals at subsequent dates, for their research potential and for documentation in case of legal action.

GUIDELINES FOR EFFICIENT RECORDS MANAGEMENT

1. Keep the system simple—emphasize speed, accuracy, and reliability.

2. Use standardized procedures and use them

Rule	Concerning	Name	Index Order of Units		
			Unit 1	Unit 2	Unit 3
1	Individual names	Larry M. Stewart	Stewart	Larry	M
		Mary Ann Pasquale	Pasquale	Mary	Ann
		J. V. Dickey	Dickey	J	V
2	Alphabetic order	Donald C. Lundgren	Lundgren	Donald	C
		Robert Lundgren	Lundgren	Robert	
		Robert A. Lundgren	Lundgren	Robert	A
3	Surnames	Schneider	Schneider		
		A. Schneider	Schneider	A	
		A. Mary Schneider	Schneider	A	Mary
4	Surnames with prefixes	James V. MacDonald	MacDonald	James	V
		Richard E. McClain	McClain	Richard	E
		Gordon M. VanAse	VanAse	Gordon	M
5	Firm names	Dispatch Printing Co.	Dispatch	Printing	Company
		Marquette Savings Assn.	Marquette	Savings	Association
		Tanner Office Supply Co.	Tanner	Office	Supply
6	Firm names containing individuals' names	Bracken Funeral Home	Bracken	Funeral	Home
		Chet Taft, Realtor	Taft	Chet	Realtor
		R. Collins, Signs	Collins	R	Signs
7	"The"	The Greenery	Greenery	(The)	
		The Ace Drawing School	Ace	Drawing	School
		Check the Plumber	Check	(the) Plumber	
8a	Hyphenated names	Mulligan-McCloskey Heating	Mulligan	McCloskey	Heating
8b	Hyphenated names	Joyce-Jean Ceramics	Joyce	Jean	Ceramics
		Link-Belt Power Tools	Link	Belt	Power
9	Abbreviations	AAA Rental Service	A	A	A
		St. Peters Cathedral	Saint	Peters	Cathedral
		Chas. Moore Printing	Moore	Charles	Printing
10	Conjunctions, prepositions, and firm endings	Moped Sales & Service	Moped	Sales	Service
		Sterrett & Co., Inc.	Sterrett	Company	Inc.
		A. Susol & Sons	Susol	A (&)	Sons
		Lutheran Church in America	Lutheran	Church	America

A

Figure 7–12. The basic rules of filing.

without variation — emphasize organization, efficiency, and consistency.

3. Train others in your system — be sure everyone with access to the files maintains them with the same care and concern as you do.

4. When in doubt, cross-reference — be sure the document trail is obvious, from alphabetic to numeric to subject files and within each area.

5. Schedule a definite time in the daily office routine for filing duties. A disciplined approach

11	One or two words	North East Coop. Assn.	North East	Cooperative	Association
		Northeast High School	Northeast	High	School
		Down Town Garage	Downtown	Garage	
12	Compound geographic names	New Mexico Publishing Co.	New	Mexico	Publishing
		San Francisco Publishing Co.	San	Francisco	Publishing
		East Rutherford Mills	East	Rutherford	Mills
13	Titles or Degrees	Dr. Salvatore Longo	Longo	Salvatore	(Dr.)
		John Prince, Jr.	Prince	John	(Jr.)
		Prince Edward Island	Prince	Edward	Island
14	Possessives	Frank's Cleaners	Frank	Cleaners	
		Mitchells' Grocery Store	Mitchells	Grocery	Store
15	U.S. and foreign government names	U.S. Dept. of the Air Force	United	States	Govt. (1)
		Internal Revenue Service	United	States	Govt. (2)
			Unit 4	*Unit 5*	*Unit 6*
			(1) Air	Force	Dept.
			(2) Internal	Revenue	Service
		Canadian Trade Office	Canadian	Trade	Office
16	Numbers	The 9th St. Plaza	Ninth	Street	Plaza (The)
		5th Ave. Hotel	Fifth	Avenue	Hotel
		Restaurant at 66 Park Plaza	Restaurant	Sixty-Six	Park
17	Banks, churches, organizations	First National Bank of Erie, Pa	Erie (Pa)	First National	Bank
		Trinity Lutheran Church	Lutheran	Church	Trinity
		Fraternal Order of Eagles	Eagles	Fraternal	Order (of)
		Iron Workers' Union	Iron	Workers	Union
18	Married women	Mrs. Greg Horgan (Mary Ann)	Horgan	Mary	Ann (Mrs.)
		Mrs. Jennifer L. Smith (Mrs. Theodore)	Smith (Theodore)	Jennifer	L (Mrs.)
		Mrs. Carol Rogers Miller (Mrs. James C.)	Miller (James C)	Carol	Rogers (Mrs.)

B

Figure 7–12. Continued.

guarantees that the files are current and that the medical assistant is not overwhelmed with the paper flow.

6. Use proper filing tools and supplies—the physical document flow through the office and the physical energy related to it can be minimized with preplanning and efficient work unit organization.

7. Use the right supplies for the right records and do not economize. Design the system and purchase supplies of good quality to minimize file maintenance activities. (Documents of substandard size should be attached to standard-sized paper and then filed.)

8. Examine folder contents each time the file is retrieved and before it is returned to the file

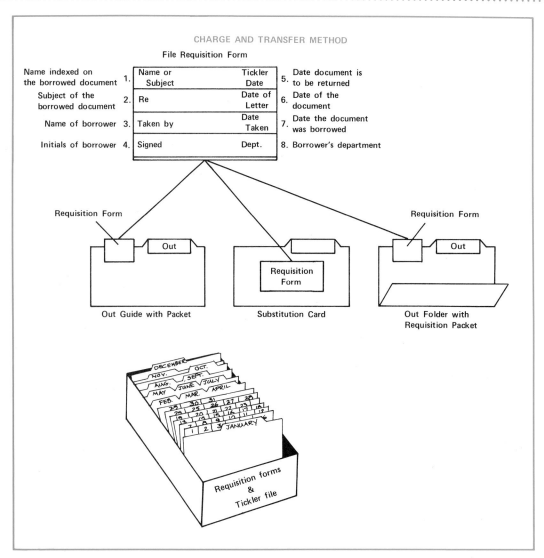

Figure 7–13. The charge and transfer method of keeping track of medical records.

cabinet. Being familiar with normal document contents reduces file search time and the chances of misfiling.

9. Maintain all facets of the system. Keep tabs and guides neat and current. Mend torn documents before refiling.

10. Organize the system for each accessibility. Active files should be at the front and center within a file cabinet, and the cabinets should be in the most active section of the work area.

11. File cabinets are for document files—do not use them to store other office equipment.

12. Emphasize physical safety. Open one drawer at a time and close the drawer immediately after use.

13. Do not cram—subdivide and cross-reference bulging files. Do not fill the drawer to capacity; doing so diminishes the neatness, order, and ease of accessibility of the system.

14. Classify documents and review them regularly.

15. Separate permanent files from active and inactive files. Regularly purge inactive records from the current files.

15. Use a well-designed color-key system. Retrieving speed and accuracy can be enhanced by file folders, guides, and labels that aid in establishing a document flow trail.

OFFICE MAINTENANCE

Another administrative organizational task assigned to the medical assistant is the supervision of maintenance for the administrative office, waiting room areas, and clinical facilities. Using the checklist approach and the equipment and supplies inventory discussed earlier, the medical assistant should include in the office procedures manual the daily, weekly, and monthly maintenance procedures specific to each area of the office unit and to the clinical areas of the practice. Most physicians employ an outside professional cleaning service. The medical assistant should collaborate with the physician to determine maintenance needs, and when and how often cleaning tasks should be completed.

In addition to supervising or coordinating the maintenance of the physical layout of the office, the medical assistant is often in charge of the library of scientific, medical, and technical materials that the physician and the office personnel use as reference documents. A card index system is the most efficient means of recording the books, journals (including those kept in the waiting room), technical monographs, pamphlets, and other materials housed in the library. The card index should include the following information: author, title, subject, publisher, year of publication, and number of pages, and editor, volume, and issue number for journals. For ease of access, the index should be cross-referenced by author, title, and subject in a manner, similar to Library of Congress listings and the Dewey Decimal System used by many medical societies. The medical assistant should review both the card index and the library materials to ensure that they are current and in good condition.

Subscriptions subject to renewal should be compiled and located in a "tickler" file in front of the card index (see Fig. 7–13). A tickler file is located in a file box or rotary file and contains pertinent information or lists that remind staff of specific tasks. Professional development materials should be added to the library, and facilities should be provided for a charge-out system so that these materials may be used frequently. As the library increases in sophistication, it may become necessary to obtain special equipment such as tape recorders, microfiche readers, and document reducers. Audiovisual materials that become part of the library holdings can then be used with ease.

PERSONNEL

The medical assistant may be asked to assist in the organization and maintenance of the office personnel file system. This task would be an advanced responsibility for the experienced medical assistant. In the large office, two different types of record keeping are usually required: individual personnel files and personnel policy statements.

INDIVIDUAL PERSONNEL FILES

A separate personnel file should be established for each medical office employee. The medical assistant should maintain this file in a confidential manner so that other office personnel do not have access to sensitive information. The file is the permanent record of the individual's employment history. It should contain pertinent information relative to promotions, pay increases, performance evaluations, training, disciplinary actions, and letters of recommendation to subsequent employers. Employee files should be stored for a reason-

able length of time (as regulated by the state) after employment has been terminated.

PERSONNEL POLICY STATEMENTS

The procedures manual outlines specific training policies enforced in the office. If the ground rules are detailed, questions regarding authority and responsibility, accrued benefits and so forth are not left to chance, and inconsistent applications are avoided. Figure 7–14 is a checklist for the subdivisions of such a personnel policy.

PATIENT TEACHING CONSIDERATIONS

Patients are oriented to the office system not only for their own needs but for those of the office staff. Each patient should understand the importance and integrity of the medical record. In addition, patients should be informed of the office policy regarding the release of information. In most cases, information is not released without the patient's written permission. Ownership of records should also be explained to avoid misunderstanding. Patients appreciate knowing the purpose of the special care their medical records receive.

RELATED ETHICAL AND LEGAL IMPLICATIONS

As was noted previously, confidentiality is both an ethical and a legal concern and is related to almost every task performed in the medical office. In handling

Administrative:	Job definitions and descriptions for each position in the office
	Hours of work
	Lunch and break periods
	Pay periods
	Job evaluation policy
	Discipline:
	probation period
	disciplinary actions
	grievance procedures
	termination procedures
Compensation:	Basic pay scale and pay increments
	Overtime pay
	Holidays
	Vacations
	Leaves of absence
	Sick pay
	Fringe benefits:
	medical insurance
	workers' compensation
	social security
	unemployment
	retirement
	profit sharing
	Professional development and training

Figure 7–14. A checklist for subdivisions of a medical office personnel policy.

patient and personnel records, protecting the patient's right to privacy is a primary responsibility. Only designated office personnel should have access to these records. In addition, the medical assistant must take care to place records out of the sight of nonauthorized individuals.

Unless information is subpoenaed by a government agency, its release from the medical record is legal only with the written permission of the patient or his or her attorney. Also, the patient has a right to read the contents of the record on request. It is important for the medical assistant to understand the legal requirements related to record handling to prevent potential litiga-

tion. As was indicated earlier, it may be useful for the office to publish its policy regarding patient records so that patients may understand their right to privacy.

SUMMARY

The challenges of organizing the office and maintaining the patient record contribute in many instances to the delivery of competent material care. The medical assistant must consistently strive to develop office practices that accomplish this objective.

DISCUSSION QUESTIONS

1. What types of office policies and procedures can be created for patients? For personnel?
2. What is the primary purpose of a patient records system?
3. What repercussions could there be if a patient's file is lost?
4. Why is a color-coded alphabetic system the "system of choice" in the doctor's office?
5. What is the difference between equipment and supplies in a medical office? What are some examples?
6. What supply items are most critical? What would happen if the office supply were depleted?

BIBLIOGRAPHY

American Medical Association: The Business Side of Medical Practice. Chicago, American Medical Association, 1989.
Humphrey DD: Contemporary Medical Office Procedures. Wadsworth, Belmont, CA, 1990.
Lane K et al, eds.: The Saunders Manual of Medical Assisting Practice. WB Saunders, Philadelphia, 1992.
Roach WF: Medical Records and the Law, ed 4. Aspen, Gaithersburg, MD, 1993.
Waters K: Medical Records in Health Information, ed 2. Aspen, Gaithersburg, MD, 1993.

PROCEDURE: Write a procedure sheet

Terminal Performance Objective: Write a procedure sheet (for a task covered in this chapter, or as assigned by the instructor) in rough draft form within 20 minutes; on instructor's approval, type final copy in time specified.

Equipment: Typewriter or word processor and printer
Typing paper
Procedures manual

PROCEDURE

1. Adopt a heading, to be used for all procedures sheets, that
   a. Identifies the task or procedure
   b. Determines who is responsible
2. Before beginning the rough draft, jot down in outline form the major points to be included.
3. Begin the rough draft from the outline. Isolate the first step and express it clearly in writing, as though you were giving specific directions. For example:
   Specific direction: Always answer the telephone politely: "Good morning—Dr. Jones's office, Cindy speaking."

4. Proceed in the same manner through each step or statement. Reread each step or statement for clarity and precision.
5. After finishing the rough draft, reread each step or statement, looking for errors and lack of cohesiveness. After the instructor approves, produce a final copy.

PRINCIPLE

1. Headings make reading and understanding easier and announce the task direction at the onset.

2. Outlines help organize the topic and subtopics into logical sequence.
3. Specific directions, as opposed to generalized instructions, are essential to clarify and standardize the steps required for a given task. General instructions may produce more than one response because different individuals may interpret them differently. Specific descriptions of actual behaviors are best. For example, regarding appropriate dress in a procedure sheet on reception techniques:
   Specific direction: "The following items should be worn: white uniform, consisting of a dress with skirt below the knees or a pants outfit, and white shoes."
   Generalized instruction: "Always look professional."
4. If each step is precisely and clearly described in as few words as possible, the main idea will be more easily understood and remembered.
5. A procedure sheet should not contain any grammatical errors. A consistent, standardized writing style promotes comprehension and retention of the material presented.

PROCEDURE: Prepare an inventory and order supplies

Terminal Performance Objective: Inventory a specified class of supplies (general office, clinical, pharmaceutical), determine the number or amount of each item required, and order the required items within the time specified by the instructor.

EQUIPMENT: File box and index cards, or notebook
Pen
Typewriter
Order blanks
Record tags

PROCEDURE

1. Assemble equipment and supplies.

2. If you use index cards, write or type the name of each item on an individual card. If you use a notebook, use a separate page for each item and use dividers with tabs to separate categories.

3. On each card or notebook page, write or type the amount on hand for that item, plus the amount needed to replenish the supply.

4. Where possible, place a reorder tag in the supply cupboard at the point at which the supply of that item is low enough to require reorder.

5. For each item that requires reordering now, mark the inventory item card or page with a tab or sticker. Place the card or page in the reorder section of the box or notebook.

6. For each card or page in the reorder section, complete the appropriate order blank or type a letter of request for that item.

7. On the card or page, type or write the date on which the order was made, plus the amount ordered. When the order is received, type in the date and amount received and return the card or page to its customary place in the file box or notebook.

8. Schedule the next inventory.

PRINCIPLE

1. Organization and planning save time and help prevent error.

2. Listing items separately allows for the flexibility needed to establish a complete inventory list.

3. Recording the amount on hand determines the amount to be reordered.

4. Reorder tags alert staff to the necessity to reorder.

5. Marking and separating the card or page sorts the items to be replenished now from those that do not require reorder at this time.

6. Requesting the item immediately prevents running out of necessary supplies.

7. Noting the order date and amount and the date received allows for tracking rate of use and delivery time.

8. Inventories should be performed regularly to ensure availability of supplies.

PROCEDURE: File a document

Terminal Performance Objective: Using the five-step process, file documents accurately, at the rate of at least one document within three minutes.

EQUIPMENT: Coding pen
File cabinet
Photocopier
Documents (patient records)
File folders

PROCEDURE

1. After assembling the equipment, inspect each document for the release marks indicating that it is ready to be filed.
2. Index the files by choosing the file folder captions under which the documents will be filed. Cross-reference, if necessary, by photocopying individual documents for filing in several folders.
3. Code each document by marking the appropriate index caption on the document to be filed.
4. Sort the documents into alphabetic order and subdivisions.
5. Store the document in the file folder and place the folder in the file cabinet.

PRINCIPLE

1. Release marks prevent the filing of documents that have not been cleared for filing.
2. Indexing ensures that the document is accessible for retrieval.
3. Coding ensures accuracy in the original filing process and in future retrieval and refiling.
4. Sorting organizes the documents for efficient filing.
5. Replacing the folder in the file cabinet completes the task of storing the document safely and ensuring its ready accessibility for future reference.

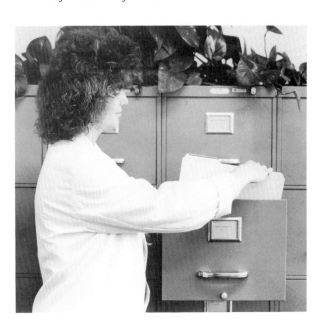

Lost, misplaced, or misfiled records may cause the patient care as well as legal problems. Following the filing rules precisely is essential.

Highlights

In Jeopardy: The Confidentiality of Medical Records

There is a growing concern among health care professionals regarding the confidentiality of medical records. Although medical care services are among the most personal types of services offered by our society, the patients' right to privacy might be in jeopardy.

The threat to maintaining confidentiality is arising from the number of legitimate requests for medical record information. Added to the list of health care professionals requiring access to patient records are government agencies, third-party payers, insurance companies, attorneys, and researchers. The growing dependency on computers and automated information systems is also contributing to the concern for safeguarding the patients' right to privacy.

Regardless of the use of computer security systems or other safeguarding protection used, the responsibility of upholding patient confidentiality continues to rest with the health care practitioners involved in caring for the patients. According to a report compiled by Healthcare Executive,* there are a number of specific actions that can be undertaken by staff members in offices and organizations that maintain medical records.

1. Limit access to patient or employee information to a selective number of staff members.
2. Develop policies for dealing with breaches of confidentiality.
3. Employ a computer security system that

has a record of reliability in safeguarding patient information and granting access to authorized personnel only.
4. Develop a policy and guidelines for the release of information to family, friends, and the media.
5. Develop a policy and guidelines for patient and employee access to their own medical records. These occurrences should be monitored by a designated staff member.
6. Instruct patients to carry emergency medical data at all times.
7. In offices dealing with substance abuse or infectious disease patients, special policies and guidelines should be implemented that ensure patient confidentiality.
8. Establish a protocol (appoint physician or staff member) for consultation regarding the release of information when questions arise.
9. Keep updated regarding the changes in government policies related to confidentiality of the medical record.
10. Educate patients about efforts (policies and procedures) employed by the office staff to ensure confidentiality.

The American College of Health Care Executives, in a public policy statement approved February 9, 1987, stated that "all health care executives have a moral and professional obligation to protect the confidentiality of patients' medical records."

As patient advocates, all health care professionals should share in this responsibility.

*From Healthcare Executive. 2 (4), July/August, 1987, with permission.

*C*orrespondence and Professional Writing

> You speak to someone face to face, but you write to someone who will not be present at your side when he reads what you have written. Therefore, written language must be even more precise and careful than spoken language.
>
> Warriner's English Grammar and Composition

CHAPTER OUTLINE

Chapter 8

Correspondence and Professional Writing

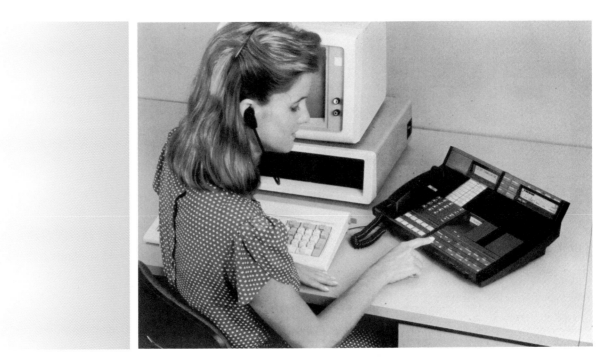

RELATED ETHICAL AND LEGAL IMPLICATIONS

SUMMARY

DISCUSSION QUESTIONS

BIBLIOGRAPHY

PROCEDURES
Write Original Correspondence

Prepare the Outgoing Mail
Sort and Open Incoming Mail
Annotate Incoming Mail

HIGHLIGHTS
Antonyms, Eponyms, and Homonyms

LEARNING OBJECTIVES

Upon completing this chapter, you will able to:

1. List the equipment and supplies necessary for letter writing.
2. List the equipment and supplies necessary for processing incoming and outgoing mail.
3. List and describe the five basic style forms for typing letters in the medical office.
4. List the seven rules that apply to letter construction.
5. Identify the component parts of a letter.
6. Identify the five letter style forms and their margin and spacing guidelines.
7. Describe the proper use of duplicate copies.
8. Describe the medical assistant's responsibilities regarding signing the physician's signature on outgoing letters.
9. Define "annotation" and explain its use.
10. Describe the situations in which the use of form letters may or may not be advantageous.
11. List the sorting and handling guidelines for incoming mail.
12. Identify four types of commonly transcribed medical records and correspondence.
13. Identify two document formats used for transcribing letters.
14. Identify two styles of chart note and the abbreviations used with each style.
15. List various medical transcription reference books.
16. List 12 instructions for preparing a manuscript.

PERFORMANCE OBJECTIVES

Upon completing this chapter, you will able to:

1. Compose original letters.
2. Type letters written in the block, semiblock, full block, hanging indentation, and simplified forms.
3. Sort and annotate incoming correspondence.
4. Proofread and edit writing samples.
5. Prepare envelopes for optical scanning and special delivery requirements.
6. Select postage classes and determine postage rates.
7. Transcribe the physician's dictation verbatim using correct abbreviations, grammar, punctuation, spelling, and terminology.
8. Proofread transcribed reports and obtain signatures and initials as appropriate.
9. Correct composition using proofreading marks and abbreviations.
10. Arrange for a meeting or for the physician's travel to a meeting.

DACUM EDUCATIONAL COMPONENTS

1. Maintain confidentiality [in letter writing and mail processing] (1.4A).
2. Receive, organize, prioritize, and transmit information (2.7).
3. Use medical terminology accurately and compose written communications using correct spelling, grammar, and format (2.10A–C; 2.11A–B).
4. Screen and process mail (3.1A,D).
5. Type and transcribe accurately (3.5A–C).
6. Prepare and maintain medical records (5.1A,B).
7. Determine the needs for documenting and reporting special mailing and facsimile communications and apply computer concepts to office practices (5.2H; 3.1C).

Glossary

Annotating: Highlighting the main points or ideas within a document by underlining or by making marginal notes

Certified Mail: Mail posted with an additional fee charged for a receipt that proves it was sent

Chronologic: According to time sequence

Correspondence file: A chronologic collection of copies of sent documents, typed but not placed within the regular patient files or project files

Cue notes: Informal notes collected by the letter composer during discussion of the message with the sender

Express mail: A system of quick deliveries offered by the US Post Office

Microcomputer: A small computer suitable for desktop or small office use

Postage meter: A device that can produce a gummed stamp of any designation. Replaces the need to stock several kinds of stamps.

Return receipt request: A request, accompanied by a fee to the US Post Office, for a receipt from the person who gets the mailing

Signature stamp: A rubber stamp constructed from a sample of a person's signature

In most medical offices, the medical assistant is responsible for processing both incoming and outgoing mail. By assuming responsibility for this task, the medical assistant enables the physician to concentrate more time on the essential aspects of patient care. The quality of outgoing written communications and the efficiency of internal mail handling affect both the image and the success of the medical practice. The experienced medical assistant is especially skilled in handling these responsibilities; independently answering requests by patients, insurance companies, and others; and supervising the routing of incoming mail and the postage and handling of outgoing materials.

ESTABLISHING THE OFFICE ROUTINE FOR LETTER WRITING AND MAIL HANDLING

In many offices a system for processing incoming and outgoing mail is described in the procedures manual. In offices without a procedures manual, or with one that does not include mail handling and letter writing, the medical assistant may suggest the inclusion of these procedures. Most offices have a large volume of incoming and outgoing correspondence that is important to the medical and legal management of patient care. A well-organized system, accepted and used correctly by the office staff, is protection against misplaced incoming mail, unacknowledged deadlines or requests, badly written outgoing letters, and mismanaged patient records. The major concerns in establishing efficient systems are to acquire the appropriate equipment and supplies, and when possible, to adhere to a specified time for letter writing and mail handling. Deciding who will write letters, who will open what mail, and how the mail will be processed is essential to the efficient management of these tasks.

EQUIPMENT AND SUPPLIES

Several equipment and supply items are necessary for the efficient operation of an office communication system. The medical assistant is often responsible for ordering and maintaining the equipment and ensuring a continuing inventory of supply items.

TYPEWRITER OR WORD PROCESSOR

One necessary item is a typewriter or word processor appropriate for the needs of the office. Given the rapid advancement of computer technology, many physicians are replacing the traditional typewriter with either word processors or microcomputers with word processing capabilities. The text editing and storage memory features of these devices make them an increasingly common choice. The technology of the microcomputer and word processor provides tremendous labor-saving opportunities in medical practice because corrections and editing do not require devices such as correction fluid or correction tape. In addition, because editing precedes printing the copy, each typed sheet gives no evidence of error. All work can be saved and stored in the computer or on disks for future reference. Regardless of the system selected, it is important that the machines themselves be reliable and easily serviced. A broken typewriter or word processor can be a major disruption in time management for the medical office. If available, a service contract with a provision for back-up equipment, usually purchasable at additional cost, is recommended to avoid such interruptions.

TYPING AREA FURNISHINGS

A desk or table of proper height and a comfortable chair are also important to the system because the medical assistants, particularly those whose work is largely administrative, spend the greater percentage of time at work seated at the desk. The chair should be padded and have wheels or rollers attached to the legs to allow movement from the typing area to another part of the table. The American Medical Association (AMA), in its *Planning Guide for Medical Facilities*, recommends approximately 25 to 30 square feet of desk area to accommodate a business computer system, including word processing capabilities and a chair for the operator. In addition, ample drawer and shelf space is usually needed to accommodate equipment and supplies and make them readily accessible.

STATIONERY

The selection of an attractive and functional letterhead or logo, along with appropriate paper quality, projects the office image. This image may, in fact, have a greater impact on the perception of the office practice than the message itself. Most physicians simply choose a style of print for a letterhead, an increasing number of small offices are using graphics, such as line drawings of the office building, and logos, such as symbols or pictures, to create an intended image and market the practice. High-quality paper should be selected in white or a light color. Stationery should be ordered both with and without the letterhead because second and third sheets of letters are typed on plain paper. Regardless of letterhead style, the names of the physicians or group, the specialty, and the address and telephone number of the practice should be included.

POSTAGE METER OR SUPPLY OF STAMPS

If large-volume mailing is required, the use of a postage meter will save time and labor. A postage meter, such as the one shown in Figure 8–1, prints its own stamp or imprints postage of any price designation or postal class. Metered mail can hasten delivery because it eliminates the need for canceling and postmarking at

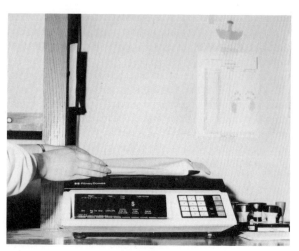

Figure 8–1. A postage meter.

the post office. The post office charges a monthly or quarterly rental fee for the key that operates the meter. The date on the meter is changed daily. Because the medical office must purchase and maintain the postage meter, these devices are used only by offices that are large enough to sustain a high volume of mail. Most offices keep a supply of stamps or stamped envelopes on hand. A systematized routine, such as a weekly task assignment, should be established to ensure that a supply of postage is available at all times.

ENVELOPES

Depending on the kinds of mailings that are ordinarily processed by the office, the medical assistant should maintain a supply of various envelopes and mailing packets. If a very large volume of mail is sent in standard (No. 10) envelopes, it would be advisable to have these printed with return addresses to match the stationery. Suppose the physician uses two sizes of stationery, the standard 8½ by 11 inches and the executive (monarch) 7¼ by 10 inches. The two sizes of envelopes needed in large supply are the No. 10, which is 4½ by 9½ inches, and the No. 7 (monarch), which is 3⅞ by 7½ inches. The postal service requires that an envelope be rectangular, at least 3½ inches high, at least 5 inches long, and at least the thickness of a postcard. The color of the stationery and envelopes should be light enough for use by the postal service's optical scanners.

ZIP CODE AND STATE ABBREVIATION DIRECTORIES

For a nominal fee, a local and national zip code directory can be obtained from the local post office and displayed in a prominent place. Proper zip coding facilitates the efficient handling of all mail. It may be useful for the medical assistant to inquire about the new "zip code plus four" system, a nine-number system designed to make deliveries to urban areas more specific and efficient. Some medical offices may qualify for postage discounts if they conform to the expanded requirements of the nine-digit zip code system.

SPECIAL STAMPS

The medical assistant should use at least two different types of rubber stamp: a changeable date stamp so that incoming mail can be dated, and a "Confidential" stamp so that physicians or other professionals can receive sensitive mail without its being opened and read by assistants. The changeable date stamp can serve double duty by stamping the chart notes sheet for patients scheduled for a visit. It may also be useful to have stamps designating various mailing categories.

OTHER EQUIPMENT AND SUPPLIES

Each office should have an accurate postage scale for weighing letters and packages to determine the appropriate postage. A sharp letter opener, a regular and a medical dictionary, and a supply of post office–approved sealing tape for securing packages is also needed. Packages secured with Scotch-type tape or string are often rejected. In addition, typical office supplies — paper, pens, business forms, and filing materials — must be maintained.

LETTER WRITING

The role of the medical assistant is clearly that of innovator, information gatherer, and facilitator. The more responsibilities the medical assistant can successfully assume for the business management of the practice, such as letter writing, the closer physicians can come to realizing their goals for patient care. Although the skills of an accurate and proficient typist are undeniably important, the medical assistant should also possess expertise in composing medical correspondence, including subscription renewals, equipment orders, travel arrangements, and payment requests.

For example, the physician should be able to say, "Send a letter to the Rotary Club and tell them I will speak at the luncheon meeting on July 12 at noon on 'Current Developments in Cardiology.'" The medical assistant would respond by making notes of the major points (date, time, subject), and then constructing a letter for the physician's approval and signature. This approach saves the physician valuable time and relieves him or her of routine letter-writing duties, with the exception of reviewing and signing the letter.

To write letters competently, the medical assistant must understand the basic aspects of composing correspondence. Since several writing styles and techniques are available, the medical assistant should be aware of alternatives and assist physicians in selecting those that most appropriately reflect their needs. The style guide for letter writing, published by the AMA, should also be consulted to ensure appropriate style selection and punctuation.

LETTER STYLES AND FORMATS

The typed style and format, or physical presentation, of the message is as important as the content in written communication. Regardless of appropriate content and correct grammar and spelling, a typed copy that is nonprofessional in appearance cancels the positive effects of the well-written message. The overall format and presentation provide a letter "picture," or projection, of the office that either adds to or detracts from the written message. Letter style and format are discussed here because many medical assistants compose letters on the word processor or on a microcomputer with word processing capability. The screen provides design and correction capabilities, and the need for handwritten draft is eliminated. There are four basic styles of business letter:

1. Block
2. Modified block
3. Modified block with indented paragraphs (also known as modified semiblock)
4. Hanging indentation
5. Simplified

These forms are illustrated in Figures 8–2 through 8–7.

The modified block and modified block with paragraph indentation (semiblock) styles are conventional and project a traditional or conservative image. The full block form (Fig. 8–3) is a newer "hybrid" form that is generally favored because of its margin consistency. The hanging indentation form has achieved great popularity with sales and purchasing firms, and although it is rarely adopted by physicians, the medical assistant is likely to see it on many incoming letters. The simplified form is popular with corporate executives. It conveys a feeling of warmth and efficiency (eliminating needless rules and procedures), and typically expresses a sense of informality. Most physicians who use the simplified form do so because of the added advantages of brevity and clarity.

Other stylistic choices include the use of punctuation alternatives for parts of the letter not included in the body, such as the salutation. In open punctuation, no punctuation appears at the end of a salutation or similar line unless the line ends with an abbreviation. Simplified and full block letters frequently are associated with open punctuation. Closed punctuation, rarely used today, ends each line outside the body of the letter with a comma or a period. Mixed or standard punctuation (inconsistent) is most common in medical practice and is used appropriately with full block, modified block, and semiblock letter styles. The objective in determining which letter style to use is always to select the style that best projects clarity and a professional image, while being easy to read.

THE BUSINESS LETTER

To the letter writer, the selection of words is as important as the use of color is to the artist. Carefully composed, the letter reflects a multilevel message combining feelings, information, and visual appeal.

The following seven rules apply to business letter construction. Each is a powerful aid to the prospective letter writer.

1. Use cue notes. Cue notes are notes taken before writing to identify the major points to be expressed in the letter. For example, the physician may request that the medical assistant write a letter to Dr. Jones thanking him for the patient referral and explaining that he will receive the results of the consultation by the end of the month. Cue notes assist in letter organization and clarity.
   Notes. To: Dr. Jones
   Re: Thank you for referral of Mrs. J. Albertes. Will send results by end of the month.

```
                    S. R. SELLARO, D.O., INC.
                       GENERAL PRACTICE
                        ANESTHESIOLOGY
                    306 WEST ELEVENTH STREET
                        ERIE, PA. 16501
                          ——
                   TELEPHONE 814 - 455-1311


                                              January 17, 1993




Mr. P. J. Browning
214 West Elm Street
Erie, Pennsylvania 16513

Dear Mr. Browning:

Thank you very much for the invitation to speak with the Rotary Club of Erie.
I have been affiliated with Rotary Clubs for several years, and I am honored
that you would ask me.

My choice of a topic for your gathering would be, "Sports Medicine."  I have
been interested in this area for several years, and believe that some of the
most recent developments could be of use to many of your members.

I understand that the meeting will be held at the Chambers Restaurant, at
12:00 noon on the 13th of March.

                         Sincerely yours,



                         S. R. Sellaro, D.O.

SRS:mk
```

Figure 8–2. Block form for business letter.

2. Establish an effective beginning. The most common error in letter writing is failure to introduce the topic adequately in the first paragraph. The quality of the letter often improves as the writing progresses. A corrective technique is to rewrite the first paragraph after the entire letter is completed. Because the purpose of the first paragraph is to gain the reader's attention, the topic should be introduced in the first four sentences.

3. Be brief and precise. The letter should be as short as possible without jeopardy to the content. The medical assistant should attempt to convey the message with precision. Wordiness clouds the message, forcing the reader to sort through the verbiage for the main idea. The medical assistant should write a rough draft from the cue notes and recheck it for wordiness before writing the final draft.

4. Avoid use of the first or second person. Although there are circumstances in which the first or second person may be used in a personal letter, it is usually preferable to write in the third person. Avoiding the use of "I," "we," or "you" whenever possible adds a sense of objectivity and professionalism. For example, it is better to say "It has been determined . . ." than to say "I (or We) have determined. . . ." This style is, however, a matter of preference. In use with the simplified form is a more direct, informal style of writing using the first and second person.

5. Use proper grammar and punctuation. Errors in grammar and punctuation project a negative public relations image. Spelling errors, sentence fragments, and misused words and punctuation suggest incompetence in all aspects of the medical practice. Although inaccurate, this percep-

S. R. SELLARO, D.O., INC.
GENERAL PRACTICE
ANESTHESIOLOGY
306 WEST ELEVENTH STREET
ERIE, PA. 16501

Telephone 814 - 455-1311

January 17, 1993

Mr. P. J. Browning
214 West Elm Street
Erie, Pennsylvania 16513

Dear Mr. Browning:

Thank you very much for the invitation to speak with the Rotary Club of
Erie. I have been affiliated with Rotary Clubs for several years, and
I am honored that you would ask me.

My choice of a topic for your gathering would be, "Sports Medicine." I
have been interested in this area for several years, and believe that
some of the most recent developments could be of use to many of your
members.

I understand that the meeting will be held at the Chambers Restaurant,
at 12:00 noon on the 13th of March.

Sincerely yours,

S. R. Sellaro, D.O.

SRS:mk

Figure 8–3. Full block form for business letter.

tion is easily acquired, especially when the letter is the initial contact. A dictionary and a comprehensive guide to grammar should be kept at the work area for reference. Proofreading the rough draft for errors is imperative. (It may be helpful to consult "Punctuation Patterns in Medical Correspondence," found in Appendix 1.)

6. Use professional terminology, but write clearly. Medical terminology must be used where appropriate, but the use of uncommon vocabulary throughout a letter should be avoided. Clarity depends on word choice. The letter should be professional in tone but not deliberately complex. The reader should not need a dictionary to interpret the message.

7. Close with a paragraph that suggests action. The purpose of the final paragraph is to motivate the reader to act when a response is needed. The closing paragraph should clearly indicate the urgency of the response and the form it should take (a call, a visit, a return letter).

LETTER MECHANICS

Because the quality of their work reflects on the office image, medical assistants must ensure that each outgoing letter is mechanically perfect. The top and bottom margins should be well planned so that the letter is centered on the paper. Each line should be contained within the proper margins.

Preferences for spacing and margin designs vary. The following guidelines are commonly used:

Margins: A minimum of 1 inch on either side of the body (10 spaces for pica type, 12 spaces for elite). At least 2 inches at the top of the paper, and at least 1 inch at the bottom.

ORTHOPEDIC SURGICAL ASSOCIATES, INC.

Joseph K. Lane, M.D.
Reeves R. Wiley, M.D.
Timothy J. Welder, M.D.

1210 Hospital Drive   690 Northern Parkway
Professional Medical Building   Suite D
Glen Burnie, MD   21061   Columbia, MD   21043

December 10, 1993

Mrs. Patricia R. Smith
120 Holly Drive
Annapolis, MD   21403

RE: Candace Smith

Dear Mrs. Smith:

You will be pleased to know that your daughter Candace's laboratory tests have all returned with negative results. A follow-up appointment is not needed for six months.

We have found that Bay County General Hospital offers Special Child Activity classes designed specifically for patients with your daughter's diagnosis. Enclosed is a brochure describing the program. We would encourage you to enroll her in this program, if at all possible.

Please call our office next May to arrange for an appointment in June for Candace.

Sincerely,

Joseph K. Lane, M.D.

JKL/smt

cc: Richard M. Rodgers, M.D.
Enclosure

Figure 8–4. *Modified block form for business letter.*

Spacing: Depending on the form used, indenting five spaces before beginning each paragraph is universally accepted. Letters are usually single-spaced between lines and double-spaced between paragraphs.

Typing and spacing errors should be double-checked before the letter is removed from the typewriter or printer. When typed on a conventional typewriter, all corrections should be made neatly, and strikeovers should never appear on the finished copy. Other letter mechanics include rules relating to parts of letters, as follows (Fig. 8–8):

Dateline. The dateline is typed on line 15 or, depending on the size of the letterhead, two or three lines below the last line of the letterhead. The month, day, and year are written in full rather than abbreviated. The name of the month is written first, followed by the day and year.

Ordinal numbers, such as *1st, 2nd,* or *3rd,* are not commonly used.

Inside address. The inside address usually includes two or more lines with the name and address of the person to whom the letter is directed. The US Postal Service prefers that the address be limited to 3 to 4 lines. These lines begin flush with the left margin. Courtesy titles (Ms. or Mr.) should be used cautiously. Although it is appropriate to use Dr., Mr., Ms., or Miss before a name, eliminating courtesy titles and placing academic degree titles after the name may be more appropriate. Do not use both types of titles together; use only one or the other. *Examples:* Dr. June Smith; June Smith, M.D.

Salutation. The introductory greeting (Dear Mrs. Smith:, Dear Dr. Smith:) is typed flush with the left margin on the second line below the last line

Figure 8–5. Semiblock, or modified block, form for business letter; note the indented paragraphs.

of the inside address and is followed by a colon. (In open punctuation a colon would not be used.)

Subject line. When the letter is written in reference to a patient, the patient's name is usually included in the first line and is considered part of the body of the letter. This subject line begins on the second line below the salutation. It can be indented, centered, or started flush with the left margin. The use of the word "Subject" is a matter of preference. *Examples:* Subject: Ann Carnes; Subject: ANN CARNES.

Body of letter. The body of the letter begins two lines below the subject line if this is used, otherwise two lines below the salutation. The first line of each paragraph may be indented five spaces, or flush with the left margin, depending on the letter style.

Complimentary closing. The closing should reflect the same formality as the salutation. If "Dear Mrs. Jones" is the salutation, an appropriate closing might be "Sincerely" or "Cordially."

Typewritten signature. The typed signature is placed on the fourth line directly below the complimentary closing to allow adequate space for the written signature.

Reference initials. Reference initials identify the author and transcriptionist of the letter and are typed flush with the left margin on the second line below the typed signature. The author's initials are capitalized and the transcriptionist's are lower case. *Example:* MAF:dlw.

Special notations. If the letter includes an enclosure, the word "Enclosure" is typed on the first

S. R. SELLARO, D.O., INC.
GENERAL PRACTICE
ANESTHESIOLOGY
306 WEST ELEVENTH STREET
ERIE, PA. 16501

TELEPHONE 814 - 455-1311

January 17, 1993

Mr. P. J. Browning
214 West Elm Street
Erie, Pennsylvania 16513

Thank you very much for the invitation to speak with the Rotary Club of
    Erie. I have been affiliated with Rotary Clubs for several years,
    and I am honored that you would ask me.

My choice of a topic for your gathering would be, "Sports Medicine." I
    have been interested in this area for several years, and believe
    that some of the most recent developments could be of use to many
    of your members.

I understand that the meeting will be held at the Chambers Restaurant,
    at 12:00 noon on the 13th of March.

                            Sincerely yours

                            S. R. Sellaro, D.O.

SRS:mk

Figure 8–6. Hanging indentation form of business letter.

or second line below the reference initials. The number of enclosures is specified (e.g., Enclosure 3). When copies of the letter are sent to other individuals, a "cc" (carbon copy), or "xc" (extra copy) notation is made in the same manner as for enclosures. *Example:* cc: C. Joy, M.D. When both are used, the copy notation is typed below "Enclosure." Because actual carbons are rarely used anymore, the "xc" notation is gaining in popularity. When more than one copy is required, the names of the individuals are either alphabetically ordered or listed according to rank. The notation "bcc" (blind carbon copy) is used if copies are distributed without the list appearing in the original letter. The "bcc" notation and the recipient names are typed on the copies. The practice of blind copying is no longer advised and its use should be discouraged.

Second page heading. When the letter is continued beyond the first page, the heading of the second and subsequent pages is typed on the seventh line from the top of the page and includes the name of the addressee, the page number, and the date (Fig. 8–9). Several acceptable variations, appear below:

1. Charles Joy, M.D. -2- April 27, 19xx
2. Charles Joy, M.D. Page 2 April 27, 19xx
3. Charles Joy, M.D. Page 2 April 27, 19xx
   Subject: Ann Carnes

The body continues on the third line below the heading or on the tenth line from the top of the

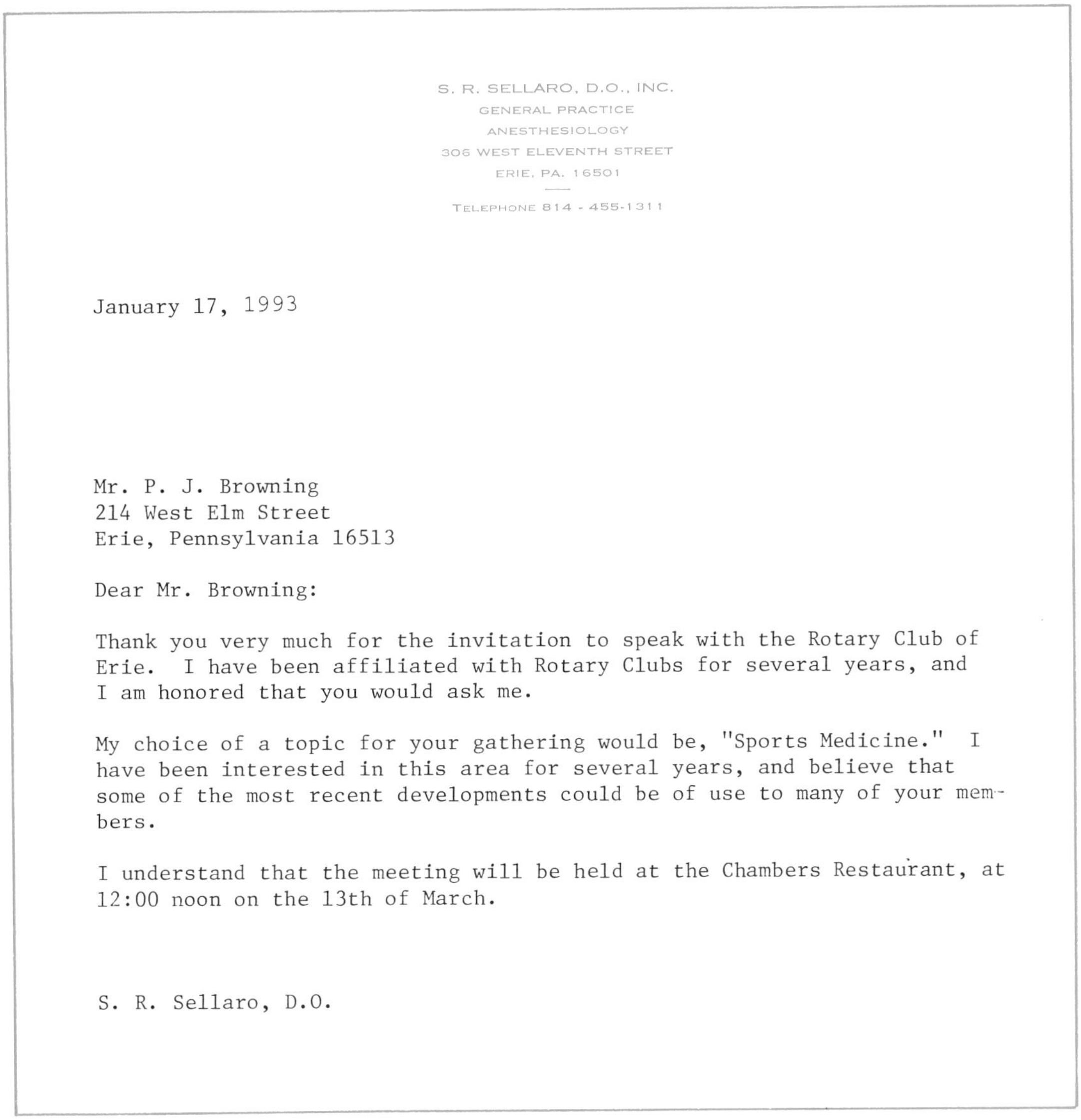

S. R. SELLARO, D.O., INC.
GENERAL PRACTICE
ANESTHESIOLOGY
306 WEST ELEVENTH STREET
ERIE, PA. 16501

TELEPHONE 814 - 455-1311

January 17, 1993

Mr. P. J. Browning
214 West Elm Street
Erie, Pennsylvania 16513

Dear Mr. Browning:

Thank you very much for the invitation to speak with the Rotary Club of Erie. I have been affiliated with Rotary Clubs for several years, and I am honored that you would ask me.

My choice of a topic for your gathering would be, "Sports Medicine." I have been interested in this area for several years, and believe that some of the most recent developments could be of use to many of your members.

I understand that the meeting will be held at the Chambers Restaurant, at 12:00 noon on the 13th of March.

S. R. Sellaro, D.O.

Figure 8–7. Simplified form of business letter. (Note that in the simplified form the subject line may replace the salutation. Example: "Speaker for Rotary Club Meeting" instead of "Dear Mr. Browning.")

page. A second page is not appropriate unless there are at least two lines to carry over.

DUPLICATE COPIES

Because of the potential importance of medical office correspondence, the medical assistant must pay meticulous attention to the creation and proper filing of duplicate copies of all correspondence. If a typewriter is used, a carbon copy or photocopy of each document should be made for subsequent storage in the appropriate file. As was mentioned earlier, most physicians' offices use the newer technology of reproducing the original document rather than using carbon paper. With computer and word-processing capabilities, it is usually more economical to print a second copy of the document than to photocopy it.

In the presentation of the final document for signing,

only the original (or originals if documents are being sent to several individuals) must be signed. File copies remain unsigned.

The document copies should be placed carefully in appropriate files. Most practices file patient-oriented documents in the patient record, create special files for projects such as research or journal writing, and place the remaining correspondence in a chronologic subject file labeled "Correspondence." The procedure that outlines and summarizes the steps required in writing original correspondence is included at the end of this chapter.

THE PHYSICIAN'S SIGNATURE

Many physicians prefer to have the medical assistant relieve them of signing routine documents and corre-

```
                         S. R. SELLARO, D.O., INC.
                          GENERAL PRACTICE
                            ANESTHESIOLOGY
                        306 WEST ELEVENTH STREET
                            ERIE. PA. 16501
                                  ──
                        TELEPHONE 814 - 455-1311




        DATELINE ------------>  January 17, 1993




Mr. P. J. Browning      <-------------- INSIDE ADDRESS
214 West Elm Street
Erie, Pennsylvania  16513
                                                SUBJECT LINE
                                                      │
Dear Mr. Browning:    <------------- SALUTATION       │

Thank you very much for the invitation to speak with the  Rotary  Club  of
Erie.  I have been affiliated with Rotary Clubs for several years,  and  I
am honored that you would ask me.

My choice of a topic for  your  gathering  would  be,  "Sports  Medicine."
I have been interested in this area for several years,  and  believe  that
some of the most recent developments could be  of  use  to  many  of  your
members.

I understand that the meeting will be held at the Chambers Restaurant,  at
12:00 noon on the 13th of March.

         COMPLIMENTARY CLOSE--------> Sincerely yours,



         TYPED SIGNATURE------------> S. R. Sellaro, D.O.

SRS:jc  <------- REFERENCE INITIALS
```

Figure 8-8. The parts of a letter. (This example business letter is in modified block form.)

Mr. P.J. Browning

Page 2

January 17, 1993

Figure 8-9. Standard heading for the second page of a letter or report.

spondence. The medical assistant should discuss this issue with all physicians in the office and endeavor to understand their preferences. Although the handling of the physician's signature is clearly a matter of physician preference, the medical assistant can follow certain guidelines in determining responsibility in this matter.

RESTRICTIONS

Some documents cannot be signed by anyone but the physician. These include patient correspondence, advice to patients, referral and consultation reports to colleagues, letters to professional associations, notes to the medical file, correspondence to hospital officials or other physicians, personal letters, and medical reports to insurance companies. Other correspondence, such as nonmedical insurance paperwork, supply orders, hotel reservations, patient notifications, and subscription orders, may be signed by the assistant with the assistant's signature.

SIGNATURE STAMPS

One procedure for handling the mechanical problem of writing individual signatures on each letter is to obtain a stamp made from a sample of the physician's signature. Signature stamps are usually not expensive and can be obtained from most printing or office supply vendors. Because the stamp could be misused, it should be secured in a locked drawer. Signature stamps have restricted use. They may be used to replace original signatures for writing and endorsing checks, and for completing forms, such as supply or "return-to-work" forms. Under no circumstances should a signature stamp be used on letters, reports, or correspondence composed by the physician or the medical assistant.

THE REPRESENTATIVE SIGNATURE

If the physician authorizes the practice, the medical assistant can (under appropriate circumstances) sign the physician's name in his or her own handwriting. It is not necessary to attempt to duplicate the actual signature. The proper procedure after signing for the physician is to initial the signature with the first and last initials of the actual signer (the medical assistant), as is shown in Figure 8–10. Another alternative is for the medical assistant to sign his or her own name in full. *Example:* Anne Lilly for M. Jones, M.D.

PROOFREADING AND EDITING

Every document mailed from the physician's office should be grammatically and mechanically perfect. To achieve this goal, every letter or document ready for mailing must be proofread. Proofreading is often the responsibility of the medical assistant. Both proofreading and editing are "art forms" that develop and improve over time. Many students get into the habit of

rushing their work and may assume that misspelled words or poor grammar will not detract from the "content of the work." This attitude is never acceptable in the medical office. Correspondence containing incorrect grammar or poor spelling projects a negative image of the medical office. Proofreading and editing usually involve scrutinizing sentence structure and checking for correct dates, correct spelling of names, and typographic errors.

The changes that the medical assistant makes in the letter should aid the recipient in interpreting the information precisely. The medical assistant should be careful not to change the meaning or content of the sentence when correcting structure, grammar, or spelling. It is possible to purchase software that checks both grammar and spelling. If the office uses a word processor or computer, this timesaving device is invaluable.

Time and patience are required for checking documents by hand. Each document must be carefully read and reread. If time permits and a particular document is crucially important, a reading from another person in the office can be helpful. Another reading may not be feasible if patient confidentiality is an issue, however.

Proofreading marks are often used to facilitate corrections on the rough draft. They can be used to mark letters or manuscripts and are universally understood by proofreaders preparing the work for final copy. Figure 8–11 illustrates proofreading marks in common use.

FORM LETTERS

Certain types of letters are used repeatedly in office practice. Most physicians use form letters to meet routine needs. The form letter is a timesaving device that can be readily applied to uniform situations. Its disadvantage is that most form letters can immediately be recognized as such, and the recipient may feel that he or she has been treated impersonally.

The decision concerning which form letter to use and when to use it should be made in consultation with the physician. To a large extent this decision may be dictated by the office workload. A series of form letters may be required to resolve difficulties in time management.

Form letters can be adopted for letters of collection, information regarding professional fees, request letters (e.g., for drug samples or reprints), and some referrals. Commonly used form letters should be placed in the procedures manual.

"FILL-IN" FORM LETTERS

For letter-writing problems that are repeated and predictable, the "fill-in" form may be the best solution. Common uses are notifying patients of test results and scheduling appointments. Figure 8–12 is an example of a fill-in form letter. The medical assistant should develop a series of these "fill-in" letters to be completed and mailed as needed. As was indicated, there are sev-

S. R. SELLARO, D.O., INC.
GENERAL PRACTICE
ANESTHESIOLOGY
306 WEST ELEVENTH STREET
ERIE, PA. 16501

TELEPHONE 814 - 455-1311

January 17, 1993

Mr. P. J. Browning
214 West Elm Street
Erie, Pennsylvania 16513

Dear Mr. Browning:

Thank you very much for the invitation to speak with the Rotary Club of
Erie. I have been affiliated with Rotary Clubs for several years, and I
am honored that you would ask me.

My choice of a topic for your gathering would be, "Sports Medicine."
I have been interested in this area for several years, and believe that
some of the most recent developments could be of use to many of your
members.

I understand that the meeting will be held at the Chambers Restaurant, at
12:00 noon on the 13th of March.

S. R. Sellaro/jc
S. R. Sellaro, D.O.

Figure 8–10. *Example of a letter with a representative signature. In this case, Joyce Cooper (jc) has signed for Dr. Sellaro.*

eral logical uses for form letters. However, when used exclusively or nonselectively, they can fail to project the desired image or to obtain results when action is necessary. The needs of the office practice, and ultimately the physician's preference, dictate which situations warrant a form letter.

SEMI-FORM LETTERS

A modified approach to form-letter writing is useful for those letters that are repeated but not in their exact forms. This approach uses the "semi-form letter." Once the medical assistant had prepared a letter that promises to be useful, a copy should be made and filed as a model for future letters of similar intent. A recommended approach to developing such a file is to use a subject-divided notebook. The subject file might include letters of recommendation, inquiry, consultation

acknowledgement, and other common types of correspondence. After the medical assistant has developed a series of each basic type of letter, one or more of each type may be used as a guide to the construction of new letters as they become necessary. Although the semi-form letter is neither as fast nor as efficient as the basic form letter, it is a compromise that retains originality and saves a substantial amount of time.

AUTOMATING FORM LETTERS

If the office uses a word processor or computer, form or semi-form letters can be stored on disks for easy editing and adjusting. Storing form letters on a special disk allows the medical assistant to choose the most appropriate form letter, modify it to the specific situation, personalize the address, salutation, and closing, and print it as an original document. All form letters can

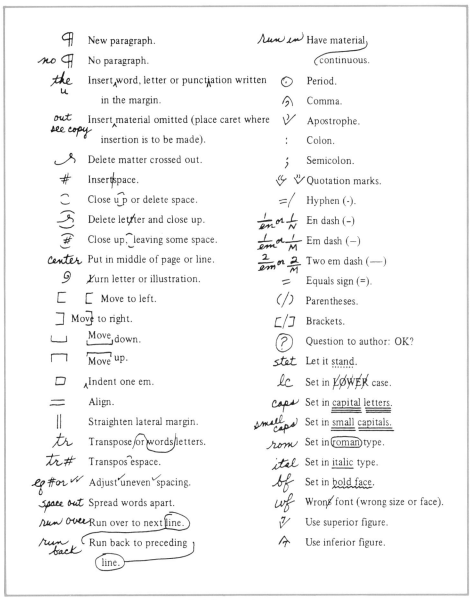

Figure 8-11. Proofreader's marks.

be prepared electronically, removing the impersonal effect inherent in other methods (see Chapter 11).

ELECTRONIC FACSIMILE COMMUNICATIONS

The facsimile (fax) machine can transmit and receive written documents immediately. The machine, called the *transceiver,* is usually a compact desktop digital unit used with public-switched telephone networks. Newer computers may also be equipped internally with fax capabilities. Documents can be immediately transmitted from one fax location to another by entering the recipient's full telephone number on the keypad of the machine. The cost of each local or long-distance trans-

mission is usually the same as that of a local or long-distance telephone call.

Document reception can be automatic or manual. If one telephone line (called a "dedicated" line) services the fax unit only, the unit automatically receives the fax transmission. The machine is programmed to answer after a set number of rings and can then receive documents. However, if a fax machine and a standard (voice) telephone share a line, a fax call must first be answered, as if to start a conversation. When the fax tone is heard, the machine must be manually started and the telephone handset hung up.

The use of the fax machine requires additional precautions to prevent the risk of unauthorized disclosure. The American Health Information Management Association (AHIMA, formerly the American Medical Records

Robert P. Green, M.D.
843 Cherry Street
Erie, PA 16503
(814) 456-1212

To:

It has been _____ months since your last physical examination.
Please call the office to make an appointment at your earliest convenience.

Sincerely,

R. P. Green, M.D.

Figure 8–12. A sample fill-in form letter.

Association) recommends that each facility use written policies for faxing patient information.

Access to patient information by unauthorized persons must be prevented. Except in emergency situations, AHIMA recommends obtaining a signed patient authorization to release records for *each* transmission. Whenever possible, original medical information should be used, or photocopies should be mail delivered. Instructions for faxing clinical data should specify whether the faxed material is to be destroyed after use or returned to the sender. AHIMA recommends faxing patient information only to other medical facilities. Faxing information to insurance companies and other nonmedical facilities is not recommended.

Fax documents are sent and received without confidential cover, such as is available when a sealed envelope is used. The machine should be placed in an area that is inaccessible to unauthorized users, and access should be restricted to one or a few authorized users. Faxed data should not be allowed to sit in the paper tray unattended. Anyone faxing documents should include a cover page with a "receipt of information verification" statement. The recipient should be called before the transmission begins to verify that the recipient will be present and to request the return "receipt."

A facility correspondence log should record each transmission sent or received. The original cover sheet is kept in the patient's file as a record of faxed data. If a fax transmission fails to reach the recipient, the recipient's fax telephone number should be checked against the telephone number on the internal logging system of the machine. If the fax was misdirected, a request should be faxed to the wrong number asking that the documents just received be destroyed. A misdirected fax incident report should be completed for permanent record.

Documents received should be immediately removed from the tray. The number of pages should be counted and compared with the number of pages noted as sent on the cover sheet. The faxed document is then sealed in an envelope and delivered to the intended recipient.

Because the medical record is a legal document and the official record of patient care, fax documents should be accepted and used only if they are clear, complete, accurate, and received in a timely manner. Because thermal fax paper deteriorates, retained records should be photocopied and the photocopy filed in the medical record. Faxed medication and treatment data orders must be signed by the physician before transmission, and then countersigned at a later date if the fax document is retained in the medical record.

Facsimile capability has revolutionized the way businesses communicate with one another. In medical practices, patient diagnostic reports can be received and filed the day the reports are prepared. Authorizations and medical records can be transmitted to help physicians make immediate decisions concerning a patient's emergency treatment. As the popular acceptance and use of fax communication spreads, equipment prices will go down and the cost advantage of faxing over forms of rapid mail delivery, such as overnight express, will become ever greater.

PROCESSING THE MAIL

Mail processing refers to sorting and routing incoming mail and selecting the method of delivery for outgoing mail. The role of the medical assistant is to supervise, develop, and improve the system for the efficient and effective management of this process.

Once a letter is written, the medical assistant must determine the method of mailing. Several mailing alternatives are available. The selection of an appropriate method depends on the type of mailing, necessity for proof of mailing, constraints of time, cost, availability of equipment such as postage meters, and often the physician's preference.

POSTAGE AND DELIVERY OF OUTGOING MAIL

The medical assistant is usually expected to be the office resource person for matters of postage and delivery and is often asked questions such as "What is the fastest way to get it there?" or "How much will it cost?" The business of postage and delivery is competitive and dynamic. Therefore, it is important for the medical assistant to stay current regarding delivery policy and cost, including federal postal services and rates, and those of private competitors such as Federal Express and United Parcel Service (UPS). A poster listing all services, rates, and descriptions is available from the post office and can be displayed in the office for quick reference. In addition, many cities have local companies that specialize in short-distance quick delivery. In an emergency, local courier companies and messenger services offer fast delivery service to nearby destinations.

Postal Classes

Outgoing letters sent by the physician can be organized to facilitate expediency. The decision of which class to assign to the letter depends on the importance of the content and possible deadline restrictions.

1. *First class.* Any item, including large packages and odd-sized envelopes, may be sent first class. First class is what the term conveys — the post office's "first class." Most ordinary letters are sent first class. The envelope is sealed and the correct first-class postage is affixed. Typewritten reports are also designated first class. Other examples include postcards and handwritten letters and materials.
2. *Second class.* Newspapers, magazines, and journals registered at the post office are designated second-class mail. Special rates are charges for these items. Journals and magazines sent by the office are more expensive than those mailed by the publisher.
3. *Third class.* This classification includes books and catalogues of 24 or fewer bound pages, manuscript copy, identification cards, circulars and other printed materials, and all other matter weighing less than 8 ounces that is not sent first or second class. Special rates apply to bulk mailing, and the post office should be consulted.
4. *Fourth class.* This classification is reserved for all merchandise and materials not included in the other classifications, such as films and books of more than 24 pages. Because postal regulations vary, the post office should be consulted when questions arise. Handbooks that explain mailing procedures and list current rates are available from the post office on request.
5. *Combination mail.* Combination mailing is used for letters or reports attached to items such as x-rays, which are mailed third class. The letter has a higher class designation and is mailed in combination with the lower-classed mail (the x-rays). When the report or letter is attached in this manner, it must have its own postage, address, and return address and must be marked "First Class" or "Letter Enclosed." The letter can also be enclosed in the package with both the first and third class postage appearing on the outside of the package and the outside marked "First Class Mail Enclosed."

Express and Priority Mail

The US Postal Service offers a quick delivery service, available 7 days a week for packages up to 70 pounds, called Express Mail. Next-day delivery and insurance (up to a specified value; check with the Post Office) are included in the fee for this service. The Postal Service also offers Priority Mail, described as "second-day service between all major business markets and three days everywhere else." The basic rate for Priority Mail, which covers packages weighing up to 2 pounds or as much material as can fit into a "flat-rate envelope," was about $3.00 in 1994. Larger packages can be sent by Priority Mail, at higher rates according to weight. Private companies, such as Federal Express, UPS, and DHL, also offer priority overnight (delivery next business morning), standard overnight (delivery next business afternoon), economy two-day, and special freight services. DHL offers the above services with the exception of the economy "second day delivery."

Insurance

It is possible to insure any piece of domestic mail for a nominal cost. The post office offers a standard fee schedule and an additional registry system for maximum security. In addition, privately owned competitors, such as UPS, offer this service. Some carriers automatically insure up to a certain amount, but may require specific wrapping requirements for breakable items to be eligible for damage claims.

Protective Designations

The US Postal Service offers several services designed to protect mailed materials. Three of these services — certificate of mailing, certified mail and registered mail — provide additional security. A *certificate of mailing* proves that an item was mailed. It does not provide proof of receipt or insurance coverage for loss of damage. A certificate of mailing is useful when it is necessary to prove that a document was mailed within a specific period or before a stated deadline. *Certified mail* provides a mailing receipt, and a record of delivery is kept at the recipient's post office. A return receipt to provide the sender with a record of delivery can be purchased for an additional fee. Certified mail is most often used to ensure that patients have received bills, or that important documents, medical reports, manuscripts, or x-rays have gone to the proper authorities. *Registered mail* is the most secure service offered by the post office. Registered mail provides insurance coverage for valuable items and is controlled from the point of mailing to the point of delivery. This service should be reserved for mailing items of tangible value, such as gifts or items that can be replaced in case of loss or damage. Postal insurance may be purchased on registered mail up to $25,000.

Return receipt service is also available when a package is sent express mail or cash on delivery, or is insured for at least $50. The return receipt is the sender's proof of delivery and includes the signature of the recipient and the date received. Except when sending express mail, the sender using return receipt service may request *restricted delivery.* Restricted delivery is made only to the addressee rather than to a company or to someone authorized in writing to receive mail for the addressee.

Preparing for Optical Scanning

The post office has developed universal systems for scanning mail optically. The post office scanners automatically read envelopes and sort them according to geographic designation. Optically scanned mail is delivered more efficiently. The post office has issued guidelines for typing both addresses and return addresses on envelopes in preparation for optical scanning. The medical assistant must follow these guidelines (Fig. 8–13).

1. The first line of the three-line name and address must be typed at least 2 inches from the top of the envelope. This requirement applies to No. 10 and No. 7 envelopes. Nothing should be typed on the bottom 5/8 inch of the envelope.

Left and right margins should be at least 1/2 inch. Addresses should not exceed four lines.
2. Everything in the address is capitalized and all punctuation is eliminated.
3. Room, suite, apartment, and building numbers are typed immediately after and on the same line as the street address.
4. On the third or fourth line of the address, which contains the city, state, and zip code, the city should not be abbreviated unless using the full name would expand the last line to more than 26 spaces.
5. A standard two-letter code is used to abbreviate the names of the states; for example: PA (Pennsylvania); SD (South Dakota). No punctuation is permitted. The list of standard abbreviations for cities is available from the post office.

Enclosures

The medical assistant is expected to insert documents and other materials neatly and properly into mailing envelopes. As was mentioned, the letter should always indicate any enclosures. Letters are inserted with all pages properly folded. Standard and monarch stationery are folded in thirds starting from the bottom and inserted in the appropriate size envelope from the bottom up. To insert a standard (8½ by 11) paper into a

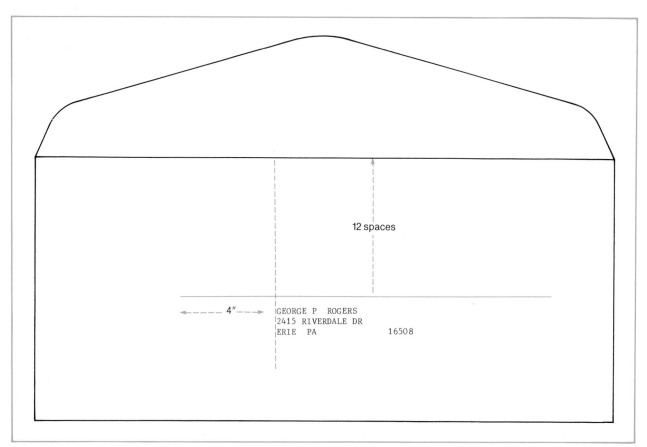

Figure 8–13. The optical scanning layout.

smaller envelope, fold first in half (top to bottom) and then in thirds.

Nonstandard items can be enclosed in various envelopes or boxes. If the office keeps using a particular size, it may be useful to ask a packaging salesperson or office supply house for advice regarding the best type and price of packaging for special needs. Packages containing breakable items are marked "Fragile." Items enclosed in envelopes that should remain flat are marked "Do Not Bend."

Many medical offices use the services of large testing laboratories for analysis of patient samples. These laboratories usually have containers specifically designed for mailing these samples. X-rays sent in the mail must receive special packaging attention to avoid damage en route. Stiff cardboard backing is usually placed alongside the x-ray in the mailing envelope. The envelope is marked "Do Not Bend" above the address, on the reverse side, and below the stamp. Special x-ray mailing envelopes may be purchased from x-ray supply companies.

Confidential Mail

Certain items are so sensitive that the physician may not want them to be opened by assistants en route to the final receiver. In such cases it is appropriate to stamp or type "Confidential" or "Personal" on the front and to the left of the address on the envelope.

The procedure related to preparing outgoing correspondence for mailing is included at the end of this chapter.

INCOMING MAIL

The first concern in handling incoming mail is sorting. Sorting can be categorized according to the action required. A general sorting guide is to open the mail in the following order, when possible:

1. Special delivery letters (mailgrams)
2. Patient payments (checks from patients or insurance companies)
3. First class mail
4. Periodicals and newspapers
5. All other materials, such as drug samples

The medical assistant assumes the responsibility of opening all mail and directing it to the addressee unless it is addressed to the physician and marked "Personal" or "Confidential." The medical assistant must assemble a letter opener, paper clips, a stapler, transparent tape, and a date stamp before opening the mail. Envelopes should be stacked facing the same direction and opened as follows:

1. Pick up a corner of the envelope and tap the outer top edge with your fingertips to avoid damaging the contents when using a letter opener.
2. Slide the letter opener along the top edge. Open all envelopes.

3. Remove the contents of the envelopes. Envelopes can be discarded if the return address appears on the letter.
4. Using a date stamp, stamp the date received in the upper right corner of the letter.
5. Check for enclosures, and staple or clip them to the letter. Read the letter to check for the word "Enclosure." If it is missing, note this on the letter.
6. Sort according to response required: letters the physician handles and those the medical assistant handles.
7. Payments are recorded immediately in the day's receipts.
8. Insurance forms are placed in a particular place for later attention.
9. Drug samples are placed in a designated area in the drug cabinet.

The physician's preferences help to determine the mail-handling process. However, certain types of mail are routinely handled by the medical assistant or the physician.

1. Mail not requiring the physician's attention and handled by the medical assistant. This category refers to mail addressed to the medical assistant directly, and to certain mail addressed to the physician, such as advertisements for office supplies, payments for office visits, and so forth. Complete mail handling by the medical assistant consists of opening, reading, and following through appropriately. Once the mail is identified as appropriate for the medical assistant to open, the action taken is recorded on the letter itself in the form of a notation above the date. If a letter is opened by error, write "Opened in Error" across the envelope and initial it.
2. Mail that requires the physician's attention. Mail that requires the physician's attention can be sorted by the medical assistant. Examples of such mail include all mail pertaining to patient diagnosis and treatment; mail from hospital officials regarding policy, procedures, notices of business meetings, and requests for consultation; and letters pertaining to legal matters. Letters relating to patients are attached to the patient record and placed with the other mail on the physician's desk. Using the patient record as reference, the physician can more effectively and efficiently interpret and respond to the mail.

Please refer to the procedure *Sort and Open Incoming Mail* at the end of this chapter for the summary of steps required in organizing and processing incoming mail.

Annotation

Annotation is the term applied to identifying and isolating the key points in a letter. It saves the physician's time and prevents valuable information from being overlooked. Annotation involves underlining important words or phrases and writing notes in the margin. Not all letters require annotation. For instance, mailings pertaining to the patient record and discussing diagnosis and treatment are not annotated. The physician reads these letters in their entirety. It is usually appropriate to annotate notices of business meetings and other business-related mail. Also, letters and documents that are to become a permanent part of the patient record should not be annotated. Discretionary judgment regarding which letters may be annotated develops with experience. Consulting with the physician to learn his or her preference in mail handling and annotation is recommended. When in doubt, the medical assistant should not annotate.

Figure 8–14 illustrates an incoming letter and its annotation by a medical assistant, using the principles and procedures (Annotate Incoming Mail) described at the end of this chapter.

Establishing Priorities for Incoming Mail

Proper handling of incoming mail requires deciding the order of informational importance and the immediate form of action required:

1. *Most important.* This mail should be brought to the physician's attention daily and should be placed on top of the stack. Personal letters, of course, would take precedence. Other types of mail requiring the physician's daily attention include results of laboratory tests and letters from other physicians regarding patient management.
2. *Potentially important.* Some correspondence addressed to the physician may be of potential

---

January 20, 1993

Adam Williams, M.D.
110 Perry Square
Townsville, PA 14502

Dear Dr. Williams:

    As you know, the AMA is preparing for its next convention. We are recruiting guest lecturers and workshop facilitators. You were referred to our office by Dr. Paul Brown as an expert in the field of gerontological medicine. We invite you to submit a proposal for a workshop. Please send an outline and other materials that would assist the committee in their determination of the compatibility of your work with our intent. Enclosed please find information describing the workshop sessions. Contact our office if we can be of further assistance. We look forward with great anticipation to your response and are hopeful that you will join us as a workshop facilitator.

    Sincerely,

    John Adams, M.D.
    Director of Continuing Education
    American Medical Association

JA/mf
Enclosure

A

Figure 8–14. (**A**) A sample letter of the type commonly received in a medical office. (**B**) The same letter, annotated by the medical assistant.

usefulness, but not of immediate concern. Journals and notifications of meetings can be delivered to the physician less frequently and stacked below the items of most importance.

3. *Unimportant.* Mail such as supply catalogs, descriptions of new products, and other miscellaneous items can be disposed of, or if potential use is anticipated, placed in a designated area for future reference.

The medical assistant can handle incoming mail effectively and efficiently developing an organizational system such as the one described in this section.

Forwarding Mail

The physician planning an extended absence may ask that critical items be forwarded for review. It is possible to either collect several days' correspondence before mailing or forward mail daily. If the physician has not requested daily forwarding, the medical assistant should be alert for important documents and consider forwarding them immediately. Special postage designations should be selected for mail forwarding to ensure the safe and timely receipt of all documents.

SPECIAL MAIL-HANDLING SITUATIONS

Certain mailing situations require special handling procedures. They are listed below.

Requesting address correction. When it is necessary to obtain a new address, "Address Correction Requested" should be written under the return address. The post office charges a small fee for the service in the form of a postage due stamp. The post office will forward first class mail to the new address and send a card with the

---

Rec. Jan 29th

January 20, 1993

Adam Williams, M.D.
110 Perry Square
Townsville, PA 14502

Note: dates on brochure conflict with your scheduled vacation time.

Dear Dr. Williams:

Re: As you know, the AMA is preparing for its next convention. We are recruiting guest lecturers and workshop facilitators. You were referred to our office by Dr. Paul Brown as an expert in the field of gerontological medicine. We invite you to submit a proposal for a workshop. Please send an outline and other materials that would assist the committee in their determination of the compatibility of your work with our intent. Enclosed please find information describing the workshop sessions. Contact our office if we can be of further assistance. We look forward with great anticipation to your response and are hopeful that you will join us as a workshop facilitator.

Sincerely,

John Adams, M.D.
Director of Continuing Education
American Medical Association

JA/mf
Enclosure

B

Figure 8–14. *Continued.*

postage due stamps and the new address to the sender.

Recalling mail. If for any reason it is necessary to recall the mail and stop its route to the addressee, the sender must file a written application with a copy of the envelope addressed identically to the one being recalled. When the mail has already left the local post office, the local postmaster can attempt to recall letters at the sender's expense. The postmaster telegraphs the postmaster at the letter's destination and requests its return.

Tracing lost mail. Mail can be traced more efficiently when a receipt of delivery is issued. If the receipt has not been acknowledged after a reasonable length of time, the post office is notified and a trace requested. First class mail can be traced, but the attempt is less likely to be successful. A special written form available at the post office may be required for tracing letters and packages.

TRANSCRIPTION

The transcription or typing of medical reports, chart notes, and letters is an important part of the daily routine in the physician's office. These documents assist the physician in coordinating patient care. They contribute to office efficiency and provide an invaluable support system for the physician.

Medical documents are vital to patient treatment and must be handled with care and skill. The result of poorly produced transcription is an incomplete, misleading, and possibly erroneous medical record. Patient care can be jeopardized and communication disrupted. Therefore it is imperative that the medical assistant become a proficient transcriptionist. Like all medical records, the physician's dictation is an extremely important part of the patient's permanent record. Because all medical documents are confidential, dictation should be transcribed promptly. The transcribed report should be complete, accurate in all details, readily accessible, and systematically organized.

The following is a list of the most commonly transcribed medical documents.

1. *Letters.* Written correspondence provides communication with other physicians and members of the patient's health care team and can convey important information to the patient. In addition, the physician may dictate personal letters to be transcribed.
2. *History and physical examination report.* The history and physical examination report is a detailed record of the patient's present and past medical history, with the findings of the physical examination. It may include laboratory data, an impression or diagnosis, and a plan for treatment. It is usually dictated after a new patient's initial office visit or as part of a consultation.

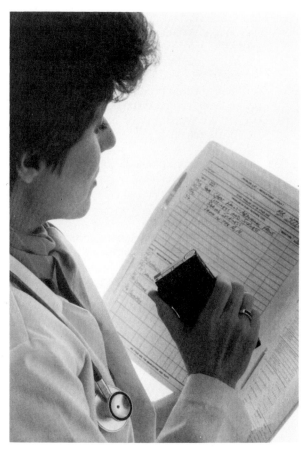

Many physicians prefer to dictate notes for the patient's chart. (Courtesy of Harris Lawes Business Products.)

3. *Chart notes.* Each office visit must be recorded in the patient's chart. Many physicians prefer to dictate information about current medical problems, findings, and treatment.
4. Consultation. A consultation occurs after a patient has been seen and examined at the request of a referring physician. The physician dictates a detailed report consisting of history, physical examination findings, laboratory data, impression or diagnosis, and other relevant information. The transcribed report is then sent to the referring physician.

TRANSCRIBING THE REPORT

After dictation is completed, the physician wraps an accompanying paper indicator strip around the cassette or places the cassette in a preprinted envelope (Fig. 8–15) and completes the dictation date and topics. The cassette is then given to the transcriptionist.

A tape should contain dictation from only one date. The oldest dictation should be transcribed first and the most recent dictation last. An exception to this rule is a *stat*, or priority, report, which must be transcribed immediately. The *stat* report takes priority over other work. The transcriptionist locates and transcribes the

Date of Dictation		Stat	Chart	Letter	Consult	☐ Side A
Dictating Physician						☐ Side B

Patient/Topic
1. _____
2. _____
3. _____
4. _____
5. _____
6. _____
7. _____
8. _____
9. _____
10. _____

☐ Stat reports only completed   Date _____
☐ Tape partially done including Patient # _____ Date _____
☐ Tape completed, reports awaiting doctor's review
☐ All reports transcribed and reviewed.   Tape may be erased.

Figure 8–15. *Sample preprinted envelope for an audiocassette with dictation.*

priority report, then returns the cassette to its original place according to the date dictated.

Confusion can arise when more than one person performs transcription. A system should be developed that readily indicates the transcription status of each cassette. It may be helpful to use preprinted envelopes to store the cassettes until transcription is completed. As each item is transcribed, a notation is made in the box provided on the envelope.

Sometimes the medical assistant may encounter words or phrases that cannot be understood or located in reference books. If the dictating physician is unavailable to supply the needed information, a blank space is left in the report. The size of the blank should be roughly based on the estimated number of syllables in the unclear word. A small colored slip of paper can be clipped to the report with a notation of where the missing word occurred and what it sounded like. The cassette tape containing that report should not be erased until all blanks in the report have been completed. All blanks should be filled in before the physician signs the report.

When the report has been transcribed completely, the cassette tape can be erased and returned to the physician for re-use.

HISTORY AND PHYSICAL EXAMINATION REPORTS

Various formats are acceptable for transcribing history and physical examination reports. Some involve extensive tabulation to line up the headings and the body of the report. The simplest format for transcription, however, is the run-on format, which follows a simple paragraph style without indentation or tabulation (Fig. 8–16). Every history and physical examination report requires a physician's signature.

CONSULTATION REPORTS

The format for a consultation report is determined by the dictating physician and falls into one of two basic categories. The report can be addressed to the referring physician in a letter with the necessary information included in the body of the letter. It also can be dictated in the form of a history and physical examination report with an accompanying cover letter. A physician's signature is required at the end of every consultation report.

CHART NOTES

Two basic formats are used in transcribing chart notes. The *present illness format* uses the same categories as the history and physical examination report, but in abbreviated form: *chief complaint* becomes *CC*, *history of present illness* becomes *HPI*, and so forth. Figure 8–17 illustrates this chart note format.

The second format is a SOAP note. Figure 8–18 is an example of a SOAP note, the problem-oriented system abbreviation for *S*ubjective, *O*bjective, *A*ssessment, and *P* components of a progress note (see Chapter 16).

Initials should be typed and signed below each entry added to the patient's chart regardless of the format used. The physician's initials in capital letters are followed by a slash and then by the medical assistant's initials in lowercase letters. The medical assistant must initial in ink next to the typed initials. The physician, after reviewing the transcribed report for completeness and accuracy, should also initial in ink next to the typed initials (Fig. 8–19). If the chart entry is inserted by the medical assistant (e.g., a notation that an insurance

HISTORY AND PHYSICAL REPORT

SMITH, JULIENNE ANN   DATE: 4-10-93

CHIEF COMPLAINT: "Chest pain while I am resting."

HISTORY OF PRESENT ILLNESS: The patient is a 60-year-old white female with a long history of hypertension and a previous inferior wall myocardial infarction. She has experienced exertional angina and one-block claudication since then. Most recently, symptoms have increased to include chest pain at rest for which she takes nitroglycerin 1/150 gm one tablet sublingually p.r.n. for pain. She needs to be evaluated for this unstable angina.

PAST MEDICAL HISTORY: The patient had a cholecystectomy in 1975 and an MI, as mentioned above, in 1983. She had the usual childhood diseases without sequelae. She had 3 normal spontaneous vaginal deliveries followed by a total abdominal hysterectomy in 1969 for uterine fibroids. She has an allergy to SULFA drugs.

SOCIAL HISTORY: The patient is a widow, living with the oldest of her 3 daughters in Maryland. She denies tobacco use. She is a social drinker.

FAMILY HISTORY: The patient's father died of a myocardial infarction at the age of 65. The patient's mother died of uterine cancer. All children are living and well. The patient has no siblings.

REVIEW OF SYSTEMS: Negative, except as mentioned in History of Present Illness.

PHYSICAL EXAMINATION: The patient is a well-developed, well-nourished, white female in no acute distress. The vital signs were stable with blood pressure of 150/100. HEENT exam was within normal limits. The lungs revealed bibasilar rales. Cardiac exam revealed a normal S1 and S2 with a Grade 2/6 systolic murmur. The extremities showed pitting edema of the feet. Cranial nerves II–XII were intact.

PLAN: Mrs. Smith's hypertension is not under control at the present time, and I am increasing her diuretic to Lasix 80 mg 1 PO q.i.d. and placing her on potassium supplementation. I am also recommending that she be scheduled to undergo a cardiac catheterization some time in the near future. In the meantime, she will continue to take her nitroglycerin on a p.r.n. basis.

_____
Alfred P. Daniels, M.D.

APD: smt

Figure 8–16. *Example of a medical history and physical examination report, in the run-on format.*

FLANAGAN, Michael   Age 82
3-17-93

CC: Shortness of breath, insomnia, weakness
HPI: Dyspnea on exertion for last 2–3 days
PE: BP 150/100. Cardiac exam reveals systolic murmur
DX: Congestive heart failure
Plan: 1.   Admit to hospital
       2.   Sodium-restricted diet and diuretic   JLT/st

Figure 8–17. *Example of a chart note in the HPI format.*

FLANAGAN, Michael   Age 82
3/17/93

S: Complaining of shortness of breath, insomnia, weakness. History of dyspnea on exertion for the last 2–3 days.
O: BP 150/100. Cardiac exam revealed systolic murmur.
A: Congestive heart failure.
P: 1.   Admit to hospital.
      2.   Sodium restricted diet and a diuretic.

James L. Triecher
James L. Triecher, M.D.

JLT/st

Figure 8–18. Example of a chart note in the SOAP format.

form was sent), only the typed and signed initials of the medical assistant need appear.

Chart notes may be typed verbatim, or the physician may instruct the medical assistant to condense each note to conserve space in the patient's chart. Narrow margins (1/2 by 1 inch) are commonly used for chart entries. Phrases rather than complete sentences are commonly used. These are examples of how a chart note can be condensed.

THE PHYSICIAN SAYS:

This is a chart note on Grace Stoffer. She is a 47-year-old woman who came into the office today, June 10, 1993, complaining of rectal bleeding, which has been intermittent for the past 2 months. The patient states that she has bright red blood after a bowel movement. She says she has lost 15 pounds.

YOU TYPE:

STOUFFER, Grace   Age 47

6/10/93

HPI: Rectal bleeding, intermittent for past 2 mo. Bright red blood after BMS. Has lost 15 lb. JKL/ST

THE PHYSICIAN SAYS:

Today's date is February 22, 1993, and this is a chart note on Norman Richards, a 14-year-old white male, who came in today with a history of a yellow discharge in the right ear and a sore throat for the past 2 days. The physical exam showed his tonsils to be inflamed and there was purulent material on the tympanic membrane of his right ear. The diagnosis was tonsillitis and otitis externa. I have given him a prescription for erythromycin 400 milligrams every 4 hours. I will see him back in 1 week. Thank you. End of dictation.

YOU TYPE:

RICHARDS, Norman   Age 14   Race: Caucasian

2-22-93

HPI: Yellow discharge A.D., sore throat $\times$ 2 days.

PE: Tonsils inflamed. Purulent material on TM of A.D.

DX: Tonsillitis and otitis externa.

RX: Erythromycin 400 mg q4h.

PLAN: Return visit in 1 wk. JKL/ST

10/7/93   Pt. scheduled for cyst removal at Bay County General on 10/7/93   ST

Figure 8–19. Example of a chart note entry, initialed by the dictating physician.

Chart notes, although condensed and containing many abbreviations, are an essential part of the medical record. As such, they require as much attention to detail as any formal report or letter.

DEALING WITH TRANSCRIPTION VARIABLES

The medical assistant must be able to transcribe every type of report or letter encountered, and to understand different voices, pronunciations, and dictation speeds. Once the report type has been identified and the proper format selected, the medical assistant can begin transcribing.

As the medical assistant listens to the dictation, some of the words or phrases in the report may not be distinct. The physician dictating may have a foreign accent, the tape may contain too much static, or the physician may be speaking too quickly. In each case the medical assistant must evaluate the problem and find a solution so that the report can be accurately transcribed. This type of problem solving is an important skill for the medical assistant to learn. Each physician and each report present unique challenges and variables. The medical assistant must be able to identify the problem and quickly effect a solution.

Table 8–1 lists some problems the medical assistant may encounter with dictation and provides some suggested solutions.

PROOFREADING

No discussion of transcription can be complete without mention of the essential skill of proofreading. Of all the transcriptionist's skills, proofreading, or checking for accuracy, may be the most important. Although a rapid transcribing speed is desirable, an error-filled report is useless. The rule to follow is "Accuracy first, speed second." Although speed is important, a report that requires much correction time is, in the end, not cost effective. The medical assistant should strive for both accuracy and speed.

USING MEDICAL REFERENCE MATERIALS

The scope of medical transcription encompasses far more than the medical assistant can learn in any introductory course in medical terminology. Because new and unfamiliar words are encountered daily in transcription, reference resources are essential.

Well-worn, well-marked reference books are the sign of a knowledgeable and competent transcriptionist. A current English language dictionary (Webster's, American Heritage, Random House, etc.) and style and grammar books are obviously essential references. However, the vast and constantly changing field of medicine requires additional references dealing with terminology specific to medicine and its specialty areas.

Following is a listing of quality reference books:

I. General medical dictionaries and word guides

Table 8–1

DICTATION PROBLEMS AND THEIR SOLUTIONS

Problem	Solution
Unfamiliar word heard in dictation	Consult reference books for correct word identification and spelling.
Garbled word; cannot be found in reference book	Increase or decrease speed control on the transcriber and listen to the word again.
	Redirect the audio signal to the speaker and listen again.
	Ask another person to listen to tape.
	Leave a blank and continue transcribing. Listen for same word to be repeated.
Dictator speaks too rapidly, running words and phrases together.	Use the speed control on the transcriber to decrease dictation speed.
	Phonetically write out the phrases that are slurred together; separate the syllables to try to form words.
Words are mumbled, as if dictated from a distance.	Increase the tone control on the transcriber.
	Clean the recording heads in the transcriber with a special cassette tape made for this purpose.
Static obscures dictator's words.	Decrease the tone control on the transcriber.
Dictator is speaking with a foreign accent; cannot be understood.	Obtain a copy of a similar report dictated by the same physician; compare words and phrases.
	Identify the dictator's accent and English words that cause trouble, then substitute the correct sound to help identify the word. *Examples:*
	"Weins" becomes "veins";
	"History of pleasant illness" becomes "History of present illness";
	"No acoo deestriss" becomes "No acute distress";
	"Piscal exam" becomes "Physical exam."

A. Alphabetic listing
Dorland's Illustrated Medical Dictionary, edition 27. WB Saunders, Philadelphia, 1988.
Stedman's Medical Dictionary, edition 25, Williams & Wilkins, Baltimore, 1990.
Thomas CL (ed): *Taber's Cyclopedic Medical Dictionary*, ed 17. FA Davis, Philadelphia, 1993.
B. Listing according to medical specialties
Sloan SB: *The Medical Word Book: A Spelling and Vocabulary Guide to Medical Transcription*, edition 3. WB Saunders, Philadelphia, 1991.
C. Terms not included in other sources
Pyle V: *Current Medical Terminology*. Prima Vera Publications, Modesto, CA, 1988.
Willey J: *Glossary of Medical Terminology for the Health Professions*. Slack, Thorofare, NJ, 1988.
II. Drug reference books
A. Listing by both generic and brand or trade name
Billups NF: *American Drug Index*. JB Lippincott, Philadelphia (annual publication).
DeLorenzo B: *Pharmaceutical Terminology*. Slack, Thorofare, NJ, 1988.
B. Several listing formats
Physicians' Desk Reference, edition 40. Medical Economics Company, Oradell, NJ (annual publication)
1. White pages — by trade or brand name
2. Yellow pages — by generic name
3. Pink pages — by drug category
III. Style and grammar reference books
Diehl MO and Fordney MT: *Medical Transcription Guide Dos and Don'ts*. Philadelphia, WB Saunders, 1990.
Diehl MO and Fordney MT: *Medical Typing and Transcribing Techniques and Procedures*, edition 3. WB Saunders, Philadelphia, 1991.
Tessier D and Pitman SC: *Style Guide for Medical Transcription*. American Association for Medical Transcription, Modesto, CA, 1985.

USING DRUG REFERENCE RESOURCES

Drug reference books are an invaluable aid to the transcriptionist. It should be noted that very new drugs, most nonprescription drugs, and experimental drugs still pending approval by the FDA will not be listed. A *current* drug reference should be available in the office so the majority of new and common drugs can be easily referenced.

Drugs are listed either by generic name or by brand or trade name. The first letter of a generic name drug is not capitalized, but the first letter of a brand or trade name drug is always capitalized. A single drug may have several brand names, as each is produced by a different manufacturer.

The medical assistant should *never* guess at the spelling when typing the names of drugs. Incorrectly

spelled drug names can confuse and possibly harm the patient if one drug is mistakenly prescribed for another. Continued medical treatment depends on accurate notation of drugs previously prescribed.

Many drug names sound alike. The following examples illustrate how easily one drug can be mistaken for another:

Imuran (a chemotherapeutic agent)
Enduron (a diuretic and antihypertensive agent)
Orinase (an oral antidiabetic agent)

When unsure of the spelling of any drug, the medical assistant should look it up in a drug reference book and read the accompanying indications for use to see if it fits the medical context of the dictation.

HELPFUL HINTS FOR MEDICAL REFERENCE

When looking up the spelling of a medical word, the medical assistant should remember that many have Latin, Greek, or French origins that may make their pronunciation quite different from their spelling. Table 8–2 shows several examples.

Although the physician's office may have some reference texts, many transcriptionists prefer to build their own personal library of reference materials. When the reference books belong to the transcriptionist, new words can be added in the margin or circled in the text with colored ink, important pages can be dog-eared, and in general, the reference books can be personalized to facilitate quick word location. Also, if the medical assistant changes jobs, the library of personalized reference books can be taken to the new office.

In addition to using reference books, some transcriptionists find it helpful to compile a list of commonly used words or phrases that pertain to the medical specialty of the office. The list can be taped to a wall for quick reference. The spelling of all the words on the list must be checked and verified.

Some transcriptionists keep an alphabetical word notebook in which they list new words, words with difficult spellings, and so on. A small address book with tabbed pages for each alphabet letter works well for listing words.

Reference materials are an invaluable aid to the medical assistant who does transcription in the office. The

Table 8–2

PRONUNCIATION OF SOME MEDICAL TERMS

Term	Pronunciation	Derivation
Bruit	Brwe	French
Debridement	Day breed maw	French
Diverticula	Die ver tick u la	Latin
Xiphoid	Zif oid	Greek
Ptosis	Toe sis	Greek

transcriptionist must be responsible and use them frequently.

MANUSCRIPT PREPARATION

Perhaps more than other professionals, physicians in office practice are charged with the responsibility of sharing their learning experiences with their colleagues. Advances in the art and science of medicine are vitally important in competent medical care. Many physicians regularly prepare manuscripts that are usually submitted for journal, rather than book, publication or for presentation at a professional meeting.

The medical assistant may be required to help in preparing these manuscripts by proofreading for grammatical errors, offering editorial and stylistic support, and organizing and typing the work. A manuscript is a written draft of a paper for publication. It is a rough draft in that the organization and content of the work must be refined and revised. More than one draft is frequently necessary to produce a well-organized and well-written manuscript. To assist the physician with this process, the medical assistant must understand the style and format expectations for scientific manuscripts.

RESPONSIBILITIES

Obviously, the credibility of a research paper or report would be suspect if the writing quality, grammar, spelling, or punctuation were in any way deficient. Therefore, the medical assistant should examine the paper carefully for editorial integrity and make necessary corrections without changing meaning or content. Table 8–3 is a guide to medical writing abbreviations, and Figure 8–10 shows the commonly used proofreader's marks. In addition, the Appendix contains sev-

Table 8–3
MEDICAL WRITING ABBREVIATION GUIDE

Correct Form	Incorrect Form	Rule
Figure 11 illustrates . . .	Fig. 11 illustrates . . .	Avoid beginning a sentence with an abbreviation
The lesion (Fig. 11) was superficial.	The lesion (Figure 11) was superficial.	Words placed in parentheses may be abbreviated.
Fever, headache, and related signs were present.	Fever, headache, etc. were present.	Avoid use of "etc." in sentences and lists.
Smith and coworkers found that . . .	Smith et al. found that . . .	Avoid use of "et al." to indicate a group of persons except in listing references.
The test took 35 minutes.	The test took 35 min.	Spell out units of time unless they appear in parentheses or in tables.
Nearly 90 percent of the patients experienced relief.	Nearly 90% of the patients experienced relief.	Spell out "percent" unless it appears in parentheses or in tables.
General Medical Supply	Gen. Med. Supply	Avoid abbreviating company names unless the abbreviation *is* the official company name, such as CIBA; 3M Company; TRW; IBM.
Article IV, Section II	Art. IV, Sec. II	Laws and bylaws are written in full when referred to for the first time. Subsequently they may be abbreviated.
prn; GI; IV	p.r.n.; G.I.; I.V.	Current practice favors omission of periods in medical abbreviations.
Escherchia coli	*E. coli*	Names for microorganisms may be abbreviated only after a first reference in full.
Professor; General; Senator; Reverend	Prof.; Gen.; Sen.; Rev.	With the exception of Ms., Mrs., Mr., and Dr., full titles are used for business letter salutations. Titles may be abbreviated in envelope blocks and inside addresses.
JAMA; N. Engl. J. Med. (in references)	Journal of the American Medical Association; New England Journal of Medicine	Names of journals are abbreviated in reference lists, but are written in full in sentences. (Example: Nelson, M.A.: Intra-arterial blood pressure. N. Engl. J. Med. 303:35–56, 1982.)

eral useful references for manuscript preparation: punctuation patterns, medical abbreviations, common medical prefixes and suffixes, and a glossary of Latin medical words.

In proofreading a manuscript, consistency of markings is important even if original rather than standard proofreading marks are used.

ORGANIZING THE MANUSCRIPT

The author of a manuscript usually proceeds through a series of written drafts before submitting the final draft for publication.

Each draft is typed to allow the author to visualize the corrected text and make further modifications. The written draft process is actually a refinement process. With each draft, the writing style, content, grammar, word usage, and other related writing characteristics are evaluated and improved.

To facilitate the reading of each draft, the draft is typed, using double-spacing. Some authors prefer different-colored typing paper to distinguish between the first, second, third, and final drafts. The final draft will be organized and typed according to specific guidelines set forth in a manuscript guide published by the journal or book company that has solicited the manuscript.

TYPING THE MANUSCRIPT

General directions for typing the manuscript are as follows:

1. Use a word processor if possible. Corrections are easily made and proofreading is facilitated by screen projection.
2. Use good-quality white bond 8½- by 11-inch paper.
3. Use double-spacing throughout the manuscript, including the abstract, references, and other sections.
4. Number the pages consecutively beginning with the title page (using arabic numerals), and place the number in the right corner (top or bottom) of each page.
5. Type the beginning of each section on a separate page.
6. Type on one side of the paper only.
7. Leave margins of 1 to 1½ inches at the top, bottom, and sides.
8. Avoid hyphenating words at the ends of lines.
9. Indent the beginning line of each paragraph five spaces.
10. Type the title on the first page in capital letters. However, use the capitalization style preferred by the journal for headings and subheadings.
11. Make photocopies.
12. Send the number of required copies to the journal. Retain several complete copies in the office file.

REPRINTS

The physician-author may have received, through previous publication, requests for reprints (printed copies of an article) and letters of interest. The medical assistant files the names of interested individuals and automatically sends them reprints from subsequent articles. A special enclosure card is attached to the reprint. Other physician-authors may prefer to write a short letter or simply write "With the Author's Compliments" on the envelope.

ASSISTING THE PHYSICIAN IN PREPARATION FOR ORAL PRESENTATIONS AND MEETINGS

PREPARING MANUSCRIPTS FOR ORAL PRESENTATION

Not all of the physician's writing is intended for publication. The physician may lecture, give speeches, or present addresses at conferences. The medical assistant proofreads and types these papers using many of the manuscript preparation guidelines. Papers for oral presentation are double spaced and typed in large type when it is available, or in capital letters if they are preferred. Word processors have several type styles (fonts) available.

Usually the physician has time restrictions for the delivery of the presentation, and the medical assistant may assist in timing the speech. For instance, the physician may be required to speak for 30 minutes. He or she may time the speech by reading it aloud. However, another method of approximating the time required is to count the number of typed pages on which 200 to 250 words appear. Each page can usually be read in approximately 2 minutes. If there are 20 pages each containing 200 words, 40 minutes would be required for presentation.

ORGANIZING MEETINGS

Selecting the Meeting Date and Time

The medical assistant's role in arranging for meetings and travel includes setting up meetings at the physician's request. The physician should inform the medical assistant of the purpose of the meeting, the names of the participants, and the desired date and time. The medical assistant must then consult the physician's office appointment book and the meeting and travel calendar.

To manage the physician's schedule, the medical assistant should write the physician's meeting and travel appointments on a calendar designed solely for this purpose. This calendar should duplicate the physician's own meeting and travel calendar and should include the following information:

❏ Date
❏ Title or purpose of the meeting
❏ Time
❏ Place

Changes must be made on both the medical assistant's and the physician's calendars.

The medical assistant then informs the physician of the available dates and times and learns the length of the meeting and the physician's preferences regarding the place. On selection of the appropriate date and time, the medical assistant then organizes the meeting.

Organizing the Meeting

If the physician initiates the meeting, the medical assistant may be responsible for organizing and coordinating it and must proceed through the following steps:

1. Reserve the selected meeting place, specifying the date, the time, and length of the meeting. Travel distance, ease of access, adequate interior space, adequate lighting and ventilation, and available parking facilities must all be considered. It may be necessary to visit the facility to verify the appropriateness of the accommodations.
2. Inform the participants of the meeting, specifying the date, the time, and the place. This step can be accomplished by telephone or correspondence (letter or postcard), depending on the nature of the meeting (small groups or conference) and the time available before the meeting date. Regardless of how the participants are informed, the medical assistant should request that they notify the office by an appointed date to confirm their attendance.
3. Prepare and type the agenda, and obtain other required materials, such as folders and handouts (reprints, budget sheets, etc.), at the physician's request.
4. Discuss with the physician the need for special equipment, such as slide and overhead projectors, writing supplies, microphones, podium, and blackboard.
5. Discuss with the physician the need for refreshments, meals, or other amenities.
6. Complete all arrangements a minimum of 2 weeks in advance of the meeting date.
7. Call the contact person at the selected meeting place to inquire about last-minute changes, such as room reservations, menu variations, and so forth.
8. Make the required travel arrangements for the physician according to his or her preference.

ARRANGING TRAVEL

The medical assistant may be responsible for organizing the physician's itinerary and arranging transportation and hotel accommodations.

In arranging transportation, the medical assistant usually enlists the services of a travel agent. The medical assistant usually uses a credit card account number to charge the tickets and requests that they be mailed to the office. Obviously, before transportation plans can be completed, the medical assistant must consult the physician. Generally the medical assistant considers the following factors in selecting transportation:

❏ Physician's preference (e.g., coach or first class airline travel)
❏ Cost
❏ Reliability
❏ Waiting periods (e.g., between flights)
❏ Potential weather problems
❏ Time schedule between arrival and attendance at meeting or conference
❏ Handling of baggage (weight requirements, carry-on luggage, etc.)

When arranging flight travel with the assistance of the travel agent, the medical assistant must be cautious in reserving flights that cannot be canceled and refunded. Also, in discussing transportation alternatives with the travel agent, the medical assistant should inquire about special rates and discounts for specified reservation times, such as a month or several weeks in advance. The travel agent will reserve a rental car or limousine if one is requested. *The Official Airline Guide* (Rueben H. Donnelley Publications, 200 Clearwater Dr., Oak Brook, IL 60521) is a subscription magazine that provides updated information on flight schedules, fares, services, and car rentals.

The travel agent may obtain hotel accommodations, or the medical assistant may select the hotel and personally make the necessary arrangements. To become acquainted with the hotel accommodations available in a particular area, the medical assistant may use one of several options. If the physician is a member of a travel or auto club, the club's office can provide assistance and make recommendations. The physician may also have personal preferences. Another alternative is to refer to the *Hotel and Motel Red Book* (American Hotel Association Directory Corp., 888 Seventh Avenue, New York, NY 10019), which lists accommodations, rates, services, and telephone numbers. American Express also provides hotel reservation services. In the absence of such assistance, the medical assistant would telephone a local reputable chain hotel and ask for reservations in another city.

If time permits, the medical assistant should request written confirmation from the hotel to ensure room reservation. When making reservations, the reservation clerk should be advised of the physician's arrival time. The following physician preferences would be considered in obtaining accommodations:

❏ Room size (one room or a suite)
❏ Number of persons
❏ Special features (exercise facilities etc.)

- Access or distance to meeting place, restaurants, golf courses, and so forth
- Cost range

Available hotel reservation selections should be discussed with the physician before the arrangements are completed.

Foreign Travel

Foreign travel requires planning months before the departure date because, in addition to transportation and hotel accommodations, the physician must obtain a passport. Passport applications are available from post offices, passport offices (in several US cities), or from travel agents. Photographs (two identical color or black and white front views, 2½ square inches) are required and must accompany the application. It is required that all individuals applying for passport privileges appear in person. The current passport can be renewed by mail if it has been obtained within the last 8 years.

The physician may request that the medical assistant learn what is needed in addition to the passport to travel in a particular country. Some countries require a visa, which is written permission or endorsement on the passport by appropriate authorities (the local consulate) indicating approval. Some countries also require a valid international certificate of vaccination. An international driving permit may be required. The medical assistant can contact a visa agency (located in Washington, DC and other major cities) for assistance in obtaining a passport and processing the visa.

The Itinerary

An itinerary is a typed list of completed travel plans in chronologic order (Fig. 8–20). The medical assistant retains a copy and gives the physician the original and copies for family members.

The itinerary should include

- Heading with name of physician, dates, and destination
- Detailed schedule for each day, including times, places, arrivals, and departures
- Addresses and telephone numbers of meeting place, hotels, car rental agencies, and so forth

The itinerary verifies travel arrangements. The medical assistant retains a copy in the office travel folder for necessary reference.

The Travel Folder

For future reference, the medical assistant keeps a travel folder for each destination to which the physician travels. It would contain copies of hotel reservation confirmations, transportation information, the itinerary, and other related documents.

The medical assistant also prepares for the physician a travel folder containing transportation information

and tickets, hotel reservations, confirmation letter, itinerary, list of travelers' check amounts and serial numbers, credit card numbers, and other related documents.

Summary of the Steps Required for Arranging Travel

1. Learn the physician's travel preferences.
2. Obtain and confirm transportation.
3. Obtain and confirm hotel accommodations.
4. Prepare the itinerary.
5. Record travel arrangements in the appointment book.
6. Reschedule patients if necessary.
7. Assemble maps (if a car has been rented).
8. Arrange for travel funds.
9. Prepare a travel folder for the physician.
10. Assemble conference or meeting materials (copies etc.)
11. Check the practice coverage with the physician.
12. Notify the answering service of the dates of the physician's coverage, and provide the names of the covering physicians.

PATIENT TEACHING CONSIDERATIONS

Letter writing should be considered as a method for instructing and informing patients of new policies, services, or fees. Although it may appear costly, mailing actually may be cost effective because of the positive public relations and the indirect advertising obtained for the practice.

Dentists and some physicians use postcard mailings to alert patients of check-up due dates. These mailings illustrate the use of marketing techniques in medical practice. To *market* means to sell or exhibit an image for the purpose of attracting or continuing to satisfy the consumer. Physicians are beginning to use mailings and newsletters to instruct patients, and are marketing their practices in the process.

RELATED ETHICAL AND LEGAL IMPLICATIONS

Letter writing and mail handling have legal implications. Letters can be used as legal evidence in malpractice suits. For instance, a letter to a patient, as a follow-up to a consultation, that describes the diagnosis and treatment plan can be used for litigation if misstatement or omission exists. Whereas the physician is responsible for writing the consultation letter precisely and thoroughly, the medical assistant is responsible for proofreading and typing the letter accurately. Also, blind copies (mentioned earlier) should not be distributed because their use raises ethical and legal concerns.

The medical assistant should consult the procedures manual to check the content and style of certain letters required in the practice of medicine, such as the letter stating the physician's withdrawal from caring for a particular patient. If a letter of withdrawal is not writ-

TRAVEL ITINERARY
Thomas Leonardi, M.D.
Chicago, IL
AMA Conference
October 10–12, 1993

Monday, October 10	7:30 AM (EST)	Depart Erie International Airport Continental Flight No. 295 Non-Stop Coach (1) Non-Smoking (B-2) Breakfast Served
	8:10 AM (EST)	Arrive Chicago O'Hare International Limousine Service to Hotel (Airport Limo) Accommodations: Hemsley Hotel 2528 Harbor Dr. (801) 216-1550 Single Room Harbor Overlook
	10:00 AM	Meeting Registration Hotel Lobby
	10:30–12:00	Conference
	12:00	Luncheon with Harold Shiels, M.D. (He will pick you up) Dr. Shiels phone number: (801) 206-4495
	1:30–4:30	Conference
	5:30	Conference Buffet
Tuesday, October 11	9:00–12:00	Conference
	12:00	Luncheon with Rochelle Whit (801) 264-1110 at The Regency (two blocks from hotel) (801) 200-4500
	2:00–6:00	Conference
	7:00	Dinner with Carl Rein, M.D. In his name at 2420 Oakmont (801) 267-1441 (He will arrange for limo pickup)
Wednesday, October 12	9:00–12:00	Conference
	12:30	Hotel Limo to Airport
	2:00 (CST)	Depart Chicago International Continental Flight No. 401 Non-Stop Coach Non-Smoking (D-3)
	2:37 (EST)	Arrive Erie International Airport

Figure 8–20. A sample travel itinerary.

ten, the physician can be sued for patient abandonment. Malpractice issues are thoroughly discussed in Chapter 3.

A common occurrence in the medical office that generates legal concern is an inquiry made regarding the patient record. The medical assistant should be aware that most legitimate inquiries from insurance companies and attorneys are made in writing and must be accompanied by the patient's written authorization to release information. The written authorization is filed in the patient record, and a response to the inquiry is made in writing by the physician when appropriate, or with his or her supervision and signature on the materials mailed. Of course, medical assistants are ethically and legally bound to keep all information regarding the

patient confidential. Therefore, extreme caution and a sensitivity to related legal issues must be exercised.

SUMMARY

The physician expects the medical assistant to type, proofread, and edit letters, route incoming mail, and oversee the postage and delivery process. In addition, the medical assistant is expected to compose letters, handle routine correspondence, and sign noncritical documents for the physician. To accomplish these tasks effectively and efficiently, the medical assistant must acquire the skills described in this chapter and must develop discretionary judgment regarding the various aspects of mail handling. Many aids are available to help the medical assistant in carrying out these responsibilities. For instance, the *Post Office Manual* can be purchased from the Superintendent of Documents (US Government Printing Office, Washington, DC, 20402). This manual describes postal services, identifies those best suited for each situation, and lists the procedures for

handling special problems. Other informative publications are available from the local post office without charge.

With experience, the medical assistant will become proficient at letter writing and mail handling and can perhaps design new in-office systems for more efficient mail management.

DISCUSSION QUESTIONS

1. Of the mail typically received by a physician, which items would be the most important to call to his or her attention daily?
2. Discuss the importance of accurate editing and proofreading for business letters.
3. Discuss the pros and cons of form letters and the typical reactions to them.
4. Describe the steps you would take if you had a package to mail and were unsure of the fastest and safest delivery method.
5. In which ways is the fax order similar or dissimilar to the order recorded in ink or by typewriter and signed in ink? To the telephone order?

BIBLIOGRAPHY

American Medical Association: AMA Planning Guide For Medical Facilities. American Medical Association, Chicago, 1986.
Conditions of Participation for Hospitals, Code of Federal Regulations. Title 42, Chapter IV, Part 482, Sections 482.24(c)(d) and 482.23(c)(2)(Subpart C).
Diehl MO and Fordney MT: Medical Typing and Transcribing Techniques and Procedures, ed 3. WB Saunders, Philadelphia, 1991.
Feste L: Guidelines for faxing patient health information. The Professional Medical Assistant, May/June 1992.
Fordney MT and Diehl MO: Medical Transcription Guide: Dos and Don'ts. WB Saunders, Philadelphia, 1990.
Iverson C: AMA Style Guide, ed 18. Williams & Wilkins, Baltimore, 1989.
Roach WH et al: Medical Records and the Law, ed 2. Aspen, Gaithersburg, MD, 1993.
Sabin W: Gregg Reference Manual, ed 6. McGraw-Hill, New York, 1985.
Tessier C and Pitman SC: Style Guide for Medical Transcription, Modesto, 1985.
Williams R. (ed): Legality of Optical Storage: Admissibility in Evidence of Optically Stored Records, Section 5, 7–24. Cohasset Association, Chicago, 1987.
Williams RM, Baker LM, Marshall JG: Information Searching in Health Care. Slack, Thorofare, NJ, 1992.

PROCEDURE: Write original correspondence

Terminal Performance Objective: Within the time specified by the instructor, and given cue notes on the recipient, purpose, and contents of a message, compose and type a rough draft of the letter. After the rough draft is approved, prepare a final copy ready for signature.

EQUIPMENT: Typewriter, or word processor and printer
Stationery, including carbon paper and correction accessories if a typewriter is used
Reference books
Cue notes
Pad and pencil or pen

PROCEDURE

1. Assemble materials.

2. Begin to draft the letter. Use the cue notes to outline and organize the main ideas.

3. Choose the appropriate letter format. Begin typing or composing the letter on the word processor with the date in the appropriate space.

4. Type or input the name and address of the recipient in the appropriate space, according to the chosen format.

5. In the appropriate space after the inside address, place the salutation:
"Dear Mr../Ms./Dr. _____:"

6. Type or input the body of the letter: the letter's purpose and the required response, if any. Avoid wordiness and grammatical errors.

7. Type or input an appropriate closing, for instance: "Sincerely,/Yours truly,/Cordially,."

8. Proofread the draft, and if necessary retype the letter. If office procedures require carbon copies of letters, be sure to make a carbon copy at this time.

9. With the letter still in the typewriter (or on the word processor screen), make a final check for typing errors (typos). Read from bottom to top and right to left.

10. If you are not making a carbon copy, make a photocopy of the letter for filing.

11. Obtain the physician's signature in ink.

PRINCIPLE

1. Having adequate working space and materials results in efficient use of time and resources.

2. A rough draft allows sufficient thought and planning and reduces error.

3. The date is extremely important because a letter, once written, is a historic document that may be needed for legal or other reference.

4. The "inside address" (the name and address on the letter itself) is necessary for filing and future reference.

5. A salutation is required in almost all letter formats.

6. The body consists of an introduction, a message, and a closing. Word choice and clarity are important assets to the reader's understanding. Knowing the nature of the message and the identity of the recipient are integral to successful composition.

7. The closing should convey appropriate feeling on the part of the supposed author, that is, the physician.

8. Checking for errors in spelling, punctuation, word choice, and sentence structure helps maintain the office reputation for professionalism.

9. It is easier to make corrections while the paper is in the typewriter. Reading out of context makes typos easier to spot.

10. An outgoing correspondence file is a valuable reference and source of proof.

11. The physician's signature attests to his or her approval of the letter and personalizes the message.

PROCEDURE: Prepare the outgoing mail

Terminal Performance Objective: Prepare outgoing correspondence for mailing at a rate of 30 seconds per piece.

EQUIPMENT: Postage machine
Postage or optical scanner
Outgoing mail marker

PROCEDURE

1. Assemble equipment.
2. Check each envelope for enclosures; check each letter for indications that there should be an enclosure.
3. Sort the outgoing mail according to postal class.
4. Determine what special handling, if any, is required.

5. Mark or stamp outgoing items as required.

6. Affix postage using a postage meter, or use an optical scanner on specially prepared envelopes.
7. Replace the equipment in the designated storage locations.
8. Deliver the mail to the post office or place it in the designated area of the office for pickup.

PRINCIPLE

1. Organization and planning save time.
2. Checking prevents omission of required enclosures.

3. Sorting determines which postal rate applies to each piece of mail.
4. Various letters or packages may require such special handling as priority mail, overnight delivery, protective designation (certified or registered), or insurance coverage.
5. Packages or letters may be marked "Fragile" (breakable items); "Do Not Bend" (x-rays); or "Confidential" (not to be opened by anyone other than the addressee).
6. Affixing postage prepares the outgoing correspondence for mailing.
7. Keeping equipment in its designated place maintains organization and accessibility.
8. Sending out or dropping off the mail completes the task and ensures delivery.

PROCEDURE: Sort and open incoming mail

Terminal Performance Objective: Sort and open incoming mail at a rate of 30 seconds per item.

EQUIPMENT: Incoming mail
Letter opener
Paper clips
Stapler
Transparent tape
Date stamp

PROCEDURE

1. Assemble supplies and equipment.

2. Sort through the mail and place in the following categories: special delivery (mailgrams); first class mail; journals; periodicals and newspapers; all other materials; personal or confidential mail.
3. Place mail marked "Personal" or "Confidential" on the physician's desk.
4. Stack envelopes facing in the same direction.
5. For each envelope (one at a time), pick up a corner and tap the outer top edge with your finger.
6. Using a letter opener, slide the opener along the top edge.
7. Remove the contents of the envelope. Sort the contents (according to the physician's preference):
   A. Mail requiring the physician's attention
   B. Patients' payments for services and other correspondence handled by the medical assistant and not requiring the physician's attention
8. Discard the envelope if the return address appears on the letter.
9. Using a date stamp, stamp the date received in the upper right corner of the letter.
10. Check for enclosures and staple or clip them to the letter. Read the letter to check for the word "enclosure." If the enclosure is missing, note this on the letter.
11. When sorting and opening are completed, check the correspondence requiring the physician's attention to determine whether the patient record should be attached for reference.
12. Assemble all payment checks and record the day's receipts immediately after replacing supplies and equipment and placing sorted mail in designated areas.

PRINCIPLE

1. Organization and planning save time and help ensure accuracy.
2. Mail will be opened and processed according to categorization.

3. The medical assistant does *not* open personal or confidential mail addressed to the physician.
4. Stacking uniformly saves time and effort.
5. Tapping the envelope avoids damaging the letter during opening.
6. Use of a letter opener is the most convenient and efficient method of opening the mail.
7. Sorting saves time for the physician and staff and ensures proper attention.

8. Efficient organization saves time and effort.

9. The date received is essential information for future reference and follow-up.
10. Keeping track of enclosures prevents losing, misplacing, or omitting important information.

11. Checking patient-related correspondence saves the physician's time and effort and ensures proper attention to patient care.

12. Recording receipts immediately prevents loss and error.

PROCEDURE: Annotate incoming mail

Terminal Performance Objective: Annotate correspondence typically received in a medical office at the rate of 5 minutes per one-page letter.

PROCEDURE

1. Place the date received in the top margin. *Example:* Rec. 1/19/82.

2. Read the letter and underline or bracket important points. *Example:* Thank you for the Re: Consultation referral on Mrs. Nancy Jones. I started Mrs. Jones on a regimen of Indovin tablets and a low purine diet.

3. Note any action to be taken in the upper right margin. If no action is to be taken, underline the body of the letter. *Example of action to be taken:* Reply necessary.

4. Attach supplemental material or patient's file where appropriate. *Example:* With a letter relating any findings, a patient's complete file should be attached.

PRINCIPLE

1. The identification of the date received is helpful in future referencing. The dateline typed on the letter may reflect inaccurately the date on which the letter was actually mailed.

2. Because the objective is to highlight important information for the physician, the format used should be consistent. In the example, "Re" denotes the main topic. The physician's attention is immediately drawn to the underlined words, eliminating the need for re-reading the letter.

3. Notes regarding action assist the physician in organizing work activities. The note immediately acquaints the physician with the nature of the letter.

4. The physician can better interpret the content of the letter when pertinent materials are attached.

HIGHLIGHTS
Antonyms, Eponyms, and Homonyms

For medical transcriptionists, antonyms, eponyms, and homonyms are the "troublesome trio" of medical language.

Antonyms are words that have the opposite meaning of other words. Antonyms may be represented by a whole word, a prefix, or a suffix. The words "good" and "bad" are antonyms.

Eponyms are adjectives that describe certain medical procedures, diseases, and anatomic parts. Eponyms are derived from surnames of individuals associated with the procedure, disease, or body part because of related research or discovery. An example is *Korotkoff sounds*, which refers to the sounds heard when blood pressure is recorded. These sounds were first identified by a Dr. Korotkoff. Another example is *Berger's disease*, a kidney disorder first researched and identified by a Dr. Berger. An eponym can be easily recognized because the name is capitalized— *Bell's* palsy, *Colles'* fracture.

Homonyms are words that are pronounced similarly but differ in spelling and meaning. Examples are "weak" and "week", and "their" and "there."

Table 8–4 lists examples of antonyms, eponyms, and homonyms frequently encountered by the medical transcriptionist.

Awareness of this "troublesome trio" will help ensure accuracy in transcriptions. To increase your vocabulary, use a dictionary to learn the meaning of unfamiliar words in the lists in Table 8–4.

To obtain answers to questions related to the use of correct grammar, either check your grammar book or call your local grammar hotline.

Table 8–4

ANTONYMS, EPONYMS, AND HOMONYMS FREQUENTLY ENCOUNTERED BY THE MEDICAL ASSISTANT

Antonyms	Eponyms	Homonyms
Prefixes	Addison's anemia	arteriosclerosis/arteriostenosis
ab—away from	Babinski's reflex	auscultation/oscillation
ad—toward	Bell's palsy	cite/site
ecto—outside	Berger's disease	dysphagia/dysphasia
ento or	Bright's disease	fascial/facial
endo—within	Cheyne-Stokes respiration	glans/glands
hypo—below	Colles' fracture	loose/lose
hyper—above	Koch's bacillus	mucous/mucus
macro—large	Korotkoff sounds	peritoneal/perineal
micro—small	Romberg's sign	radical/radicle
	Stensen's duct	vesical/vesicle
Suffixes		
-ectomy—excision		
-tomy—incision		
Whole Word Antonyms		
stasis—blood flow; stoppage		

*T*elephone Management

> The telephone is the most powerful tool for creating first contact impressions. People will not always remember what was said, but will never forget how what was said affected them. . . .
>
> Einstein Consulting Group

CHAPTER OUTLINE

Telephone Management

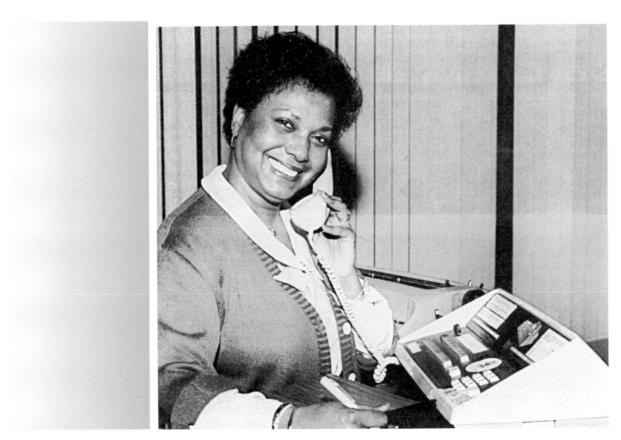

LEARNING OBJECTIVES

Upon completing this chapter, you will be able to:

1. State the techniques for answering incoming telephone calls and the correct elements involved in the telephone greeting, telephone handling, and telephone closure.
2. State the various elements of telephone etiquette when using the various types of telephone equipment.
3. Develop an appropriate telephone personality using tact, courtesy, and selective listening skills.
4. Distinguish between the types of incoming calls that can be handled by the medical assistant and those that require referral to a physician or other health personnel.
5. List the types of patient encounters that require special handling and discretionary judgment.
6. List four principles for resolving conflict and facilitating effective telephone interaction.
7. List key questions to ask patients that will help the medical assistant organize, abstract, and record the telephone call.
8. List the guidelines that will facilitate efficient placement of a variety of local, long distance, and conference calls and use of telephone answering machines, answering services, or mobile communications.

PERFORMANCE OBJECTIVES

Upon completing this chapter, you will be able to:

1. Evaluate problem care via the telephone by analyzing patient complaints, recording relevant data, and presenting accurate, safe, and effective advice.
2. Manage the caller on hold with a minimum of delay.
3. In a simulated medical office setting, correctly place a caller on hold.

DACUM EDUCATIONAL COMPONENTS

1. Receive, organize, prioritize, and transmit information (2.7).
2. Use proper telephone technique (2.8).
3. Interview the patient by telephone (2.9).

Glossary

Audible: Loud enough or otherwise able to be heard
Discretionary judgment: Intuition and knowledge used to arrive at conclusions and decisions
Disposition: The final result or conclusion of an action
Enunciation: Clear pronunciation of words
Interaction: The meeting and verbal exchange between two or more persons, for example, patient and medical assistant
Nonverbal cues: Facial expressions and other facets of body language that convey meaning
Personality: The inner person; the part of psychologic essence that energizes behavior
Public relations: Conscious image projection to the general public
Screening: An assessment or sorting of phone calls that results in categorization for appropriate handling

The telephone is a communication and public relations tool essential to the operation of the medical office. It is the most common link not only between patient and physician, but also between the physician's office and all other offices associated with health care delivery.

It is the telephone voice that initially creates images and expectations of the office staff and the physician. In medical practice, effective telephone management is directed toward presenting a positive image and satisfying the needs and expectations of the caller. Certain techniques and procedures are appropriate for handling telephone calls received in the medical office. The calls received are typically frequent, unanticipated, and disruptive, and interfere with the completion of the tasks at hand. They therefore require professional management. This chapter discusses causes of frustration in telephone management, describes methods for dealing with related problems, and presents the skills that enable the medical assistant to represent the office professionally through telecommunications.

NONVERBAL COMMUNICATION PROBLEMS

The most immediate problem in telephone management is that the speaker cannot be seen. Nonverbal cues such as facial expressions, which are helpful in conveying the message, are unavailable.

To test the importance of nonverbal communication, close your eyes momentarily while talking with a friend or listening to a classroom lecture. When you reopen your eyes, you will be amazed at the diversity and quantity of information being transmitted. When the eyes are closed, communication awareness is lessened. Facial expression, hand and body movements, and other nonverbal cues are all helpful in interpreting the spoken word. The message is interpreted not only through what is being said, but also through judgments concerning feelings about what is said. The medical assistant must learn to function without the aid of these nonverbal cues in accurately giving and receiving messages over the telephone.

Advertisers learned this lesson when they extended their focus from radio to television audiences. It is now rare for an advertising agency to design a commercial that can be used both on radio (without nonverbal cues) and on television (with nonverbal cues).

Clear speech, a projection of positive attitudes, appropriate choice of words, an assertive style, and knowing when to ask closed- versus open-ended questions are variables to be considered in developing an effective technique and pleasant telephone personality.

DEVELOPING AN APPROPRIATE TELEPHONE PERSONALITY

A telephone personality is a reflection of one's own personality. However, because of the limitations of the telephone, a pleasant, well-mannered personality may be more difficult to express over the telephone than in person. Projecting a positive, cooperative attitude to the caller requires consideration of the following factors, all of which influence the development of a telephone personality appropriate for medical office practice:

Enunciation. Speaking clearly over the telephone is especially important. Because the individual cannot be visualized, correct interpretation of the message depends on hearing the words precisely. Activities such as chewing gum, eating, and propping the telephone between the ear and shoulder hinder proper enunciation.

Pronunciation. Incorrect pronunciation of words can also detract from correct interpretation of the message and can cause serious misunderstanding. Listening carefully to experienced medical assistants and consulting a dictionary are helpful for learning to pronounce unfamiliar words. Generally, however, unfamiliar words should be avoided.

Distinctiveness. Even if properly pronounced, words can be misunderstood because several letters of the alphabet sound alike. It may be necessary at times to ask the caller to spell a word, particularly a name. When clarifying the word, it is common practice to state the letter and then a word that begins with the letter. *Examples:* D as in dog, V as in Victor, M as in man, N as in Nancy. The letters most frequently confused are b-d, d-t, b-p, f-s, b-v, m-n, c-z, and p-t.

Expressiveness. Talking at a moderate rate and volume helps the caller to understand what is being said. In addition, although not visible, facial expressions and gestures vitalize the conversation. Smiling over the telephone helps a telephone voice to sound pleasant. Good posture is also an important consideration in expressing a positive attitude toward the caller. Sitting straight helps the voice sound stronger and enthusiastic.

Courtesy. Using commonly courteous words such as "please" and "thank you" conveys to the caller that the answerer is a well-mannered professional. Courtesy is expressed by projecting an attitude of helpfulness, apologizing for delays or errors, using the person's name during the conversation, and being tactful when it is necessary to refuse the caller's request. Also, requesting rather than demanding is courteous and elicits the caller's cooperation more readily. Such phrases as "What's your name?" or "Repeat that, I didn't get it." sound abrupt and impolite compared with "May I have your name, please?" or "Would you please repeat that information?" When ending the conversation, it is courteous to say "Thank you for calling" and to let the caller hang up first.

Attentive listening. Giving the caller full attention is a difficult task in the medical office, where so much distraction is present, such as patients and staff at or near the desk, other telephones ringing, and business machines operating. The medical assistant must develop selective listening skills through practice. Selective listening is the ability to tune out distractions and focus full attention on the telephone conversation. Attention focused on the caller reduces the likelihood of misinterpretation or asking the caller to repeat the message. In addition, interrupting the caller to speak to another person should be avoided unless it is absolutely necessary. It may convey to the caller that the matter being discussed is unimportant to the listener.

In essence, a telephone personality should express one's own natural traits of enthusiasm, cooperation, and pleasantness. Awareness of the factors discussed enhances the projection of an appropriate telephone personality in the medical office.

TELEPHONE ANSWERING TECHNIQUES

HANDLING THE EQUIPMENT

The telephone should be answered promptly—whenever possible, by the second ring. The telephone receiver should be removed gently from its cradle with the nondominant hand (the left hand in right-handed persons), freeing the dominant hand to write messages. The telephone is held with the receiver on the ear and the mouthpiece placed directly in front of and approximately 1 inch from the lips. From this position the voice is clear and audible. Propping the telephone between the ear and the shoulder interferes with voice clarity and hampers the precise pronunciation of words because the jaw cannot move freely. The medical assistant can handle accidental occurrences, such as dropping the telephone or banging it against an object while picking it up, by apologizing to the caller and then identifying the office.

HANDLING THE IMMEDIATE RESPONSE

The immediate response to the call should be an appropriate greeting in accordance with the discretion of the physician. The major telephone companies, most of which provide telephone etiquette courses for their clients, prescribe the following basic techniques in the order given:

1. Identify time of day and express cordiality. When you pick up the phone, begin by saying "Good morning" or "Good afternoon."
2. Identify the office by name. *Examples:* "Dr. Smith's office," "Drs. Smith and Jones," or "Orthopedic Associates." Sometimes physicians

prefer "Doctor's office," particularly when a call comes in on a private line.
3. Identify the person speaking. *Example:* "Miss Black speaking."
4. Express willingness to assist the caller. *Example:* "What may I do to help you?" The patient or caller is assured of the medical assistant's interest.
5. Close the conversation appropriately. *Examples:* "Thank you for calling. Goodbye." "I'll expect to hear from you, then, by the 29th of this month." "We will look forward to seeing you on November 11. Goodbye."

The procedure for managing telephone calls is given in detail at the end of this chapter.

PLACING THE CALLER ON HOLD

The medical assistant should place a caller on hold only when it is necessary and only after identifying the office and waiting for a response to "May I please put you on hold?" or "Will you please hold?" If the caller's response is "Yes, I can hold," the medical assistant thanks the caller and states, "I will return in a few minutes." Asking "Will you please hold?" provides the caller with the choice of holding or calling back. The medical assistant's courtesy elicits the caller's cooperation. Most people are irritated when a call is answered by "Hold, please" or "I have to put you on hold." Providing callers with alternatives promotes their acceptance of holding.

The hold should not exceed 90 seconds. If it does, the medical assistant returns to the caller and asks "Can you continue to hold? It will be a few more minutes." The caller is again given a choice and is reassured that he or she has not been forgotten. If the caller on hold must wait beyond 3 minutes, or indefinitely, the medical assistant should apologize to the caller by saying, "I'm sorry, Mrs. Jones. Rather than continuing to keep you on hold, could I return your call?"

In this instance as in all other telephone conversations, ending the call pleasantly is essential to leaving the caller with positive feelings. Such closing statements as "Thank you for your patience. Goodbye." are more pleasing than "Sorry about this," or "We're just so busy today," or "Don't worry, I'll get back to you." The procedures that summarize and outline the steps required in placing a caller on hold and managing the caller are included at the end of this chapter.

INCOMING CALLS

A telephone system essentially has two functions: to respond to emergency calls and to provide administrative information, including making appointments. Approximately 40% of incoming calls concern administrative assistance; the remaining 60% require immediate attention.

EMERGENCIES

Chapter 10 covers routine appointment scheduling handled by the medical assistant. The information in this chapter enables the medical assistant to schedule an appointment for the patient on the basis of screening techniques specifically designed to determine the purpose and urgency of the office visit. Certain symptoms indicate that the caller is experiencing an emergency. Rather than scheduling an appointment, the medical assistant puts the call through to the physician immediately. If the physician is not in the office, the medical assistant obtains the patient's name and address (or location) and informs the caller that an ambulance will be sent to transport the patient to a hospital or medical center. The patient's name, location, and telephone number should be obtained as early as possible because the patient may be cut off. It is important to stay calm and mentally alert when an emergency call comes in to the office. Symptoms that should be treated with emergency care include

1. *Severe pain anywhere in the body.* Be especially alert for severe chest pain, with or without shortness of breath and nausea. These symptoms characterize heart attack (myocardial infarction).
2. *Profuse bleeding from any body orifice or surface.* Profuse bleeding is heavy and is often characterized by a continuous outpouring of blood. The caller may refer to this event as "hemorrhaging."
3. *Severe difficulty breathing.* The caller may make statements such as "Can't catch my breath," "Can't breathe," or "Can't get any air."
4. *Loss of consciousness.* The caller may state that the patient "passed out" or "can't be awakened."
5. *Severe vomiting or diarrhea.* Be alert to continued episodes of vomiting or diarrhea, particularly in children or the elderly, who experience more serious complications because they become dehydrated easily.
6. *Temperature over 102° F (38.9° C).* In either adults or children, high fever can lead to serious complications and constitutes an emergency whether or not there are accompanying symptoms. (An ambulance is called either if the physician has first been notified and suggests such action or if he or she cannot be reached.)

Each of these situations will be further discussed in the clinical chapters of this text.

ROUTINE CALLS FROM PATIENTS

Patients call the medical office for many predictable reasons, such as to

1. *Obtain administrative information*
   A. Schedule an appointment
   B. Inquire about fees and services
   C. Inquire about billing or insurance

2. *Resolve a care-related problem*
   A. Clarify instructions
   B. Inquire about laboratory results
   C. Obtain medication refills
   D. Report on progress regarding illness or treatment
   E. Ask questions about illness or treatment.

Appointment Scheduling

The medical assistant who receives calls for nonemergency problems must decide whether to

1. Offer home-management advice
2. Schedule an appointment for the same day
3. Refer the call elsewhere.

The medical assistant must be able to exercise independent and informed judgment. He or she must decide whether a patient should be seen immediately; as soon as possible during the current office hours; the same day (in the afternoon if the morning is booked), or later in the week or month.

The medical assistant must safely sort out many incoming calls and advise the callers. Many calls can be handled by the medical assistant; others require referral to the physician. Table 9–1 clarifies the processing of incoming calls. (The policy and procedures manual should include instructions regarding the processing of these calls. Typical guidelines are listed below.)

Training in telephone skills and patient management is an important strategy in the quality of telephone management and triage (sorting cases according to severity). Patients call when the physician is out of the office or caring for other patients. If the person entrusted with telephone management is inadequately trained or makes errors in judgment, unnecessary office visits may be scheduled and patients requiring emergency treatment may be overlooked.

Inquiries Regarding Fees and Services

The caller may request information regarding the availability of services or the physician's fee schedule. The medical assistant can handle these calls when policies are clear and the physician has given approval. In some instances, the medical assistant may ask the caller's name and number and record the inquiry. The physician then returns the call.

Requests for Clarification of Instructions

The medical assistant may, when knowledgeable, assist the patient in understanding the instructions given. Often the patient is referred to the clinical medical assistant who was present during the office visit and who may have instructed the patient. The medical assistant or the physician returns the call.

Table 9-1
REFERENCE GUIDE FOR INCOMING CALLS

Type of Call	Handled By	Handled How and When
Patient emergency	Medical assistant (interrupts physician)	Physician talks to caller immediately.
Appointment scheduling	Medical assistant	Medical assistant schedules appointments as incoming calls occur.
Fees, services, billing, and insurance	Medical assistant when possible. If necessary, medical assistant may refer to or consult with physician.	Medical assistant attempts to resolve questions at time of call or return call. Physician returns call if necessary.
Clarification of instructions	Medical assistant or physician (depending on specific situation)	Medical assistant may handle at time of call, or physician or medical assistant may return call.
Laboratory results	Physician, or medical assistant with physician's approval	Physician returns call for abnormal results. Medical assistant usually gives normal results at time of call or returns call.
Medication refill	Medical assistant with physician's approval	Medical assistant takes message, checks with physician, returns call to patient, and calls pharmacy.
Report on progress regarding illness or treatment	Medical assistant	Medical assistant takes message and informs physician. Medical assistant or physician may return call.
Personal calls for medical assistant	Medical assistant	Medical assistant informs caller of office policy and returns call during off-duty hours.
Personal calls for physician	Medical assistant or physician	Medical assistant follows physician's instructions. May put family members through to physician when instructed to do so.
Treatment of illness	Physician	Medical assistant takes message. Physician or medical assistant instructed by physician returns call.
Unidentified caller for physician	Medical assistant	Medical assistant instructs caller to write to physician.
Physician's professional associates	Physician	Medical assistant puts calls through to physician unless otherwise instructed.
Patient's family	Medical assistant or physician	Medical assistant may call if appropriate. When necessary, medical assistant takes message and physician returns call.
Medical and nonmedical business	Medical assistant or physician	Medical assistant handles whenever possible by returning calls or after checking with physician. In some instances, it may be appropriate for physicians to call back.

Inquiries Regarding Laboratory Test Results

In many medical offices, the medical assistant informs the patient of normal laboratory results following the physician's interpretation of these results and his or her direction to inform the patient. The physician, however, communicates abnormal results and explains what they mean. Again, the policy and procedures manual is instructive regarding the processing of these calls.

Inquiries Regarding Billing or Insurance

Billing and insurance are usually handled by the medical assistant. Because of the nature of the patient's questions or concerns, the medical assistant may need to return the call promptly after reviewing the patient's records.

Requests for Medication Refills

Patients frequently call the office to obtain prescription refills. The medical assistant records the necessary information and attaches the call notation to the patient's record for the physician's attention. Depending on the preference of the physician, either the medical assistant or the physician calls in the prescription refill to the pharmacy.

Progress Reports Regarding Illness or Treatment

Physicians often instruct their patients to call back to report their progress or to relate the effectiveness of the medication or treatment prescribed. The medical assistant records the information in the patient record and attaches a notation to the record for the physician's consideration. The medical assistant or the physician may then make a return call according to the physician's judgment.

Questions Regarding Illness or Treatment

The medical assistant can best handle questions pertaining to the patient's illness or treatment (e.g., "Should I still be feeling like this?" or "I'm getting dizzy spells. Could it be from the pills?") by recording the information and attaching the notation to the patient's record for the physician's attention and return call.

OTHER TYPES OF ROUTINE CALLS

Occasionally, patients may call to request the name of a physician in another specialty. The policy and procedures manual usually contains a referral list. Common practice is to give the caller at least two from which to choose. Obviously, the names must be approved by the medical assistant's physician-employer.

The processing of all calls depends ultimately on the policies established by the physician in collaboration with the office staff. These should be recorded in the policy and procedures manual, and where necessary, the procedures should be described.

CALLS THAT REQUIRE SPECIAL HANDLING

At times the medical assistant encounters calls from patients who are angry, need reassurance, consistently canceling appointments, or have other innumerable needs. The medical assistant, in handling these calls, relies on his or her background in communication skills and psychology. Discretionary judgment comes with experience. However, certain guidelines help the medical assistant to manage these special instances effectively.

THE ANGRY CALLER

The major objective in handling an upset or angry caller is to resolve the caller's anger positively. Helpful techniques for relating to the angry caller include remaining calm, not returning the anger, and conveying understanding and interest. These techniques are discussed in Chapter 4 and can apply to telephone management. Examples of statements that express interest and understanding are "Mrs. Smith, I can understand why you're angry. Let's try to work this out together. Now as I understand it. . . ." and "Mrs. Smith, I know you're upset. I want to help, but I need to ask you a few questions so I can better understand the situation." Most important in these statements is not the words themselves, but the attitude conveyed.

Some principles for resolving conflict are helpful in determining appropriate responses:

1. Allow the caller to express angry feelings without interruption. Do not take the patient's anger personally. Stay calm and resist the reflex to react. Separate the person from the situation and avoid the accusation–defense–reaction cycle.
2. Acknowledge the caller's viewpoint: "I can understand your frustration." If possible, identify an area of agreement: "Yes, I agree that we should have notified you earlier." However, take care to discern acceptable areas of agreement and to consider the legal implications of the response.
3. Direct the communication to problem solving as quickly as possible: "Let's work together to solve this problem." "In what way can I help?"
4. Use closure and follow-up to reinforce resolution of conflict: "I will check that for you and call you tomorrow in the late morning. Will that be convenient?"

THE CALLER WHO NEEDS CONTINUAL REASSURANCE

Some patients call the office repeatedly to discuss the progress of an illness, ask questions concerning the illness or treatment, or clarify instructions. Although it is common practice for patients to call regarding these matters, some patients need reassurance in addition to information. To help the patient, the medical assistant must identify the patient's need for clearer instructions, schedule an appointment with the physician to discuss concerns, or respond kindly and patiently to each call. In some instances, these individuals are persistent talkers and may have to be interrupted with, "Before we hang up, I just wanted to say that I will discuss this with the doctor." Any comment that suggests terminating the conversation is appropriate.

The physician should be consulted about dealing with repeat callers. Without some strategy for handling such calls, these patients can become dependent on the medical assistant for continued reassurance and can consume an unreasonable amount of time. Solutions should be considerate of the patient's needs with regard to medical law and ethics.

THE CALLER WHO REPEATEDLY CANCELS APPOINTMENTS

Appointments canceled with insufficient or no notice disrupt schedule management. Obviously, cancellations are an expected occurrence and are not usually troublesome. However, patients who cancel repeatedly require special attention. If a patient consistently makes and then cancels the appointment, the reason could be an overcrowded schedule or the individual's resistance, fear of the examination itself, or fear of the results. The medical assistant should discuss his or her perception with the physician. A practical method for dealing with a patient who cancels consistently is to schedule the patient at the end of the day, preferably for the last appointment. The cancellation is then less disruptive.

PERSONAL CALLS FOR THE MEDICAL ASSISTANT

Other calls that may be troublesome are calls from the medical assistant's own friends and family. Usually friends and family are cooperative and respond favorably to statements such as, "You know I would love to talk to you, but I can't talk during office hours. Can I call you back at noon or after work?" Accepting personal calls during office hours is not in keeping with the expected standard of professional behavior. The medical assistant should avoid the situation by alerting friends and family in advance that telephone conversations during office hours are not permitted.

SCREENING OF MEDICAL AND NONMEDICAL CALLS

Screening is a procedure in which the caller is asked specific questions. The caller's response to these questions helps to determine how and by whom the call is to be handled. The choice of questions is related to specific categories of call. Office policy should dictate how calls are to be screened.

REQUESTS BY IDENTIFIED CALLERS TO SPEAK TO THE PHYSICIAN

A common problem in telephone screening is dealing with the caller who, regardless of the purpose for calling, asks to speak to the physician. The medical assistant's response to the caller must initially convey the message, "The doctor is with a patient. May I help you?" Word choice is crucial. Note the difference between the foregoing response and the statement, "The doctor is busy now." Both responses carry the same meaning. The first, however, allows the caller to accept

the situation gracefully, rather than prompting a reaction such as, "The doctor is busy doing what? He's too busy for me?" Nonthreatening responses produce the best results.

The medical assistant may occasionally receive calls in which the callers misrepresent their identity or intentions in asking to speak to the physician. On occasion, salespersons respond to the medical assistant's request in the following manner:

> *Medical* "Could you please tell me the pur-
> *Assistant:* pose of your call?"
> *Salesperson:* "This is Ron Miller. I have the physician's financial portfolio ready and am calling to discuss it with him."

Many patients who ask to speak to the physician actually want to schedule appointments or to discuss a change in symptoms, the progress of an illness, or laboratory results. The medical assistant must safeguard the physician's time with the office patient already receiving attention. The physician is interrupted and a call put through only when screening reveals that the call requires this action.

Other callers requesting to speak to the physician are the physician's family, friends, and professional associates; the patient's family; individuals requesting confidential information; and medical and nonmedical business callers.

1. *Personal callers.* Calls from the physician's family and friends are handled according to the physician's preference. Most often, physicians prefer not to have the call put through immediately. The medical assistant informs the physician, who returns the call later.
2. *Professional associates.* Calls from other physicians are usually put through immediately. Other related health professionals (e.g., pharmacists, hospital staff nurses, and laboratory technologists) who ask to speak with the physician are put through frequently. These callers recognize the physician's responsibility to office patients and usually do not request to speak with the physician unnecessarily. Again, the physician's preference for handling these types of calls influences their management.
3. *Patient's family.* Calls from a patient's family are usually not immediately put through to the physician. Instead, the individual's name and phone number and the purpose of the call are recorded for the physician's reference in returning the call. Occasionally, family members unable to speak with the physician may ask the medical assistant for confidential information regarding the patient. The medical assistant must, of course, refuse and encourage the individual to speak with the physician.
4. *Individuals requesting confidential information.* Friends, insurance agents, the media, and other interested individuals may also request,

but not receive, confidential information. Exceptions are individuals representing institutions to which the patient has been admitted, or the offices of physicians to whom the patient has been referred. Their requests for information from the patient's record may be satisfied if the caller is first checked for credibility. One way to check credibility is to ask the caller the social security number or birth date of the patient; another is to record the caller's name and number and call back. When returning the call, verify the institution and the caller's identity.

5. *Medical and nonmedical business callers.* Certain calls from the pharmacy, laboratory, or other medical facilities can be handled either by the medical assistant or by a return call from the physician. For instance, calls from the pharmacy regarding refills are not immediately put through to the physician. The message is recorded and the physician returns the call.

Calls from the laboratory regarding test results are handled by the medical assistant. Test results are written on forms available for this purpose. The medical assistant pulls the patient's record, attaches the results, and places the record appropriately for the physician's review.

The medical assistant handles nonmedical business calls independently; by calling back after consulting with the physician; or by arranging a return call from the physician. The approach to the call is decided according to the caller, the caller's intent, and the immediacy of the matter. For instance, calls from the physician's attorney stating a need to speak with the physician are most likely put through if, after the medical assistant's initial response of "The doctor is with a patient," the attorney still insists on speaking with the physician.

Other appropriate responses to nonmedical business callers include, "The doctor will review the message and will contact you," "Please send literature for the doctor to review," and "I will call you back if the doctor would like an appointment scheduled."

The medical assistant should treat all calls carefully, should never speak rudely to the caller, and should review all nonpatient calls with the physician before discarding the messages.

In this and all telephone-handling situations, the medical assistant's discretionary judgment is shaped by practice, by observing experienced medical assistants, and by reading related literature such as the journal *The Professional Medical Assistant.*

Requests by Unidentified Callers to Speak to the Physician

The medical assistant asks unidentified callers to identify themselves and state the purpose of the call. If this request is denied, the approach to handling the call depends on the established office policy recorded in the procedures manual. A common approach is to suggest

that the unidentified caller write a letter to the physician and mark it "Personal."

The medical assistant's major responsibilities in telephone screening are to avoid interrupting the physician, and to independently handle calls that do not require the physician's attention; decisions regarding medical care and decisions that exceed the parameters of the medical assisting profession should be made by the physician.

OBTAINING THE CORRECT MESSAGE

The next step after the medical assistant greets the caller is to learn the purpose of the call. The caller may, without direction, state the purpose of the call.

Medical Assistant: "Good morning, Dr. Jones's office, Cindy speaking."
Patient: "Cindy, this is Ralph Evans, and I'd like to make an appointment."

Often, however, the message must be sorted and interpreted. An example follows of a conversation in which the purpose is unclear.

Medical Assistant: "Good morning, Dr. Jones's office, Cindy speaking."
Patient: "Yes, well I wanted to speak to the doctor. I haven't felt well lately, and I don't know if I should talk to him or maybe just make an appointment. I was in last month and I. . . ."

In addition to the screening techniques that determine how and by whom the call is handled, certain guidelines can be used to determine the needs of the patient by helping the caller to state his or her purpose clearly. The medical assistant's goal in communicating with the caller is to interpret the message accurately.

The following guidelines facilitate effective telephone interaction:

1. *Establish calmness.* When either responding to or initiating the call, use a calm voice to reassure the patient and prepare you to receive the message accurately.
2. *Maintain calmness and patience.* The caller may be agitated and in a hurry to tell you something. Listen attentively. Do not interrupt unless it becomes necessary, for instance, when the caller speaks at great length.
3. *Restate the question or concern.* Attempt to summarize the issue and to clarify it for both yourself and the caller. Summarize by stating the major points, providing the opportunity for the patient to correct misunderstanding. *Example:* "Mrs. Jones, I will leave a message for the doctor that you are still having headaches, that you have finished your medication, and that you wanted to ask the doctor if your prescription should be refilled."

4. *Obtain the correct name and telephone number.* If one or two critical numbers or letters in a message are misunderstood, it costs time and energy later. Be certain to repeat these items carefully. When recording names that may be confusing, repeat the letters as you write: "R as in Robert, P as in Paul," and so forth. You may need to ask the caller to spell his or her name.

5. *Record the message.* Keep a message pad close to the phone so that the patient's name, phone number, message, and directions to the physician can be recorded without delay. Never trust your memory; write everything down.

It may become necessary to ask the caller to state the purpose of the call when other techniques fail. In other instances, such as when the caller wants to speak with the physician, it is appropriate to directly ask the purpose of the call.

Caller: "I would like to speak to the doctor."
Medical Assistant: "Could you please tell me the purpose of the call?"

While obtaining the message through verbal response, the medical assistant must take notes to record the call, its purpose, and how it will be handled. Abstracting the message by recording meaningful notes requires practice. The discussion that follows is helpful in developing this skill.

ABSTRACTING THE MESSAGE

Obviously, the entire telephone message cannot be written out exactly as the caller conveys it. Call slips with carbons are most often used for recording telephone messages (Fig. 9–1). They provide limited space for writing the message itself. While listening to the caller, the medical assistant must abstract and record the message. *Abstracting* refers to isolating key points and recording the purpose of the call precisely and concisely on the call slip. For the following example, the medical assistant has the call-slip pad and a pen assembled and is ready to write.

Medical Assistant: "Good morning, Dr. Jones's office, Cindy speaking."
Patient: "Hi, Cindy. I'd like to speak to the doctor."
Medical Assistant: "May I ask who's calling, please?"
Patient: "Oh, sure. This is Mrs. Michaels."
Medical Assistant: "Mrs. Michaels, I'm sorry, but the doctor is with a patient. May I help you?"
Patient: "Well, maybe you can. I don't know what to do. I was in last week, last Wednesday actually, and the doctor gave me these pills. Well, I went to him because my stomach was upset and these pills don't seem to be helping any. He said something about trying

Figure 9–1. A telephone message form.

them first and if they didn't help then maybe getting a stomach x-ray. I don't know. I'm just getting disgusted. I've not felt well for a month."

The medical assistant, while listening, has written the following in the spaces provided on the call slip: the patient's name, date, and time of the call, and "States medication prescribed last Wed (9/1) for stomach 'hasn't helped.' Questioning what to do. Asks if x-ray should be scheduled per your suggestion." The medical assistant also signs the call slip for the physician's reference. If "Return Call" is printed on the slip, the medical assistant checks the space provided to alert the physician. The medical assistant then instructs the patient that the physician will call back. (The medical assistant may call back at the physician's request to schedule an x-ray.) The call slip is then attached to the patient record and placed with the physician's phone messages.

Proficiency at abstracting telephone messages requires practice. Certain key questions can facilitate the task.

1. *What is the purpose of the call?* Why is the caller making this call? What is the *major* concern? Is the caller conveying feelings as well as words? What is the tone of voice? The medical assistant can attempt to answer in one sentence

the question, "What does the caller want?" or "What is the caller really asking?"

2. *What are the caller's expectations?* What does the caller want the physician, the medical assistant, or another member of the staff to do? What does the caller want to have happen? When? How?

3. *What is the caller's reaction to the medical assistant's response?* Does the caller seem satisfied with the response? Does the caller understand what will be done? Does the action meet expectations?

Referring back to the example: Mrs. Michaels made the call to inform the doctor that she was not feeling any better (1). She wanted to know if she should have an x-ray (2). She is satisfied that the doctor will call her back (3).

The above statements are explicit (readily ascertained and obvious). Mrs. Michaels is also communicating frustration. She wants to feel "better." Furthermore, she most probably wants immediate action. Although Mrs. Michaels did not make these statements, she implied them in the tone of the conversation. Abstracting is a necessary skill in clinical medical assisting as well. The medical assistant must enter precise, concise notes pertaining to vital signs and presenting symptoms on the patient record.

As with all skills, the medical assistant's skill level and confidence will develop and improve with each step through professional training: in the classroom, on externship, and finally during employment following certification.

RECORDING THE CALL

Most physicians prefer to have certain types of calls noted in the patient record. These calls may come from patients reporting on their progress, questioning or protesting some aspect of medical care, or expressing anger concerning any aspect of office practice or medical treatment. The medical assistant notes the date, time, and initials of the recorder. Recording the call directly on the patient record in addition to leaving a telephone message slip for the physician ensures competent, comprehensive treatment and protection against litigation. The medical assistant should quote patient statements, when it is appropriate to do so, rather than record information imbued with value judgments.

Example

INCORRECT RECORDING

Patient called upset and angry about how long she had to wait to be seen by the doctor. She tends to be impatient and volatile and was unable to be calmed. She wanted the physician to know her feelings.

CORRECT RECORDING

12/18/87 Patient called at 10:45 a.m. regarding the length of time she waited before being seen by the physician. Stated: "I wasted an hour and a half of my time . . . I'm thinking of changing doctors." The reason for the delay was explained. Patient was assured that the physician would be informed of her call. Mary Franzeze.

Attention to correct methods of recording messages on the patient record is the best protection against malpractice claims.

ORGANIZING TELEPHONE MESSAGES

As was previously mentioned, call slips are specially designed for recording telephone messages. They can be purchased from a medical forms supply house. The form should provide space for recording the following information:

1. Name of the person receiving the call
2. Date and time the call is received
3. Name and phone number of the caller
4. Message
5. Action required
6. Signature of the person who answered the call

Most call slips are designed with carbon copies and come in a tear-out telephone message format (Fig. 9–2). One copy is attached to the patient record and placed with other call slips and patient records for the physician's attention. Another copy is usually left in the record book at the medical assistant's desk. The medical assistant checks the call slips before leaving for the day to make sure calls have been returned. Patient records used to respond to the call are refiled. All incoming and outgoing calls to patients should be recorded in the patient record.

OUTGOING CALLS

The medical assistant's telephone responsibilities include outgoing calls. The medical assistant may place a variety of local and long-distance calls, arrange for conference calls, and organize a storage system for commonly used telephone numbers.

PLACING CALLS

Medical assistants place many calls to patients, suppliers, and other medical offices. Adherence to the following guidelines will facilitate efficient telephone use.

1. Choose a time to call that is convenient to both the medical office and the person who is being called.
2. Before placing the call, pinpoint its purpose and objectives.
3. If complex information is to be exchanged during the call, make notes before and during the call for later reference.

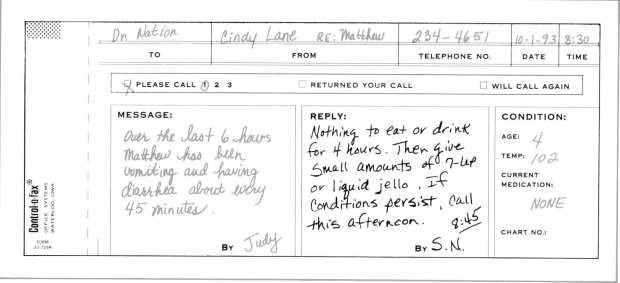

Figure 9–2. A tear-out telephone message form, which provides a permanent record of the telephone call in the form of a telephone log. (Courtesy of Control-o-fax.)

4. Begin by identifying the name of the office and stating your own name.
5. Clearly state the purpose of the call.
6. Record all pertinent information, including names, dates, and numbers.
7. Repeat critical information to check for accurate listening and recording.
8. Close the conversation cordially. Use such closing statements as "Thank you. Goodbye." or "Thank you. I will get back to you by next Friday. Goodbye."

DIRECT DIALING

To avoid directory assistance charges, the medical assistant should look up outgoing numbers in the telephone directory. Additional local directories and directories for other areas are usually available at no charge. If the exact spelling of a business or supplier name is unknown, the number can be checked under the specific heading in the yellow pages. If someone has recently moved, dialing the old number may produce a recording of the new number without directory assistance.

When directory assistance must be used, the medical assistant should give the operator full information. Up to two numbers can be requested for each directory assistance charge. Each telephone company publishes the number of directory assistance calls allowed each month at no charge (usually three or four calls). Charges apply even to unpublished or unlisted numbers and to those the operator cannot find. Additional charges include an operator handling charge for calls placed through the operator (by dialing 0). Operator assistance is free from most pay telephones, from hospital telephones, and for 800-number assistance. Callers can also receive credit or a refund from the telephone company by dialing 0 after a reached wrong number or poor connection.

LONG-DISTANCE CALLING

Increased competition and electronic sophistication have made long-distance dialing common and affordable. The medical assistant should maintain a directory of area codes. If the telephone number of a party in another city is unknown, the medical assistant should dial directory assistance in that city (1-Area code-555-1212). For "800" service numbers, dial 1-800-555-1212.

It is also important to remember that time zones vary throughout the country. A call placed from an office in Ohio at 9 AM, for example, would ring at 6 AM in California. Long-distance dialing is discounted between 5 and 11 PM Sunday through Friday, and is least expensive between 11 PM and 8 AM every day, all day Saturday, and Sunday between 8 AM and 5 PM. The cost of station-to-station dialing is lower than that of person-to-person or operator-assisted dialing, and is usually worth the risk of dialing station-to-station and not reaching the desired party. If the likelihood of reaching a particular individual is small, however, a person-to-person call is justified. The person-to-person call is most expensive and should be reserved for reaching a particular person or extension in a company or government agency. The caller should check before dialing to determine whether there is an 800 listing. Person-to-person calls are placed by dialing 0 followed by the number. Several telephone companies provide specialized long-distance call services. Services should be compared and selected according to how they best accommodate the physician's particular needs. Long-distance telephone companies can be contacted as follows:

AT&T	1-800-222-0400
MCI	1-800-333-1000
US Sprint	1-800-877-6000
RCI	1-800-836-8080
Allnet	1-800-783-2020

SPECIALTY OPERATORS

Specialty operators handle overseas and conference calls. The medical assistant can arrange such a call by dialing 0 and requesting connection with the appropriate operator.

The conference operator, for example, can arrange for a large number of persons from several locations to speak with each other simultaneously. Many physicians use this service to consult with other physicians regarding complicated cases and to discuss other professional issues.

FREQUENTLY CALLED NUMBERS

It is useful to develop a simple and flexible system for referencing commonly called telephone numbers. Laboratories, other medical offices, pharmacies, and other frequently used numbers should be cross referenced and filed. This practice will save time required to look for numbers continually in the directory as well as reduce costs for directory assistance.

Because medicine is a dynamic field, the file must be flexible. New numbers are frequently added and old numbers purged. Several commercial directory systems are available to accommodate this procedure. It may be helpful to obtain telephone directories listing departments, staff physicians, and support personnel for each hospital or medical center where the physician is affiliated or has staff privileges.

TELEPHONE SYSTEMS AND EQUIPMENT

Although it is the medical assistant's skills that ultimately create an effective phone system, the choice of equipment can affect calling efficiency. Telephones and related equipment are becoming more sophisticated and less expensive. The level of competition for both telephone hardware and services such as long-distance calling is increasing dramatically. The medical assistant must remain current regarding changes by the local telephone company and competing electronics dealers to learn of the latest developments in both services and equipment.

The final choice of telephone systems depends on the type of practice, the type of call most frequently received and placed, and the size and complexity of the medical practice.

TYPES OF TELEPHONES

Almost all offices (including medical offices) have replaced the older-style rotary dial telephone with push-button equipment. There are two important reasons for this trend. The push-button telephone is faster and more accurate. The typical business telephone is used hundreds of times per day, and the touch-tone telephone makes the office system compatible with several evolving telephone services, including those provided by competing long-distance companies. Another consideration is the size and capacity of the telephone. Few medical offices can use a single telephone. Instead, the typical small or medium-sized office uses a multiline telephone, such as a six-button telephone (Fig. 9–3) or a ten-button telephone. These instruments allow for several telephone lines in the office, intercom capabilities within the office, and the capacity to place a caller on hold. In addition, the multiline system allows for conference calls. The intelligent placement of several telephone sets within the office complex, including treatment rooms and the physician's own private office, can maximize the efficiency of the overall system.

Most telephone companies and their competing electronic supply houses provide consultants on a no-fee basis who evaluate specific office needs and make recommendations.

LARGE-OFFICE SYSTEMS

In large office complexes, a small switchboard system, such as is shown in Figure 9–4, may be appropriate. Costly hardware and procedures are required to operate even the smallest switchboard. The hardware and procedures should not become overly complicated.

TELEPHONE ACCESSORIES

Many features and accessories can be added to the office systems. Many physicians use speaker phones, which allow the individual to talk without holding the receiver and to have the incoming call amplified. Many speaker systems can be also used as office intercommunication devices. This feature allows the physician to speak to persons in other areas of the office complex.

Some telephones have redial and memory features. A redial system allows the caller to place the outgoing call on hold in case there is a busy signal. As soon as the destination does not ring busy, the call goes through and the caller is signaled, thus saving the time required for several redials. A memory capacity allows the telephone to be programmed for commonly called telephone numbers, so that the entire number does not have to be dialed each time it is called.

Some medical offices provide headsets with microphones to leave the medical assistant's hands free during calls. Many available headsets are remote and wireless, allowing the wearer to move freely while talking.

THE ANSWERING SERVICE

There are two general approaches to after-hours telephone services. The most widely used method is the professional answering service, which answers the tele-

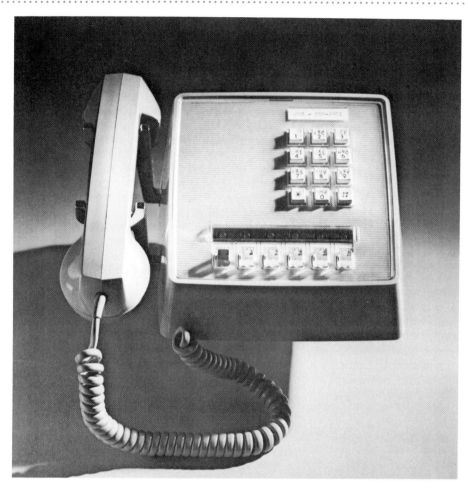

Figure 9-3. A six-button telephone. (Courtesy of GTE.)

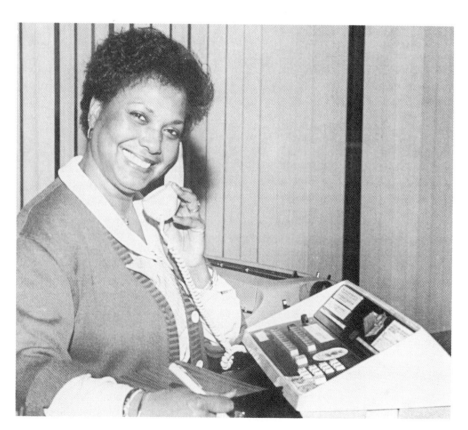

Figure 9-4. A small switchboard. (Courtesy of GTE.)

phone and takes messages when the office is closed or when no one is on duty. Many types of services are available from these agencies. They range from a predetermined few hours of coverage per week to 24-hour, 7-day comprehensive programs that may include answering for the office during working hours after a designated number of rings. Services may be contracted in different ways. The service answers the telephone under the office number, or the patient may call a different number for after-hour and emergency situations handled by the answering service. The advantage of a professional service is that a person, rather than a machine, listens to callers and interprets the message. If a patient has a serious problem, the answering service may attempt to reach the physician at home.

A second, less desirable and less frequently used alternative is a tape-recorded message that allows space and time for patients to leave messages on the answering machine. For cases requiring immediate care, the message must include the name and telephone number of the physician or another physician on call. Answering machines of this type are inexpensive and widely available.

MOBILE COMMUNICATIONS

Some physicians prefer to have a direct line of communication with the office so that they can be reached or can contact staff members. Both mobile telephones and personal paging devices make direct communication possible. Mobile phones may be installed in automobiles or boats. If the physician is in a designated area with a telephone, a call-forwarding feature on the office switchboard can transfer calls to that location or directly to an office telephone.

Another mobile device is the personal pager (beeper) (Fig. 9–5), which is available from most utilities and communication service companies. The physician activates an electronic device that can be comfortably carried in a pocket. If an emergency arises, the medical assistant can dial a predetermined number that activates a beeper in the pocket device. The physician then goes

to a telephone and dials the office. Other paging systems are activated by an answering machine. After hearing the message, the caller dials his or her own telephone number and activates the message system by hitting the pound (#) sign. The physician can then redial the caller's number.

PATIENT TEACHING CONSIDERATIONS

The telephone can be used to teach and advise patients. Some physicians schedule telephone call-in hours during which patients can speak to them directly. This practice is most frequent in pediatric medicine. Patients can also be instructed and encouraged to call the office concerning business matters during the hours when the physician is not seeing patients.

A brochure that introduces the patient to the medical office can contain such information. Tactful wording is necessary so that the patient feels that the policy best serves his or her needs. Patients should be informed that the call "is welcomed any time during office hours but can usually be given concentrated attention and be more quickly processed when visiting patients are not in need of the medical assistant's attention." As always, the physician's preference dictates policy.

Patients can also be instructed in using the telephone more effectively. For instance, patients should be told to have a pencil and pad available for writing instructions and to keep frequently used emergency numbers near the telephone for quick reference. In case of illness, patients should take their temperatures before they call. Handouts discussing the well-stocked medicine cabinet are useful for saving time during home management advice.

RELATED ETHICAL AND LEGAL IMPLICATIONS

The patient's right to privacy is both an ethical and a legal concern in all aspects of medical practice. Telephone calls can interfere with this right.

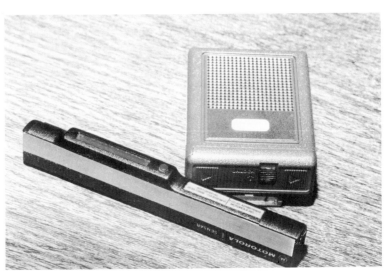

Figure 9–5. A doctor's beeper. (Courtesy of GTE.)

One instance in which this right may be breached occurs when the medical assistant places a call to the patient. If it is necessary to reach the patient at work, the medical assistant should not identify the call as coming from the physician's office unless speaking directly to the patient. Only if the patient has given permission should this information be revealed. Without a release from the patient, the physician can be sued for invading the patient's privacy.

Another legal concern is related to the return-call procedure. The time of return calls should not be specified unless the situation is urgent. The patient should be informed that the physician will return the call. If necessary, the medical assistant can advise the patient to expect the call in the early or late morning, afternoon, or evening. Stating an exact time implies a binding contractual agreement. It is most important to follow through and honor the return call in as little time as possible.

In addition, medical assistants must be aware that patients may ask their advice concerning treatment over the telephone, particularly if the physician is unavailable. It is *illegal* for the medical assistant to diagnose or prescribe treatment. In addition, the medical assistant must avoid reassuring statements that are unfounded, such as "I'm sure the doctor will find out exactly what's wrong."

Other legal concerns are related to recording calls and giving information to patients over the telephone. Although not all administrative calls from patients are noted in the patient record, all calls received from patients who are reporting progress or complaining about some aspect of care should be recorded to protect against legal action. In addition, medical assistants should record only calls they themselves receive. Medically important telephone conversations should be recorded and filed in the patient record in chronologic order and retained permanently.

Information recorded through a telephone call is admissible in a court of law. Several cautionary measures can improve the quality of patient care and reduce liability.

1. Develop written policies for questions, decisions, and advice presented to patients over the telephone. Clarify who is responsible for what.
2. Develop written step-by-step questions and guidelines for each symptom commonly encountered. These guidelines should include symptoms, decision guidelines, and home management advice.
3. Routinely train and evaluate all staff involved in telephone management.
4. Record information that is "smarter, not longer."
5. Maintain a "low threshold" for appointments. Although there are no hard-and-fast rules, the safest action is to schedule any patient who is worried.
6. Discuss risk management issues (legal implications) with all staff.

A legal concern associated with giving information to the patient relates to inquiries regarding laboratory results. Although the medical assistant can inform patients of results interpreted by the physician, it is never permissible to assume that results within the normal range can readily be shared with the patient. The medical assistant must first obtain the physician's approval.

Another area of legal concern relates to information given the answering service as to where the physician can be reached when the office is closed. If such information is not forthcoming, the physician can be sued for patient abandonment. It is the medical assistant's responsibility to inform the service of the physician's whereabouts, and to check the service for messages when the office opens in the morning and at other times during the workday (such as lunchtime) when the service is in operation.

SUMMARY

The medical assistant is often expected to be the office resource person for telephone handling and equipment. It is therefore important for the medical assistant and the physician to establish a working understanding of the medical assistant's responsibility in processing calls. (Apart from legal limitations, the physician's preference dictates these responsibilities.) Most physicians value a medical assistant with the initiative to investigate new equipment, improve systems, and exercise discretionary judgment in telephone communications.

The procedure manual should contain a description of telephone procedures that includes guidelines for placing telephone calls, the type of calls to be placed, and the identification of the individual responsible for the task.

DISCUSSION QUESTIONS

1. Identify several communication problems related to telephone use.
2. Define "telephone personality" and list several characteristics.
3. List four types of calls the medical assistant handles independently. Give reasons why.
4. Explain why screening is an important part of telephone communications.
5. List the essential components of the telephone message.

BIBLIOGRAPHY

Books
General Telephone Company: GTE Telephone Courtesy Handbook. Department of Public Relations, Erie, PA, 1992.
Hospitality Telephone Skills Workshop Materials. The Einstein Consulting Group, Philadelphia, 1985.
Katz H: Telephone Medicine Triage and Training. Slack, Thorofare, NJ, 1990.

Videos
American Media: Handling Incoming Calls. American Media, Des Moines, 1985.
American Media: Telephone Courtesy Pays Off. American Media, Des Moines, 1985.
American Media: Dealing with People on the Telephone. American Media, Des Moines, 1985.

PROCEDURE: Manage telephone calls

Terminal Performance Objective: Evaluate problem care via the telephone by analyzing patient complaints, recording relevant data, and presenting accurate, safe, and effective advice (within the professional parameters of medical assisting and according to the physician's direction), within a reasonable time period.

EQUIPMENT: Tape recorder and audio cassette
Telephone record forms and pencil

PROCEDURE

1. Answer within two rings.

2. Extend greeting and identify the office and speaker:
   a. "Good morning . . ."
   b. "Doctor Goodman's office . . ."
   c. "Ms. Johnson speaking . . ."
   d. "May I help you?"
3. Obtain the caller's name and telephone number.

4. Obtain the caller's information:
   a. Time and date
   b. Complaint or purpose of the call
5. Offer assistance:
   a. Appointment
   b. Referred to _____
   c. Home care advice (according to physician's instruction)
      Independent _____
      Consulted with _____
   d. Patient to return call
      Yes _____
      No _____
   e. Description of advice:
   f. Message for physician to call back:
      Degree of urgency:
      How soon call is expected:
6. Record the information gathered and outcome in steps 3 to 5.

7. Close the call by repeating to the caller the decisions and disposition of the call and end with a cordial expression of good-bye.

PRINCIPLE

1. Ringing telephones are a source of irritation to everyone.

2. The greeting provides the caller with the information required to proceed with the conversation and sets a tone that is pleasant and professional. Giving your name shows the willingness to take responsibility for the call.

3. Using the caller's name shows you are giving full attention to the phone call and enables you to call the caller back should the telephone disconnect.

4. Accurate history taking is necessary for relevant advice and disposition. Questioning the caller directs the caller to provide the required information.

5. Details of assistance enables the physician to be able to review details of telephone instructions and to change or modify patient instructions. Any advice (medical) given to the patient should be guided by the physician's written instructions and follow established protocol. This caution is necessary to avoid malpractice suits or other legal consequences.

6. Medically significant calls should be documented in the medical record. Written notes assure accurate message interpretation and avoids having the caller repeat information.

7. A friendly closing leaves the caller feeling well-received and aids in reducing caller anxiety and dissatisfaction.

PROCEDURE: Manage a caller on hold

Terminal Performance Objective: Manage the caller on hold with a minimum of delay and within a reasonable time period.

EQUIPMENT: Tape recorder and audio cassette
Telephone record forms and pencil

PROCEDURE

1. Answer within two rings.

2. Extend greeting and identify the office and speaker:
   a. "Good morning . . ."
   b. "Doctor Goodman's office . . ."
   c. "Ms. Johnson speaking . . ."
   d. "May I help you?"
3. Obtain the caller's name and telephone number.

4. Ask "Will you hold the line please while I _____?"

5. Return to the caller every 60 seconds.

6. Thank the caller for waiting.
7. Apologize for delays.
8. Offer to call back, if possible
   OR
9. Proceed with or transfer the call.

PRINCIPLE

1. Ringing telephones are a source of irritation to everyone.
2. The greeting provides the caller with the information required to proceed with the conversation and sets a tone that is pleasant and professional. Giving your name shows the willingness to take responsibility for the call.
3. Using the caller's name shows you are giving full attention to the phone call and enables you to call the caller back should the telephone disconnect.
4. Asking only "Will you hold please?" or saying "Hold please," does not give the caller the chance to respond if he or she cannot hold.
5. Frequent communication informs the caller as to the status of the call and reassures the caller that she or he is not forgotten.
6. The caller will be less dissatisfied with having to wait.
7. Every caller considers his or her call important.
8. The caller has the option whether or not to continue holding.
9. A friendly closing leaves the caller feeling well-received and aids in reducing patient anxiety and dissatisfaction.

PROCEDURE: Place a caller on hold

Terminal Performance Objective: In a simulated medical office setting, place a caller on hold correctly within 15 seconds.

EQUIPMENT: Telephone with hold function

PROCEDURE

1. Answer the telephone by greeting the patient and identifying the office and yourself.

2. Ask the patient, "Will you hold, please?" and wait for the response.
3. If a call cannot be put through after a short time (60–90 seconds) return and inform the caller that the line is still in use: "Will you continue to hold?" If time permits, obtain the caller's number in case the call is cut off.
4. Return to the caller with "Thank you for waiting," and proceed with the transfer.

PRINCIPLE

1. The correct procedure for answering the telephone should be followed consistently. This initial response presents the caller with information necessary to proceed with the call.
2. Waiting for the response gives the caller an option. It may not be possible for the caller to hold.
3. Waiting a maximum of 90 seconds reassures the caller that he or she is not forgotten and makes the wait more acceptable.

4. Speaking to the caller before transferring removes possible confusion and extends courtesy, which helps the caller to be less dissatisfied with having to wait.

HIGHLIGHTS

Telecommunication Services of the Future

Throughout the United States, a new movement in telecommunications connecting physician's offices with hospitals is gaining momentum.

In an effort to contain and reduce their own cost of telephone systems, hospitals and medical centers are purchasing multidimensional telecommunications services and charging physicians a fee for using and participating in the system. Digital telephone switches and computer branch exchanges can receive and route telephone calls and computer information.

Hospitals that purchase a high-volume package of services from the telecommunications vendor can decrease long-distance costs and attract and retain physicians who find quicker access to test results (through a telephone system that connects the physician's office with the hospital), thus promoting positive patient relations.

In many such telecommunications systems, physicians telephoning from the office can access the hospital's telephone system and computers to retrieve critical information from the laboratory, radiology, pharmacy, and medical records departments. Patients calling physicians at the hospital are transferred by the hospital operator directly to the physician's office. Systems equipped with a voice mailbox system function as answering machines and paging systems.

The hospital manages the telecommunications system like a nonprofit business, usually billing physicians on a monthly basis. Physicians using these systems find them affordable because of the features offered, although they may find the cost somewhat higher than that of telephone service provided by local utility companies.

According to Mark McDougall, associate director to the Healthcare Information and Management Systems Society, the changeover to an integrated telephone and data communications system is inevitable. Becoming familiar with telecommunications system vocabulary will help dispel the technology's mystique.

TELECOMMUNICATION SYSTEMS GLOSSARY

Call detail recording: A system that records the caller's name, date, time, and number called (similar to a telephone company's long-distance report).

Electronic message service: A system that records messages on a computer system. They can be retrieved by using a special code number, calling the operator, or obtaining a printout at a terminal point.

Facsimile machine: A system that sends images of printed pages over telephone lines to another facsimile machine.

Radio paging: A system that sends voice messages or written messages or a tone, all of which are received by a portable pager.

Switch: A computer system that routes telephone calls between telephones. The system can be operated by a key (electromechanical) switch or a digital switch.

Voice-data integration: A system that enables telephone (voice) and computer data to be received and routed over the same wiring system.

Voice mail: A computer system that records telephone messages (an answering machine); the user can record and send or receive messages by dialing a code number.

> Patients' needs will be better served if health professionals see their own actions and choices not only in the context of the 15 minute visit but rather in the setting of the patient's lifetime.
>
> Naomi Remen, MD
> *The Human Patient*

CHAPTER OUTLINE

APPOINTMENT SCHEDULING SYSTEMS
  Time-Specified Scheduling
  Open Hours Scheduling
  Wave Scheduling
  Modified Wave Scheduling
  Double Booking
  Categorization Scheduling

THE APPOINTMENT BOOK
  Essential Information
  Size and Placement
  List of Standard Procedure Times
  Extended Times for Patients with Special
    Needs

SCHEDULING GUIDELINES
  Limited and Shared Resources
  Recorded Appointment Information

PATIENT CONSIDERATIONS IN APPOINTMENT
    SCHEDULING
  Scheduling the Physical Examination
    Appointment
  Accommodating Patient Needs
  Appointment Screening
  Motivating Patients

WELCOMING THE PATIENT
  The Greeting
  New Patient Orientation and Registration

PLANNING FOR UNANTICIPATED DISRUPTIONS
  Physician Delays
  The Acutely Ill Patient
  Accepting Referrals
  Walk-Ins
  Cancellations and No-Shows
  Buffer Time

REFERRAL TO OTHER FACILITIES
  Scheduling Surgery
  Hospital Admission Certification
  Second Surgical Opinions
  Instructing the Patient

THE NEXT APPOINTMENT AND THE
    APPOINTMENT CARD
  Follow-up Calls

RELATED ETHICAL AND LEGAL IMPLICATIONS

SUMMARY

DISCUSSION QUESTIONS

BIBLIOGRAPHY

PROCEDURES
  Organize the Appointment Book
  Schedule an Appointment
  Record Patient Cancellations and Missed
    Appointments
  Schedule a Referral

HIGHLIGHTS
  Stress, Work, and Health

Chapter 10

Organizing and Coordinating Appointments

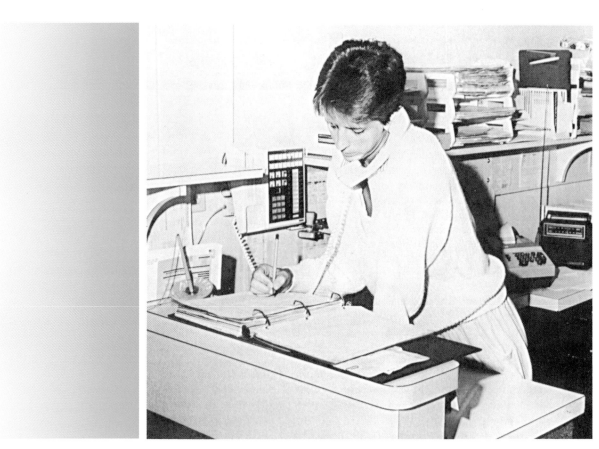

LEARNING OBJECTIVES

Upon completing this chapter, you will be able to:

1. List and describe the various scheduling systems.
2. State the standard times required to complete common office procedures.
3. List the essential information required to schedule an appointment.
4. List and describe the procedural steps for scheduling new appointments and follow-up visits.
5. List the conditions that should be considered emergencies, those that require immediate appointments, and those that require same-day appointments.
6. Describe the importance of public relations and first impressions in enhancing the reputation of the physician and the physician's office.
7. Describe the appropriate handling of patient-canceled and physician-canceled appointments for both routine and ill patients.
8. Describe the medical assistant's role in scheduling physician referrals and appointments for services outside the office.
9. State the legal implications of the appointment book in cases of canceled appointments and of urgent decisions.

PERFORMANCE OBJECTIVES

Upon completing this chapter, you will be able to:

1. Schedule new and established patient appointment times, accounting for office priorities and patient needs and preferences.
2. Determine when a patient should be seen in the office for immediate care, and when an emergency exists.
3. Arrange immediate transportation and referral to an emergency care facility.
4. Complete a patient sign-in and registration form.
5. Handle unanticipated disruption of appointments, such as patient cancellations, no-shows, and physician delays.
6. Refer patients to other facilities for admission, surgery, further diagnosis, or follow-up care.
7. Place follow-up calls to patients to inquire about progress and compliance with treatment.

DACUM EDUCATIONAL COMPONENTS

1. Schedule and monitor appointments (3.2A–K).
2. Determine needs for documentation and reporting (of all internal and referred appointments and results) (5.2H).
3. Follow established policy in initiating or terminating medical treatment (5.4A–C).
4. Exercise efficient time management (6.6A).
5. Orient patients to office schedules and appointment procedures (7.1A,B).

Glossary

Acute condition: condition that is not a life-threatening (emergency) situation but should be treated promptly
Block scheduling: filling preset intervals (usually 15 minutes) on a physician's daily schedule sheet
Buffer time: "free" time slots during the day's schedule
Disease: a pathologic process with characteristic signs and symptoms that usually requires specific treatment
Emergency patients: patients whose medical conditions necessitate immediate care
Essential information: information required for proper scheduling: patient's name, complaint, time of onset, duration, and patient's telephone number
Hemorrhage: sudden, profuse, and excessive bleeding
Illness: a condition that deviates from a normal state
No-show: a patient who fails to appear for a scheduled appointment
Prompting: explaining clearly to patients what is expected of them
Sign: objective physical evidence of disease or dysfunction
Symptom: any indication of disease or illness perceived by the patient

The complexity of medical practice, combined with the demand for expanded physician's services, has increased the need for an efficient appointment-scheduling system. The traditional approach to scheduling appointments in the medical office is being challenged by the development of urgent and immediate care centers, which offer physician availability without appointment. In most of these centers, physicians are accessible to walk-in patients from early morning to very late evening 7 days a week. Limited office hours or extended waits are not as acceptable to patients today as they were in the past. Patients' expectations for health care have evolved beyond the treatment of acute illness. Illness prevention and maximum wellness are additional health goals characteristic of many contemporary patients.

While scheduled hours are still more common than nonscheduled office hours in office practice, the pressure of competing scheduling arrangements increases the emphasis on optimal use of office resources and efficient management of the physician's and the patient's time. Physicians need sufficient time to provide comprehensive care to each patient. However, they must receive a sufficient number of patients economically feasible to maintain the practice.

Patients, by contrast, want to be seen on time. In addition, they want the assurance that they have been allotted adequate contact with the physician. Considering both the patient's and the physician's needs in adopting a method of appointment scheduling is necessary but difficult.

The most common practice for scheduling individual appointments balances both the patient's and the physician's needs. This practice, called *blocking method,* is a time-specified approach to preplanned appointments. *Blocking* means segmenting and allotting specific times for patient care in the appointment book.

This method allots time both for visits scheduled in advance and for same-day, unscheduled visits, such as for acute illness. Scheduling parameters are shaped by the physician's preferences, the type of specialty, the facilities, the size and type of staff, and the needs of the typical patient. Although scheduling alternatives are discussed, this chapter emphasizes time-specified scheduling and presents information that the medical assistant needs to know in order to develop appointment management skills. The techniques of appointment scheduling are related to time management, which is one of the most pervasive concerns of the office staff.

APPOINTMENT SCHEDULING SYSTEMS

TIME-SPECIFIED SCHEDULING

The time-specified approach is most widely used for appointment scheduling in medical offices. In this method, each time frame printed on the appointment sheet must be scrutinized for accountability. The time-specified method uses the physician's time efficiently while providing competent, comprehensive care to patients. Obviously, the use of time on the appointment sheet must be organized and planned in advance to accommodate patient and nonpatient appointments, emergencies, facility and staff availability, and unpredictable disruptions.

The time interval between appointments is a matter of physician discretion. Appointment books are typically blocked in 15-minute time segments. Patients requiring more than 15 minutes would have an arrow extending from below their name and through the required number of segments. For instance, a patient scheduled for a complete physical examination may require four segments (1 hour). One of the advantages of planned appointments is that when the system is operating efficiently, the physician and the staff do not experience the stress of being rushed to catch up, and the patient feels assured of receiving adequate attention.

Example

10:15 Evelyn Jones — Pap smear
10:30
10:45 John Carter — back pain
11:00 Cindy Lee — premarital exam

OPEN HOURS SCHEDULING

The only scheduling required for open hours is the decision of when to open and close the office. This method was the first used by physicians. Patients are seen by the physician on a first come – first served basis. As the demands for the physician's time changed, individualized appointments became common practice. However, in some geographic areas, open hours are regaining popularity. As was previously mentioned, health care facilities, such as urgent care centers based in various outreach locations, are providing immediate care for acute illness without appointments and are attracting a significant patient population. Because these facilities offer 10- to 12-hour, 7-day-a-week physician availability, patients appear willing to accept "open hours" and expect to wait to be seen by the physician. Obviously, the open hours approach is heavily weighted toward the patient's needs, allowing optimum flexibility. The disadvantage, of course, is the potential inefficient use of the physician's time. Most physicians in private practice are reluctant to return to this mode of scheduling.

WAVE SCHEDULING

Wave scheduling is a type of appointment planning that allows more flexibility than structured, time-segmented allotment. In wave scheduling, several patients are scheduled in a specific period (usually 1 hour). Patients are instructed to arrive on the hour and are seen in the order of their arrival. The rationale for this method is the belief that 15-minute segments are too confining. Although the physician may still see four patients in 1 hour and the average is still 15 minutes, some patients require more, others less, than the 15-minute segment. The wave method allows for these variations. A major disadvantage is the confusion that results when each patient learns that the others were scheduled for the same time. The medical assistant must take care not to schedule too many lengthy procedures in 1 hour because doing so may delay the physician, the office staff, and the patient. Therefore, unless they have received an advance letter or brochure describing the policies of the practice, most patients will not find wave scheduling as palatable as the time-specified approach.

Example

    10:00 Evelyn Jones — Pap smear
          John Carter — back pain
    10:30 Cindy Lee — premarital exam

MODIFIED WAVE SCHEDULING

The modified wave is a type of scheduling that combines the time-specified and wave approaches. Patients are instructed to arrive at the office in planned intervals within the designated hour. Many alternatives are available for scheduling. For instance, one patient may be scheduled at 9:00, another patient at 9:20, and a third at 9:40. Another example is the scheduling of three patients in 30 minutes at 10-minute intervals. The second half hour can be used for catching up or for seeing only two patients. The risk of confusion that exists with the wave method also applies to the modified wave.

Example

    10:00 Evelyn Jones — Pap smear
    10:10 John Carter — back pain
    10:30 Joe Smith — BP check
    10:45 Next scheduled appointment

DOUBLE BOOKING

The practice of scheduling patients for the same appointment time is called *double booking*. Double booking is used in the wave scheduling alternative previously discussed. Scheduling patients for the same appointment time risks a decrease in satisfaction. Patients may suspect the staff of "herding in" as many patients in as short a time as possible and without sufficient personal attention. For this reason, time-specified scheduling continues to remain the standard practice.

Example

    10:00 Evelyn Jones — Pap smear
          John Carter — back pain
    10:15 Paul Andrews — skin rash
          Jean Smith — abdominal pain

CATEGORIZATION SCHEDULING

Categorization scheduling is another modification of the time-specified approach. Specific procedures are scheduled in certain time frames. For example, the phy-
sician may request that the medical assistant schedule all routine physical examinations in the morning or on two mornings a week. Another example is a pediatrician's office that schedules all sick children at the same period (e.g., 8:30 to 11 AM) to keep them separate from healthy children scheduled for well-child visits. This type of scheduling better prepares the physician for certain types of diagnostic procedures and can accommodate his or her personal mental and physical energy expenditures.

THE APPOINTMENT BOOK

Although some offices schedule appointments by computer, the appointment book is still the method of choice. Regardless of the method used, the scheduling guidelines apply to the recording of appointment data.

In most offices, the first step in implementing a scheduling system is to acquire an appropriate appointment book. Figure 10–1 shows an example of a standard appointment book sheet. Spiral-bound or looseleaf appointment books are available to meet the physician's advance scheduling needs for 1 year. Single pages may contain column space for 1 day or 1 week (five columns) and may be spread across two pages. If special needs exist, such as scheduling for a large number of physicians or a space on the sheet for special information, alternatives are available. Figure 10–2 is an example of a specialized appointment sheet for a three-physician office. Medical supply houses offer a wide variety of styles and formats to meet these individualized needs.

Regardless of style or format, however, essential information must be recorded on all appointment sheets. In addition, before a particular scheduling system is chosen, the office staff must consider several other factors, such as the size and placement of the book, time allowance for particular procedures, and other organizational concerns. (Refer to the Procedure, "Organize the Appointment Book," on page 202.)

ESSENTIAL INFORMATION

The office scheduling sheets must provide adequate space for recording the following data:

1. *Who.* The name of the person making the appointment
2. *Why.* The purpose of the appointment
3. *When.* The time designated for the office visit
4. *Duration.* The length of time needed for the visit
5. *Additional information.* The patient's home and work telephone numbers in case of cancellation or change in schedule, or if the patient is new.

The medical assistant should note additional tests to be done that day, such as an x-ray, before the patient sees the physician. The patient should come 30 minutes before the appointment to allow time for the tests.

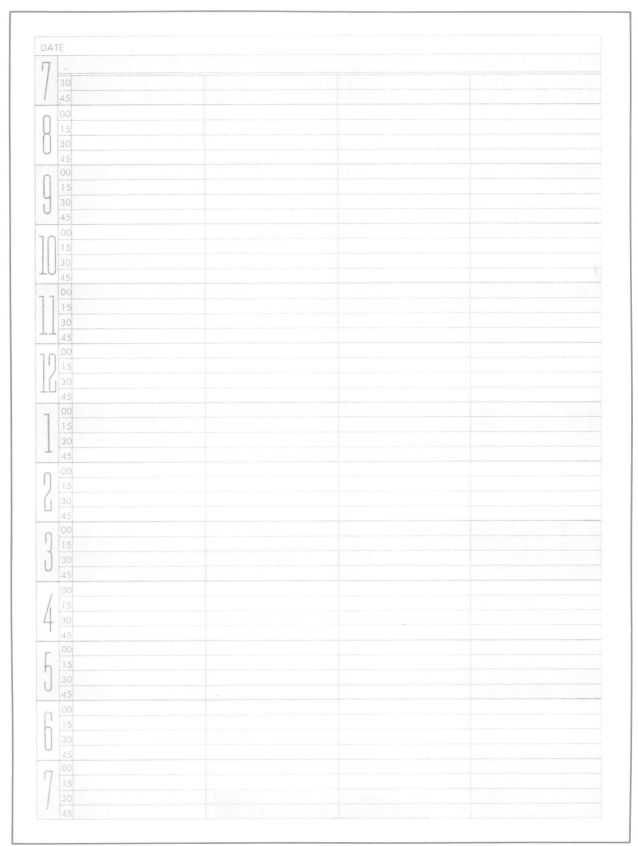

Figure 10–1. A standard appointment sheet.

Month _____

Date _____

Day _____

	Dr. Smith	Dr. Jones	Dr. Brown
8:00	At State University		
8:15	— — —		
8:30	— — —		
8:45	— — —		
9:00	— — —	Hospital Rounds	
9:15	— — —	— — —	
9:30	— — —	— — —	
9:45	— — —	— — —	
10:00			
10:15			
10:30			
10:45			
11:00			
11:15			
11:30			
11:45			
12:00			
12:15			
12:30			
12:45			
1:00			

Figure 10–2. A specialized appointment sheet.

Certain formats require that all time frames on the sheet be accounted for by either markings or written information. The principles and procedures for recording essential information are presented at the end of this chapter.

SIZE AND PLACEMENT

Although the size of the appointment book depends on the scheduling demands of the practice, it should fit in a specific space on the medical assistant's desk and should open flat for writing ease. Filled appointment books are placed in a storage area and are not destroyed because of their potential importance as legal documents in litigation proceedings.

LIST OF STANDARD PROCEDURE TIMES

A list that contains the average times required to complete common office procedures is particularly useful. Table 10–1 is an example. This list has two important uses. First, the medical assistant can use it to determine the time required for specific types of appointments, such as Pap smears. Second, the list can identify procedures that may cause scheduling problems.

For example, a review of past schedule data may show that days with a large number of physical examinations caused delays and excessive waiting periods. Such data might indicate that time allowances for physical examinations should be reevaluated. (Please refer to the procedure for evaluation of office waiting periods discussed in Chapter 5.)

By working with the physician in formulating a list of procedure times, and through periodic reevaluation, the medical assistant can help to minimize scheduling difficulties.

EXTENDED TIMES FOR PATIENTS WITH SPECIAL NEEDS

Some patients, such as the elderly or handicapped, may require more office time than others. The list of

Table 10-1
GUIDE TO ESTIMATED TIMES FOR COMMON MEDICAL OFFICE PROCEDURES*

Procedure	Time in Minutes
Allergy testing	30
Cast change	30
Complete physical examination	30-60
with electrocardiogram	15+
Dressing change (with drain)	15
Hypertension follow-up	10-15
Minor surgery	30-60
Office visits†	
Brief	5-10
Intermediate (for acute illness)	15-20
Extended	30+
Patient teaching session/conference	30-60
Pelvis and pap test	15-30
Prenatal checkup	15-30
Replacement suturing	30
Suture removal	10-20

*The times given are approximate and may be adjusted to accommodate physician preference and patient needs.

†The intermediate visit is the most common. These breakdowns reflect standard manual record-keeping categorizations.

standard times could include the names of patients known to require more time and a notation of the reason.

SCHEDULING GUIDELINES

The major objectives of determining required time are to maximize the physician's time and to accommodate patient needs. Therefore, it is important to gather and evaluate basic information before organizing the day's appointments.

1. Assess the different types of appointment scheduled (physical examinations, treatment, tests). Some physicians may prefer, for example, to schedule all routine examinations in the morning because they can be postponed easily if the physician is delayed.
2. As was previously discussed, an estimate of the time required for each common type of appointments is necessary for effective planning (e.g., complete examination: 60 minutes; treatment: 15 minutes, etc.). The medical assistant, with the collaboration of the physician, estimates time allotments for procedures.
3. The handling of acute illnesses and emergencies also requires planning. It is common for patients to call with problems requiring immediate attention. Therefore, most physicians prefer to schedule blocks of time for same-day visits.

The medical assistant should discuss these considerations with the physician before adopting a scheduling plan, and the specifics should be described in the procedures manual.

Besides helping to organize the appointment system, the medical assistant assumes responsibility for monitoring it. Monitoring includes determining the length of time each appointment requires and whether the time allotted for emergency cases is adequate or excessive. These procedures are particularly important if patients routinely wait longer than is reasonable for their appointments. There may also be frequent time lags in the physician's day when no appointments are scheduled. The actual time required for various kinds of appointments may differ from the predicted time. The physician must rely on feedback from the medical assistant concerning these conditions. To help the physician participate in maintaining patient flow and schedule, the medical assistant should post a typed list of all patients and the purpose of their visits in the order of their expected arrival, or give the list to the physician at the beginning of office hours. The physician's preferences, the availability of staff and facilities, and the accommodation of patients' needs can harmonize if the appointment plan is monitored continuously.

LIMITED AND SHARED RESOURCES

Another scheduling guideline is to assess the use of available resources. The office may house a particular resource, such as a special examination room or therapeutic device, which because of constant use causes problematic disruptions in patient flow. This consideration is particularly relevant when the medical assistant schedules appointments for several physicians who share office facilities and equipment.

If sharing facilities becomes a recurring problem, the medical assistant can anticipate and prevent the difficulty by including a separate scheduling category in the appointment book. Figure 10-3 illustrates a scheduling arrangement for a situation involving a limited facility.

RECORDED APPOINTMENT INFORMATION

Essential information is usually recorded in pencil. However, some physicians may prefer that black ink be used to protect against potential legal problems because ink is less likely to be erased. A red pen may be used to indicate that a patient is new. Essential information can be recorded in pencil and a red N placed after the new patient's name. Corrections, such as appointment cancellations, are made with a black pen rather than a pencil. The major objectives in recording information are to write legibly and neatly and to include pertinent information.

Some patients will make appointments in person at the time of the office visit. However, most appointments are scheduled over the telephone. In any case, the medical assistant must record meticulously all the required information according to the guidelines listed below.

Month _____

Date _____

Day _____

	Dr. Smith	Dr. Jones	Ultrasound Machine
8:00			
8:15		Green, Lois 412-6190	
8:30		(Back Pain)	Dr. Jones: Mrs. Green
8:45			
9:00			
9:15			
9:30			
9:45			
10:00			
10:15			
10:30	Brown, Jim 417-2014		
10:45	(Tennis Elbow)		Dr. Smith: Mr. Brown
11:00			
11:15			
11:30			
11:45			
12:00			
12:15			
12:30			
12:45			
1:00			

Figure 10-3. A limited facilities appointment sheet.

1. *Patient's name.* Record the full name, written or printed clearly, with the last name entered first in the space provided. The full name is necessary because several patients may have the same surname, particularly in family medicine practices:

   9:30 Evans, Ralph (Sr.)
   9:45 Evans, Raymond
   10:00 Evans, Ralph (Jr.)

2. *Reason for visit.* Note the purpose of the visit in the book, using universally accepted abbreviations. Abbreviations most frequently used in appointment scheduling are as follows:

N & V	Nausea and vomiting
CPE or CPX	Complete physical examination
I & D	Incision and drainage
PAP	Pap smear
ROV	Return office visit
B/P	Blood pressure check
S/R	Suture removal
P & P	Pap smear and pelvic examination

   (Other abbreviations used in medicine are contained in the Appendix.)

3. *Telephone number.* Both home and work numbers should be recorded in case the appointment must be changed. The letter *H* should precede a home number, and *W* a work or business number. Even if it is unnecessary to record both telephone numbers for all patients in a particular practice, it is useful to record both numbers for all new patients.

4. *Time of appointment.* The patient's name should be entered next to the appropriate time.

5. *Length of appointment.* Knowledge of time al-

lowance for specific office procedures is required to estimate the time needed for a particular appointment. The medical assistant should insert the schedule guide for procedures and their approximate times, with an example of a blocked sheet, in the inside cover of the appointment book for convenient access (see Table 10–1).

Figure 10–4 illustrates appointment blocking. Mrs. Jones is scheduled for 30 minutes for her annual physical examination, and Mr. Brown is coming in for a postsurgical checkup. Mr. Brown's visit will take only 15 minutes. Note that Mrs. Jones's name is followed by an arrow that indicates a need for the 8:15 to 8:30 time slot.

Time-segment accountability is the essence of schedule blocking. The appointment sheet contains 15-minute spaces. Therefore, a patient who needs a 45-minute appointment at 10:00 AM is written into the 10:00 space, and an arrow is drawn through the next two spaces (see Lois Peters in Fig. 10–4). Because there is no arrow under Joyce Martin in Figure 10–4, the 9:00 AM slot is available for scheduling. Not all physicians prefer the use of 15-minute segments, which assumes that patient visits will average 15 minutes. In addition to acquiring familiarity with the mechanics of appointment scheduling, the medical assistant may follow general scheduling guidelines that facilitate responsiveness to the needs of the patient and the physician. The Procedure, "Schedule an Appointment," on p. 203 summarizes these guidelines.

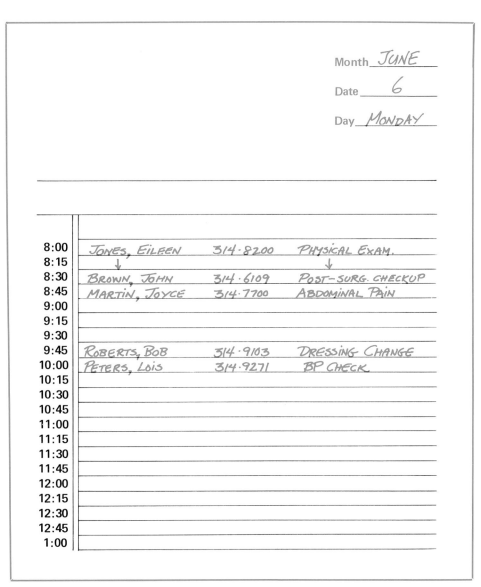

Figure 10–4. Proper appointment entries.

PATIENT CONSIDERATIONS IN APPOINTMENT SCHEDULING

SCHEDULING THE PHYSICAL EXAMINATION APPOINTMENT

Many patients request appointments for routine physical examination. Although this type of appointment does not take precedence over an emergency or acute condition, the patient should not be made to wait for an unreasonable length of time either in the waiting room or the examination room. Understanding the motive for the physical examination request is an important consideration in assigning an appointment time. The request for a physical examination may reflect either the patient's interest in obtaining regular checkups or a concern related to a particular problem. The appointment may be for a return visit suggested by the physician. It is important to remember that an appointment including a physical examination for the first visit may require additional time. If the patient is not experiencing any specific problems and has not been asked to return within a certain period, it is accepted practice to schedule a physical examination within 4 to 6 weeks.

ACCOMMODATING PATIENT NEEDS

Although a logical system of appointments may be established, flexibility and an understanding of the needs of individual patients must govern its application. In certain instances, patients cannot be scheduled within the structured appointment times. The physician must decide how to accommodate the patient's schedule and must provide guidelines that are applicable in such situations. These guidelines should be detailed in the procedures manual.

Patients are often reluctant to state their purpose in requesting an appointment. In this instance, the medical assistant must say, for example, "Mr. Jones, having a general idea of why you wish to see the doctor will help me to schedule an adequate amount of time for your appointment."

The medical assistant should direct the patient in choosing an appointment time. Awareness of special needs is important in making appointments. For instance, a disabled patient may require a longer appointment time. Other patients with special needs are those scheduled for diagnostic or laboratory tests, or for procedures that require fasting or other special preparation. For such a patient, a late afternoon appointment would not be appropriate. Also, a patient requesting an appointment for a second opinion before surgery is given scheduling priority. Priority is also given to patients referred by other physicians. When possible, such patients are seen within 24 hours. The medical assistant should also consider the time required to obtain results of laboratory, radiologic, or other diagnostic tests scheduled outside the office.

Patients who are busy professionals themselves may prefer early morning appointments or may wish to be scheduled at other times when waiting is minimized. Time-constrained patients can be instructed to call the office an hour before the appointment to determine whether office visits are running late. Calling in advance can reduce the irritation of a long wait. The medical assistant should encourage nonpatients, usually walk-ins, to make an appointment. Unless the nonpatient is presenting an emergency or acute illness, a full schedule should not be altered.

APPOINTMENT SCREENING

The medical assistant must use prudent judgment in protecting the health and convenience of the patient and maintaining the efficient operation of the office. If the patient is experiencing an emergency, the medical assistant either notifies the physician, or in appropriate circumstances, encourages the patient to obtain emergency treatment in a hospital, medical center, or emergency care center.

Patient screening, discussed in Chapter 9, is necessary to determine the urgency of the patient's need to see the physician that same day. All office staff should be trained in telephone and appointment guidelines on an ongoing basis. Established guidelines should indicate what questions the medical assistant asks the patient to reveal the nature of the symptoms.

The medical assistant must also be aware that degrees of severity often distinguish an acute illness from an emergency. Examples of conditions that require evaluation include but are not limited to:

Emergencies (Life Threatening) Requiring Immediate Evaluation

1. Acute allergic reaction with respiratory difficulty
2. Convulsion in progress
3. Convulsion that has stopped
4. Drug overdose or poisoning
5. Coma or unconsciousness with or without injury
6. Diabetic reaction
7. Uncontrollable bleeding
8. Drowning or near-drowning
9. Penetrating wounds of the chest or stomach
10. Behavior changes following head injury
11. Severe chest pain
12. Severe pain anywhere
13. Excessive bleeding from anywhere in the body (e.g., vagina, open wound, surgical site)
14. Dizziness
15. Forceful nausea, vomiting, or diarrhea lasting more than 24 hours
16. Inability to move a body part, or stiff neck and ill appearance
17. Difficulty in breathing or asthma attack
18. Sudden change in any condition
19. Laceration or suspected fracture
20. Head injury, even if there are no symptoms or only mild symptoms, such as disorientation or mild headache

21. Injury following any fall from a high place
22. Very sudden illness or illness that appears serious
23. Acute allergic reaction without respiratory symptoms

Conditions Requiring Same-Day Evaluation

1. Unusual discharge from body orifices, such as blood in urine or vomitus
2. Fever that lasts more than 24 hours
3. Earache
4. Rash
5. Sore throat
6. Swollen glands
7. Skin infections
8. Pain or burning with urination
9. Symptoms not improving
10. Pain in abdomen, joints, or muscles.

An understanding of illness, disease, and the related symptoms learned in the clinical component of the medical assistant program enables the medical assistant to recognize the difference between acute illness and emergency. For instance, pain anywhere must always be evaluated for emergency. After screening a patient who has chest pain and learning the onset, location, intensity, and duration of the pain, the medical assistant recognizes that an emergency exists. When the physician is not available, the medical assistant refers the patient to an emergency care facility and arranges transportation if it appears advisable to do so. When the physician is in the office, he or she is interrupted immediately.

Another patient may call complaining of diarrhea. When screened, the patient states that he has been noticing it for 3 weeks and that it has occurred approximately five times. No bleeding or pain is present. This situation does not represent an emergency. The medical assistant, however, schedules an appointment as soon as possible.

MOTIVATING PATIENTS

No matter how efficient the mechanical aspects of the office scheduling system, the behavior of patients affects its operation. Confused, late, or absent patients wreak havoc in the best-organized systems. It is the medical assistant's role to motivate and educate patients in this regard.

As each appointment is scheduled, the medical assistant gently reminds the patient of the expected or optimum arrival time. The medical assistant might say, "We would appreciate it if you could be in the office a few minutes before your scheduled appointment." Patients who habitually arrive late can be scheduled at the end of the day, when there is less chance of disrupting scheduling flow. In addition to gentle reminders and schedule manipulation, the medical assistant can elicit patient cooperation by explaining the importance of keeping appointments and being on time. These explanations

can be printed in brochures that describe the practice. Patients are also more motivated to be on time for appointments when they are seen on schedule and their own time constraints are respected.

The medical assistant can help ensure the patient's cooperation by thanking patients for their promptness when it is appropriate to do so. For instance, when a patient enters the office on time, it is reinforcing to thank him or her for being on time: "Good morning, Mr. Davis. You are right on time for your appointment." It is also useful to be clear and direct in scheduling visits. The medical assistant might end a scheduling conversation with a statement such as, "We will see you in the office before 2:00 PM on Thursday, April 2nd."

Under no circumstances should the medical assistant be short or discourteous to a patient. Negative reinforcement can only complicate the already difficult problem of scheduling. The medical assistant should thank the patient who is positive and cooperative. If not, the medical assistant should either say nothing or choose a positive response.

Examples

NEGATIVE RESPONSE

You know, Mrs. Jones, by coming in late you set us all behind and we can never catch up. It's not fair.

POSITIVE RESPONSE

Mrs. Jones, I know how difficult it is to be on time, but your coming late creates some scheduling problems for our office. Can I help in some way? Perhaps there are times that would be more convenient for you.

WELCOMING THE PATIENT

Patients form initial impressions of the medical office as a consequence of their first interaction with the medical assistant. The medical assistant's initial behavior sets the tone for the patient's visit by influencing the patient's opinion about the visit. In addition, patients entering the office base their positive or negative judgments on the appeal of the physical surroundings. The patient generalizes judgments about the medical assistant and the physical surroundings to the competence of the physician and other staff members. If new patients or others visiting the office are made to feel welcome and comfortable, and the pleasantness of the surroundings creates a positive effect, the patient feels at ease with the decision to come to this physician. Patients expect their needs to be met by a competent and caring physician and staff. Their satisfaction is reflected in their cooperation with medical treatment, which both benefits the patients themselves and serves the best interests of the practice in promoting a positive image. Marketing and sales literature has demonstrated consistently that patients who are well treated and satisfied act as press agents. Dissatisfied patients, however, may discontinue the services of a particular physician regardless of his or her medical expertise, thereby detracting from a positive public image. More important, the dissatisfaction and anxiety caused by initial mistreatment may interfere with the medical effectiveness of the diagnostic and treatment regimen.

The medical assistant can function positively as the sales and marketing agent for the office by extending courtesy and goodwill, and by projecting enthusiasm and a genuine concern for the patient. As an effective marketing representative, the medical assistant helps to ensure the continued financial success of the entire practice, and consequently the job security of the office staff.

In welcoming the entering patient, the medical assistant has the first opportunity to influence that patient's judgment concerning the practice. New patients require an orientation to the office. Because medical assistants are on duty day after day, they feel at ease in the office and may forget how intimidating and foreign it can seem to patients, particularly new ones. A patient may be sick or in pain and may be nervous, irritable, and uncommunicative. Even under the best of circumstances, the patient is probably taking time from a busy schedule, missing opportunities to do other important things, and concerned about paying medical bills. The medical assistant must remember that the purpose of the medical office and its staff is to meet the needs of each person who enters, including the patient's family, friends, and others.

Patients should not receive the impression that paperwork, or a conversation with another staff member or a personal telephone call, is more important than their arrival. The medical assistant must make a concerted effort to greet every person who arrives in the office and to use empathy when welcoming each patient. To deal successfully with patients, the medical assistant must be aware of their frustrations and must act as a host or hostess even if the patient is an unwilling guest.

THE GREETING

Each person who arrives at the medical office should be acknowledged. In an office where people could easily enter unnoticed, instructions to sign in on arrival should be posted. The medical assistant can greet patients as they come to the desk to sign in. When the medical assistant is talking on the telephone or engaged in conversation with another person at the desk, a smile or nod can acknowledge the patient signing in. As soon as possible, the medical assistant should face the patient and offer an appropriate greeting.

Example

"Mrs. Jones, hello. I'm sorry I was on the phone when you came in."

The medical assistant should avoid asking the patient "How are you today?" or "How are you feeling?" The patient may feel uncomfortable answering these questions in the public waiting room. Also, the medical assistant probably does not have time for a lengthy conversation and should therefore take care when asking leading questions or making comments. However, it would be appropriate to provide a realistic assessment of the waiting period, such as "The doctor will be ready for you shortly," or some other comment based on the medical assistant's knowledge of the patient. In addition to greeting the patient, the medical assistant should also acknowledge and welcome other persons accompanying the patient.

The medical assistant's greeting should be brief and limited but not rushed. If the physician is late, the greeting could also include a truthful explanation of any office or scheduling problems (the air conditioning is malfunctioning, the physician is late because of an emergency, etc.). When stating that the physician is delayed, however, the medical assistant should not elaborate on the reason beyond providing a clear explanation when it is appropriate.

As has been mentioned, the medical assistant should, if possible, begin the day's schedule by making a list of the patients expected, and by noting new patients and becoming familiar with their names and the reasons for their visit. Addressing patients and other visitors by name indicates that their visits have been anticipated. In addition, the medical assistant can then consult the sign-in sheet to check the order of arrivals and note any missed appointments. The sign-in sheet (Fig. 10–5) should be labeled with the physician's name if there is more than one physician in the practice.

NEW PATIENT ORIENTATION AND REGISTRATION

For persons visiting the office for the first time, the medical assistant follows the greeting with an explana-

Date _____
(Please Sign In Below)

1. _____
2. _____
3. _____
4. _____
5. _____
6. _____
7. _____
8. _____

Figure 10–5. An office sign-in sheet.

tion of office policy. Information may include the days and hours when the office is open, prescription refill policy, telephoning, the handling of emergency situations, appointment scheduling procedures, insurance processing, and preferred methods of payment. Some offices mail brochures or letters with this information to new patients before their first visit. In such cases, it is good policy to ask at the first visit if the patient received the information and if there are any questions. Many physicians, however, prefer that patients read these materials at the time of the first visit.

The medical assistant also obtains the new patient's data at this time. Nonmedical patient data is usually recorded on a patient registration form (Fig. 10–6).

One method of collecting the data is to give the patient the forms with a pen and clipboard, explain what is needed, and request that the patient fill out the forms. This method frees the medical assistant to perform other tasks and lessens the chance of information error. The registration form or card is then placed in a file box or file wheel (Fig. 10–7) for ready access. Preferences for appointment times and other special notations can also be written on the patient registration card. In addition to the correct spelling of the patient's name, the medical assistant can note a phonetic spelling, particularly for names that are difficult to pronounce.

PLANNING FOR UNANTICIPATED DISRUPTIONS

No matter how carefully scheduling is maintained, the nature of medical practice creates a number of scheduling problems. Causes of unanticipated delays include the physician's hospital and professional responsibilities, patients who are late for their appointments or cancel minutes before, referrals from other offices, and emergency visits. Because delays occur in every medical office, they should be expected and accommodated. However, all unanticipated visits except emergency cases should be scheduled around existing appointments.

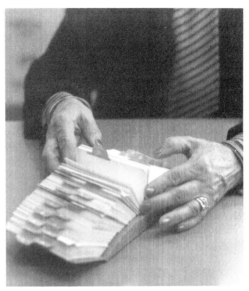

Figure 10–7. File wheel for patient registration cards.

PHYSICIAN DELAYS

Most physicians have responsibilities outside the medical office, such as patient hospital visits, hospital staff meetings, and surgical schedules. These out-of-office responsibilities must be worked into the office scheduling system. Figure 10–8 illustrates a procedure for blocking the times that the physician will be out of the office. The block of time should include travel time to and from the hospital or other destination.

Because the treatment of hospital patients or the completion of a surgical procedure may take precedence over the physician's office responsibilities, the physician will sometimes be late for office visits. If the physician will be delayed for an extensive period, it is important to tell the patients. Usually a delay of 10 minutes is considered reasonable.

As was previously mentioned, in this era of competitive medicine, the physician must be attentive to patient needs. Working people do not have time for extended

Last Name   First

Address _____

_____

Phone   W_____   H_____

Employer _____

Insurance _____

Spouse _____   Children _____

Figure 10–6. A patient registration and intake card.

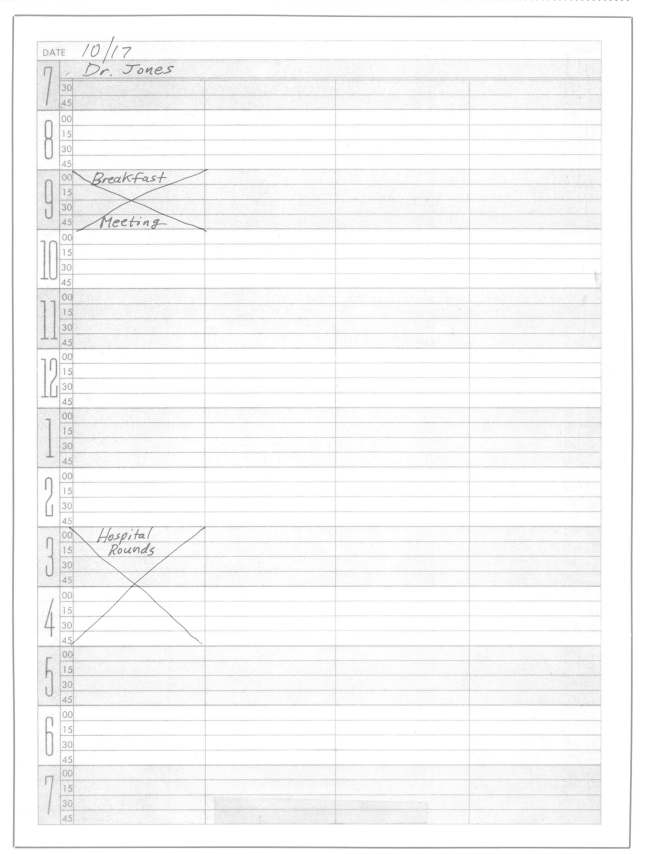

DATE _10/17_

7 . Dr. Jones
    30
    45

8   00
    15
    30
    45

9   00 Breakfast
    15
    30
    45 Meeting

10 00
    15
    30
    45

11 00
    15
    30
    45

12 00
    15
    30
    45

1   00
    15
    30
    45

2   00
    15
    30
    45

3   00 Hospital
    15   Rounds
    30
    45

4   00
    15
    30
    45

5   00
    15
    30
    45

6   00
    15
    30
    45

7   00
    15
    30
    45

Figure 10–8. The appointment sheet should indicate blocks of time (including travel time) during which the physician is out of the office or otherwise unavailable for seeing patients.

delays. Although most medical office visitors realize that there may be a reasonable delay, telephoning patients to inform them of longer delays, when possible, is a necessary and courteous service that is usually well received. Also, informing patients when they arrive that their appointments are delayed can temper their annoyance, particularly when they are given the opportunity to reschedule. Emergency occurrences that cause long waits are understandable if they are infrequent. If, however, long delays become the rule rather than the exception, it may be useful to reevaluate the appointment management system.

The physician's involvement in professional societies and community organizations also places demands on appointment management. The physician may leave the office regularly to attend meetings, conferences, and other professional functions. The medical assistant must note these commitments in the appointment book to avoid scheduling patients during this time and to remind the physician of the commitment.

The medical assistant should review the appointment book with the physician at least once each week to advise him or her of upcoming commitments and to allow time for adjustments. The physician's awareness of how time is being allocated can identify objectives and foster cooperation.

THE ACUTELY ILL PATIENT

As was mentioned earlier, patients who report symptoms of acute illness are usually seen immediately or on the same day that the call is received. The medical assistant must schedule open times in advance to accommodate acutely ill patients.

The frequency of acute illness depends on the type of medical practice. If such calls occur rarely (as might be the case in a general surgeon's office), they can be worked into the regular patient flow and given preference. If, however, these calls are frequent and occur daily, as in a family medical practice, it is necessary to expand the number of open time frames. If, by asking specific questions, the medical assistant determines that the patient is acutely ill and must be seen that day, an appointment is scheduled in a block designated for acute illness. If all time slots are filled, the medical assistant can check with the physician and call the patient back regarding the designated time.

If, however, the patient is already scheduled and is seeking an earlier appointment because of convenience, the medical assistant should encourage the patient to keep the previously scheduled time. If the illness or condition is not acute and the patient is not scheduled for an appointment, the medical assistant schedules the patient at the earliest available time that is convenient for the patient.

As a courtesy, some offices create a "tickler list" of patients who desire earlier visits. In case of a cancellation, the persons on this list can be contacted.

When a particular patient's need for a same-day appointment is questionable, there are several possible responses:

1. A brief note including the patient's name and symptoms brings the problem to the physician's attention. The medical assistant can call back and inform the patient of the physician's decision, and the appointment can be scheduled accordingly.
2. For reference, the medical assistant can use a relatively detailed guide to common acute problems and symptoms. This guide should be inserted in the appointment book or strategically posted at the desk in addition to being included in the procedure manual.
3. The physician's experience is the ultimate basis for decisions regarding appointment scheduling.

ACCEPTING REFERRALS

Other offices may regularly send patients for examination or treatment. As a courtesy to other physicians who make these referrals, the medical assistant should make every effort to schedule the referred patient promptly (within 24 hours of the referral, when possible). The medical assistant notes the referral in the appointment book and subsequently in the patient record for reference so that the physician can acknowledge the referral or write a letter of appreciation to the referring physician.

Another type of referral is the patient referral: one patient refers another. Although an effort is made to schedule the appointment promptly, the referred patient is not given special preference. However, the office should acknowledge the referral by sending an appreciation card to the referring patient.

WALK-INS

Occasionally, patients or nonpatients walk in and request an immediate appointment with the physician. In handling these situations, the medical assistant must be tactful and fair. If no emergency exists, the medical assistant informs the visitor that the physician is seeing patients and that the day is completely scheduled. After obtaining pertinent data and determining the reason for the visit, the medical assistant may offer to schedule an appointment in the next available space. It may be appropriate to record the visitor's name and number and instruct the visitor that the physician will telephone later. The medical assistant, with the physician's approval, may also suggest that the patient go to the nearest immediate care center and make a follow-up appointment with the office physician. Obviously, discretionary judgment is necessary. The approach to this situation must depend on the identity of the visitor, the reason for the appointment request, and the physician's preference.

CANCELLATIONS AND NO-SHOWS

Advance-notice cancellations and missed appointments (no-shows) occur regularly in medical practice.

Patients who cancel occasionally should be thanked for their courtesy in notifying the office. Even short notice is better than none, allowing the medical assistant to call patients whose names are on the "tickler list" or the physician to catch up if the office is running behind schedule.

When a patient fails to keep an appointment, the medical assistant should make a note on both the schedule and the patient's chart. All no-shows and cancellations are identified in the appointment book by "no-show," "NS," or "failed to show," or, for patient-canceled appointments, "canceled." These notations are entered above the patient's name on the appointment sheet. If another appointment is scheduled, the date and time are noted in the appointment book. All no-shows and appointments canceled by patients or the physician should be recorded in the progress notes section of the patient record by day, date, and appointment time. Careful documentation is the best protection against legal claims. The medical assistant should record all attempts to reach the patient and any refusal by the patient to reschedule.

If a patient complaining of a headache is scheduled for examination but does not keep the appointment, the patient cannot successfully claim that any subsequently developed health problem is due to malpractice or abandonment if his or her failure to keep the appointment is on record. If a patient's appointment is not rescheduled and the patient prefers to reschedule at another time, the notation "w/c" ("will call") should be written in the appointment book after the patient's name and a notation made in the chart notes. The Procedure, "Record Patient Cancellations and Missed Appointments," on page 204 lays out the steps of this process.

It is sometimes necessary for the physician to cancel appointments with patients. If cancellation occurs on the day the appointment is scheduled, the medical assistant telephones the patient and reschedules the appointment. Because of legal concerns, the physician must be careful to cancel only nonurgent appointments or to refer urgent visits to another physician rather than delay attention.

When the physician cancels in advance, the medical assistant again telephones the patient and reschedules. If the patient cannot be reached, the medical assistant may send a letter by certified mail informing the patient of the cancellation and giving rescheduling instructions. The mail receipt is filed in the patient record.

BUFFER TIME

Many physicians find that no matter how meticulously the staff carries out the scheduling system, unanticipated difficulties cause overscheduling. Because of this problem, it is common practice to leave several periods unscheduled and to block them out in the appointment book. Usually, these buffer times are divided between morning and afternoon. These allotted times prevent the physician from running behind schedule. If there are constant delays and excess waiting periods,

the office should increase the time allotted for referrals, acute illness, and buffer periods. If, however, idle gaps occur between scheduled appointments, these allowances should be reduced.

REFERRAL TO OTHER FACILITIES

Occasionally, the physician must refer office patients to other facilities for clinical tests, consultations with other physicians, hospital admission, and often surgical procedures. The medical assistant usually makes the arrangements in cooperation with the patient.

First, the medical assistant consults the patient regarding his or her personal schedule and preferences. Information is then relayed to the referral office or the hospital, and the patient is kept informed.

In arranging a hospital or medical center admission, the medical assistant gives the following information to the admission secretary:

1. Patient's full name
2. Social security number
3. Address
4. Telephone number
5. Type of accommodation desired
6. Most recent prior admission
7. Admitting diagnosis
8. Age
9. Admitting physician's name
10. Occupation and insurance information, if requested

It is good practice to request the admission secretary send a copy of the admitting form to the office for the patient record. In scheduling a patient for diagnostic tests in a medical facility, the medical assistant gives the patient's name, address, and telephone number, the purpose of the examination, and other pertinent details as requested. In addition, the medical assistant informs the patient of any special preparation required and provides any available printed material that specifically details the particular procedure. The procedures and principles for scheduling referrals are outlined in the Procedure on page 205.

SCHEDULING SURGERY

The physician may determine that the patient requires surgery. The steps for scheduling surgery depend on the need. When the need for surgery is urgent, the first consideration is reserving time in the surgery department schedule. When the surgery is elective (preplanned and not urgent), the patient's scheduling preferences are considered along with the available period in the surgery department and the surgeon's schedule.

When an appropriate time has been determined, the medical assistant calls the surgery department secretary or officer in charge to reserve the time and the room, and often to arrange for the anesthesiologist. The surgery department representative requires the following information:

1. Day and time options approved by the physician
2. Type of surgery
3. Time required for the surgery
4. Patient's full name
5. Sex and age
6. Telephone number
7. Surgeon's name and names of assistants
8. Any special requests made by the physician, such as the type and amount of blood to be prepared if a transfusion should be necessary.

The patient may also be asked to complete a preadmission form. Some medical centers require this form to ensure that all admission records are processed before the actual date of admission. Depending on diagnostic-related group guidelines, patients may or may not be admitted the day before surgery. The medical assistant must be careful to coordinate these dates precisely.

HOSPITAL ADMISSION CERTIFICATION

In most cases, if a patient is to be admitted to the hospital, the reasons and planned length of stay must be reviewed and certified by the patient's insurance carrier. If precertification is not obtained, covered expenses may be reduced as much as 25%. The patient initiates the process by contacting the insurance carrier. In cases of emergency, the patient or the patient's family must contact the insurance carrier within 48 hours after admission. When a proposed hospitalization or treatment is reviewed and approved by the insurance carrier, the patient receives a *notice of pretreatment review*, or *preadmission certification*. A copy is also sent to the physician.

If medical complications prolong the patient's stay beyond the certified period, a *continued stay review* must be submitted for recertification before the patient's last certified day. This system encourages the earliest and most sound date of discharge, thus reducing unnecessary hospital stays and expenses.

If a patient is covered under a health maintenance organization or independent practice association the plan must provide or authorize all services. Inpatient services not covered by these plans require preadmission certification and continued stay review. Noncompliance may result in a reduction or denial of benefits. For network plan coverage, the participating primary care facility is responsible for initiating precertification and continued stay reviews.

SECOND SURGICAL OPINIONS

It is common for physicians to have different opinions about a patient's need for surgery. Many insurance carriers now encourage patients to seek second opinions, and pay 100% of the cost. Some insurance carriers require a second opinion for certain nonemergency, elective surgeries. Whether or not the second surgeon agrees with the first opinion, the insurance carrier pays for the second opinion and may pay regular benefits for noncosmetic procedures. If the patient has an elective

surgical procedure without seeking a second opinion, the insurance carrier may reimburse the patient at only 50% for covered surgeon fees or otherwise reduce the patient's benefits.

INSTRUCTING THE PATIENT

Patients often have questions and concerns regarding visits to hospitals and other offices. They ask important questions regarding impending procedures. The medical assistant should make every attempt to answer questions honestly. If the medical assistant does not know the answer, the patient should be referred to the physician or other appropriate resource person. Anxiety regarding a referral is common. Therefore, obtaining answers to questions is an effective way to increase the patient's confidence and diminish anxiety. Procedure and treatment brochures to prepare and educate the patient are often available from referral facilities.

Patients may be provided with preprinted referral slips that contain spaces for the name, address, telephone number, and check-in time for admission or outpatient procedures. For hospital admission, the same slip could list the personal items patients may bring with them.

Patients scheduled for diagnostic procedures or surgery should know what to expect. Although preparations differ for diagnostic procedures, certain expectations are routine for surgical procedures:

1. A chest x-ray, laboratory tests, and an electrocardiogram, if these tests have not been already performed
2. A visit from the anesthesiologist
3. Fasting and special skin preparations
4. Bowel preparations, if necessary

When the patient knows what to expect, anxiety is often reduced. The medical assistant should communicate verbal instructions carefully and not depend solely on the preprinted material to educate the patient and alleviate concern.

THE NEXT APPOINTMENT AND THE APPOINTMENT CARD

If possible, patients should be encouraged to make the next appointment before leaving the office. This practice eliminates the inefficiency of additional telephone calls and allows the medical assistant to speak directly with the patient. Some patients resist because of personal scheduling difficulties and must call back. Patients requiring frequent visits should be always scheduled on the same day and at the same time of day to help them remember appointment times.

Most physicians keep a supply of appointment cards on hand; such as the one shown in Figure 10-9. The card should contain the preprinted instruction, "If unable to keep your appointment, kindly give 24 hours' notice." Appointment cards may have pertinent instruc-

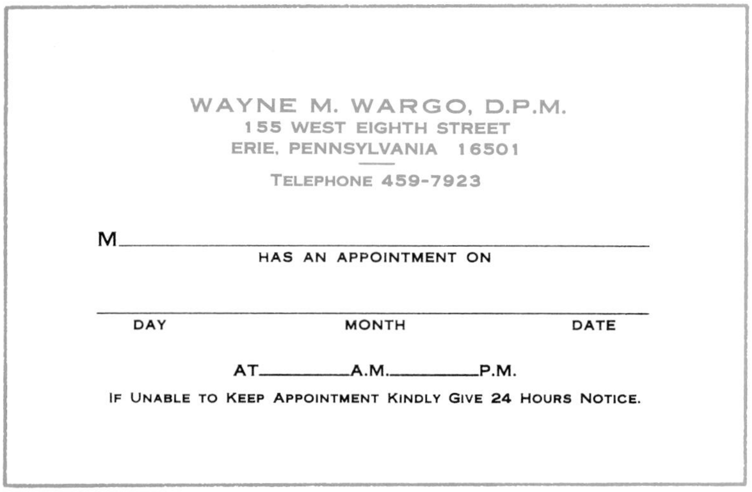

WAYNE M. WARGO, D.P.M.
155 WEST EIGHTH STREET
ERIE, PENNSYLVANIA 16501
TELEPHONE 459-7923

M_____
HAS AN APPOINTMENT ON

_____
DAY   MONTH   DATE

AT_____A.M._____P.M.
IF UNABLE TO KEEP APPOINTMENT KINDLY GIVE 24 HOURS NOTICE.

Figure 10–9. A typical appointment card.

tions printed on the back, such as a map, a list of substituting physicians on call in the physician's absence, or an explanation of the office policy regarding canceled appointments. Some offices require a minimal charge for cancellations without advance notice. If this policy is followed, it must be posted or printed on the back of the appointment card to let patients know in advance that there is a charge. However, most offices

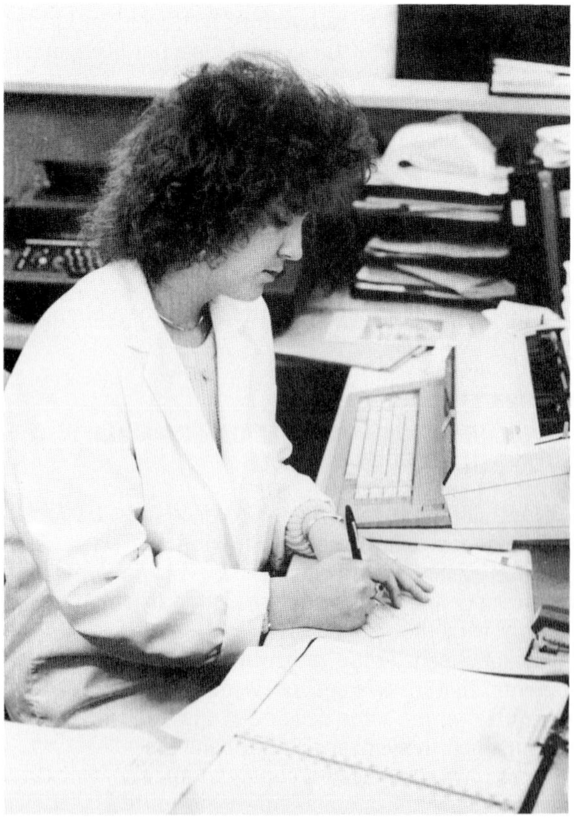

Scheduling the patient's next appointment and completing the appointment card before the patient leaves the office save both the patient and the staff time by eliminating the need for scheduling over the telephone.

do not follow this policy because it is difficult to collect the money and this approach can cause ill will.

FOLLOW-UP CALLS

The practice of making follow-up calls to check on the patient's progress, although relatively new in medicine, has become a powerful marketing tool for promoting patient loyalty. Follow-up calls have become commonplace in 24-hour community care centers, medical centers, and hospitals that offer special services such as ambulatory surgery. The office telephones the patient the day after the office visit or a treatment program has been completed, and again several days or weeks later. The medical assistant inquires about the patient's progress and asks if there are any questions or problems. Asking "Have you had any additional difficulties?" or "Do you have any questions?" is appropriate.

The physician may wish to create a priority list for follow-up calls. Obvious inclusions in this category would be:

1. Patients who have had extensive procedures
2. Patients who seem unsure of what is expected
3. Patients who are seriously ill or in pain
4. New patients.

Individual practices might include other categories. These techniques and others, such as sending new patients "Thank you" notes, increase patient satisfaction and the overall effectiveness of the medical practice in securing and maintaining a practice. Similar "thank you for your referral" notes can be designed for established patients. These marketing approaches add a human touch and go a long way toward making patients feel they have decided well in choosing their medical care.

RELATED ETHICAL AND LEGAL IMPLICATIONS

There are several legal concerns related to appointment scheduling. The first pertains to the appointment book. As was previously discussed, the appointment book is a legal document that accounts for the physician's time and contact with patients. All deviations from an originally scheduled appointment, such as cancellations and no-shows, should be noted in the appointment book, and no-shows should be charted.

Physician-canceled appointments should also be noted and a notation made that the appointment was rescheduled (*Example:* Resch. 10/9). In addition, when the physician is unable to see patients for personal or professional reasons, another physician of equal competence and expertise in the same specialty must substitute. A physician who does not arrange for coverage may be liable to litigation on the grounds of negligence and abandonment (leaving the patient unattended).

If appointment transactions such as patient cancelations and no-shows are not well documented in the appointment book, and especially in the patient record, a patient may claim that the physician did not offer an appointment and thereby caused subsequent health problems. Therefore, the medical assistant must meticulously record scheduling transactions in the appointment book and on the patient record, noting the date, his or her initials, and the outcome (such as rescheduling).

Another legal concern pertains to patient screening. The medical assistant must use extreme caution regarding scheduling decisions for an acutely ill patient or one who is experiencing an emergency. It is the physician's legal responsibility to see patients who are experiencing emergencies or acute illnesses. Again, an acutely ill patient who was refused an appointment could bring charges of abandonment and neglect.

Ethically, the medical assistant must treat all patients equally in attempting to schedule the most convenient times. It is unethical to schedule patients too closely and to engage in chronic overbooking. Judging the authenticity of the patient's stated need to see the physician is also unethical. The medical assistant must accept the patient's stated purpose for the visit at face value rather than attempting to analyze or second-guess the patient.

Prolonged patient waits present an ethical problem. The ethics of the practice objectives must be scrutinized when patients consistently wait for unreasonable periods before being seen by the physician. Is patient flow being compromised for the sake of financial gain? Is the patient's time perceived to be less important than that of the office staff? These questions can begin the process of self-examination for the medical office staff.

Patients who require follow-up calls also provide concern for potential legal actions and ethical considerations. For instance, in the case of a patient who underwent minor office surgery, failure to check on that patient's progress the day after surgery could result in a claim of negligence or malpractice.

SUMMARY

The medical assistant is responsible for the efficient management of physician and patient time. The blocking, or time-specified, method of organizing and planning appointments is the most frequently used and generally adheres to time management principles appropriate for the medical office. Although the medical assistant may follow specific guidelines in scheduling appointments, maintaining flexibility in the scheduling plan is necessary to meet patient needs rather than the rigid demands of the clock. The information presented in this chapter should enable the medical assistant to understand the complexity of appointment scheduling and encourage an awareness of the underlying goals.

The medical assistant is the physician's public relations agent. Careful and considerate treatment of patients provides the difference, as patients perceive it, between adequate and excellent care. While the physician is examining and treating patients, a technically demanding task in itself, it is the medical assistant who must greet patients, minister to their needs, answer their questions, and ensure that they comprehend instructions. This function of the medical assistant is critical to the financial success of the office and the delivery of competent care.

DISCUSSION QUESTIONS

1. What are the most important characteristics of an appointment book or appointment sheet?
2. Discuss how you felt when you were last kept waiting in a medical office.
3. What strategies could minimize the annoyance of a long office wait?
4. In which situations should a patient be seen immediately?
5. Give an example of a patient call that would justify immediate emergency action.
6. Why is welcoming the patient an effective means of positively influencing patient satisfaction?
7. Why are patients often anxious when referred to another office?
8. What factors cause unanticipated delays in a medical office?

BIBLIOGRAPHY

American Medical Association: Medicolegal Forms with Legal Analysis. The Association, Chicago, 1990.
Humphrey DD: Contemporary Medical Office Procedures. Wadsworth, Belmont, CA, 1990.
Katz H: Telephone Medical Triage and Training. Slack, Thorofare, NJ, 1990.
Lewis M and Warden CD: Law and Ethics in the Medical Office Including Biomedical Issues, ed. 2, FA Davis, Philadelphia, 1988.

PROCEDURE: Organize the appointment book

Terminal Performance Objective: Organize the appointment book according to predetermined variables (such as the physician's scheduled absences) with 100% accuracy within a reasonable time.

EQUIPMENT: Appointment book
Pen
Red pencil (or other markers)
List of physician's preferences and schedule

PROCEDURE

1. Check date if it is preprinted, or write in.

2. Block (cross out) the times the physician will be unavailable for appointments, including meetings, conferences, and travel time.

3. Block out time frames in the amount of time reserved for acutely ill patients calling and requiring medical attention the same day. Consistently use the special markings selected by the staff for this purpose.

4. Write the particular reasons for the physician's absence beside the blocking marks. Include conferences, meetings, luncheons, and other events.

PRINCIPLE

1. Checking day, date, and time printed or written on the sheet prevents errors, saves time, and helps to maintain an orderly appointment book.

2. By blocking out these times, the medical assistant avoids confusion and knows precisely when appointments may be scheduled. For instance, the office may open at 8 AM, but the first appointment may be routinely scheduled for 9 AM.

3. Planning for acutely ill patient visits and scheduling time frames in advance ensures smoother patient flow and reduces waiting periods for scheduled patients.

4. When the medical assistant is aware of the physician's scheduled commitments, he or she may remind the physician of the event and monitor patient flow more closely to enable the physician to be on time for the engagement. In addition, the medical assistant should be aware of necessary travel time and potential delays in the physician's return.

PROCEDURE: Schedule an appointment

Terminal Performance Objective: Schedule an appointment after determining if and when a patient should be seen in the office; make the determination and appointment with 100% accuracy within a reasonable time.

EQUIPMENT: Appointment book
Pen
Red pencil (or other marker)

PROCEDURE

1. Ask the patient why he or she wants to make an appointment; ask when the patient is not available.

2. Offer at least two choices, if available; state the day, date, and time.

3. After the patient chooses a time, repeat the choice to the patient.
4. Record the appointment in the appointment book and (if the patient is in the office) on an appointment card.
5. Close with a phrase expressing anticipation of the next visit, and specify the date.

PRINCIPLE

1. Knowing the purpose of the visit enables the medical assistant to make a reasonable estimate of the time required. Asking about availability indicates a willingness to accommodate the patient's needs and gives the patient the opportunity to eliminate inconvenient times.
2. Offering choices enables the patient to choose a convenient time and demonstrates the importance of the patient's input.
3. Repetition confirms the appointment and avoids error.

4. Immediate recording helps prevent errors or omissions.
5. Friendly confirmation expresses appreciation for advance scheduling and provides further verification of the date.

PROCEDURE: Record patient cancellations and missed appointments

Terminal Performance Objective: Record a patient cancellation and a patient no-show with 100% accuracy within a reasonable time.

EQUIPMENT: Appointment book
Pen
Patient record

PROCEDURE

1. Record the cancellation or no-show in the appointment book by writing "no-show" or "canceled" above the scheduled appointment. If a new appointment is scheduled, record the day, date, and time of the new appointment in the appropriate space.
2. Record the cancellation or no-show in the patient record.
3. If a new appointment is scheduled, write the day, date, and time in the patient record in the progress notes section. *Example:* Patient canceled appointment. (Indicate if the appointment was canceled by the physician.) 2/25/89. Rescheduled for 3/15/89.
4. Telephone a patient who has missed an appointment to inquire if he or she would like to reschedule. *Example:* "Dr. Green asked me to call you to inform you that you missed your appointment this morning. Would you like to reschedule?"
5. If the patient would rather call back than reschedule, write "w/c" in the patient record, noting that patient was called and asked to reschedule.

PRINCIPLE

1. Recording all scheduling information provides a permanent legal record.

2. Recording missed appointments provides a record for the physician.
3. Careful documentation is the best protection against legal claims.

4. A telephone call provides the patient who accidentally missed an appointment with the opportunity to reschedule, and demonstrates the physician's concern.

5. Documentation helps provide legal protection against charges of negligence or abandonment.

PROCEDURE: Schedule a referral

Terminal Performance Objective: Schedule an appointment for a patient who is being referred to another physician. Make the appointment according to predetermined specifications, with 100% accuracy, within a reasonable time.

EQUIPMENT: Telephone
Pen
Tablet
Physician's orders
Patient record
Special instructions for patient preparation

PROCEDURE

1. Assemble next to the telephone sheets containing the following information:
   A. Name of patient, patient's telephone number, and other personal data required
   B. Name and telephone number of the referral facility (diagnostic facility, medical center, etc.)
   C. Purpose of the appointment
   D. Date
   E. Special physician instructions for the patient, referral facility, or both
2. Call the referral facility, provide the necessary information, and schedule the appointment, giving the patient's name (and other information); and the specific purpose of the appointment (e.g., procedure); obtain any special patient instructions.
3. Call the patient to provide the necessary information: time, date, place, special instructions.

4. Give the patient the appointment information, and provide an opportunity to repeat instructions.
5. Record the calls to the patient and the facility on the patient record (date, time, procedure or purpose, etc.).

6. Marking the patient record or other designated area (such as tickler file) as a reminder that a report from the referral facility is pending.

PRINCIPLE

1. Assembling the required information promotes efficient use of time and helps prevent error.

2. Referral facility time frame must be accommodated prior to informing the patient of the date, time, and special instructions.

3. The patient can only cooperate in preparing for the appointment when essential information has been provided.
4. Repetition reinforces the mutual understanding between the patient and the medical assistant.
5. Documentation is required for both legal and medical considerations, and gives the physician a record of implemented orders.
6. Noting the pending report provides continuity of care and maintains a check for patient compliance.

HIGHLIGHTS
Stress, Work, and Health

Several medical and psychological researchers have identified stress as a major health care problem. There are two primary reasons for growing concern related to the ill effects of stress and the increased attention it is receiving within the medical industry. First is the clinical fact that stress has been linked with a number of health-related diseases, including cardiovascular disease. The second and perhaps more compelling issue is the fact that stress itself seems to be caused by conditions that are common in the health care professional's work environment. A paradox exists in that the working conditions in medical settings, including the medical office, tend to create one of the health problems that the medical profession is in business to eradicate.

Stress can be simply defined as the body's natural reaction to what it considers a threat. In the early days, the stress reaction provides a biologic safety valve. Early humans, sensing danger from the environment, received a charge from the body's hormonal systems. Adrenaline was pumped from the body, respiration increased, and several other natural mechanisms were engaged to prepare for either a fight or a flight. Modern society has moved out of the jungle and no longer confronts grave physical dangers, but the mechanism has remained. Now, however, the body generally looks for psychologic rather than physical threats. Therefore, when a patient is annoying or you have a conflict with a fellow staff member, the same hormonal process is activated. Blood pressure, pulse, and respiration increase. All metabolic activity accelerates.

Stress is primarily a nonintellectual function. Telling yourself that you will not be "bothered" by a ringing telephone or a growing workload probably will not help. For self-protection, the body will continue to activate its traditional stress mechanisms. The factors linked with stress at work include dealing with people, a lack of control over outcomes, changing workloads, technical complexity, deadlines, critical issues, and ambiguity or uncertainty over events. These conditions are typical in the health care industry. Not surprisingly, researchers have learned that medical personnel are at significant risk for stress and its ill effects.

The short-term symptoms of stress are dysfunction in accomplishing daily work-related tasks. Persons experiencing stress are likely to have reduced job satisfaction, lowered productivity, loss of creativity, and inability to deal with people. Often, these symptoms of stress lead to a situation in which individuals feel that they have little or no self-worth, thus compounding the stress-related problem. Long-term effects of stress may result in symptoms such as tiredness, irritability, eating and sleeping disorders, drinking problems, and an array of other factors that may be debilitating.

These symptoms, both short and long term, can culminate in emotional and physical illness. There is no simple cure for the stress of a difficult job. However, modifications of lifestyle and personal approach to confronting stressful situations can be helpful:

1. Balance activity with rest and obtain sufficient sleep.
2. Eat a well-balanced diet without skipping meals.
3. Manage your time effectively by prioritizing, organizing, writing things down, and following through.
4. From time to time throughout the day, slow down, close your eyes for a moment, and try to calm yourself. Breath slowly and deeply, collect yourself, and stretch your muscles. Try some progressive relaxation, relaxing first your feet, then your ankles, and so forth.
5. Exercise moderately and regularly.
6. Learn more about stress management by reading texts and articles about becoming aware of and coping with stress.

If you recognize that you are at risk as a result of stress, you may be better able to guard against the potentially debilitating effects of your work. By being able to manage stress effectively in your work environment, as a health professional you will be a better resource to patients needing assistance in their own stress management.

*B*usiness Machines and Computers in the Medical Office

> Business machines can add an "extra pair of hands" to the busy medical office.
>
> — Sharon Vance

CHAPTER OUTLINE

LEARNING OBJECTIVES

Upon completing this chapter, you will be able to:

1. Identify the common uses of the adding machine or calculator in the medical office.
2. Describe the six steps for word-processing a written document.
3. Name the five features of copying machines and list the advantages of each.
4. List the potential uses and advantages of computers in the medical office.
5. State the ways in which the needs of the office might determine its requirements for new equipment.
6. Describe the steps involved in developing a purchase proposal.
7. Describe the types of equipment warranties and maintenance agreements.

PERFORMANCE OBJECTIVES

Upon completing this chapter, you will able to:

1. Transcribe dictated material with 100% accuracy in the final draft, within a reasonable time.
2. Proofread a transcribed letter, achieving 100% accuracy after editing, within a reasonable time.

Chapter 11

Business Machines and Computers in the Medical Office

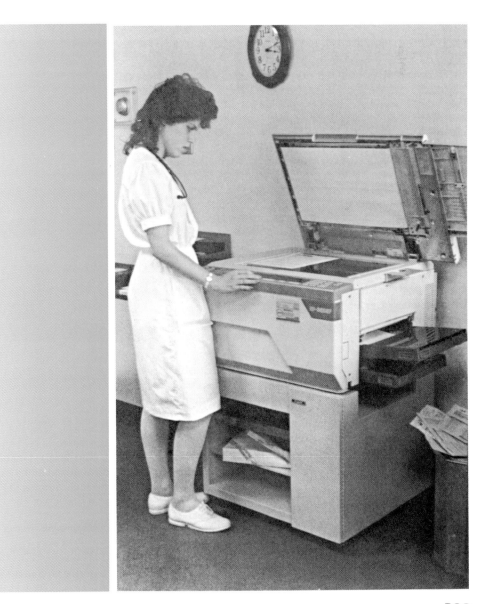

DACUM EDUCATIONAL COMPONENTS

1. Receive, organize, prioritize, and transmit information (using computers and other business machines) (2.7 A–C).
2. Perform basic secretarial skills (using typewriters and word processors) (3.1A).
3. Perform basic secretarial skills (as in [2], and maintain office equipment, such as the 10-key calculator, adding machine, or photocopier) (3.1C).
4. Apply computer concepts for office procedures (3.4A–E).
5. Operate and maintain facilities and equipment safely (6.2A–D).
6. Evaluate and recommend equipment and supplies for the practice (6.4A–D).

Glossary

Central processing unit (CPU): the "brain" of a computer that carries out the programmed instructions

Cost justification: supporting information showing that benefits from the purchase of a new machine or the upgrading of an existing machine will warrant the acquisition price

Default: preset values used in operations or calculations; the user can change and save other values

Directory: list of the file names on a disk or on a menu

Electronic mail: information output using a telephone and a modem

Extension: a suffix to a file name preceded by a period (.) and having one, two, or more characters; an extension defines or identifies a type of file more specifically

File: related data stored as a single unit on a floppy disk or fixed disk

File name: a unique name on a specific floppy disk or in a single fixed disk directory that enables the computer system to find specific information; a file name is usually one to eight characters long and may have an optional short name, or extension

Function keys: the gray keys on the keyboard that combine a series of commands into a single keystroke

Hardware: the physical components of a computer system

High-density disk: a disk whose data is more tightly packed than that on a single density disk, allowing the storage of more material in the same physical disk

Interface: exchange of information between the computer and the user or between two computer components

Memory: the part of a computer that stores information

Menu-driven software: software that allows the user to choose from a menu shown on the screen, replacing the need to know DOS (Disk Operating System) commands

Remote access: a mode in which the user can control unattended computer terminals in another location

Reprographics: reproduction or duplication of documents

Software: programmed instructions that tell a computer what to do and how to do it

Terminal: the keyboard and display portion of a computer system

Utility program: preset commands that make the operation of a computer easier, faster, and more "user friendly"

Word processing: the use of test-editing equipment to produce a typewritten document

The medical assistant is responsible for the operating wide array of business machines in the medical office. The medical assistant must become familiar with the applications of business machines and should explore new ways to effectively integrate the use of office equipment into daily routines.

The typewriter has long been a mainstay in the medical office. Many models and capabilities are available today. In addition to new typewriter technology, new technology exists for duplicating and transcribing, and computers play an increasingly important role in record keeping and financial transactions.

Not all offices need the full range of machines and options discussed here. However, the medical assistant must be sufficiently familiar with them to make informed recommendations to the physician, who usually makes the final purchasing decisions according to the research and needs of the office personnel.

THE TRANSCRIBER

All transcribers contain certain features. However, some older models still in use may not provide all the

Table 11-1
STANDARD TRANSCRIBER FEATURES

Feature	Points to Remember	Feature	Points to Remember
Volume control	Beginning transcriptionists tend to keep volume higher than necessary, which distorts sound. Volume must be adjusted for each transcription.	Headphone	Excludes extraneous office sounds. Maintains confidentiality.
		Foot pedal control	Permits hands to remain on keyboard. Pedal parts are easily confused.
		Erase control	Provides cleaner tape erasure. Easy to accidentally erase.
Tone control	Increased treble accentuates consonants, making dictation clearer. Excessive treble causes static. Excessive bass muffles consonants.	Indicator strip	Used to locate priority dictation or note special item. Marks on strip do not always line up with beginning of report.
Speed control	Speeds slow speech Slows rapid speech Separates words Matches dictation speed with transcription speed.	Voice-activated sensor	Produces gap-free dictation. Eliminates need to hold microphone.
		Insert control	Added dictation does not need rerecording or erasing.
Audio speaker control	Can clarify words Disrupts office environment. Compromises confidentiality. Should be used only briefly.	Scanning	Facilitates rapid identification and location of all dictation on cassette.
		Cassette tape	Some standard-size transcribers can be adapted to accept cassettes. Can become worn with prolonged use, resulting in poor sound reproduction.
Automatic backspace control	Rewind tape slightly when it stops, then restart it. Set control's to meet transcribing needs so no words are missed.		

features listed in Table 11-1. Proper use of the transcribing unit can greatly increase transcription speed. The controls should be adjusted to produce the clearest dictation possible at a rate that matches but never overwhelms transcription speed.

To become familiar with the transcriber, the medical assistant can take a cassette, and as it plays, manipulate the controls to determine the effect of each on the dictated sound. In addition to the controls for *On, Stop, Rewind, Fast forward, and Play* found on standard tape recorders, standard features of most transcribers are shown in Figure 11-1.

RESOURCES

1. *Equipment manual.* The equipment manual contains detailed descriptions of specific equipment and explains all functions and special features. This illustrated booklet is the transcrip-

tionist's most valuable reference. The manual also provides important information regarding proper care and cleaning, repair telephone numbers, stock numbers, and sources for authorized parts and accessories.
2. *Equipment manufacturer.* If the equipment manual is missing, the medical assistant should call or write to the manufacturer and request a copy. When purchasing new equipment, the office staff should insist that the sales representative explain the equipment thoroughly.
3. *Office personnel.* The medical assistant should request instruction from other office employees who are proficient in using the equipment.

SPECIAL EQUIPMENT FEATURES

Several machines have built-in timesaving devices that can increase transcription speed and accuracy. The

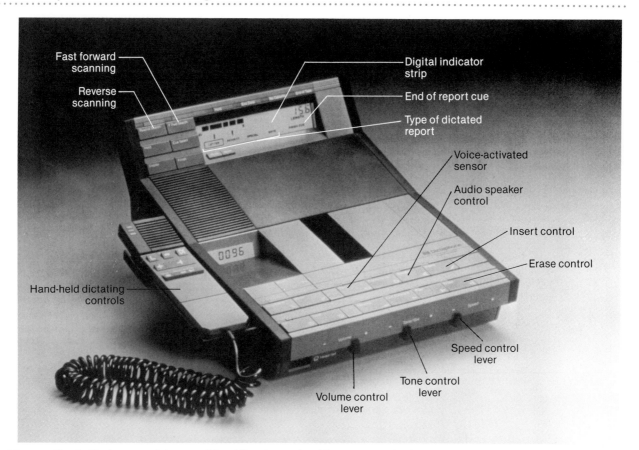

Figure 11–1. Desktop model transcribing/dictation unit with many standard and special features. (Courtesy of Dictaphone Corporation.)

following timesaving devices are found on various pieces of equipment:

1. Automatic speller
2. Electronic memory
3. Automatic error correction
4. Automatic dictation insertion
5. Units combining dictation equipment, transcribers, and multifunction telephones (Fig. 11–2).

The Procedure on page 225 outlines the process of transcribing dictation; the Procedure on page 226 covers the crucial proofreading step.

ADDING MACHINES AND CALCULATORS

Every medical office needs a machine that can perform arithmetic functions. Today's adding machines and calculators are computerized, smaller, and faster and can perform more complex calculations than their predecessors (Fig. 11–3). Calculators are now available in many sizes, with different capabilities, functions, and data storage features, and at various prices. With the correct software, the computer can perform adding machine and calculator functions.

DETERMINING NEEDS AND USES

The staff must identify the needs of the medical office before purchasing an adding machine or calculator. Needs vary from office to office, but most medical offices need the following:

1. Basic arithmetic functions of addition, subtraction, multiplication, and division. Speed and accuracy enhance the efficiency of jobs such as totaling patient charges and payments on the day sheet, totaling bank deposits, calculating payroll deductions, determining patient account balances as charges are made or payments received, and determining the correct change due a patient.
2. *Printed record of calculations.* A printed record verifies the accuracy of the numbers entered when long strings of numbers are calculated.
3. *Ability to retain a constant.* If employees are subject to a 2% local income tax, for example, the machine should be able to hold the 2% figure for repetitive calculations.
4. *Accumulation of totals (Memory capacity).* The machine should be able to add the deductions columns of the payroll register and accumulate the column totals so that the grand

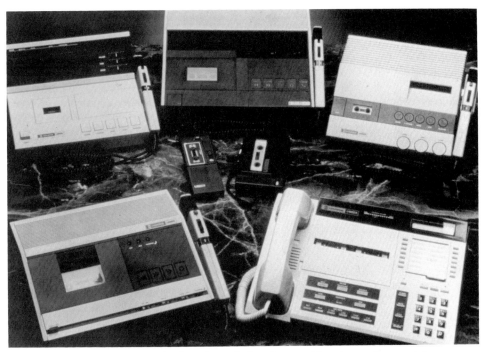

Figure 11–2. Multipurpose units combine the functions of dictation machine, transcriber, and, in some cases, telephone. Note the hand-held recorders in the center of the photograph. (Courtesy of Harris/Lanier Business Products.) 1903

total of deductions is immediately available without the need to reenter the column totals.

5. *Percentage calculations (Financial analysis functions).* Some offices perform more extensive calculations.

The best way to identify the calculation needs of a medical office is to compile a list of all calculations performed routinely and explore the ways in which a calculator could add to office efficiency.

EQUIPMENT FEATURES

Although adding machines and calculators come in a wide variety of sizes, shapes, and capabilities, they all include the basic 10-key format shown in Figure 11–4. The center row is the *home key row*. The index, third, and fourth fingers are placed on the home keys, which must be memorized before numbers can be entered quickly. Once the keys are mastered, quick entry of numbers increases office efficiency.

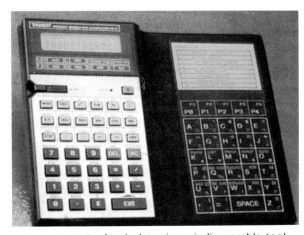

Figure 11–3. A calculator is an indispensable tool.

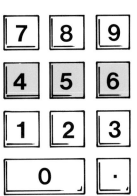

Figure 11–4. Typical adding machine or calculator keypad. Home key row is 4-5-6.

The medical assistant should read and understand the operations manual for the office adding machine or calculator. If a manual is not available in the office, the manufacturer can provide a copy. The manual lists the available functions, provides step-by-step procedures for each, and provides tips for maintenance and troubleshooting. Operations manuals should be stored in a location convenient to the machine user.

WORD PROCESSORS

In word processing, text-editing equipment puts words into a chosen format that can be reproduced as a printed document. Word processing includes the following steps:

1. *Input.* Input is the entry of information into memory. It can originate as recorded dictation, a note from the physician, or any item that requires a written record.
2. *Editing.* Editing is the manipulation or rearranging of the input data into the required format. Letters containing typographic errors, for example, are unprofessional output documents and should not be mailed.
3. *Verification (Proofreading).* The document should be proofread to verify accuracy of information and format and to ensure correct spelling.
4. *Printing.* After all required corrections and changes have been made, the printer produces a paper document, or hard copy. This documentation or correspondence can then be appropriately processed.
5. *Approval.* The person who originated or dictated the data must signify approval by signing or initialing the document.
6. *Delivery.* The finished product must be routed to the intended user. For example, letters should be mailed, and notes concerning patients should be affixed to their charts.

DETERMINING NEEDS AND USES

The medical office processes large amounts of data. Factors unique to the office should be identified before the equipment comparison process begins. Specific office requirements could include

Mail merge capabilities, from a database to envelopes, letters, and mailing labels

Name labels for patient charts or billing

Transcription of treatment notes or other patient information

Letters to physicians, insurance companies, or other authorized persons concerning patient care

Insurance forms

Occasional miscellaneous correspondence and reports.

Issues include whether the physician dictates notes for patient charts, whether name labels are typed for patient charts, whether insurance forms are typed or handwritten, and whether printing forms can save costs.

In addition to word processing, computers may be used to store and update business records, handle accounts receivable and accounts payable transactions, store and maintain patient and mailing lists, complete medical insurance forms, provide a cross-index of insurance coding numbers, or perform numerical computations. A medical office considering the addition or upgrading of a computer system must identify computer capabilities and compatibilities. Some questions to be considered are: Will the computer be used only for word processing, or will it also be used for maintaining accounts receivable, accounts payable, and inventory levels? Should the computer be used for financial analysis or demographic analysis? Should the computer be used to maintain patient records?

Even if patient records are maintained by computer, patient charts are still necessary. Charts provide valuable hard copy of stored information. If patient records were maintained only on the computer, the physician could not access patient information if the computer was "down" (not functioning properly). Without hard copy of forms or patient records, work can come to standstill.

Many types of computer are available. It is extremely important for the medical office staff to know how they want the computer system to function for them. How many people will need access to the system? How much room is available for the hardware? Is the hardware compatible with medical practice software? How much money is the physician willing to invest in the system? Questions such as these must be decided even before a computer sales representative is contacted.

EQUIPMENT FEATURES

Machines available for word processing range from the basic electric typewriters with limited memory through word processing software programs to sophisticated, independent word processing systems.

The most widely used office word processing equipment is the basic electronic typewriter, such as the IBM Selectric. Typewriters today come in a wide range of models with various features. Many typewriters use correction tape, which reduces the correction of typographic errors to a mere keystroke. The newer line of computerized typewriters "remember" whole lines or paragraphs so that errors can be corrected easily. Typewriters with memory can store frequently used words and phrases, and some models can store form letters. Other advantages include quiet operation, decreasing cost, and energy savings (Fig. 11–5).

Computerized systems offer speed of operation and

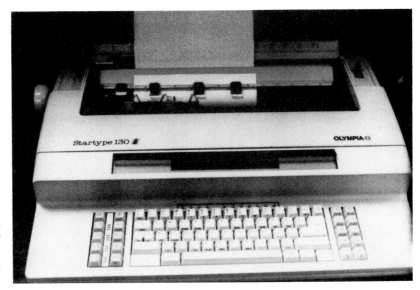

Figure 11–5. The electric typewriter has been updated by the addition of such word processing features as memory storage and the ability to check spelling.

ease of correcting or editing copy. Many word processing systems contain a dictionary, which corrects spelling errors with a keystroke. Frequently used words may be added to the dictionary listing. Repetitive items, such as collection letters and appointments reminders, may be stored on disks and reused without retyping. An advantage of this feature is the ability to create new forms, especially when low usage discourages commercial printing. Infrequently used forms could be input and individually printed as the need arises.

In addition, the medical assistant should explore the potential cost savings of printing frequently used forms on the computer printer rather than commercially. Various forms that could be designed and computer printed include forms for history and physical examination, initial patient information, billing letters, and various accounting needs. In all these forms, the categories are already there, and the medical assistant simply inputs the patient information. The medical assistant should compile a list of all repetitive tasks and determine whether computer-generated forms could increase office efficiency in each case.

As technology continues to advance, and the price of word processing systems continues to decline, more and more medical offices will find such a system cost effective. The operation manual for the machine can be used for both instruction and resource. The computer keyboard is an expanded version of the typewriter keyboard. The traditional QWERTY layout of 50 keys, plus the space bar, for letters, numbers, and punctuation marks (Fig. 11–6) is augmented by function keys. The number and purpose of function keys vary from system to system. Figure 11–7 shows a close-up of the 101-key keyboard common to many kinds of personal computer.

A *display screen*, consisting of a liquid crystal display or a TV-like monitor, shows the data as it is typed.

The final element of a word processing system is the printer, which puts the word processed information on paper. Many types of printer are available. They operate at different speeds and produce print of varied quality. *Impact printers* produce type by striking (impacting) against an inked ribbon. *Dot matrix printers* use dots to form each character. *Letter-quality printers* produce characters that look like typewritten characters.

Laser printers, although more expensive, produce typeset quality print and are much faster than impact printers (Fig. 11–8).

The medical office can acquire word processing software in several ways. The easiest is to purchase generic word processing programs, such as WordPerfect or Microsoft Word, from a computer store (see Fig. 11–

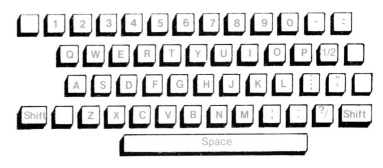

Figure 11–6. The QWERTY keyboard has been the standard layout of the keys for letters, numbers, and punctuation signs since the early days of the typewriter.

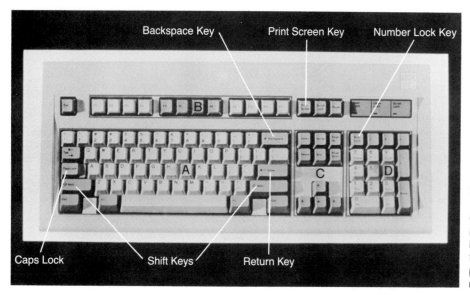

Backspace Key   Print Screen Key   Number Lock Key

Caps Lock   Shift Keys   Return Key

Figure 11-7. The standard 101-key computer keyboard includes the QWERTY keyboard (A), function (B) and control keys (C) for computer operations, plus a numerical keypad (D). (Courtesy IBM Corporation.)

12). Recent developments include programs specially designed for medical practice.

REPROGRAPHICS

Most medical offices use some kind of copying machine. Copying machines have largely replaced, the use of carbon paper to create document copies. Like many other business machines, copying machines have become substantially more sophisticated and simultaneously less expensive. The modern medical office could not carry out many of its essential business functions without a copier (Fig. 11-9).

DETERMINING NEEDS AND USES

Typically, an office duplicating machine is used to copy correspondence, technical documents, journal ar-

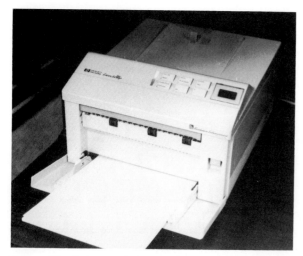

Figure 11-8. Laser printers produce typeset-quality print quickly and quietly.

ticles, billing forms, insurance forms, tax and financial documents, and patient instructions.

As with other decisions involving business machines, the first step before shopping for a copier is to determine the office requirements (Table 11-2). The medical assistant determines what office processes and procedures could be streamlined for increased efficiency and for cost savings. Also, the medical assistant should compile a "wish list" of functions and uses for equipment. It is important that the end must justify the means; in other words, that the machine must be able to pay for itself through increased efficiency and saved time. In addition, the practical considerations of noise, room temperature, and paper storage should be considered in regard to machine placement. Operators or codes may be designated for review of machine use and codes may be assigned to protect them from misuse or abuse.

EQUIPMENT FEATURES

Plain paper copiers (Fig. 11-10) use a process in which a photograph of the document is heat imprinted onto the paper. The technical advantage is that the process uses ordinary paper, even regular office stationary letterhead, labels and colored paper. Copiers vary in the numbers of pages copied per minute. While a high-speed copier (see Fig. 11-9) may cost more initially, savings in operation time and paper price may offset the cost if the work load requires a large amount of daily photocopying.

Copiers offer various optional functions in addition to basic quality and speed of duplication:

1. *Collating and front-back functions.* If the office routinely copies multipage documents, the collating function may be an important purchasing consideration (Fig. 11-11). This function compiles multipage documents and arranges each by page, saving time and effort. Copiers with a collating function generally cost more, and the added cost must be weighed against

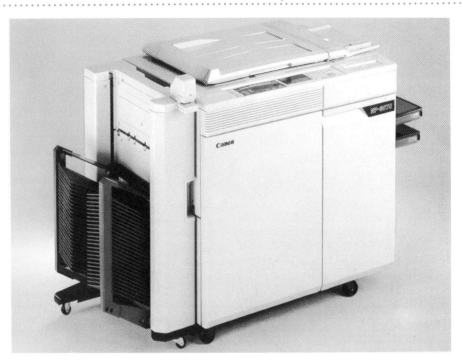

Figure 11-9. High-speed copiers can duplicate at the rate of 70 copies per minute. (Courtesy of Canon USA, Inc.)

possible savings. Copying on both sides of the page can save on paper costs. However, not all machines have this function. The time it takes to reload pages manually or transfer copies to another feed mechanism can offset the additional cost of a partially automatic paper feed feature. If it is office policy to routinely print front and back copies from originals, a fully automatic system is important.

2. *Adaptation to various paper sizes.* Many copiers accept both standard-size paper (8½ by 11 in) and legal-size paper (11 by 14 in). If bills are copied, the copier also must accept billing-sized paper.

3. *Automatic feed.* Some copiers have a built-in automatic feed mechanism, whereas others may require an automatic feed attachment. Some copiers have neither capacity. This function allows the operator to place a stack of documents (such as patients' bills or insurance forms) in the machine at once; the machine automatically feeds one at a time through for copying. If many documents are often copied at once, this function becomes an important feature.

4. *Number of copies.* Some copiers limit the number of copies that can be designated, such as allowing a choice of 1 to 99 copies. If more than 99 copies are desired, the operator must copy the first 99, then reset the machine to copy the rest. If the office makes numerous copies of the same document, this feature is important.

One last consideration is the overall capacity of a copier. Inexpensive desktop models are built for occasional, single-copy use. If the office copies great quantities of material daily, heavier-duty machines will long outlast smaller, cheaper models. The sales representative should collect information on the numbers of

copies produced per day and per year, the types of documents copied routinely, and both the current uses and future intended uses of the machine. Many service contracts and warranties are limited to a maximum number of copies per month or year. If copy activity exceeds the usage stated in the contract, the copier

Table 11-2

CHECKLIST FOR IDENTIFYING OFFICE BUSINESS MACHINE NEEDS*

Checklist Items	Examples
Type of machine	Copier, computer, etc.
Functional requirements	What it must do
Number of uses per day	Number of copies, laboratory tests, etc.
Time for processing desired	How many copies per minute, etc.
Output desired	Letters on letterhead stationery, laboratory report on self-stick paper, insurance claims, daily cash receipts, etc.
Other features desired	Built-in correction tape on typewriter, continuous feed attachment for copier, etc.
Space or size limitations	Available space
User percent of operation	Each employee's anticipated machine use

* Checklist should be completed by all employees. The complete lists should be compiled and used in preparing a needs assessment report.

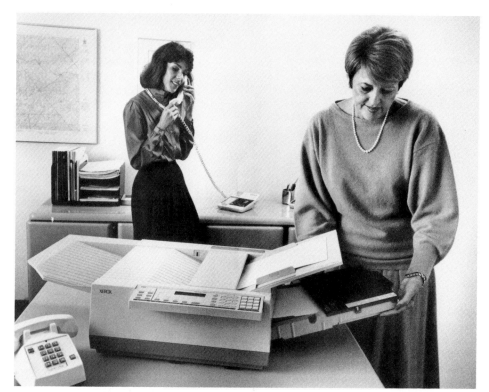

Figure 11-10. Plain-paper copiers duplicate documents using thermal transfer; they can use many kinds and sizes of paper. (Courtesy Xerox Corporation.)

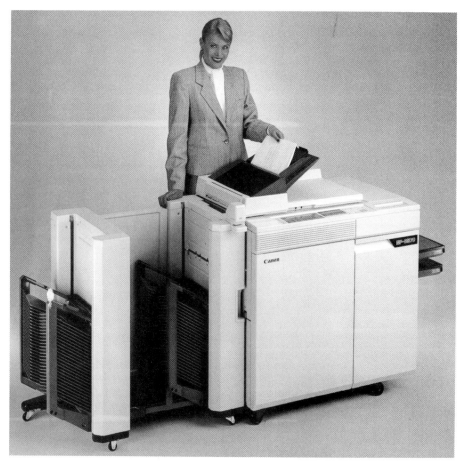

Figure 11-11. Automatic collation is a time-saving feature available on some copiers. (Courtesy Canon USA, Inc.)

company will not honor the warranties and service purchased with the equipment.

The sales representative should provide the staff with detailed operation and maintenance instructions and leave copies of an instruction booklet for future reference. It is also advisable to place the operating instructions booklet in a prominent place for easy access.

DEVELOPING A PURCHASE PROPOSAL

The first step in proposal development — requesting and justifying the expense of a piece of machinery — is to identify all the ways in which the machine could be used. This assessment includes both current and project uses. The office staff should be creative and explore various possibilities for procedural changes, formatting approaches, and other office functions that could be streamlined for increased efficiency. The more uses that can be identified or projected, the smaller the cost per unit. Every employee in the office should contribute to this usage composite. Each employee has his or her own perspective and ideas about how the machine could be used. There is no better resource for information than the employee who will actually use the equipment. That employee is aware of existing problems, can identify the status of work flow, and is therefore a valuable resource.

Once the needs have been delineated, product research can begin. The medical assistant should contact representatives or request product information from as many sources as possible. The data collected (brochures, price listings, memos of conversations with salespersons, etc.) should all be organized in a folder or looseleaf binder for ready access. This data collection helps to compare products and identify the available equipment function capabilities. These various capabilities should be considered according to their possible uses in the office. Again, input from every employee is necessary.

Next begins the process of comparing the prices and various features of each company's equipment. These data are compared both with each other and with the list of identified needs and uses. This process eliminates some products quickly. In the end there should be a first, second, and third choice ranking of equipment that seems most suitable. The lowest price is not the sole indicator for choice. Often it is possible to be "penny wise and pound foolish" if selection is based on cost alone and excludes all other features or potentials.

The results of all activities so far are compiled into a needs assessment listing and cost justification report. This report should be mathematical and requires research for completion. The justification must include all projected savings that could result from the machine purchase, including costs of time (salary), supplies, and procedures. Also included are all the additional expenses that could be incurred, such as copier paper, toner, floppy disks, printer paper, cassette tapes, ribbon, and ink jets. These items are categorized as *nondurable goods*. Justification should always include all possible acquisition costs of both durable (equipment) and nondurable goods.

The final step in proposal development requires that the staff agree on and submit their choice of equipment to the physician along with the ensuing rationale for the choice. The physician makes the final purchasing decision.

Sometimes the best decision is to do nothing or to lease equipment. In most instances the product will continue to improve and the price will come down. A purchase that is not justifiable now may become realistic for consideration in 6 to 12 months.

TROUBLESHOOTING

Most manufacturers and business machine dealers provide customers with a troubleshooting guide. This guide lists possible causes for a machine malfunction. For instance, most guides direct the user to check the power source if a machine does not function. A power cord that is not completely plugged in may prevent power from reaching the machine. Another example is checking the connection of the earphones to the transcription unit if no sound can be heard. Such examples may sound simplistic, but the troubleshooting checklist can save the physician a significant amount of money. Paying the service call fee and delaying office work to have the repair person secure a loose connection is neither efficient nor cost effective.

MAINTENANCE AND REPAIR OF BUSINESS MACHINES

Business machines in a medical office are often used daily or even continuously. Any business machine operates more efficiently and lasts longer with proper care. The operations manual provides instructions for daily care and cleaning, and suggestions for minimizing problems, for instance, use of dust covers, static electricity pads, and electric isolation lines.

All machines require service or repair at some point. The medical assistant can contribute to the longevity of the machines through proper care and cleaning and recognition of potential problems. The telephone number of the company repair service should be kept current and on file.

WARRANTIES AND SERVICE CONTRACTS

Generally, new machines are covered by a warranty for a certain period after purchase. A warranty offers the buyer assurance that the manufacturer will repair or correct any machine failure free of charge during the time specified. Some machines are covered by an extended warranty for certain parts. When the warranty period has expired, the owner must pay the cost of maintenance and repair.

Improper care or abuse may nullify the warranty or service contract. For example, spilling coffee inside the new typewriter could be considered abuse or negligence, and the repair cost would not be covered.

Many business machine dealers and some independent companies offer an additional service contract on business machines. A service contract is an agreement between the owner and the service provider. The owner pays a sum of money, and the service provider agrees to provide service for a specified time. If no service contract has been purchased, the physician must pay for each service call made to the office and for any parts or labor required.

Service contracts generally include periodic cleaning, lubrication, and inspection. The contract may include the replacement of worn out or defective parts, or may include only the labor cost and stipulate that the buyer pay for needed parts. This type of preventive maintenance is thought to decrease the number of machine breakdowns.

ELECTRIC SAFETY

The medical assistant should be aware of potential office hazards. Frayed electric cords or broken plugs should be reported and repaired as soon as possible. Multiple machines plugged into the same outlet or cords stretching across open floor space could cause serious injury. Any possibly hazardous situation should be discussed and a solution implemented. Employees and patients deserve a safe office.

MEDICAL OFFICE COMPUTERS

Because the amount of work and the need for documentation in the medical office have grown dramatically over the past few years, it has become essential to process medical and financial information efficiently and accurately. Quality assurance now requires the documentation of all services and charges involved in patient care. The computer provides this important aspect.

MEDICAL INFORMATION

One important use for the computer is to provide the physician with comprehensive (interpretive) reports, which contain diagnostic information needed to establish or rule out a particular diagnosis or to indicate any abnormalities. Many laboratory and hospital information systems provide interpretive reports that list ranges of normal values, flag abnormal values, and arrange data in an accessible and readily understandable format.

At one time, the only computers with enough computing power, speed, and memory storage space were the large *mainframe computers*. These room-sized machines were too costly and specialized for all but the largest medical facilities. However, the development of the *microprocessor* changed computers. Microprocessors, or chips, are extremely small assemblies of electric circuits necessary for computer operation and memory.

Microprocessors have increased power, speed, and memory storage. They have made the *personal computer* (PC) an affordable option.

Figure 11–12 illustrates the basic PC. The setup consists of a keyboard, central processing unit (CPU), and monitor (a television-like unit that displays the data). Most PC systems are also attached to a printer. Such a system can run by itself or can be linked to a local area network that allows all the machines in the medical office to communicate with each other and to share access to information.

Systems are now available to deliver medical information, billing information, and patient information to the physician in a timely manner so that the patient receives the greatest benefit at the lowest cost.

The machinery—keyboard, CPU, printer, and monitor—is known as *hardware*. The computer programs that tell the computer what to do and how to do it are called *software*. Both hardware and software continue to improve at a dizzying pace. Several systems especially designed for medical offices are available. Such systems handle all patient records, medical information, and billing, insurance, and financial data to help physicians and staff to deliver the best possible medical care at the lowest possible cost. Most medical facilities are now or will soon be computerized.

Larger libraries, particularly those affiliated with universities, operate computer-search services. The National Library of Medicine offers the computerized retrieval service entitled MEDLARS (Medical Literature Analysis and Retrieval System), which is available at libraries in medical centers, hospitals, and universities. The institutions participating in this system house terminals connected by telephone line to computers at the National Library of Medicine. In addition to compilation of references in books and articles, MEDLARS has access to databases including Medline (biomedical referencing), TOXLINE (toxicology), Chemline (dictionary of chemical substances), and Cancerlit (cancer literature).

The National Library of Medicine also produces *Index Medicus*, a monthly publication that indexes the

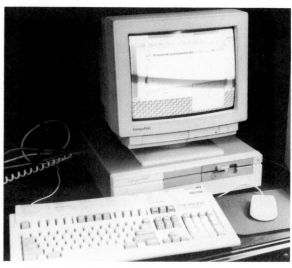

Figure 11–12. A desktop personal computer.

world's leading biomedical literature by author and subject. The physician may request a search for all articles pertaining to a particular topic or by a certain author. In response to the programmed request, the computer supplies a printed list of all the articles in question. A computer search is the most accurate and comprehensive method of reviewing the titles of all articles published during a particular period. The total cost is related to the nature of the search. For example, the more journals are requested, the more costly is the search.

INTRAOFFICE COMMUNICATION

The computer can be used to store and generate information regarding office policies, mission statements and objectives, and medical philosophy in general, both for patient education and employment purposes. Procedure manuals with information about standard operational procedures, Occupational Safety and Health Administration facility requirements, and Clinical Laboratory Improvement Act (CLIA) requirements can also be stored in the system.

The computer can generate special reports and lists concerning quality control data, lists of diagnoses, abnormal laboratory tests, and maintenance records. The laboratory computer can store information on specimen requirements, standard deviations, instrument parameters, test procedures, test methods, and documentation of periodic review measures. Information regarding specimen requirements, collection, transport, and processing can be stored in easily accessible form.

In practice management, computers can produce prompt, reliable reports to manage patient demographic information, billing systems, and the more complex management of patient medical information. A well-designed computer system should improve medical record keeping, patient care planning, budget planning, and the general operation of the office.

SOFTWARE PROGRAMS

Office software may be generally categorized into three types: spreadsheet, word processing, and database programs. A *spreadsheet* is an electronic worksheet, containing numbers and formulas in columns and rows, that calculates mathematical relationships among numbers. Spreadsheets are used mainly to produce budgets, profit and loss statements, and other cash flow reports. Spreadsheets can also be used for technical reports that involve time and numeric variables or trends.

Word processing software manipulates, edits, writes, and prints text. Refer to the foregoing text and also to Chapter 8, which describes the uses of word processing for business correspondence and professional writing.

A *database* is a collection of data, either numeric or textual, that is keyed in (input) and stored (saved) to ultimately produce powerful demographic and analytic reports. Each database has a specific format that allows future additions and alterations as the activities and needs of a medical practice change.

A software program, like a file cabinet, contains files. A *file* consists of related information (data) that is stored on a removable or fixed disk. Each file or program contains navigational directories, commands selected by menu options or function keys, and the data (individual records). The individual records contain fields that, when filled, ultimately represent the total information that can be retrieved and printed as hard copy reports and records. Hard copy reports are placed in the patient record and considered official (legal) records.

Menus

A menu is an optional function offered by the program. A cursor is moved to the option of choice on the menu. Menus are most useful when choices are limited and for persons new to the computer. The keyboard is used to enter alphanumeric (letters and numbers) and numeric data into the computer. American Standard Code for Information Interchange (ASCII) is the universal coding system that allows one program to read and understand other programs.

Most newer software programs are based on *relational* database programming. Relational programs allow the user to enter information in one area of the database and to use and retrieve that information while working in other files of the same program. A relational database spares the user the time and effort of repetitive information entry.

Principles of Data Entry

To enter or retrieve data, the computer must be told where to enter or search for information. The user enters this information by keying in the location of a file. To locate a file, a series of commands, or file specification, must be entered in the following order: (1) the drive letter that contains the file, (2) the directory or subdirectory that contains the file, and (3) the name of the file, including a file extension; for example:

$$C: MEDPROG\backslash CODE.dtf$$

Once a file has been retrieved, subdirectories and commands are available as menu selections. Data can be input and output either by command line entry (typing commands) or by menu selection. Some screens are for display only; data entry is not possible. Data entry screens contain fields that are filled in whenever "Insert," "New," "Edit," "Find," or similar commands are used. Some typical commands are as follows:

Director (search) commands:

Insurance	Billing	Diagnoses	Doctors	Hosp	Lab
Employees	Reports	Procedures	Meds	Patients	
Appointment	Patient List				

Data entry (field) commands

New   Retrieve   Edit   Next   Previous   Save   Delete
Print   Batch   Exit

A SAMPLE MEDICAL OFFICE DATABASE PROGRAM

Medical office database programs usually have four basic sets of data files.

Patient Files

Patient files contain the name, address, and insurance information of all the patients in a practice. A patient file is the computer equivalent of the patient information form and patient ledger card. The patient file can generate ledgers, statements, specific patient reports, and a full or partial list of the patients in the practice. With specific codes, patient files can be cross-referenced to a particular physician in a multi-physician practice, a particular diagnosis, a drug study, or a special situation, such as a listing of patients with disabilities. The patient file format can be designed to include as little or as much information as the physician and office staff desire.

With experience, a new services rendered record (SSR) file can be entered in minutes. Once the medical assistant has entered the diagnosis and procedure codes and the patient and insurance information, most of the data entry is done. When an established patient comes into the office, new information pertaining to that visit can be entered in seconds. The computer automatically retrieves the necessary insurance, diagnosis, and procedure code information, and the vital statistics on the patient. A sample of a patient file follows. Many other optional fields can be created.

First Name:	Jane
Last Name:	Harrison
Patient Codename:	HarriJane (automatic)
Sex:	F
Physician:	JA
Referring Physician:	R. Davis
Family Physician:	K. Burton
Diagnosis:	CHF
Code (automatic):	411
Description (automatic):	Congestive heart failure
Insurance:	MC (Medicare)
Policy Number:	123456789A
Insured's Name:	Frank Harrison

Code Files

Procedure and diagnostic code files contain the various codes and the charge for each procedure. These codes are entered as a first step in converting from a manual system, and are updated as codes or office requirements change. The information in these files automatically interfaces with the patient files.

Procedure code files include medical procedure codes (Current Procedural Terminology 4, or CPT-4), a brief description of the services, and their charges. A typical office usually needs 25 to 100 procedure codes. An example is shown below:

CPT-4 code:	99212
Internal code description:	OVB
Description:	Office Visit, Brief
Regular fee:	$20.00

In certain states, some offices are required to include additional codes, such as auxiliary and modifier codes. The procedure code database can be designed to accommodate as many pieces of information (screen fields) as are needed by the office.

Diagnostic procedure codes include the International Classification of Diseases 9, Clinical Medicine (ICD-9-CM) codes for commonly encountered diagnoses, the names and addresses of hospitals and other medical care facilities, and the names of referring physicians. Examples of procedure files with ICD-9-CM codes are:

ICD-9-CM code:	411
Internal code description:	CHF
Description:	Congestive Heart Failure

ICD-9-CM code:	599
Internal code description:	UTI
Description:	Urinary Tract Infection

Services Rendered Record Files

Services rendered record files make up the bulk of the database. Thousands of records are created over time in this file. A new record is created each time a patient charge is entered for an office visit or hospitalization. In a relational database, each time a new SSR is entered, information is automatically accessed from the patient file and the two code files. If information is changed in any file, it is automatically reflected in the other three files.

The SSR file is used to enter the type of service rendered with each patient contact:

Type of Place:	O (Office)
Date from:	9/1/94 Date To: (hospitalizations)
Diagnosis today:	UTI
Description (automatic):	Urinary Tract Infection
Procedure(s):	OVB
CPT code (automatic):	99212

	Date	Procedure code (automatic)	No. of visits	Charge (automatic)
1.	9/1/94	OVB	1	$20.00
2.	9/1/94	ECG	1	$30.00

A billing file can be opened in a subdirectory under the SSR file. The computer can calculate patient receivable fees and determine how an insurance carrier might calculate payment, if the physician accepts assignment. Fees, approved fees, insurance carrier reimbursement, and the amount to bill the patient can be accessed automatically and used to print automatic monthly bills.

Date	Procedure code (automatic)	No. of visits	Charge (automatic)
1. 9/1/94	OVB	1	$20.00
2. 9/1/94	ECG	1	$30.00

Total (automatic):		$50.00
Approved (determined by carrier):		46.35
Source of payment:	MC	
Carrier reimbursement (in this case, 80% of $46.35):		37.08
Patient responsible for balance:	No___ Yes__X__	
Amount to bill patient (automatic):		$ 9.27

The billing file can electronically bill insurance carriers (such as Medicare or Blue Shield), print health insurance claims forms, and print patient statements.

Reports and Appointments

The relational database can be used not only for analytic and financial functions, but to create printed reports under a "Reports" option. This option permits systematic auditing of the financial state of the practice, overdue accounts, late third-party payments, and monthly trends.

A good software package should also include an electronic appointment system. Most appointment systems are located under a subdirectory of the patient file. The appointment calendar is retrieved by month and then by date. The date selected is displayed with time slots. The medical assistant selects the appointment time and enters the patient's code name in the time slot. The information can be printed each day as both the appointment log and the activity day sheet. In addition, the electronic appointment system can be used to initiate patient follow-up or recall.

THE MEDICAL ASSISTANT AS THE BUSINESS MACHINE RESOURCE PERSON

The medical assistant can help the physician by serving as a business machine resource person. This role requires a knowledge of available business machines, their capabilities and uses, and information sources, and the ability to compare and evaluate the various machines. The resource person also must be able to justify any proposed cost of updating or replacing equipment by calculating the useful life of the proposed machine against the current and projected needs and growth of the practice.

KEEPING UP WITH OFFICE TECHNOLOGY

Establishing regular contact with business machine vendors is one way to stay informed of the latest technology. Although salespeople are most familiar with the products they sell, they also are aware of the latest developments in the industry. Also, many magazines and newsletters are devoted to the latest developments in business machines. Some of these publications are specifically aimed at smaller business operations. Some medical publications, such as *Medical Economics* or *The Professional Medical Assistant*, provide information on current medical office technology. All resource information should be placed in a notebook or file so that it is all in one place and easily accessible.

SUMMARY

Most physicians have little time to devote to "state-of-the-art" advances in business machines. As a result, the medical assistant must assume a broad responsibility in this area. It is not enough simply to understand the nature and operation of the equipment being used in the office. The medical assistant must be committed to keeping up with advances in business machine technology, and must consider their possible office application. When the medical assistant has identified a product that seems to be potential valuable to the office, he or she should bring this information to the attention of the physician. Steps in developing a proposal to purchase new equipment, upgrade or replace existing equipment, or add to current equipment include

1. Identification of needs and desires
2. Product research
3. Comparison of prices and capabilities
4. Needs assessment and cost justification
5. Recommendation of preferred machine and rationale for the recommendation
6. Presentation of information as a report to the physician.

DISCUSSION QUESTIONS

1. What are some common uses of the adding machine or calculator in the medical office?
2. List and explain the six steps in a word processing system.

3. List some common typing requirements in a medical office.
4. Name and describe the two basic processes that copiers use to duplicate documents.
5. What are some items that should be considered in determining office copying needs? Briefly explain or describe each item listed.
6. What are the two parts of an office computer system? Explain.
7. Define the following terms:
   a. Microprocessor
   b. Memory
   c. Central processing unit
   d. Additional storage
   e. Printer
   f. Program
   g. Backup
8. Do all computer printers produce the same style and grade of printing? Explain.
9. Discuss the role of the business machines resource person in the medical office.
10. Describe the difference between a warranty and a service contract.
11. List and describe the steps in developing a proposal for the purchase or updating of a medical office business machine.

PROCEDURE: Transcribe dictation

Terminal Performance Objective: Transcribe dictated material with 100% accuracy in the final draft, within a reasonable time.

EQUIPMENT: Dictation tape
Dictation machine
Typewriter or word processor
Paper (plain for draft, letterhead stationery for final)
Dictionary and other references (grammar, medical terminology) as needed
Correcting tape or liquid (if typewriter is used)

PROCEDURE

1. Assemble equipment and supplies.
2. Turn on the dictation machine and insert paper in the typewriter or turn on the word processor (or computer).
3. Set the volume, tone speed, and controls on the dictation machine according to your needs.
4. Set the spacing, margins, type set, and so forth on the typewriter or word processor.
5. Type the letter draft and proofread it.

6. Correct errors and type the final copy.

7. Turn off the machine and obtain the physician's signature. Send the letter or document to the intended recipient.

PRINCIPLE

1. Organization saves time.
2. Readying equipment is one of the necessary first steps in proper completion of the procedure.

3. Setting the controls to meet your needs ensures accurate transcription.
4. Setting parameters properly ensures accurate transcription.
5. Drafting enables the transcriptionist to proofread the letter or document it for accuracy.
6. The final copy should represent the projected professional image: letterhead for letters, appropriate encasement for reports and other documents.
7. The final steps are necessary for procedure completion, physician approval, and validation.

PROCEDURE: Proofread a transcribed letter

Terminal Performance Objective: Proofread a transcribed letter, achieving 100% accuracy after final editing, within a reasonable time.

EQUIPMENT: Dictionary and other references (grammar, medical terminology) as needed
Correcting tape or liquid (if typewriter is used)

PROCEDURE	PRINCIPLE
1. Read each sentence for completeness.	1. Reading sentences prevents omissions and incompletion.
2. Check for incorrect punctuation, verb tense, word endings, and subject-verb agreement.	2. Correct grammar provides an accurate report that reads smoothly.
3. Check spelling. Do not assume or guess.	3. Spelling is essential to accuracy and prevents misinterpretation.
4. Check the correctness of the medical content in the report.	4. The medical data must agree with all facts presented, and the words must be used accurately in the text.
5. When unsure, relisten to the tape.	5. The spoken word often clarifies content and grammar errors.
6. Correct the errors, and print the letter, and place it in the designated area for the physician's signature.	6. The final steps complete the task and ensure physician approval.

HIGHLIGHTS

The Human Side of Automation

The use of machine technology in the medical office has become commonplace. Laboratory and other diagnostic equipment, computers, telecommunication systems, and multifunctional duplicating machinery coexist in contemporary medical offices. Much research has been published regarding the impact of automation on the manufacturing industry. What conclusions can be drawn from this research regarding the impact of automation on the medical office staff?

Surprisingly, many economists, sociologists, and management experts claim that rather than demeaning the worker—taking away control and responsibility from the worker—automation has, in many instances, actually increased the number and types of skills performed by individuals and has radically changed traditional work practices. Table 11–3 illustrates some of the major changes.

Automation is viewed as the catalyst for these changes because technology has required individuals to learn new skills, renew their commitment to the organization, and assume greater responsibility for error-free task performance.

Ironically, health care professionals have been engaged in the practice of these "new" concepts for decades. Functioning as multiskilled practitioners and team members, health care professionals appear to adapt well to technological advances. By comparison, 15 years ago, fewer than 24 United States manufacturing plants were organized into a teamwork-managerial structure. Today, several hundred business offices and factories are organized in a fashion representative of the new concepts described in Table 11–3. Perhaps, by the very nature of their work, health care professionals have initiated the humanizing of automation.

For health care professionals, automation presents new challenges and the opportunity to upgrade skills,

Table 11–3

CHANGING ORGANIZATIONAL APPROACHES*

Assumptions Regarding Workers

Old Concept	New Concept
Workers expect to be paid for work but do not expect to achieve increasing responsibility.	Workers desire challenges, increasing responsibility, and autonomy.

Job Design

Old Concept	New Concept
Work is compartmentalized, narrowly defined. Individuals responsible for few specialized tasks.	The nature of work requires multiskilled team members who combine their talents toward achieving common objectives.

Organization and Management Style

Old Concept	New Concept
Pyramid, autocratic organization and management style. Worker has little input. Supervisors maintain power and control.	Workers have input, democratic, few layers of authority. Power to implement change shared among workers.

*From Special Report. Management Discovers the Human Side of Automation. Business Week, September 29, 1986, with permission.

increase responsibility, and expand role expectations. Health care professionals may continue to lead the way in approaching automation with openness and a sense of adventure rather than with fear and resistance.

Unit 3

*F*inancial Management

The chapters in this unit focus on the management of financial responsibilities in medical office practice. The medical assistant is required to carry out all financial interactions precisely. The knowledge and skills essential to performing these tasks include banking, billing, accounting, and insurance processing. In addition, competent financial management requires the medical assistant to observe the policy of confidentiality and to be informed about other ethical and legal issues, which are also addressed in these chapters.

This unit represents another of the many facets of medical assisting. The medical assistant is a professional member of the medical office team who manages all business functions of the practice efficiently and effectively and whose role is crucial to the financial solvency of the practice.

Unit Objectives

Upon completing this unit, you will be able to:

1. Describe the procedure for check writing and statement reconciliation.
2. Demonstrate the procedures related to banking functions, including check writing, completing bank deposit slips, and reconciling the bank account.
3. List the essential components of billing and collection policies.
4. Describe and explain a physician's fee schedule.
5. Demonstrate the use of the pegboard system to post charges.
6. List the components of the accounting equation and describe the function of each component.
7. List and describe the major types of insurance program encountered in the medical office.
8. Demonstrate the procedures related to insurance processing.
9. Identify the legal considerations associated with filing insurance claims.

> No matter how routine the procedure, ultimately what will be remembered is our treatment of people rather than our efficiency in completing the task.
>
> Mary Ann Borgia, RN

CHAPTER OUTLINE

LEARNING OBJECTIVES

Upon completing this chapter, you will be able to:

1. Identify and describe the three types of medical practice organization.
2. Describe three types of bank account and the advantages of each.
3. Describe the procedure for check writing.
4. Describe five situations that cause the bank statement to differ from the checkbook balance.

Chapter 12

Banking and Financial Procedures: Bookkeeping I

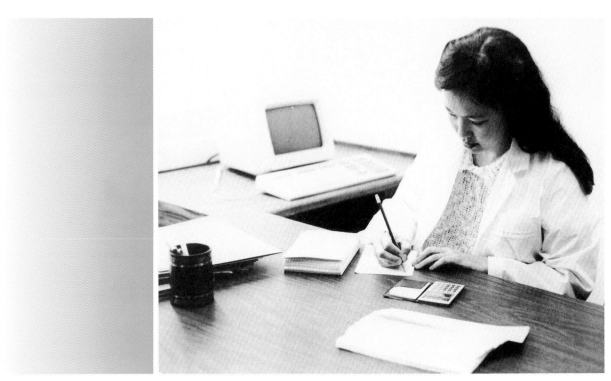

PERFORMANCE OBJECTIVES

Upon completing this chapter, you will be able to:

1. Calculate interest earned on money deposited in interest-bearing accounts.
2. Complete a deposit slip and prepare checks for deposit.
3. Prepare checks for payment of office expenses.
4. Reconcile a bank statement balance to the checkbook balance.

DACUM EDUCATIONAL COMPONENTS

Maintain records for accounting and banking purposes (process payments, and balance financial records) (8.6A – D).

Glossary

Asset: possession of value; typical assets include cash, amounts receivable from patients, inventory, equipment, and prepaid rent

Certified or cashier's check: check for which a bank guarantees sufficient money in the account to cover it

Check: written order from the checking account owner to the bank authorizing the bank to pay a certain amount to a specified recipient

Corporation: legal entity, created by the state, whose owners have a transferable interest represented by shares of capital stock

Endorsement: signature on the back of each check or money order by the person to whom it is made out

Interest: an amount of money paid to a depositor by a bank or other financial institution for the use of the depositor's money

Liabilities: due debts; typical liabilities include amounts due to suppliers, and amounts due to creditors for loans and mortgages

Nonsufficient funds: lack of money to cover a check as the result of an overdraft (check amount greater than the amount on deposit)

Partnership: business or enterprise created by a voluntary association of two or more persons who carry on the activities of a firm as coowners operating for a profit

Professional association: group of like professionals with common goals and objectives

Service charge: fee levied by a bank for handling and maintaining an account

Sole proprietorship or single proprietorship: individual business or enterprise owned entirely by one person

Many physicians engage experts such as bankers, accountants, and business advisors to assist in decisions affecting the business management of their medical practice. However, the daily financial activities are usually the responsibility of the medical assistant. As in other areas, the medical assistant must establish skill in and realize the importance of managing financial matters.

The level of sophistication of the office's general business practices reflects both the size of the practice and the orientation of the physician. In any case, the medical assistant plays an important role in carrying out the office financial policies.

TYPES OF MEDICAL PRACTICE ORGANIZATION AND THEIR LEGAL IMPLICATIONS

There are three forms of business organization for office practices: single proprietorship, or single-physician practice; partnership; and professional corporation. The form of organization determines whether approval is required from state agencies, how the profits are distributed, who makes decisions affecting employees of the practice, who makes other management and financial decisions, whether the owners are legal agents of the firm, and who assumes the legal responsibilities and liabilities.

SINGLE PROPRIETORSHIP

The simplest form of medical practice to organize and operate is the single proprietorship, or single-physician practice. The physician is in total control and makes all financial, administrative, and medical decisions. All income remaining after expenses are paid belongs solely to the physician. If the practice fails, the physician suffers the total loss.

When operating a single-proprietorship practice, the physician is *personally* liable for all debts incurred by the practice. The physician's personal and business financial operations should be kept separate to facilitate accurate recording of the business operations. If the practice becomes unable to pay its debts, the personal assets of the physician may have to be used for payment. The life of the practice depends solely on the physician. If the physician becomes unable to practice, the office will not continue to operate.

PARTNERSHIP

In a partnership, the ownership of the medical practice is divided among two or more physicians who agree to share their financial resources and medical talents. Although a partnership may be an oral agreement, a written contract between the partners provides the legal framework for decisions concerning each partner's sphere of authority, share of profits, financial contributions; the distribution of losses; practice management structure; and what should be done if one of the partners dies. By pooling resources in a group practice, physicians can extend their medical skills and financial resources beyond what each could manage individually. The assets of a partnership are not owned by specific individuals, but belong to the group. Income after expenses is distributed to all partners as stated in the partnership contract. Property purchased for the group by any partner becomes the property of all partners jointly. If the partnership dissolves, the partnership agreement determines how the practice assets are to be distributed regardless of the initial investment amount.

Partnerships have several disadvantages. Legally, one partner may speak for all the partners. Thus, all partners are legally responsible for the decisions of each one. For example, if one partner signs a contract to purchase a computer system for the office, the partnership is bound to honor the contract. Another disadvantage of the partnership is its limited life. A partnership is dissolved whenever a partner leaves the practice for any reason, such as withdrawal, bankruptcy, incapacity, or death. Also, admission of a new partner dissolves the previous contract. A new contract must be established if the operation of the practice is to continue with minimal interruption.

Partners in a general partnership are subject to unlimited liability. If a general partnership is unable to pay its debts, the partners must contribute sufficient personal assets to pay the debts of the partnership. To escape the unlimited liability of a general partnership, some practices organize as *limited* partnerships, in which liability is limited to the amount of investment in the practice.

PROFESSIONAL ASSOCIATIONS OR CORPORATIONS

The third form of medical practice organization is the professional association, or professional corporation. A corporation is formed under state law and has its own legal identity separate from the physicians comprising the practice. The physicians are paid a salary, as are the other employees of the practice. A corporation has the right to buy and sell property, make contracts, borrow money, and go to court, all in its own name. A corporation is held fully responsible for its debts, and if the bills cannot be paid, the property of the physicians is protected. Many physicians use this type of medical practice organization as a way of limiting personal liability. However, the physicians are still personally liable for any malpractice claim.

In some instances, a corporation may provide tax advantages and increased benefits from certain pension, profit-sharing, life insurance, and health insurance plans. As a result, the use of the designation *PC* (professional corporation) or *PA* (professional association) after a physician's name has become increasingly common. However, larger corporations must pay income taxes on their profits. In addition, the owners must include most of the dividends earned on profits in their personal income subject to taxation. As a result, the profits of a corporation are taxed twice—once to the corporation and once to the owners.

TECHNICAL ASPECTS OF MONEY

Medical practice income is based on the concept of the time value of money. The medical assistant should have a basic understanding of this phenomenon. During daily office business operations, large amounts of cash and checks flow into and out of the "cash box." To operate the financial policies of the practice effectively, the medical assistant needs a working knowledge of various types of bank account and of the dynamic nature of money itself.

CASH MANAGEMENT

Two basic principles sustain the management of cash.

1. Money in the office cash box is less valuable than money invested and earning interest or dividends.
2. Money in hand is worth more than money that will be acquired later.

It is important not to let large amounts of money (either cash or checks) accumulate in the office. Beyond the immediate security concerns, it is good business to move the money as quickly as possible to a bank or other financial institution.

INTEREST

Money not needed for payment of immediate bills should be deposited in an account that will earn interest. Interest is usually expressed as a percentage rate and is calculated by the following formula:

$$\text{Interest} = \text{Principal} \times \text{Percentage rate} \times \text{Time}$$

(time is expressed as a fraction of a year)

For example, if $5000 is deposited and left in the account for 60 days at a 7% interest rate, after 60 days the $5000 has earned $58.83 in interest. This simple interest is calculated as follows:

$$\text{Interest} = \$5000 \times 7\% \times \frac{360}{60}$$

(a year is considered 360 days)

Interest may also be compounded, or interest paid on the interest already earned. In the example, the principal for the second 60-day period would be $5058.33 rather than the original $5000. Interest can be compounded at various times as determined by bank policy. Obviously, interest compounded daily yields the most income.

TYPES OF BANK ACCOUNT

REGULAR CHECKING ACCOUNT

Most medical practices maintain a regular checking account. A regular checking account does not pay interest but offers availability and flexibility. The bank may reduce or eliminate its charge for handling a regular checking account if a minimum balance is maintained.

Depositing all money into a regular checking account also provides a mechanism for recording financial transactions. Office records may periodically be compared with bank statements to ensure accuracy.

INTEREST-EARNING CHECKING ACCOUNT

A sufficient amount of money to meet routine and recurring expenses should be kept in a regular checking account. The rest can be invested. Many medical practices maintain a second checking account that earns interest. Money is periodically moved from the interest-earning to the regular checking account. Most interest-earning checking accounts have some constraints, such as a maximum number of checks that may be written during a specified period, a limit on the

dollar amount of any check drawn on the account, or a minimum balance requirement. This type of checking account may be used to pay bills that occur infrequently, such as yearly insurance premiums.

SAVINGS ACCOUNTS

The medical practice may have a savings account in addition to checking accounts. Money also may be invested in potential earnings vehicles such as stocks, bonds, or real estate.

Although the physician must consult with business advisors to determine the types of account the practice will maintain, the medical assistant must be aware of the different types of account available. The medical assistant is usually expected to keep the records of the accounts and to perform various office banking functions.

DEPOSITS

An important advantage of depositing all money into one account is that the record of that account can be compared with the office intake record.

DEPOSIT SLIPS

The bank provides depositors with forms called *deposit slips* or *deposit tickets* to list the amounts being deposited. The deposit slips are preprinted with the name, address, and account number of the practice. The medical assistant completes the deposit slip by filling in the date and the amount of currency and coin to be deposited, and listing each check by bank number and source (patient or third-party payer).

CURRENCY AND CHECKS

Currency and coins should be sorted by denomination and placed in wrappers provided by the bank. Checks and money orders must be endorsed before they are deposited. There are several types of endorsement: open, limited, and restrictive. Open endorsements, shown in Figure 12–1, should never be used because they enable anyone to cash the check. Limited endorsement (Fig. 12–2) is usually used for third-party checks. For example, Mrs. Jenks, a patient, receives a check from her daughter for $50.00, the amount Mrs. Jenks owes the physician. If Mrs. Jenks uses that check to pay the physician, she must complete a limited endorsement on the back of the check (see Fig. 12–2). Restrictive endorsements (Fig. 12–3) should be used in the physician's office, including the words "For deposit only" and the physician's account number. This type of endorsement makes it impossible for anyone other than the bank to cash the check. A restrictive endorsement may be handwritten, but usually a rubber stamp is used to facilitate the procedure. The restrictive endorsement should be stamped on all checks and money orders in

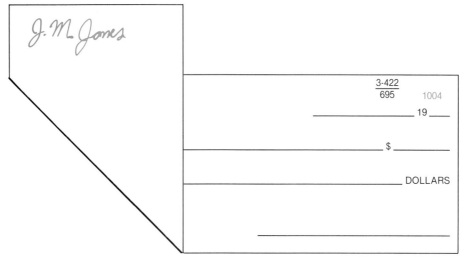

Figure 12–1. Open endorsement of a check.

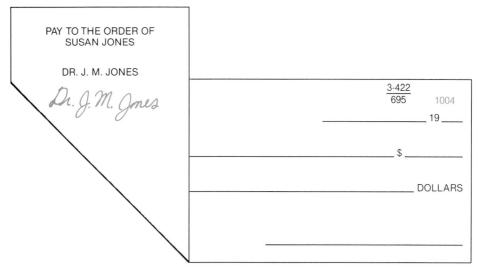

Figure 12–2. Limited endorsement of a check.

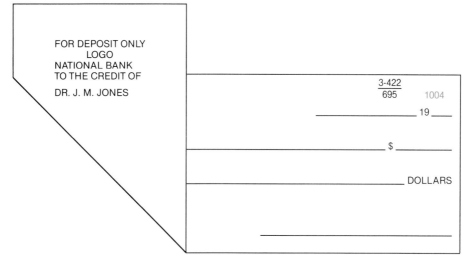

Figure 12–3. Restricted endorsement of a check.

the office at the time they are received—immediately. Endorsements are stamped on the back of the check and next to the check's printed statement "pay to the order of" (the left side of the check). If the back of the check designates a special area for the endorsement, it is important to stamp or sign the endorsement within the preprinted space.

After the deposit slip has been filled out, the checks endorsed, and the money wrapped, the amounts on the deposit slip are totaled. The deposit slip (Fig. 12–4), along with the cash and checks, is then taken to the bank.

DEPOSIT RECEIPTS

After receiving the currency, checks, and deposit slip, the bank teller gives the depositor a receipt indicating the date and total amount of the deposit. The amount shown on the receipt should be the exact amount totaled on the deposit slip. On returning to the office, the medical assistant should staple the bank receipt to the office duplicate copy of the deposit ticket. Doing this provides proof of the transaction for the physician's accounting records.

At times the medical assistant may be unable to get to the bank during regular banking hours. In this case, the deposit may be placed in the night deposit drop at the bank. The bank then mails the deposit receipt. The duplicate deposit ticket should be held until the deposit receipt is delivered to the office.

CHECKS

REVIEWING CHECKS WRITTEN BY PATIENTS

When accepting a patient's check, the medical assistant should examine it to ensure that it has been filled out correctly (Fig. 12–5). If the patient has written "Paid in full" on the face of the check, the account balance should be examined immediately to make sure it will cover the check. Accepting a check with this notation can mean writing off any balance due on the account. If the patient has written a future date on the face of the check, the check is said to be *postdated* and should not be deposited until the specified future date arrives. If a postdated check is accidently included with the day's deposits, the bank will probably process the check, and may be returned marked "Insufficient funds." In general, the medical office should refuse to accept postdated checks from patients. The office also should not give change for checks written for more than the amount owed. If such a check were accepted, it would deplete the office cash supply and eliminate the possibility of an audit trail from the patient's payment on the ledger card to the check recorded on the deposit slip.

CHECK WRITING

To ensure that the physician's financial records provide a complete and accurate summary of all financial

Figure 12–4. A bank deposit ticket.

transactions, payments for office expenses should always be made by check. Checks should always be completed in ink, typewritten, or the amount perforated onto the check by a small machine called a checkwriter. The intent is to make it very difficult, if not impossible, for anyone to alter name of the payee (the party named on the check) or the amount of the check (Fig. 12–6).

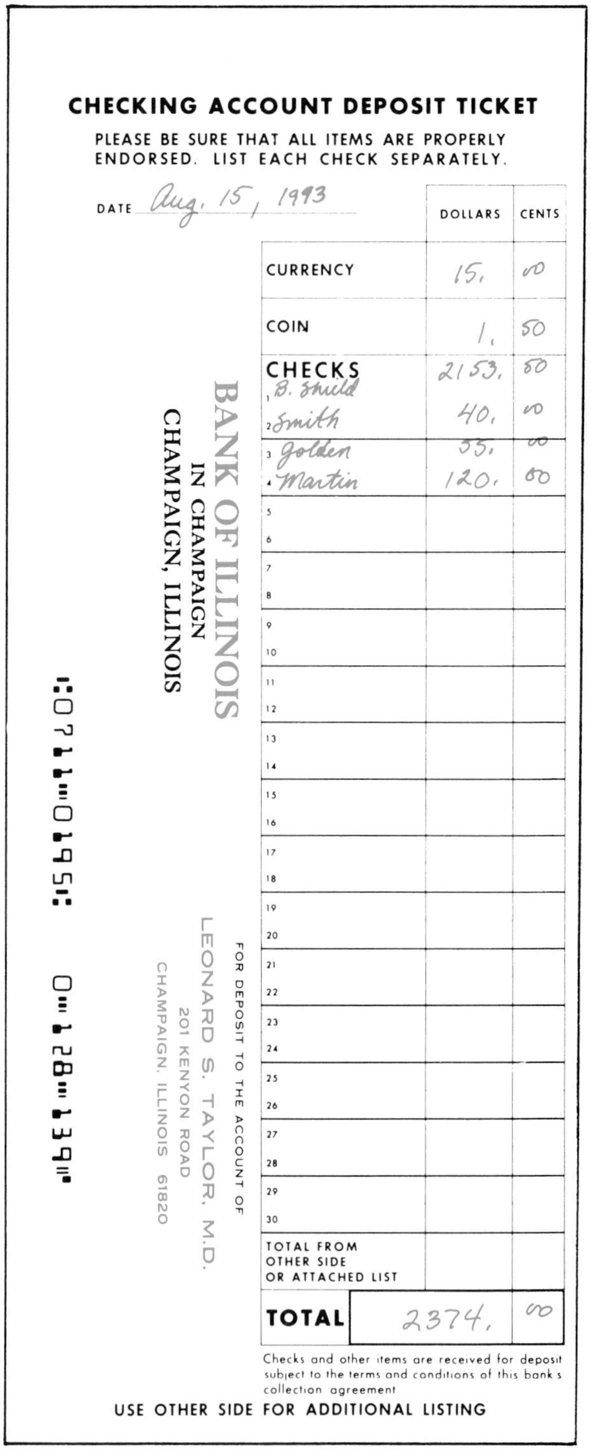

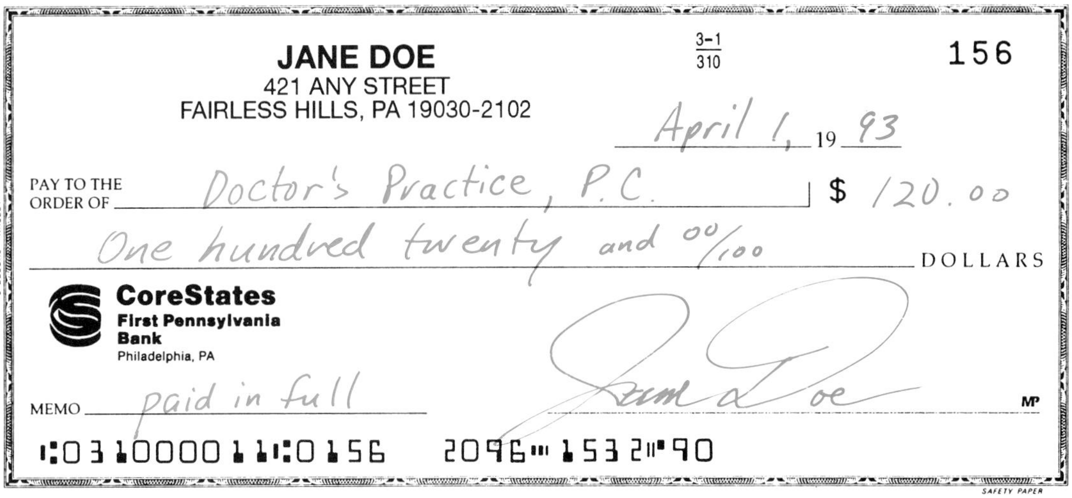

Figure 12-5. Immediately upon receipt of each personal check, verify the accuracy of the areas indicated in color.

The practice may use a checkbook or a pegboard system with checks and check registers (Fig. 12–7). In either case, before any check is written, the balance in the account should be up to date on the check stub or the check register. Each deposit should be added to the previous balance, and each check should be subtracted from the balance as it is written. In a checkbook with stubs, the stub should be completed before the check is written. The stub should contain the check number, the date, the name of the payee and the reason for payment (Fig. 12–8). All information on the stub must be complete and accurate because it is used to record the payment in the physician's accounting records. If a pegboard system is used, carbonized forms allow the necessary information to be entered on the check and the register at the same time. To note the reason for payment, the amount of the check may be entered in a special column on the register for that type of expense. The new balance also may be entered in the space provided on the register.

The number of the check is an important control feature. Sequential numbering ensures that unauthorized checks are not written. It also eases the job of sorting bank-processed checks.

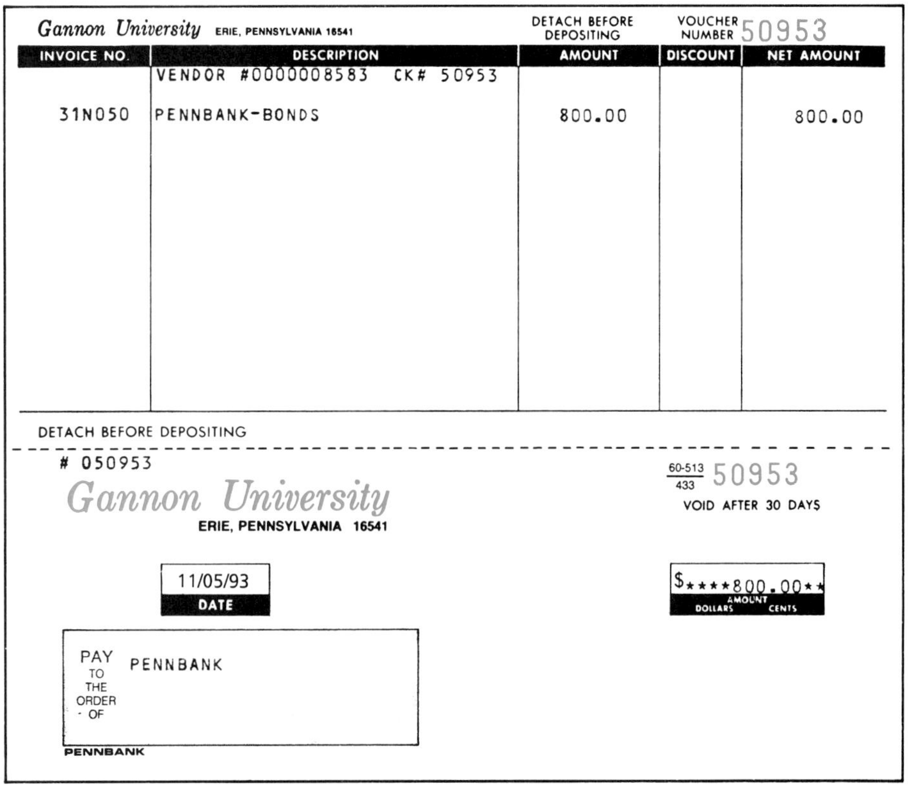

Figure 12-6. Expense check prepared with a checkwriter.

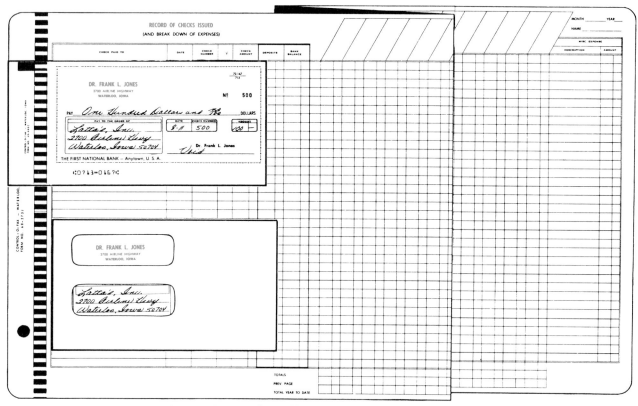

Figure 12-7. Pegboard system for writing and recording checks. (Courtesy Control-o-fax.)

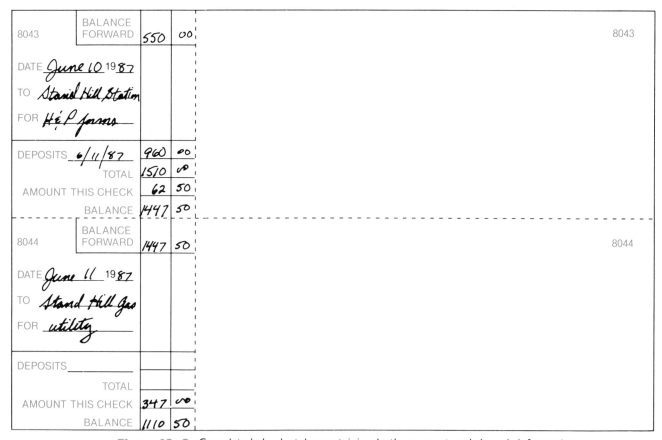

Figure 12-8. Completed check stubs containing both payment and deposit information.

The medical assistant should take care to review checks for printing errors. If an error is made in preparing a check, "VOID" should be written in large letters across the face of the check so that it may not be used again. Voided checks should be retained with other banking records to account for all checks.

The check should be prepared in the following manner:

1. Write the date and name of the payee.
2. Enter the amount of the check in the space beside the payee's name using the numerical format. Make sure that the decimal point is in the correct place.
3. Write the amount of the check below the payee's name. Begin at the extreme left of the space provided (to prevent alterations) and enter the dollar amount of the check in words followed by "and" (representing the decimal point); then enter the cents as a fraction of 100. Draw a line through any remaining blank space to prevent alterations.
4. Detach the check and give it to the physician to sign along with the bill or invoice being paid.
5. Send the check to the payee after it is signed.

The procedure for *preparing a check for payment of an office expense* is included at the end of the chapter.

LOST OR STOLEN CHECKS

Occasionally, a check may be lost or stolen after it has been issued. The medical assistant should examine the records to verify that a check was sent. If a reason-

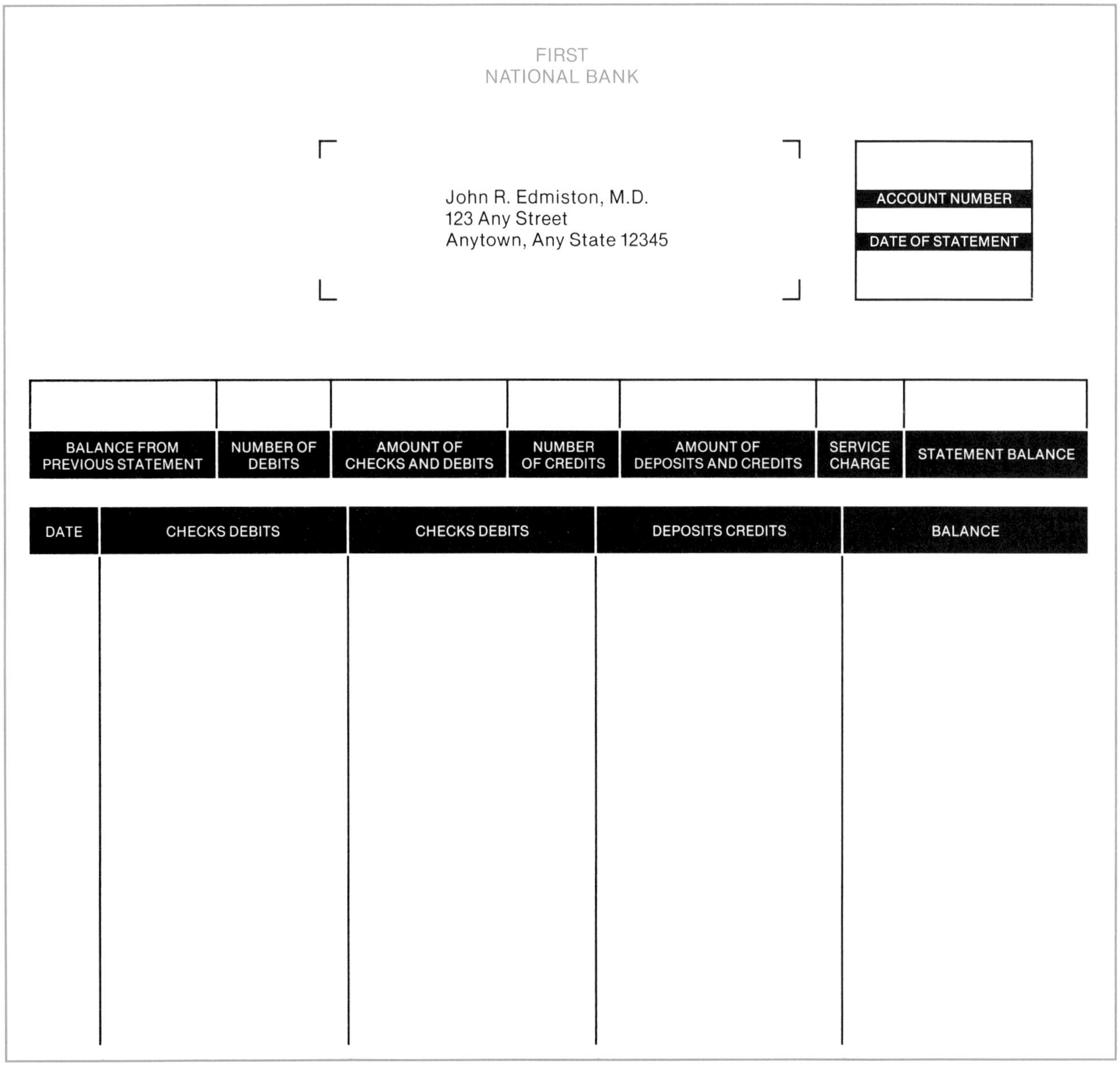

Figure 12-9. Bank statement.

able time (7 days) has elapsed, it can be considered lost. The medical assistant should contact the bank to make sure the check has not been presented for payment. If not, a "stop payment" order should be executed, authorizing the bank not to make payment if the check is presented. The bank charges for this service, but it is better to pay the service fee than to have two checks presented to and paid by the bank. The stop payment notice should be attached to the check stub or retained with other banking records. The amount of the check should be added to the current checkbook balance. A new check can then be issued to replace the one lost.

CANCELED CHECKS

An issued check eventually is returned to the bank on which it was originally drawn. After the bank has paid out funds for the check, it is returned to the medical office as a *canceled check* with a statement listing the deposits for that period, any bank charge deducted during the period, and a final balance in the account as of the date of the statement (Fig. 12–9).

SPECIAL CHECK TYPES

The physician may occasionally find it necessary to use a special kind of check for transactions. Some government tax units do not accept a personal check in payment of tax obligations. The physician may use a cashier's check or a certified check. A *cashier's check* is purchased from a bank. It is guaranteed by the bank and written on the bank's own checking account. A

certified check is one of the physician's regular checks that is verified and stamped by the bank before being used. Bank certification verifies that the amount shown on the check has been set aside and guarantees the validity of the check.

BANK STATEMENT RECONCILIATIONS

Usually, the balance shown on a monthly bank statement is different from the balance for the same date in the office checking account records. Possible reasons are:

1. *Outstanding checks*, or checks that have been written and subtracted in the checkbook but have not yet been presented to the bank for payment. The bank statement balance would be higher than the checkbook balance.
2. *Deposits in transit*, or deposits added in the checkbook that occurred after the date of the bank statement preparation. The bank statement balance would be lower than the checkbook balance.
3. *Errors*, made either by the medical assistant in the checkbook arithmetic or by the bank.
4. *Bank charges*, deducted by the bank for service, check imprinting, a stop-payment order, and so forth. The bank statement balance would be lower than the checkbook balance.
5. *Dishonored checks*, or checks deposited by the practice but refused payment because the patient did not have enough money on deposit to

```
                        DR. J.M. JONES
                      BANK RECONCILIATION
                        AUGUST, 1984

BALANCE PER BANK STATEMENT                                      $796.00

    + Deposits In Transit
          August 30                        $250.00
          August 31                         550.00              800.00
                                                               1596.00

    − Outstanding Checks
          #151 Aug. 30                      800.00
          #152 Aug. 30                      400.00            − 1200.00

    = Adjusted Bank Balance                                    $396.00

BALANCE PER CHECK BOOK                                         $410.00

       □ Service Charge                                           4.00
       □ NSF Check                                               10.00

ADJUSTED CHECKBOOK BALANCE                                     $396.00

PREPARED BY: Meg Green
DATE: Sept. 2, 1993
```

Figure 12–10. Bank reconciliation is used to adjust the checkbook balance.

cover the check. The bank states the reason for the dishonored check. In the case of nonsufficient funds (NSF), the bank statement balance would be lower than the checkbook balance. The medical assistant should notify the patient that the check has been returned. NSF checks may be redeposited one more time at the patient's request. At the time of redeposit, the check amount is subtracted from the original deposit. If the patient sends a new check, the original check is returned to the patient and the amount added to the patient's account balance.

To account for the differences between the cash balance on the bank statement and the cash balance in the checkbook, the medical assistant must make calculations involving both balances. This process is called *reconciling the figures*. A bank reconciliation (Fig. 12–10) should be prepared to show the reasons for the differences. Many banks provide a reconciliation form on the reverse of the bank statement, but a separate statement can be prepared. Because both the bank statement balance and the checkbook balance usually need adjustments, the reconciliation process changes both figures, which must work out to equal amounts. The Procedure on page 243 describes the process of reconciling a bank statement.

SUMMARY

The banking and financial issues discussed in this chapter, if properly managed, can increase the profitability of a medical office significantly. The medical assistant may be responsible for handling day-to-day banking and financial matters, but it is the physician's responsibility to make major financial decisions for the practice. The medical assistant should attempt to gain further knowledge in the areas introduced in this chapter to make the greatest possible contribution to the office. Additional education in accounting and finance can facilitate this objective.

DISCUSSION QUESTIONS

1. List the three types of medical practice organization and briefly discuss each.
2. What are the two basic principles underlying cash management?
3. What are certified checks? What are cashier's checks?

PROCEDURE: Prepare a check for payment of an office expense

Terminal Performance Objective: Prepare a business check for payment of an office expense with 100% accuracy within a reasonable time.

EQUIPMENT: Checkbook
Workbook application exercises
Workbook case studies

PROCEDURE

Complete the check stub as follows:
1. Write the date and name of payee.
2. Write the amount of the check.
3. Write the description of the check or other accounting reference number.

4. Subtract the amount of the check from the previous balance.
5. Enter the new checkbook balance.

Complete the check as follows:
6. Write the date and the name of the payee in ink.

7. Enter the amount of the check in the space beside the payee's name using the numeric format of dollars followed by cents. Take care that the decimal point is in the correct place.
8. Write the amount of the check below the payee's name. Begin at the extreme left of the space provided and enter the dollar amount of the check in words.
9. Continue the entry with the word "and" and then enter the cents as a fraction of 100.
10. Draw a line through any remaining blank space.

11. Detach the check and give it to the payor (the physician) to sign along with the bill or invoice being paid.

PRINCIPLE

3. The description of the check or some other identifying accounting reference is necessary for completing the accounts payable journal. Expenses are charged to specific accounting ledgers.

6. Writing in ink makes it difficult for anyone to alter the payee's name. Checks are usually honored only for 6 months or less.
7. The bank uses the numeric entry as a first determination of the amount of the check. A misplaced decimal point could result in a check-cashing error.

8. Beginning the entry on the extreme left prevents alterations in front of the wording.

9. "And" represents the decimal point in writing.

10. Filling any blank space prevents alterations after the wording.
11. An attached bill or invoice is a reference to justify the writing of the check and is mailed with the payment.

PROCEDURE: Reconcile a bank statement balance and the checkbook

Terminal Performance Objective: Account for and correct any differences between the cash balance on the bank statement and the cash balance in the checkbook, with 100% accuracy and within a reasonable time.

EQUIPMENT: Checkbook stubs
Canceled checks
Deposit receipts
Bank statement
Workbook application exercises
Workbook case studies

PROCEDURE

Checks and Deductions Update

1. Arrange the canceled checks returned with the bank statement in numeric order.

2. Include any voided checks.

3. Compare each check amount with the corresponding stub amount, accounting for all check numbers.

4. Compare each stub amount with each check amount appearing on the bank statement. Make check marks to indicate agreement.

5. Correct any stub amount that differs from the statement amount (if the statement is correct) and correct the balance forward.

6. List and total all outstanding checks (checks that have not been returned). Check the previous month's bank reconciliation.

7. Enter any checks listed on the statement but not shown in the checkbook, subtract the amounts, and correct the balance forward.

8. Enter any service charges, other bank charges, and dishonored checks not shown in the checkbook, subtract the amounts, and correct the balance forward.

Deposits and Credits Update

9. Arrange the deposit receipts in chronologic order.

10. Include any receipts for loan advances or other credits and stopped payments.

11. Compare each deposit receipt with the corresponding checkbook stub, accounting for all deposits.

12. Compare each deposit receipt with each deposit amount appearing on the bank statement.

13. Correct any stub deposit that differs from the deposit receipt and statement amount and correct the balance forward.

PRINCIPLE

1. Check sorting speeds accounting. If the statement displays checks in numeric order, steps 1 and 3 may be eliminated.

2. Bank statements display an asterisk (*) to help locate missing check numbers (checks paid from previous statements, void checks, and checks written but not yet paid).

3. Even if the check amount and bank statement agree, the amount on the stub may be entered incorrectly. Comparing checks with stubs determines whether the discrepancy originated with the checkbook or with the bank.

4. Comparing the stubs with the bank statement ensures the amounts agree and keeps track of the accounts.

5. Errors should be corrected before the reconciliation is prepared.

6. Outstanding checks make the bank statement balance higher than the checkbook balance. Checks may be outstanding from a previous statement period.

7. Checks not entered in the checkbook make the bank statement balance lower than the checkbook balance.

8. Additional bank charges not entered in the checkbook make the bank statement balance lower than the checkbook balance.

9. Deposit receipt sorting speeds accounting. if the statement displays deposits in chronologic order, steps 9 and 11 may be eliminated.

10. Bank statements display additional credits, such as automatic loans, interest, check reversal, payments stopped, and electronic transfers.

11. Even if the deposit receipt amount and bank statement agree, the amount on the stub may be entered incorrectly. Comparing receipts with stubs determines whether the discrepancy originated with the checkbook or the bank.

12. Comparing receipts with the bank statement ensures that the amounts agree.

13. Errors should be corrected before the reconciliation is prepared.

PROCEDURE

14. List and total all outstanding deposits (deposits that have not been credited). Check the previous month's bank reconciliation.
15. List and add any deposits listed on the statement but not shown in the checkbook and correct the balance forward.

Reconciliation

16. Record the new bank statement balance.
17. Add the total outstanding deposits.
18. Subtract the total outstanding checks.
19. Compare the adjusted bank statement balance with the checkbook balance. The balances should agree.
20. Enter the date of the reconciliation and initial the document.

PRINCIPLE

14. Outstanding deposits make the bank statement balance lower than the checkbook balance. Deposits may be outstanding from a previous statement period.
15. Deposits not entered in the checkbook make the bank statement balance higher than the checkbook balance.

HIGHLIGHTS
What Is a Bank?

Like medicine, banking has changed dramatically in the past decade. Banking is now a marketing-oriented, modern business that resembles a McDonalds' restaurant or a department store, with a full array of advertising, slogans, signs, and promotions. Why have these changes occurred so rapidly?

Years ago, people regarded banks as institutions, like churches or schools. There was a vague notion that banking was connected with federal or state government. Banks, as a rule, did not engage in overt acts of competition, such as advertising or promotion. Some individuals still persist in this view of banking.

During the past 10 years, however, deregulation of banking by government agencies created a new business environment. Banks are now clearly businesses that must succeed on their own merits. In addition to this new competitive environment, other financial institutions (brokerage houses and savings and loan institutions, for example) can now offer services that have traditionally only been offered by banks (and vice versa). The stage was set for some stiff competition.

Essentially, then, the modern bank is a business in which professional bankers offer products (formerly called "services") such as checking accounts, savings accounts, car loans, lines of credit, charge cards, and so forth. Each bank struggles to offer a wide array of attractive and profitable products so that it can be a viable business. The bank takes a client's money, invests it in the financial market, and returns a bonus (interest) to the client. For the bank to succeed, it must make enough profit on the difference between the interest that it earns by investing and the interest due customers to pay all of its bills. Naturally, the bank must also attract enough client's to provide monies to invest.

New promotions and competition provide substantial opportunities for taking advantage of bank discounts on loans, checking, and other services. A consumer of banking services may actually bank at several institutions. In contrast, however, it is desirable to build a long-term relationship with one bank and developing a working relationship with a banker who can be trusted for advice and counsel. At the banking supermarket, the wise individual needing banking services takes time to shop, compare services, weigh the needs and values of each, and learn as much as possible about the actual differences among banks before pledging loyalty.

> Good communication between patients and the medical practice is the basis for a sound credit and collection policy.
>
> Sharon Vance

CHAPTER OUTLINE

LEARNING OBJECTIVES

Upon completing this chapter, you will be able to:

1. List the components of the new patient information form.
2. Compare the advantages and disadvantages of extending credit and receiving payment at the time of service.
3. List and describe each component of the pegboard (one-write) system.
4. List four situations in which a patient's account balance might be adjusted.
5. Explain how aging patient accounts can provide valuable information about collection goals and efforts.
6. Describe the methods of notifying patients of their overdue accounts.
7. Describe the changes in the billing cycle and recording of payments for accounts turned over to a collection agency.
8. Describe and explain a physician's fee schedule.
9. Describe two special patient problems encountered in fees collection.
10. List five federal laws regulating credit and collections.
11. List three ways to enlist the courts as a resource for the collection of accounts.

246

Chapter 13

*B*illing and Collections: Bookkeeping II

PLEASE RETURN THIS FORM TO THE RECEPTIONIST

PREVIOUS BALANCE	NAME

A. OFFICE VISITS

1.Initial New Patient - New Illness: $ _____
☐ Limited ☐ Intermediate ☐ Comprehensive
90010   90015   90020

2.Established Patient _____
☐ Limited ☐ Intermediate ☐ Extended
90050   90060   90070

3.☐ Complete Physical   90080 _____
4.☐ Special Exam: Work-School-Ins

B. INJECTIONS & IMMUNIZATIONS:
907 _____
907 _____

C. EKG   93 _____

D. PATHOLOGY:
1.☐ Pap Smear   88150 $ _____
2.☐ Tissue _____

E. HOSPITAL CARE: (_____)
Name

1.Admit w/Hist. & Phy. __/__/__
☐ Intermediate ☐ Comprehensive
90215   90220

2.Daily Care # ____ @$ ____   90260 _____

M T W T F S S

3.Discharge __/__/__   90292 _____

4.Emergency Room: __:__ A/P ____ hrs.
☐ During Ofc. Hrs. ☐ After Ofc. Hrs.
99065   99064

RETURN: ____ Days ____ Weeks ____ Months

F. CONSULTATION: __/__/__ $ _____
Ref. _____
Phy. _____
1.☐ Intermediate 2.☐ Extensive 3.☐ Comprehensive
90605   90610   90620

G. SURGICAL ASSIST: _____
Primary Surgeon

H. LABORATORY

1.☐ UA	81000	10.☐ K-Blood	84132	
2.☐ CBC	85022	11.☐ Thyroid Pro.	82756	
3.☐ Hct.	85014	12.☐ Na-Blood	84295	
4.☐ Hgb.	85018	13.☐ Pro. Time	85610	
5.☐ Glucose	829	14.☐ SMA #	800	
6.☐ Tolerance	82951	15.☐ Preg. tests	86006	
7.☐ T. Cult.	87060	16.☐ Mono test	86300	
8.☐ U. Cult.	87086	17.☐ Sed Rate	85651	
9.☐ BUN	84520	18.☐ Gram Stain	87205	

Other
Lab. _____

I. OTHER SERVICE - SURGERY - X-RAY

DIAGNOSIS: ☐ Continuing Treatment of Previous Diagnosis _____

NEXT APPT. ____ ____ ____ ____ AM/PM
Day Month Date Time

Date of Service _____
ATTENDING PHYSICIAN'S STATEMENT
AMA Current Procedural Terminology, 4th Edition
Patient: _____

J. MATERIALS: _____

PATIENT DISABILITY STATEMENT
☐ Illness   ☐ AM
Onset of ☐ Injury __/__/__ ☐ PM
☐ Disabled ☐ Partially Disabled
__/__/__ thru __/__/__
O.K. to return to ☐ Work ☐ School ☐ P.E. __/__/__
I hereby authorize payment directly to the physician whose name appears on this form.

TOTAL CHARGE $ _____

IRS# 99-2220115
SMITH and JONES
Professional Corporation
3070 W. Airline Highway Anytown, U.S.A. 50704
Telephone 234-4651
☐ Wilbur C. Smith, M.D.   ☐ Raymond J. Jones, M.D.
SS# 265-50-1023   SS# 234-14-7728
BS# 7992   BS# 8213

89-12-0529   2100

PERFORMANCE OBJECTIVES

Upon completing this chapter, you will be able to:

1. Identify the party responsible for a patient's debt and prepare a new file with the patient information form, photocopies of the patient's insurance card, and a photocopy of the first check tendered for payment.
2. Check credit references and explain the grounds on which credit may be refunded.
3. Communicate fee information to patients and explain the payment plans and necessary paperwork for each type of credit arrangement.
4. Request payment from patients.
5. Prepare fee reduction agreements.
6. Enter services, fees, and payments on the day sheet and patient ledger card.
7. Prepare itemized statements.
8. Prepare an age analysis to keep up to date on overdue accounts.
9. Prepare and mail various types of collection letters.
10. By telephone or in person, follow government regulations pertaining to credit checks and debt collection to ensure that the physician's policies are uniform, fair, and nondiscriminatory.

DACUM EDUCATIONAL COMPONENTS

1. Use manual bookkeeping systems (for accounts receivable) (8.1A–E).
2. Manage accounts receivable (8.4A–G).
3. Maintain records for accounting and banking purposes (8.6A–C).

Glossary

Aging schedule: Patient account balances listed by number of days due or overdue, most recent payment date, and special notes about the account
Cash flow: Receipt of money by the practice
Charges: Amounts owed by patients for services rendered by the physician
Litigation: Payments made to the medical office by patients or third parties
Third party: Any person, insurance company, or government agent other than the patient or the patient's family who pays all or a portion of the patient's account

One of the most difficult and sensitive aspects of office management is the collection of fees owed by patients. Given the time value of money, it is obviously to the physician's advantage to collect the full fee for services when they are rendered. To alert patients to this policy, many physicians post a small sign in a conspicuous area of the office stating, "All services should be paid for in full at the time of service unless other arrangements have been made in advance." The patient is then prepared for the visit and is not embarrassed or irritated when payment is requested at its conclusion.

Although patients are requested to pay at the time the service is rendered, there are many instances when partial or no payment is made. If the physician has agreed to participate in an insurance plan and will be paid 100% of the fee directly by an insurance company or other third party, the patient makes no payment at the time of service. For instance, patients do not pay when they are seeking an insurance-reimbursable second surgical opinion, hold a policy under the Veterans Administration payment plan, or have been treated for

injuries covered under a workers' compensation plan. For patients covered by Health Maintenance Organization (HMO) copayment plans, only the patient portion of the fee (usually $5 or $10) should be collected.

In offices that display "payment at the time of service" signs, the physician may choose not to participate in a particular plan, in which case the patient assumes the responsibility for processing the insurance form. The patient must complete the form and send it to the insurance company. In this instance, the patient is expected to pay at the time the service is obtained and is then reimbursed by the insurance company. In other instances when the fee cannot be collected at the time of service, the bill and a mailing envelope should be given to the patient to encourage immediate payment. In still other instances, fees are collected through routine monthly billing. Regardless of the particular payment plan the office chooses, it is often the responsibility of the medical assistant to tactfully inform all patients of the payment policy. New patients should be informed of this policy before the first visit.

Although there are advantages to each payment plan

(physician or patient insurance processing), payment at the time of service is preferable in terms of the time value of money and predictable cash flow. In addition, this policy relieves the office staff of the burden of collection, which may involve numerous telephone calls and letters to the patient.

Some physicians may prefer to extend credit. The medical assistant should understand thoroughly the physician's philosophy concerning credit. Many physicians allow the medical assistant a great deal of latitude in making credit decisions, whereas others insist on reviewing each decision. In either case, the medical assistant plays a significant role in fee collection.

COLLECTION OF INFORMATION

All new patients should be required to complete a patient information sheet. This form should include the patient's full name, current address and telephone number, date of birth, social security number, business address and telephone number (for both husband and wife), name and address of the nearest relative not living in the immediate household, and the names of both former physicians and those currently providing care. The form should also include the patient's medical insurance information. If the patient has insurance coverage, it is wise to photocopy both sides of the insurance card and attach the copies to the information form. This information assists in the preparation of the patient's medical and financial records. For credit checks and insurance collection purposes, the patient must sign an authorization for release of information on the form. Figure 13-1 is a sample form.

EXTENDING CREDIT

When credit is extended to a patient, credit information on the patient information form should be checked as soon as possible, and always before the credit agreement is decided. Credit checks can be conducted through credit bureau companies or credit bureaus operated by medical association (local Bureaus of Medical Economics). These resources usually maintain information on borrowers and may even record specific patient ratings and repayment habits to doctors and dentists. Typical credit information should include:

1. The patient's address and moving habits
2. Verification of employment
3. The patient's approximate salary
4. Ratings and reports on the patient's payment habits
5. Unusual information, such as bankruptcy history or change of name

It is also important to extend credit to the correct person. If a person other than the patient is to be responsible for medical services, the correct name, address and employment information should be obtained.

If this person (the third party) is not with the patient at the time of service, the third party should be contacted to verify his or her willingness or obligation to pay the fees. If the third party is not legally responsible for payment of services, a signed statement of responsibility should be obtained. If the third party is an insurance carrier, the patient's insurance card should be photocopied, and the patient should sign the release and authorization portions of the insurance claim form. (See Chapter 15, "Insurance Processing.")

Credit information must be kept confidential. The data obtained cannot be released to any other physician, agency, or company. If an insurance carrier, such as Medicare, requires information about a patient's payments, balance, or credit arrangements, this information cannot be released without the patient's signed consent.

Credit cards can be used as a means of extending credit. However, credit card memberships can be costly to both physicians and patients. Credit card companies charge fees (usually 1%–7%) dependent on the volume of business charged. Such a financing plan may result in interest charges to the patient, thereby increasing the cost of medical care.

Banks, credit associations, and some medical associations offer financing for medical care. In these cases, the physician may deduct from the total office fee the interest fees that the patient has paid to the bank or association. When other financing is not available or feasible, the physician and the patient can initiate an installment agreement. (See the "Legal Implications" section in this chapter.)

THE PEGBOARD SYSTEM

The medical office must maintain accurate and complete records regarding services received by patients (charges) and payments made by patients or third parties (receipts). Many physicians use the *pegboard system* to maintain accounting records efficiently and accurately.

The pegboard system consists of a flat writing surface with a series of evenly spaced pegs along its left edge. Pegboard forms are specially designed, with left-sided perforations that are held in place by the pegs and line up all the underlying forms. As information on the top form is completed, the pressure-sensitive paper transfers the same information to all copies below. (Refer to Chapter 12 for a description of pegboard check-writing systems.)

This "one-write" system generates all the financial records needed for each transaction with a single entry transferred onto the various other forms through the use of pressure-sensitive noncarbon paper. Basic pegboard systems are available for accounts receivable (patient receipts and payments) and for accounts payable (office purchases and payroll).

When used for patient accounts, the pegboard system simultaneously generates a daily earnings summary, a deposit slip, a ledger card, and a patient charge

MEDICAL RECORD INFORMATION

NAME _____

HOME ADDRESS _____

HOME PHONE _____ BIRTHDATE _____ DRIVERS LIC. # _____

SOC. SEC. # _____ AGE _____ MARITAL STATUS _____

OCCUPATION _____ EMPLOYER _____

EMPLOYER ADDRESS _____ PHONE _____

NAME OF SPOUSE _____

SPOUSE EMPLOYER _____

ADDRESS _____ PHONE _____

NAME, ADDRESS, AND PHONE OF NEAREST RELATIVE NOT LIVING IN

IMMEDIATE HOUSEHOLD:

    NAME: _____

    ADDRESS: _____

    PHONE: _____ RELATIONSHIP _____

NAMES OF OTHER PHYSICIANS CURRENTLY PROVIDING CARE

_____

_____

_____

MEDICAL INSURANCE COMPANY

    COMPANY _____ POLICY # _____

_____

_____

Information on this card may be released to appropriate agents for purposes of confirmation of credit rating and for matters pertaining to insurance collection.

Signed _____ Date_____

Figure 13-1. New patient information sheet.

and receipt slip. A single entry records the data on all four of these source documents.

When used for payments, the pegboard system records a cash payment journal entry, a voucher, and a check. As the check is completed, simultaneous voucher proof of supplier expenditures and disbursements categorizes cash expenditures.

Payroll is accomplished by a single entry for each employee that is recorded simultaneously on a payroll journal, an employee earnings record, an employee earnings statement, and a payroll check with a voucher stub.

Several pegboard systems are available. The type to be used is determined by the needs of the individual practice. The basic concept is the same for all the available systems, but the specifics require training in the use of the one chosen.

See the procedure for posting charges and payments using the pegboard system at the end of this chapter.

RECORDING CHARGES IN THE PEGBOARD SYSTEM

The medical assistant should complete the information on the patient ledger card heading when the patient is seen for the first time. The patient's name and address are typed in the space provided. This card is used to prepare monthly bills.

When the patient arrives at the office, the medical assistant prepares and attaches a charge slip, or superbill (Fig. 13-2), to the front of the patient's chart. The physician completes the information on the forms and returns it to the medical assistant at the conclusion of the office visit. Either the physician or the medical assistant enters the dollar amount on the charge slip, using the physician's fee schedule. (The *fee schedule* is a price list for all procedures and supplies used to treat a patient and should be kept current.) Figure 13-3 shows a sample physician's fee schedule. Patients should be informed that a fee schedule is available upon request.

After the charges have been entered and totaled, the charge slip, or superbill, is placed over the correct line on the pegboard. The medical assistant must make sure it lines up with the correct line on the daily log underneath. The patient ledger card (Fig. 13-4) is then placed between the two forms. Thus, when the information is written on the top form, it is entered simultaneously on the patient account card and the daily log (Fig. 13-5).

PLEASE RETURN THIS FORM TO THE RECEPTIONIST

PREVIOUS
BALANCE   NAME

A. OFFICE VISITS
1. Initial New Patient - New Illness: $ _____
   ☐ Limited   ☐ Intermediate   ☐ Comprehensive
   90010   90015   90020
2. Established Patient
   ☐ Limited   ☐ Intermediate   ☐ Extended
   90050   90060   90070

3. ☐ Complete Physical   90080 _____
4. ☐ Special Exam: Work-School-Ins _____

B. INJECTIONS & IMMUNIZATIONS:
                                       907___ _____
                                       907___ _____

C. EKG _____   93___ _____

D. PATHOLOGY:
1. ☐ Pap Smear   88150 $ _____
2. ☐ Tissue _____

E. HOSPITAL CARE: (_____)
                          Name

1. Admit w/Hist. & Phy. ___/___/___   _____
   ☐ Intermediate   ☐ Comprehensive
   90215   90220

2. Daily Care # _____ @$ _____   90260 _____
   ___/ ___/ ___/ ___/ ___/ ___/ ___/
    T   T   W   T   F   S   S

3. Discharge ___/___/___   90292 _____
                                          A
4. Emergency Room: ___:___ P _____ hrs. _____
   ☐ During Ofc. Hrs.   ☐ After Ofc. Hrs.
   99065   99064

RETURN: _____ Days _____ Weeks _____ Months

F. CONSULTATION: ___/___/___ $ _____
Ref. _____
Phy. _____
   1. ☐ Intermediate 2. ☐ Extensive 3. ☐ Comprehensive
      90605   90610   90620
G. SURGICAL ASSIST: _____
                          Primary Surgeon
H. LABORATORY
1. ☐ UA   81000 _____ 10. ☐ K-Blood   84132 _____
2. ☐ CBC   85022 _____ 11. ☐ Thyroid Pro. 82756 _____
3. ☐ Hct.   85014 _____ 12. ☐ Na-Blood   84295 _____
4. ☐ Hgb.   85018 _____ 13. ☐ Pro. Time   85610 _____
5. ☐ Glucose   829 _____   14. ☐ SMA # _____ 800 _____
6. ☐ Tolerance 82951 _____ 15. ☐ Preg. tests 86006 _____
7. ☐ T. Cult. 87060 _____ 16. ☐ Mono test   86300 _____
8. ☐ U. Cult. 87086 _____ 17. ☐ Sed Rate   85651 _____
9. ☐ BUN   84520 _____ 18. ☐ Gram Stain   87205 _____
Other
Lab. _____

I. OTHER SERVICE - SURGERY - X-RAY
_____
_____
_____
                    ☐ Continuing Treatment
DIAGNOSIS: of Previous Diagnosis _____
_____

NEXT _____ AM
APPT. Day Month Date Time PM

Date of Service _____
ATTENDING PHYSICIAN'S STATEMENT
AMA Current Procedural Terminology, 4th Edition
Patient: _____

J. MATERIALS: _____

PATIENT DISABILITY STATEMENT
   ☐ Illness   ☐ AM
Onset of ☐ Injury ___/___/___   ☐ PM
   ☐ Disabled   ☐ Partially Disabled
   ___/___/___ thru ___/___/___
O.K. to return to ☐ Work ☐ School ☐ P.E. ___/___/___
I hereby authorize payment directly to the physician
whose name appears on this form.

TOTAL CHARGE $ _____

IRS# 99-2220115
SMITH and JONES
Professional Corporation
3070 W. Airline Highway Anytown, U.S.A. 50704
Telephone 234-4651
☐ Wilbur C. Smith, M.D.   ☐ Raymond J. Jones, M.D.
SS# 265-50-1023   SS# 234-14-7728
BS# 7992   BS# 8213

89-12-0529   **2100**

Figure 13-2. Example of a charge slip ("superbill") in a "one-write" pegboard system.

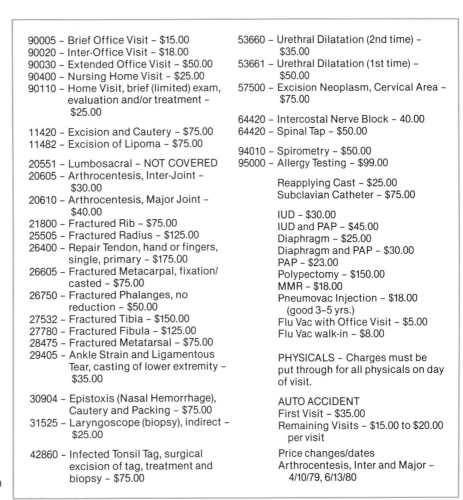

90005 – Brief Office Visit – $15.00
90020 – Inter-Office Visit – $18.00
90030 – Extended Office Visit – $50.00
90400 – Nursing Home Visit – $25.00
90110 – Home Visit, brief (limited) exam, evaluation and/or treatment – $25.00

11420 – Excision and Cautery – $75.00
11482 – Excision of Lipoma – $75.00

20551 – Lumbosacral – NOT COVERED
20605 – Arthrocentesis, Inter-Joint – $30.00
20610 – Arthrocentesis, Major Joint – $40.00
21800 – Fractured Rib – $75.00
25505 – Fractured Radius – $125.00
26400 – Repair Tendon, hand or fingers, single, primary – $175.00
26605 – Fractured Metacarpal, fixation/casted – $75.00
26750 – Fractured Phalanges, no reduction – $50.00
27532 – Fractured Tibia – $150.00
27780 – Fractured Fibula – $125.00
28475 – Fractured Metatarsal – $75.00
29405 – Ankle Strain and Ligamentous Tear, casting of lower extremity – $35.00

30904 – Epistoxis (Nasal Hemorrhage), Cautery and Packing – $75.00
31525 – Laryngoscope (biopsy), indirect – $25.00

42860 – Infected Tonsil Tag, surgical excision of tag, treatment and biopsy – $75.00

53660 – Urethral Dilatation (2nd time) – $35.00
53661 – Urethral Dilatation (1st time) – $50.00
57500 – Excision Neoplasm, Cervical Area – $75.00

64420 – Intercostal Nerve Block – 40.00
64420 – Spinal Tap – $50.00

94010 – Spirometry – $50.00
95000 – Allergy Testing – $99.00

Reapplying Cast – $25.00
Subclavian Catheter – $75.00

IUD – $30.00
IUD and PAP – $45.00
Diaphragm – $25.00
Diaphragm and PAP – $30.00
PAP – $23.00
Polypectomy – $150.00
MMR – $18.00
Pneumovac Injection – $18.00 (good 3–5 yrs.)
Flu Vac with Office Visit – $5.00
Flu Vac walk-in – $8.00

PHYSICALS – Charges must be put through for all physicals on day of visit.

AUTO ACCIDENT
First Visit – $35.00
Remaining Visits – $15.00 to $20.00 per visit

Price changes/dates
Arthrocentesis, Inter and Major – 4/10/79, 6/13/80

Figure 13-3. Example of a fee-for-service schedule.

MARCH MEDICAL GROUP
A PROFESSIONAL CORPORATION
14950 MARCH AVENUE
SANTA ROSA, CA. 94950
TELEPHONE 545-4500

| DATE | REFERENCE | DESCRIPTION | CHARGE | CREDITS | | CURRENT BALANCE |
				PAYMENTS	ADJ.	
		BALANCE FORWARD ⟶				

PLEASE PAY LAST AMOUNT IN THIS COLUMN ⬅

THIS AREA FOR SERVICE CODES

OV—Office Visit   X—X-Ray   ROA—Received on Account
C—Consultation   NC—No Charge   TC—Telephone Consultation
EX—Examination   INS—Insurance   FA—Failed Appointment

Figure 13-4. Patient ledger card.

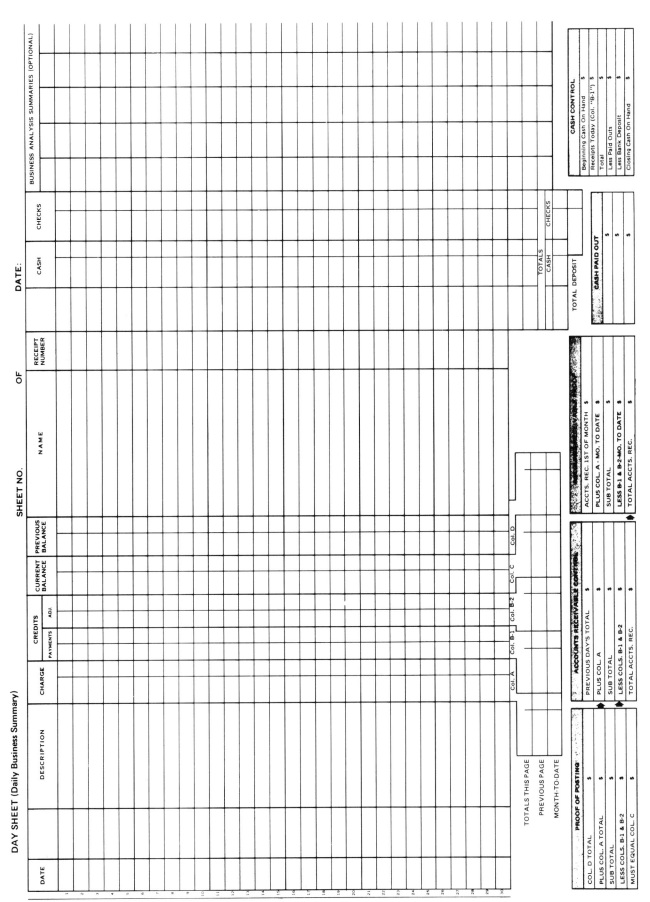

Figure 13–5. Daily log.

If a patient is charged for services rendered outside the office (surgery, house calls, etc.), it is necessary to prepare a charge slip (superbill) in the manner indicated above. The source document for such a transaction may be a prepared form or merely a slip of paper on which the physician has written notes. Surgeons sometimes maintain a "surgery book"—a notebook or logbook that lists each surgery performed, the patient's name, the date, and the charge.

RECORDING PAYMENTS IN THE PEGBOARD SYSTEM

When a patient makes a payment, the proper entry must be recorded on the patient ledger card. When payment is by check, the patient's canceled check serves as the receipt, so it is not necessary to prepare another. When a patient makes a cash payment after the date of service, the medical assistant should complete a pegboard receipt and give it to the patient.

Often, insurance companies send payments for several patients at the same time. The company sends one check with a list of those patients included in the payment. The list of payments should be separated by patient and totaled to make sure the check amount is correct. Then the amounts may be recorded on each patient's account card and the daily log.

The Procedure section at the end of this chapter summarizes the steps required to post charges and payments using the pegboard system.

DAILY TOTALS

At the end of every day, the columns on the daily log should be totaled and proofed. A format for proofing is generally provided at the bottom of the daily log, but usually it is as follows:

Previous balance
+ Charges added today
− Payments received today
− Adjustments (To determine the balance of the adjustment column *on the daily log,* the credits are added and the debits are subtracted.)
= New balance

Most daily logs provide this format for accounts receivable control at the bottom of the page. The total from the previous page plus today's charges, minus today's payments, gives a new accounts receivable balance (see Fig. 13–5). This balance (the running balance) is entered on the next day's log as the previous total. The running balance should equal the total of all patient account cards in the patient ledger. Agreement is usually automatic in the one-write (pegboard) system. If the account card balance is less than the accounts receivable control balance, an account card is probably missing. If the account card balance is greater than the accounts receivable control balance, duplicate ledger cards may exist for one or more patients.

FEE ADJUSTMENTS AND CANCELLATIONS

Most pegboard systems include a column headed "Adj." This column is the adjustments (see Fig. 13–5). This column may be used to handle refunds of overpayments, reductions in accounts for various reasons, and nonsufficient funds (NSF) checks. The pegboard system uses only the ledger card and the daily earnings page; there is no need for a patient charge slip, unless the adjustment is taken at the same time as a charge or payment. Below are explanations and examples of the more common adjustments necessary.

1. *Overpayments.* Occasionally, an insurance company sends payment for a bill that the patient has already paid. In this case, the payment is recorded as usual, and the patient account card then shows a credit, or negative balance, in the current balance column. When the practice writes a check to refund this overpayment to the patient, the amount is added in the adjustments column to return the balance to zero.

2. *Reductions in accounts.* The physician may decide to reduce or eliminate an amount owed for various reasons, including professional courtesy to a colleague. On reviewing a case, the physician also may reduce the amount owed by a patient. If a patient declares bankruptcy or the physician believes the amount owed is too small to warrant action by a collection agency, the amount may be written off. A fee should never be reduced to obtain quicker payment or reduce collection efforts. As a consequence, patients may then believe that the physician's original charge was inflated. Charges in excess of the amount allowed by Medicare also must be subtracted from patient accounts. Physicians sometimes accept any insurance payment as a fee if the patient's financial situation falls below certain levels.

3. *Collection agency payments.* When accounts are turned over to a collection agency, the physician no longer bills the patient and the patient rarely pays at the office. Normally, the patient pays the collection agency directly, and the physician receives a statement and check from the agency monthly. For each account on which payment has been made, the agency keeps its fee and remits only the excess to the physician. However, the physician must reduce the patient account by the total amount the patient paid the agency. For this purpose, the amount received by the physician is recorded in the payment column, and the difference between this and the total amount paid by the patient is entered in the adjustments column. This total amount is then subtracted from the previous balance to arrive at the new balance.

4. *Nonsufficient funds checks.* When the bank returns a check because the patient did not have adequate money on deposit, the patient

owes the physician the amount of the check. When the physician's office first received the check, the amount was subtracted from the patient's account, so now it must be added to that account. The amount must be entered in the adjustments column and added to the old balance.

In patient refund and NSF situations, each adjusted amount is a reversal of payment (an *addition* to the previous balance). In overpayments and account reductions, the adjusted amounts are reversals of charges (subtractions). Normally, the amount entered in the adjustment column is a subtraction, or credit, as if a payment has occurred. When a situation (debit or recharge) requires an addition to the balance, the amount is also entered in the adjustment column, but in a circle or parentheses. (The addition procedure is the reverse of the procedure for the balance column.)

BILLING

Because it is not always possible to collect fees at the time of service, there are always outstanding fees. Patients with outstanding balances should be billed monthly, even if an insurance claim is pending. Monthly billing keeps the patient informed of the status of the account. However, if the physician has agreed (for example, if he or she has contracted as a Medicare provider), the third-party payment is the total that can be collected. For example, patients participating in state medical assistance programs cannot be billed for the difference between the physician's charges and the copayment received. Balances remaining after copayment on this type of account must be "adjusted," or subtracted from, on the patient's ledger card.

STATEMENT PREPARATION

The patient's statement can be prepared in several ways, depending on the physician's preference and the methods available.

1. *Individual statements.* An individual statement is prepared by hand or typed from the information on the patient ledger card (see Fig. 13–4). It is mailed to the patient in a manually addressed envelope. This method is time consuming and impractical for offices processing a large number of statements.
2. *Photocopied statements.* The photocopy method of statement preparation is very common. The patient ledger card is photocopied. The copied statements are folded to fit special "window" envelopes, thus eliminating hand-addressed envelopes.
3. *Independent billing services.* Independent accounts receivable management firms prepare and mail all patient statements. Their fees can be expensive, and the service requires the re-

moval of patient financial records from the office while statements are being prepared. However, in larger medical offices, the advantage of eliminating this clerical task may justify the use of the service.
4. *Computerized billing.* As medical offices become increasingly computerized, automatic preparation of patient statements has become common. Instead of photocopying each patient's account, the medical assistant instructs the computer to print statements from the accounts. The computer-generated statements must still be folded and placed in envelopes, but this form of billing can save the medical assistant much time and effort. On-line computer billing in insurance companies eliminates stationery and mailing costs and allows for quicker payment to the physician.

BILLING SCHEDULE

Physicians' offices should have a regular billing schedule. Some offices prefer to bill immediately after a service is rendered; others bill twice a month; some bill every 3 weeks. If billing is monthly, the statements should be mailed before the end of the month so they can be included in patients' monthly budgets. If billing is twice a month, the statements should reach patients before the 15th and before the end of the month. If billing is computerized, statements are usually generated daily after each data entry.

If a large number of statements are sent each month, the office may use *cyclic billing,* in which portions of the statements are mailed out at various times during the month. For example, patients whose last names begin with *A* through *H* would be billed on the 6th, *I* through *Q* on the 16th, and *R* through *Z* on the 26th. This system eliminates the burden of preparing and mailing all statements on one day, and also spreads out the receipt of money over the entire month. Cyclic billing is useful for maintaining an even cash flow.

AGING OF ACCOUNTS

It is accepted that not all patients pay their bills on time. At some point, overdue accounts may require further action. The *aging schedule* determines which patient accounts must be followed up. An aging schedule is simply a record of all patient account balances, when the charges originated, the most recent payment date, and any special notes concerning the account. This information is taken from the patient ledger cards. The medical assistant should use this information to prepare an aging schedule each month.

Figure 13–6 shows a typical aging schedule. The balance column shows the total amount due the physician. The next five columns indicate when the charges originated. The last payment column indicates the most recent payment date. The explanation column lists details of the account status, such as what action has been

PATIENT	BALANCE	0–30 DAYS	31–60 DAYS	61–90 DAYS	91–120 DAYS	OVER 120 DAYS	LAST PAYMENT	EXPLANATION
ALEXANDER, A.B.	$ 500.00	250.00	250.00					REMINDER NOTICE SENT
FINNEY, J.P.	675.00		375.00	300.00				2ND NOTICE
McMULLIN, G.R.	1780.00					1780.00	MARCH 1	COLLECTION AGENCY
BRAGGINS, C.L.	350.00	350.00						BLUE SHIELD FILED 7-22

Figure 13–6. Aging schedule. The total of the balance column must equal the total of the other amount columns added together.

taken, notes on telephone contacts, patient assurances, and insurance pending.

An analysis of the aging schedule provides the physician with valuable information. Trends in length of time outstanding, amounts collected, and insurance claims outstanding emerge. It is also possible to determine the collection percentage by dividing the total amount collected on the accounts during the current billing cycle by the total balance column. It is generally accepted that a 100% collection is unrealistic and that collection rates of 95% to 98% are excellent.

Collection rates vary according to the type of practice. The American Medical Association provides figures on desired and actual collection rates for various types of practice.

THE COLLECTION PROCESS

COLLECTION NOTICES

Patients should receive the first billing notice at the end of the month in which the charge occurred. Many patients pay all or most of the balance on receipt of this first statement. Including a colored, preaddressed payment envelope for the patient's convenience has been proven to be an effective collection tool.

If payment is not received, the second billing should initiate the collection policy. The second statement may include a reminder notice. This notice may be a sticker or a handwritten note asking the patient to pay the balance due. Office supply dealers carry various color-coded stickers with preprinted messages such as "Final Note," "Please Pay," and "Past Due." Use of these preprinted messages can save considerable time.

If payment is not received within 30 days of the second notice, the third bill may include a stronger note urging the patient to either pay or contact the office if there is a problem. Depending on the practice, the third or fourth billing may contain a final notice, giving the

patient a last chance to pay the outstanding balance. This notice may be a preprinted sticker, a handwritten note, or even a personal letter from the physician (Fig. 13–7). It includes information as to what further collection steps will be taken if no payment is received. For instance, the office may inform the patient that the account will be turned over to a professional collection agency or an attorney.

TELEPHONE COLLECTIONS

At some point in the collection process, the medical assistant may be asked to contact the patient by telephone concerning the overdue bill. This method is quick and effective for communicating with patients about treatment charges. The medical assistant should listen attentively to the patient's explanation of why the payment is in arrears, should inquire about when payment can be expected, and should notice whether the patient expresses any dissatisfaction with either the treatment received or the charges. The medical assistant should notify the physician immediately of any patient's dissatisfaction so that steps may be taken to alleviate potential litigation.

The conversation should close with the patient's agreement to pay. The medical assistant should make detailed notes during the conversation. The notes should be written on the back of the patient's ledger card, attached to the ledger card, or filed in a special "Collection Notes" file. This financial information should not be included in the patient's medical file.

AVAILABLE COLLECTION RESOURCES

If the patient does not pay after a final notice has been sent, the account may be placed with a collection agency or the physician's attorney for further collection efforts. The attorney may seek help from the court in collecting the account.

Smith and Jones Professional Corporation
3070 W. Airline Highway
Anytown, U.S.A. 50704
April 15, 19____

Mr. Clinton Rogers
1308 Nice Street
Anytown, U.S.A. 50704

Dear Mr. Rogers,
  It has been brought to my attention that your bill in the amount
of $ 157.00_____ is past due.
  As you know, the cost of providing medical care to you is high,
and I cannot continue to provide service without payment. I am,
therefore, asking that you pay this bill within 10 days. If I do not
hear from you within that time, I will be forced to turn your account
over to a collection agency. Of course, if you have already sent
payment, please accept my thanks and disregard this notice.
  I look forward to hearing from you.

                                   Sincerely,

                                   Wilbur C. Smith, M.D.

Figure 13–7. Letter written by a physician requesting payment of an overdue bill.

COLLECTION AGENCIES

Use of a collection agency should be a last resort, and the physician should review each patient account flagged for collection agency handling before the account is placed. Using a collection agency involves the loss of both the patient's goodwill and practice revenue. Many collection agencies charge up to 50% of the patient's account balance as their fee. However, if all efforts by the office staff have been unsuccessful, the potential receipt of even half the outstanding balance may justify the use of a collection agency.

The collection agency must be chosen carefully. Many agencies are privately owned and operated, and some specialize in medical accounts. Additionally, some medical associations operate collection agencies for their members. The medical assistant should investigate the agency's collection practices and reliability, and should check any agency under consideration with the local Better Business Bureau and with state and national organizations of credit agencies. The medical assistant should evaluate the agency's philosophy and operational methods; most agencies invite potential clients to visit their offices and see the service in operation. The medical assistant should request references,

and if possible, interview other physicians who use that agency. Such inquiries provide information concerning ethics, promptness, and efficiency. Physicians must be careful in choosing a collection agency because that agency will represent them to the public.

Once an account has been turned over to a collection agency, the physician has signed over responsibility for monitoring payment and may not send any further bills to the patient. The collection agency makes reports periodically on activity concerning all accounts. When an account is turned over to the agency, the medical assistant may be asked to provide the agency with pertinent information concerning each account. If the patient contacts the physician's office to discuss the account after it has been turned over to the collection agency, the medical assistant should instruct the patient to contact the agency for further discussion concerning the account. If the practice receives payment on an account that has been turned over to the collection agency, the payment should be recorded and the agency notified immediately.

The physician receives a monthly statement from the collection agency listing the total amount collected, the total amount remitted to the office, and the fees due the agency. The collection agency generally deducts its payments, but the medical assistant must deduct the total amount paid (the agency portion and the physician's portion) from the patient's account.

SPECIAL PROBLEMS

SKIPS

Occasionally, a patient moves and leaves no forwarding address. Patients who use this tactic are commonly referred to as "skips." Tracing skips may either be easy or impossible. Some potential sources of aid in locating a skip include the telephone company, which can provide information about new telephone listings; other physicians who have treated the patient; the patient's bank; or the patient's friends, neighbors, or relatives. It is good practice to photocopy the first check submitted by each new patient so that the banking information will be on file when "skips" occur. In this situation the patient information record may prove invaluable; information such as a driver's license number may help in the tracing process. If a skip cannot be located with a reasonable amount of effort, the account should be tagged for placement with a collection agency.

BANKRUPTCY

Another special problem arises when patients file for bankruptcy. There are two types of bankruptcy: straight bankruptcy, which is covered by Chapter 11 of the Bankruptcy Law; and wage earner's bankruptcy, which is covered under Chapter 13 of that law. If a patient files for straight bankruptcy, he or she comes under direct protection of the court, and all collection procedures must cease. When the physician is notified that a patient has filed a bankruptcy petition, he or she is informed of the court proceeding date and must either attend the proceeding or file a written proof of claim. Because physician's fees are not backed by collateral, the physician generally is one of the last creditors to be paid out of the debtor's assets. The physician very seldom receives any money allocation from the court. If a patient files for wage earner's bankruptcy, he or she agrees to pay a fixed amount to the bankruptcy referee, from whom all creditors then receive distributions. Although the total amount each creditor receives through this plan may not be the total amount due from the debtor, creditors may not garner wages or in any way proceed against the debtor who is under a wage earner's plan.

WRITE-OFFS

Although several resources for collection are available, some physicians choose simply to "write off," or cancel, the amount owed by a patient. Write-offs often happen if the account balance is minimal and the cost of collection efforts exceeds the amount owed.

A write-off may be due to the expiration of time during which a legal collection suit may be filed against a patient. Statutes of limitation set a specific time limit for the collection of overdue accounts. The statutes vary by state and type of account.

An *open-book account* is the type physicians use most often. The time of an open-book account runs from the date of the last entry for a specific illness. For patients with chronic illnesses, it is almost impossible to set time limits. Another type of account is based on a written contract. When a written contract exists, the time runs from the date of the last installment or the single due date. The last type of account is the *single-entry account,* which is usually used for small amounts and one-time treatment, such as in an emergency. The usual statute of limitations for debt collection is three years, but some states may have shorter statutes for single-entry accounts.

CLAIMS AGAINST ESTATES

If a patient has died, the full amount of the bill should be submitted to the patient's estate. This bill should be sent by certified or registered mail so the physician has proof of receipt by the estate. If there is no response within 10 days, or if the estate rejects the bill, the physician may file a claim against the estate with the county clerk in the county of probate of the will. If the court accepts the physician's claim, written notification is sent. The payment may, however, be delayed by the probate process. If the physician chooses to cancel or reduce the fee, a registered letter of condolence with the offer to adjust the fee should be sent to the patient's family. The letter is sent so that the family will not think the physician made the adjustment because of faulty action on his or her part.

PATIENT TEACHING CONSIDERATIONS

As was indicated previously, patients should be informed regarding payment-for-service policies as early as the telephone call for the first appointment. The patient should know, in addition to when payment is expected for service, how to make payment (by check, cash, or credit card) and the consequences of late or nonpayment. Usually, this information is included in the patient brochure or welcome letter mailed to new patients before the first visit.

Fee collection is a sensitive issue and must therefore be handled nonthreateningly, both verbally and in writing, to elicit patient cooperation. Nonetheless, it is essential to orient the patient clearly to payment expectations. Informed patients can prepare to meet these expectations and make responsible decisions regarding medical care.

RELATED ETHICAL AND LEGAL IMPLICATIONS

The medical office should establish a policy regarding past due accounts. This policy should be applied to all patient accounts in a timely and consistent manner. The older a bill becomes, the harder it is to collect.

During the collection process, the medical staff must take care to protect the rights of the patient. Federal and state laws exist to protect the consumer (the patient) from unscrupulous collection practices. For legal reasons, the office staff should never threaten or promise a collection procedure that cannot or will not be carried out. Below are brief descriptions of the statutes governing credit and collections.

1. Truth in Lending Act, or Regulation Z of the Consumer Protection Act. Requires full written disclosure regarding the finance charges for large payment plans involving four or more installments, excluding a down payment. The disclosure must take place at the time credit is extended to the consumer (patient). Whether or not there is a financing charge, this written agreement must contain the items outlined in Fig. 13–8. This regulation does not apply, however, if the consumer agrees to pay in one sum or in less than four payments and then decides independently to make drawn-out partial payments.
2. Fair Credit Reporting Act. Provides guidelines for reporting and collecting credit background information and updates. It allows consumers (patients) to learn the nature and substance of information collected about them by credit reporting agencies, and to correct and update erroneous information.
3. Guide Against Debt Collection Deception (Federal Trade Commission). Provides collection guidelines for creditors, and provides the consumer (patient) with protection from fraudulent and deceptive tactics.

4. Notice on Use of Telephone for Debt Collecting (Federal Communications Commission). Outlines specific times when calls can be made, and prohibits calling at odd hours (after 8 PM, for example), threatening phone calls, and other harassment. States and localities may have additional statutes concerning the use of the telephone for debt collection. The medical assistant should be familiar with any applicable local and state laws or regulations.
5. Equal Credit Opportunity Act. Prohibits discrimination in granting credit. To prevent accusations of credit discrimination, it is important to obtain detailed credit information from the consumer (patient) before performing any services. Once the credit information is obtained, it should be checked with a credit bureau as soon as possible. The credit bureau will verify data such as the patient's residence and moving history, employment, and the consumer's approximate salary, and will give reports on how the consumer pays bills, and any other relevant information, such as history of bankruptcy or name changes. If the data are satisfactory, credit is extended. If the consumer has a poor credit rating, credit may be denied on that basis.
6. Fair Collection Practices Act. Provides guidelines for determining fair and just collection steps for creditors.

All of these laws are important because they provide the legal framework within which the medical assistant must execute the physician's collection policy.

A collection resource available to the physician is litigation. The physician may elect to seek payment through small-claims court, which is part of county government. In some states, small-claims courts deal only with claims limited to $500 or $1000. There are no juries or lawyers, and the costs are usually minor. Precise procedures, forms, times, and other rules must be observed. The necessary information concerning small-claims court in any particular county is available through the small-claims court office.

The physician may choose to have an attorney file suit against a patient, especially for larger account balances. The medical assistant should never threaten a lawsuit unless the physician has given permission for such action. If the lawsuit is decided in favor of the physician, some states allow the patient's wages to be garnered for payment of the debt.

Fee adjustments and cancellations can result in malpractice suits, especially when a patient dies. In other cases, the patient may not pay a fee even after the physician has agreed to reduce it. Unless there is a witnessed, written agreement that specifically states "without prejudice" and includes specific time limits for payment, the physician forfeits the right to collect the original fee if the patient does not pay the reduced fee. The physician should consider malpractice statutes of limitation before filing a collection suit with the courts.

REQUIRED ITEMS FOR REGULATION Z

1. Must be discussed at the time the agreement is first reached between patient and physician.

2. Agreement must be put in writing.

3. Written agreement must contain:

   A. Total amount of the debt

   B. Amount of the down payment

   C. Date each payment is due

   D. Date the final payment is due

   E. Amount of each payment

   F. Finance charges

   G. Interest rate expressed as an annual percentage

4. Patient and physician must both sign the agreement.

5. Patient and physician retain a copy for their records.

Figure 13–8. The Truth in Lending Act requires full disclosure of these items whenever a physician and patient arrange for payment of a fee in four or more installments.

It is advisable to wait until this time has elapsed before suing a patient.

SUMMARY

Because the medical assistant usually administers and implements the physician's collection policies, he or she must thoroughly understand the physician's philosophy regarding payment for service and fee collection. The medical assistant educates the patient as to charges and payment options, requests payment tactfully, records payment received accurately, and participates sensitively in collecting late fees.

More than any other area of medical assisting, these billing and collection procedures can justify the cost of the medical assistant to the physician. As administrator of the billing and collection policies, the medical assistant plays a crucial role in the financial solvency of the physician's practice and serves as the communication link between the physician and the patient.

The collection system outlined in this chapter should provide for an open, honest, and responsible relationship among the office staff, the physician, and the patient. The physician assumes the responsibility of providing high-quality medical treatment for a fee. The patient accepts treatment with the promise to pay the physician for services rendered. Both the patient and the physician can benefit from an association marked by mutual appreciation and courtesy.

DISCUSSION QUESTIONS

1. List two reasons why medical offices should try to collect fees at the time of service.
2. List and discuss four methods of statement preparation used in medical offices.
3. When is the best time to mail monthly statements to patients? Defend your answer.
4. Explain cyclic billing. Why is it used?
5. What resources are available to the physician in collecting debts?
6. List and describe the two types of bankruptcy.

BIBLIOGRAPHY

Anderson HR, Caldwell JR, Needles BE Jr: Principles of Accounting, ed 4. Houghton Mifflin, Boston, 1990.
Foster G, Horngren CT: Cost Accounting, ed 7. Prentice-Hall, Englewood Cliffs, NJ, 1991.
Skousen FK, Smith J: Accounting, ed 11. College Division, South-Western Publishing, Cincinnati, 1992.

PROCEDURE: Use the pegboard system for posting charges and payments

Terminal Performance Objective: Post a series of charges and payments with 100% accuracy within the time specified by the instructor.

EQUIPMENT: Pegboard
Pen
Calculator
Daysheet
Receipts
Ledger cards
Balances

PROCEDURE

1. Assemble supplies and equipment.

2. Prepare the pegboard for daily posting by placing a daysheet on the board. Place the overlapping blank receipts over the pegs. Align the top receipt with the first line of the daysheet.

3. Write the balance from the previous day in the designated space on the daysheet.

4. Insert the ledger cards of the patients to be seen today under the receipts. Insert the first ledger card under the first receipt.

5. Write the patient's name, date, receipt number, and existing balance from the ledger card in the spaces provided on the receipt.

6. Detach the charge slip from the receipt and clip it to the patient record. Return the ledger cards to the designated location.

7. At the end of the patient's visit, the patient hands you the slip. Accept the returned slip and write the fee (refer to fee schedule) for procedures marked by the physician.

8. Match the charge slip number with the receipt of the same number.

9. Replace the ledger card under the receipt. Enter the service code number and fee on the spaces provided on the receipt.

10. If the patient makes a payment, record the amount and enter the new balance in the spaces provided.

11. Give the completed receipt to the patient for his or her own records and insurance processing.

12. Replace the ledger card in the file. Repeat the steps described above for each patient seen by the physician on this date.

13. At the day's end, total all columns on the daysheet. Write in pencil.

14. After the calculations are checked, write the totals in ink.

15. Enter total of accounts receivable in the accounting journal.

PRINCIPLE

1. Organization and planning save time and help prevent error.

2. Proper alignment of receipts with the daysheet prevents error.

3. Carrying over the previous day's balance helps keep accounts accurate.

4. In the pegboard system, one-write entry posts the record to the receipt ledger and daysheet simultaneously.

5. The information from the ledger card is necessary for correct billing.

6. Detaching the charge slip prepares it for the physician's entry of services performed.

7. The fee charged must be compatible with the service performed.

8. Matching the charge slip and receipt numbers prevents error in billing.

9. Recording information simultaneously facilitates the one-write system.

10. Recording payment immediately provides an accurate and updated financial statement.

11. The patient must retain a copy of the receipt for future reference and validation of charges and payment.

12. Replacing the ledger card completes the task and avoids losing or misplacing valuable records.

13. Calculating totals is a necessary step in determining total charges, payments, and balances for that date. Numbers are temporarily written in pencil to check calculations and erase errors.

14. Writing in ink provides a permanent record.

15. Entering the total in the accounting journal completes the daily accounting cycle.

HIGHLIGHTS

Fee-Setting Strategies for Medical Office Practice

Typically, the physician's fee schedule reflects the fees that other physicians in the area and specialty charge for services and that are in accordance with third-party reimbursement. Several factors may have an impact on the present fee-setting strategies, causing change and requiring the attention of the administrative medical assistant. In the medical office, these factors include cost containment programs and the contemporary movement away from charge-based reimbursement toward disease-related reimbursement. In the hospital, these factors include the presence of controls related to the appropriate and effective use of personnel, equipment, and facilities.

According to Thomas W. Reinke, MBA, David H. Glusman, CPA, and William C. Garrow, MBA, CPA, in an article on financial management appearing in the January 1988 issue of *Pennsylvania Medicine*, certain pricing concepts used in industries and other settings may be relevant for medical office practice. These involve targeting income, negotiating payment rates, and determining the profitability of third-party participation. Instead of determining desired income, most practices increase fees when striving to increase income.

TARGET INCOME

In targeting income, the following steps must be followed:

1. *Selecting the price segment.* Physicians may have to determine where they want to position themselves (whom they want to serve, where, and what services will be provided) and then determine the appropriate fee structure.
2. *Selective increasing of the fees for certain services.* The fee increases, to target income, should reflect the variations in third-party reimbursement (insurance providers) rather than occur across the board. Different services should receive different fee increases. For instance, in-patient services are likely to be more fully covered by insurance providers, whereas outpatient services (medical office charges) are less fully covered. Fee increases in either area would depend on the coverage and volume of each service. Dollar increases may not be appropriate for medical office fees.

NEGOTIATED RATE PAYERS

Negotiated rate payers include health maintenance organizations, preferred provider organizations, and other prepaid plans in which the physician is contracted to supply certain services. In order to increase the amount for higher payment or change the service mix (types of services offered) or to become the sole provider, the physician must negotiate with the administrators of the plan.

THIRD-PARTY PARTICIPATION

The physician may, as another alternative to traditional fee-setting, decide not to participate in third-party reimbursement. Although there may be some merit in this approach for certain practices, depending on the specialty and geographic location, government regulations may forbid the physician's adoption of this income increase alternative. For example, Medicare now requires that nonparticipating physicians notify their patients in writing that they do not accept Medicare as full payment, and that they inform the patients of the pricing differences for certain surgical procedures.

PATIENT CONSIDERATIONS

Today's patients are more price conscious, and the impact of a fee increase on the patient's satisfaction with the practice must be considered. Marketing research has demonstrated that a consumer's perception of the fee is more significant than the actual fee. However, patients are often willing to pay a higher fee when actual time spent with the physician is increased and satisfying, waiting time has been minimized, or convenient appointment times are available.

Favorable responses from patients are much more likely when they are informed of fee increases well in advance.

THE ROLE OF THE MEDICAL ASSISTANT

The office staff must be able to respond appropriately to patient comments regarding fee increases and must therefore be properly informed. They should know not only what to say, but how to say it. Medical assistants should also be alert to comments that signal a patient's inability to pay and should be prepared to propose solutions such as payment schedules or other plans. The staff must understand the need for a targeted income plan and the benefits to patients and to themselves. In the future of medical practice, the physician will rely more heavily on the medical assistant's input regarding management decisions. The medical assistant should remain aware of the changes occurring in the cost of medical care and fee-setting strategies.

14

Basic Accounting, Accounts Payable, and Payroll: Bookkeeping III

> Good financial record keeping provides a complete and accurate picture of the business operations of the medical practice.
>
> Sharon Vance

CHAPTER OUTLINE

LEARNING OBJECTIVES

Upon completing this chapter, you will be able to:

1. Explain the purpose of the day sheet and its relationship to the general ledger.
2. Define each element of the accounting equation.
3. List the steps in the accounting cycle.
4. Differentiate the procedures used to determine the accuracy of accounts in the general ledger from those used for the accounts receivable ledger.
5. List the procedures purchasing and paying invoices.
6. Apply the general Fair Labor Standards Act requirements to overtime pay and employee time off from work.
7. List the withholding taxes and employee contributions required by law.

Chapter 14

Basic Accounting, Accounts Payable, and Payroll: Bookkeeping III

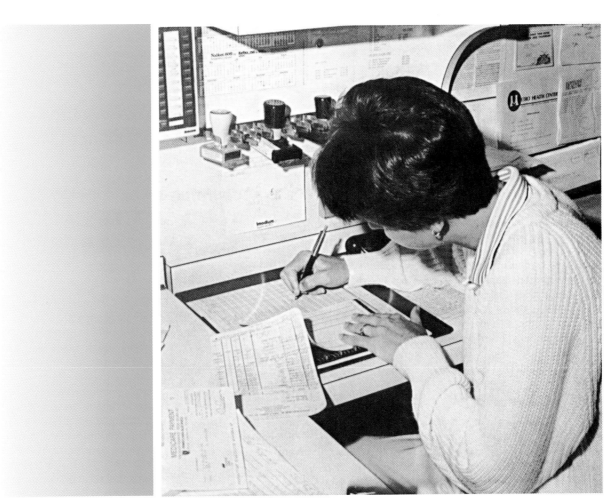

PERFORMANCE OBJECTIVES

Upon completing this chapter, you will be able to:

1. Prepare a trial balance.
2. Organize and maintain a petty cash system.
3. Calculate gross wages and net pay for normal working hours and overtime.

DACUM EDUCATIONAL COMPONENTS

1. Manage accounts payable (and petty cash by tracking purchase orders and paying bills) (8.5A–C).
2. Use a manual bookkeeping system (with both single- and double-entry elements) (8.1A).
3. Process employee payroll (including calculating hours, payroll deductions, and employee contributions) (8.7A–F).

Glossary

Account: Individual record of specific items in the accounting system

Accounting equation: Assets = Liabilities + Owner's equity

Assets: Anything of value used in the operation of a practice

Balance sheet: Financial statement indicating the financial position of the practice at a particular time

Capital equipment: Broad term that may include a variety of items, although it usually refers to operating machines or purchases greater than a set amount (e.g., $300 or $500) other than expendable supplies

Credit: In double-entry bookkeeping, the amount that is recorded on the right side of an account, usually representing increases in monetary resources; in each journal entry the credit side must equal the debit side; the right side of an account

Debit: In double-entry bookkeeping, the amount that is recorded on the left side of an account, usually representing increases in anything acquired for the intended use or benefit of a business; in each journal entry, the dollar amount of the debit must be equal to the dollar amount of the credit; debits are recorded on the left and presented first; the left side of an account

Disbursements: Money paid out by the practice

Equity: The physician's investment in the practice

Ledger: Record of all accounts used in the practice

Liabilities: Amounts owed to creditors

Receipts: Money taken in by the practice

Source document: Written information providing the basis for an entry in the accounting records

Transaction: Financial activity or event in which something of value is exchanged for something of equal value

---

The physician must have complete and accurate records of the medical treatment rendered to patients, and complete and accurate financial records that summarize the business operations of the medical practice. The accounting process is the means by which a business measures

1. What comes in
2. What goes out
3. What properties remain
4. The equities of the owners and creditors in what is left over.

Accounting is the process of recording various business events, called *transactions*, expressed in monetary terms, grouped into related categories and summarized into financial reports. The two most common financial reports are the *balance sheet*, which indicates the physician's financial position at a particular time, and the *income and expense statement* (sometimes called a *profit and loss statement* or *operating statement*), which shows the operating results of the practice during a specific period. Accounting is the means by which the physician measures the profitability and solvency of the practice, weighs alternative courses of action, discovers significant trends in treatment, and estimates which events may have a positive or negative impact on the practice in the future.

OUTSIDE SERVICES

The medical assistant usually is responsible for preparing basic personnel and patient forms for accumulating, recording, and summarizing data. Management, accountants, taxing authorities, and the physician all use these forms. This process is called *bookkeeping* and differs from accounting by recording only the financial data on the forms selected, and in accordance with the procedures established, by the accountants. It is assumed that the physician uses an external accounting service to review the accounting process and to prepare the financial reports and tax summaries. Because physicians' legal and financial responsibilities have increased, they rely extensively on business management and accounting services to handle business affairs. Large health maintenance organizations (HMO) and clinical practices may have their own accounting departments to perform these functions internally.

Most accounting firms offer instruction courses for the physician's office personnel. The medical assistant should use these outside sources for training in the basic accounting skills needed to prepare and coordinate information with the accountant, for answers to questions, or for making procedural changes to update the physician's financial records. The essential steps in developing an office bookkeeping system are listed below.

1. Design forms for the original recording and the final summarizing of data that are in keeping with the size and type of office practice.
2. Develop a written office accounting procedure manual.
3. Establish a policy reinforcing the use of approved accounting procedures.
4. Chose the devices needed, such as a one-write pegboard system, ledger cards, or computers, to mechanize the routine recording and summarizing of functions.
5. Train personnel capable of making the necessary decisions.

THE ACCOUNTING EQUATION

Transactions that occur in a practice fall into three categories: assets, liabilities, and equity. These three categories form the major headings of the balance sheet.

Assets are valuable resources that are owned. For example, office assets could include furniture, instruments, medical equipment and supplies, examination tables, and even pencils and other stationery supplies.

Liabilities are debts owed by the practice. Examples of liabilities are the electricity bill, charges for medical and stationery supplies, taxes, and the mortgage or rent.

Equity is the difference between the assets of the practice and the claims against these assets. Equity is the investment that the physician has in the practice.

The *accounting equation* states that the total of the properties (assets) equals the sum of creditors' claims (liabilities) and the claims of the owner. This concept can be expressed by the following equation:

$$Assets = Liabilities + Owner's\ equity$$

The two sides of this equation must be equal at all times. Practice activities or financial events (transactions) change the amounts in the equation, but the total on the left must always equal the total on the right.

THE ACCOUNTING CYCLE

The major function of an accounting firm is to accumulate the data from business papers (checks, invoices, etc.), summarize the data, and present periodic reports of the physician's operation and financial condition. This process is called the *accounting cycle.* The accounting cycle consists of five steps:

1. Analyze transaction or source documents to determine accounts affected.
2. Record source document information in a journal.
3. Transfer journal information to the general ledger accounts (posting).
4. Prepare a trial balance to prove debit and credit equity of all the general ledger accounts.
5. Prepare an income and expense (profit and loss) statement and a balance sheet (financial condition statement) using the trial balance information.

The accounting cycle can be summarized as:

transactions → journal → general ledger → accounts → financial statements

IDENTIFYING TRANSACTION TYPES

Transaction information is considered a *source document.* A source document is any document that provides the information needed to record the transaction. Source documents include utility bills, patient payments for services, patient charge slips, insurance company payment checks, check stubs, loan payments, or invoices for stationery supplies.

JOURNAL RECORDING

Financial data are recorded twice: once in the original journal entry and again when the amounts are posted to the general ledger accounts. Transactions recorded in the journal are considered the first formal entry in the accounting system. Use of a journal provides:

1. A chronologic record of all transactions
2. A list of all debits and credits in one place
3. Complete information about the transaction

that can be easily recorded in the separate ledger accounts

4. A means of locating and correcting errors

Various types of journals are used in accounting systems according to the needs of the business. The medical assistant might be responsible for several types of journals, including an accounts receivable, an equipment and supplies payment, a payroll, and a cash receipts journal.

Journal entries comprise three lines: the account name to be debited, with the amount written in the debit column; the account name to be credited, indented slightly, with the amount written in the credit column; and an explanation line, which gives details of the transaction (Fig. 14–1). Each transaction is recorded in the journal as it occurs. This process is called *journalizing the transaction*. The debit and credit columns in the journal should be totaled to establish their equality. The debits and credits should be equal. If the totals are not equal, the error must be located and the necessary corrections made.

GENERAL LEDGER

The collective record of individual accounts (summarizing the effects of transactions for each account) makes up the *general ledger*. Whereas the journal contains a daily record of all transactions, the general ledger groups accounts together in categories (by titles). This process groups all the changes in each account category for a certain period, and eventually computes a final balance for each category. Under a double-entry bookkeeping system, in each journal entry, the dollar amount of the debit (left side) must equal the dollar amount of the credit (right side) (see Fig. 14–1). Each transaction has two sides, and the recording entry must reflect both. If an account is to be debited, the journal entry must show the appropriate title and amount to the left; the offsetting credit must be placed to the right. Each entry is actually an equation: debits equal credits.

Because equality applies to the parts, the whole must

also be true. The sum of the debits must equal the sum of the credits after all dollar amounts have been transferred from the journal to the general ledger. The major advantage of the double-entry system is its capacity to disclose arithmetic error through inequality. A single-entry system, which most physicians use, records only one side of a transaction and provides no check on the mathematical accuracy of the final balances. All transactions pertaining to one account can be found in one place. The general ledger thus contains journal information but rearranges it to provide information in the forms required for category and balance summary. In the double-entry system, the journal entries are recorded in the proper accounts and in the appropriate ledger, either daily or at some other specified time. As was mentioned earlier, this process is called *posting*.

CREATING ACCOUNTS

An account is established for each category of asset, liability, and owner's equity. The simplest account form is called a *T-account* because of its shape (Fig. 14–2).

The accounts are grouped into categories and numbered for easy identification. The normal sequence of numbering is: (1) assets, (2) liabilities, (3) owner's equity, (4) revenue, and (5) expenses. A cross-listing of all ledger accounts with their respective account numbers is called a *chart of accounts* (Fig. 14–3).

ACCOUNTS RECEIVABLE

The medical assistant is responsible for recording the accounts receivable transactions. This important general ledger account must be recorded daily and submitted at least monthly. Each time the physician provides medical care to a patient, revenue is created. The physician's cash assets increase, or if payment is delayed, accounts receivable increases. A patient's promise to pay the physician is considered an asset and falls into the accounts receivable category in the general ledger. It is not feasible to record every individual patient charge and payment in the general ledger for the following reasons:

	JOURNAL			Page /
DATE	**ACCOUNT TITLE AND EXPLANATION**	**POST. REF.**	**DEBIT**	**CREDIT**
Oct. 19	Utilities		300.00	
	Cash			300.00
	Sand Hill Gas Co. (Bill paid)			

Figure 14–1. Journal headings and an example of a journal entry.

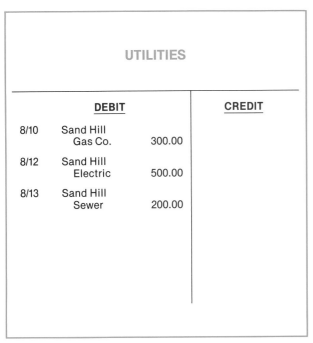

UTILITIES			
	DEBIT		**CREDIT**
8/10	Sand Hill Gas Co.	300.00	
8/12	Sand Hill Electric	500.00	
8/13	Sand Hill Sewer	200.00	

Figure 14–2. Example of a T account.

1. Errors would be difficult to find.
2. Balances owed by individual patients would be difficult to determine.
3. Preparing monthly bills to patients would be burdensome.
4. Itemized statements for insurance purposes could not be prepared easily.

Recording and reporting accounts receivable, therefore, are greatly simplified when only one account in the general ledger summarizes all patient accounts (see Chapter 13). This method requires a subsidiary, or secondary, ledger (day sheet) in which a separate account is kept for each patient. The day sheet provides a means of keeping financial records on patients in one place. At any time, if the balances of all the accounts in the patient ledger are added together, they must equal the balance shown in the control account in the general ledger (see Chapter 12, Fig. 12–4).

TRIAL BALANCE

After each account in the general ledger has been verified, the general ledger information is summarized in a *trial balance,* which confirms the accuracy of the entries and posting. A trial balance lists each account and balance contained in the general ledger. The debits must equal the credits. If the two are equal, the account balance is verified.

If the total of the debit column in the trial balance does not equal the total of the credit column, the cause must be located and corrected. The first step is to determine the amount of the discrepancy, which may give a clue to the problem. Some common errors are listed below.

1. *An account balance was omitted.* If the amount of the discrepancy is $200, for example, the accounts in the ledger should be examined to see if there is an account with a $200 balance.
2. *An amount was recorded on the wrong side of the trial balance or the wrong side of an account.* If the discrepancy is easily divisible by 2, an amount that was to be a debit may have been entered as a credit, or vice versa. The account balances should be checked for such an error. Also, the transactions posted from the journal to the ledger should be checked.
3. *Digits were transposed.* A transposition is a reversal of digits of a number, for example, $450 instead of $540. If an error of this type

CHARTS OF ACCOUNTS	
Asset accounts	101 through 199
Liability accounts	201 through 299
Owners equity accounts	301 through 399
Income accounts	401 through 499
Expense accounts	501 through 599

JOHN EDMISTON, M.D. CHART OF ACCOUNTS

Assets	
101	Cash
102	Acct Rec – Susan Shapper
103	Acct Rec – Office space rental
104	Medical equipment
105	Office equipment

Liabilities	
201	Acct Payable – Cope Bank
202	Acct Payable – Bess Office Supply Co.

Owners Equity	
301	John Edmiston, capital

Income	
401	Textbook royalties

Expenses	
501	Rent expense
502	Salary expense
503	Utility expense

Figure 14–3. Chart of accounts.

involves only two digits, the amount of the error, in this case $90, is divisible by 9.

4. *A slide has occurred.* A slide occurs when a number is written with the decimal point in the wrong place, for example, $1450 instead of $145. The amount of this error is also divisible by 9 ($1450 - 145 = 1305 \div 9 = 145$).

If more than one error has occurred, the amount of the difference between the trial balance column totals does not indicate where the error lies. In that case, the numbers should be checked in reverse order: first the trial balance totals, then the account balances, and finally the journal entries.

Erasers and correction fluid have no place in correcting accounting records. Instead, a line should be drawn through the incorrect item and the correct information entered above or to the side. The accounts contained in the trial balance can easily be identified as balance sheet and income statement accounts. Once the trial balance is completed, it is possible to compile the income statement and balance sheet. It is assumed that the final year-end financial statements will be prepared by the physician's accountant or another outside firm because special items must be considered at year's end. The procedure for determining the trial balance is included at the end of this chapter.

INCOME STATEMENT

The income statement is prepared first because the net income or net loss is used in compiling the balance sheet. The income statement (Fig. 14–4) is also called a *profit and loss statement* and produces a net income or net loss. The income statement is prepared periodically,

usually monthly. The form consists of a header, an income section, an expense section, and a net income or net loss section.

When a patient pays for services rendered, or an insurance company sends a reimbursement check, the amount is considered an asset and is recorded on the income statement. The statement lists expenses owed for the indicated period. The expenses are subtracted from the income. The amount remaining indicates the financial profit gained or the loss incurred during the specified period; in other words, it indicates the financial status of the practice.

BALANCE SHEET

The main reason for recording the financial information of any business is to facilitate periodic reporting. The financial report that shows the amount and nature of the assets, liabilities, and owner's equity at a specific time is called the *balance sheet.* The balance sheet shows the current financial condition of the physician's practice. It does not, however, give information concerning the way that the operation of the practice has affected the owner's equity. Therefore, another financial statement, called the *income statement,* is usually prepared. This statement reports the total income received by the practice and the total expenses that make that income necessary.

The balance sheet has three components: the heading, which contains the date of the analysis; the liability side (the right); and the asset side (the left). Figure 14–5 illustrates a balance sheet showing how income from professional fees increases owner's equity, whereas expenses of the practice decrease it.

JOHN EDMISTON, M.D.
Income Statement
For the month ending May 30, 19_____

Income

Blue Cross reimbursement	2,000.00	
Patient Accounts Payment received	3,000.00	
Sale of ENT instruments	1,000.00	
Total Income		6,000.00

Expenses

Utility expenses	500.00	
Salary expenses	3,000.00	
Mortgage expenses	1,000.00	
Total Expenses		4,500.00
		——————
Net income		1,500.00

Figure 14–4. Example of an income statement.

JOHN EDMISTON, M.D.
Balance Sheet
May 20, 19____

ASSETS		LIABILITIES	
Cash	3,000.00	Accounts Payable	
		Sand Hill Gas Co.	1,000.00
Medical			
Supplies	7,000.00	Betty Corporation	7,000.00
Medical		Owners Equity	
Equipment	3,000.00	John Edmiston, capital	5,000.00
Total	13,000.00	Total	13,000.00

Figure 14–5. Example of a balance sheet.

PURCHASING

Included in the management of the physician's financial transactions is the control of cash payments, or *disbursements*. The physician needs verification of payments for goods and services received. The medical assistant must maintain complete and accurate financial records. General ledger accounts created for the expenses of a business may include accounts payable, supplies on hand, prepaid rent, car, accumulated depreciation on capital equipment, and payroll. The medical assistant is usually responsible for "keeping the books" on this information and for providing, at least monthly, a summary of this information to the accountants.

ORDERING SUPPLIES

In larger medical offices, purchase of needed items may require a purchase requisition. This formal request is given to the appropriate person for processing. Every office should have one authorized person who is responsible for purchasing. Often, this purchasing responsibility is delegated to the medical assistant. The medical assistant may be allowed to decide on purchases or may require the physician's approval for purchases exceeding a specific dollar amount. Quality, price, and service are important factors to be considered in choosing a supplier. The medical assistant should make a notation of each order to facilitate follow-up.

RECEIVING SUPPLIES

When an order arrives, the goods actually received should be checked against the packing slip and the original order to make sure that all items are included. If the goods received do not match the items listed on the packing slip, the medical assistant should contact the supplier so the order or the account can be corrected.

PAYING INVOICES

The supplier sends an invoice, or bill, requesting payment for the goods or services purchased by the physician (Fig. 14–6). When the invoice is received, it should be compared with both the original order and the packing slip to verify that it is correct. If the invoice is correct, it may be processed for payment.

To pay an invoice, the medical assistant prepares a check for the exact amount and gives it to the physician to sign along with the original order, packing slip, and invoice. The date of payment, check number, and check amount are written on the invoice so it will not be paid twice. After being signed, the check and supplier copy of the invoice are mailed to the supplier. The physician's copy of the invoice, along with the order note and packing slip, is filed with other paid invoices according to the filing system.

RECORDING PAYMENTS

Disbursements can be entered into the accounting records in several ways, depending on the accounting system used. If a combination journal or general journal is used, the check stubs from the practice checkbook become the source documents for recording the transaction. If the pegboard system is used, the disbursement record serves as the journal. (Refer to Chapters 12 and 13 for discussion of pegboard systems.) The purchasing procedure is summarized below.

1. One authorized person should be in charge of purchasing to ensure that only supplies and services actually needed are ordered.

JIM'S TRANSCRIPTION SERVICE
10 BRENNEN STREET
ANYTOWN, MISSOURI 12345

Invoice No. 6789

To: John Edmiston, M.D.
121 Beach Ave.
Oyster Cove, MO 54321

ORDER NO.	DATE	SHIPPED VIA	NO. PKGS.

NO. PAGES	DESCRIPTION	UNIT PRICE	AMOUNT
		TOTAL DUE	

Figure 14-6. Example of a supplier invoice.

2. High-quality goods and services should be ordered at the best possible prices, with shelf life considered when necessary.
3. Orders placed should be recorded to monitor prompt service or receipt of goods.
4. Shipments received should be checked against packing slips to verify that all goods have been received.
5. Invoices should be verified for mathematical accuracy and checked against the original order and packing slip to ensure that only goods and services actually received are paid for.
6. Invoices should be paid in a timely manner. Payment should be noted immediately on invoices to prevent double payment. Paid invoices should be kept on file.

PETTY CASH

It is not practical to use checks for small transactions. The office should maintain a petty cash fund for such payments. The physician determines the types of payments and the dollar amounts that can be paid from petty cash. The money is kept in a locked box or drawer.

A payment from the petty cash fund requires a written receipt. Special forms, called petty cash vouchers

(Fig. 14-7), are kept with the cash. When petty cash is used for payment, the information on the petty cash voucher is completed and signed by both the person issuing and the person receiving the money. The voucher information should include date, amount, reason for expenditure, signature of the person issuing the money, and signature of the person receiving the cash.

PETTY CASH

No._____

Date _____ 19 ___ $_____
For _____
_____
Charge to account _____

_____   _____
Received By   Approved By

Figure 14-7. Petty cash voucher.

The completed voucher is placed in the petty cash box as expenditure verification.

When the fund requires replenishing, the vouchers are totaled. This total added to the remaining cash should equal the total of the original fund. The vouchers are classified according to type, such as delivery expense, postage expense, or expense for office supplies. These vouchers are the source documents for entry of expenses into the accounting records. A check to replenish the cash is written for the exact amount of the totaled vouchers. If the pegboard system is used, the amounts for each type of expense are entered on the disbursement record as the check is written. If the pegboard system is not used, the vouchers verify the journal entry. Each type of expense requires a debit, and the amount of the totaled vouchers is credited to cash. The vouchers are then canceled by writing the date and fund-replenishing number on each. The check is cashed, and the money is added to the petty cash fund. A petty cash book, or petty cash disbursements record, also may be used to keep a running total of the petty cash spent (Fig. 14–8). The procedure for preparing and recording the petty cash voucher is included at the end of this chapter.

PAYROLL

Federal, state, and local laws require records of all salaries and wages paid to employees. The payroll tasks include calculating the amount of wages or salaries paid and amounts deducted from employees' earnings. Other payroll tasks involve writing checks with numerous deductions, tracking data for payroll taxes, and filling out payroll tax forms. The physician is required by law to keep payroll data for 4 years.

Employee earnings are either salaries or wages, plus other indirect forms of payment, such as paid time off and employee benefit and service programs. A salary is a fixed amount paid to an employee on a regular basis regardless of the number of hours worked. Wages are based on a specific rate per hour, day, or week. In incorporated practices the physician is considered an employee of the corporation and receives a paycheck. The payroll is the total direct and indirect earnings of all employees for a pay period. A separate record, called the *employee's earnings record,* is kept for each employee (Fig. 14–9). A list of all employees and their earnings, deductions, and other information is called

PETTY CASH REGISTER
From June 1 to June 30, 19____

DATE	VOUCHER NO.	PAID TO	FOR	AMT.	BALANCE
		Bal. Brought Frwd.			2.25
		Replenish Fund		25.00	27.25
6/2	32	Post Office	Mail Package	1.25	26.00
6/3	33	Nicole's Hardware	Door Keys	3.00	23.00
6/6	34	Jim's Office Supply	Tape & Pens	7.00	16.00
				End of Month Balance	

Figure 14–8. Example of a petty cash register using a running total.

NAME					SOC. SEC. NO.			DEPENDENTS		YEAR

ADDRESS	BIRTH DATE	DEDUCTIONS
JOB TITLE	PAY RATE
EMPLOYED / TERMINATED	
SPOUSE	REASON	RECORD OF CHANGES
PHONE		

DATE	RATE

EMPLOYEE	CHECK NUMBER	PERIOD ENDING	REGULAR	EARNINGS	TOTAL	FICA	FED. TAX	DEDUCTIONS			NET PAY	CUMULATIVE FICA

1ST QTR — QUARTER TOTAL / TOTAL-TO-DATE

2ND QTR — QUARTER TOTAL / TOTAL-TO-DATE

3RD QTR — QUARTER TOTAL / TOTAL-TO-DATE

4TH QTR — QUARTER TOTAL / TOTAL-TO-DATE

Control-o-fax® OFFICE SYSTEMS WATERLOO, IOWA
FORM NO. 50-390 E

Figure 14-9. Employee earning record. (Courtesy of Control-o-fax.)

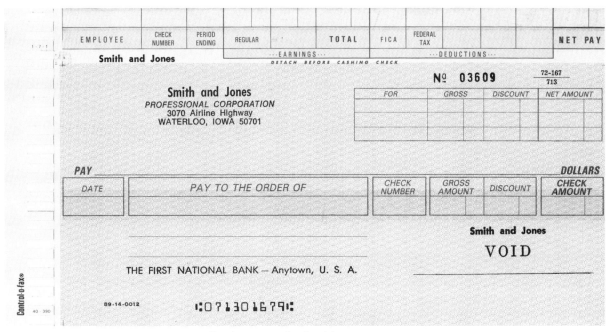

Figure 14-10. Employee paycheck with attached payroll information.

the *payroll register.* The payroll register is used as the source document for recording the payroll.

Each employee must receive a pay statement for each pay period. This information is frequently printed on the stub of the employee's paycheck (Fig. 14-10). The check provides monetary compensation for services rendered, and the stub shows how that compensation was calculated. The data on the stub reflect exactly what has been recorded in the payroll register and the employee's earnings record. The procedure for payroll transactions is given at the end of this chapter.

Fair Labor Standards Act

The Fair Labor Standards Act regulates the number of hours employees may work, establishes a minimum wage, and outlines requirements concerning overtime pay. The act requires the employer to record the number of hours worked by each employee. A time book or time card is the most widely used recording format (Fig. 14-11). Overtime premiums are generally paid to nonexempt employees for any work they do on the six and seventh days in a scheduled work week. Employees exempt from the Fair Labor Standards regulations are eligible for overtime pay only under special situations. They are usually not compensated for overtime.

Nonexempt employees are paid one and one-half times their normal hourly rate (time and a half) for all hours worked beyond the normal eight during their scheduled work day. For the sixth consecutive day of the work week, employees are paid one and one-half times the normal rate for each hour worked. On the seventh consecutive work day, they are paid twice the normal rate (double time) for each hour worked. On a company-approved holiday, employees are paid double

time plus normal holiday pay for each hour worked. Part-time, nonexempt employees are usually paid overtime premiums if they exceed 8 hours in a day or 40 hours in a week.

Any unpaid time off from work can affect the calculation of the total number of work hours in a week and can easily affect overtime eligibility. For example, an employee receiving 4 hours off without pay on a Thursday morning to visit the dentist may make up the time on the same day by working an extra 4 hours in the afternoon. However, an employee asked to make up the hours on a Saturday should receive 4 hours of overtime

TIME CARD				
DATE	IN	OUT	REG. HRS.	O.T. HOURS
			Total	Total

Figure 14-11. Employee time card.

pay if that Saturday is the sixth or seventh consecutive work day.

Make-up time for missed work should be approved in advance. Under the government regulations, an employee is under no obligation to make up time. The legal limits on how many hours an employee can work in a day, or how many days in a week, must be considered because unpaid time off from work can result in overtime eligibility.

WITHHOLDING TAXES

All employers are required by law to withhold (deduct) federal, state, and local (if applicable) income taxes from an employee's gross earnings. The employee's gross pay (total amount earned) is more than the net, or take-home pay, actually received. Deductions also include FICA (Federal Insurance Contributions Act, or Social Security) and voluntary deductions, such as health care, dental care, life insurance, and retirement plans. An employee's net, or take-home, pay is calculated by subtracting all taxes withheld and all voluntary deductions. In addition to employee deductions, employers make certain contributions for each employee: FICA, FUTA (Federal Unemployment Contribution Tax), Medicare, and SUI (State Unemployment Insurance).

The employer's tax and business liabilities increase (accrue) at each payroll period. These liabilities represent employer payroll taxes and contributions set aside for quarterly tax deposits and benefit premium payments. The balance sheet should disclose fully the company's liability for payroll-related items owed but not yet paid. Therefore, liability accounts owed for payroll-related liabilities should be created.

Each time payroll checks are prepared, the medical assistant should record the liability increases to each account. At least four accounts should be set up: deductions withheld from employee earnings, employer payroll taxes, employee retirement pension plans, and employees medical insurance. These liability accounts track both employee withholdings and employer contributions because the employer owes and must eventually pay all these amounts.

At each payroll period, the medical assistant must record each deduction, the amount withheld from paychecks, and each payroll expense in the business checking account, and must transfer each transaction as a debit to the appropriate liability account and a credit to cash. Later, taxes withheld on behalf of employees, accrued employer payroll taxes, expenses for medical insurance, and pension plan contributions will be paid and the liability accounts decreased (credited) by the amount paid.

FEDERAL INCOME TAX

The amount of federal income tax withheld is determined by wage-bracket tables provided in the Internal Revenue Service (IRS) *Circular E Employer's Tax Guide* and by state and local income tax units. The tables are revised yearly and can be obtained through contacting these offices. The guides contain separate withholding tables for single and married employees. The tables base the amount of tax to be withheld on the total taxable wages and the number of exemptions that the employee has listed on the Federal Withholding Allowance, or W-4 form.

SOCIAL SECURITY TAX

The second required federal deduction is social security, or FICA, tax. The social security benefits program was established by the Federal Insurance Contribution Act of 1935. The physician and the employee pay FICA tax in matching amounts. Both the tax rates and the ceiling for gross earnings subject to tax are given in the IRS *Circular E Employee's Tax Guide*. FICA deductions support the old-age, survivors, disability insurance (OASDI), and Medicare programs. Before 1991, the FICA matching amount was reported as a single percentage (e.g., 7.65%). Law now requires the Medicare tax portion to be reported separately. For wages paid in 1992, the OASDI rate is 6.2% and the Medicare portion is 1.45%.

UNEMPLOYMENT COMPENSATION TAX

The employer is required to pay federal and state unemployment compensation taxes. In some areas, these taxes may be imposed on the employer only and therefore do not affect the employee's pay. In other areas, these taxes are shared by both the employer and the employee. The taxes are imposed as a percentage of the total gross earnings.

THE W-2 FORM

The employer is required to prepare and distribute a wage and tax statement (Form W-2) to each employee no later than January 31 of each year. This statement lists summary earnings data for the preceding calendar year, gross wages, and all FICA, state and local income taxes, and all voluntary deductions withheld. The information for the W-2 form is obtained from each employee's earning record.

TAX REMITTANCE

The taxes withheld from the employee's earnings and the employer's tax contributions must be remitted to the appropriate taxing authorities. The payroll register contains the information required to complete tax remittance forms and prepare the journal entries to record these transactions.

Information from the payroll register (Fig. 14–12) is used to generate a payroll journal (Fig. 14–13). All deductions are recorded as liabilities, or amounts owed by the employer to various agencies. With the payroll

For the week ending 1-29-93

Employee Name	Earnings Through	Hourly Rate	Regular Hours	Regular Earnings	OT Hours	OT Earnings	Total Gross	Subject to Unemp.	Subject to FICA	Subject to Med	FICA Taxes	Medicare Taxes	Federal Inc Taxes	Health Insur	Total	Net Pay	Check No.
Smith	0.00			6000.00			6000.00	6000.00	6000.00	6000.00	372.00	87.00	733.25	48.00	1240.25	4759.75	421
Jones	0.00			6000.00			6000.00	6000.00	6000.00	6000.00	372.00	87.00	1786.59	45.00	2290.59	3709.41	422
Durr	800.00	7.50	40.00	300.00			300.00	300.00	300.00	300.00	18.60	4.35	38.00	6.00	66.95	233.05	423
Blake	1200.00	5.00	40.00	200.00			200.00	200.00	200.00	200.00	12.40	2.90	23.00	4.00	42.30	157.70	424
Totals				12500.00			12500.00	12500.00	12500.00	12500.00	775.00	181.25	2580.84	103.00	3640.09	8859.91	

Figure 14-12. A payroll register.

register as an information source, the employer's FICA tax liability should be entered in the journal. To determine this amount, it is necessary to multiply the total of the "Subject to FICA" and "Subject to Medicare" columns by the current rate. In our example, this would be $12,500.00 times 0.765, or $956.25. The journal entry would be as follows:

Payroll tax expenses $956.25

Employer's FICA tax payable $775.00

Medicare tax payable $181.25

The debit is to an account called "Employer Tax Expense" because the employer's portion of FICA is a tax imposed on the total payroll.

As was stated earlier, federal income taxes, employee FICA taxes, employer FICA taxes and state and local unemployment taxes (if applicable) usually are remitted monthly. The tax payment due date, however, is determined by the total amount of the taxes owed. Complete tax information can be found in the IRS *Circular E Employer's Tax Guide.* The proper amount is deposited monthly in a qualified federal depositary institution. This institution usually is a nearby bank. A Federal Tax Deposit form is completed and given to the bank with the payment. Figure 14-14 shows a sample form.

Whatever accounting method is used, source documents must first be recorded in some permanent, standardized financial description, complete with reference guides (audit trails) that provide a means of reconstructing the transaction later. Second, the data must be classified into groups of similar transactions to save processing time and to summarize like kinds of transactions. Frequently, this classification process requires indexing or coding methods similar to those discussed in connection with file management. When the classified data have been sorted by common characteristics, the computation procedures, or processing, may then be performed. The final step, or summary, results in a printed report that organizes and condenses the data to clarify any decisions that must be made.

AUDITING AND TAXES

The physician usually arranges for an accountant or financial service to review the financial records of the practice at least yearly. *Auditing* is the reviewing of financial data to verify accuracy and completeness. The medical assistant responsible for bookkeeping must provide the required financial records and answer questions about the accounting system used.

COMPUTERIZED ACCOUNTING

Accounting and bookkeeping computer programs can be cost effective by relieving the medical assistant of repetitive, time-consuming tasks. The program uses built-in tax tables to calculate gross pay and all taxes and other deductions. It then writes the paycheck and voucher stub, records the transaction in the checking account, and keeps track of tax liabilities. Even if all accounting functions in the office are computer generated, however, the medical assistant must have a basic knowledge of accounting principles.

Various commercial businesses also provide bookkeeping, accounting, and payroll services. A complete accounting package or a single component can be purchased.

RELATED ETHICAL AND LEGAL IMPLICATIONS

Federal, state, and local tax laws regulate not only tax payments, but the reporting of wages and incomes. These laws must be followed carefully. Individual state requirements vary. It is important to understand clearly the data and forms required and the timetable for payment remittances. Penalties for late deposits and filings can be severe.

Any time the employer's signature is required on a legal document, that document can be signed only by the employer. It may *not* be signed by anyone in the employer's place.

The employer is required to keep up-to-date records of employee earnings and deductions, and of earnings,

PAYROLL JOURNAL ENTRY

Salaries Expense	$12,500.00
Federal Income Taxes Payable	2,580.84
Employees FICA Taxes Payable	775.00
Employees Medicare Taxes Payable	181.25
Health Insurance Payable	103.00
Cash	8.859.91

Figure 14-13. A payroll journal entry.

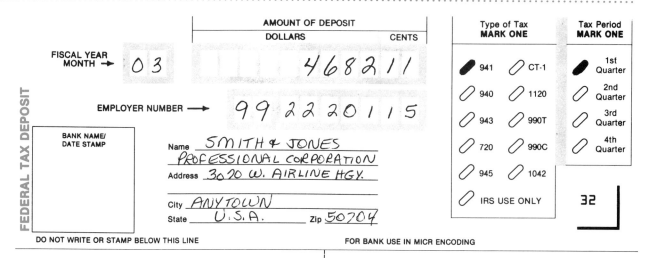

Figure 14–14. A federal tax deposit form.

income, salaries, and disbursements. Every 3 months, the employer must submit employee withholding payments plus an equal amount as the employee's contribution to FICA and Medicare. Additionally, the employer must complete and submit a quarterly federal tax return.

As was stated previously, federal law requires the employer to provide each employee with a Wage and Tax Statement (form W-2) no later than January 31. The employer can be fined or prosecuted for noncompliance.

SUMMARY

The accounting system is perhaps the single most abused aspect of the typical physician's office practice. Most physicians are inexperienced and essentially uninterested in designing or maintaining good accounting procedures. This area, then, is another in which the medical assistant may become an invaluable asset to the medical office. As a knowledgeable resource person, the medical assistant can relieve the physician of the mechanical burdens of recordkeeping and accounting and can maintain the accuracy and efficiency of those functions.

DISCUSSION QUESTIONS

1. Discuss each element of the accounting equation. What effect does revenue have on the equation? Payment of expenses?
2. List the steps in the accounting cycle and briefly describe each. Trace the payment of the telephone bill through the accounting cycle.
3. Explain an accounts receivable subsidiary ledger (day sheet). How does receipt of payment on account from the patient affect the subsidiary and general ledgers?
4. What procedure determines the accuracy of the accounts receivable balance in the subsidiary ledger? If the total of the schedule of accounts receivable does not match the balance of the accounts receivable in the general ledger, what steps would you take in looking for the error?

BIBLIOGRAPHY

Anderson HR, Caldwell JR, Needles BE Jr: Principles of Accounting, ed 4. Houghton Mifflin, Boston, 1990.
Foster G, Horngren CT: Cost Accounting, ed 7. Prentice-Hall, Englewood Cliffs, NJ, 1991.
Skousen FK, Smith J: Accounting, ed 11. College Division, South-Western Publishing, Cincinnati, 1992.

PROCEDURE: Prepare a trial balance

Terminal Performance Objective: Confirm the accuracy of the general ledger entries and postings, and verify the status of the general ledger account by determining the trial balance with 100% accuracy within the time specified by the instructor.

EQUIPMENT:　General ledger
Calculator
Pen

PROCEDURE

1. Assemble supplies and equipment.

2. Check to be certain each account in the general ledger is verified.

3. List each account title in the general ledger, along with the balance for that title.

4. If a discrepancy exists, determine the amount and cause of the error.

5. Correct the error by drawing a line through the incorrect item and entering the correct information above or to the side.

6. Date the verification of the trial balance and prepare the income statement or balance sheet from the trial balance accordingly.

PRINCIPLE

1. Organization and planning save time and help prevent error.

2. The accuracy of the trial balance depends on initial verification of accounts.

3. Listing titles and balances verifies the account balance. The total of the items in the debit columns should equal the credits.

4. The purpose of the trial balance is to verify the balance or to identify and correct errors. (See the chapter text for common errors.)

5. Neat corrections ensure clarity, legibility, and legal protection.

6. Using an updated trial balance keeps accounting records current.

PROCEDURE: Prepare and maintain a petty cash account

Terminal Performance Objective: Prepare and record petty cash vouchers with 100% accuracy within the time specified by the instructor.

EQUIPMENT: Petty cash record forms
Petty cash vouchers
Disbursement record
Checks
Expenditure list

PROCEDURE

1. Assemble the necessary equipment and supplies. The instructor will specify the amount of money in the petty cash fund.
2. Write a check to "Petty Cash" or "Cash" for the amount specified.
3. Record the beginning balance in the "Miscellaneous" column of the disbursement record.
4. For each entry on the expenditure list (which represents money withdrawn from the petty cash fund for which a receipt is not available), prepare a petty cash voucher.
5. Record each voucher on the petty cash record form. Calculate the new balance and enter it in the designated space on the form.
6. After making vouchers for all the entries on the expenditure list, subtract the last balance from the original petty cash amount (beginning balance) to find out the amount required to restore the fund to the beginning balance.
7. Total the petty cash entries according to the accounts to which they apply, and enter those totals in the appropriate columns in the disbursement record.
8. Record the dollar amount (the amount of the check) added to the fund.
9. Record the new balance in the petty cash record.

PRINCIPLE

1. Organization and planning save time and help prevent error. In an actual medical office, the physician determines the size of the petty cash fund.
2. Writing the check establishes the petty cash fund.
3. Recording the beginning balance also records the original petty cash amount.
4. The vouchers serve as receipts.

5. Keeping a running balance tells you when to replenish the fund.
6. The sum of the vouchers and the current balance should always equal the beginning balance. In the actual medical office, the medical assistant would replenish the petty cash fund regularly or when necessary.
7. Categorizing, totaling, and recording disbursements help to avoid error.
8. Accurate and immediate recording reduces the chance for error.
9. Recording the new balance keeps the record current.

PROCEDURE: Complete payroll transactions

Terminal Performance Objective: Using the textbook and workbook application exercises, calculate payroll deductions, issue payroll checks, enter each transaction into the proper account, and balance the distribution columns with the checks written.

EQUIPMENT: Employee earning records
Employee time cards
Payroll register
Disbursement record or payroll journal
Payroll checks with payroll information
Calculator

1. Set up payroll expense categories:

Category	Type	Description	Tax-Related
Payroll	Expns	Payroll transaction	Y
Comp FICA	Sub	Employer contribution	Y
Comp FUTA	Sub	Employer contribution	Y
Comp MCARE	Sub	Employer contribution	Y
Comp SUI	Sub	Employer contribution	Y
Comp HEALTH	Sub	Employer contribution	Y
Comp LIFE	Sub	Employer contribution	Y
Gross	Sub	Compensation to employee	Y

Comp—compensation; Expns—expenses; FICA—Federal Insurance Contribution Act; FUTA—Federal Unemployment Contribution Tax; MCARE—Medicare; Sub—category; SUI—State Unemployment Insurance.

2. Set up liability accounts:

Account	Description
Payroll—FICA	FICA contributions
Payroll—FUTA	Federal unemployment tax
Payroll—FIT	Federal income tax
Payroll—MCARE	Medicare contribution
Payroll—SUI	State Unemployment Insurance
Payroll—SIT	State income tax
Payroll—HEALTH	Health insurance
Payroll—LIFE	Life and disability insurance

3. Calculate total hours worked from the employee's time card.
4. Calculate time and a half and double time from the employee's time card.
5. Enter the total hours on the payroll register under the appropriate columns.
6. Using the employee's pay rate on the earnings record, multiply the hours by the rates for regular time and overtime.
7. Enter the total gross taxable earnings in the appropriate column. Subtract any pretax benefits (benefits not taxable as income), such as health care programs.
8. Using the *Circular E Employer's Guide* and the employee's earnings record, calculate the federal income tax withholding on taxable income by marital status and number of exemptions.
9. Using the *Circular E Employer's Guide* and the employee's earnings record, calculate the FICA (6.2%) and Medicare employee tax withholding (1.45%).
10. Using state tax guides, calculate the state and local (if applicable) income tax withholding by marital status and number of exemptions.
11. Using federal and state guidelines, calculate the employer's FUTA and SUI contributions, if applicable, and post to employer account.
12. Enter any employee deductions, such as life insurance and disability.
13. Calculate the net pay.
14. For FICA and Medicare taxes, enter the amount withheld from the employees in the employer FICA contribution and Medicare columns.
15. Enter any other items, such as FUTA and SUI contributions, and any other employer contributions.
16. Complete the check stub with the employee's name, date, and pay period. Enter the gross taxable pay as a positive amount, withholdings and deductions as negative amounts, and the net pay on the stub.
17. Write the payroll check for the net pay amount.
18. Transfer each deduction to the appropriate liability account, where the transfer will increase the tax or benefit liability.

HIGHLIGHTS
The Use of Plastic Money in Medical Office Practice

As physicians become more concerned about the business aspects of their offices and move toward developing more convenient ways of allowing patients to pay their fees, the use of major credit cards in payment for health care services in the medical office is increasing. It is therefore important that the medical assistant understand the basics of the credit card, or "plastic money," system of payment.

From the vantage point of the physician, there are two advantages to using credit cards: marketing and financial. From the marketing perspective, a charge card makes it easier for the patient for pay for services. With the charge card alternative, patients who might otherwise be reluctant to schedule an important appointment, or who would find it difficult or inconvenient to arrange payment, can simply charge the services. Research has indicated that charge cards increase sales and payment for all kinds of businesses and services.

The financial motivation is that the charge card shifts the responsibility for accounts receivable and for debts away from the physician and to a third party (usually a bank). Once a medical service is charged on a major credit card, the physician is assured of receiving payment immediately. Any difficulties in collection or involving the credit of the person who has made the charge become the responsibility of the credit card agency.

Naturally, this convenience is not without cost. Physicians who use credit cards are charged a percentage of the fee for the service provided to the patient, and they pay that percentage to the third party agent who handles the charge transaction. For example, if the patient places a $100 payment on the credit card, the third party (credit card agency) may credit the physician's account with $97. The physician is charged $3 for the transaction. The amount charged the physician is often negotiable and depends to a large extent on the current economy and the market

leverage of the particular physician requesting the service. A very large office with a substantial cash flow, for example, might secure a slightly lower rate than a smaller practice with less volume. Generally, the percentage charged the physician's office ranges from 1% to 5%.

One operational inconvenience is that each credit card company has a limit beyond which a charge requires authorization. Many medical services exceed this limit. If a fee is higher than a charge card limit, the medical assistant must call a special telephone number to request an authorization number. Unless this number is affixed to the transaction receipt, the bank will not ensure the transaction.

Questions regarding the credit card payment system can be answered by the representative of the third party (bank), that is, the account owner. Information about charge services is also available from almost any lending institution. In most cases, the place to begin discussion of credit card use for the payment of medical office services is the bank or other institution that handles most of the other office accounts.

In the charge card–oriented economy, the inclusion of charge services is another way of offering convenience to the patient. Although some communities perceive the use of credit cards for the payment of health care services to be unprofessional and inappropriate, such use appears to be increasing. Concern has been expressed regarding inflated charges for medical services to help offset the cost to the physician. However, in today's competitive climate of medical office practice, some physicians choose to accept major credit cards and to pay the handling fees without inflating the cost of health care services. They believe that the small percentage charged by the bank is well worth the increase in revenue and the reduction of problems often associated with the collection of accounts receivable.

Chapter 15

Insurance Processing

CHAPTER OUTLINE

Chapter 15

*I*nsurance Processing

Blue Shield ®

06/01/
EFFECTIVE DATE

JOHN F. DOUGH   B

111 22 3333
SUBSCRIBER'S I D NO

7654321   N123
GROUP NO

Enter the letter and number in
the arrow PLUS the subcriber's
identification or membership number in the usual place on the claim
form. (Note: The number inside
the arrow and the ID card will vary
by Blue Shield Plan.)

N123

READ INSTRUCTIONS BEFORE COMPLETING OR SIGNING THIS FORM

TYPE OR PRINT   ☐ MEDICARE   ☐ MEDI-CAL   ☒ STANDARD

PATIENT & INSURED (SUBSCRIBER) INFORMATION		
1 PATIENT'S NAME (First name, middle initial, last name) John F. Dough	2 PATIENT'S DATE OF BIRTH 1 , 1 , 40	3 INSURED'S NAME (First name, middle initial, last name) John F. Dough
4 PATIENT'S ADDRESS (Street, city, state, ZIP code) 123 Main Street New York, New York 00000	5 PATIENT'S SEX MALE ☒ FEMALE	6 INSURED'S I.D. NO., MEDICARE NO. AND/OR MEDICAID NO (include any letters) 111 22 3333
	7 PATIENT'S RELATIONSHIP TO INSURED SELF SPOUSE CHILD OTHER X	8 INSURED'S GROUP NO (Or Group Name) N123 7654321
9 OTHER HEALTH INSURANCE COVERAGE Enter Name of Policyholder and Plan Name and Address and Policy or Medical Assistance Number None	10 WAS CONDITION RELATED TO A PATIENT'S EMPLOYMENT YES ☐ X NO B AN AUTO ACCIDENT YES ☐ X NO	11 INSURED'S ADDRESS (Street, city, state, ZIP code) 123 Main Street New York, New York 00000
12 PATIENT'S OR AUTHORIZED PERSON'S SIGNATURE (Read back before signing) I Authorize the Release of any Medical Information Necessary to Process this Claim and Request Payment of MEDICARE Benefits Either to Myself or to the Party Who Accepts Assignment Below SIGNED	DATE	13 I AUTHORIZE PAYMENT OF MEDICAL BENEFITS TO UNDERSIGNED PHYSICIAN OR SUPPLIER FOR SERVICE DESCRIBED BELOW SIGNED (Insured or Authorized Person)

285

LEARNING OBJECTIVES

Upon completing this chapter, you will be able to:

1. List and describe the major types of medical insurance programs encountered in the medical office.
2. Define the terms *breach of confidentiality* and *fraud* as they apply to filing insurance claims.
3. Define *HMO, PPO, IPA,* and *IPP.*
4. Differentiate between inpatient and outpatient service.
5. List and describe the five government-mandated insurance programs and the eligibility requirements for each.
6. Describe the general attitudes of the successful health care worker who specializes in insurance-form processing.
7. Describe the filing procedures and deadlines for government-mandated programs and Blue Cross–Blue Shield programs.
8. List the reasons for which claims may be rejected and explain the procedure for appealing claim payments that are not within the expected payment range.
9. Describe the precautions the medical assistant should take to avoid filing incorrect or incomplete claims.
10. Identify the legal considerations associated with filing insurance claims.

PERFORMANCE OBJECTIVES

Upon completing this chapter, you will be able to:

1. Process patient claims using the Health Care Financing Administration (HCFA) 1500 claim form in mailable quality without errors that could result in claim rejection.
2. Process workers' compensation reports.
3. Process insurance payments and write-offs.
4. Select Current Procedural Terminology (CPT), International Classification of Diseases 9, and Evaluation and Management codes from customized procedure and diagnostic code lists.

DACUM EDUCATIONAL COMPONENTS

1. Analyze and use current third-party guidelines for reimbursement (8.3).
2. Implement current procedural terminology (CPT and ICD-9 coding) (8.2).

Glossary

Allowable charges: maximum dollar amount of charges approved for reimbursing under Medicare or a schedule of benefits regardless of the amount charged by the physician

Assignment of benefits: authorization by the patient to allow the insurance plan to pay benefits directly to the physician

Authorization to release information: written permission given by the patient or the patient's representative authorizing the release of medical information to an insurance company; this signed release is required to avoid breach of confidentiality

Benefits: the amount the insurance company pays for specific medical procedures covered by the policy

Claim: a request for payment of medical expenses covered by the insurance policy

Coinsurance: the portion of any medical bill that the patient pays—usually 20% to 25% of the charge; also called *copayment*

Coordination of benefits: sharing of benefits responsibility among multiple insurance plans

CPT code: Current Procedural Terminology code (see the procedure codes section in this chapter)

Diagnostic code: the code number assigned to a specific diagnosis

Deductible: the amount a patient must pay for covered charges during a calendar year before a plan will make any payments

Explanation of benefits: voucher attached to the payment check listing the benefits that were paid and explaining why portions of the fees were excluded from payment

Fiscal agent or fiscal intermediary: an insurance company designated by the federal or state governments to process claims payments for Medicare, Medicaid, and Civilian Health and Medical

Continued

Program of the Uniformed Services (CHAMPUS); fiscal agent contracts are awarded through competitive bidding

ICD code: International Codes for Diagnosis (see the procedure codes section in this chapter)

Precertification: payment approval for the purpose and length of a hospital stay before the patient is actually admitted; also called a *prior approval form*

Procedural code: a code number assigned to a specific procedure or service in one of the three coding systems

Prior authorization: approval of payment for treatment or referral based on the treatment plan submitted to an insurance company or government program before treatment begins or before the patient sees a specialist

Provider: physician or other supplier of medical services or equipment

Reasonable allowable charges or approved fee: the usual and prevailing fee for a medical service; accounts for variations among geographic regions, the complexity of professional skills required, and other pertinent factors

Resource-based relative value study: basis of a procedure coding system, used by workers' compensation and some other insurance plans, based on the skill, time, and cost of each service

Funk and Wagnall's dictionary defines insurance as "Protection against risk, loss, or ruin by a contract in which an insurer or underwriter guarantees to pay a sum of money to the insured in the event of some contingency such as death, accident, or illness, in return for the payment of a premium." There are many types of nonmedical insurance (life, household, professional liability, etc.). However, medical insurance (payment for treatment of illness and injury in the medical setting) is the sole subject of this chapter.

Approximately 85% of the physician's income is paid by some form of medical insurance. Insurance benefits are paid when a patient files a claim; or the claim is filed by the medical office. For example, the law now requires that Medicare claims be filed by Medicare providers (physicians, laboratories, etc.). In offices that require the patient to file for other types of insurance reimbursement, the medical assistant gives the patient a billing statement that includes the applicable diagnosis, a list of the services rendered with their identifying codes, and the individual fees for service. Most offices, however, prefer to maintain tighter control over accounts receivable and process all types of claims. An additional benefit of insurance billing by the office is favorable patient response. Many patients experience difficulty with filing and are pleased when the staff assumes this responsibility for them. Regardless of who files the claim form, the medical assistant must have the knowledge and skills to complete it or to assist the patient in doing so.

MEDICAL INSURANCE OPTIONS

There are three options for medical insurance benefits:

1. Government-sponsored programs, financed and regulated by the federal or state government for specific groups of people. This chapter discusses the four government programs that the medical assistant must manage in the office:

Medicare, Medicaid, Civilian Health and Medical Program of the Uniformed Services and Civilian Health and Medical Program of the Veterans Administration (CHAMPUS/CHAMPVA), and workers' compensation.

2. Group-sponsored or individual policies purchased through commercial insurance companies.

3. Fixed, prepaid fee plans with contracted health care providers, obtained either individually or through a group.

MEDICARE

Medicare is the federally funded health care program instituted by the US Congress and administered by the Health Care Financing Administration (HCFA). Originally designed to help senior citizens pay for medical care, the Medicare Act was expanded in the 1970s. Now it covers medical costs for eligible patients of any age with end-stage renal disease (ESRD) requiring treatment by dialysis or kidney transplant, for organ donors, and for patients with total disability lasting longer than 29 months. In 1983, amendments implemented Diagnosis-Related Groups (DRG), a new payment plan for hospital services. In 1989, the Omnibus Budget Reconciliation Act (OBRA 89) set new requirements for Medicare claims filing and changed the appearance of the Medicare card.

In 1992, amendments to Social Security included a prospective payment plan for most Medicare inpatient (hospital) services in the United States. The payment plan offsets the rising costs of health care by imposing fixed amounts paid for patient care. The fixed amount paid per patient is based on the classification, or grouping, of patients according to their medical diagnosis. A DRG reimbursement is based on the premise that similar medical diagnoses should generate similar hospitalization costs. For example, all patients admitted for an appendectomy should be charged the same fee regardless of the actual hospital costs. If the actual hospital bill is less than the DRG reimbursement, the hospital may keep the difference. If the bill is greater than the DRG reimbursement, however, the hospital must absorb the difference.

There are approximately 481 DRGs. They are classified first by major diagnostic categories, then as either medical (M) or a surgical (S) cases. Examples are shown below:

Major Diagnostic Category 18: Infectious and Parasitic Diseases

DRG #	Type of Case	Title
415	S	Surgical procedure for infectious and parasitic diseases
416	M	Septicemia, 17 years of age or older
417	M	Septicemia, 0 to 17 years of age
418	M	Postoperative and posttraumatic infections (complications)
419	M	Fever of unknown origin, age older than 69 and/or cc*
420	M	Fever of unknown origin, age older than 69 without cc.

*cc—comorbidity or complication.

With the passage of OBRA 89, the Congress empowered the HCFA to develop a reimbursement system for Medicare Part B (medical insurance) based on a relative value. The result of this mandate is the resource-based relative value system (RBRVS) designed to control the spending for Medicare Part B services. The system, developed by researchers at Harvard University, is being implemented over 6 years beginning in 1992. It will establish a more logical basis for physician payment and will slow the rise in spending for all physician services, but particularly in certain specialties. The system will regulate

1. Professional services by physicians
2. Services and supplies connected with physicians' services
3. Outpatient physical and occupational therapy
4. Diagnostic x-rays and other diagnostic tests
5. X-ray, radium, and radioisotope therapy, including technicians' materials and services.

MEDICARE ELIGIBILITY

Medicare is a two-part program. Part A (hospital insurance) covers inpatient hospital services, outpatient diagnostic services, some posthospital care, and care received in an extended care facility. Part B (medical insurance) must be purchased by the patient and covers physician charges for inpatient and outpatient services, outpatient diagnostic services, drugs administered by the physician, ESRD and home health care, and prescription medical supplies. Part B, however, does not cover some items, including:

1. Routine physician examinations and tests directly related to those examinations (the patient must have an active diagnosis or injury for these services to be covered)
2. Examinations for the sole purpose of prescribing eyeglasses or hearing aids
3. Immunizations, with the exception of pneumococcal vaccinations or vaccinations administered to prevent infection following an injury
4. Cosmetic surgery, except when it is necessary to repair an accidental injury
5. Nonprescription drugs

Eligibility for Medicare benefits is determined by the Social Security Administration because everyone who is eligible for social security is automatically enrolled in Part A. Persons eligible for Part A may enroll in Part B by paying a monthly premium. Persons older than 65 and not eligible for Medicare (workers who have not worked enough to qualify for social security or who did not participate in the Social Security program) may enroll by paying for both Part A and Part B. Additionally, blind and otherwise disabled persons of any age, and dependent widows or widowers between ages 50 and 65, may qualify (Fig. 15–1).

MEDICARE BILLING

Medicare billing for Part A is completed by the hospital or other treating institution. Part B billing is completed by the physician's office staff. The Medicare program is a copayment plan with an annual deductible fee. Generally, Medicare pays the participating physician 80% of approved or allowable charges after the patient has paid the deductible fee. The patient is responsible for the remaining 20% of the allowable charges.

Medicare reimburses either the patient or the physician directly. If the physician is to be paid directly, the patient must sign the "assignment of benefits" section of the Medicare claim form. The patient agrees to give, or "assign," the payment to the physician, and Medicare pays the reimbursement with a check made out in the physician's name.

Physicians may formally enter into a provider agreement with Medicare and become participating physicians, or they may choose not to participate. Patients seen by Medicare-participating physicians pay only the annual deductible fee and the 20% copayment (also called *coinsurance*) of the charges allowed to the physician. Allowable charges may or may not be as high as the physician's fee, but the allowable charge is the combined maximum amount reimbursable by both Medicare and the patient to the physician. After payment of the deductible fee and the 20% copayment, participating physicians do not bill Medicare patients for more than the 80% of the amount allowed and paid by Medicare, regardless of the actual service amount. This type of agreement is called *accepting assignment*. The physician agrees to accept the Medicare check as payment in full for the remaining balance. An example follows:

How To Determine If Your
Patient Is Entitled To Medical Benefits

The Department of Social Security issues a Medicare card to every person who is entitled to Medicare benefits.

This card identifies the Medicare beneficiary and includes the following information:

    Name (exactly as it appears on the Social Security records)
    Medicare Health Insurance Claim Number (HICN)
    Sex
    Date of entitlement
    Type of benefits to which beneficiary is entitled under the Medicare program
    Enrollee's signature

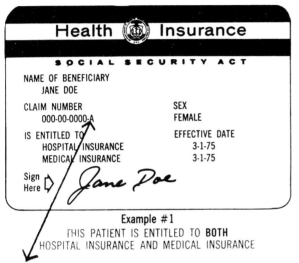

Example #1
THIS PATIENT IS ENTITLED TO **BOTH**
HOSPITAL INSURANCE AND MEDICAL INSURANCE

Code letter at end of ID number means:
A = Breadwinner
B = Spouse
D = Widow of deceased breadwinner
    (and so on with many other
    check letters)

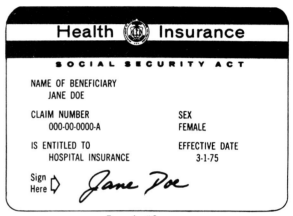

Example #2
THIS PATIENT IS ENTITLED TO HOSPITAL BENEFITS ONLY
THERE IS NO ENTITLEMENT FOR MEDICAL BENEFITS

Retired railroad workers' ID will
begin with code "WA"

These claims are mailed to:

    Travelers Insurance Company
    P.O. Box 30050
    Salt Lake City, UT 84125

Figure 15–1. Medicare ID card.

Actual charge	$375.00
Medicare allowable charge (for the particular service)	$275.00
Minus deductible (in this case, the annual deductible has been previously met)	−0
Medicare 80% payment (80% of $275)	220.00
Patient 20% payment due (20% of $275)	+55.00
Total paid by Medicare *and* the patient:	$275.00
Credit adjustment to the patient account	$100.00

Patients may be billed the actual service amount, however, for any services not covered by Medicare, provided that the patient is informed in advance that the service is not covered.

Patients treated by nonparticipating physicians personally pay the physician the total limiting charges (the charges set by Medicare for nonparticipating physicians) and then apply for Medicare reimbursement. The patient may or may not assign benefits to the physician. If the patient does not assign benefits to the physician, the patient receives the Medicare check for 80% of the allowable charges, minus the annual deductible if it has not been met, and then is personally responsible for paying the physician the total limiting charge. An example follows:

Actual charge	$375.00
Medicare limiting charge (for the nonparticipating physician)	$275.00
Minus deductible (in this case, the annual deductible has been previously met)	−0
Medicare 80% payment (80% of $275)	220.00
Medicare payment to the patient	220.00
Patient copayment (20% of $275)	+55.00
Balance due from the patient	$375.00

Nonparticipating physicians are not required to take Medicare benefit assignment unless a patient is also a recipient of Medicaid benefits.

MEDICARE COORDINATION OF BENEFITS

If the patient is covered by another health insurance program, payments from the other plan may be coordinated so that the patient receives payments for up to 100% of the eligible medical charges. Before billing, the medical assistant must use established insurance industry guidelines to determine which is the primary plan and which is the secondary plan. For example, Medicare is the secondary carrier for a patient 65 to 69 years of age who is still employed and covered by an employer's group health plan. In this case, the patient can submit expenses unpaid by the group plan to Medicare for coordination of benefits. However, if a retired person older than 65 carries individual medical insurance in addition to Medicare coverage, the additional insurance is the secondary plan and integrates benefits with Medicare, the primary plan. *Integration* refers to the assumption by the other health plan of charges remaining after Medicare has paid its allowable charges.

Some patients purchase supplemental "medigap" insurance to help pay for inpatient and outpatient deductibles fees and services not covered by Medicare. In such cases, Medicare must be billed first and an Explanation of Benefits (EOB) form copied and attached to the supplemental insurance claim form for submission. The EOB is an attachment, or voucher, to an insurance company check explaining what benefits were paid and why certain items were excluded (see Figs. 15–2 and 15–3).

THE OMNIBUS BUDGET RECONCILIATION ACT OF 1989

The Omnibus Budget Reconciliation Act of 1989 (OBRA 89) has imposed certain requirements on Medicare claims filing. Effective September 1, 1990, all physicians, participating or nonparticipating, submit to Medicare all claims for covered services provided to the Medicare beneficiaries.

Physicians may not charge the beneficiary for preparing and filing the claim. To be considered for payment, all Medicare claims must be filed by December 31 of the year following the year in which the services were rendered. Claims submitted by participating physicians are usually processed and paid within 17 days; if not, Medicare usually pays interest to the physician. Physicians who fail to submit claims for Medicare beneficiaries may be subject to a penalty of up to $2000 for each violation. Nonparticipating physicians are not allowed to bill patients for the entire charge of a service, as federal regulations limit the maximum allowable actual charge to Medicare patients.

The medical assistant must be prepared to process Medicare claims and assist patients with their filing forms. Figure 15–4 is a sample of a frequently used form for all types of health insurance claim. In filling out such forms, the medical assistant must be able to provide

1. Diagnosis and ICD codes (see Fig. 15–4, item 21)
2. Complete billing information, including CPT code, description of service rendered, and the charge for that service (item 24).
3. Mailing address of the local fiscal intermediary.

The insurer who uses the universal form affixes the company logo and address of the form. When the form is used to make a Medicare claim, no logo or address is attached.

To process Medicare claims, the medical assistant should be able to provide the following information:

1. The name and address of the regional fiscal agent for Medicare
2. The name and phone number of the regional fiscal agent's provider representative.

In addition, the medical assistant should keep available a current copy of *Your Medicare Handbook*, published by the Social Security Administration and available at all local Social Security offices.

MEDICAID

In 1965, the US Congress mandated that each state establish a program to assist certain groups of people with payment of medical expenses. This program is called Medicaid (Medi-Cal in California) and is part of the Title 19 Social Security Act. The federal government provides each state with an equitable amount of money to fund this health care program. Individual states are free to extend benefits beyond the stated minimums if they are willing to pay the cost of these extensions from the state treasury. Persons eligible to receive benefits under this program may include those receiving welfare assistance, low-income persons who

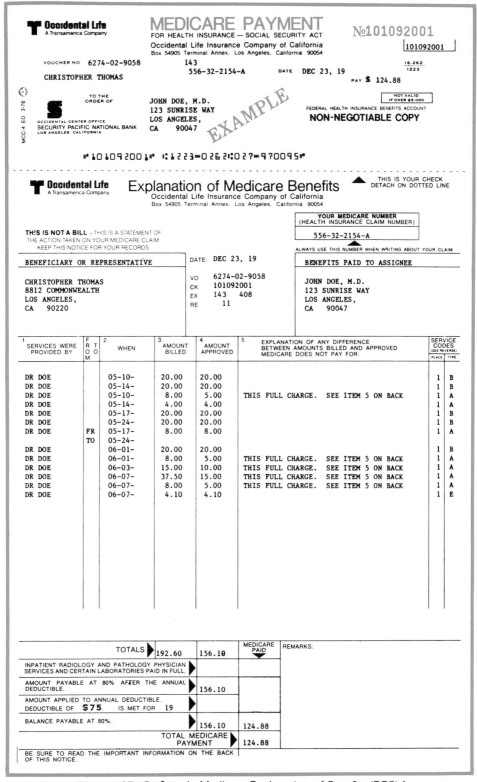

Figure 15-2. Sample Medicare Explanation of Benefits (EOB) form.

BLUE SHIELD of California

P.O. BOX 3637, SAN FRANCISCO, CA 94119 (415) 445-5151
P.O. BOX 92945, LOS ANGELES, CA 90009 (213) 642-5600

PATIENT'S NAME	GROUP NO	SUBSCRIBER NO.	CLAIM NO.	PROVIDER OF SERVICES	MO	DAY	Y
JONES MARY	9900-000	R12345678	0278258000000	SMITH JOHN	09	21	87

A CLAIM HAS BEEN RECEIVED FOR THE SERVICES SHOWN BELOW. IT HAS BEEN PROCESSED
IN ACCORDANCE WITH THE BENEFITS OF THE SUBSCRIBER'S BLUE SHIELD HEALTH PLAN

EXPLANATION OF BENEFITS

FOR THE CLAIM RECEIVED ON   9/15/78

JONES MARY A.
123 Main Street
Downtown, Ca. 92349

PHYSICIAN MEMBER - YES   9148292

SERVICES BILLED	PROC. NO.	DATES OF SERVICE FROM MO	YR.	DAY	TO DAY	NO. OF SERVICES	AMOUNT BILLED	MAX. CONTRACT AMOUNT PAYABLE BY BLUE SHIELD	UNPAID AMOUNT	CODE	AMOUNT PAID
HOME/OFFICE	9000C	09	01			01 0	15 00		15 00	1	00
LABORATORY	81000	09	01			01 0	5 00	5 00			5 00
RADIOLOGY	71020	09	01			01 0	20 00		20 00	2	00

UNPAID CODE EXPLANATION

1   THIS SERVICE IS NOT A BENEFIT OF THE BASIC COVERAGE.   SUPPLEMENTAL BENEFITS MAY APPLY -
SUBSCRIBER SHOULD SUBMIT BILL WITH SUPPLEMENTAL CLAIM FORM FOR REVIEW.

2   X-RAY SERVICES NOT RELATED TO A SPECIFIC ILLNESS OR INJURY ARE NOT A BENEFIT OF THE
FEDERAL EMPLOYEE PROGRAM.

BLUE SHIELD
of California

720 CALIFORNIA ST   •   SAN FRANCISCO, CA 94108
5959 W CENTURY BLVD.   •   LOS ANGELES, CA 90045

PAID TO

JOHN SMITH, M.D., INC.
777 MEDICAL CENTER DRIVE
DOWNTOWN, CA 92349

PROVIDER NO	CHECK NO.		
00A123450	**9148292**		
MO	DAY	YEAR	PAY DOLLARS	CENTS
09	21		$*******5	00

*******5*DOLLARS**00*CTS

NOT
NEGOTIABLE

Figure 15-3. Sample Blue Shield EOB form.

PLEASE
DO NOT
STAPLE
IN THIS
AREA

HEALTH INSURANCE CLAIM FORM

	PICA					PICA	

1. MEDICARE   MEDICAID   CHAMPUS   CHAMPVA   GROUP HEALTH PLAN   FECA BLK LUNG   OTHER   1a. INSURED'S I.D. NUMBER   (FOR PROGRAM IN ITEM 1)

☐ (Medicare #)   ☐ (Medicaid #)   ☐ (Sponsor's SSN)   ☐ (VA File #)   ☐ (SSN or ID)   ☐ (SSN)   ☐ (ID)

2. PATIENT'S NAME (Last Name, First Name, Middle Initial)

3. PATIENT'S BIRTH DATE   MM   DD   YY   SEX   M ☐   F ☐

4. INSURED'S NAME (Last Name, First Name, Middle Initial)

5. PATIENT'S ADDRESS (No., Street)

6. PATIENT RELATIONSHIP TO INSURED   Self ☐   Spouse ☐   Child ☐   Other ☐

7. INSURED'S ADDRESS (No., Street)

CITY   STATE

8. PATIENT STATUS   Single ☐   Married ☐   Other ☐

CITY   STATE

ZIP CODE   TELEPHONE (Include Area Code)   (   )

Employed ☐   Full-Time Student ☐   Part-Time Student ☐

ZIP CODE   TELEPHONE (INCLUDE AREA CODE)   (   )

9. OTHER INSURED'S NAME (Last Name, First Name, Middle Initial)

10. IS PATIENT'S CONDITION RELATED TO:

11. INSURED'S POLICY GROUP OR FECA NUMBER

a. OTHER INSURED'S POLICY OR GROUP NUMBER

a. EMPLOYMENT? (CURRENT OR PREVIOUS)   YES ☐   NO ☐

a. INSURED'S DATE OF BIRTH   MM   DD   YY   SEX   M ☐   F ☐

b. OTHER INSURED'S DATE OF BIRTH   MM   DD   YY   SEX   M ☐   F ☐

b. AUTO ACCIDENT?   PLACE (State)   YES ☐   NO ☐

b. EMPLOYER'S NAME OR SCHOOL NAME

c. EMPLOYER'S NAME OR SCHOOL NAME

c. OTHER ACCIDENT?   YES ☐   NO ☐

c. INSURANCE PLAN NAME OR PROGRAM NAME

d. INSURANCE PLAN NAME OR PROGRAM NAME

10d. RESERVED FOR LOCAL USE

d. IS THERE ANOTHER HEALTH BENEFIT PLAN?   YES ☐   NO ☐   *If yes*, return to and complete item 9 a-d.

READ BACK OF FORM BEFORE COMPLETING & SIGNING THIS FORM.
12. PATIENT'S OR AUTHORIZED PERSON'S SIGNATURE I authorize the release of any medical or other information necessary to process this claim. I also request payment of government benefits either to myself or to the party who accepts assignment below.

SIGNED _____ DATE _____

13. INSURED'S OR AUTHORIZED PERSON'S SIGNATURE I authorize payment of medical benefits to the undersigned physician or supplier for services described below.

SIGNED _____

14. DATE OF CURRENT: MM   DD   YY   ◄ ILLNESS (First symptom) OR INJURY (Accident) OR PREGNANCY(LMP)

15. IF PATIENT HAS HAD SAME OR SIMILAR ILLNESS. GIVE FIRST DATE   MM   DD   YY

16. DATES PATIENT UNABLE TO WORK IN CURRENT OCCUPATION   MM   DD   YY   FROM   TO   MM   DD   YY

17. NAME OF REFERRING PHYSICIAN OR OTHER SOURCE

17a. I.D. NUMBER OF REFERRING PHYSICIAN

18. HOSPITALIZATION DATES RELATED TO CURRENT SERVICES   MM   DD   YY   FROM   TO   MM   DD   YY

19. RESERVED FOR LOCAL USE

20. OUTSIDE LAB? $ CHARGES   YES ☐   NO ☐

21. DIAGNOSIS OR NATURE OF ILLNESS OR INJURY. (RELATE ITEMS 1,2,3 OR 4 TO ITEM 24E BY LINE)

1. ⌊___ . __⌋   3. ⌊___ . __⌋

2. ⌊___ . __⌋   4. ⌊___ . __⌋

22. MEDICAID RESUBMISSION CODE   ORIGINAL REF. NO.

23. PRIOR AUTHORIZATION NUMBER

24. A DATE(S) OF SERVICE						B Place of Service	C Type of Service	D PROCEDURES, SERVICES, OR SUPPLIES (Explain Unusual Circumstances) CPT/HCPCS	MODIFIER	E DIAGNOSIS CODE	F $ CHARGES	G DAYS OR UNITS	H EPSDT Family Plan	I EMG	J COB	K RESERVED FOR LOCAL USE
From MM	DD	YY	To MM	DD	YY											
1																
2																
3																
4																
5																
6																

25. FEDERAL TAX I.D. NUMBER   SSN ☐ EIN ☐

26. PATIENT'S ACCOUNT NO.

27. ACCEPT ASSIGNMENT? (For govt. claims, see back)   YES ☐   NO ☐

28. TOTAL CHARGE $

29. AMOUNT PAID $

30. BALANCE DUE $

31. SIGNATURE OF PHYSICIAN OR SUPPLIER INCLUDING DEGREES OR CREDENTIALS (I certify that the statements on the reverse apply to this bill and are made a part thereof.)

SIGNED _____ DATE _____

32. NAME AND ADDRESS OF FACILITY WHERE SERVICES WERE RENDERED (If other than home or office)

33. PHYSICIAN'S, SUPPLIER'S BILLING NAME, ADDRESS, ZIP CODE & PHONE #

PIN#   GRP#

(APPROVED BY AMA COUNCIL ON MEDICAL SERVICE 8/88)   **PLEASE PRINT OR TYPE**   FORM HCFA-1500 (12-90),   FORM RRB-1500 FORM OWCP-1500

CARRIER → / PATIENT AND INSURED INFORMATION / PHYSICIAN OR SUPPLIER INFORMATION

Figure 15-4. Universal insurance form.

are medically needy but not disabled, those receiving aid to dependent children, and blind and disabled persons. Often, this program covers foster children and adopted children who have birth defects. Eligibility and benefits vary greatly, and final determination is made by the individual state. Basic covered services include the following:

1. Inpatient hospital care (limited to 12 inpatient days per year)
2. Outpatient services (limited to 12 outpatient visits per year and when medically indicated)
3. Laboratory and x-ray services
4. Skilled nursing facility care
5. Early diagnostic screening and treatment for children younger than 21
6. Family planning services

Physicians who accept Medicaid patients automatically agree to accept state reimbursement as payment in full for all covered services. Some states have cost-share programs that require the patient to pay a small, specified amount for each office visit, prescription drug, or both. In these states, the amount to be collected from the patient is specified on the patient's Medicaid enrollment or identification card. The patient cannot be billed for the difference between the physician's normal fee for services and the Medicaid-approved fee. Patients can be billed *only* for any procedure not covered by Medicaid. Some states require that certain patients pay a predetermined dollar amount of medical expense each month before they become eligible for Medicaid assistance.

The medical assistant must ask the Medicaid patient for proof of eligibility each time the patient comes to the office for treatment. Eligibility may change from month to month, depending on the family income or circumstances. All states have established acceptable proofs of eligibility in the form of cards, tickets, coupons, stickers, labels, and so on. Often, these must be attached to the service report claim for billing. Fiscal intermediaries require the claim to be properly identified with current eligibility proof.

In addition, certain procedures, such as nonemergency surgery, require prior authorization before treatment can begin. This authorization must be obtained in writing. Preliminary authorization can often be obtained from the local Medicaid official by telephone. The telephone authorization must then be followed up with the written request.

Most Medicaid claims are filed on the HCFA 1500 claim form. However, several states have been granted waivers to use specially designed forms for filing if they have direct electronic data system computer access.

States have individual deadlines for accepting claims. These deadlines vary from 60 days to 1 year from the date that services were rendered. Claims reaching the fiscal intermediary after the cutoff date are not considered for payment.

The medical assistant should maintain a resource file that contains frequently used Medicaid information. This information could be kept on cards in a file box or drawer, in a looseleaf binder, or by any system that permits frequent updating. The information should include the following:

1. Name and address of offices where potential Medicaid clients can apply for assistance
2. Name, address, and telephone number of the local Medicaid administrative offices
3. Name, address, and telephone number of the fiscal intermediary's administrative offices
4. Medicaid-covered services available locally
5. Information on local eligibility identification
6. Local rules concerning prior authorization of services

COMBINED MEDICARE AND MEDICAID PROGRAM, CROSSOVER CLAIMS, DUAL RECIPIENTS, AND MEDI-MEDI CLAIMS

Individuals who meet the eligibility requirements for both the Medicare and Medicaid programs are known as *crossover clients, dual recipients,* or *Medi-Medis.* These claims are billed on the HCFA 1500 form unless the state has been granted a waiver to use its own specially designed form. Figure 15–5 illustrates areas for special consideration when a crossover claim form is completed.

After Medicare processes the claim, it is transferred to the Medicaid office for further processing. The physician receives payments from each approved claim, one from Medicare and one from Medicaid. Once both payments have been received, the medical assistant adjusts the ledger for any differences between the total amount paid on the claim and the amount charged by the physician.

MILITARY AND VETERANS ADMINISTRATION PROGRAMS

In the 1950s, the federal government initiated a military-oriented medical program currently called the Civilian Health and Medical Program of the Uniformed Services (CHAMPUS). This program covers the dependents of active-duty and retired military personnel. A corollary program is the Civilian Health and Medical Program of the Veterans Administration (CHAMPVA). In 1973, additional programs were established to cover the surviving spouses and dependent children of persons who died as result of military service, and those of veterans who were totally and permanently disabled as a result of military service. These programs cover the cost of medical care obtained in the civilian community because it is either unavailable at the local military health facility or not covered by either CHAMPUS or CHAMPVA.

All nonemergency inpatient care sought in a civilian hospital must have prior authorization from CHAMPUS if the program is to assume responsibility for payment. This prior authorization form, called a nonavailability statement, or Form DD 1251, is obtained from the

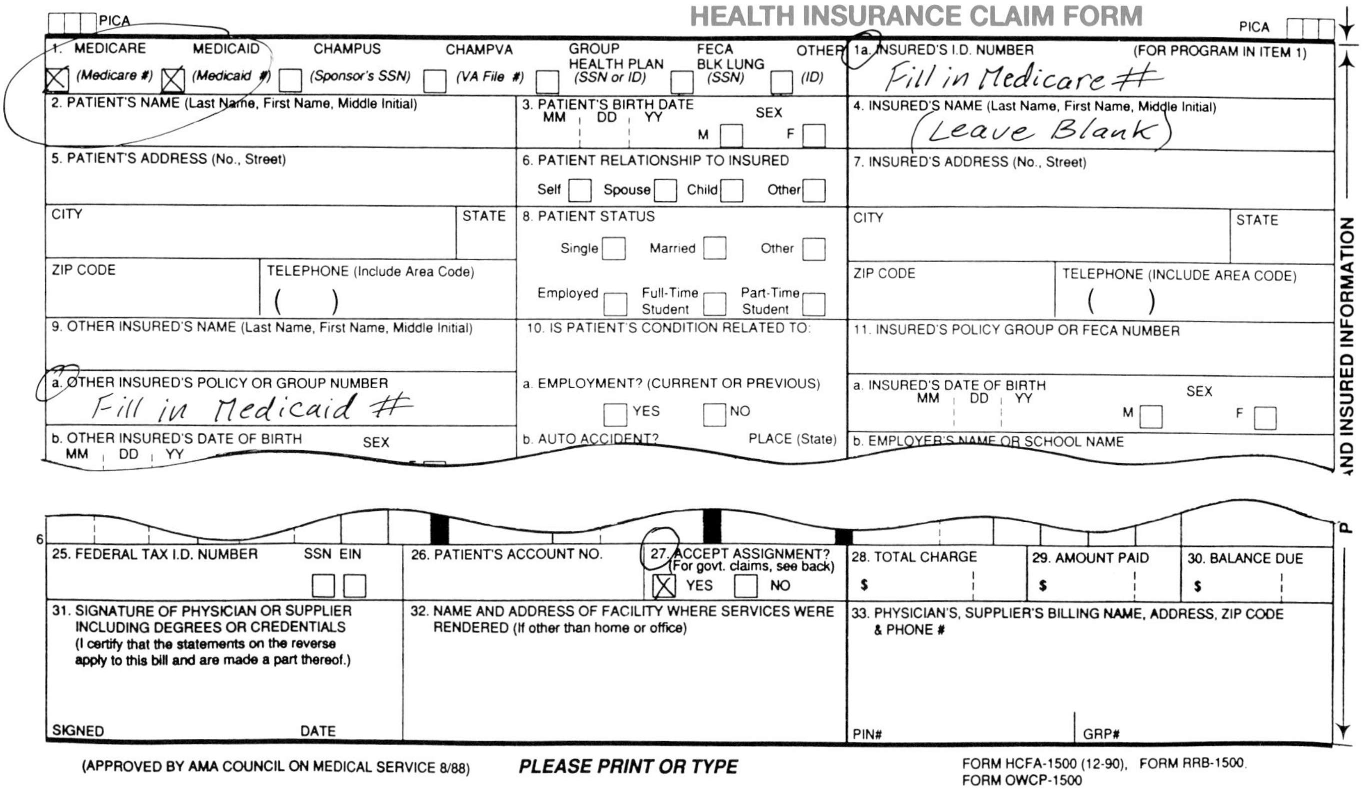

HEALTH INSURANCE CLAIM FORM

(Handwritten on form: "Fill in Medicare #", "Leave Blank", "Fill in Medicaid #")

1. Top of Form — Check the Medicare box
2. Box 4 — Leave blank
3. Box 1A — Type in the patient's Medicare ID #
4. Box 9A — Type in the patient's Medicaid ID #
5. Box 7A — Check the "yes" box. (If Yes is not checked, the Medicare portion is sent to the patient and the Medicaid portion is not paid.)

Figure 15–5. Areas for special consideration when completing a crossover claim.

dependents' administrative officer at the local military medical facility (Fig. 15–6). Authorization is waived if the patient lives more than 40 miles from a military medical facility that could render the care, or if an accessible facility is temporarily unable to handle the case.

A copy of the form must be attached to the first claim filed for payment by CHAMPUS. Claims filed for continuation of this "authorized civilian medical care" do not need to have copies of the statement attached. CHAMPVA recipients and users of the outpatient por-

tion of either program do not have to obtain prior authorization.

The fiscal intermediary who services the billing area employs representatives who can help the medical assistant with billing and eligibility problems. The intermediary's office usually issues periodic bulletins to keep the medical office apprised of changes in billing procedures or available services.

Physicians may elect to participate in CHAMPUS/CHAMPVA on a case-by-case basis. This type of participation is different from participation in certain other

NONAVAILABILITY STATEMENT
DEPENDENTS MEDICAL CARE PROGRAM
(AR 40-121, SECNAV INST 6320.8A, AFR 160-41, PHS GEN CIR NO 6)

(This Statement is Issued for your Immediate use)

THE ISSUANCE OF THIS STATEMENT MEANS:

1. The medical care requested is not available to you at a Uniformed Services facility in this area.
2. If you receive medical care from civilian sources and such care is determined to be authorized care under the Medicare Program, it will be paid for by the Government to the extent that the program permits.
3. If you receive medical care from civilian sources and it is determined that all or part of the care is not authorized under the Medicare Program, THE GOVERNMENT WILL NOT PAY for the unauthorized care.

The determination of whether medical care you may receive from civilian sources is authorized for payment cannot be made at this time because this determination depends, among other things, upon the care you actually receive. Further, no statement regarding your condition or diagnosis made hereon will be considered in any way determinative as to whether care rendered for such condition is payable under the Medicare Program.

The use of this statement is subject to the conditions and limitations set forth in the regulation issued under the Dependents' Medical Care Act as codified in 10 U.S.C. 1071-1085.

This form must be presented with your Uniformed Services Identification and Privilege Card (DD Form 1173), identified below, when you obtain civilian medical care.

DEPENDENT. SPOUSE OR CHILD, RESIDING WITH SPONSOR

DEPENDENT'S LAST NAME - FIRST NAME - MIDDLE INITIAL

UNIFORMED SERVICES IDENTIFICATION
AND PRIVILEGE CARD (DD FORM 1173)

CARD NUMBER | EXPIRATION DATE

PREFIX | NUMERICAL | SUFFIX

DEPENDENT'S ADDRESS *(Complete mailing address)*

SPONSOR MEMBER OF UNIFORMED SERVICES ON ACTIVE DUTY

SPONSOR'S LAST NAME - FIRST NAME - MIDDLE INITIAL

BRANCH OF SERVICE

☐ ARMY ☐ NAVY ☐ AIR FORCE

SERVICE NUMBER | GRADE OR RANK

☐ MARINE CORPS ☐ PUBLIC HEALTH

☐ COAST GUARD ☐ COAST & GEODETIC SURVEY

ORGANIZATION AND OFFICIAL DUTY STATION

REMARKS

STATION AT WHICH PERMIT ISSUED | DATE ISSUED

GRADE OR RANK, AND POSITION OF ISSUING OFFICER | SIGNATURE OF ISSUING OFFICER

DISTRIBUTION *(Three signed copies of this statement will be furnished the dependent for distribution as follows):*
DEPENDENT *(Original copy)* ATTENDING PHYSICIAN *(Duplicate copy)* CIVILIAN MEDICAL FACILITY *(Triplicate copy)*

Figure 15–6. CHAMPUS nonavailability statement (DD1251).

programs, which must be on an all-or-nothing basis. A physician who agrees to participate must sign the claim form, submit it for billing, and write off any amounts greater than those CHAMPUS allows. The patient is always responsible for any copayment or deductible fee due under the program. The physician receives payment directly from the fiscal intermediary.

If the physician does not participate, the patient completes and submits the top half of CHAMPUS Form 500 or 501 (a duplicate of HCFA Form 1500), attaches the physician's itemized statement to it, and submits it to the fiscal intermediary for direct reimbursement (Fig. 15–7).

The government fiscal year begins October 1 and ends September 30. Claims must be received 1 year from the end of the year in which services were rendered.

The medical assistant should obtain, maintain, and keep current the following resource information pertaining to CHAMPUS/CHAMPVA:

1. Name and telephone number of the local health care benefit advisor
2. Name and address of the regional fiscal agent
3. Name and address of all local government health care facilities
4. Name, address, and telephone number of the local service representative from the fiscal intermediary

WORKERS' COMPENSATION

Workers' compensation, another congressionally mandated program, has established minimum state requirements to cover the employers' cost of on-the-job injury or illness. It allows individual states to exceed the federal benefit standards at their own expense. This program was initiated because regular medical insurance companies do not cover job-related illness or injury.

The physician must file a Doctor's First Report of Occupational Injury or Illness when a patient seeks the physician's care for a job-related illness or injury. Patients must be seen by a physician within 24 hours of the injury or illness. The filing time for the report varies from state to state, but most states require filing within 72 hours of the patient's initial visit. Copies of the report are required for

1. The employer's compensation insurance carrier
2. The employer
3. The state compensation board
4. The patient's medical file.

Figure 15–8 shows a copy of a report form.

Patients must report job-related illness or injury to the employer before seeking medical care. It is the responsibility of the medical assistant to ask the patient to see whether this has been done and to obtain the name and address of the employer's insurance carrier.

Because the Doctor's First Report of Occupational Injury or Illness is not a billing form, all bills for authenticated work-related injuries or illnesses must be submitted to the compensation carrier. Bills should be filed with the carrier every 30 days during active treatment until the entire cost has been paid. To maximize payment, the medical assistant must itemize and use code descriptors for each service rendered or supply used. Physicians who accept workers' compensation cases agree to accept the compensation carrier's approved fees as payment in full. Patients are not billed for any unpaid portion of the account. There are no deductible fees or copayment obligations. The patient is, however, responsible for any bill rejected by the workers' compensation board. The patient has the right to appeal any rejected bill, and any dispute surrounding the claim is taken to the local workers' compensation appeals board.

Basic workers' compensation benefits may include the following:

1. Medical treatment (both inpatient and outpatient medical and surgical care, drugs, prostheses, reasonable transportation, etc.)
2. Temporary disability income (a weekly wage loss benefit)
3. Permanent disability income (a weekly or monthly cash benefit)
4. Death benefits (burial allowance and cash benefits for dependents of fatally injured workers)
5. Rehabilitation benefits

The compensation laws require that any requests for medical records contain *only* information related to the treatment of the work-related illness or injury. When a patient seeks medical care for a work-related illness or injury from his or her regular attending physician, a separate workers' compensation chart and ledger card must be established. The medical assistant must flag both the charts and the ledger cards to indicate that two charts and two ledger cards exist for this patient. The physician and office personnel must take extra care to ensure that all entries are made on the proper file or ledger.

The report must cover the following areas:

1. How the patient was injured: slipped, fell, was struck by object, and so forth
2. Object: Struck by, cut with, knocked down by, fell onto, and so forth
3. Body part injured: Head (which part), arm (which side, which part), finger, hand (which part), multiple body parts, and so forth
4. Injury: Cut, contusion, bruise, fracture, sprain, abrasion, concussion, and so forth
5. Date and time: Date and exact time of injury
6. Patient's complaints: Symptoms (the extent of injury or illness)
7. Physician's diagnosis: Should include specific reasons why conclusions were reached

CHAMPUS/CHAMPVA CLAIM FORM

For services or supplies provided by civilian sources except Institutions

Read cover instructions and the back of this form before completing and signing!

Form Approved
OMB No.
022-RO382

Patient/Sponsor Information (Items 1 through 18 to be completed by the beneficiary/patient or sponsor)

1. PATIENT'S NAME (Last name, First name, Middle initial)

2. PATIENT'S DATE OF BIRTH
MONTH   DAY   YEAR

7. SPONSOR'S NAME (Last name, First name, Middle initial)

3. PATIENT'S ADDRESS (Street, city, state, ZIP code)

4. PATIENT'S SEX
☐ MALE   ☐ FEMALE

8. SPONSOR'S SOCIAL SECURITY NO. OR VA FILE NO.

9. VA STATION NO.

PHONE NO. (Include area code)

6. PATIENT'S RELATIONSHIP TO SPONSOR
☐ SELF   ☐ SPOUSE
☐ NATURAL or   ☐ STEPCHILD
   ADOPTED CHILD
OTHER (Specify):

10. SPONSOR'S DUTY STATION OR ADDRESS FOR RETIREES

5. MILITARY/VA IDENTIFICATION CARD

CARD NO.

ISSUE DATE
MONTH   DAY   YEAR

EFFECTIVE DATE
MONTH   DAY   YEAR

EXPIRATION DATE
MONTH   DAY   YEAR

15. IS CONDITION WORK RELATED?
☐ YES ☐ NO

PHONE NO (Include area code)

11. SPONSOR'S BRANCH OF SERVICE

12. SPONSOR'S GRADE/RANK

14. DO YOU HAVE OTHER HEALTH INSURANCE? ☐ YES ☐ NO
IF YES, ENTER NAME OF OTHER PLAN OR PROGRAM:

MILITARY SERVICE RELATED?
☐ YES ☐ NO

☐ USA   ☐ USAF   ☐ USMC   ☐ USN
☐ USCG   ☐ USPHS   ☐ NOAA   ☐ VA

AUTOMOBILE ACCIDENT RELATED?
☐ YES ☐ NO

13. SPONSOR'S STATUS
☐ ACTIVE DUTY   ☐ RETIRED   ☐ DECEASED

ADDRESS

CITY   STATE   ZIP

16. INPATIENT/OUTPATIENT CARE
☐ OUTPATIENT   ☐ INPATIENT-EMERGENCY ☐ INPATIENT HOSPITAL-OUTSIDE 40 MILE RADIUS
☐ INPATIENT-SKILLED NURSING FACILITY   ☐ INPATIENT-OTHER
☐ INPATIENT HOSPITAL-WITHIN 40 MILE RADIUS (ATTACH DD FORM 1251)

14a. TYPE OF COVERAGE:
☐ EMPLOYMENT (GROUP)   ☐ MEDICAID   ☐ STUDENT PLAN
☐ PRIVATE (NON-GROUP)   ☐ MEDICARE   ☐ OTHER:

17. DESCRIBE CONDITION FOR WHICH YOU RECEIVED TREATMENT. IF AN INJURY, NOTE HOW IT HAPPENED.

14b. OTHER IDENTIFICATION NUMBER

14c. EFFECTIVE DATE
MONTH   DAY   YEAR

14d. OTHER PROGRAM THROUGH EMPLOYMENT?
EMPLOYER NAME:

18. SIGNATURE OF PATIENT OR AUTHORIZED PERSON, CERTIFIES CLAIM INFORMATION AND AUTHORIZES RELEASE OF MEDICAL OR OTHER INSURANCE INFORMATION. READ INSTRUCTIONS AND BACK OF THIS FORM BEFORE SIGNING.

SIGNED: DATE:

RELATIONSHIP TO PATIENT:

Physician/Other Provider (Items 19 through 33 are to be completed by the physician or other provider.)

19. NAME, ADDRESS & PHONE NO. OF REFERRING PHYSICIAN

20. NAME & ADDRESS OF FACILITY WHERE SERVICES RENDERED (other than home or office)

☐ PRIVATE PRACTICE or   ☐ UNIFORMED SERVICES

21. PROVIDER OF SERVICES
☐ ATTENDING PHYSICIAN
☐ OTHER:

22. HOSPITALIZATION INFORMATION
MO   DAY   YEAR   MO   DAY   YEAR
ADMITTED   DISCHARGED

23. LAB WORK OUTSIDE YOUR OFFICE?
☐ YES ☐ NO   CHARGES:

24. DIAGNOSIS, SYMPTOM OR NATURE OF ILLNESS OR INJURY, RELATE DIAGNOSIS TO PROCEDURE IN COLUMN "D" BY REFERENCE TO NUMBERS 1, 2, 3, or DX CODE

1.
2.
3.

25.A. DATES OF SERVICE MO/DAY/YEAR	B* PLACE OF SERVICE	C PROCEDURE CODE IDENTIFY:	D. DESCRIBE PROCEDURES/SUPPLIES FOR EACH DATE. SUBMIT REPORT EXPLAINING UNUSUAL SERVICES OR CIRCUMSTANCES	E DIAGNOSIS CODE	F CHARGES	LEAVE BLANK

26. PATIENT'S ACCOUNT NO.

29. PHYSICIAN'S OR OTHER PROVIDER'S NAME, ADDRESS, ZIP CODE & PHONE NO. (INCLUDING AREA CODE)

G. TOTAL CHARGES
$

30. AMOUNT PAID BY BENEFICIARY
$

31. AMOUNT PAID BY OTHER INSURANCE
$

27. PROVIDER'S SOCIAL SECURITY NO.

32. AGREEMENT TO PARTICIPATE (READ BACK OF THIS FORM)
☐ YES   ☐ NO

28. PROVIDER'S EMPLOYER I.D. NO.

33. SIGNATURE OF PHYSICIAN OR OTHER PROVIDER (READ BACK OF THIS FORM BEFORE SIGNING)

PROVIDER NO.

SIGNED: DATE:

*PLACE OF SERVICE CODES

1 — (IH) — INPATIENT HOSPITAL	4 — (H) — PATIENT'S HOME	7 — (NH) — NURSING HOME	A — (IL) — INDEPENDENT LABORATORY
2 — (OH) — OUTPATIENT HOSPITAL	5 — (DCF) — DAY CARE FACILITY (PSY)	8 — (SNF) — SKILLED NURSING FACILITY	B — (OF) — OTHER MEDICAL/SURGICAL FACILITY
3 — (O) — DOCTOR'S OFFICE	6 — (NCF) — NIGHT CARE FACILITY (PSY)	9 — (AMB) — AMBULANCE	C — (RTC) — RESIDENTIAL TREATMENT CENTER

CHAMPUS FORM 500 JUNE 1978

0 — (OL) — OTHER LOCATIONS

D — (STF) — SPECIALIZED TREATMENT FACILITY

Figure 15-7. CHAMPUS Form 500.

DOCTOR'S FIRST REPORT
OF
OCCUPATIONAL INJURY OR ILLNESS

AGRICULTURE AND SERVICES AGENCY
DEPARTMENT OF INDUSTRIAL RELATIONS
DIVISION OF LABOR STATISTICS AND RESEARCH
P. O. Box 965, San Francisco, Calif. 94101

Immediately after first examination mail one copy **directly** to the Division of Labor Statistics and Research. Failure to file a report with the Division is a misdemeanor. (Labor Code Section 6413.5) Answer all questions fully.

☞ A. INSURANCE CARRIER

Do not write in this space

1. **EMPLOYER**
2. Address (No., St. & City)
3. Business (Manufacturing shoes, building construction, retailing men's clothes, etc.)

4. **EMPLOYEE** (First name, middle initial, last name)   Soc. Sec. No.
5. Address (No., St. & City)
6. Occupation   Age   Sex
7. Date injured   Hour   M. Date last worked
8. Injured at (No., St. & City)   County
9. Date of your first examination   Hour   M. Who engaged your services?
10. Name other doctors who treated employee for this injury

11. **ACCIDENT OR EXPOSURE:** Did employee notify employer of this injury?   Employee's statement of cause of injury or illness:

12. **NATURE AND EXTENT OF INJURY OR DISEASE** (Include all objective findings, subjective complaints, and diagnoses. If occupational disease state date of onset, occupational history, and exposures.)

13. X-rays: By whom taken? (State if none)
    Findings:

14. Treatment:

15. Kind of case (Office, home or hospital)   If hospitalized, date   Estimated stay
    Name and address of hospital
16. Further treatment (Estimated frequency and duration)
17. Estimated period of disability for: Regular work   Modified work
18. Describe any permanent disability or disfigurement expected (State if none)

19. If death ensued, give date
20. **REMARKS** (Note any pre-existing injuries or diseases, need for special examination or laboratory tests, other pertinent information.)

Name   Degree   { PERSONAL SIGNATURE OF DOCTOR }
    (Type or print)
Date of report   Address (No., St. & City)

FORM 5021 (REV. 1)   *Use reverse side if more space required*

Figure 15-8. Worker's compensation form.

Claims cannot be processed until the Doctor's First Report of Work Injury is received. The injury date and claim number (when available) should always appear on any correspondence concerning the injury. The billing must include these data along with the name of the patient and the name of the patient's employer.

The medical assistant should keep current information concerning compensation cases readily available. This information should include the following:

1. Address for the state and federal compensation boards or commissions
2. State deadlines for filing Doctor's First Report of Occupational Injury or Illness
3. Current guidelines and fee schedule as published by the state workers' compensation carriers

GROUP PROGRAMS AND PLANS

There are two types of group programs. The first is employer sponsored (car dealers, school districts, industrial organizations, local power and water companies, retail department store chains, professional sports teams, private firms and businesses, local and county government agencies, suppliers of medical care, etc.) or union sponsored (retail clerks, meat cutters, textile workers, carpenters, plumbers, etc.). The second is sponsored by other organizations or associations (medical assistants' associations, lodges, clubs, societies, or fraternal organizations). Group officials determine which insurance company, health maintenance organization (HMO), or individual practice association (IPA) becomes the insurance carrier for the group, and also determine the specific benefits or exclusions of the plans. Participants may often have more than one option. For example, a large organization or union may offer prepaid medical insurance in an HMO, IPA, Blue Cross/Blue Shield plan, or private indemnity program. During the open enrollment period or at the time the employee is hired, the policy holder selects the plan. Some previously available plans may be canceled, with

new choices available after union negotiations. Small organizations generally have a single plan available for the group, and the group itself may help to select the plan.

MAJOR MEDICAL PLANS

Group major medical plans include both basic medical insurance and catastrophic coverage for costs of illness and injury beyond those covered in the basic medical portion. The employee and the employer may share the cost of the insurance (the premium) or the employee may pay 100% of the premium. These plans usually have annual individual and family deductible fees and require the employee to share the medical expenses, such as in an 80%-20% copayment agreement, up to a predetermined maximum cost. The plan pays 100% of all remaining eligible expenses in any calendar year.

Features of a major medical plan usually include hospital precertification. If precertification is required, the insurance plan must certify the reason for and planned length of the stay. If medical complications might prolong a hospital stay, the plan must be notified before the last designated day for recertification. Many plans require and pay for second opinions.

Many patients consider the freedom to choose a health care provider to be the most important feature of a major medical plan. Most plans include standard benefits, such as inpatient and outpatient psychiatric care, hospice care, well-baby care, and prescription discounts. Table 15–1 summarizes a typical major medical plan.

INDIVIDUAL POLICIES

A person who is not eligible for medical coverage through a group plan or a government program must apply to one of the many commercial insurance companies marketing individual medical insurance policies. Individual policies are usually the most expensive types

Table 15–1

FEATURES OF A TYPICAL GROUP MAJOR MEDICAL INSURANCE PLAN

Option		
Deductible fee (annual)	Individual	$300, $600, or $1000
	Family	$600, $1200, or $2000
Coinsurance	Employer/Employee	75%/25%
Maximum out-of-pocket expense (excluding deductible)	Individual	$1250
	Family	$2500
Precertification required		Yes
Second surgical opinion		100% deductible
Plan maximum		Unlimited
Obstetric coverage		Unlimited

of health insurance available. Group plans are required by the Continuation of Benefits Reconciliation Act (COBRA), to provide health care continuation coverage to employees when employment ends, or to employee spouses who become divorced or separated. COBRA plans are temporary extensions of health care coverage at the full group rate cost. Full group rate costs to the individual include both the employer's and the employee's contribution, plus an administrative fee. The extension period for individual policies under a group plan is 18 to 36 months, depending on the qualifying event.

CONTRACT VARIATIONS FOR GROUP OR INDIVIDUAL PLANS

When medical insurance coverage is obtained through a group or individual plan, the patient may have to decide between a plan that uses only contracted health care providers and one that allows freedom of choice in selecting a health care provider. Two general styles of restricted or preferred provider plans are (1) HMOs and (2) IPAs or IPPs.

HEALTH MAINTENANCE ORGANIZATIONS

An HMO is a group of practitioners within a self-contained corporation who share treatment space in the corporation buildings and provide a wide range of medical care for a fixed periodic payment. Ancillary services (laboratory, physical therapy, pharmacy, x-ray, central supply, etc.) may be located either in the facility or elsewhere. All routine medical care must be provided by members of the practice group. Exceptions are emergency care obtained at a local hospital, and emergency or nonemergency care received when the beneficiary is traveling outside the HMO service area. A client seeking nonemergency care away from home must contact the HMO for authorization before receiving care to obtain reimbursement for that care.

In return for fixed, prepaid fee, or *capitalization*, the HMO provides medical care for the participant and covered members of the family, regardless of the nature and number of services, through specified doctors participating hospitals. HMO plans are usually less expensive than group hospital and medical benefits under a major medical plan. A copayment agreement with the participant is usually a small rate payable when services are reduced, such as $5 or $10 per office visit or $5 per prescription or prescription refill. Referrals outside the HMO require prior approval from the HMO.

INDIVIDUAL PRACTICE ASSOCIATIONS AND INDIVIDUAL PROFESSIONAL PLANS

The IPAs and IPPs are composed of individual private practitioners who have contracted to provide medical care to members of the IPA or IPP groups for a specific fee per service. The members are not bound together in a corporate practice, facilities are not shared, and ancillary services are not centralized. Every subscriber must select a primary care physician who is responsible for coordinating medical care for that subscriber. As in the HMO plans, the subscriber must obtain prior authorization from the primary care physician before seeing a specialist, whether or not that specialist belongs to the plan, and within 48 hours of receiving emergency medical care from noncontracted providers, to obtain full reimbursement.

Specific hospitals contract with HMOs, IPAs, and IPPs for inpatient and outpatient care. All three types of plans have instigated cost-containment features resulting in premiums that cost considerably less than those for plans offering unrestricted choice of physicians. The major disadvantages to these restricted plans are (1) the lack or limited choice of participating physicians and (2) the need for prior authorization for a patient to see a specialist not belonging to the group, whether locally or outside the area covered by the plan. In duplicate coverage these service plans usually provide secondary coverage.

BLUE SHIELD AND BLUE CROSS PROGRAMS

The Blue Cross program originated in Texas during the Depression as a prepaid hospitalization plan. The American Hospital Association quickly endorsed the new medical insurance concept and marketed it to all the states. Several years later, a prepaid health plan called Blue Shield was established to cover physicians' charges for office visits and surgery. For years many people have had the misconception that Blue Cross and Blue Shield are a single insurance plan. This misconception arose when employers issued a single insurance identification card to their employees indicating that coverage included both plans. Usually, only Blue Shield is billed for physicians' services when patients have the combined plans. Blue Cross is billed by the hospital.

Most Blue Shield claims must be sent to the regional Blue Shield office where the policy originated. It is important to check the back of the subscriber's identification card for the correct mailing address.

In the late 1960s, large nationwide companies requested national coverage for their employees, and the Blue Shield permanent reciprocity program was developed. These plans are easily identified by the large red double-headed arrow on the subscriber's identification card. A capital N and a three-digit number are printed inside this arrow; they must be copied on the claim form during billing. The reciprocity plan claim form is sent to the local Blue Shield office (Fig. 15–9).

The medical assistant should instruct patients in the correct procedure for obtaining reimbursement for office visits. All claims should be filed no later than 1 year after the services were rendered. Reimbursement varies with the plan. In one method, the patient pays the physician and then applies for reimbursement from Blue Shield. In the second method, the physician files the claim and the patient is billed for any uncovered services after payment has been received from Blue

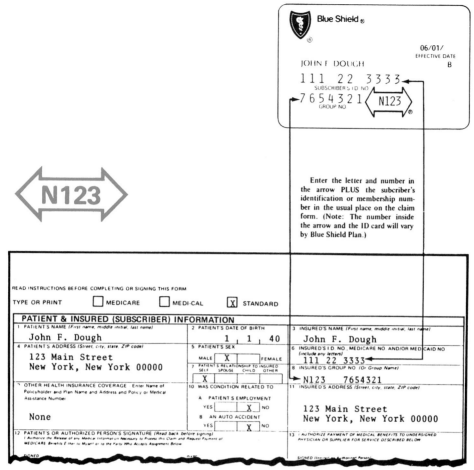

Figure 15-9. The large double-headed arrow on a Blue Shield subscriber's card indicates that his or her policy is part of a Blue Shield permanent reciprocity plan.

Shield. There are variations on these methods for reimbursement. For instance, physicians may become "members" of Blue Shield by signing a contract of participation with the regional corporation. A participating physician agrees to accept the local Blue Shield–determined fee, along with any applicable deductible fees and copayments, as payment in full under policies written by the local corporation.

All basic claims are filed on either a Blue Shield service report form or the HCFA Form 1500, depending on the requirement of the local corporation. Claims filed with a Blue Shield corporation based outside the local area should be filed on the HCFA Form 1500. (In Fig. 15-10, the areas blocked off are those not required in billing Blue Shield.) The patient obtains supplemental major medical forms from the employer or the local Blue Shield billing office. Provider representative departments are available to help with claim problems.

The medical assistant should keep the following information readily available and current:

1. Address and telephone number of the local Blue Shield office
2. Name and telephone number of the local Blue Shield professional representative

3. List of covered services for all local large Blue Shield plans
4. Preferred billing methods and claim forms used locally
5. Limits and provisions of the local reciprocity agreement

PREPARING AN INSURANCE CLAIM FORM

Most insurance companies and the federal and state government fiscal intermediaries accept the HCFA 1500 (12-90) claim form. The medical assistant must check the claim form identification numbers at the lower left corner to be sure that the 12-90 version is being used.

The claim form is divided into two sections. The top section is headed "Patient and Insured (Subscriber) Information," and the lower section is headed "Physician or Supplier Information." Some medical assistants ask the patient to complete the top portion of the form, but the medical assistant always completes the bottom portion (Fig. 15-11). Many insurance companies use electronic scanners. Claim forms are printed with a non-

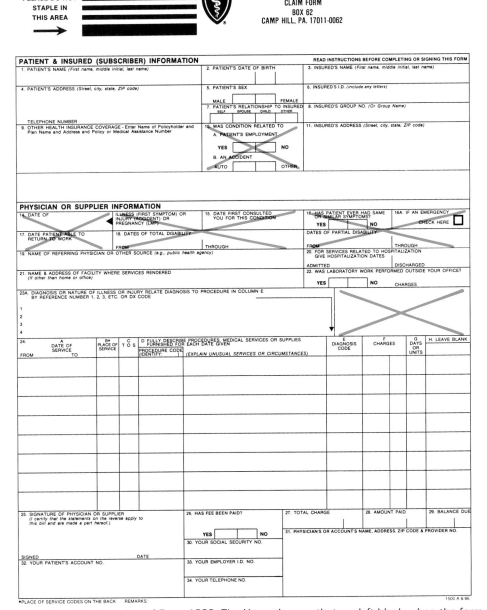

Figure 15-10. The Blue Shield version of Form 1500. The Xs mark areas that are left blank when the form is completed.

scannable red ink, so that the scanner reads only the typed information. All the data requested by the insurance company must be typewritten; handwritten information cannot be scanned.

The medical assistant should check the appropriate designated program box on the top line of the claim form directly under the heading "Health Insurance Claim Form." If the claim does not fall under the five government programs listed, the "Other" box is checked and the name of the insurance company typed in the blank space next to the heading. It is helpful to include the mailing address of the insurance company in the same box.

Each numbered box contains a specific prompt for information to be typed in that space. For example,

Item 1a indicates that a CHAMPUS claim needs both the sponsor's and the patient's social security numbers even if the patient is a minor. Furthermore, the Federal Employee Compensation Act (FECA), which covers work-related injury claims from federal workers, requests that the patient's (not the subscriber's) social security number appear in Item 1a (Fig. 15-12).

SPECIAL COMPANY INSURANCE FORMS

When a patient brings in a special company form that does not follow the HCFA 1500 format, the medical assistant should do the following:

1. Check to be sure that the patient or subscriber

PATIENT COMPLETES AND SIGNS FIRST 13 ITEMS

PLEASE DO NOT STAPLE IN THIS AREA

HEALTH INSURANCE CLAIM FORM

PICA

1. MEDICARE MEDICAID CHAMPUS CHAMPVA GROUP HEALTH PLAN FECA BLK LUNG OTHER 1a. INSURED'S I.D. NUMBER (FOR PROGRAM IN ITEM 1)
(Medicare #) (Medicaid #) (Sponsor's SSN) (VA File #) (SSN or ID) (SSN) (ID)

2. PATIENT'S NAME (Last Name, First Name, Middle Initial)
3. PATIENT'S BIRTH DATE MM DD YY SEX M F
4. INSURED'S NAME (Last Name, First Name, Middle Initial)

5. PATIENT'S ADDRESS (No., Street)
6. PATIENT RELATIONSHIP TO INSURED Self Spouse Child Other
7. INSURED'S ADDRESS (No., Street)

CITY STATE
8. PATIENT STATUS Single Married Other Employed Full-Time Student Part-Time Student
CITY STATE

ZIP CODE TELEPHONE (Include Area Code) ( )
ZIP CODE TELEPHONE (INCLUDE AREA CODE) ( )

9. OTHER INSURED'S NAME (Last Name, First Name, Middle Initial)
10. IS PATIENT'S CONDITION RELATED TO:
11. INSURED'S POLICY GROUP OR FECA NUMBER

a. OTHER INSURED'S POLICY OR GROUP NUMBER
a. EMPLOYMENT? (CURRENT OR PREVIOUS) YES NO
a. INSURED'S DATE OF BIRTH MM DD YY SEX M F

b. OTHER INSURED'S DATE OF BIRTH MM DD YY SEX M F
b. AUTO ACCIDENT? PLACE (State) YES NO
b. EMPLOYER'S NAME OR SCHOOL NAME

c. EMPLOYER'S NAME OR SCHOOL NAME
c. OTHER ACCIDENT? YES NO
c. INSURANCE PLAN NAME OR PROGRAM NAME

d. INSURANCE PLAN NAME OR PROGRAM NAME
10d. RESERVED FOR LOCAL USE
d. IS THERE ANOTHER HEALTH BENEFIT PLAN? YES NO If yes, return to and complete item 9 a-d.

READ BACK OF FORM BEFORE COMPLETING & SIGNING THIS FORM.
12. PATIENT'S OR AUTHORIZED PERSON'S SIGNATURE I authorize the release of any medical or other information necessary to process this claim. I also request payment of government benefits either to myself or to the party who accepts assignment below.
SIGNED ___ DATE ___
13. INSURED'S OR AUTHORIZED PERSON'S SIGNATURE I authorize payment of medical benefits to the undersigned physician or supplier for services described below.
SIGNED ___

MEDICAL ASSISTANT COMPLETES APPLICABLE ITEMS 14 THROUGH 33

14. DATE OF CURRENT: ILLNESS (First symptom) OR INJURY (Accident) OR PREGNANCY(LMP) MM DD YY
15. IF PATIENT HAS HAD SAME OR SIMILAR ILLNESS. GIVE FIRST DATE MM DD YY
16. DATES PATIENT UNABLE TO WORK IN CURRENT OCCUPATION FROM MM DD YY TO MM DD YY

17. NAME OF REFERRING PHYSICIAN OR OTHER SOURCE
17a. I.D. NUMBER OF REFERRING PHYSICIAN
18. HOSPITALIZATION DATES RELATED TO CURRENT SERVICES FROM MM DD YY TO MM DD YY

19. RESERVED FOR LOCAL USE
20. OUTSIDE LAB? YES NO $ CHARGES

21. DIAGNOSIS OR NATURE OF ILLNESS OR INJURY. (RELATE ITEMS 1,2,3 OR 4 TO ITEM 24E BY LINE)
1. ___ 3. ___
2. ___ 4. ___
22. MEDICAID RESUBMISSION CODE ORIGINAL REF. NO.
23. PRIOR AUTHORIZATION NUMBER

24. A DATE(S) OF SERVICE From To MM DD YY MM DD YY | B Place of Service | C Type of Service | D PROCEDURES, SERVICES, OR SUPPLIES (Explain Unusual Circumstances) CPT/HCPCS MODIFIER | E DIAGNOSIS CODE | F $ CHARGES | G DAYS OR UNITS | H EPSDT Family Plan | I EMG | J COB | K RESERVED FOR LOCAL USE

1
2
3
4
5
6

25. FEDERAL TAX I.D. NUMBER SSN EIN
26. PATIENT'S ACCOUNT NO.
27. ACCEPT ASSIGNMENT? (For govt. claims, see back) YES NO
28. TOTAL CHARGE $
29. AMOUNT PAID $
30. BALANCE DUE $

31. SIGNATURE OF PHYSICIAN OR SUPPLIER INCLUDING DEGREES OR CREDENTIALS (I certify that the statements on the reverse apply to this bill and are made a part thereof.)
SIGNED ___ DATE ___
32. NAME AND ADDRESS OF FACILITY WHERE SERVICES WERE RENDERED (If other than home or office)
33. PHYSICIAN'S, SUPPLIER'S BILLING NAME, ADDRESS, ZIP CODE & PHONE #
PIN# GRP#

(APPROVED BY AMA COUNCIL ON MEDICAL SERVICE 8/88) **PLEASE PRINT OR TYPE** FORM HCFA-1500 (12-90), FORM RRB-1500. FORM OWCP-1500

Figure 15–11. When using the universal health claim form (Form 1500) to file a claim, the patient may fill out part of the form while the medical assistant fills out the rest.

A FOR CHAMPUS CLAIMS, ENTER AN "X" IN THE CHAMPUS SQUARE IN BOX 1
AND ENTER THE SPONSOR'S SS NUMBER IN BOX 1a.

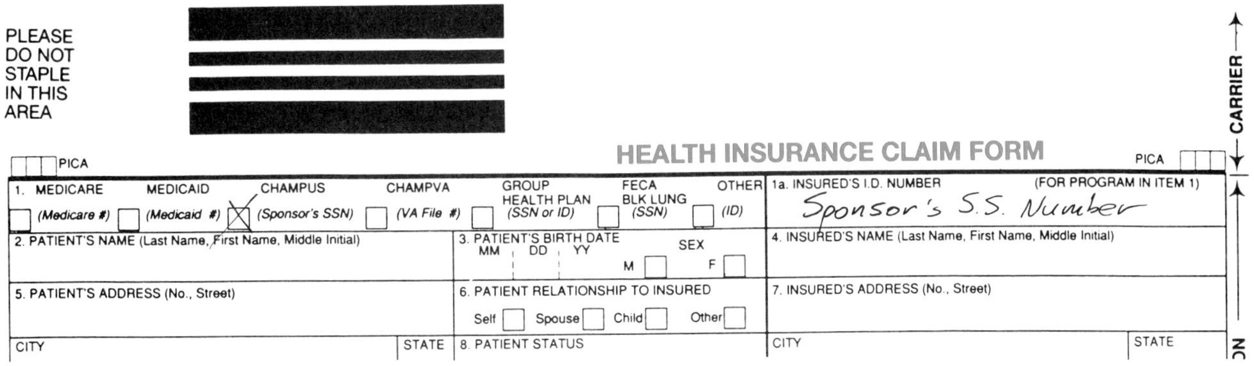

B FOR FECA CLAIMS, ENTER AN "X" IN THE FECA SQUARE IN BOX 1
AND ENTER THE FECA ID NUMBER IN BOX 1a.

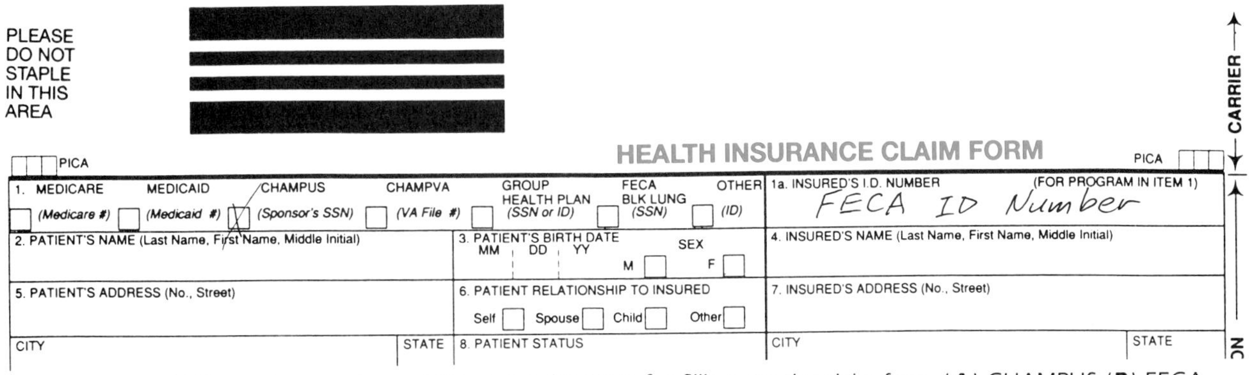

Figure 15–12. Different insurers have different requirements for filling out the claim form. (**A**) CHAMPUS (**B**) FECA.

has completed the employee or insured portion of the form.

2. Have the patient sign the authorizations for release of information and release of benefits to the provider on both the special company form and a copy of HCFA Form 1500. These authorizations are items 12 and 13 on the HCFA form.

3. Review the information in the provider portion of the company form to see if HCFA items 14 through 18 must be answered, and look for any questions not on the HCFA form.

4. Answer any questions on the company form that are not on the HCFA form.

5. Complete the HCFA form. Answer items 14 through 18 if they appear on the company form.

6. Copy both forms for the patient's records.

7. Staple the HCFA form to the company form and forward both to the insurance company.

All completed information should be carefully proofread to ensure its accuracy. Correct information is essential for the claim to be processed rapidly. If the company uses an optical scanner, even a typographical error can cause the claim to be rejected and returned to the office for corrections. A returned form results in payment delay.

CODING FOR INSURANCE CLAIMS

Originally coding was developed to assist in the organization of medical records for retrieval, research, and education. Today coding has become a part of government regulation for government insurance programs, such as Medicare and Medicaid, and for many private insurance companies as well. Despite the burdens that government regulation may impose, coding facilitates claim processing, and if done correctly, the amount and timeliness of payment awarded the physician.

Several different coding systems are used in insurance processing:

- ◼ *The California Standard Nomenclature* (CSN) (now rarely used)
- ◼ *Physician's Current Procedural Terminology* (CPT), published annually by the American Medical Association
- ◼ *The Health Care Procedural Coding System* (HCPCS), mandated by Congress for Medicare claims and updated annually
- ◼ *The International Classification of Diseases, Adapted, Revision 9, Clinical Modification* (ICD-9-CM, or ICD-9), published by the World Health Organization, with an *Official Authorized Addendum to ICD-9-CM* published each October.

It is extremely important to know exactly how to use these code books. Directions accompany each section of each book and should be followed precisely. The medical assistant should study each code book carefully to be completely familiar with each set of directions at billing time.

Because coding is revised annually, the medical assistant responsible for coding should attend at least one CPT and one ICD-9 class each year. In addition, it is essential to read the newsletters and bulletins prepared by Medicare and insurance companies, and the subscription services offered by coding book publishers, throughout the year. Failure to keep up to date could result in loss of income to the physician.

PROCEDURE CODES

Procedure codes are numbers that have been established and assigned to describe precisely every procedure performed and every service rendered by medical practitioners and their staffs.

The CSN and the CPT codes use five-digit codes and two-digit modifiers. HCPCS adds an alphanumeric system and local modifiers. Figure 15–13 shows representative samples of the CPT codes. Modifiers indicate that a standard procedure has been altered. For instance, −78 indicates that the patient returned to the surgery department for a related procedure during the postoperative period; −50 indicates that surgery is bilateral. The lists of modifiers should be studied because they increase or decrease the value of the service.

Government insurance programs (federal and state) and private insurance companies require CPT coding of all procedures submitted on claim forms. Otherwise, claims are suspended until further information is submitted or are rejected entirely.

The code for a visit with the physician indicates not only the level of care the patient received, but also where it was given (office, hospital, emergency department, home, or nursing facility), and whether the patient was new or established.

Codes may be accompanied by a brief description of the type of visit or the type of procedure performed. For example, after the code "99201" is entered, a brief description follows: "99201—Office visit, new patient." Because several codes exist for office visits alone, the medical assistant must be sure that the code selected describes precisely what procedure the physician performed.

DIAGNOSTIC CODES

Diagnostic codes have been established and assigned to describe precisely every disease, condition, problem, or diagnosis currently recognized. ICD-9 is recognized as the international standard for diagnostic coding. Figure 15–14 is part of a page from an ICD-9 coding manual.

The ICD-9 uses three-digit codes, with a fourth digit added when more detail is required regarding the cause, site, or manifestation of a disorder. Frequently, a fifth digit is added for even greater specificity.

ICD-9 coding is required on all Medicare claims, whether the physician is participating or not. Most private insurance companies also require ICD-9 diagnostic codes in addition to procedure codes. Through computer cross-checking, insurance companies compare the diagnostic codes with procedure codes stated on the claim form to determine whether the procedure is "medically necessary for prudent treatment of the patient's diagnosis, as it is stated on the claim form."

The complete set of ICD-9 books comprises three volumes, but only the first two are used routinely in the physician's office. Volume 1 lists conditions by code number and is organized into 17 chapters by body system. Volume 1 also contains two supplementary classifications ("Factors Influencing Health Status and Contact with Health Service," called *V codes,* and "External Causes of Injury and Poisoning," called *E codes*).

Volume 2 is organized into three sections: (1) "Index to Diseases and Injuries," (2) "Table of Drugs and Chemicals," and (3) "Index to External Causes of Injuries and Poisonings" (used with Volume 1, E codes). Within each section, the conditions or diseases are listed alphabetically. Volumes 1 and 2 are cross-referenced for each code.

Commercially published code books may be preferred over the traditional volumes. Commercial manuals include special hints and enhancements designed specially to help with coding for the medical office. This information includes:

1. Codes that should never be used
2. Codes that may result in delayed, reduced, or rejected claims
3. Codes that require additional information.

Selecting the proper codes requires using the patient's medical record and ledger card. The diagnosis

OFFICE X-RAY

Spine AP/Lat survey	72010
Cerv. spine AP & Lat	72040
Chest (2 views)	71020
Thoraco lumb. spine	72080
Sacroiliac 3 views	72202
Sacrum/coccyx	72220
Pelvis, complete	72190
Hip unilat comp.	73510
Clavicle	73000
Shoulder 3 views	73030
Humerus	73060
Elbow	73080
Forearm	73090
Wrist	73110
Wrist with navic	73110
Knee A/P and Lat	73560
Knee 3 views	73562
Tib/FIB	73590
Ankle	73610
Foot	73630

OUTPATIENT SURGERIES AND PROCEDURES

Appendectomy	44950
Breast Bx.-Exc	19120
Aorto/fem bypass	35546
Arthroscopy	
knee, diagnostic	29870
knee removal foreign body	29874
knee, debridement and shaving	
articular cartilage	29877
Arteriography	75718
Cardiac catheterization, left heart	
retrograde	93510
injection procedure	93544
imaging supervision	93555
Cardiovascular stress test	93017
Cholecystectomy	47600
w/cholangiograms	47605
w/open expl. common duct	47610
Laparoscopic chole. w/exploration	
common duct	56342
Colectomy w/colostomy	44140
Echocardiography, real time	93307
+Doppler echo. pulsed wave	93320
+Doppler colorflow	93325
Exc. exostosis/olecranon	24120
Femoropopliteal embolectomy	34210
Ing. hernia rep.	49505
Muscle biopsy	20206
CPR	92950
Cardioversion	92960
Laminectomy; first lumbar,	
decompression	63030
cervical	63020
Surgical assistant	-80

PROFESSIONAL SERVICE LABORATORY

BUN	84520
CBC with differential	85022
General health panel	80050
Hb	85018
Hct	85014
K-blood	84132
KOH/NACI	87220
Multichannel/panel	800__
Na-blood	84295
Obstetric panel	80055
Occult blood	82270
PAP (outside lab)	88150
Pro-time	85610
SED rate	85651
Strep throat/kit	87082
Torch antibody panel	80090
U. cult	87086
U/A without microscopy	81001
Venipuncture	36415
Wet mount	87210

PROCEDURES

All supplies	99070
Audiometry screen	92551
Biopsy	11100
Addt'l lesion	11101
Cryosurgery for acne	17340
Ear irrig. cerumen removal	69210
ECG tech. & prof.	93000
Endometrial Bx.	58100
Excision benign	11__
Excision malignant	116__
I & D abscess	10060
Nail removal	11750
Proctosigmoidoscopy, flexible	45330
Skin repair - complex	131__
Lac. repair - simple	120__
Spirometry	94010
Strapping	292__

Figure 15-13. Samples from the CPT code lists.

CIRCULATORY SYSTEM

442 Other aneurysm

Aneurysm (rupture) (cirsoid) (false) (varicose)
Aneurysmal varix

Excludes: arteriosclerotic cerebral (437)
arteriovenous (747.6, 747.8)
coronary (412)
heart (412)
ruptured cerebral (430)

443 Other peripheral vascular disease

443.0 Raynaud's syndrome

Raynaud's:
disease
gangrene
phenomenon (secondary)

443.1 Thrombo-angiitis obliterans (Buerger's disease)

443.2 Chilblains

Dermatitis congelationis
Pernio

443.8 Other

Acrocyanosis
Acroparesthesia:
simple (Schultze's type)
vasomotor (Nothnagel's type)
Erythrocyanosis
Erythromelalgia

Excludes: frostbite (991.0–991.3, E901)
immersion foot (991.4, E901)

443.9 Unspecified

Intermittent claudication
Peripheral vascular disease NOS
Spasm of artery

Excludes: spasm of cerebral artery (435)

ICD-9-CM diagnoses codes

Abdominal angina; Mesenteric artery syndrome; Chronic vascular insufficiency of intestine 5571	Acute bronchitis and bronchiolitis 466
Abnormal involuntary movements 7810	Acute conjunctivitis 3720
Abnormal loss of weight 7832	Acute delirium, not drug induced 2930
ABO incompatability 6562	Acute dilation of stomach 5361
Abruptio placentae; Placenta previa; Antepartum hemorrhage 641	Acute hysterical psychosis 2981
	Acute glomerulonephritis; Acute nephritis... 580
Abscess of anal and rectal regions 566	Acute laryngitis and tracheitis; Epiglottitis; Croup 464
Abscess of lung 513	Acute myocardial infarction 410
Achalasia and cardiospasm 5300	Acute myocarditis; Pericardial effusion..... 422
Achlorhydria 5360	Acute nasopharyngitis; Cold; U.R.I.......... 460
Acidosis (metabolic, respiratory) 2762	Acute nephritis; Acute glomerulonephritis... 580
Acne rosacea 6953	Acute pericarditis 420
Acne vulgaris (pustular, cystic, etc) 7061	Acute pharyngitis 462
Acquired deformities of foot and ankle 7367	Acute polyneuritis, infective; Guillain-Barre syndrome 3570
Acquired deformities of toes 735	Acute prostatitis 6010
Acquired hemolytic anemias 283	Acute pulmonary edema, not cardiac 5184
Acute alcoholic intoxication 3030	Acute pulmonary heart disease; Acute cor pulmonale 415
Acute and subacute endocarditis, bacterial.. 4210	
Acute bowel infarction; Mesenteric thrombosis; Intestinal gangrene 5570	Acute pyelonephritis; Acute pyelitis........ 5901
	Acute renal failure 584

Figure 15–14. Sample page from an ICD-9 coding manual.

must be validated by the medical record. For coding documentation, the medical record should contain the following:

- ❏ Chief complaint
- ❏ Present history with details of illness
- ❏ Type of examination performed
- ❏ Laboratory and diagnostic values and findings
- ❏ Diagnosis or complaint
- ❏ Detailed description of treatment

Insurance companies use only the coding on the claim form to determine whether a procedure is medically necessary for the "prudent treatment of the patient." However, the insurance company may request to see medical records. If a procedure was not documented, the company does not acknowledge it. Records must back up the coding to ensure that the physician always receives the maximum reimbursement. If the medical assistant cannot decide which code to use, the physician makes the final selection.

Miscoded claim forms can cause some or all procedures submitted to be declared "uncovered benefits" because the procedure coded was not medically necessary for treatment of the diagnosed disorder. Coding for procedures that were not performed may result in claims of insurance fraud against the physician, with fines and penalties up to $2000.

MEDICARE EVALUATION AND MANAGEMENT CODES

As part of the standardization of Medicare policies under OBRA 89, HCFA established the new uniform Evaluation and Management coding system for physicians' services. These codes will replace the former CPT physician visit codes by renumbering the CPT 90000 code range to a 99000 range. The new E and M 99000 codes must be used on all Medicare claims. HCFA publishes a cross-reference guide to old and new coding.

The new E and M codes are based on three key components of medical care: history, examination, and medical decision making. In addition, the system includes the contributory factors of counseling, coordination of care, and the severity of the problem; and a time factor for all services rendered directly by the physician to the patient or the patient's family.

Component 1: Patient history. Four types of histories are recognized:

- ❏ Problem focused: Chief complaint, brief history of present illness or problem
- ❏ Expanded problem focused: Chief complaint, brief history of present illness; system review of presenting problems
- ❏ Detailed: Chief complaint, extended history of present illness; extended system review; past, family, and/or social history included
- ❏ Comprehensive: Chief complaint, extended history of present illness; complete system review; complete past, family, and/or social history

Component 2: Type of examination. Four types of examination are recognized:

- ❏ Problem focused: Examining only the affected body area or organ system
- ❏ Expanded problem focused: Examining the affected body area or organ system and other symptomatic or related organ systems
- ❏ Detailed: Extended examination of the affected body area and other symptomatic or related organ systems
- ❏ Comprehensive: Complete single-system specialty examination or complete multisystem examination

Component 3: Medical decision making. Medical decisions are recognized and defined as:

- ❏ Straightforward
- ❏ Low complexity
- ❏ Moderate complexity
- ❏ High complexity

The three contributory factors are defined as

1. Counseling with the patient and/or the patient's family regarding any of the following:
   - ❏ Diagnosis and prognosis
   - ❏ Informed consent (risks and benefits of treatment options)
   - ❏ Instruction and follow-up care
   - ❏ Compliance and risk factor follow-up
   - ❏ Patient and family education
2. Coordination of care in other facilities, such as hospitals, emergency departments, and nursing facilities
3. Seriousness of presenting problem. Five levels of problem are recognized:
   1. Minimal
   2. Self-limited or minor
   3. Low severity
   4. Moderate severity
   5. High severity

Time

Time inclusion as a separate factor is new. The time factor assists in selecting the most appropriate level of service. *Time in the office* is the time that the physician typically spends face to face with the patient, the patient's family, or both. *Time for hospital care* is the time the physician spends in the patient's unit and at the bedside. *Face-to-face time* is time the physician spends with the patient only. Face-to-face time with the medical assistant, to obtain a history, for instance, is not included in the code used for the office visit or consultation.

Same-Day Service Coding

In general, the visit descriptors contain the phrase "per day," referring to all services provided on that day. The code should reflect all services provided on that day *for related problems*. There are exceptions if, for example, two visits in one day are for unrelated problems, or if a patient does not need critical care initially but requires it later in the day. If multiple services are performed in one day for related problems, reporting two or more management service codes would be considered duplicative. The following situations, while not entirely inclusive, can be used as starting guidelines:

If a patient seen in the office is admitted to a hospital on the same date, the office services must be "rolled up" into the initial hospital care code.

If a patient is seen in the office at 3:30 PM and admitted to the hospital at 2:00 AM the next day, both the office visit and initial hospital care may be reported because the phrase "same date" refers to calendar dates rather than to 24-hour periods.

If a patient is admitted to the hospital and discharged on the same day, only the appropriate code for initial hospital inpatient services may be used.

If a physician performs a hospital visit and a hospital discharge on the same day, only the hospital discharge code is used for the final day of the hospital stay.

Evaluation and management services in a nursing facility on the same date are "rolled up" into the initial nursing facility care code, even if the physician saw the patient first in the office or an emergency department. If a nursing facility patient is admitted to the hospital and the physician saw the patient in both places on the same day, only the initial hospital inpatient service code may be used.

Emergency and Critical Care Codes

Time is deliberately not included in the emergency department visit codes because emergency situations have too many variables. If a patient is admitted to the hospital through the emergency department, all physician's services provided in conjunction with the admission are considered part of the initial hospital care when performed on the same date as the admission. A physician who treats a patient registered in the emergency department of a hospital may use emergency department services codes.

Critical care codes are intended for all critical care services that require the constant attention of the physician. Critical care includes treatment for cardiac arrest, shock, bleeding, respiratory failure, and postoperative complications. Critical care is usually given in an intensive care unit, respiratory care unit, or emergency department. Noncritical procedures (e.g., joint reduction, casting, and bladder tapping) are not included in the critical care codes and should be reported separately.

If an office visit is for a true emergency, appropriate office codes must be used. Emergency department codes may not be used if the patient is not treated in an organized hospital-based facility. However, nonemergency services performed in the emergency department normally are designated by lower-level emergency codes. Office codes should be used if the patient is seen in the emergency room as a convenience to the physician.

Consultation

If the physician assumes responsibility for patient care following a consultation, the initial consultation should be reported using the appropriate consultation code. Subsequent visits are then reported as established patient office visits or subsequent hospital care, depending on the setting.

A new patient is defined as one who has not received any professional services from the physician within the past 3 years. If, in a multiphysician practice, a physician in the same specialty has seen and billed a patient within 3 years, the patient is considered "established." A physician consultation may result in a consultation with another physician in the same group practice.

Medical Assistant Duties

One specific E and M code, 99211, is defined as "Office or other outpatient visit for the evaluation and management of an established patient, that may not require the presence of a physician." This code can be reported if a physician's employee performs a limited service that does not require the supervision of a physician. However, this code cannot be reported in addition to other E and M services performed *by the physician* on the same day.

Payment for Technical Components of Services

The Omnibus Budget Reconciliation Act of 1990 (OBRA 90) prohibits Medicare payment for the physician's interpretation of electrocardiograms (ECG) performed in conjunction with a visit or consultation. The technical component (performance) of the ECG may be billed if the ECG is performed in the physician's office.

In general, new-physician reimbursement is at a decreased percentage for the first 4 years of practice. There are exceptions to this rule.

Although medical supplies are generally considered a part of practice expense and the physician cannot request separate payment, payment for supplies is allowed if certain procedures are performed in the physician's office. These allowable procedures are listed in the CPT code book. The cost of drugs is excluded from the fee schedule and is paid according to the purchase price or the wholesale price, whichever is lower. Injections performed in conjunction with a visit cannot be billed separately. If no E and M service occurs at the time of an injection, payment is based on the appropriate CPT code. Chemotherapy is billed as a separate procedure.

PROCESSING INSURANCE PAYMENTS

Insurance claim reimbursement is based on four criteria: (1) Usual, customary, and reasonable (UCR), (2) the Medicare Resource-Based Relative Value Scale (RBRVS), (3) fee schedules, and (4) diagnosis-related groups (DRGs).

REIMBURSEMENT DETERMINATION

The UCR fee is determined by comparing the actual fee charged by a physician with the fees charged by other physicians in the same geographic area and specialty. The *usual fee* is the fee charged by the physician submitting the claim. The *customary fee* is the fee charged by other physicians. The *reasonable fee* may not match the usual or the customary fee, but can be accepted if it accounts for any unusual circumstances, such as additional skill or time required for the service. Some UCR plans require physicians to accept UCR payment as payment in full, whereas others do not.

The RBRVS system bases fees on the conversion factors that indicate the relative value of the service performed. Procedures are coded with relative value units that reflect the skill and time required, the geographic location of the practice, and the overhead cost of each service. From the codes, the unit values are converted on a scale to dollar amounts and represent the new RBRVS fee schedule. (A fee schedule is a list of accepted payments for services decided in advance by an insurance plan.) Medicare reimburses 80% of the fee schedule amount; the patient is responsible for the other 20%. While the RBRVS system is being phased in (1992 to 1996) and depending on the historic geographic UCR payment, physicians will be reimbursed according to either the RBRVS schedule or a blend of RBRVS and UCR. In 1996, reimbursement will be based totally on the RBRVS fee schedule. Fee schedules may be based on the UCR and RBRVS experience of other insurance companies.

EXPLANATION OF BENEFITS

Regardless of the plan, insurance payments sent directly to the physician should be accompanied by an Explanation of Benefits (EOB) form (Fig. 15–15), which details how the insurance payment was calculated and why any procedure was declared an "uncovered benefit." This document explains any deductible fees and copayments for which the patient is responsible. It may also advise the physician of any portions to be "written off" because of the physician's participation in the insurance plan. The medical assistant should review each EOB before posting the check to be sure that all procedures submitted on the claim form were processed and that the amount allowed for each procedure is within the expected payment range.

If the insurance payment is lower than expected, the medical assistant should compare the procedures listed on the EOB with those listed on the office copy of the claim. If a processing error by the insurance company is suspected, the medical assistant must request a correction. The medical assistant should copy the office copy of the billing form; copy the EOB, highlighting the procedure in question; and write a brief note requesting that the billing be reviewed. The same process applies to a procedure that is not reimbursed because it was "incompatible with the diagnosis" when in fact it was medically necessary. A copy of a pathology report, discharge summary, or operative report accompanying the original billing often forestalls these misunderstandings.

If the payment was due to an error on the original claim form, the medical assistant should submit a corrected claim and send a copy of the EOB with a request for reconsideration of the data. If the error was due to a surgery coding error, a copy of the operative report is attached. If the error was due to an omission of one or more procedures from the claim form, no additional documentation is needed.

Blue Cross, Blue Shield, Medicare, CHAMPUS/CHAMPVA, IPAs, IPPs, and Medicaid (Medi-Cal) often process claims in batches. One check combines payments for all claims submitted by the physician or physician group during the specified period (weekly, semimonthly, or monthly). In these cases, the EOB accompanying the payments lists all claims processed during the current period. Each claim is listed separately on the EOB, with a full accounting of how payment was determined on each claim. The medical assistant should ensure that the total amount of the check agrees with the combined amounts credited as payment for each claim, and should verify claims as described above for the individual EOB (Fig. 15–16).

PATIENT TEACHING CONSIDERATIONS

The medical assistant must be well informed in all aspects of insurance billing. This is necessary not only for processing claim forms and directing them to the proper agency, but also to help the patient deal with medical insurance complexities. The medical assistant is not permitted to interpret the patient's actual policy or extent of coverage. The patient must consult his or her employer's personnel office for a group plan, or the company representative for an individual plan. However, the medical assistant may help the patient in many other ways. Examples would include explaining the claim form and what information is required, explaining the importance of providing the office with the identifying eligibility form for Medicaid, outlining the CHAMPUS/CHAMPVA or Medicare basic program, and advising the patient of the difference between Medicare parts A and B. The medical assistant must also teach patients to be accurate in completing their forms when they themselves bill the insurance company to obtain payment for services. The essential information for billing includes the proper diagnosis and diagnosis code, the dates and places of service, the procedure

BLUE SHIELD of California

P O BOX 3637, SAN FRANCISCO, CA 94119 (415) 445-5151
P.O. BOX 92945, LOS ANGELES, CA 90009 (213) 642-5600

PATIENT'S NAME	GROUP NO	SUBSCRIBER NO.	CLAIM NO.	PROVIDER OF SERVICES	MO.	DAY	Y
JONES MARY	9900-000	R12345678	0278258000000	SMITH JOHN	09	21	87

A CLAIM HAS BEEN RECEIVED FOR THE SERVICES SHOWN BELOW. IT HAS BEEN PROCESSED
IN ACCORDANCE WITH THE BENEFITS OF THE SUBSCRIBER'S BLUE SHIELD HEALTH PLAN

EXPLANATION OF BENEFITS

FOR THE CLAIM RECEIVED ON   9/15/78

JONES MARY A.
123 Main Street
Downtown, Ca. 92349

PHYSICIAN MEMBER - YES   9148292

SERVICES BILLED	PROC. NO.	DATES OF SERVICE FROM MO	YR.	DAY	TO DAY	NO. OF SERVICES	AMOUNT BILLED	MAX. CONTRACT AMOUNT PAYABLE BY BLUE SHIELD	UNPAID AMOUNT	CODE	AMOUNT PAID
HOME/OFFICE	9000C	09	01			01 0	15 00		15 00	1	00
LABORATORY	81000	09	01			01 0	5 00	5 00			5 00
RADIOLOGY	71020	09	01			01 0	20 00		20 00	2	00

UNPAID CODE EXPLANATION

1   THIS SERVICE IS NOT A BENEFIT OF THE BASIC COVERAGE. SUPPLEMENTAL BENEFITS MAY APPLY -
SUBSCRIBER SHOULD SUBMIT BILL WITH SUPPLEMENTAL CLAIM FORM FOR REVIEW.

2   X-RAY SERVICES NOT RELATED TO A SPECIFIC ILLNESS OR INJURY ARE NOT A BENEFIT OF THE
FEDERAL EMPLOYEE PROGRAM.

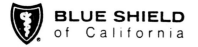

BLUE SHIELD
of California

720 CALIFORNIA ST • SAN FRANCISCO. CA 94108
5959 W CENTURY BLVD. • LOS ANGELES. CA 90045

PAID TO

JOHN SMITH, M.D., INC.
777 MEDICAL CENTER DRIVE
DOWNTOWN, CA 92349

PROVIDER NO	CHECK NO.
00A123450	**9148292**

MO	DAY	YEAR	PAY DOLLARS	CENTS
09	21		$*******5	00

*******5*DOLLARS**00*CTS

NOT NEGOTIABLE

Figure 15-15. An explanation of benefits (EOB) statement from Blue Shield.

Notice of Payment

Provider
MELVA WEEKS, M.D. 1002 Cesaro Court, N.W. Washington, D.C. 20013

Blue Shield.

Medical Service of D.C.
550 12th Street S.W.
Washington D.C. 20024

Physicians' Service:
Washington   479-6560
Maryland   479-6570
Virginia   479-6580

Date	3/1/82
Physician or Hospital Number	XXXX
Page	01

Patient's Name		ID Number	Claim and Patient Number (If Applicable)	Date of Service						Type of Service	Provider Charges		Allowed Benefits		Amount Paid		Payment		Remarks Code	Physici Numbe
Last	First			From			To				$	¢	$	¢	$	¢	Code	Percent		
				M	D	Y	M	D	Y											
JONES	CELIA	R23478138 PAT #	2012195711 37192	1	3	82	1	3	82	SURG	100	00	70	00	56	00	R	80		
HARRIS	S.	123567890	2003175430	1	2	82	1	2	82	EFA	35	00	35	00	35	00	P	100	****	
ROBERTS	SUE	165342800	2020134890	1	16	82	1	30	82	RAD	60	00	50	00	50	00	C	100	****	
ROBERTS	SUE		2020234890	1	16	82	1	16	82	SUR	200	00	125	00	125	00	C	100		
FRANK	JOAN	F21247983	211241374	2	5	82	2	8	82	SUR	80	00	60	00	3	00	M			
WISE	MARY	065319217	2075175132 NOT PROVIDED	3	15	82	3	15	82	SUR	30	00	21	00	21	00	1	100		
OATS	BILL	577134214 PAT #	2071101133 178244	2	24	82	2	24	82	SUR	20	00	9	00	9	00	B	100		
PARKS	EARL	R07113842	2040171235	12	4	81	12	4	81	INJ	25	00	6	04	6	04	AK		****	
QUEEN	JOHN	R13411321 PAT #	2009195703 3429622	1	15	82	1	15	82	LAB	44	00	39	00	31	25	R	80		
SAMUELS	DON	R01781140	2012177249	12	9	81	12	9	81	MED	89	50	14	00	14	00	AP		****	
SAMUELS	DON	R01781140	2012277249	12	9	81	12	9	81	SUR	426	50	85	30	85	30	MP		****	
TUSCON	JOHN	175342100	2099185346	2	8	82	2	8	82	SUR	75	00	75	00	75	00				
TUSCON	JOHN	175342100	2099185346	2	8	82	2	8	82	SUR	75	00	50	00	50	00CR				3401
WHITE	DONNA	081254344	2095123456 NOT PROVIDED	1	23	82	1	23	82	LAB	30	00								0433

0433	BASIC COVERAGE EXCLUDES OBSTETRICAL SERVICES
3401	THIS IS AN ADJUSTMENT OF A PREVIOUSLY PAID CLAIM

Payments indicated by asterisks(••••) in Remarks Code field represent payment in full.

4C6-5696   Rev. 11/80

See Participating Handbook for explanation of Codes and Method of Appeals.

TOTAL	$460 59	CHECK NUMBER	234567

Figure 15–16. A combined explanation of benefits (EOB) from Medicare.

codes, and the individual cost of each service. Other patient instruction may include checking the EOB with the patient to ensure that all benefits have been paid properly, and instructing the patient on follow-up inquiries for improperly paid claims.

LEGAL AND ETHICAL IMPLICATIONS

Medical assistants who have the responsibility of filing medical insurance claims should be aware of two important legal issues: breach of confidentiality and fraud.

CONFIDENTIALITY

Breach of confidentiality is the unauthorized release of confidential patient information to a third party (a person other than the patient, physician, or staff members). A written consent to release medical information must be obtained from the patient, parent, or legal guardian before a claim form can be completed. After the patient signs a release (authorization for release of medical information) on a master claim form, a photo-

copy of the form should be placed in the patient's record, and another copy should be attached each time the insurance is billed to the company. All claims filed within the dates stated on the release form should have the words *signature on file* typed on the claim form in box 12 (Fig. 15–17).

A signed release of information is restricted to information necessary for processing a particular insurance claim. The medical assistant must verify that anyone calling the office about a claim is legitimately entitled to that patient's information. To verify the legitimacy of a caller, the medical assistant could pull the copy of the claim from the file and ask the caller to read the wording in question from the original claim. Another method for verification is asking to return the call. Bona fide insurance clerks will readily provide the company phone number. The switchboard operator will identify the company when the medical assistant returns the call. If the caller objects to these verification procedures, the medical assistant should refuse to give any information over the telephone. The caller should be asked to submit the request in writing on company stationery, specifying exactly what information is needed. Signed releases and official letters requesting

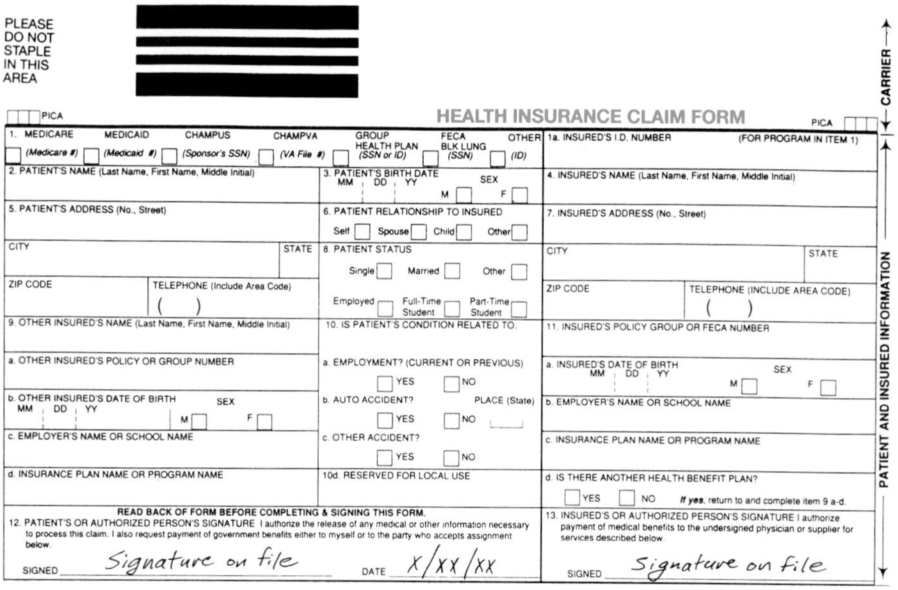

Figure 15-17. Claim marked "signature on file."

information prove that breach of confidentiality or invasion of privacy has not occurred.

FRAUD

Fraud is the deliberate misrepresentation of facts. The patient may ask that the date of services, the description of procedures, or the diagnosis on a claim be changed. If, for example, the date of a service is changed, the patient may collect undue benefits. A change of diagnosis could result in collection when the actual disorder was excluded from the patient's policy. Patients may also request a copy of their year's billing and ask that any insurance payments listed on the ledger be omitted from the typed statement. In these instances, the patient's objective may be to obtain an inflated medical deduction on income tax or to collect from a second insurance company. The medical assistant must tell the patient firmly but politely that the records will not be altered or adjusted in any way.

Another situation that could involve the medical assistant is a request that a diagnosis not entered on the patient's record be entered on the claim form. Compliance with this request constitutes fraud by deliberate misrepresentation of the facts. All insurance companies have the right to audit medical records and ledgers at any time, and the medical assistant is responsible for seeing that they are true and accurate.

The medical assistant should be aware that participating physicians have signed a contract to accept the insurance company's maximum fee as the total fee to be billed for covered services. The patient may not be billed for any amount on the claim form greater than the insurance company's allowable fee. Exceptions, of course, include authorized deductible fee and coinsurance. The patient may be billed for the physician's total fee for any *uncovered* services.

The procedure for processing an insurance claim form is detailed at the end of this chapter.

SUMMARY

This chapter provides techniques for prompt and accurate claim processing. These techniques can be summarized as follows:

1. Photocopy insurance identification cards at the first visit; photocopy Medicaid identification cards at the first visit of each month.
2. Record all patient identifying information accurately.
3. Be particularly careful about transferring identifying numbers (social security, policy or member numbers, address, and age and birthdate).
4. Check to be sure that the release form is signed or that a copy of a release of information form is on file.
5. Secure an assignment-of-benefit signature if this is the office policy.
6. Enter information for only one patient on a claim form.
7. Use the proper ICD-9-CM, CPT, CSN, or HCPCS code for each procedure billed.
8. Do not list several procedures as one unless the codes permit this.
9. List injections; state injectable material and the amount given.
10. If there are multiple visits on the same day, state the time of day for each visit.

11. Make a copy of the claim form for referrals, whether to or from another provider of service, and keep the copy on file.
12. Attach reports, such as operative reports or discharge summaries, that assist in processing complicated claims.
13. Enter the physician's actual fee regardless of payment expected.
14. Process claims immediately.
15. Secure the signature of the provider on those claims that require it.
16. Date and initial the forms you prepare.
17. Make a chart and ledger card notation when the insurance form is mailed.
18. Make and keep a carbon or photocopies of all forms.

These techniques, if practiced precisely, result in patient satisfaction, quick receipt of third-party payments, and a well-managed cash flow in the office.

DISCUSSION QUESTIONS

1. Discuss the skills and attitudes that the medical assistant should possess for insurance processing.
2. Describe the code books used in insurance billing and discuss the importance of their accurate use.
3. Name the form that is used for the Medicare, Medicaid, and CHAMPUS/CHAMPVA fiscal intermediaries.
4. Discuss the various legal ramifications that the medical assistant must consider in insurance billing.
5. Describe the steps you should take to ensure that your billing was clean and accurate.
6. Define the term *participating physician.*
7. List the most important aspects of the workers' compensation program report forms.

BIBLIOGRAPHY

American Association of Medical Assistants: A User's Guide to the Resource Based Relative Value Scale. American Association of Medical Assistants, Chicago 1992.
American Medical Association: CPT-4 1992. American Medical Association, Chicago, 1991.
Gylys B: Computer Applications for the Medical Office. FA Davis, Philadelphia, 1991.
Lane K (ed): The Saunders Manual of Medical Assisting Practice. WB Saunders, Philadelphia, 1992.
ICD-9-CM International Classification of Diseases, revision 9, ed 4, vols 1–3. Clinical Modification, 1992. Practice Management Information Corporation, Los Angeles, 1992.
Kotoski GN: CPT Coding Made Easy: A Technical Guide, ed 2. Aspen, Gaithersburg, MD, 1992.
RBRVS Fee Schedule: A Plain English Guide, Part B News. Federal Register 56:227, November 25, 1991.

PROCEDURE: Process an insurance claim

Terminal Performance Objective: Process patient claims using the HCVA Form 1500, in mailable quality and without errors that may result in rejection, within a reasonable period.

EQUIPMENT: Patient medical history
Patient registration form
Patient superbill or ledger card

PROCEDURE

1. Check the applicable program box.

Patient and Insured (Subscriber Information):

2. Complete items 1-5.
   a. Last name first
   b. Use 6-digit dates, for example, 05-23-50, for all entries.

3. Complete item 6. Include any letters or suffixes that appear with the number.

4. Complete items 7-11.
   a. If the patient is covered by a health plan, the group number is on the patient's insurance card.
   b. List all other plans the patient has reported to the office or list "none."
   c. Include the patient's telephone number.
   d. Have the patient sign item 12. If the patient has not signed the form, write "signature on file" or "release attached."
   e. Have the patient sign item 13.

   f. If the insurance company requires its own form, have the patient sign the plan form and attach it to Health Care Financing Administration (HCFA) Form 1500.

Physician or Supplier Information:

5. Write "N/A" for items 14-18.

6. Complete items 19-23.
7. Complete items 23, 1-4. Specifically list
   a. Principal diagnosis and International Classification of Diseases (ICD) 9 code
      b. Each secondary diagnosis and ICD-9 code.

8. Complete items 24, A-G.
   a. Use 6-digit dates
   b. Look for place of service codes on the back of the form.
   c. Enter the CPT code for and the description of each charge for service. List each service individually.

PRINCIPLE

1. Checking the box indicates the insurance plan being billed.

3. The patient number, usually the social security number, is the beneficiary's individual identification number. The letter describes the patient's membership in the program.
4.
   a. In a group plan, the patient's first reference number is the group number.
   b. It is necessary to know all the patient's plans for the purpose of coordinating benefits.

   d. Forms must include the patient's signature as permission to release medical records.

   e. The patient's signature on item 13 authorizes the insurance company to pay the claim benefits directly to the physician. Some companies require their own forms to be on file in addition to HCFA Form 1500.

5. Items 14-18 are in cases relating to accident and injury (e.g., worker's compensation) or pregnancy.

7. Correct listing and coding establish that the condition is covered and has been treated in a timely manner. The principal and secondary diagnostic codes may change under special patient circumstances (modifiers) that require special services and reports or additional procedures and treatments.

   b. Place of service codes indicate where the services were performed.
   c. Services may include, but not be limited to, procedures, treatments, diagnostic tests and procedures, medical and surgical supplies, injections and drugs, laboratory tests, and materials.

PROCEDURE

    d. Cross-reference by entering the diagnosis number 1–4 from item 23 above, or enter the ICD-9 code again for each service.

    e. Enter the fee posted on the ledger card for each service.

    f. Enter the number of times each service was rendered, if more than once.

    g. Type of service codes are on the back of the form. List only one code per line.

    h. Leave item 24H blank.

9. Complete items 25–27.

    a. Have the physician sign the form or use a facsimile signature stamp. Initial the box.

    b. If the physician is a participating plan provider, check "yes" to accepting the assignment of benefits.

    c. Add up the charges and check the totals against the patient's ledger card.

10. Skip items 28–30.

11. Complete item 31. Stamp or write the provider information, including the identification number.

12. Complete item 32 if the office uses a numbering system for filing patient accounts.

13. Enter the physician's federal identification number (the license number) under item 33.

14. Review the entire form for errors and omissions.

15. Have the form signed.

16. Photocopy the form and place the copy in the patient's file.

17. Mail the claim to the appropriate carrier.

PRINCIPLE

    d. Cross-referencing justifies why the particular service was performed.

    e. All procedures must be itemized individually.

    h. Item 24H is filled in by the insurance company.

    a. A signature must appear on all claims. Initials identify who prepared the form.

    b. If the assignment is accepted, the physician agrees to accept the allowable charges as payment in full.

    c. Checking the total charges ensures that the full charge is submitted whether or not the patient has already paid a portion of the fee.

10. The insurance company has not made any prepayment to the physician. The balance due reported to the insurance company should equal the total charges on the patient ledger card.

11. The identification number is the physician's license number, which is issued by the state and is required by the Internal Revenue Service. This number is also used to keep track of the physician's income.

12. The number in item 32 provides a billing cross reference for computer use.

13. Each physician in a group practice has a separate tax identification number.

14. Errors and omissions may result in decreased payment or denial of benefits.

15. Each form must have the physician's signature.

16. If a claim is lost or rejected, the copy will provide a means of tracking the claim.

17. Timely submission usually results in a 15- to 17-day processing period and quicker payments.

Section II

Clinical Procedures

Unit 4

Clinical Responsibilities

The chapters in this unit focus on clinical medical assisting skills, which pertain to preparing the patient for examination and assisting patient and physician during patient examination and treatment. The assistant must anticipate the physician's needs as to the type of examination, the specific equipment needed, and the extent of assistance required by the patient. This requires judgment based on a reasonable understanding of physical examinations, the methods and equipment used, and the related role of the medical assistant.

The first logical step in patient care is to determine the nature of the patient's problem; in most cases, this requires a general or specific physical examination. The adequately prepared medical assistant should be able, upon learning the reason for a patient's visit, to prepare the examination room and equipment and to provide assistance during the examination as required.

Once the physical examination has been completed, the next step is treating the patient. The physician will choose the appropriate treatment modalities. The medical assistant will be expected to provide knowledgeable support to the physician and guidance to the patient. To function successfully in the clinical setting, the medical assistant must perform the role of facilitator. Integration of the knowledge and skills essential to this role is the goal of this unit.

Unit Objectives

Upon completing this unit, you will be able to:

1. Describe the techniques for obtaining and recording the patient interview.
2. Explain and demonstrate the technique for obtaining and recording vital signs.
3. Describe how to prepare the patient for examination.
4. Describe the medical assistant's role in assisting with the general physical examination, as well as with each of the specific examinations.
5. Recognize nutrition and diet therapy as a treatment alternative, and describe need assessment and patient teaching associated with therapeutic diets.
6. Understand basic pharmacologic concepts and how they relate to drug administration and demonstrate the administration of medications.
7. Identify instruments required to perform medical office surgery and describe tray setup and patient preparation for minor surgery.
8. Explain the role of rehabilitative medicine in treatment.
9. Describe common medical office emergencies and treatment responses.
10. Perform clinical procedures related to medical office practice.
11. Construct a dietary modification plan.
12. Follow OSHA standards in performing clinical procedures.

> **I**t is as important to know the person who has the disease as to know the disease the person has.
>
> Sir William Osler

CHAPTER OUTLINE

LEARNING OBJECTIVES

Upon completing this chapter, you will be able to:

1. Identify the elements of the source-oriented and problem-oriented medical records.
2. Explain the purpose and types of information needed for each element or section of the patient history.
3. Apply interview methods for collecting data for each section of the narrative history, initial database, and subjective, objective, assessment, and plan (SOAP) note.
4. Identify and apply the guidelines for effective documentation.
5. Describe the characteristics of ineffective documentation.
6. Discuss the legal implications of the patient history and interviewing process.

PERFORMANCE OBJECTIVES

Upon completing this chapter, you will be able to:

1. Obtain accurate and full information from the patient related to the patient's past health and present conditions for the physician's use in creating a health care plan.

320

Chapter **16**

*P*atient History and Physical Assessment

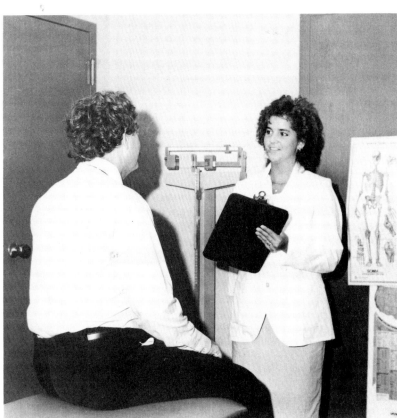

2. Record the data using clear and concise language and appropriate terminology on a source-oriented or problem-oriented medical record.

DACUM EDUCATIONAL COMPONENTS

1. Interview and take a patient history (4.6)
2. Interview effectively (2.9)
3. Use medical terminology appropriately (2.10)
4. Maintain confidentiality (1.4)
5. Assist the physician with examination and treatments (4.8)
6. Document accurately (5.1)

Glossary

Assessment: Questions regarding the patient's current health status which are asked at the beginning of each office visit
Documentation: Accountable recordkeeping
Health: State of physical, mental, and social well-being
History: Systematic, thorough discussion and recording of all relevant past medical data that may affect current or future patient care
Sign: A physical change in the body apparent to the physician on objective assessment or that can be measured scientifically
Symptom: A physical change in the body apparent only to the patient experiencing the physical change

The first and most fundamental step in the clinical process is the patient interview. Its purpose is to collect data that will enable the physician to develop a plan of care. The interview is organized into two parts: the history and the physical assessment.

The *history* is a logically organized discussion and recording of prior health status and significant medical events that may or may not affect the current diagnosis or treatment. Two formats exist for documenting this information: source-oriented narrative entries or the problem-oriented initial database with SOAP notes.

The *source-oriented* format of organization is the more traditional of the two. The history, progress notes, nutritionist's notes, laboratory notes, and so forth, are located separately within the patient's record. The *problem-oriented* system organizes records from the entire health team in one area under each of the patient's problems. The *SOAP format* prescribes four focal points for discussing the patient: Subjective, Objective, Assessment, and Plan. Policies and procedures vary for collecting and recording this information.

Generally, the source-oriented history is taken at the time of the first visit, placed in the patient record, and updated with narrative notes during subsequent visits and treatments. In the problem-oriented medical record (POMR), the patient history is a part of the initial database and updated with SOAP notes during subsequent visits and treatments.

The *physical assessment* consists of questions regarding the patient's current health problem and takes place at the beginning of each office visit. Whereas the history includes the comprehensive collection of data from three holistic domains—physical, psychological, and social—the physical assessment, as the name implies, considers solely the physical aspects of the patient's health. Unlike the physician's physical examination, however, the physical assessment does **not** lead to a medical diagnosis. Rather, it alerts the physician to areas of deviation from normal, places actual or potential problems in perspective, and oftentimes points the physician in particular directions.

During the physical assessment, the patient relates specific complaints (symptoms), concerns, or the particular reason for the visit. (Specific complaints as they relate to body parts and systems also are described in Chapters 20 and 21, Specific Physical Examinations, Parts I and II.) The physical assessment process also documents progress or deterioration of the patient's condition since the last visit.

The components and general aspects of the patient record have been discussed in Chapter 6, Establishing the Patient Record. This chapter focuses on the characteristics of effective documentation and presents the skills of obtaining and recording the patient history and physical assessment. This procedure is described in detail at the end of the chapter.

The medical assistant's role in each is to assist the physician in acquiring the information necessary to determine the patient's diagnosis or progress. Each physician decides in advance the extent of the medical assistant's role in gathering a careful and complete history. The medical assistant may also be responsible for initiating the physical assessment and collecting designated data. Using the medical assistant's documented interactions with the patient as a starting point, the physician most likely will obtain further information.

Although the history and physical assessment are discussed separately, they generally appear together in the medical record. Each medical facility develops its own forms and specifies the grouping and location of the data in the patient's record.

THE PATIENT HISTORY

Basically, there are three approaches for obtaining information regarding the patient's past health status: the physician-only approach, the physician-team approach, and the patient self-directed approach. A discussion of these will help clarify the medical assistant's role.

Some physicians prefer to interview the patient and obtain the history themselves. They believe that the patient should provide information only once, directed to the physician. This method describes the physician-only approach to the patient history.

Other physicians maintain that "two heads are better than one." They believe that a history initiated by the medical assistant and expanded by the physician is more likely to focus on critical information and save the physician's time. Standardized checklist forms are available that direct the questioning and provide space for documentation. In the physician-team approach just described, the medical assistant precedes the physician and plays a cooperative role in gathering information.

In the patient self-directed approach, the patient responds to a written questionnaire aimed at uncovering the patient's health history. Several standardized forms are available for this purpose. This approach saves both the physician's and the medical assistant's time, but it has some drawbacks. Patients often find this method impersonal. Responses are often too brief or limited, and the questions are subject to individual interpretation. Figure 16–1 is an example of a questionnaire used to obtain the patient's history. Medical assistants functioning within the patient self-directed framework serve as patient facilitators and resource persons, providing whatever assistance the patient requires to interpret the questions and complete the forms.

Perhaps the most critical aspect of obtaining patient information relates to patient confidentiality and privacy. Many patients have concerns or reservations about revealing the details of their past health history. Thus, all interviews should be conducted privately in an area removed from office traffic (usually in the examination room).

CONTENT OF THE PATIENT HISTORY

The general medical history is obtained during the patient's first office visit. Data collection techniques vary slightly, depending on whether the information is collected using the traditional source-oriented system of recordkeeping or the POMR (see Chapter 6).

In the source-oriented system, the information is organized and recorded as follows:

1. *Patient history.* The history begins with the patient's chief complaint (CC) and present illness (PI), then progresses to the patient's general health condition, past medical history, family health history, and a profile of the patient's personal and social life and well-being. The history is always *subjective* and therefore should be recorded from the patient's point of view rather than as observed by the interviewer.
2. *Physical examination.* Recorded by the physician, this information confirms the patient's history, permits the observation of findings not reported in the history, and provides *objective* information about the patient's current health problem and general state of health. This portion of the patient's record may also include a provisional (probable) diagnosis or a final diagnosis, diagnostic tests ordered, and the treatment plan.
3. *Laboratory data.* This section constitutes an additional source of *objective* data and includes any type of testing, such as laboratory tests, x-rays, or electrocardiograms.

In the problem-oriented system, the patient's record is organized so that specific problems are numbered, defined, and then referred to throughout the record. Major components include the following:

1. *Initial database.* The initial database consists of the patient's complete health, family, and social history; the physical examination; the physician's assessment; patient profiles gathered from other physicians or health care providers; and available laboratory data.
2. *Problem list.* The problem list is a numbered list of past and present medical, social, environmental, and psychological problems. Derived from the initial database, this list serves as a permanent index to the patient's record.
3. *Progress notes.* Each progress note begins with a specific problem and its number and then for each entry continues as follows:

S = Subjective data (patient history)
O = Objective data (physical examination and laboratory findings)
A = Assessment (provisional or final diagnosis)
P = Plan (further diagnostic test, treatment plan, patient teaching plan, etc.)

The following two entries are also sometimes used and make up what is termed the "SOAPIE" note:

CASE #		PATIENT'S NAME	
ADDRESS _____ INSURANCE _____		DATE _____	NO. OF CHILDREN _____
TEL. # _____ REFERRED BY _____	OCCUPATION _____	AGE SEX	SMWD

NOTE: THIS IS A CONFIDENTIAL RECORD OF YOUR MEDICAL HISTORY AND WILL BE KEPT IN THIS OFFICE. INFORMATION CONTAINED HERE WILL NOT BE RELEASED WITHOUT YOUR PERMISSION.

LIST YOUR CHIEF COMPLAINTS & SYMPTOMS

1. _____
2. _____
3. _____
4. _____
5. _____

PAST ILLNESSES

HAVE YOU EVER HAD?	Yes	No
Measles	Yes	No
Duodenal Ulcer	Yes	No
Scarlet Fever, Scarletina	Yes	No
Diphtheria	Yes	No
Smallpox	Yes	No
Pneumonia	Yes	No
Tuberculosis	Yes	No
Pleurisy	Yes	No
A Murmur of the Heart	Yes	No
Heart Disease	Yes	No
Arthritis or Rheumatism	Yes	No
Bone or Joint Disease	Yes	No
Neuritis, Neuralgia	Yes	No
Bursitis, Sciatica	Yes	No
Polio, Meningitis	Yes	No
Bright's Disease	Yes	No
Kidney Stone	Yes	No
Kidney Infection	Yes	No
Recent Weight Gain	Yes	No
Recent Weight Loss	Yes	No
Weight now _____ 1 Yr. Ago _____		
Maximum _____ Minimum _____		

CIRCLE ALL ANSWERS	Yes	No
Anemia	Yes	No
Jaundice	Yes	No
Easy Bleeding	Yes	No
Epilepsy	Yes	No
Migraine Headache	Yes	No
Diabetes	Yes	No
High Blood Pressure	Yes	No
Low Blood Pressure	Yes	No
Nervous Breakdown	Yes	No
Hay Fever	Yes	No
Asthma	Yes	No
Hives, Eczema	Yes	No
Boils, Frequent	Yes	No
Colds, Frequent	Yes	No.
Allergies	Yes	No
Allergies to Drugs	Yes	No
Which Ones _____		
Smoke Cigarettes	Yes	No
How many _____		
Drink Moderately	Yes	No

DO YOU HAVE ANY OF THESE SYMPTOMS?

	Yes	No
In General, do you feel Bad?	Yes	No
Your appetite is Poor?	Yes	No
Trouble with Swallowing	Yes	No
Hoarseness	Yes	No
Sore Throat	Yes	No
Chills or Fever	Yes	No
Any Eye Disease, Impaired sight	Yes	No
Any ear disease, Impaired hearing	Yes	No
Any nose, sinus, mouth trouble	Yes	No
Fainting Spells	Yes	No
Loss of Consciousness	Yes	No
Convulsions	Yes	No
Paralysis	Yes	No
Dizziness	Yes	No
Severe headache	Yes	No
Depression	Yes	No
Anxiety, Nervousness	Yes	No
Hallucinations	Yes	No
Enlarged Glands	Yes	No
Enlarged Thyroid or Goiter	Yes	No
Underactive Thyroid	Yes	No
Overactive Thyroid	Yes	No
Skin Disease	Yes	No
Chronic Cough	Yes	No
Chest Pain	Yes	No
Angina	Yes	No
Spitting up Blood	Yes	No
Night Sweats	Yex	No
Shortness of Breath	Yes	No
Palpitations or fluttering of heart	Yes	No
Swelling of hands, feet, ankles	Yes	No
Varicose Veins	Yes	No
Bladder Infection	Yes	No
Albumin, Sugar, Pus, or Blood in Urine	Yes	No
Difficulty in Urination	Yes	No
Abnormal Thirst	Yes	No
Abdominal Pain	Yes	No
Indigestion	Yes	No
Liver Enlarged	Yes	No
Fried Fatty Food Intolerance	Yes	No
Gall Bladder Disease	Yes	No
Colitis	Yes	No
Hemorrhoids	Yes	No
Rectal Bleeding	Yes	No
Constipation	Yes	No
Diarrhea	Yes	No
Change in Bowel Habits	Yes	No
Insomnia	Yes	No

SURGERY

OPERATIONS	HOSPITAL	YEAR
1.		
2.		
3.		
4.		

HOSPITALIZATIONS

FOR WHAT ILLNESS

1.		
2.		
3.		
4.		

FAMILY HISTORY

	IF LIVING AGE	ILLNESS	IF DECEASED AGE	CAUSE
Father				
Mother				
Sisters				
1.				
2.				
3.				
Brothers				
1.				
2.				
3.				

WOMEN ONLY   MENSTRUAL HISTORY

Age at Onset _____

Regular   Yes _____ No _____

Cycle _____ days (from start to start)

Usual Duration _____ Days

Heavy _____ Medium _____ Light _____

Date of Last Period _____

How Many Pregnancies _____

How Many Children _____

How Many Miscarriages _____

Complications of Pregnancy _____

DID OR DOES YOUR MOTHER, FATHER, SISTER OR BROTHER HAVE

	Yes	No
Diabetes	Yes	No
Heart Trouble	Yes	No
High Blood Pressure	Yes	No
Epilepsy	Yes	No
Stroke	Yes	No
Hemophilia or Blood Diseases	Yes	No
Gout	Yes	No
Duodenal Ulcer	Yes	No
Rheumatic Fever	Yes	No

FORM S-41776

Figure 16-1. Questionnaire for patient. (Courtesy of E. Gary Lamsback, M.D.)

PHYSICAL EXAMINATION: TEMP. ____ PULSE ____ RESP. ____ B.P. ____ HT. ____ WT. ____   LABORATORY FINDINGS:

GENERAL APPEARANCE _____

SKIN _____ MUCOUS MEMBRANE _____

EYES: VISION _____ PUPIL _____ FUNDUS _____

EARS: _____

NOSE: _____   DATE

THROAT: _____ PHARYNX _____ TONSILS _____

CHEST: _____ BREASTS _____

HEART: _____

LUNGS: _____

ABDOMEN: _____

GENITALIA: _____

RECTUM: _____

PELVIC: _____

EXTREMITIES: _____ PULSES: _____

LYMPH NODES: NECK _____ AXILLA _____ INGUINAL _____ ABDOMINAL _____

NEUROLOGICAL: _____

DIAGNOSIS: _____

_____

_____

TREATMENT: _____

_____

DATE			SUBSEQUENT VISITS AND FINDINGS	B.P.	WGT.
MO.	DAY	YR.			

PATIENT'S NAME

Figure 16–1. Continued.

= Actions taken (treatments or teaching completed)

E = Evaluation (statement of patient outcomes or progress, usually used to begin the next progress note)

The following is a sample progress note:

SAMPLE POMR PROGRESS NOTE

#4 GASTRIC ULCER

S: Pt has felt well since she was seen 3 mo ago, except for pain in reaction to certain foods and hunger. She takes her medication, knows its name and dosage. She follows a diet that has no fried or spicy foods. She thinks she is losing weight — her "clothes are looser."

O: P 78, regular; Wt 82.5 kg (182 lb); BP 132/88 R arm lying, 124/82 R arm, standing. Bowel sounds normal, abdomen soft and nontender

A: Medication controlling problem fairly well. Weight down 2.3 kg (5 lb). Patient takes her medication; however, her diet contains a lot of aggravating foods, even though she states she has reduced contraindicated foods. She seems motivated to lose weight now that her clothes are looser. She needs to know about spacing meals and snacks to prevent hunger and prepared foods that will aggravate her condition. Will continue same medication. Patient will need annual blood work and ECG in 2 mo.

P: 1. Diet instructions: Pt will call to set appt with nutritionist.
2. Continue same medication: Tagamet 300 mg qid.
3. Return visit in 2 mo for annual physical and blood work.
4. ECG next visit.

I: Patient given following instructions:

1. Nutritionist's name and telephone number.
2. Prescription for Tagamet.
3. Appointment for annual check-up and ECG.
4. Prescription for blood work.

These basic components comprise the traditional health history and initial database format of the POMR. Figure 16–2 also provides examples of forms used in the POMR system.

IDENTIFYING INFORMATION

The first part of the recorded history most often consists of identifying information that generally describes the patient's behavior, general appearance, and interpersonal skills. This information is gathered in two parts: the relevant demographic data, and a brief patient profile, written in a narrative format. The medical assistant may obtain the demographic date; however, the physician generally writes the narrative or dictates a descriptive narrative and the initial physical findings for transcription by the medical assistant.

This initial narrative may be called the "social history" or the "history and physical" (H&P) and is obtained by the physician during the first visit for use as reference in subsequent visits. Such data help the physician "key in" on the patient's emotional state and personal habits, both of which contribute to the patient's overall health status.

Although some physicians do not obtain or include the H&P in the patient's office record, hospital accreditation agencies require this information for inclusion in the medical records of all hospitalized patients. Many physicians maintain this practice in the office as well.

Examples

DEMOGRAPHIC DATA:

Name. George Adams
Birth Date. March 12, 1951
*Marital Status.** Married
Children. Darlene (16), Harry (12), Albert (6)
Occupation. High School Teacher — Math
Education Level. Master's degree

EXCERPT FROM A DESCRIPTION NARRATIVE

Patient Profile: George teaches math at Central High, and appears to enjoy his work. In addition, he is the school's head basketball coach. During the summer, George paints houses for extra income. His wife works part time as a substitute teacher. The entire family engages in his favorite hobbies of camping and fishing. His father was a factory worker; his mother, a housewife.

In a holistic approach, the H&P portion of the interview provides information about the patient's psychological, sociocultural, developmental, and spiritual characteristics. Psychosocial characteristics include the behaviors and emotions of the patient, as well as the patient's communication skills, intellectual performance, support systems, and self-image. Sociocultural characteristics include educational background, financial situation, recreational activities, neighborhood, cultural influences, family heritage, marital status, occupation, and primary language. Developmental characteristics include growth and maturation, the patient's current developmental stage, and the effects of the patient's current health status on the attainment of developmentally appropriate goals.

---

*Marital status is often referred to under social status.

A

ALLERGY:

NAME_____ Age_____ 1st Visit_____

Prob. No.	Problem—Active	Date of Onset	Date Entered	Manner in which problem was treated and resolved	Date Resolved

Date   /   /   PHONE CALL

NAME OF PATIENT:_____   **PHONE:**_____

PERSON CALLING:_____   **PHONE:**_____

PROBLEM:

ALLERGIES:
PHARMACY: PHONE:

	MEDICATION	DOSE	DISP	DIRECTIONS	REFILLS
1.					
2.					
3.					

BILLING OF HOSPITAL PATIENTS

Name of Patient	Date of Admission	Date of Discharge	Date Dr. turned into the office	Date Charged	Date Billed	Date Pmt. Rec.	Amt. Bill

PROGRESS NOTES

INITIAL H&P:_____.   SEE ORANGE BOOK OR H&P SHEETS.
                                        SEE PROBLEM LIST ON INSIDE COVER.

PROBLEM #	PLAN

Figure 16–2. Examples of forms used in the problem-oriented medical record (POMR) system. (Courtesy of Joseph M. DeFranco, M.D.)

B

LABORATORY

Name_____

Date	Test

Date	Test

X-RAYS

Name_____

Date	Test

Date	Test

LETTERS

Name_____

Date	

Date	

Figure 16–2. Continued.

BASIC HABITS (SOCIAL HISTORY)

The purpose of the social history is to identify the patient's personal habits and to gain insights regarding the subsequent connections between medical problems and the patient's lifestyle. The following aspects are usually included:

1. *Diet and nutrition.* What kinds of food are preferred? How often? How much?
2. *Patterns of weight.* Is the weight satisfactory to the patient? Is it stable? If it fluctuates over the years, by how much?
3. *Exercise.* Does the patient engage in regular exercise? How much? How often? What type?
4. *Smoking.* If the patient smokes, how much and what type of materials (pipes, cigars, cigarettes)?
5. *Drinking.* What kind of alcoholic beverages are used, and in what quantity? How much water is consumed daily?
6. *Sleeping.* Does the patient have regular sleeping habits? If so, how many hours per day?
7. *Drugs.* Which legal or illegal drugs are used on a regular basis (including vitamins, aspirin, and so forth)?

FAMILY HISTORY

Because the tendency to develop certain diseases has been linked to familial or hereditary predisposition, the physician will want to know the family's health history. For instance, if the father ultimately died of heart failure, it would be useful to know if he was overweight and if he smoked or exercised on a regular basis.

The patient is asked to list the health habits, illnesses, and diseases of both parents, siblings, and maternal and paternal grandparents. Age and cause of death, when appropriate, are also recorded.

PAST ILLNESSES

The patient is asked to provide a record of all past illnesses, diseases, surgeries, and injuries. The list should include usual infant and childhood diseases (with approximate dates), immunizations, incidence of pneumonia, hospitalizations, surgical procedures, chronic conditions such as arthritis, hay fever, allergies, and drug sensitivities (with approximate date of onset). The female patient is asked to list the onset of menstruation (menarche), menstrual cycle history, and the number and date of pregnancies and their outcome (normal delivery, and so forth). Allergies, especially due to drugs, should be labeled in red on every page of the patient's record.

SELF-PERCEPTION

Some physicians are interested in learning the patient's own perception of his or her general health status. An open-ended question (see Chapter 4, Understanding and Communication with Patients and Their Families) such as—"How would you describe your general health at this time?"—is asked and the response recorded. The patient's perspective provides useful information for the physician and may be valuable in determining a diagnosis and designing a treatment regimen. For example, responding to the question above, a male patient may state: "This is the first time I ever had pain like this. I'm not a complainer, and have had other aches and pains . . . but nothing like this." The patient is attempting to impress upon the physician the severity of the pain. From the patient's perspective, although not verbalized, he perceives himself as being in poor health because of the experience of intense pain and because of his focus on the pain.

PHYSICAL ASSESSMENT

The physical assessment includes a thorough description of the health problem that has motivated the patient to seek health care, and the physician's evaluation of each body system.

CHIEF COMPLAINT AND PRESENT ILLNESS

The CC and PI should be gathered first and recorded chronologically, beginning with the onset of the problem. A good way to begin recording the physical assessment is: "The patient was well until . . ." and include the following:

1. *What is the CC?* Encourage the patient to begin the interview by relating the CC in his or her own words. Avoid asking the patient if the pain is severe or dull and avoid using descriptive terms in questioning because these might influence the patient in the choice of words.
2. *What is the history of this illness?* Prompt the patient to relate chronologically how the CC became problematic (onset) and to list the associated events or symptoms.
3. *How long has the complaint been present?* Help the patient express the duration of the illness accurately.
4. *In what physical area is the problem localized?* Assist the patient in describing the specific location affected. If more than one area is involved, how do these interact?
5. *How are the symptoms progressing?* Ask the patient probing questions such as: "Are the symptoms moving throughout the body? Did the trouble develop suddenly or slowly?"
6. *What is the character of the symptoms?* Direct the patient to describe the nature of the complaint in terms of severity: discomfort, dull ache, severe pain, and so forth. Do these symptoms come and go suddenly or slowly?
7. *How is the complaint related to activity?* Help the patient to determine if the problem may be linked with a particular activity such as sleeping, eating, or walking.

Once these seven major questions have been answered, the physical assessment continues by discussing two general issues. First, what, if any, treatment has been attempted in the past, either by other physicians or by the patient; and second, what is the general physical, psychological, and social impact of the present health problem. The physician usually performs this latter phase of the assessment, and the information is recorded for further study by the physician and for subsequent inclusion in the patient's file. As previously mentioned, some physicians prefer to use a standardized questionnaire such as the one shown in Figure 16–3. Others may record assessment data on a form of

Patient_____ Date_____

Interviewer_____

1. Chief Complaint:

2. History:

3. Length of Complaint:

4. Physical Area Affected:

5. Progress of Symptoms:

6. Character of Symptoms:

7. Problems with Basic Activities:

8. Miscellaneous:

Figure 16–3. *A standardized interview form.*

their own design or place information from the interview in a specific location in the patient record. In any case, the method of presentation is optional so long as the reader can understand the material and the data is placed in an accessible, clearly marked location.

REVIEW OF SYSTEMS

The review of systems (ROS) is the final step of the physical assessment. It consists of the history and current evaluation of each of the major body systems and any associated symptoms. These include the following:

1. *Head.* Headaches, pains, tension
2. *Eyes.* Visual problems, strain, drainage, tearing, pain
3. *Ears, nose, and throat.* Hearing problems, drainage, dizziness, ringing in ears, pain, congestion, sinus problems, hoarseness, difficulty swallowing, epistaxis
4. *Mouth.* Dental or gum disease, sores, bleeding
5. *Cardiovascular system.* Palpitations, dizziness, exhaustion, pain, high or low blood pressure, peripheral edema
6. *Respiratory system.* Shortness of breath, breathing irregularities, asthma, discharge or cough
7. *Urinary system.* Voiding habits, discharges, frequency, pain, odor and color of urine
8. *Gastrointestinal system.* Dietary habits, weight changes, stomach disorders, indigestion, hunger pains, nausea, types of stools, regularity of bowel movements, hemorrhoids, bleeding
9. *Menstrual cycle.* Interval, regularity, discharge
10. *Neurological system.* Dizziness, weakness, sporadic loss of coordination, tremors, changes in memory or difficulty in concentrating
11. *Psychological assessment.* State of mental health, nervousness, symptoms of distress
12. *Musculoskeletal system.* Pain, deformity, immobility, swelling
13. *Skin.* Rashes, hives, itching, bleeding, sores, burns

During the ROS, the patient's attention should be directed to that particular system under review, and questions should be asked relating to the history, evolution of symptoms, and present condition of each. The physician or the medical assistant, as directed by the physician, may make the following sample inquiries:

Examples

Physician: "Now that we have some information about your urinary system, what can you tell me about your stomach and bowel habits? Why don't you begin by discussing your day-to-day eating habits and how your stomach reacts to various foods."

Patient: "Well, I used to eat quite a lot, but lately I've had to cut down because I'm watching my weight. I can eat just about anything I want with the exception of fried foods, which seem to give me indigestion."

Physician: "Exactly which foods do this to you?"

Patient: "Well, I've noticed that fried potatoes and meats, especially hamburgers, cause quite a bit of stomach pain."

Physician: Does this happen every single time you eat fried foods?"

Patient: "I would say about 80 percent of the time."

Physician: "How about your bowel habits?"

Patient: "Well, I seem to be quite regular with normal stools. I rarely have trouble with diarrhea or constipation."

Physician: "Do you ever experience nausea? Have you had any trouble with hemorrhoids? Do you have problems with indigestion? . . ."

When the patient's responses trigger a particular concern, the physician will focus on the response in an attempt to gain as much insight as possible about the patient's symptoms.

OBSERVATION AND INTERVIEWING

The interview establishes the physician-patient relationship. Lying at the heart of the interview is a mutual concern for the patient's well-being. The therapeutic relationship that ensues becomes the foundation for subsequent health education and counseling involving both the patient and the patient's family.

The first step of the interview is the introduction. The medical assistant should introduce herself or himself in a way that clarifies the reason for the interview. Next, the medical assistant should communicate a sense of trust and confidentiality, to reduce the patient's feelings of anxiety and helplessness, and discuss the patient's concerns about the personal nature of the information being shared. Finally, the medical assistant should convey an attitude of competence and professionalism. When concluding the interview, the medical assistant should thank the patient for his or her cooperation and indicate what the rest of the visit will entail.

Interview sources include the patient, family, a significant other, and physician-team members. The patient's health record is another good source of health information. When the patient is critically ill, disoriented, confused, mentally handicapped, or very young, the family or a significant other become the primary sources for obtaining accurate information.

Regardless of the interviewing format preferred by the physician, the medical assistant can benefit from an understanding of basic interviewing skills. The attitude of the interviewer should be professional and interested. Adding eye contact, appropriate touching, and attentive listening can help the patient feel comfortable while being interviewed. Visual assessment of patient comfort is also helpful. Does the patient appear to be at ease? Is the patient visibly ill or otherwise distressed? The medical assistant's observation of the patient's posture, grooming, clarity of expression, and other attributes may assist the physician to determine the diagnosis. These observations, if the physician prefers, may be summarized and noted on the patient record by the medical assistant. A discussion of specific verbal interviewing tactics follows.

VERBAL TACTICS

The most common medium for interviewing is verbal communication. These eight interviewing guidelines can assist the interviewer in obtaining pertinent information.

1. *Be nonjudgmental.* The continuity of a conversation between a medical assistant and a patient can be destroyed when the medical assistant offers judgments. Whether positive or negative, judgments by the interviewer interfere with the objectivity of the information-transfer process. Negative feedbacks tends to stifle the patient, whereas positive feedback may prompt the patient to continue onto meaningless tangents. The medical assistant needs to listen, ask probing questions, and record answers when appropriate but never pass judgment or condemn a patient for health care beliefs or practices.

Example

Patient: "Whenever I'm hungry at night, I have a bowl of ice cream with chocolate syrup."

Incorrect Response: "Well, you know that you'll never lose weight like that."

Correct Response: If dietary habits are the object of questioning, the medical assistant might ask: "How often do you eat at night?", or no response may be necessary.

2. *Use short, probing questions.* On occasion, it may be necessary for the medical assistant to interrupt the patient to clarify important points or to slow the process of relating critical events so that the information can be absorbed. The best approach is to use brief, probing questions such as "Excuse me, but . . .

could you clarify that?"
could you describe that more specifically?"
how often did it happen?"
how did you feel about it?"

These probes serve to provide needed structure in the dialogue. In addition, they provide a kind of verbal feedback that assures the patient the medical assistant is listening.

At times it is also appropriate to ask open and closed questions. The methods of stating questions to elicit certain responses were discussed in Chapter 4, Understanding and Communicating with Patients and Their Families. By way of review, statements such as "Describe the pain" are open ended, permitting the patient to discuss specific problems freely, without limits or direction. On the other hand, closed questions produce predictable, directed responses: "Where is the pain?" or "How long have you had the pain?"

3. *Listen and respond with interest.* The assessment interview provides an excellent opportunity for establishing the patient's trust and forms the basis for future interactions. During the process of probing, the medical assistant should demonstrate interest in the patient. This can be accomplished by adding phrases such as "That's very interesting" or "I'm not sure that I understood" to the probes that were previously discussed.

The medical assistant should be supportive and listen without offering false reassurance. Listening requires silence and attention, which encourages patients to verbalize. Momentary silence can also be used to slow the pace of the interview and provide the opportunity for the medical assistant to make notations.

Occasionally, general leads should be offered. Statements such as "Continue, please" or "And then what happens?" help to maximize verbal responses.

4. *Use simple questions that the patient will understand.* The patient is relatively untrained in medical terminology and office procedures. When phrasing questions the medical assistant should use language and structure that the patient can easily understand.

5. *"Mirror" the patient's important statements.* During the course of discussion, the patient will ultimately focus on health-related events of critical importance. These are the most important aspects of the description and contain particular information that must be recorded and transmitted to the physician. To ensure the accuracy of this information, the medical assistant should attempt to "mirror" the patient's statements by stopping the conversation and repeating the information to the patient as follows: "Am I correct in saying that . . .," or "So, you *do* feel . . ."

Example

Patient: ". . . and every time that I eat red meat during a meal, I wake up during the evening with a severe stomach ache."

Medical Assistant: "Just a moment. Let me see if I understand you. Each time you eat red meat, you are awakened during the evening because of stomach pain?"

6. *Seek clarification.* The medical assistant may use statements as "I'm not sure what you mean" to encourage the patient to offer further explanation.

7. *Verbalize the implied.* To avoid inaccurate interpretation based on inference, the medical assistant can direct the patient to verbalize specifically.

Example

Patient: I suppose these headaches are from working at that place.

Medical Assistant: Work is very stressful?

8. *Summarize.* Summarization provides a useful check for accuracy and completeness. Once the data has been collected, verify the information with the patient. An experienced interviewer can conduct an assessment interview in 10 to 20 minutes. While all of the barriers to communication discussed in Chapter 4 also apply to interviewing, advice and excessive repetition specifically impede the interviewing process. Advice may be illegal or unethical, and although repeating or mirroring the patient's comments is sometimes useful, overuse of this technique may be irritating to the patient.

PINPOINTING THE CHIEF COMPLAINT AND PRESENT ILLNESS

Identifying the patient's overriding problem requires the gathering of accurate data during the patient interview. To focus on a single problem or concern, the medical assistant should develop skills that lead to the "pinpointing" of specific symptoms or other important medical clues. Pinpointing is the process of moving language from the general to the specific. A pinpointed statement is one that is clear and precise. The following is an example of a patient description that has been changed from a general to a more useful "pinpointed" perspective:

Example

General: "It seems I have always had headaches as long as I can remember. I must use a ton of aspirin every year."

Pinpointed: "I have been bothered by frequent headaches. For example, during the past 2 weeks, I have had six headaches. Three of these were so severe that I had to take three aspirin to get relief."

Converting a patient's vague and generalized statements into pinpointed descriptions assists the physician in understanding both the nature and severity of a particular problem. In most cases, once patients begin to grasp the nature of the pinpointing process, they will automatically begin to do their own pinpointing, thus facilitating the medical assistant's task.

Pinpointing should be used whenever the patient begins to describe an important symptom or a related event. If the patient is not able to remember specific details accurately, the medical assistant should ask the patient to keep a record of such events in the future. This type of record can provide valuable information about the frequency of certain symptoms as well as the circumstances under which the symptoms occur. In addition to lending focus to patients' descriptions of symptoms, pinpointing also helps eliminate meaningless or emotional expletives and exaggeration.

Example

Meaningless: "It seems like I always have a cold."

Meaningful: "I have had a sore throat and nasal congestion at least six times this past year."

The medical assistant must gently but persistently guide the patient toward specific, accurate, and quantified descriptions. To assist patients in pinpointing, the medical assistant can use "who, what, where, when, and how" questions to classify patient statements. The approach should be time-efficient without giving the patient an impression that there is a "rush" to get finished.

CHARTING (WRITING) PATIENT ASSESSMENTS

As previously discussed, the medical assistant may be delegated the tasks of recording parts of the complete history and physical assessment. Once the information has been collected, the medical assistant should document the interview immediately by making notations in the patient record. Guidelines for recording the patient's description of symptoms and other information related to the purpose of the visit are presented below. With practice and experience, the medical assistant will recognize proper and improper charting in the patient record and will become more adept at making appropriate notations.

PATIENT QUOTES

Charting includes language that appeals directly to the senses, such as quotes. The written record of the patient's own description of symptoms may consist of pertinent word-for-word statements enclosed in quotes. For example, if the patient states that the pain "comes and goes," and when asked for details, explains that the pain "seems to occur after eating certain foods and when I get hungry," the written record should reflect only the second statement in quotes, as it better describes "comes and goes." Use quotes only when clarity would otherwise suffer. Therefore, the proper charting for these statements would be:

> States she experiences pain "after eating certain foods and when I get hungry."

OBSERVABLE DATA

In addition to using patient quotes, the medical assistant must also report what she or he sees, hears, feels, or smells in terms as close as possible to the actual experience. Exactness as to the frequency, duration, and severity of a symptom's occurrence is also required for the physician to determine the correct diagnosis and treatment plan. Standard medical terms and abbreviations (Table 16–1) should be used. For example, the patient states that the pain has "a way of coming and going and seems to be around the stomach area." The patient is pointing to an area below the umbilicus. "It's always there, but it feels like a knife going in and out when it gets worse. It usually happens in the late evening. It's been like that almost every day for 2 weeks now." The proper charting would be:

> Sharp intermittent pain in the hypogastric region, usually worsening in the late evening for the past 2 weeks. Other times pain is duller but persistent.

BRIEF NOTATION

The medical assistant's notes must be concise. Therefore, the notations should reflect only the focal point and not the patient's word-for-word descriptions (unless a direct quote provides a better context for the problem, as stated above). The patient often elaborates with unnecessary information and may become diverted in conversation. These are natural tendencies in conversation. The medical assistant's responsibility is to select and record relevant information to conserve the physician's time.

In the foregoing examples, the words "present" or "noted" would be redundant—only the observations are reported. In the second example, "hypogastric" and "intermittent" are accepted medical terms to describe the location and frequency of pain. Complete sentence structure is not necessary. However, relevant information should never be sacrificed for brevity.

JUDGMENTAL STATEMENTS

The medical assistant's notations in the patient record should be confined to the recording of data associated directly with the purpose of the visit and the

Table 16–1

HISTORY AND PHYSICAL ASSESSMENT ABBREVIATIONS

1°, 2°	Primary, Secondary
BP	Blood pressure
$\bar{c}$	with
CC	Chief complaint
CV	Cardiovascular
Dx	Diagnosis
E	Evaluation
FH	Family history
GI	Gastrointestinal
Gravida	Pregnant woman
GU	Genitourinary
H&P	History and physical
HEENT	Head, eye, ear, nose, and throat
HBP	High blood pressure
Hx	History
I	Intervention
Ⓛ	Left
MSX	Musculoskeletal
P	Pulse
Para	Viable births
PE	Physical examination
PH	Past history
PI	Present illness
POMR, POR	Problem-oriented medical record, Problem-oriented record
Px	Problem
R	Respiration
Ⓡ	Right
ROM	Range of Motion
ROS	Review of systems
$\bar{s}$	Without
SH	Social history
SOAP	Subjective, Objective, Assessment, Plan
T	Temperature
T&A	Tonsillectomy and adenoidectomy
UCD	Usual childhood diseases
URI	Upper respiratory infection
UTI	Urinary tract infection
XR	X-Ray
=	Equal
≠	Unequal
>	Greater than
<	Less than
↑	Increase
↓	Decrease
−	Negative
+	Positive
#	Number, pound, has been given or done
♂	Male
♀	Female

listing of symptoms. Statements or nonverbal responses that reflect important feelings or facts are often made to the medical assistant and should be recorded for the physician's reference. If a patient winces in pain when placed in a certain position, the medical assistant should record:

> Winced and frowned when placed in the recumbent position.

Rather than record the patient is "in pain," the medical assistant records the visible evidence of pain.

The medical assistant should always avoid using the words "appears" or "seems," since these terms indicate that the observer is unsure of the observation. Entries such as "tolerated the procedure well" are meaningless. If there are no details to discuss, do not include them. Other redundancies include "cool to the touch" and "brown in color." Concentrate on presenting sufficient data in the fewest possible words such as "cool" or "brown." Avoid recording judgmental statements or conjecture concerning the patient's personality or behavior such as "confused" or "depressed." Labeling mental states communicates little but the writer's attitude. Describing behaviors is more effective. For example, the patient starts to cry when she mentions the bruises.

> *Improper charting.* Patient appears upset.
> *Proper charting.* Crying and stating that . . .

Other common judgments are "good" and "normal." The actual observation which leads to this type of conclusion should be substituted, such as "pain-free" or "not bleeding." Finally, the absence of a particular symptom can be as important as its presence. Therefore, the medical assistant should note in the chart the absence of drainage, shortness of breath, dizziness, nausea, vomiting, or any other problem.

WRITING STYLE

Chart notes should be easy to read. Information that is not easy to read is not easy to understand. Sentences should be short with capitals and periods. Like items should be clustered, and new ideas should start on a new line. Stringing ideas together with commas and dashes obscures the message. Ditto marks should never be used and blank spaces should be lined out to avoid suggesting that information has been omitted. Subjects, verbs, and prepositions that are obvious or grammatically understood should also be omitted.

PROOFREADING

Chart notes must be proofread for errors and omissions. If an omitted word needs to be added, a carat (^) should be used to record the omitted material. The entire record, as well as any additions, should be written in ink and include the initials of the writer. To delete an unnecessary word, a single line is struck over the word and the deletion is initialed. Never "white out" an entry. Incorrect spellings that could confuse the reader should be corrected or deleted and replaced. Unless there is a policy otherwise, use standard proofreader's marks.

TIME, DATE, AND INITIALS

Accountability for charting the date, time, and procedures is the responsibility of the medical assistant. All narrative reporting and notations made in the patient's record must be initialed by the medical assistant with the time and date. In this way the physician will know who has written the notes if there should be a need for further discussion (there may be more than one medical assistant). Moreover, initialing provides legal protection for the medical assistant and the physician.

Do not chart before the fact; record all notes promptly. Timely documentation decreases the likelihood that important information will be missing, inaccurate, or unclear.

PATIENT TEACHING CONSIDERATIONS

The patient is more willing to cooperate and provide information when the purpose and method of the interview have been clearly explained. Throughout the interview process, the medical assistant actually teaches the patient how to respond, what the medical assistant and physician need to know, and the role this information will play in planning the patient's health care regimen.

Standardized patient history forms in which the patient records basic health information should not be given to the patient without explanation and direction. When the patient has finished filling out the form, the medical assistant should check it for completeness and answer any questions the patient may have regarding information requested on the form. Too often, a patient is given a form and left alone to complete it. The patient history is too valuable a diagnostic tool to be left in the patient's hands without providing assistance.

RELATED ETHICAL AND LEGAL IMPLICATIONS

Confidentiality is the foremost concern related to obtaining and recording information. The patient has both an ethical and a legal right to privacy. Not only should the patient be interviewed in a private area, but the history or interview should be discussed in the office only when necessary as it relates to patient care. Confidential patient information should never be discussed outside the office.

Another important legal concern that has been touched on in other chapters and is discussed in detail in Chapter 3, Medical Law and Ethics, is the method of charting. Documenting care is as important legally as giving the care. Omissions are a major factor leading to lawsuits, but both omissions and inclusions are potentially damaging. For instance, if care that was given and should have been recorded is not recorded, it did not happen under law, and the physician may later be unable to prove having met standards of quality care. Careful, precise language and legible writing is the obvious protection against legal claims.

In addition to what is or is not recorded and the method of recordkeeping, another concern for the medical assistant is that information recorded under his or her signature falls within professional practice guidelines for medical assisting. The medical assistant must be particularly careful to avoid recording conjecture or value statements or implying diagnosis. For example, the following statement should be avoided, as it is value-laden and based on conjecture: "Patient does not appear well-groomed and seems upset about her illness." A more appropriate notation would be: "Patient states: 'I don't even care how I look anymore. It's not just being sick that's bothering me. It's my husband's reaction.'"

The method of making corrections of the medical record is discussed here and in Chapter 3. Specifically, additions or changes should be made by careful word

insertion or drawing a single line through an error and writing the correction above and placing the writer's initials and date alongside, as follows:

Sunday
Takes an OTC sleeping aid every ˄ ~~night~~. MAF
1/6/93

The medical assistant may wish to consult other texts that, although written primarily for nurses, discuss documentation guidelines from a legal perspective.

SUMMARY

The medical assistant is partially or completely responsible for obtaining and recording patient information in the clinical setting. This chapter presented guidelines that can aid in accomplishing these tasks effectively. The information obtained becomes part of the patient's permanent record—a legal document that serves as a history of the care the patient received and that enables the physician to provide the patient with continuous, comprehensive, and competent care. Patient comfort and privacy are foremost to the success of the process.

DISCUSSION QUESTIONS

1. What kinds of information are necessary for the following sections of the patient health history? Why are they necessary?

Identifying information
Chief complaint
History of present illness
Past medical history
Family history
Review of systems

2. What information does the problem-oriented medical record (POMR) initial database contain?
3. What is a patient interview? When does it occur? What information is obtained?
4. Discuss the proper methods of recording information on each section of the patient history, initial database, and progress notes.
5. Why should value statements be avoided when recording information in the patient history?

BIBLIOGRAPHY

Coulchan, JL and Block, M: The Medical Interview: A Primer for Students of the Art. FA Davis Co, Philadelphia, 1992.
Doenges, ME and Moorhouse, MF: Nurse's Pocket Guide: Nursing Diagnosis with Interventions, 3rd ed. FA Davis Co, Philadelphia, 1991.
Griffith, J and Ignatavicius, D: The Writers Handbook: The Complete Guide to Clinical Documentation, Professional Writing, and Research Papers. Research Applications, Inc, Baltimore, 1986.
Hogstel, M and Keen-Payne, R: Practical Guide to Health Assessment. FA Davis Co, Philadelphia, 1993.
Kettenbach, G: Writing S.O.A.P. Notes. FA Davis Co, Philadelphia, 1990.
Schwartz, MH: Textbook of Physical Diagnosis: History and Examination. WB Saunders Co, Philadelphia, 1989.

PROCEDURE: Interview the patient to obtain and record a history and physical assessment

OSHA STANDARDS:

Terminal Performance Objectives: Obtain from patients accurate and full information related to past health and present conditions for the physician's use in creating a health care plan.
Record the data using clear and concise language and appropriate terminology within 10 to 20 minutes.

EQUIPMENT: Tape recorder and audio cassette
Patient history form (source-oriented or problem-oriented record)
Workbook Application Exercises
Workbook Case Studies

PROCEDURE	PRINCIPLE
1. Select a private, quiet, and comfortable environment.	To help the patient resolve any anxieties or concerns about the personal nature of the information and to establish an atmosphere for listening.
2. Prepare for the interview by reviewing the objective of the interview and deciding who is the most reliable source of information (e.g., if not the patient, then which family member?)	To focus upon the facts, other sources may be necessary.
3. Call the patient by name, introduce yourself, and explain the procedure and its purpose.	To identify that you have the correct patient and to encourage cooperation.
4. Use terminology the patient will understand. Speak slowly, clearly, and distinctly.	The patient is untrained in medical terminology and medical procedures.
5. Ask about the patient's chief complaint first.	To let the patient feel purpose and expediency in the interview.
6. Immediately record information during the history and assessment as follows:	To provide accurate and complete information without relying on memory after the interview.

Health History

  a. Demographic data
  b. Basic habits
    1. Diet
    2. Exercise
    3. Smoking
    4. Drinking
    5. Sleep
    6. Drugs
  c. Family history
  d. Past history and illnesses
    1. Dates
    2. Times
    3. Durations of hospitalizations, illnesses
    4. Immunizations

Assessment

  e. Chief complaint and present illness
  f. Self-perception
  g. Review of systems
    1. Eyes, ears, nose, throat, mouth
    2. Cardiovascular
    3. Respiratory
    4. Urinary
    5. Gastrointestinal
    6. Menstrual cycle

PROCEDURE

    7. Neurologic
    8. Psychological assessment
    9. Musculoskeletal
   10. Skin

7. Listen attentively.

8. Respond with interest and concern.

9. Use eye contact.

10. Gather information using the various interview approaches:
   a. Neutral, open-ended questions
   b. Nonjudgmental responses (by accepting what the patient says)
   c. Short, probing closed questions to clarify
   d. General leads
   e. Placement of events in time and sequence
   f. Restatement for clarification
   g. Single-point focusing
   h. Verbalization of the implied
   i. Mirroring responses
   j. Pinpointing
   k. Summarization

11. Assess the patient's attitude during responses.

12. Take notes and record information accurately and legibly.

13. Upon completion of the session, provide the patient with the opportunity to ask questions and instruct and prepare the patient for the phases of examination which follow.

14. Thank the patient for his or her cooperation.

15. Proofread and then place the completed information in the patient record and route the patient record to the next appropriate area.

PRINCIPLE

To communicate trust and encouragement of the patient's cooperation.
Sensitivity encourages the patient to express feelings.
To help the patient feel comfortable during the interview.
Questioning approaches vary depending on what information is desired.

Attention to nonverbal cues helps to modify the approach and pinpoint information.
Accurate documentation is essential to the physician's assessment of the patient's health status.
Patients are usually more cooperative and comfortable when they know what to expect and can ask questions.

To express friendliness and display professional mannerisms.
To notify the physician that the interview has been completed.

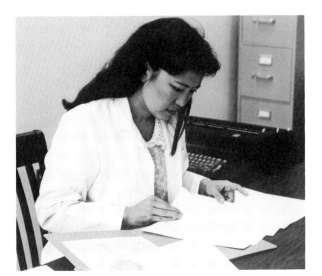

HIGHLIGHTS

Freedom of Information . . . The Past and the Present

Until the passing of recent legislation (Freedom of Information Act), patients have not had the right to see or obtain copies of their own medical records unless they initiated a lawsuit. In the medical office in the past, many physicians refused the patient access to their medical records. Some physicians were reluctant to permit the patient to read the medical record for fear that the patient would be anxious or confused or would not know the meaning of the physician's charting notes and diagnostic findings. Still another motivation for the physician's resistance was the concern that patients would be given fuel to add to the already seemingly out of control fire made of increasing numbers of malpractice suits. Likewise, hospitals did not release medical records to patients without the permission of the attending physician because they felt that physicians owned the medical records and that they, the hospital staff, were merely custodians.

The rethinking of medical record ownership has been brought about by changes in legislation. In 1973, the report by the Commission on Medical Malpractice recommended that the information contained in the medical record be accessible to patients without their seeking the aid of an attorney. During that same year, the 1973 US Privacy Protection Study Commission urged states to enact legislation permitting patients not only access to their own medical records but the right to make corrections as well.

Today, such access has been granted. Not only has legislation been enacted that gives patients the right of ownership of the information in medical records, but also enacted are regulations pertaining to controls related to fees for duplication, timing of responses, and recourse if response is denied.

At the present time, a physician refusing the patient access to the medical record would have to prove that he or she is exercising the Doctrine of Professional Discretion in doing so. Under this doctrine, the physician may determine that the patient's emotional health would be adversely affected if access is granted. If the patient challenged such a decision, the courts would decide the validity of the physician's action. The Doctrine of Professional Discretion is usually applied by physicians treating patients who are mentally or emotionally ill.

While the laws have been changed, the debate over ownership continues. The current debate focuses on some peripheral issues of ownership: How should the information be made accessible? Should patients actually maintain their own set of records?

The Freedom of Information regulations and the related complex controversies directly affect everyone working in the health care industry. Health care professionals, recognizing this fact, should keep abreast of updated changes and opposing views in order to participate in formulating fair regulations that are considerate of both the patient's and the physician's rights.

Chapter 17

Vital Signs

> S timuli from the internal and external environment impact upon the person causing biophysical responses. It should be remembered, however, that people are much more than biophysical beings.
>
> C. Hames
> Concepts of Helping

CHAPTER OUTLINE

Chapter 17

*V*ital Signs

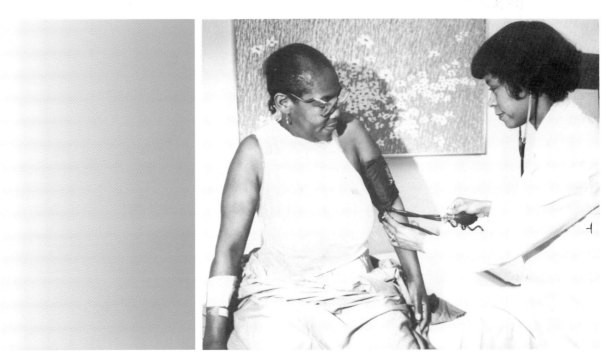

Measure Rectal Temperature of a Child
Measure Axillary Temperature of an Adult
Manage a Situation in Which a
    Thermometer Is Accidentally Broken
Measure and Assess Radial Pulse
Measure and Assess Apical Pulse
Measure and Assess Respiration
Measure and Assess Blood Pressure

Determine Orthostatic Variations in Blood
    Pressure
Measure Height and Weight

HIGHLIGHTS
    Bloodborne Facts: Holding the Line on
        Contamination

LEARNING OBJECTIVES

Upon completing this chapter, you will be able to:

1. State the purpose for measuring the vital signs.
2. Explain the physiology pertaining to each of the vital signs.
3. State adult and pediatric normal values and their ranges for each vital sign measurement.
4. List the variables affecting each of the vital signs, and describe how each of these measurements is influenced by these variables.
5. List and describe the four characteristics of pulse.
6. List and describe the four characteristics of respiration.
7. State the importance of obtaining and recording height and weight.
8. Use temperature conversion charts accurately.
9. Describe how to properly apply infection control procedures to the care equipment used in obtaining the temperature, blood pressure, and height and weight.

PERFORMANCE OBJECTIVES

Upon completing this chapter, you will be able to:

1. Measure and record oral, rectal, and axillary Fahrenheit temperatures of adults and children.
2. Convert Fahrenheit measurements to the Celsius scale.
3. Clean the work area or flush a patient's oral cavity after an incident involving a mercury spill with fragments of glass, and record the incident in the patient chart and on an incident report.
4. Measure, assess, and record radial and apical pulses and respirations.
5. Measure, assess, and record blood pressure measurements for the patient in the lying, sitting, and standing positions.
6. Measure and record height and weight.

DACUM EDUCATIONAL COMPONENTS

1. Apply principles of aseptic technique and infection control (4.1).
2. Take vital signs (4.2).
3. Prepare and maintain examination and treatment area (4.6).
4. Prepare patients for procedures (4.7).
5. Assist the physician with examinations (4.8).
6. Document accurately (5.1).

Glossary

Anthropometric: *measuring the growth of tissue and bones*
Assessment: *analysis and evaluation of the status or quality of a particular condition or subject*
Basal: *in body physiology, pertaining to the lowest possible level*

Continued

Disoriented: state of mental confusion
Diurnal: pertaining to daytime
Inverse: reversal of normal relationship
Metabolism: physical and chemical processes by which the human body is maintained
Physiology: the basic processes underlying the functioning of organisms
Sclerotic: hardening of a part

The accurate measuring and recording of vital signs is a major responsibility of the medical assistant. This task requires a thorough understanding of the physiologic aspects of the vital signs, height, and weight and their physical characteristics. This chapter introduces these concepts to the medical assistant student. The discussion is divided into five distinct sections: (1) body temperature, (2) pulse, (3) respiration, (4) blood pressure, and (5) height and weight.

The vital signs, also known as *cardinal signs*, are measurements that indicate the state of health of the human body. "Vital" comes from the Latin word *vita*, meaning life. The vital signs are indications of the condition of life. In a state of well-being, all of the vital signs — body temperature, pulse rate, respiratory rate; blood pressure; height and weight, including skinfold thickness — fall within an average range. Although the more traditional categorization of vital signs does not include height and weight, the relationship of these signs to wellness has received increasing attention, and their inclusion as part of the physical assessment of the patient has become accepted practice. The abbreviations TPR and BP refer respectively to *T*emperature, *P*ulse, *R*espiration, and *B*lood *P*ressure. In a state of ill health, the measurement of any of the vital signs may vary. The degree of variation depends on the cause, with measurements occurring below or above the average range. Factors other than disease, such as environmental changes, activity, and emotional state, influence fluctuations. Together with the patient history, the results of laboratory and other clinical tests, and the physical examination, vital signs enable the physician to determine the diagnosis.

INTRODUCTION TO INFECTION CONTROL

Whereas medial *asepsis* (techniques of cleanliness to prevent the transmission of harmful or disease-causing microorganisms) is discussed later in Chapter 24, the basics of infection control is introduced here because of its importance to each clinical procedure in the medical office.

Handwashing is the most significant infection control for the medical assistant. The medical assistant should wash the hands before obtaining vital signs, preparing the patient for the physical examination, and placing hands on the patient during examination and treatment. Handwashing is a cleaning, rather than a sterilizing

procedure. In nonsterile procedures, an object or the skin is cleaned to reduce the number of pathogenic (disease-causing) microorganisms. In sterile procedures, measures must be taken to provide *surgical asepsis*. This includes absolute sterilization, whereby all microorganisms are killed and the object is totally free of their contamination. Ungloved hands can never be sterile.

Because the medical assistant moves from one patient to another, assisting with examination and treatment procedures and assembling instruments, the potential for cross-contamination is significant. Therefore, the medical assistant must become habituated to washing his or her hands in the correct manner before and after each patient contact and after each potentially infectious situation, such as after removing gloves used for handling contaminated materials.

The wearing of gloves reduces the chance of cross-contamination coming into contact with patient blood and body fluids or handling other contaminated materials. Other environmental safety work area restrictions include:

1. Carefully dispose of contaminated materials, such as urine, feces, and respiratory secretions, by placing them in a plastic bag with an orange or orange-red biohazard symbol (Fig. 17–1), tightly closing the bag, and disposing of it immediately as local regulations require.
2. Place specimens that could puncture a container within a puncture-resistant secondary container.
3. If outside contamination of the primary container occurs, place it within a secondary container to prevent leakage.

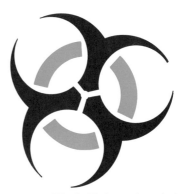

Figure 17–1. Biohazard symbol.

4. Keep the examination table and the room and furniture free from dust and dirt, and decontaminate work surfaces after any contamination and at the end of each day.
5. Teach patients to cover their noses and mouths when coughing and sneezing, and immediately dispose of paper tissues in a biohazard container.
6. Do not eat, drink, apply cosmetics or lip balm, smoke, or handle contact lenses; use discretion in wearing jewelry with the uniform, as crevices (particularly in rings and bracelets) are areas where pathogens collect.
7. Do not keep food and beverages in refrigerators, freezers, or near any area where blood and other potentially infectious materials are present.
8. Conduct all procedures in a manner that minimizes splashing, spraying, splattering, and generation of droplets of blood or other potentially infectious materials.

These suggestions serve to orient and alert medical assisting students to the importance of infection control and its application in the procedures of obtaining vital signs and assisting with the physical examination. Other suggestions and further discussion are included where appropriate throughout the text.

OCCUPATIONAL SAFETY AND HEALTH ADMINISTRATION BLOODBORNE PATHOGENS EXPOSURE CONTROLS

The clinical procedures at the conclusion of this chapter and those presented throughout the text include important symbols to assist the medical assistant in complying with the Occupational Safety and Health Administration (OSHA) guidelines to control bloodborne pathogen exposure. Universal blood and body fluid precautions, called simply *universal precautions*, are intended to prevent skin puncture and mucous membrane and nonintact skin exposures of health care workers to bloodborne pathogens and other potentially infectious materials. These controls include the following:

1. The classification of body fluids to which universal precautions apply
2. The use of protective barriers (clothing, shields)
3. The correct selection and use of gloves
4. Waste management

Universal precautions means that all blood or other potentially infectious materials must be considered infectious regardless of the perceived health status of the patient or coworker. To address the four specific control measures listed above, each procedure listed in this text contains symbols that represent the controls applicable to that procedure. The symbols are listed as "OSHA Standards" at the beginning of each procedure.

When OSHA Standards symbols are listed, it is assumed that the student has familiarized herself or himself with their meanings and can integrate the precautions into the procedure even though they are not further discussed within the procedure and principles narrative itself.

The OSHA Standards symbols are intended to alert the student to the universal precautions at the onset of each procedure. Table 17–1 explains the OSHA Standards symbols used throughout this book. The explanation for these standards are also listed on the inside back cover of this text for continued quick reference.

BODY TEMPERATURE

Body temperature represents the balance maintained by the body between heat lost and heat produced. Body heat is described in terms of heat units called *degrees*. Body temperature is derived from a process called *metabolism*, which refers to the chemical and physical changes occurring inside or outside the body that produce heat (Table 17–2). A healthy person's temperature varies during the day depending on these internal and external factors, with the maximum temperature occurring between 5:00 PM and 7:00 PM.

In the unhealthy person, illness upsets the metabolic process and disturbs the amount of heat being produced. In most bacterial disease processes, the metabolic activity is increased, thus increasing body temperature. While the physiology of the fever mechanism is not well understood, it is generally believed that the infective organisms (foreign proteins) affect the hypothalamus, which in turn sets the body's thermostat at a higher temperature. Thus, fever is thought to be the body's defensive reaction against disease, as heat is believed to inhibit the growth of some bacteria and viruses.

Periods of growth also affect metabolic rate. In infants and children, metabolism is increased owing to the great expenditure of energy required for early growth and development and the general immaturity of the heat-regulating system, which is more responsive to chemical and physical changes than that of adults. In addition, infants and children experience rapid heat loss across their body surface area, which is large relative to blood volume and tissue mass. The phenomenon is characteristic of the inverse relationship of metabolic rate to body size.

The heat regulatory system, which consists of skin receptors activated in the hypothalamus of the brain, monitors the balance between heat produced and heat lost. Heat is both produced and lost continuously during life. The mechanisms of heat regulation are extremely effective in maintaining temperature balance. When the body overheats, the nervous system processes the message and activates a cooling system called *perspiration*. Perspiration is the excretion of moisture through the pores of the skin. The nervous system causes superficial blood vessels on the skin to dilate, allowing more blood to reach the surface and

Table 17-1

SYMBOLS FOR OSHA BLOODBORNE PATHOGEN EXPOSURE CONTROLS
APPLICABLE TO CLINICAL PROCEDURES

  OSHA exposure categories applied to specific tasks as follows:

 Tasks that involve exposure to blood, body fluids, or tissues, or that carry a potential for spills or splashes. Appropriate protective measures should be used *every time.*

 Tasks that involve no exposure to blood, body fluids, or tissues in the normal work routine, but exposure or potential exposure may occur in certain situations. Appropriate protective measures should be used in these situations.

 Tasks that involve no exposure to blood, body fluids, or tissues. Appropriate protective measures are *not* necessary.

 Washing hands after a procedure.

 Washing hands before and after a procedure.

  Disposable sharp equipment that must not be bent, recapped, removed, sheared, or purposely broken. Equipment should be disposed of in a rigid, leakproof, puncture-resistant container that is color-coded orange or orange-red or labeled with the orange-red biohazard sign.

 Reusable sharp equipment that must be placed immediately, or as soon as possible, after use into appropriate sharps containers. The containers used to receive contaminated equipment must be puncture-resistant, leakproof, and color-coded orange or orange-red or labeled with the orange-red biohazard sign.

 Masks, goggles, or face shielding is required as protection whenever splashes, spray, splatter, or droplets of blood or other potentially infectious materials may be generated and eye, nose, or mouth contamination can reasonably be anticipated.

 Protective clothing, such as laboratory coats, gowns, or aprons, is required as protection whenever splashes, spray, splatter, or droplets of blood or other potentially infectious materials may be generated and clothing contamination can reasonably be anticipated.

 Biohazard bags must be used to discard materials containing blood or other potentially infectious materials. The bags must be leakproof and color-coded orange or orange-red or labeled with the orange-red biohazard sign.

 Decontamination requires using a bleach solution or Environmental Protection Agency–registered germicide. All contaminated work surfaces must be decontaminated after completion of procedures and immediately, or as soon as feasible, after any spill of blood or other potentially infectious materials (as well as at the end of the work shift) if the surface may have become contaminated since the last cleaning

 Gloves must be worn when it is reasonably anticipated that there will be hand contact with blood, other potentially infectious materials, nonintact skin, and mucous membranes. Gloves are not to be washed or decontaminated for reuse and are to be replaced as soon as practical when they become contaminated, or if they are torn or punctured or their ability to function as a barrier is compromised. *Utility* gloves may be decontaminated for reuse provided that the glove is intact and able to function as a barrier. *Examination* gloves are used for nonsterile procedures. *Sterile* gloves are used for minor surgery and other sterile procedures. (See also Chapter 24, Medical Office Surgery, for gloving procedures).

release heat. Since the blood is cooled in this manner, the body's temperature is likewise lowered.

Heat is also lost through water vapor in the lungs during expiration, and through urination. When moisture from all of these sources (including perspiration) evaporates, heat is released, and the body is cooled.

Other causes of heat loss are external. Environmental changes that subject the body to high temperatures raise the temperature of the blood, which in turn signals the hypothalamus to activate the heat-losing

center. Impulses are sent to sweat glands, and perspiration and cooling of the skin results.

When fever is experienced, superficial blood vessels closest to the skin constrict. The small papillary muscles at the base of the hair follicle also constrict and "goosebumps" form. Shivering and chills occur and heat is manufactured. Theoretically, shivering continues to occur and promote heat until the thermostat setting (by foreign proteins) is reached.

When more heat is produced than is lost, the body

Table 17–2

FACTORS AFFECTING BODY TEMPERATURE

Rate Increased	Normal Conditions	Rate Decreased
Exercise, physical activity (up to 105°F [40.6°C])	Activity	Decrease muscular activity
Late afternoon, early evening (4 PM to 6 PM)	Diurnal variants	Sleep, early morning (1 PM to 4 AM)
Active digestion	Food intake	Fasting, starvation
Increased room temperature, warm seasons	Environment	Decreased room temperature, cold seasons
Increased blood pressure	Blood pressure changes	Decreased blood pressure
Increased pulse and respiration	Metabolic changes	Increased perspiration, urination, defecation
Increased thyroid hormone, adrenalin	Hormonal changes	Decreased thyroid hormone, adrenalin
Newborns, active children, growth spurts	Age	Older adults
Blood vessel constriction	Cardiovascular changes	Blood vessel dilation
Ovulation, pregnancy	Emotions	Mental depression, grief
Stress, anxiety, fear, self-consciousness		
Bacterial infections, some viruses, degenerating body tissues	Illness	Some viral infections
Brain tumor or trauma	CNS injury	Fainting, CNS injury
Severe dehydration	Disease processes	Mild dehydration
Hyperthyroidism		Hypothyroidism
Allergic drug reactions	Drugs	Antibiotics, antiinfectives, antipyretics

CNS = central nervous system.

temperature is above normal, or elevated. Conversely, when more heat is lost than is produced, the body temperature drops below the normal range.

NORMAL BODY TEMPERATURE

The normal range for oral temperatures of resting adults is from 97°F to 100°F (36°C to 37.8°C). *Oral temperature* refers to the temperature of the oral cavity when the mercury tip of the oral thermometer is placed under the tongue and held in place for 3 to 5 minutes. Electronic thermometers register in 5 to 10 seconds or are removed from the patient's mouth when an audible sound is heard. Average oral temperature is usually considered to be 98.6°F (37°C). Many active children have temperature readings slightly above 100°F (37.8°C). In the elderly, normal temperature often falls to slightly below 97°F (36°C).

Rectal temperature measurements are usually 1°F or 1°C higher than the oral equivalent (on both Fahrenheit and Celsius scales, the longest lines on the thermometer represent 1° of temperature). The average normal rectal temperature is 99.6°F (37.5°C). A newborn's normal temperature ranges from 97.7°F to 99.5°F (36.5°C to 37.5°C). *Rectal temperature* refers to the temperature in the anal canal when the mercury tip of the rectal thermometer is inserted in the rectum and held in place for 2 to 4 minutes.

The average normal axillary temperature is 97.6°F (36.4°C). *Axillary temperature* refers to the temperature of the axilla (armpit) when the mercury tip of the thermometer is placed in a dried underarm area and

held in place for 10 minutes. The average axillary temperature is usually considered to be 1°F lower than oral temperature.

It takes a longer time to obtain the axillary temperature because, unlike the oral and rectal orifices, the armpit is not a closed orifice. Furthermore, there is no superficial vascularization in the armpit, whereas the oral and rectal orifices do have superficial blood vessels that readily supply heat.

CHARACTERISTICS OF FEVER

Fever (*pyrexia*) is a body temperature of over 100°F (37.8°C) in the resting child or adult. Fever, in itself, is not an illness but a sign that the body's defense mechanism is working properly to fight infection.

Children have less precise temperature regulation and higher normal temperatures than adults. Infants have higher basal temperatures than children. Children in the 1- to 5-year age group may experience febrile convulsions. Evidence indicates that these seizures are set off by the rate of temperature rise rather than the degree of fever. A febrile convulsion usually occurs very early in an illness and before it is known that a fever is present.

Prolonged high fever without fluid replacement causes dehydration. *Dehydration* (the excessive loss of moisture) is characterized by a flushed appearance, dry skin, and abnormal cramping and is always an emergency. Fever, even at 104°F (40°C) levels lasting for several days, is rarely harmful or dangerous to the brain; however, untreated, abnormal prolonged high fevers (105°F [40.5°C]) can cause irreversible brain damage or death.

TREATMENT OF FEVER

Treatment for uncomplicated fever may include the following measures:

1. Drink plenty of fluids (approximately 12 cups per day), provided kidney and cardiac functions are normal.
2. Wear lighter clothing (provided it does not cause chills).
3. Keep clothing and bed linens dry.
4. Eat well-balanced meals.
5. Discontinue exercise or strenuous activities.

Contrary to popular belief, sponging provides only temporary relief of fever and is therefore only recommended for relief of symptoms when a fever is over 103°F (39.5°C). If the physician orders sponging, a wet cloth or sponge should be briskly rubbed over the patient's arms, legs, and trunk to let the water evaporate from the skin surfaces. The principle of sponging is to increase heat loss through evaporation. Plain water at room temperature should be used. Alcohol, cold water, and ice water should not be used because they cause shivering and constriction of surface blood vessels, which in turn raises body temperature. Immersing the body in water or covering with washcloths impedes evaporation and should not be done. Sponging should be done only for 15 to 20 minutes, while waiting for the first dose of an antifever medication to take effect. Sponging should be discontinued if shivering occurs.

In general, fever alone can cause listlessness, and mechanically lowering the fever can make the patient feel better. On the other hand, if the patient does not feel any ill effects from the fever itself, treatment for minor elevations is often not necessary. What is important is to identify the cause of the fever and to treat it.

Antifever medications can benefit the patient. Aspirin may be prescribed *EXCEPT for chickenpox or any influenza-like illness.* Research indicates a possible connection between the administration of aspirin for acute febrile illnesses and Reye's syndrome. Reye's syndrome is a potentially fatal disease of children almost always associated with a previous viral infection, especially influenza type B and chickenpox (although at least 14 other viral infections are known to have preceded the onset of Reye's syndrome). Once thought a rare disease, Reye's syndrome is believed to be a major cause of death in children over the age of one. Acetaminophen (Tylenol, Tempra) is as effective a fever reducer as aspirin and may be used safely in place of aspirin in acutely febrile patients.

FEVER TERMINOLOGY

Certain terms are used to characterize body temperature and its various phases. These terms are described

Table 17–3
TERMS USED TO CHARACTERIZE BODY TEMPERATURE

Fever. Elevated body temperature beyond the normal range. Pyrexia and hyperthermia are synonyms for fever.
Hypothermia. Subnormal body temperature.
Febrile. Adjective pertaining to fever; feverish. "The child is febrile."
Afebrile. Adjective form denoting that fever is not present. "The child is afebrile."
Onset. Also termed *invasion.* Refers to period when fever begins.
Continuous. Temperature remains constantly elevated, with variations usually not exceeding 1°.
Defervescence. Fever subsides or disappears.
Intermittent fever. Fluctuations of body temperature between periods of subnormal temperature and fever.
Remittent fever. Temperature fluctuates several degrees above normal levels but does not return to normal levels between these periods of fluctuation.
Subsiding. Phase of fever when temperature is returning to normal levels.
Lysis. Gradual return of elevated body temperature to normal levels.
Crisis. Sudden return of elevated body temperature to normal levels. Usually accompanied by *diaphoresis* (profuse sweating).

in Table 17–3 and visualized graphically in Figure 17–2.

THE CLINICAL THERMOMETER

A clinical thermometer is used to measure the body temperature and is calibrated in either the Fahrenheit or Celsius (centigrade) scale (Fig. 17–3). Oral thermometers have a long, slender mercury bulb, which allows the largest surface contact with tissues when the thermometer is placed under the tongue or in the axilla. A thermometer with a shorter, blunter bulb is used to obtain the rectal temperature because the shape helps to prevent injury when inserted into the rectum and the thermometer can be securely held by rectal tissue. The upper tips of rectal and oral thermometers are color-coded for ease of identification: red (rectal) and blue (oral). A security-bulb thermometer, used primarily in hospitals and medical centers, has a special shatterproof encasement to prevent breakage and may be used for obtaining a disoriented patient's temperature.

On contact with warm human tissue, the mercury in the bulb of any glass thermometer rises. When the mercury rises to equal the body temperature, it does not continue to increase. The temperature reading is obtained by referring to the calibration scale on the thermometer and noting the point reached by the mercury.

On both the Fahrenheit and Celsius scales, the longest lines on the thermometer represent 1° of tempera-

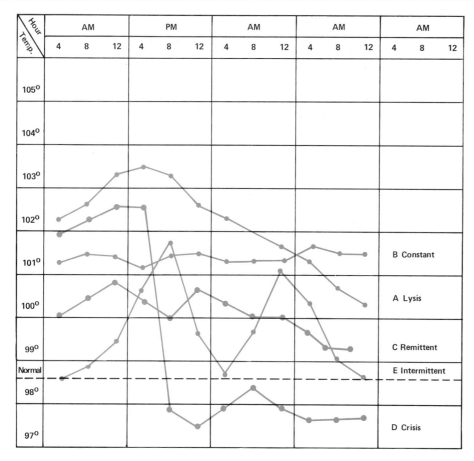

Figure 17–2. Fever categories.

ture. However, on the Fahrenheit scale, the shorter lines represent 0.2° increments, whereas on the Celsius scale they are read as 0.1° increments (Fig. 17–4). Figure 17–5 is a chart used for converting Fahrenheit to centigrade (Celsius).

Electronic thermometers (see Fig. 17–3) are also available in the centigrade or Fahrenheit scale. These are blue or red color-coded and equipped with disposable covers. They are used for obtaining both oral and rectal temperatures. A reading can be obtained in approximately 10 seconds with ± 0.2° accuracy. Although electronic thermometers are widely used in hospitals, some physicians continue to use glass thermometers in their offices.

Disposable plastic oral thermometers (used once only) are also available for obtaining body temperature. Heat-sensitive material turns dark when the thermometer is placed under the tongue for 60 seconds. An advantage of using this type of thermometer is that, because they are thrown away, cleaning is not required.

A disposable sheath is available for glass thermometers (oral or rectal). A sheath is a plastic casing which fits over the thermometer. After use, the casing is slipped off the thermometer, inside out, to avoid thermometer contamination and then discarded, thus avoiding the necessity for cleaning thermometers. Sheathed rectal thermometers must be thoroughly lubricated for patient comfort.

The newest technique for measuring body temperature is the infrared tympanic thermometer. These thermometers are able to record body temperature in 3 seconds. The instrument resembles the otoscope and uses a disposable probe cover that is the shape of an ear speculum. The advantages of using this type of thermometer include the elimination of cleaning, the avoidance of possible contamination from body fluid, and the speed with which body temperature is recorded, which is especially helpful when treating disoriented or uncooperative patients. The site is also easily accessible in adults and children.

See the procedures at the end of this chapter for detailed descriptions of how to take oral, rectal, and axillary temperatures, and of conversion between Fahrenheit and Celsius scales. The procedure for dealing with accidental breakage of a thermometer is also given.

Because oral thermometers are constructed from glass, care must be taken to avoid breakage. If breakage should occur, pieces must be carefully disposed of in a puncture-resistant container that is then closed tightly. Touching mercury should be avoided to prevent injury to the skin.

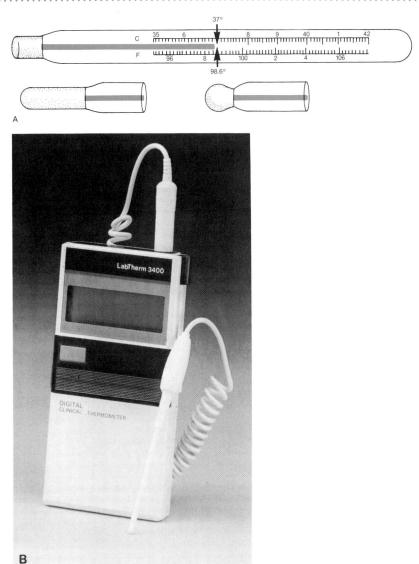

Figure 17–3. (A) A thermometer with both Fahrenheit and Celsius (centigrade) temperature scales. The blunt bulb can be used for both oral and rectal insertion. The elongated bulb (bottom, left) is found on a rectal thermometer. (From Saperstein, AB and Frazier, MA: Introduction to Nursing Practice. FA Davis, Philadelphia, 1980, p 456, with permission.) **(B)** An electronic thermometer. (Courtesy of Labtron Scientific Corporation and Villa Medical Supply.)

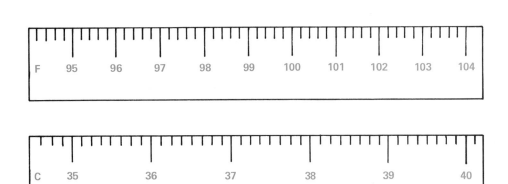

Figure 17–4. Comparison of Fahrenheit and Celsius scales.

Conversion Chart

Fahrenheit (F)	Centigrade (C)	Fahrenheit (F)	Centigrade (C)
32	0	101.3	38.5
95.0	35	102.2	39
95.9	35.5	103.1	39.5
96.8	36	104	40
97.7	36.5	104.9	40.5
98.6	37	105.8	41
99.5	37.5	106.7	41.5
100.4	38		

Convert Fahrenheit to Centigrade by subtracting 32 from the Fahrenheit reading and multiplying the remainder by $5/9$.

$$C = (F - 32) \times 5/9$$

Convert Centigrade to Fahrenheit by multiplying the Centigrade reading by $9/5$ and adding 32 to the product.

$$F = (9/5 \times C) + 32$$

Figure 17–5. Conversion chart for Fahrenheit and Celsius scales.

PULSE

The pulse beat is another vital sign that indicates the state of health of the human body. The rate and characteristics of the pulse are dynamic physiologic functions that provide clues to the condition of the cardiovascular system. Counting and interpreting pulse characteristics accurately is an integral part of the patient assessment.

Pulse can be defined as the wave of alternating expansion and relaxation of the arterial walls with each beat, or contraction, of the *left ventricle* of the heart, which carries 60 to 70 mL of blood to the aorta, thus distending the walls of the aorta and causing the pulse wave. Each time the heart beats, blood is forced into the arteries; the arteries expand as the wave of blood passes through and then return to their previous state. This wave sensation is referred to as the pulse and can be felt by lightly placing the fingertips over a superficial artery.

PHYSIOLOGY OF PULSE

The *apical pulse* is the beat of the heart with each contraction of the left ventricle and is detected with a stethoscope held over the apex of the heart. The heart is divided into four chambers (Fig. 17–6). The left ventricle is the chamber that, when filled with fresh (oxygenated) blood, contracts (pumps) and forces blood into the major artery, the aorta. From the aorta, the

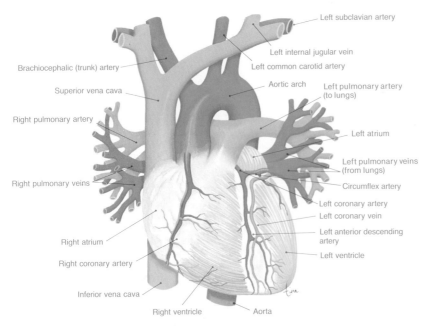

Figure 17–6. Chambers of the heart. (From Scanlon, VC and Sanders, T: Essentials of Anatomy and Physiology. FA Davis, Philadelphia, 1991, p. 268, with permission.)

blood is channeled into all of the arteries of the cardiovascular system. Therefore, normally the pulse rate in any of the arteries is the same as the actual heart rate.

The arteries are composed of an elastic muscular wall. The wall of the normal pulsating artery is soft and pliable; the abnormal artery is hard and knotty due to the loss of elasticity or inner vessel sclerotic build-up. When blood is being forced through a normal artery, the vessel stretches, increasing in size. As the left ventricle is filling and is in a state of rest, the walls of the arteries also are relaxing. The artery therefore contracts and relaxes. Atheromatous build-up (fatty deposits or plaque that has accumulated inside the vessel) makes the walls rigid and reduces elasticity. The pulse offers an assessment of the condition of the cardiovascular system.

VARIABLES AFFECTING PULSE

As with all vital signs, any change in the body's metabolism (normal functioning) will cause normal fluctuations in pulse rate (Table 17–4). Therefore, it is preferable to speak of normal *ranges* of pulse rate rather than normal pulse rates.

Disease causes fluctuations in the pulse rate and may also affect the regularity and strength of the pulsation.

The heart is a muscle and, like all other muscles in the body, is subject to the aging process. With age, the heart becomes less efficient, and the left ventricle loses contractibility, thereby becoming less forceful in its contraction and resulting in reduced cardiac output. *Cardiac output* is the amount of blood pumped from the left ventricle into the aorta per minute. Because the amount of blood pumped by the heart per unit of time is reduced in an older adult, the normal pulse is slower than that of a younger person.

Since metabolism influences pulse rate, it is reasonable to expect that increased physical demands on the cardiovascular system, which increase metabolism, also increase heart rate and pulse. With regular exercise, however, the heart muscle is strengthened, and the long-term effect is a *slower* pulse rate. For instance, the average resting pulse rate of an athlete may be 56 beats per minute, and this rate is within normal bounds for a well-conditioned athlete.

With strong emotions, the metabolism and heart rate may increase, causing a corresponding increase in pulse rate. During stress, certain substances, including epinephrine (adrenaline), are released in the body, stimulating the whole human mechanism to accelerate. Feelings of fear, anger, or excitement are catalysts in the process. Because of this relationship between stress and

Table 17–4

FACTORS AFFECTING THE RANGE OF PULSE RATES AND RATES OF RESPIRATION

Rate Increased	Normal Conditions	Rate Decreased
Exercise, physical activity (short term)	Activity	Long-term exercise and conditioning
Sudden standing	Postural changes	Lying down, poor posture
Late afternoon, early evening	Diurnal variants	Sleep
Active digestion	Food intake	Starvation
Heat, increased CO_2 in blood, high altitudes	Environment	Cold, decreased CO_2 in blood
Decreased blood pressure	Blood pressure changes	Increased blood pressure
Increased metabolism	Metabolic changes	Decreased metabolism
Increased thyroid hormone, adrenalin	Hormonal changes	Decreased thyroid hormone, adrenalin
Infancy to adulthood	Age	Older adults
Blood vessel dilation	Cardiovascular changes	Blood vessel constriction
Pregnancy	Reproductive	
Stress, anxiety, fear, self-consciousness	Emotions	Mental depression
Most infections, fever	Illness	
Acute or sudden pain, hemorrhage	Pain and injury	Unrelieved, severe pain
Shock	CNS injury	Untreated shock, coma Brain injuries (stroke, skull fracture)
Atherosclerosis	Diseases processes	Kidney damage
Hyperthyroidism		Hypothyroidism
Acute or chronic cardiovascular disease		Certain types of heart disease
Chronic lung disease		
Anemia, edema, circulatory disorders		
Drugs that increase heart rate: atropine, ephedrine, nicotine	Drugs	Drugs that decrease heart rate: digitalis, CNS depressants
Acute poisoning	Poisoning	Late-stage poisoning

CNS = central nervous system.

metabolism, the vital signs, which include the pulse, are measurable indicators of the level of physiologic and psychological stress.

CHARACTERISTICS OF PULSE

Pulse has several major physical characteristics: rate, rhythm, volume, and condition of the arterial wall. A pulse rate (numeric value) alone is an inadequate determination of pulse as a vital sign. Judgments regarding other characteristics are also necessary, and a discussion of those follows:

1. *Rate*. This characteristic of the pulse refers to the number of beats per minute. The usual adult pulse rate ranges from 60 to 90 beats per minute. A pulse rate of 80 is considered to be the clinical average. Clinical averages for non-adults are as follows: infants, 100 to 160 beats per minute; children ages 1 to 7, 80 to 120 beats per minute; children over age 7, 80 to 90 beats per minute. Adolescents range from 60 to 100 pulse beats per minute. Elderly adults range from 60 to 90 pulse beats per minute. Well-conditioned athletes may have pulse beats averaging 50 to 70 beats per minute.
2. *Rhythm*. The term used to describe the pulse tempo. The pulse should have a regular pattern of beats occurring in a smooth, evenly paced sequence. Irregular patterns are referred to as arrhythmias.
3. *Pulse volume (force)*. Refers to the palpable strength of the beat. When the pulse is counted, the wavelike sensation of blood pulsating through the artery can be described as weak, strong, thready, full and bounding, or alternating between strong and weak pulsations. The normal pulse should feel full and strong and be easily palpated, or felt, by gentle pressure of the fingertips to one of the pulse sites. Sometimes, the pulse cannot be felt at all.

   To avoid terms that are vague and subject to misinterpretation, some hospitals and medical offices use a more objective scale for reporting the force of a pulse. Table 17–5 is the scale for classifying pulse strength.
4. *Condition of arterial wall*. In addition to the volume (force) of the pulse, the texture of the wall of the artery can be determined when obtaining the rate and rhythm. Normal texture is smooth and soft; abnormal texture is described as knotty or hard.

ARRHYTHMIAS

The term *arrhythmia* refers to an absence of rhythm caused by an irregular contraction of the cardiac muscle. The prefix "a" signifies without, and "rhythm" signifies movement that can be measured.

Cardiac arrhythmias are not necessarily abnormalities. Certain arrhythmias, such as premature ventricular

Table 17–5
SCALE FOR REPORTING PULSE STRENGTH

0	Pulse not palpable
+1	Difficult to palpate; weak and thready, easy to obliterate with slight pressure
+2	Requires light palpation; but once located, stronger than +1
+3	Normal; easy to palpate, not easily obliterated (low arterial tension soft and elastic arterial wall elasticity)
+4	Strong, bounding; easily palpated, difficult to obliterate (high arterial tension, hard and inelastic arterial wall)

contractions (commonly referred to as PVCs) and tachycardia, may be considered normal in the healthy functioning heart. Usually, however, when an arrhythmia is detected, the physician first attempts to rule out the presence of heart disease rather than presume normal heart function. Arrhythmia is never a disease in itself but rather a potential sign of cardiac dysfunction. The medical assistant must be acquainted with the terminology and patterns of arrhythmias because he or she may be the first—and perhaps the only—person who discovers the occurrence of an arrhythmia during the routine procedure of obtaining the vital signs (Table 17–6). The medical assistant should immediately report the detection of any suspected arrhythmia to the physician, so that the physician can then proceed to assess the nature and seriousness of the finding.

PULSE SITES

Pulse readings may be obtained anywhere on the body where the artery is near the body surface and lies over a bone. The most common pulse reading is taken at the radial pulse, so named because the radial artery that is palpated to obtain the pulse rate lies over the radius bone at the wrist. Two fingers are gently applied to this site to feel the pulsations. The radial pulse is favored because it is easily accessible and most comfortable for the patient. (See procedures at end of chapter.)

The carotid, brachial, dorsalis pedis, femoral, temporal, and popliteal arteries (Fig. 17–7) may also be used for obtaining the pulse rate and characteristics. The carotid artery is the large artery that arises from the base of the neck on either side of the trachea (windpipe). By exerting gentle pressure under the chin and slightly to the side of the neck, the carotid pulse can be detected. The brachial artery is located in the antecubital space of the arm (at the bend of the elbow) and is used to obtain the blood pressure reading. The popliteal pulse is located in the crevice behind the knee. The dorsalis pedis artery is located on the upper aspect of the foot, along an imaginary line extending from the groove formed between the big and second toe. (This pulse may be congenitally absent). The femoral artery is located in the flexible area of the hip (groin) between

Table 17–6
TERMS USED TO DESCRIBE ABNORMAL CARDIAC PATTERNS

Tachycardia. Arrhythmia characterized by rapid but regular heart and pulse rates in excess of 90 beats/min. Tachycardia is normally produced during periods of exercise. When occurring at rest, it may be related to stress. Tachycardia may also be linked with diseases such as coronary artery disease.

Bradycardia. Arrhythmia characterized by slow heart and pulse rates usually below 60 beats/min. Bradycardia can be a normal byproduct of athletic development. An athlete may have a resting heartbeat of 56 beats/min because of the strength and efficiency of each contraction.

Extrasystole. Arrhythmia characterized by extra contractions (systoles), or beats. After the heart beats normally, a premature contraction follows with a slight pause before the next beat. This irregularity of rhythm causes the individual to experience the pulse sensation of a skipped beat. Occasional occurrence may be normal and temporary or may be associated with cardiovascular disease.

Atrial fibrillation. An atrial rate that may be more than 400 beats per minute and unable to be counted. This arrhythmia is associated with diseases such as myocardial infarction and hyperthyroidism.

Ventricular fibrillation. A ventricular rate that may be above 350 beats/min and unable to be counted. This condition usually results in circulatory failure.

Heart block. An extremely serious arrhythmia where impulses are not transmitted from the atria of the heart to the ventricles, and therefore, the ventricles seek their own rhythm. The heart and pulse rates are excessively slow, perhaps 30 to 40 beats/min.

the thigh and the abdomen. The temporal pulse, located on either side of the face in the temple area, is easily palpated and evaluated. These pulse sites, although seldom used by the medical assistant for obtaining pulse measurements, are most often evaluated by the physician performing an examination to assess the presence of pulse irregularities that may indicate peripheral vascular disease.

Another pulse site, the apical pulse (the heartbeat detected by placing a stethoscope over the heart) is the site of choice for assessing the pulse rate of an infant or young child. In an infant or young child, the pulse may be difficult to find in the extremities and can be more easily lost while counting owing to the child's movement. In addition, the apical pulse should be taken in any patient with suspected arrhythmia. (See the procedure at the end of this chapter for a step-by-step description of how an apical pulse is taken.)

RESPIRATION

The vital sign that represents the general state of the respiratory system is termed *respiration*. Together with temperature and pulse, respiration is an essential measurement in the standard TPR procedure. Respiration is the term used to designate the movement of air into the lungs and alveoli and the removal of carbon dioxide from the blood through the tracheobronchial tree.

PHYSIOLOGY OF RESPIRATION

Respiration has both internal and external phases. External respiration (*expiration*) refers to the exchange of oxygen and carbon dioxide that takes place in the lungs. Internal respiration (*inspiration*) refers to the exchange of these substances taking place in the tissues during the chemical process of metabolism. Thus, the medical assistant, in obtaining the rate and characteristics of respiration, is evaluating two respiratory movements in breathing since inspiration (drawing air into the lungs) and expiration (forcing air out of the lungs) together represent one act of respiration.

The respiratory center in the brain is located in the medulla oblongata. This center is affected by the nervous system and impulses initiated elsewhere in the body, as well as by the body's temperature and the chemical composition of the blood flowing through the brain's center. Impulses are sent from the respiratory center of the brain and travel down the spinal cord to the nerves that control the diaphragm and the intercostal muscles. Here, chemical and reflex signals aid the neural mechanisms that control breathing by enabling the body to adapt respiration to change in metabolism.

Chemical control is achieved mainly by the amount of carbon dioxide in the blood, which directly affects the respiratory center of the brain. Ventilation rate and depth increases automatically as the amount of carbon dioxide increases in the arterial blood. Thus, even though humans can send voluntary messages to the brain to "hold the breath" or "breathe slowly," voluntary control is still limited. It is not lack of oxygen but excess of carbon dioxide that causes the person to breathe again. On the other hand, prolonged rapid breathing, such as hyperventilation, results in a reduced amount of carbon dioxide in the blood caused by excessive excretion of carbon dioxide through the lungs. Immediate treatment involves having the patient breath into a paper bag to replace the carbon dioxide "blown off" during hyperventilation. Along with chemical control, specialized centers in the pons initiate and regulate the involuntary function of breathing during sleep and other periods when breathing becomes an automatic process.

Inspiration occurs when impulses from the respiratory center stimulate the diaphragm to contract. When the diaphragm contracts, abdominal organs move downward and forward, and push the ribs upward and outward to facilitate lung expansion. Expiration occurs when the lungs, chest wall, and diaphragm return to the relaxed position. Respiration is affected by most of the same variables that affect the other vital signs (see Table 17–4).

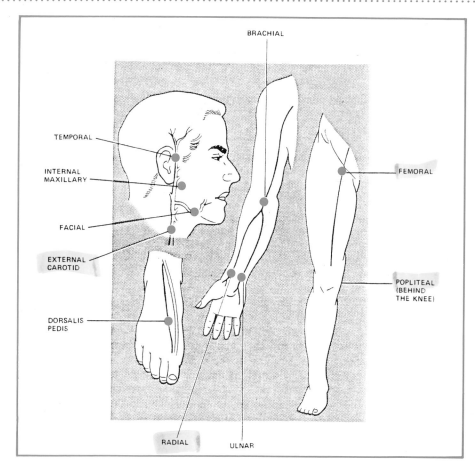

Figure 17-7. Pulse sites. (From Saperstein, AB and Frazier, MA: Introduction to Nursing Practice. FA Davis, Philadelphia, 1980, p 481, with permission.)

CHARACTERISTICS OF RESPIRATION

The characteristics of respiration affected by the mechanics of respiration are rate, rhythm, depth, and audibility. A description of these follows:

1. *Rate.* The rate of respiration is the number of breaths (one cycle of inspiration and expiration) per minute. The ratio of one respiration to four pulse beats is usually expected when the patient is at rest. The normal rates or averages based on age are as follows:

Age	Rate per Minute
Infants	30 to 60
1 to 7 years	18 to 30
Adult	12 to 20
Older Adult	Gradually increasing

2. *Rhythm.* A regular, even breathing pattern is considered normal for adults and children. The normal breathing pattern for infants, however, is irregular. Voluntary breath-holding or involuntary and automatic interruptions in the breathing pattern, such as sighing, are also considered normal.

3. *Depth.* The depth of respirations refers to the amount of air being inhaled and exhaled. When the patient is at rest and when no abnormality is present, respirations have a consistent depth, with the chest expanding and contracting at a normal rate with even depth. By contrast, when exercising, the breath may be more rapid and shallow but easily discernible. Rapid, shallow breathing also occurs in some disease states, and chest movement may be almost imperceptible.

4. *Audibility.* Normally, there are no noticeable breath sounds during the breathing process, with the exception of snoring. In certain diseases, particularly of the respiratory system, breath sounds may become noisy. When referring to noisy respirations, the term *stertorous* is applied. An individual with blockage of the nasal passageway may have stertorous breathing. Other descriptive characteristics of breathing are represented by use of specific terminology. *Rales* is the term used to denote abnormal sounds produced by the flow of air through liquid in the smaller air passages (fine rales) or in the larger air passages (course rales) and audible only by auscultation with a stethoscope. *Rhoncus* (singular), *rhonchi* (plural), are dry, coarse rales in the air passages that resemble either wheezing or snoring sounds. *Wheezing* is

another descriptive characteristic pertaining to breath sounds and is associated with noise experienced during difficult breathing.

TERMINOLOGY OF BREATHING PATTERNS

Table 17–7 lists certain terms used to denote special types of breathing patterns that are not disease conditions in themselves but merely describe a disruption of the normal breathing pattern. In these terms in Table 17–7, the suffix "pnea" refers to breathing.

When an individual cannot inspire enough oxygen to supply all of the body's cells with oxygenated blood, the normal pink skin coloring, particularly around the lips and on the nail beds, is replaced by a bluish tinge. The bluish tinge represents the increased level of carbon dioxide that is present in the blood and is termed *cyanosis*. The respiration terms discussed above are those

Table 17–7
TERMS USED TO DESCRIBE BREATHING PATTERNS

Eupnea. Normal effortless breathing.

Dyspnea. Labored breathing characterized by an increased effort to inhale and exhale. Rate and depth are often increased. In some disease states, dyspnea occurs only on exertion.

Apnea. Signifies a temporary rather than permanent cessation of breathing. *Sleep apnea* is a condition in which there are short, temporary periods of apnea occurring during sleep.

Orthopnea. Condition in which individuals with certain diseases affecting the heart and lungs can breathe comfortably only in the upright or sitting position.

Hyperpnea. An increased depth of respirations which may or may not include an increased rate. Hyperpnea follows strenuous exercise or can accompany conditions associated with increased rate and depth of respiration (see Table 17–4).

Hyperventilation. An abnormally prolonged rapid and deep breathing, usually associated with an acute anxiety. Symptoms include faintness, some degree of apprehension, and heart palpitations. Hyperventilation may also be caused by central nervous system disorders, or by drugs that increase the sensitivity of the respiratory centers, such as salicylates.

Hypoxia. Broad term meaning diminished oxygen to the body. Symptoms include dyspnea, rapid pulse, fainting, and mental disturbances. Angina pectoris (localized chest pain) is due to hypoxia because of a decreased supply of O_2 to the heart muscle.

Aerophagia. The act of swallowing or gulping air that results in rapid and irregular breathing.

Cheyne-Stokes Respiration. Breathing that may occur in patients approaching death. This condition is characterized by respirations gradually increasing in rapidity, subsiding, and then ceasing for prolonged period (up to 50 sec) before beginning again (alternating apnea and hyperventilation).

frequently encountered by the medical assistant in the office setting. The procedure followed for measuring and assessing respiration is given at the end of this chapter.

BLOOD PRESSURE

The measurement of blood pressure is yet another vital sign of major significance to the patient's diagnosis and treatment. In fact, because high blood pressure (hypertension) is often asymptomatic (without symptoms), it is common practice to obtain a blood pressure reading for all patients each time they visit the office, regardless of the purpose for the visit. (TPR readings are usually obtained only for patients with suspected infection or other specific conditions, and for those receiving complete physical examinations).

The medical assistant must have a thorough knowledge of the blood pressure physiology and must be competent in the procedural skills to obtain an accurate measurement, to facilitate the physician's goal for patient care and to answer the patient's questions regarding blood pressure.

PHYSIOLOGY OF BLOOD PRESSURE

Blood pressure indirectly measures the amount of force, or pressure, exerted on the walls of the arterial blood vessels as the blood pumped by the heart is pushed through these arteries (Fig. 17–8). The *cardiac cycle* (pump cycle) is the term used to refer to the two phases of the heartbeat: contraction and relaxation. Blood pressure measures the pressure in the arteries during both phases. Systole is the phase of cardiac contraction. *Systolic blood pressure* measures the pressure in the arteries when the left ventricle of the heart contracts. Diastole is the phase of cardiac relaxation. *Diastolic blood pressure* measures the pressure in the arteries when the left ventricle is at rest.

NORMAL BLOOD PRESSURE

Blood pressure is measured in millimeters of mercury (mm is the abbreviation for millimeter; Hg is the chemical symbol for mercury). Although blood pressure varies with age, in the average adult at rest, the arterial blood most commonly exerts enough pressure to raise a column of mercury to the height of 120 mm during systole and 80 mm during diastole. The normal range extends from 110/70 to 140/90 mmHg.

The average arterial pressures (systolic/diastolic) for various age groups are as follows:

Newborn	50 to 52/25 to 30
6 years	95/62
10 years	100/65
16 years	118/75
Adult	120/80
Older Adult	138/86

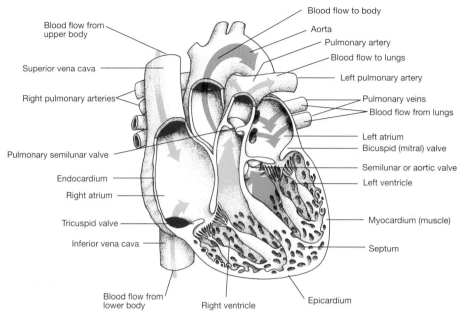

Blood flow from upper body
Superior vena cava
Right pulmonary arteries
Pulmonary semilunar valve
Endocardium
Right atrium
Tricuspid valve
Inferior vena cava
Blood flow from lower body
Right ventricle

Blood flow to body
Aorta
Pulmonary artery
Blood flow to lungs
Left pulmonary artery
Pulmonary veins
Blood flow from lungs
Left atrium
Bicuspid (mitral) valve
Semilunar or aortic valve
Left ventricle
Myocardium (muscle)
Septum
Epicardium

Figure 17–8. Diagram of the blood flow through the heart and major blood vessels. (Adapted from Gylys BA and Wedding ME: *Medical Terminology: A Systems Approach*, ed 2. FA Davis, Philadelphia, 1988, p 149.)

CARDIOVASCULAR FACTORS AFFECTING BLOOD PRESSURE

Certain physiologic and external factors influence the blood pressure (see Table 17–8). Specific *cardiovascular* factors affecting blood pressure include:

VOLUME Volume is the amount of blood in the arteries. An increase in blood volume increases blood pressure, and vice versa. For example, an individual who has been injured in an accident and is hemorrhaging will have a lowered blood pressure because the volume of blood has decreased. Because the left ventricle is not filling to full capacity, the volume of blood (cardiac output) lessens with each contraction, and thus the pressure in the vessels drops.

PERIPHERAL VASCULAR RESISTANCE This term refers to the resistance of the arteries to the flow of

Table 17–8
FACTORS AFFECTING BLOOD PRESSURE

Rate Increase	Normal Conditions	Rate Decreased
Exercise, physical activity (short term)	Activity	Relaxation
Lying, legs elevated	Postural changes	Sudden standing, postural changes
Late afternoon, early evening	Diurnal variants	Sleep, early morning
Increase adrenalin	Metabolic changes	Decreased adrenalin
Older adults	Age	Birth to adulthood
Right arm (3 to 4 mmHg higher)	Cardiovascular changes	Left arm (3 to 4 mmHg lower)
Late pregnancy, postpuberty males, postmenopausal women	Reproductive	Middle pregnancy
Stress, anxiety, fear, worry (hypertension)	Emotions	Mental depression, grief (hypotension)
Obesity	Nutrition	Starvation, anemia
	Illness	Dehydration, infections, fever
	Pain	Intense pain
Increased arterial blood volume	Blood volume	Decreased arterial blood volume (hemorrhage)
Increased intracranial pressure	CNS	Shock, fainting, collapse, CNS disorders
Atherosclerosis, arteriosclerosis hyperthyroidism, renal disease, liver disease, heart disease	Disease processes	Cancer, hypothyroidism, approaching death, weak heart, massive heart attack
Caffeine, stimulants, nicotine	Drugs	Antihypertensives, diuretics, narcotic analgesics, antiarrhythmias

blood. The diameter of the artery determines the degree of resistance: *the smaller the diameter, the greater the resistance.* For example, an individual with *atherosclerosis* (fatty deposits lining the walls of the blood vessels) or *arteriosclerosis* (rigid vessel walls) will have an increased blood pressure because of the narrowed diameter of the vessel.

The diastolic pressure provides an important indicator of the condition of the vessels because the left ventricle is at rest during the diastolic phase. An increased diastolic pressure, therefore, means that even though the heart is relaxed, the vessel pressure is greater than normal, indicating the probability of a disease that causes the narrowing of vessels.

CONDITION OF THE HEART MUSCLE The condition of the heart muscle is an important factor related to blood volume. A strong, forceful pump works efficiently and tends to normalize blood pressure. A weakened heart muscle has the reverse effect.

VESSEL ELASTICITY *Elasticity* refers to the capacity of the vessel to alternately expand and contract. An example of a vessel condition resulting in flow of elasticity and thus increased resistance to blood flow and increased blood pressure is arteriosclerosis (hardening of the arteries).

BLOOD PRESSURE TERMINOLOGY

The following terms are commonly used to describe the specific measurements related to blood pressure:

HYPERTENSION A systolic reading above 140 mmHg with a diastolic reading above 90 mmHg is considered to be above normal and is termed *high blood pressure*, or *hypertension*. One or both readings (systolic and diastolic) can be elevated in hypertension. The diagnosis of hypertension, however, is never made on the basis of one reading. Rather, the blood pressure pattern, ideally taken about the same time of day in a regular sequence (daily or weekly), is examined to determine a conclusive diagnosis. Frequent blood pressure screening is essential for uncovering abnormally high readings, which then become suspect for hypertension.

HYPOTENSION A systolic reading below 100 mmHg or 95 mmHg with a diastolic reading below 70 mmHg (some authorities say 60 mmHg) is considered to be below normal. This reading may indicate *low blood pressure*, or *hypotension*. One type of hypotension is orthostatic hypotension. Orthostatic hypotension may occur when a person quickly changes position from a supine to an upright position or stands for a prolonged period of time.

VENOUS PRESSURE Although the medical assistant *never* obtains measurements of venous pressure or central venous pressure, the probability of exposure to these terms warrants their discussion. *Central venous pressure* is the pressure of blood in the superior vena cava. *Venous pressure* is the pressure of blood in the veins. Normal values for central venous pressure are 5 to 10 cm H_2O. Obtaining central venous pressure is a procedure not routinely performed. Under normal con-

ditions, arterial pressure is considered to be a conclusive determinant of the state of health of the heart and blood vessels.

PULSE PRESSURE The difference between systolic and diastolic pressures is an extremely important measurement in diseases and trauma of the neurologic system, especially the brain. The average pulse pressure is 40 mmHg (the difference between a systolic pressure of 120 and a diastolic pressure of 80; a ratio of 3:2:1). This difference (*pulse pressure*) provides information on the condition of the arteries. Conditions such as atherosclerosis and cerebral vascular accident (*stroke*) greatly increase pulse pressure.

EQUIPMENT FOR MEASURING BLOOD PRESSURE

The stethoscope and the sphygmomanometer are the instruments used to obtain a blood pressure reading. The stethoscope is used to listen to the sounds of the blood in the artery. Although a stethoscope with a bell-shaped end is preferred to detect blood pressure sounds, a stethoscope with a round end, called a *diaphragm*, is more commonly used because the diaphragm covers a greater area and is easily secured in place. Sound is conducted to the ears by the two pieces of tubing that end in earpieces. The flexible rubber tubing connects to the metal neck piece to which the rubber earpieces are attached. The earpieces are turned slightly forward and placed in the ear. The forward position facilitates hearing the sounds because the ear canal runs forward toward the nose. The stethoscope is not sterilized, but the ear tips can be removed and placed in disinfectant solution when necessary. Otherwise, it is cleaned after each use as described in the procedure for obtaining blood pressure.

The sphygmomanometer is the instrument used in conjunction with the stethoscope to measure blood pressure. *Sphygmo* means pulse, and a *manometer* is an instrument that measures pressure. The sphygmomanometer apparatus includes a rubber bag encased in cloth with metal hooks and eyes or Velcro adhesive strips for fastening of the cuff. Also included are a pressure gauge (manometer) and a pressure bulb that has a control valve (usually a screw or dial).

The pressure gauge can be either of the aneroid or the mercury type. In an *aneroid* gauge (Fig. 17–9), a clocklike apparatus with calibrations is used to determine the blood pressure reading. The *mercury* gauge (Fig. 17–10) is a glass column containing mercury, with calibrations on either side of the column. Both types have a numeric scale, usually ranging from 0 to 240, in increments of 10. The reading is determined by reading the number or calibration corresponding to the level of mercury at the first and last distinct sounds.

The mercury manometer is more accurate, and the measurement is more readily identified. For these reasons, it is used most frequently. Most physicians' offices have mercury manometers installed on the wall at eye level in each examination room.

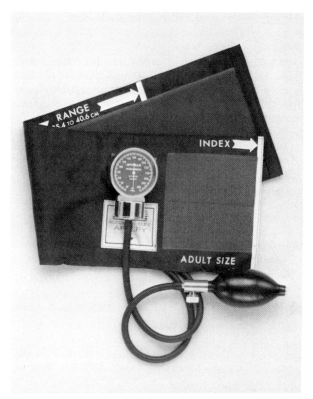

Figure 17-9. Aneroid blood pressure apparatus. (Courtesy of Labtron Scientific Corporation and Villa Medical Supply.)

The *blood pressure cuff* is the cuff containing an air-inflatable rubber bag. The cuff is snugly applied to the patient's upper arm. There are three categories of sizes to fit various individuals:

1. *Small:* for children and adults with small upper arm diameters. Cuff size variations for children are also available.
2. *Medium:* for the adult of average size.
3. *Large size:* for the obese adult.

The *pressure bulb* is a hollow rubber bulb that is used to pump air into the bag. The bulb fits into the palm of the hand, and the control valve attached to the bulb (usually a screw type) can be manipulated by the thumb and forefinger.

The principles and procedures descriptions at the end of this chapter thoroughly list each step in obtaining the blood pressure reading with the use of this equipment.

PHYSIOLOGY OF BLOOD PRESSURE MEASUREMENT

Physiologically, when this equipment is used, external pressure is being applied to the vessel by means of the inflated cuff. The air is pumped to approximately 30 mm above the patient's known systolic blood pressure in order to completely compress the artery. When the

cuff is properly positioned on the upper arm, it is level with the heart. When the cuff is inflated, blood circulation in the distal portion of the artery ceases. The heart, however, continues to pump blood into the vessel. Pressure is increased, and the vessel increases in size.

At this point, no sounds are heard through the stethoscope because there is greater pressure in the cuff than in the artery. When the cuff is gradually deflated by manipulating the control valve, blood begins to push or spurt through the artery because the cuff pressure and the artery pressure become equalized. Sounds are now audible through the stethoscope. When the bag is deflated further and the pressure in the cuff is less than the pressure in the artery, no further sounds are discernible.

The sounds heard when the cuff is being deflated have a definite beat and rhythm (pulsation), but the discernibility and volume fluctuate. There are five phases of sounds, together called the *Korotkoff sounds*, named for the physician who identified them.

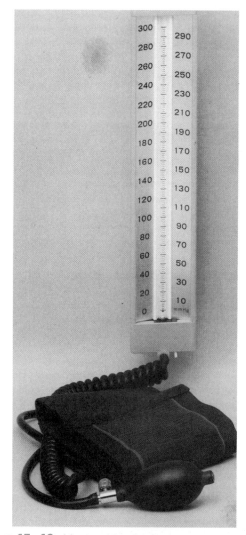

Figure 17-10. Mercury blood pressure apparatus. (Courtesy of Labtron Scientific Corporation and Villa Medical Supply.)

These sounds are heard between the systolic and diastolic levels. *It is important to note that the systolic reading corresponds to the first distinctly audible sound, and the diastolic reading refers to the last distinctly audible sound.* The sounds in between are not easily categorized or differentiated but are explained here to broaden the medical assistant's understanding of blood pressure.

As pressure declines in the cuff, the sounds of phase 1 appear as clear tappings that gradually increase in intensity. During phase 2, the sounds develop a swishing quality. If the cuff is not inflated to above the patient's systolic (phase 1) blood pressure, phases 1 and 2 can be missed entirely and phase 3 mistaken as the systolic pressure. Occasionally, phase 2 sound is termed the *auscultatory gap*. Auscultatory gaps may occur in hypertension and certain heart diseases. Phase 3 is characterized by crisper sounds that increase in volume. In phase 4, the sounds are muffled, and they disappear altogether in phase 5. In addition to obtaining and recording phases 1 and 5, the physician may also prefer that phase 4 be recorded as the "fading sound." In such instances, the recording may be noted as, for example, BP: 120/100/80.

While the Korotkoff sounds are sometimes distinctly recognizable, they are not separately measured. Again, only the first distinctly audible beat that occurs in two consecutive beats and the last distinctly audible beat compose the systolic and diastolic readings. The Korotkoff sounds are considered so that the changes in volume and quality can be anticipated and accepted as a normal occurrence.

INTERPRETATION OF ABNORMAL BLOOD PRESSURE READINGS

When a high blood pressure reading is obtained, it is advisable to permit the patient to rest and attempt a second reading shortly thereafter (15 to 20 minutes). This serves as a check on the accuracy of the first measurement and takes into account that the first reading may have been high because of the patient's anxiety. Repeating the procedure several times in the same arm may in itself elevate the pressure, however, partially because of the patient's subsequent discomfort.

The medical assistant must proceed with caution in relating the abnormal measurement to the patient requesting an interpretation of the reading. Although it is usually advisable to inform the patient of the numeric values, interpretation or diagnosis is outside the standard of practice for a medical assistant. The medical assistant would be in error to inform the patient that the reading is indicative of hypertension or hypotension. The assistant can, however, state that a diagnosis can only be made by the physician, who evaluates the blood pressure readings over a period of time, noting patterns and the presence of variables. As always, the medical assistant must exercise discretionary judgment to provide patient care of the best quality.

ERROR-PRODUCING CONDITIONS IN OBTAINING THE BLOOD PRESSURE

1. A release valve that is not tightened properly results in difficulty inflating the cuff and inability to read the mercury column accurately.
2. Deflating the cuff too slowly results in a false-high diastolic reading. Deflating the cuff too rapidly results in false-low systolic and false-high diastolic readings.
3. If the rubber bladder of the cuff is not deflated prior to obtaining a reading, this results in a loose cuff placement.
4. A cuff that is applied too loosely does not exert an adequate amount of pressure on the vessel and results in inaccurate high readings.
5. An air leak in the bladder delays the inflation rate and could cause a false-high reading.
6. Failure to pause for 1 to 2 minutes between retakes may result in abnormally high readings, as recovery time may be insufficient to allot a rest period for the previously constricted vessel.
7. A cuff size too large or too small to fit the patient's arm snugly will prevent the medical assistant from obtaining an accurate measurement of blood pressure since the pressure applied by the cuff in these instances is either too great or inadequate. Width of the cuff also affects the accuracy of the blood pressure measurement. A cuff that is too wide produces a false-low reading; a narrow cuff produces a false-high reading. Cuff sizes are as follows:

Newborn infants	2.5 cm (1 inch)
Children 1 to 4 years	6 cm (2.4 inches)
Children 4 to 8 years	9 cm (3.6 inches)
Adults	13 cm (5.2 inches)
Obese adults	20 cm (8 inches)

8. An inaccurate level of inflation may result in a false-low systolic reading.
9. Failure to keep the arm relaxed and at heart level may lower systolic pressure. Support the patient's arm while applying the cuff.

HEIGHT AND WEIGHT

An anthropometric measurement is a measure of various body dimensions, including weight, height, size, and proportion. Although the patient's height and weight are not routinely taken after the initial physical examination unless ordered by the physician, they are considered here along with the vital signs because they, too, are indicators of the patient's state of general health. This is particularly true of weight gain and loss.

In certain groups of patients, however, weight measurements may be routinely obtained. These include: (1) patients following special diets, to monitor potential results; (2) maternity patients, to detect weight loss or gain due to dietary habits, or weight gain possibly due to water retention (a weight gain of up to 5 lb a day may be indicative of fluid retention); (3) children, to indicate growth patterns, to detect hormonal disturbances, and to assess general signs of their state of health; (4) patients on diuretics and certain cardiac drugs; and (5) patients being treated for diabetes and congestive heart failures. Desirable weights for men and women, according to height, are given in Table 17–9.

EQUIPMENT FOR MEASURING HEIGHT AND WEIGHT

A balance scale is used to obtain both the height and weight measurements. Balance scales fall into two basic categories: mechanical and electronic. *Mechanical scales* essentially use the principle of the fulcrum, or lever, to arrive at a precalibrated set of weights that equalize the patient's total weight. *Electronic scales* (which are technically not balance scales) are increasing in popularity because the balance of weights does not need adjustment. Most electronic scales provide an immediate digital readout when the patient steps on the scale.

Both scales are equipped with a height bar. It is adjusted by lifting it above the patient's head and then gently placing the bar on the top of the head in order to obtain the correct height.

RECORDING THE DATA

If the patient's perception of the height and weight differs from the actual measurements, the patient's response may indicate a potential difficulty in body image perception. Such reactions should be noted in the patient record. The patient's statements concerning sudden or recent weight gains and losses may indicate serious disease, such as diabetes, hyperthyroidism (weight loss), or hypothyroidism (weight gain). These variations should also be noted in the patient record.

In addition to these factors, the medical assistant should keep in mind that the height of older adults may gradually decrease, often as a result of osteoporosis (increased density of the bone) and kyphosis (exaggeration of the thoracic curve of the vertebral column re-

Table 17–9
MEDIAN HEIGHTS AND WEIGHTS AND RECOMMENDED ENERGY INTAKE. RECOMMENDED DIETARY ALLOWANCES. REVISED 1989.

Category	Age (y) or Condition	Weight (kg)	Weight (lb)	Height (cm)	Height (in)	REE[a] (kcal/d)	Multiples of REE	Average Energy Allowance Per kg	Average Energy Allowance Per day[c]
Infants	0.0–0.5	6	13	60	24	320		108	650
	0.5–1	9	20	71	28	500		98	850
Children	1–3	13	29	90	35	740		102	1300
	4–6	20	44	112	44	950		90	1800
	7–10	28	62	132	52	1130		70	2000
Males	11–14	45	99	157	62	1440	1.70	55	2500
	15–18	66	145	176	69	1760	1.67	45	3000
	19–24	72	160	177	70	1780	1.67	40	2900
	25–50	79	174	176	70	1800	1.60	37	2900
	51+	77	170	173	68	1530	1.50	30	2300
Females	11–14	46	101	157	62	1310	1.67	47	2200
	15–18	55	120	163	64	1370	1.60	40	2200
	19–24	58	128	164	65	1350	1.60	38	2200
	25–50	63	138	163	64	1380	1.55	36	2200
	51+	65	143	160	63	1280	1.50	30	1900
Pregnant	first trimester								+0
	second trimester								+300
	third trimester								+300
Lactating	first 6 months								+500
	second 6 months								+500

Source: From Food and Nutrition Board, National Academy of Sciences—National Resources Council.

[a]Calculation based on FAO equations, then rounded.
[b]In the range of light to moderate activity, the coefficient of variation is ± 20%.
[c]Figure is rounded.

sulting in a hunchback, or round-shouldered appearance).

The role of the medical assistant is to accomplish the measurement and recording of height and weight accurately and with concern for the patient's sensitivities regarding these crucial health areas (see the procedures at the end of this chapter). The height and weight are recorded by using the abbreviations for height (Ht) and weight (Wt) followed by the numeric measurement.

Example:

Ht 5'9"; Wt 170 lb

The physician determines the significance of these measurements, taking into account the time of day, dress (clothing or examination gown), weight history, dietary habits, activity, and other factors specific to the individual. Customarily, the last recorded weight is used as a reference for comparison with the present measurement.

DOCUMENTATION OF VITAL SIGN MEASUREMENTS

The method of recording the numeric value of the vital signs has been noted in the specific procedural steps for each of the vital signs. However, in addition to recording the measurements, other guidelines pertaining to recording vital signs should be followed. These guidelines are applications of proper techniques for making written entries in the patient record.

Record:

1. The date and time.
2. Specifics such as left or right arm for blood pressure (if a second blood pressure measurement is taken, note the elapsed time). Pulse and respiration characteristics (such as "stertorous breath sounds" or "thready pulse") should be written after the numeric entry. Use precise medical terminology. Do not use words like "appears" or "seemed." Such assessment of vital signs is well within the scope of duties for the medical assisting profession.
3. Initial or sign in full *all* patient record notations, including vital signs. Some states require full name and title of the employee.
4. Format example:

2/21/93
BP: 120/80 (right arm); 99-90-20
Pulse irregular and thready
Counted for 3 minutes. MAF

(**Note:** in the example, "99-90-20" indicates temperature, pulse, and respiration, respectively.)

PATIENT TEACHING CONSIDERATIONS

All adult patients, and particularly parents of small children, should know how to use a thermometer to obtain temperatures safely and accurately. Pulse assessment should be taught to those patients receiving medication for cardiovascular disease. Specifically, they should receive instruction to detect and identify certain alterations in rate, rhythm, and volume.

Respiratory assessment should be taught to patients with preexisting respiratory disease to help these patients determine signs of impending complications. In addition, patients should receive instruction in preventive measures for avoiding respiratory infections, which would complicate existing respiratory dysfunctions. The medical assistant may also teach patients with specific needs how to perform breathing exercises.

Blood pressure assessment should be taught to patients concerned about developing or controlling hypertension. Patients should be informed of the risks of hypertension, how to prevent or control these risks, the role of diet and exercise, and the value of compliance with the prescribed drug therapy.

Whereas some patients have a special interest in acquiring health education relevant to their specific health needs, other patients request instruction because they wish to participate in monitoring their own health. Regardless of the patient's motive, all patients interested in health information warrant the special attention of the medical assistant–patient educator.

RELATED ETHICAL AND LEGAL IMPLICATIONS

As in the performance of all procedures the medical assistant's role with regard to obtaining vital signs, from an ethical and legal perspective, is to function within the parameters of the medical assisting profession. The medical assistant must carefully select the response to a patient asking whether his or her blood pressure reading is high or low. Patients should be informed of the measurement with the physician's consent, but the medical assistant should never venture a diagnosis. For example, a response such as "Yes, you have high blood pressure" is a statement of diagnosis and thus inappropriate. An appropriate response might be "Your blood pressure is 140/90, and although that is on the high end of the normal range, a diagnosis of high blood pressure can never be made from just one reading. The physician will answer all your questions and help you better understand how to interpret the reading."

The medical assistant must also take care to precisely record vital sign measurements. Errors in diagnosis and in treatment that are attributable, at least in part, to any error in obtaining or recording the vital signs implicate the medical assistant in any legal action the patient may pursue against the physician.

SUMMARY

Vital signs are the body's own health barometers and are an important aspect of almost every visit to the physician's office. Respiratory rate, rhythm, depth, and audibility, as well as height and weight, are generalized representations of the state of health of the individual. Since obtaining these measurements is a primary function of the clinical medical assistant, medical assistants must have confidence in their theoretic and practical expertise. Understanding the physiologic principles behind these measurements and the reasons for obtaining and recording these measurements is imperative to the development of confidence and professional competence.

DISCUSSION QUESTIONS

1. Why are "vital signs" so named?
2. What is the significance of OSHA standards? How should the medical assistant apply these to medical office practice?
3. Explain why body temperature varies during the day and night. Discuss the impact of illness on body temperature.
4. Define the term *pulse volume.* How would you describe it to a patient who had to monitor his or her own pulse rate, rhythm, and volume?
5. Identify the "controls" responsible for respiration. Differentiate between voluntary and involuntary respiration.
6. Describe the cardiovascular factors affecting blood pressure. How is a diagnosis of hypertension made?
7. What is the value of monitoring an adult patient's anthropometric measurements in medical practice?
8. What major points would you include in developing a patient teaching plan for a mother who will be obtaining the temperature, pulse, and respiration of her 6-month-old infant? What cautions and information beyond the procedure would you provide?

BIBLIOGRAPHY

Guyton, AC: Human Physiology and Mechanisms of Disease, 5th ed. WB Saunders Co, Philadelphia, 1992.
Hemmler, RL, et al: The Human Body in Health and Disease, 7th ed. JB Lippincott Co, Philadelphia, 1992.
Scanlon, VC and Sanders, T: Essentials of Anatomy and Physiology. FA Davis Co, Philadelphia, 1991.
Warden-Tamparo, CD and Lewis, MA: Diseases of the Human Body. FA Davis Co, Philadelphia, 1989.

PROCEDURE: Measure oral temperature of an adult or a child over 3 years of age

OSHA STANDARDS:

Terminal Performance Objective: Measure an accurate oral Fahrenheit temperature, then convert to the Celsius scale within 5 minutes.

EQUIPMENT: Oral Fahrenheit thermometer, blue tipped
Thermometer sheaths
Patient form or chart
Cold water and detergent
Alcohol swab
Biohazard bag for disposal
Fahrenheit-Celsius conversion chart or the formula:
  F = (9/5 × C) + 32

PROCEDURE

Preparation

1. Hold the Fahrenheit thermometer at the end-grip, and check the bulb and stem for cracks or breaks.

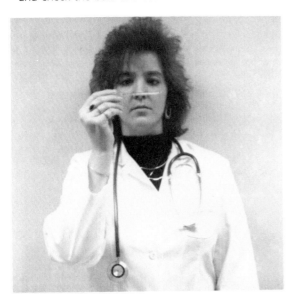

Check the mercury level.

PRINCIPLE

1. Although thermometers are made of heat-tempered glass, mercury expansion from excessive heat can cause the bulb to crack or break while in storage.

PROCEDURE   **PRINCIPLE**

2. Shake the thermometer over a soft surface with downward snaps of the wrist until the mercury column goes below 96°F (35.5°C).

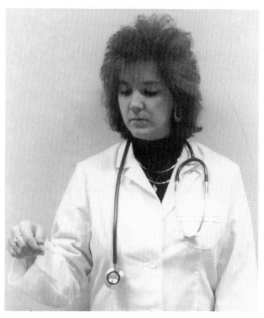

Shake down the mercury level.

3. Insert the thermometer bulb into the sheath opening at the pull-apart end of the outer wrap, sliding the thermometer in gently until it touches the opposite end of the sheath.

4. Grasp the outer wrap on each side of the perforated line, and twist hands in opposite directions until the outer wrap tears at the perforation.

5. Pull the thermometer together with the sheath tab from the outer wrap.

6. Ask the patient's name and explain the procedure.
   • Place the patient in a sitting or lying position.
   • Ask if the patient has had hot or cold liquids, eaten, exercised, or smoked within the last 15 minutes.
   • Ask the patient not to bite down on the thermometer and to avoid talking.

3,4,5. To make temperature taking more sanitary and to help protect against the possible danger of a broken thermometer.

6. To reduce the risk of error and to provide assurance to anxious patients, and:
   • To prevent the thermometer from breaking should the patient fall.
   • To wait 15 minutes if there are any outside factors that will alter body temperature.
   • To prevent a false-low temperature reading due to talking and to prevent thermometer breakage from biting down with the teeth.

PROCEDURE

7. Position the bulb carefully under the tongue so that it rests in a heat pocket.

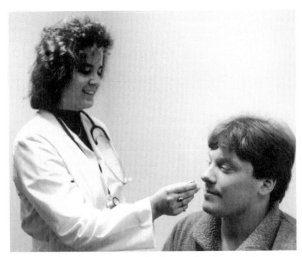

Position the thermometer in the patient's mouth.

8. Keep the thermometer in place for approximately 4 minutes (3 to 5 minutes). The lips should be closed.
9. Pull the sheath away by grasping the white tab with one hand and the end of the thermometer with the other. The sheath will turn inside out, ready to be discarded.
10. Discard the sheath into a biohazard receptacle.

Reading the Thermometer

11. Position the thermometer at eye level with light at your back and rotate the thermometer until the silver column of mercury is seen between the scale and the numbers.

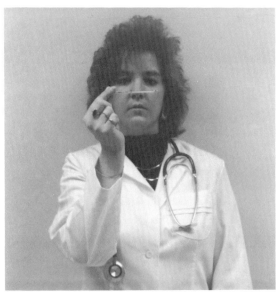

To read the thermometer, position it at eye level with the light at your back.

PRINCIPLE

7. To ensure placement in one of the two heat pockets (see diagram) and prevent placement in other areas over or under the tongue or at the back of the mouth, which may cause the thermometer to register as much as 1.2°F or 1°C lower.

8. To provide sufficient time for the mercury column to expand.
9. To protect the medical assistant from the contact of body fluids.

10. To protect others from exposure to body fluids.

11. To facilitate seeing the mercury column.

PROCEDURE

12. Read the temperature mark where the silver column ends (each scale marking represents 0.2°F).

13. Recording the reading on the designated form or chart. Include patient's name, date, and time along with the reading. The abbreviation for temperature is T. Example: date, time: T, 99.2°F/37.3°C O (orally) (initials).

Clean-Up

14. Wash the thermometer gently in cold, not warm or hot, soapy water; then rotate the thermometer while swabbing it from the end-grip to the mercury bulb with an alcohol swab.

15. Place the thermometer in a specifically designed container for clean oral thermometers. Keep thermometers out of direct sunlight and away from heat.

PRINCIPLE

12. The mercury column expansion stops where the Fahrenheit scale is equivalent to the body's temperature.

13. To prevent having to repeat the procedure or recording an error due to forgetfulness. Oral temperatures are usually 1°F or C lower than the rectal equivalent; therefore, the "O" designation is important for the physician to make the proper interpretation.

14. To prevent the mercury from expanding, a major cause of thermometer breakage, and to disinfect the thermometer before replacing it in storage.

15. To separate oral thermometers from rectal and axillary thermometers and to prevent mercury expansion from the sun or other heat sources.

PROCEDURE: Measure rectal temperature of an adult

OSHA STANDARDS:

Terminal Performance Objective: Measure and record an accurate rectal Fahrenheit temperature; then convert to the Celsius scale within 5 minutes.

EQUIPMENT: Rectal Fahrenheit thermometer, red tipped
Thermometer sheaths
"Vaseline," Petroleum Jelly, or other lubricant or prelu-
    bricated sheaths
Examination glove(s) (optional)
Disposable drape sheet
4 × 4 gauze
Cold water and detergent
Alcohol swab
Biohazard bag for disposal
Patient form or chart
Fahrenheit-Celsius conversion chart or the formula:
    $F = (9/5 \times C) + 32$

PROCEDURE

Preparation

1. Hold the Fahrenheit thermometer at the end-grip, and check the bulb and stem for cracks or breaks.

2. Shake the thermometer over a soft surface with downward snaps of the wrist until the mercury column goes below 96.0°F.

3. Insert the thermometer bulb into the sheath opening at the pull-apart end of the outer wrap, sliding the thermometer in gently until it touches the opposite end of the sheath.

4. Grasp the outer wrap on each side of the perforated line and twist hands in opposite directions until the outer wrap tears at the perforation.

5. Pull the thermometer together with the sheath tab from the outer wrap.

6. Lubricate the sheath by pressing the tube of lubricant and allowing a small amount to fall onto the sheath while rotating to obtain even lubrication. Lubricate to 1 inch above the bulb.

7. Close door to examining room.

8. Ask the patient's name and explain the procedure.

9. Assist the adult patient to assume a Sims' (side-lying) position, and cover the patient from chest to knees with a drape sheet placed diagonally. Adjust the drape sheet to expose the buttocks.

10. Separate the buttocks so that the anal sphincter is seen clearly, and insert the thermometer gently for approximately 1½ inches. Allow the buttocks to fall back into place.

11. Hold the thermometer in place for 2 to 3 minutes. Do not leave the patient for any reason before removing the thermometer.

PRINCIPLE

1. Although thermometers are made of heat-tempered glass, mercury expansion from excessive heat can cause the bulb to crack or break while in storage.

2. To avoid missing an accurate subnormal (below 98.6°F) temperature reading.

3,4,5. To make temperature taking more sanitary and to help protect against the possible danger of a broken thermometer.

6. To reduce friction and thereby facilitate insertion of the thermometer and to minimize irritation to the anal canal.

7. To prevent needless embarrassment and to maintain the patient's dignity.

8. To reduce the risk of error and to provide assurance to anxious patients.

9. To provide patient comfort and privacy and to ensure safety.

10. To prevent injury to the anal sphincter by visualizing the anal opening.

11. To prevent accidents while giving sufficient time for the mercury column to expand.

PROCEDURE

12. Place the other hand on the patient's upper hip or thigh.

13. Remove the thermometer and pull the sheath away by grasping the white tab with one hand and the end of the thermometer with the other. The sheath will turn inside out, ready to be discarded.
14. Discard the sheath into a biohazard waste receptacle.

Reading the Thermometer

15. Position the thermometer at eye level with light at your back, and rotate the thermometer until the silver column of mercury is seen between the scale and the numbers.
16. Read the temperature mark where the silver column ends.

17. Record the reading on the designated form or chart. Patient's name, date, time, and reading are included. The abbreviation for rectal is an R. Example: date, time: T, 37.3°C/99°F R (rectally) (initials).

Clean-Up

18. Wash the thermometer gently in cold, not warm or hot, soapy water; then rotate the thermometer while swabbing it from the end-grip to the mercury bulb with an alcohol swab.
19. Place the thermometer in a specifically designated container for clean rectal thermometers. Keep thermometers out of direct sunlight and away from heat.

PRINCIPLE

12. To add comfort to the patient and to remind the patient not to roll into a supine position or move the upper leg.
13. To protect the medical assistant from contact with body fluids.

14. To protect others from exposure to body fluids.

15. To facilitate seeing the mercury column.

16. The mercury column expansion stops where the thermometer's scale is equivalent to the rectal temperature.
17. To prevent having to repeat the procedure or recording an error due to forgetfulness. Rectal temperatures are usually 1°F or 1°C higher than the oral equivalent; therefore, the "R" designation is important for the physician to make the proper interpretation.

18. To prevent the mercury from expanding, a major cause of thermometer breakage, and to disinfect the thermometer before replacing it in storage.

19. To separate rectal thermometers from oral and axillary thermometers and to prevent mercury expansion from the sun or other heat sources.

PROCEDURE: Measure rectal temperature of a child

OSHA STANDARDS:

Terminal Performance Objective: Measure and record an accurate rectal Fahrenheit temperature; then convert to the Celsius scale within 5 minutes.

EQUIPMENT: Rectal Fahrenheit thermometer, red-tipped
Thermometer sheaths
Vaseline petroleum jelly or other lubricant or prelubricated sheaths
Examination glove(s) (optional)
Disposable drape sheet
4 × 4 gauze
Cold water and detergent
Alcohol swab
Biohazard bag for disposal
Patient form or chart
Fahrenheit-Celsius conversion chart or the formula:
$F = (9/5 \times C) + 32$

PROCEDURE	PRINCIPLE
Preparation	
1. Hold the Fahrenheit thermometer at the end-grip, and check the bulb and stem for cracks or breaks.	1. Although thermometers are made of heat-tempered glass, mercury expansion from excessive heat can cause the bulb to crack or break while in storage.
2. Shake the thermometer over a soft surface with downward snaps of the wrist until the mercury column goes below 96.0°F (35.5°C).	2. To avoid missing an accurate subnormal (below 98.6°F [37°C]) temperature reading.
3. Insert the thermometer bulb into the sheath opening at the pull-apart end of the outer wrap, sliding the thermometer in gently until it touches the opposite end of the sheath.	3,4,5. To make temperature taking more sanitary and to help protect against the possible danger of a broken thermometer.
4. Grasp the outer wrap on each side of the perforated line, and twist hands in opposite directions until the outer wrap tears at the perforation.	
5. Pull the thermometer together with the sheath tab from the outer wrap.	
6. Lubricate the sheath by pressing the tube of lubricant and allowing a small amount to fall onto the sheath while rotating to obtain even lubrication. Lubricate to 1 inch above the bulb.	6. To reduce friction and thereby facilitate insertion of the thermometer and minimize irritation to the anal canal.
Patient Procedure	
7. Close the door to examining room.	7. To keep the child quiet and warm.
8. Ask the adult to identify the child by name and explain the procedure to the adult.	8. To reduce the risk of error and to provide assurance to anxious parents.
9. Place the child on his or her abdomen on a firm surface. Have the adult hold onto the child during the procedure.	9. To immobilize the child and to ensure safety.
10. Separate the buttocks with one hand, and with the other hand, insert the thermometer into the rectum approximately 1 inch. Allow the buttocks to fall back into place.	10. To prevent injury to the anal sphincter by visualizing the anal opening.
11. Hold the buttocks together firmly with the thermometer lodged between the fingers of the same hand.	11. To hold the thermometer in place in case the child automatically responds by bearing down to expel the thermometer.

PROCEDURE

12. Place the other hand in the small of the child's back, keeping the elbow straight and leaning slightly on the child.

13. Hold the thermometer in place for 3 to 5 minutes. Do not leave the child for any reason before removing the thermometer.

14. Remove the thermometer while continuing to hold the child, and set it on gauze out of reach of the child.

15. Have the adult take over holding the child, and assist with diapering and dressing.

16. Pull the sheath away by grasping the white tab with one hand and the end of the thermometer with the other. The sheath will turn inside out, ready to be discarded.

17. Discard the sheath and gauze into a biohazard waste receptacle.

18. Position the thermometer at eye level with light at your back, and rotate the thermometer until the silver column of mercury is seen between the scale and the numbers.

19. Read the temperature mark where the silver column ends.

20. Record the reading on the designated form or chart. Patient's name, date, time, and reading are included. The abbreviation for temperature is T; the abbreviation for rectal is R. Example: date, time: T, 37.3°C/99.2°F R (rectally) (initials).

Clean-Up

21. Wash the thermometer gently in cold, not warm or hot, soapy water; then rotate the thermometer while swabbing it from the end-grip to the mercury bulb with an alcohol swab.

22. Place the thermometer in a specifically designated container for clean rectal thermometers. Keep thermometers out of direct sunlight and away from heat.

PRINCIPLE

12. To hold the child securely, thereby preventing injury.

13. To prevent the child from rolling off the surface and sustaining an injury while allowing time for the mercury column to expand.

14. To prevent the child from rolling off the surface or reaching for the thermometer.

15. To ensure the child's safety and warmth.

16. To protect the medical assistant from contact with body fluids.

17. To protect others from exposure to body fluids.

18. To facilitate seeing the mercury column.

19. The mercury column expansion stops where the Fahrenheit scale is equivalent to the rectal temperature.

20. To prevent having to repeat the procedure or recording an error due to forgetfulness. Rectal temperatures are usually 1°F or 1°C higher than the oral equivalent, therefore, the "R" designation is important for the physician to make the proper interpretation.

21. To prevent the mercury from expanding, a major cause of thermometer breakage, and to disinfect the thermometer before replacing it in storage.

22. To separate rectal thermometers from oral and axillary thermometers and to prevent mercury expansion from the sun or other heat sources.

PROCEDURE: Measure axillary temperature of an adult

OSHA STANDARDS:

Terminal Performance Objective: Measure and record an accurate axillary Fahrenheit temperature; then convert to the Celsius scale within 5 minutes.

EQUIPMENT: Fahrenheit thermometer, safety tipped
Thermometer sheaths
4 × 4 gauze
Cold water and detergent
Alcohol swab
Biohazard bag for disposal
Patient form or chart
Fahrenheit-Celsius conversion chart or the formula:
$$F = (9/5 \times C) + 32$$

PROCEDURE

Preparation

1. Hold the Fahrenheit thermometer at the end-grip, and check the bulb and stem for cracks or breaks.

2. Shake the thermometer over a soft surface with downward snaps of the wrist until the mercury column goes below 96.0°F.

3. Insert the thermometer bulb into the sheath opening at the pull-apart end of the outer wrap, sliding the thermometer in gently until it touches the opposite end of the sheath.

4. Grasp the outer wrap on each side of the perforated line, and twist hands in opposite directions until the outer wrap tears at the perforation.

5. Pull the thermometer together with the sheath tab from the outer wrap.

Patient Procedure

6. Close door to examining room.

7. Ask the patient's name and explain the procedure.

8. Assist the adult patient to a sitting position, and expose the axillary area with the patient's modesty in mind.

9. Dry the area with tissue or gauze, and insert the thermometer in the axilla. Instruct the patient to hold the thermometer in place by tightly pressing the arm against the chest.

10. Leave the thermometer in place for 10 minutes.

11. Remove the thermometer, and pull the sheath away by grasping the white tab with one hand and the end of the thermometer with the other. The sheath will turn inside out, ready to be discarded.

12. Discard the sheath into a biohazard waste receptacle.

PRINCIPLE

1. Although thermometers are made of heat-tempered glass, mercury expansion from excessive heat can cause the bulb to crack or break while in storage.

2. To avoid missing an accurate subnormal (below 98.6°F [37°C]) temperature reading.

3,4,5. To make temperature taking more sanitary and to help protect against the possible danger of a broken thermometer.

6. To prevent needless embarrassment and to maintain the patient's dignity.

7. To reduce the risk of error and to provide assurance to anxious patients.

8. To provide patient comfort and privacy and to ensure safety.

9. To free the area of perspiration, which will prevent the thermometer from slipping and to ensure a tight closure.

10. To give a longer time for the mercury column to expand.

11. To protect the medical assistant from contact with body fluids.

12. To protect others from exposure to body fluids.

PROCEDURE

Reading the Thermometer

13. Position the thermometer at eye level with light at your back, and rotate the thermometer until the silver column of mercury is seen between the scale and the numbers.
14. Read the temperature mark where the silver column ends.

15. Record the reading on the designated form or chart. Patient's name, date, time, and reading are included. The abbreviation for rectal is an R. Example: date, time: T, 37.3°C/99°F R (rectally) (initials).

Clean-Up

16. Wash the thermometer gently in cold, not warm or hot, soapy water; then rotate the thermometer while swabbing it from the end-grip to the mercury bulb with an alcohol swab.
17. Place the thermometer in a specifically designated container for clean rectal thermometers. Keep thermometers out of direct sunlight and away from heat.

PRINCIPLE

13. To facilitate seeing the mercury column.

14. The mercury column expansion stops where the Fahrenheit scale is equivalent to the rectal temperature.
15. To prevent having to repeat the procedure or recording an error due to forgetfulness. Rectal temperatures are usually 1°F or 1°C higher than the oral equivalent; therefore, the "R" designation is important for the physician to make the proper interpretation.

16. To prevent the mercury from expanding, a major cause of thermometer breakage, and to disinfect the thermometer before replacing it in storage.

17. To separate rectal thermometers from oral and axillary thermometers and to prevent mercury expansion from the sun or other heat sources.

PROCEDURE: Manage a situation in which a thermometer is accidentally broken

OSHA STANDARDS:

Terminal Performance Objectives: Clean the work area or flush a patient's oral cavity following an incident involving a mercury spill and fragments of glass, and record the incident in the patient chart and on an incident report.

EQUIPMENT: *Thermometer not in use:*
Utility gloves
Two index cards
Damp cloth or paper towels
Germicide
Dry paper towels
Sharps container
Biohazard bag

Thermometer in use:
Examination gloves
Emesis basin
Drinking glass
Water
Sharps container

PROCEDURE

1. Wear utility gloves.

2. Scoop up the pellets of mercury with two thin cards or still pieces of paper.
3. Dispose of the mercury pellets into a porcelain septic (toilet) bowl.
4. Sponge up the pieces of broken glass with a damp, thick cloth or paper towel.

5. Dispose of the glass and cloth or paper towels in a puncture and leakproof biohazard bag.
6. Clean the surface of the spill with a paper towel and germicide.
7. Dry the surface with clean paper towels.
8. Dispose of cleaning materials in the biohazard bag.

While the Thermometer Is in Use:

1. Wear examination gloves.

2. Instruct the patient to relax the jaw muscles, not to swallow, and to lean his or her head forward.
3. Allow the saliva to drain the fragments of glass and mercury into an emesis basin.
4. Do not probe the fragments with fingers or a swab.
5. Rinse the mouth with small amounts of water, being careful not to swallow the water, mercury, or glass fragments.
6. Repeat rinsing until all fragments of glass have been removed.
7. Assure the patient that he or she is not in danger of mercury poisoning.
8. Notify the physician to examine the patient.

PRINCIPLES

1. To prevent the mercury from forming a chemical reaction with precious metals such as gold.
2. Mercury cannot be picked up; however, it can be rolled onto another surface.
3. Mercury is a hazardous waste substance.

4. Wiping glass over a surface can scratch the surface or cause the glass to cut through the cloth or paper towel.
5. To prevent injury to others.

6. To ensure all glass and mercury is removed.

7. To prevent slipping or other injury.
8. To prevent injury to others.

1. To prevent the mercury from forming a chemical reaction with precious metals such as gold.
2. To prevent the patient from swallowing the fragments or lacerating the oral mucosa.
3. Saliva acts as a moistening agent that will flush the debris out of the oral cavity without being swallowed.
4. The glass fragments are extremely sharp.
5. Large amounts of water may trigger the swallow or gag reflex.

6. To flush away all remaining debris.

7. The mercury in a thermometer is triple-distilled, pure, and elemental and cannot be absorbed into the body.
8. The physician will examine the patient to ensure all pieces of glass have been removed.

PROCEDURE

9. Dispose of the contents of the emesis basin into a porcelain septic (toilet) bowl.
10. Thoroughly wash the emesis basin and drinking glass.

11. Chart the incident in the patient's record.
12. Complete an incident report. Example: date, time: mercury contamination caused by broken thermometer in patient's mouth. Patient: Jane Doe, 12 Main St., Anytown, NY, (800–555–1212). Patient sneezed and bit through thermometer. C. Smith, CMA, in attendance at the time of the incident. Mouth thoroughly rinsed with plain water. No evidence of any material swallowed. Patient examined by Dr. Goldman. No lacerations or mercury noted in the oral cavity. Patient discharged with no follow-up. All mercury debris contained in marked biohazard container (initials).

PRINCIPLE

9. Mercury is a hazardous waste substance.

10. To prevent mercury chemical reactions and the transfer of microorganisms to other patients and to oneself.
11. To record the incident in case of further complications.
12. To create a record of the names of the persons involved, addresses, phone numbers, accident description, nature of injury, and follow-up care.

PROCEDURE: Measure and assess radial pulse

OSHA STANDARDS:

Terminal Performance Objective: Measure, assess, and record an accurate radial pulse within 2 minutes.

EQUIPMENT: Watch with a second hand sweep.

PROCEDURE

1. Identify the patient and explain the procedure.

2. Place the patient in a sitting or lying position.
   - Sitting—bend the patient's elbow 90 degrees, support the lower arm, and extend the wrist with the palm down.
   - Lying—place the patient's arm across his or her lower chest, with wrist extended and palm down.
3. Compress the radial artery gently against the radius with the tips of the first two or three fingers.

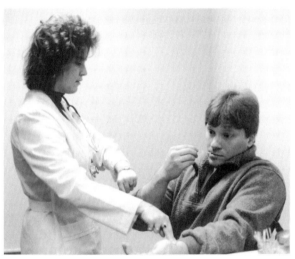

Determining temperature, pulse, and respiration (TPR).

4. Establish that the pulse is felt.

5. Count the pulsations for 30 seconds and multiply by two when the pulse is regular.
6. Count the pulsations for a full minute when the pulse is irregular.
7. Assess rhythm and strength of pulse and elasticity of the artery.

8. Record the reading immediately. Example: date, time: P, 72, +1, irregular (initials).

PRINCIPLE

1. To reduce the risk of error and provide assurance to anxious patients.
2. To fully expose the radial artery while the patient is at rest. Wait 10 to 15 minutes after physical activity.
   - To facilitate feeling the rise and fall of the chest during the evaluation of respiration.

3. To avoid distorting or obliterating the pulsation (expansion and contraction of the artery) by too much pressure. Too little pressure will not allow the pulsations to be felt.

4. Rate is determined accurately only after the pulsations are felt for a few seconds and confirmed.
5. When rhythm and volume appear normal, 30 seconds is sufficient to determine an accurate reading.
6. When rhythm and volume appear irregular, at least 60 seconds is needed to observe the irregular patterns.
7. Rhythm is normal or irregular.* Strength is 0, +1, +2, +3, or +4 (see Table 17–5). An artery is normally straight, smooth, round and elastic; in disease, the artery may be hard, cordlike, and tortuous.
8. To avoid having to repeat the procedure or recording an error due to forgetfulness. The pulse reading is usually measured and recorded after the temperature recording and before measuring and recording the respiratory rate.

---

*If arrhythmia is present, the physician may order an electrocardiogram or an assessment of the apical pulse in conjunction with the radial pulse to detect any pulse deficit. In pulse deficits, the radial pulse is usually slower than the apical pulse

PROCEDURE: Measure and assess apical pulse

OSHA STANDARDS:

Terminal Performance Objective: Measure, assess, and record an accurate apical pulse within 4 minutes.

EQUIPMENT: Watch with a second hand sweep
Stethoscope
Alcohol swab

Note: This procedure is used to confirm abnormalities detected in the radial pulse, to assess an infant's or young child's heart rate, or when the radial pulse site is inaccessible.

PROCEDURE

1. Identify the patient and explain the procedure.

2. Position the patient in a sitting or lying position.

3. Warm the bell or diaphragm of the stethoscope with the palms of the hands.
4. Place the stethoscope over the fifth intercostal space at the midclavicular line (between the fifth and sixth ribs, usually just below the nipple).

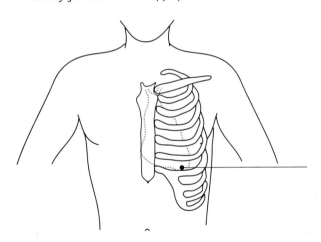

5. Count the number of heart beats occurring in 1 minute when the heartbeat is regular.
6. Count the number of heart beats for 3 minutes, and divide by three if the heartbeat is irregular. Note that the count was for 3 minutes.
7. Record the reading immediately. Example: date, time: apical pulse, 72 beats/min for 3 minutes, occasional irregular rhythm (initials).
8. Clean the earpieces and diaphragm of the stethoscope with an alcohol swab.

PRINCIPLE

1. To reduce the risk of error and provide assurance to anxious patients.
2. To ensure a more accurate reading while the patient is at rest.
3. To keep the patient comfortable during the procedure.

4. To place the stethoscope at the apex of the heart.

5. When rhythm and volume appear normal, 1 minute is sufficient to determine an accurate reading.
6. When rhythm and volume appear irregular, at least 3 minutes is needed to observe the irregular patterns.

7. To avoid having to repeat the procedure or to record an error due to forgetfulness. Recording the count as apical avoids confusion.
8. To prevent cross-contamination.

PROCEDURE: Measure and assess respiration

OSHA STANDARDS:

Terminal Performance Objective: Measure, assess, and record an accurate respiration (in conjunction with the pulse) within 2 minutes when normal findings are present or within 3 minutes when the count is extended to 1 full minute for each.

EQUIPMENT: Watch with a second hand sweep.

Note: This procedure immediately follows the counting of the radial pulse rate, and while the fingertips remain on the radial pulse, as though the pulse rate were still being measured.

PROCEDURE

1. Identify the patient (if the patient has not already been identified at the start of a pulse count).
2. Do not explain the procedure.

3. Position the patient in a sitting or lying position so that chest movement is visible, or place the patient's arm across his or her abdomen or lower chest (alternative — place your hand directly on the patient's abdomen).
4. Count for 30 seconds the rise of fall of the chest, counting each inhalation and exhalation as a single respiration.* Multiply by two.
5. Count respirations that are irregular in rhythm or abnormally slow or fast for 1 full minute.
6. Note the depth and rhythm of respirations. Record any irregularities or other characteristics that may be present.
7. Record the respirations with the temperature and pulse rate immediately. Example: date, time: T, 37°C/98.6°F (o); P 72 +1 irregular (3 min); R, 18, stertorous, shallow (initials).

PRINCIPLE

1. To reduce the risk of error.

2. Patients who are aware of their own breathing tend to become self-conscious and unknowingly or knowingly alter their usual rate.

3. In patients who are dressed or who have shallow breathing, chest movements can be almost imperceptible.

4. When the respirations are regular and the rate within normal range, 30 seconds is sufficient to obtain an accurate reading.

5. A full minute is necessary to confirm an irregular rhythm or rate deviations from the normal range.
6. Depth is shallow, normal, or deep; rhythm is normal or irregular. The character of breathing may reveal specific alterations or the presence of disease.
7. To avoid having to repeat the procedure or recording an error due to forgetfulness or confusion with the pulse rate. Some prefer to count the respiration first then the pulse rate, as the respiration rate is an easier number to remember until both procedures are completed and recorded.

---

*In an infant or young child, count respirations for 1 full minute. Young children and infants in an irregular rhythm. Respirations in infants are easier to count by using a stethoscope and continuing to observe the rise and fall of the chest or clothing over the chest.

PROCEDURE: Measure and assess blood pressure

OSHA STANDARDS:

Terminal Performance Objective: Measure, assess, and record an accurate blood pressure measurement within 2 minutes when normal findings are present or within 4 minutes if the procedure must be repeated.

EQUIPMENT: Sphygmomanometer, aneroid or mercury column
Blood pressure cuff
Stethoscope (the American Heart Association recommends the use of the bell-type to hear the low-frequency Korotkoff sounds clearly)
Alcohol swab

PROCEDURE

1. Identify the patient and explain the procedure.

2. Instruct the patient to sit for 5 minutes, legs not crossed, feet flat on the floor.

3. Palpate the brachial or radial arteries in each arm, and select either the right arm or the arm with the stronger pulse.

4. Support the forearm and palm at heart level.

5. Wrap the correct-sized cuff smoothly and snugly around the arm with the center cuff bladder over the brachial artery and the lower edge of the cuff about 1 inch above the natural crease across the inner aspect of the elbow. The tube connecting the cuff to the machine should be away from the patient's body; the tube to the inflating tube close to the body.

PRINCIPLES

1. To reduce the risk of error and provide assurance to anxious patients.

2. To relax the patient and eliminate the chance of altering blood pressure by patient exertion or venous pooling of blood in the legs.

3. To determine the arm with the higher pressure (a difference of 5–10 mm is normal).

4. To avoid a false-low reading if the arm is above heart level and to facilitate correct cuff application.

5. To ensure the correct amount of pressure will be applied over the brachial artery. The bladder should inflate directly over the brachial artery to ensure that proper pressure is applied during inflation. Tubing must be out of the way to prevent rubbing with the stethoscope, which creates interfering sounds. Cuff too wide—false-low reading; cuff too narrow—false-high reading; cuff too loose—false-high reading.

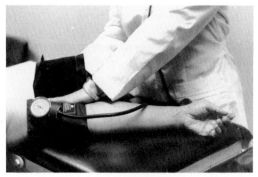

Wrap cuff around upper arm.

PROCEDURE

6. Determine the maximum inflation level by palpating the radial pulse and inflating the cuff smoothly until the pulse is no longer felt. Deflate the cuff and mentally add 30 mm to the reading at which point the pulse was obliterated.

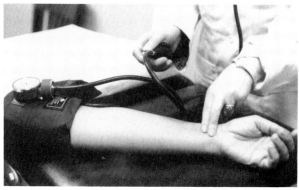

Feel radial pulse with fingertips while inflating cuff.

7. Wait 1 to 2 minutes while checking the pulse rate by taking the pulse for 30 seconds and multiplying by two.
8. Place the stethoscope into ears.

9. Palpate the brachial artery midway between the anterior and medial aspects of the arm.
10. Place the diaphragm of the stethoscope over the brachial artery firmly enough to obtain a seal, but lightly enough to avoid obliterating the artery, and without touching the cuff or the tubing.

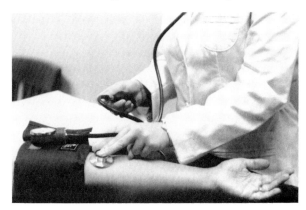

Place stethoscope over brachial artery.

PRINCIPLE

6. To prevent a false-low systolic reading due to auscultatory gap (missing the first Korotkoff sound), and to prevent potential injury to the vessel or venous congestion, resulting in a false-high reading. If a systolic pressure has been recently recorded on the patient's record, this step can be eliminated and the cuff inflated to 30 mm above the recorded systolic measurement.

7. To prevent venous congestion and false-high readings.

8. To free hands for taking the blood pressure. Earpieces should follow the angle of the ear to facilitate hearing.
9. To ensure proper location of the stethoscope. The pulse will be on the inner aspect of the arm.
10. To ensure optimal sound reception and prevent a false-low systolic and a false-high diastolic reading from poorly fitting earpieces.

PROCEDURE

11. Close the thumb valve, and squeeze the bulb so that the cuff inflates at a rapid but smooth continuous rate (7 to 10 seconds) to the maximum inflation level that was previously determined.

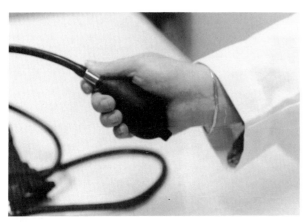

Open control valve to deflate cuff.

12. Deflate the cuff by opening the thumb valve slightly and maintaining a constant deflation rate of 2 mm per second. Listening throughout the entire range of deflation until 10 mm below the level of the diastolic reading.
13. Note the first distinctly audible pulse sound heard— the systolic pressure. Read the gauge at eye level, and remember the corresponding number on the pressure gauge.

14. Continue deflating the cuff, noting any point when a muffled or dampened sound appears.

15. Note the last distinctly audible heard—the diastolic pressure. Remember to read the corresponding number on the pressure gauge.

16. Fully deflate the cuff by opening the thumb valve and allow the remaining air to escape.
17. If the reading is not certain, wait 2 minutes and repeat the procedure.
18. Remove the equipment, and record immediately as the systolic pressure over the diastolic pressure. Example: date, time: left arm first reading, 120/80; second reading, 128/84 (initials).
19. Clean the stethoscope earpieces and diaphragm with an alcohol swab.

PRINCIPLES

11. Prevents air leak during inflation. A rapid, continuous rate prevents venous congestion and a false-high reading. Blood is now collected in the artery, and on gradual release of the cuff, will begin flowing forcefully through the vessel.

12. To prevent false readings from too rapid or slow a decline of the mercury level or the gauge needle. Too slow—false-high diastolic; too fast—false-low systolic, and false-high diastolic.
13. The first Korotkoff sound indicates the systolic pressure. Eye level prevents inaccurate readings. The blood is first able to proceed through the artery, exerting lateral pressure while moving forward in the artery and against the external pressure exerted on the vessel by the inflated cuff.

14. The fourth Korotkoff sound may be recorded in adults with hypertension and as the indication of the diastolic pressure in children.

15. The fifth Korotkoff sound is the last sound heard and indicates the diastolic pressure in adults. Blood is flowing through the brachial artery unimpeded by external pressure. Pressure in the cuff is now lower than in the artery.
16. To prevent further arterial occlusion resulting in numbness and tingling in the patient's arm.
17. To prevent venous congestion and false-high readings.

18. To avoid error. Any error in recording could potentially result in a false diagnosis or treatment.

19. Alcohol cleanses earwax lodged in the tips and reduces the chances of transmitting organisms.

PROCEDURE: Determine orthostatic variations in blood pressure

OSHA STANDARDS:

Terminal Performance Objective: Measure and record accurate blood pressure measurements for the patient in the lying, sitting, and standing positions within 10 minutes when normal findings are present or within 15 minutes if any of the readings must be repeated.

EQUIPMENT: Sphygmomanometer, aneroid or mercury column
Blood pressure cuff
Stethoscope (the American Heart Association recommends the use of the bell type to hear the low-frequency Korotkoff sounds clearly)
Alcohol swab

PROCEDURE

1. Identify the patient and explain the procedure.

2. Instruct the patient to lie down for approximately 5 minutes; then obtain the apical pulse and blood pressure.

3. Assist the patient to sit at a 90° angle. Obtain the blood pressure and apical pulse immediately.

4. Inquire about what the patient is feeling.

5. Assist the patient to stand. Obtain the blood pressure and apical pulse readings immediately.

6. Ask the patient what effect the change in position may have caused.

7. Record the blood pressure readings, the apical rates, and the patient's reactions to positional changes. Example: date, time: R/A, 118/76; AP, 68 beats/min, lying; time: R/A, 110/70; AP, 74 beats/min, sitting; time: R/A, 96/68; AP, 80 beats/min standing (initials).

8. Report questionable results to the physician immediately.

PRINCIPLES

1. To reduce the risk of error and to provide assurance to anxious patients.

2. A 5-minute waiting period allows the blood pressure to stabilize.

3. Blood pressure must be taken immediately to detect positional differences.

4. Position changes may cause the patient to feel dizzy.

5. Blood pressure and heart rate may further change when the patient stands.

6. The patient may need to rest briefly due to increased dizziness.

7. The measurements should be recorded immediately to avoid error.

8. Immediately report:
   a) Systolic changes greater than 10 mm from the lying to sitting or lying to standing position.
   b) Diastolic changes greater than 20 mm from the lying to sitting or lying to standing position.
   c) Apical pulse changes greater than 20 beats per minute from the lying to sitting or lying to standing positions.

PROCEDURE: Measure height and weight

OSHA STANDARDS:

Terminal Performance Objective: Measure and record an accurate height and weight for an adult patient within 1 minute.

EQUIPMENT: Scale
Paper towel

PROCEDURE

1. Identify the patient and explain the procedure.

2. Check to make certain both 50-lb and per-pound bar weights are on zero and that the pointed end of the bar is floating in the middle of the balance frame.
3. Place a paper towel on the footrest of the scale.
4. Lift the height bar and raise it higher than the expected level of the patient's head.
5. Instruct the patient to remove his or her shoes.
6. Instruct the patient to step on the scale and stand erect.
7. Gently lower the height bar in place, protecting the patient's head, and rest the bar on the crown of the head.
8. Leave the height bar at the measurement.

9. Move the large weight to the nearest 50-lb weight notch. (Example: Move the bar to 150 lb for a man expected to be somewhere between 150 and 200 lb.)
10. Move the smaller weight to the number that will permit the pointed end of the bar to float in the middle of the balance frame.
11. Instruct the patient to step off the scale and put on his or her shoes.
12. Add the large weight and the small weight number to the nearest $\frac{1}{4}$ lb.
13. Note the height measurement to the nearest $\frac{1}{4}$ inch.
14. Immediately record the patient's weight and height. Example: date, time: Wt, $125\frac{1}{2}$ lb; Ht, $5'5\frac{1}{4}''$ (initials)
15. Move the weight bars to zero, return the height bar to its resting position, and dispose of the paper towel.

PRINCIPLES

1. To reduce the risk of error and to provide assurance to anxious patients.
2. To ensure that the scale at zero is in balance. If not, adjust until the bar floats in the middle of the frame.

3. To reduce the chance of transmitting foot infections.
4. To avoid possible injury to the patient by the height bar.
5. Shoes would give a false-high height and weight.
6. Standing erect ensures an accurate measurement.

7. To avoid possible injury to the patient's scalp.

8. The height measurement will be recorded when the weight is recorded.
9. To ensure efficiency of time and motion.

10. The scale indicates the patient's weight when the pointer floats in the middle of the balance beam.

11. To prevent possible injury to the patient.

12. Weight is measured in $\frac{1}{4}$-lb increments.

13. Height is measured to the nearest $\frac{1}{4}$-inch increment.
14. To avoid any error in data.

15. To ready the scale for use with the next patient.

HIGHLIGHTS

Bloodborne Facts: Holding the Line on Contamination

Keeping work areas in a clean and sanitary condition reduces employees' risk of exposure to bloodborne pathogens. Each year about 8700 health care workers are infected with hepatitis B virus, and 200 die from contracting hepatitis B through their work. The chance of contracting human immunodeficiency virus (HIV), the bloodborne pathogen which causes acquired immunodeficiency disorder, with occupational exposure is small, yet a good housekeeping program can minimize this risk as well.

DECONTAMINATION

Every employer whose employees are exposed to blood or other potentially infectious materials must develop a written schedule for cleaning each area where exposures occur. The methods of decontaminating different surfaces must be specified, determined by the type of surface to be cleaned, the soil present, and the tasks or procedures that occur in that area.

For example, different cleaning and decontamination measures would be used for a surgical operatory and a patient room. Similarly, hard-surfaced flooring and carpeting require separate cleaning methods. More extensive efforts will be necessary for gross contamination than for minor spattering. Likewise, such varied tasks as laboratory analyses and normal patient care would require different techniques for clean-up.

Employees must decontaminate working surfaces and equipment with an appropriate disinfectant after completing procedures involving exposure to blood. Many laboratory procedures are performed on a continual basis throughout a shift. Except as discussed below, it is not necessary to clean and decontaminate between procedures. However, if the employee leaves the area for a period of time, for a break or lunch, then contaminated work surfaces must be cleaned.

Employees also must clean (1) when surfaces become obviously contaminated; (2) after any spill of blood or other potentially infectious materials; and (3) at the end of the work shift if contamination might have occurred. Thus, employees need not decontaminate the work area after each patient care procedure, but only after those that actually result in contamination.

If surfaces or equipment are draped with protective coverings such as plastic wrap or aluminum foil, these coverings should be removed or replaced if they become obviously contaminated. Reusable receptacles such as bins, pails, and cans that are likely to become contaminated must be inspected and decontaminated on a regular basis. If contamination is visible, workers must clean and decontaminate the item immediately, or as soon as feasible.

Should glassware that may be potentially contaminated break, workers need to use mechanical means such as a brush and dustpan or tongs or forceps to pick up the broken glass — never by hand, even when wearing gloves.

Before any equipment is serviced or shipped for repairing or cleaning, it must be decontaminated to the extent possible. The equipment must be labeled, indicating which portions are still contaminated. This enables employees and those who service the equipment to take appropriate precautions to prevent exposure.

REGULATED WASTE

In addition to effective decontamination of work areas, proper handling of regulated waste is essential to prevent unnecessary exposure to blood and other potentially infectious materials. Regulated waste must be handled with great care — i.e., liquid or semiliquid blood and other potentially infectious materials, items caked with these materials, items that would release blood or other potentially infected materials if compressed, pathologic or microbiologic wastes containing them and contaminated sharps.

Containers used to store regulated waste must be closable and suitable to contain the contents and prevent leakage of fluids. Containers designed for sharps also must be puncture-resistant. They must be labeled or color-coded to ensure that employees are aware of the potential hazards. Such containers must be closed before removal to prevent contents from spilling. If the outside of a container becomes contaminated, it must be placed within a second suitable container.

Regulated waste must be disposed of in accordance with applicable state and local laws.

LAUNDRY

Laundry workers must wear gloves and handle contaminated laundry as little as possible, with a minimum of agitation. Contaminated laundry should be bagged or placed in containers at the location where it is used, but not sorted or rinsed there.

Laundry must be transported within the establishment or to outside laundries in labeled or red color-coded bags. If the facility uses universal precautions for handling all soiled laundry, then alternate labeling or color coding that can be recognized by the employees may be used. If laundry is wet and it might soak through laundry bags, then workers must use bags that prevent leakage to transport it.

RESEARCH FACILITIES

More stringent decontamination requirements apply to research laboratories and production facilities that work with concentrated strains of HIV and HBV.

Source: From US Department of Labor, OSHA, Washington, DC.

> It is impossible to overemphasize the immense need humans have to be protected, safe, listened to, taken seriously, and understood. _____
>
> Paul Tournier, MD

CHAPTER OUTLINE

LEARNING OBJECTIVES

Upon completing this chapter, you will be able to:

1. Explain the proper procedure for gowning the patient, and demonstrate the specific techniques presented.
2. Describe the appropriate use of partial and full examination gowns.
3. List the basic examination positions, and explain when each is used.
4. Explain the proper care and disposal of reusable and disposable gowns and linens.

PERFORMANCE OBJECTIVES

Upon completing this chapter, you will be able to:

1. Assist the female patient into the lithotomy position.
2. Assist patients into the knee-chest, jack-knife, and Sims' positions.

Chapter 18

Gowning, Positioning, and Draping

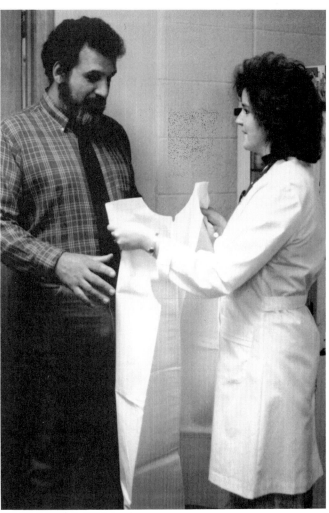

DACUM EDUCATIONAL COMPONENTS

1. Prepare and maintain treatment area (4.5).
2. Prepare patients for procedures (4.7).
3. Assist the physician with examinations and treatments (4.8).
4. Document accurately (5.1).
5. Apply principles of aseptic technique and infection control (4.1).

Glossary

Cross-contamination: carrying or transferring of microorganisms from one place or person to another place or person

Discretionary: determining the different outcomes of possible alternative choices

Pelvic Examination: examination of the contents of the pelvis, which includes the cervix and vaginal wall

Psychically: pertaining to the mind

Symptomatology: the group of perceptible changes in the body or its functions that indicates disease

---

In addition to interviewing patients and obtaining their vital signs, the medical assistant also prepares patients for examination by assisting them with gowning, positioning, and draping. The most common gowning positions and draping techniques are described in this chapter. Other positions used with specific diagnostic procedures and examinations are discussed in later chapters. Special considerations for determining the type of gowning, positioning, and draping for each patient are also presented, with emphasis placed on the patient's right to privacy and personal comfort.

These preparatory procedures are the prelude to any examination. Since most patients who visit the office require a partial or complete physical examination, the medical assistant must know and apply the proper procedures for each type of examination and use discretionary judgment to modify techniques according to the needs of the physician and patient.

GOWNING

For the physician to examine the patient, the patient must disrobe and put on a gown that will facilitate performing the procedure by exposing only the body part to be examined. Factors to be considered in determining the extent of undress and gowning required are as follows: the patient's comfort and need for privacy, the type of examination or procedure to be performed, the patient's age and sex, and the accessibility of the body part to be examined.

TYPES OF GOWNS

Gowns can be made of either cloth or paper. Cloth gowns must be laundered after each use, whereas paper gowns are disposable. The physician's preference deter-

mines the type of gown used in a particular practice setting. Also, depending on the type of examination, either a partial or a full gown may be used. *Partial gowns* cover only the shoulders, chest, and back, with street clothing worn from the waist down. *Full gowns* are at least knee length, with an opening extending the full length of the gown. They are closed by either ties or Velcro strips. Usually, all clothing is removed (underwear is sometimes an exception). The opening may be worn either in the back or in the front, depending on the physician's preference and the ease of accessibility.

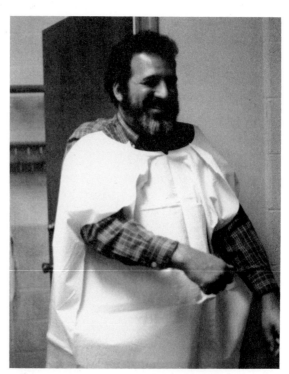

"How about if I just wear it like this?"

LAUNDRY PROCEDURES

Although soiled gowns and linens have been identified as a source of large numbers of pathogenic microorganisms, the actual risk of disease transmission is negligible. Reusable gowns and linens contaminated with blood or with potentially infectious materials should be handled as little as possible and bagged at the location where they were used. Such laundry is placed in a leakproof laundry bag marked with the biohazard symbol or color-coded orange or orange-red. Contaminated laundry must never be sorted or rinsed in the area of use.

Medical assistants who handle contaminated laundry must wear protective clothing and gloves to prevent contact with blood or other potentially infectious materials. If the laundry is being sent off site, then the laundry service should be equipped to handle contaminated laundry and to wash soiled linens according to Occupational Safety and Health Administration standards. Laundry washed on site must be washed with detergent in hot water at least 160°F (71°C) for 25 minutes.

SELECTING THE RIGHT GOWN

The medical assistant decides how to instruct the patient to disrobe and gown after giving careful consideration to the following criteria:

1. *First visit.* A patient visiting the office of an internist or family practice physician for the first time usually receives a complete physical examination. Since this type of examination involves a check of all body parts and systems, a full gown is required. Other medical specialties do not require that the patient receive a complete examination but instead require a specific type of comprehensive examination focusing on a particular part or system.
2. *Purpose of the visit.* The purpose of the visit determines the extent of disrobing and gowning that is necessary. The patient's presenting symptoms or reason for the visit gives clues as to the type of examination the physician will perform. If, for example, a patient is coming to the office because of a persistent cough, congestion, and sore throat, a partial gown is the appropriate choice because the chest, and not the lower body, needs to be exposed for examination. The medical assistant's capacity to anticipate the type of examination to be performed and, consequently, how to gown, position, and drape the patient will increase as his or her knowledge of clinical medical assisting and clinical medicine expands. Discussions in this text on the methods of examination, along with actual work experience, will help to build the medical assistant's confidence and competence.
3. *Sex and age.* The sex and age of the patient significantly help to determine the extent of

disrobing and gowning required. An adult man may not require gowning for partial examinations; an infant may not require gowning at all. Removal of upper body clothing usually will be sufficient.
4. *Individual need for privacy.* Some patients are reluctant to disrobe, and although directions are given, the patients may be resistant. All individuals have needs for privacy, but to varying degrees. When these individual variations are known and anticipated, special handling of the patient is facilitated. Allow the patient to retain clothing as desired if it will not interfere with the process of examination. If the clothing will impair access to the body part to be examined, the medical assistant must explain the necessity for removal of the clothing. If the patient continues to resist, it is usually advisable to instruct the patient to discuss the removal of clothing with the physician.

PATIENT INSTRUCTION AND ASSISTANCE

Gowning instructions should be thorough and clear to save time and relieve patient anxiety. However, the extensiveness of instruction would differ for a 4-year-old's annual examination and a 40-year-old's monthly visit. Presumably, the 4-year-old, perhaps an unwilling patient and unfamiliar with the disrobing procedures, will need more careful direction than the experienced and cooperative 40-year-old. Some patients will need assistance in disrobing. Others can be given the gown and drape sheet along with precise instructions and can then be left alone to carry out the procedure in private. Although some elderly patients may need assistance, it should not be assumed that all do. Again, the medical assistant's discretionary judgment is required. Assessing the patient's needs through observation and attention is imperative. Obviously, patients with disabled limbs caused by injury or disease, and disoriented, weak, or frail patients require assistance.

When a family member or friend accompanies the patient to the examination room, the patient should be asked if he or she prefers to disrobe alone. The medical assistant, however, when appropriate, should leave the room while the patient disrobes and gowns. Before leaving the room, the medical assistant should instruct the patient to disrobe and gown in accordance with the following considerations.

POSITIONING AND DRAPING

Positioning the patient is the responsibility of the medical assistant and an essential component of preparation of the patient for examination. Assisting the patient to assume certain positions facilitates the examination. Depending on the type of position used, certain body parts become more accessible, patient comfort becomes more obtainable, exposure is achieved, and the physician's examination of the patient is accommodated.

EXAMINATION TABLE

Most examination tables are power-operated and can be raised or lowered by pushing a button. They are well-padded and of ample width and length to support almost any size patient. Usually constructed of a vinyl material, they can be easily cleaned with a cloth and antiseptic soap after each patient's use. In cases of contamination, however, the surfaces must be cleaned with a bleach solution or other Environmental Protection Agency–registered germicide. For added sanitary protection, they are covered by a sheet of paper that extends the entire length of the table. This paper is pulled from a roll that is usually attached beneath the top of the table and secured at the bottom of the table. After each patient has left the room, the paper is torn and removed carefully with minimal movement of the paper and without holding it against clothing and discarded in a leakproof biohazard bag. The table is then recovered with fresh paper. When the table is stationary and cannot be adjusted, a step stool should be kept in the room to facilitate getting the patient up onto and down from the table.

TYPES OF POSITIONS

Many types of positions can be used during the examination, depending on the type of examination and the sex of the patient. Those discussed here are basic and are illustrated in Figure 18–1. Other positions are used in conjunction with particular medical specialties. These, however, are usually modifications of the basic positions described in this chapter.

1. *Erect standing.* Sometimes referred to as the "anatomic position," the erect standing position enables the physician to examine the patient's musculoskeletal system and complete certain aspects of the neurologic examination. In this position, the patient stands upright with arms at sides and palms turned out facing forward. He or she may be instructed to bend over, walk, or move specific body parts in a particular manner. The physician observes these movements to determine the patient's level of coordination, strength, flexibility, balance, and range of motion.
2. *Sitting.* The gowned patient sits upright on the examination table, with legs dangling over the table or feet placed on a footstool. The patient is covered by a drape sheet that extends from the

Someone having Resp. heart etc. problems

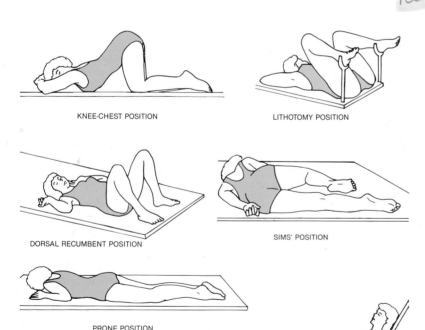

KNEE-CHEST POSITION

LITHOTOMY POSITION

DORSAL RECUMBENT POSITION

SIMS' POSITION

PRONE POSITION

FOWLER'S POSITION

SUPINE

Figure 18–1. The basic patient positions for medical examinations.

lap. The head, chest, back, and front (heart, lungs, breasts, axilla, and upper extremities) can be examined in this position. In addition, some neurologic reflex testing (such as ankle and knee reflexes) can be performed. Whenever possible, the patient should begin the office visit in the sitting position, and as the examination progresses, is then assisted in assuming subsequent positions. The reason for beginning the examination process in the sitting position is to increase the patient's physical and psychological comfort, as well as to provide for full expansion of the lungs to facilitate their examination. In the sitting position, the patient can converse more freely with the physician, and the good rapport established leaves the patient feeling that the physician has taken the time to understand the individual rather than simply treating the disorder.

3. *Supine.* The patient is lying flat on the back with arms at the sides and is covered by a drape sheet extending from under the axilla. The supine position facilitates examination of the chest, heart, abdomen, and extremities. The head and neck can be examined in this position as well as in the sitting position. Certain neurologic reflex testing is also performed in this position.

4. *Dorsal recumbent.* The patient is supine, but the legs are sharply flexed at the knees and the feet are on the table. The drape sheet is placed over the patient in a diamond-shaped fashion and then adjusted to cover and wrap each leg (with corners of the sheet) and to cover the chest and abdomen and the pubic area (with the remaining corners). When the examination is initiated, the corner covering the pubic area is lifted and turned onto the abdomen to expose the genital area. The vagina and rectum can then be examined in the female, and the rectum, in the male. In addition, the parts examined with the patient in the supine position can also be examined in the dorsal recumbent position for those patients more comfortable with knees flexed.

5. *Lithotomy.* This is the position of choice for the vaginal examination and the Pap smear procedure. It is also the position preferred when a *vaginal speculum* (an instrument used to increase the vagina's width for proper visualization) is used to perform a pelvic examination. The female patient assumes the dorsal recumbent posture, but instead of placing the feet on the table puts them in stirrups (see Fig. 18–1). The patient's knees are flexed, the buttocks are moved to the edge of the table, the feet are placed in stirrups, and the legs are spread apart. Draping is the same as in the dorsal recumbent position.

6. *Sims'.* In this side-lying position, the patient is instructed to lie on the left side with the left arm behind the body and the right arm forward, flexed at the elbow. Both legs are flexed at the knee, but the right leg is sharply flexed and positioned next to the left leg, which is slightly flexed. A drape sheet covers the patient from the breasts to the toes and is adjusted when necessary to expose the anal area. In the male, the rectum can be examined in this position, and in the female, the rectum and vagina can be examined. This position is also frequently used to administer an enema.

7. *Prone.* The patient is lying flat on the abdomen with the head turned slightly to the side. The arms can be positioned above the head and extended, or alongside the body. The back, spine, and lower extremities can be examined in this position. A drape sheet extends from the waist to the knees and is adjusted for adequate exposure when necessary.

8. *Knee-chest.* The patient is assisted into a kneeling position with buttocks elevated and head and chest on the table. Arms are extended above the head and flexed at the elbow. A small pillow can be placed under the chest to promote patient comfort, as this position is uncomfortable, particularly for an extended period of time. The rectum is examined in this position in both males and females, and specific examination procedures using a *sigmoidoscope* (an instrument used to visualize the bowel) can be performed. Draping may require the use of two sheets to cover the back and wrap the legs.

9. *Fowler's.* The patient sits on the examination table with the back supported and the legs slightly flexed on the table. A drape sheet covers the patient's legs. This position is used in particular for patients with dyspneic conditions.

10. *Proctologic jack-knife.* The knee-chest position is assumed more sharply with the use of a special table usually found in the office of a *proctologist* (a physician who specializes in diseases of the colon, rectum, and anus). Draping is the same as in the knee-chest position. Proctologic examinations are performed in this position in both male and female patients.

SELECTING THE CORRECT POSITION

The position chosen depends on the following variables:

1. *Symptomatology.* The patient's symptoms offer significant clues that can help the medical assistant in anticipating the type of examination to be performed. For example, a patient with respiratory complaints will most likely remain in the sitting position to facilitate examination of the respiratory system.

2. *Type of examination and procedure.* The patient may be scheduled for a certain type of

examination or a specific procedure. After the initial interaction between physician and patient, the medical assistant helps the patient from the sitting into the proper position. For example, a patient scheduled for vaginal examination would be assisted to assume a lithotomy position.

3. *Age and sex.* The age and sex of the patient are important considerations in positioning. For example, a rectal examination can be performed in one of the several positions listed; the position chosen would fit the age and sex of the individual.

PATIENT INSTRUCTION

The medical assistant should briefly explain the reason for assuming a particular position to the patient and give clear and precise instructions that enable the patient to assume the position with minimal assistance. As necessary, the medical assistant can provide assistance by gently placing his or her hands on the patient and directing the desired movement. (See procedures at the end of this chapter for aiding the patient in lithotomy, jack-knife, Sims', and knee-chest positions.)

Considerations for patient instruction in positioning are identical to those for gowning. It is important to emphasize, however, that handicaps or disease conditions might alter the patients' capacity to assume the desired position. Patient safety and comfort are always the highest priorities.

PREVENTING AND ALLEVIATING PATIENT DISCOMFORT

Several aspects of gowning, positioning, and draping may cause patients to feel uncomfortable physically and emotionally. Most of these discomforts are related to (1) nonselective or prolonged exposure of body parts, which may cause uneasiness and embarrassment, and (2) maintaining positions for prolonged periods, which may cause muscle spasms or pain. Although the medical assistant is not usually present during the actual examination, a female medical assistant is almost always present during the examination of a female patient by a male physician for legal considerations, which are explained later in this chapter. When medical assistants are present during examination of the patient, they assist the physician in the selective exposure of the patient and attend to the patient's comfort.

The guidelines presented below will be helpful in alleviating or preventing patient discomfort:

1. The patient should remain gowned and draped with breasts, abdomen, and pelvic area unexposed until the physician actually begins the examination. Only the body part being examined is exposed. A way of gauging the patient's

comfort with the draping process is for the medical assistant to imagine himself or herself in the place of the patient.

2. The patient should not remain in an uncomfortable position any longer than is required to complete the examination or treatment procedure. A female patient placed in the lithotomy position (see Fig. 18–1) for even a short time may experience cramping in the inner thigh area and back of the calves. If cramping occurs, the patient can be instructed and assisted in assuming a supine position (see Fig. 18–1). The medical assistant can relieve the cramp by placing the palm of one hand on the patient's knee and the palm of the other on the ball of the foot of the affected leg. By pressing down on the knee cap while simultaneously pushing up on the ball of the foot just above the arch, the cramp usually will be diminished and the positioning procedure can resume.

3. The medical assistant should be alert for ways of increasing the patient's comfort during positioning. For example, a small pillow positioned under the head can offer support and generally increases the patient's comfort. Any position can be modified to alleviate patient discomfort or to accommodate a weakened or painful body part. For example, a weakened patient unable to sit may be placed in a supine position with the head of the table elevated. If the patient complains of some discomfort during positioning, the medical assistant must use discretionary judgment in alleviating the discomfort by adjusting the position or offering support, such as a pillow to the back of a side-lying patient or placing the hands on the patient to help offer support in maintaining a certain position.

4. A drape sheet may be insufficient for keeping the patient warm while he or she waits in the examination room for the physician. Providing the patient with a blanket can increase comfort and prevent chilling. Offering water to drink or a magazine to read are also thoughtful activities patients appreciate.

PATIENT TEACHING CONSIDERATIONS

While positioning patients for examination, medical assistants can instruct them in the various uses of certain positions. For instance, the dorsal recumbent position is used by females when inserting vaginal creams or suppositories. This position, along with the side-lying (Sims') and knee-chest positions, also helps to relieve flatus (gas). As the medical assistant proceeds through the educational program, he or she will undoubtedly learn a number of other medical uses for many of the positions discussed in this chapter and will be able to share this information with patients when appropriate.

RELATED ETHICAL AND LEGAL IMPLICATIONS

Medical assistants are responsible for patients' safety in both the waiting room and the examination room. Safety related to positioning includes avoiding injury to the patient. If the medical assistant leaves a patient unattended in a position or asks a patient to assume a position while being left unattended, and the patient falls and sustains injury, the physician is legally responsible for the damages incurred. Obviously, a sick child or a debilitated or severely ill adult should never be left alone in the examination room. When the medical assistant's absence is unavoidable, a family member should be present in the examination room.

The medical assistant should also take care in positioning the patient not to inflict pain or injury. Listening to and observing the patient will help the medical assistant to be attentive to the patient's comfort.

Finally, when female patients are examined by male physicians, the female medical assistant remains in the examination room to provide legal protection for the physician in case the patient later accuses the physician of inappropriate behavior.

SUMMARY

The medical assistant's role in preparing the patient for examination includes gowning, placing the patient in the appropriate position, and draping. The assistant's responsibilities also include psychological preparation of the patient in terms of ensuring the patient's privacy and comfort, and this consideration should underlie all physical activities. As the medical assistant requires an understanding of how the physical examination proceeds and the type of examination to be performed based on the purpose of the visit and the age and sex of the patient, he or she will be better able to anticipate the physician's needs regarding gowning, positioning, and draping of the patient.

DISCUSSION QUESTIONS

Isolate the major objectives that underlie your approach to each of the following situations:

1. A patient has fractured her left arm, and it is in a cast. How would you approach gowning for a complete physical examination? Would you give any special instructions to the patient?
2. All patients coming to Dr. Jones' office are given a full gown and instructed to completely disrobe. Mrs. Smith does not remove her underwear. Describe your approach.
3. John Armstrong is 2 years old. He is visiting the doctor with symptoms of cough, congestion, runny nose, and fever. How would you prepare him for examination?
4. Mrs. Alberts is wearing a necklace and earrings. She is gowned and awaiting a complete physical examination. Would Mrs. Alberts be asked to remove her jewelry? Defend your response.
5. Mr. Pole is 76 years old and awaiting a rectal examination. Which position would Mr. Pole likely assume? Defend your response.

BIBLIOGRAPHY

Howard, A and Howard, W: Quote taken from Exploring the Road Less Traveled. Simon & Schuster, New York, 1985.
Potter, PA: Pocket Nurses Guide to Physical Assessment. CV Mosby, St. Louis, 1986.

PROCEDURE: Assist patient in the lithotomy position

OSHA STANDARDS:

Terminal Performance Objective: Assist the female patient into the proper position required for the examination of the external genitalia and for the speculum examination within 1 minute, without any discomfort to the patient or breach of patient modesty.

EQUIPMENT: Examination table with stirrups
Patient gown
Drape sheet
Wipes

PROCEDURE

1. Identify the patient and explain the procedure.

2. Instruct the patient to lie flat on her back just before the physician is ready to perform the examination.
3. Adjust the stirrups.

4. Instruct the patient to bend her knees and place her feet on the corners of the table.
5. Keeping the patient's genital area covered, instruct the patient to slide the buttocks down as close to her feet as is comfortable.
6. Place the patient's feet one at a time in the stirrups by placing one hand over the ball of the foot and cupping the ankle just above the heel with the other hand.

7. Instruct the patient to slide the buttocks further until they are at the edge of the examination table.

8. Separate the legs at the knees, and place the drape over the patient's legs so that it covers the perineal area.

PRINCIPLE

1. To reduce the risk of error and provide assurance to anxious patients.
2. To provide a comfortable first-step transition.

3. Stirrups too far away from the patient will not provide enough flexibility of the knee; stirrups too close will not allow the patient's buttocks to reach the end of the table; stirrups placed too wide or narrow will cause the hip joint discomfort.
4. Muscular strain is reduced when the position is assumed in gradual steps.
5. Again, muscular strain is reduced.

6. Stirrups support the legs and the feet. Stirrups are necessary if the speculum examination is to be performed. In body mechanics, patient limbs are moved by holding and gently manipulating joints.
7. This places the patient in the full lithotomy position and allows the greatest accessibility to the perineal area.
8. To afford privacy while increasing exposure of the perineal area.

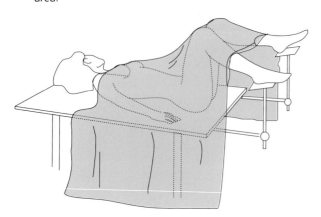

PROCEDURE

9. After the examination, instruct the patient to slide the buttocks up on the examination table to a comfortable position where the legs are extended.
10. Lift both feet out of the stirrups at the same time, and place them on the examination table.
11. When the patient is able, assist her to a sitting position.
12. Hand the patient several wipes.
13. Let the patient know when you will return, and allow the patient time alone to dress.

PRINCIPLE

9. Gradual resumption of normal positioning reduces the chance of muscle spasm.
10. Removing the feet individually increases the potential for muscular cramping in the calf.*
11. This position is most comfortable and signals the procedure's completion.
12. To remove the lubricant used during the examination.
13. Explaining what happens next diminishes patient anxiety.

*If a cramp occurs, place the leg flat on the table, and press down on the knee with the palm of one hand while pulling up the ball of the foot with the palm of the other hand.

PROCEDURE: Assist patient in the jack-knife position

OSHA STANDARDS:

Terminal Performance Objective: Assist the adult patient into the proper position required for the procto-logic examination within 1 minute, without any discomfort to the patient or breach of patient modesty.

EQUIPMENT: Proctology table
Patient gown
Two drape sheets
Wipes

PROCEDURE	PRINCIPLE
1. Identify the patient and explain the procedure.	1. To reduce the risk of error and provide assurance to anxious patients.
2. Instruct the gowned patient to lie on the table stomach down with the arms under the head. Place a small pillow under the patient's head.	2. Since the table is split to facilitate a jack-knife position, the patient's head will be lowered and the buttocks elevated. The pillow provides more comfort.
3. Place one drape sheet over the patient's legs and another diagonally over the upper body overlapping the drape sheet covering the legs.	3. To afford the patient a sense of privacy.
4. Just prior to the examination of the rectal area, fold back the upper drape to expose the rectal region.	4. Facilitates exposure of the rectal area while affording the patient the greatest degree of modesty possible in this position.
5. After the examination, assist the patient off the table.	5. The patient most likely will be unbalanced from the position.
6. Hand the patient several wipes.	6. To remove the lubricant used during the examination.
7. Let the patient know when you will return, and allow the patient time alone to dress.	7. Explaining what happens next diminishes patient anxiety.

PROCEDURE: Assist patients in the Sims' position

Terminal Performance Objective: Assist the adult patient into the proper side-lying position required for the examination of the vaginal or rectal areas within 1 minute, without any discomfort to the patient or breach of patient modesty.

EQUIPMENT: Examination table
Patient gown
Drape sheet
Wipes

PROCEDURE

1. Identify the patient and explain the procedure.

2. Instruct and assist the gowned patient to lie on the left side of the examination table. Place a small pillow under the patient's head.
3. Instruct the patient to roll the upper body further onto the side-lying position so that the patient is almost lying on the chest.
4. Sharply flex the right leg over the abdomen, and slightly flex the left leg underneath it.
5. Drape the patient.

PRINCIPLE

1. To reduce the risk of error and provide assurance to anxious patients.
2. The pillow provides comfort. The patient's buttocks should be at the long edge of the table.

3. This position facilitates examination of the rectal area.

4. This further facilitates examination of the rectal area.

5. To provide the patient with a sense of modesty.

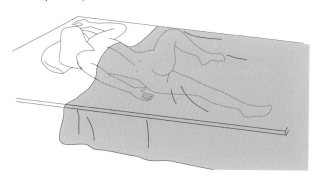

6. Just before the examination of the rectal area, fold back the drape corner to expose the anal region, and place a towel under the buttocks.
7. After the examination, assist the patient to a sitting position and then off the table to dress.
8. Hand the patient several wipes.
9. Let the patient know when you will return, and allow the patient time alone to dress.

6. Facilitates exposure of the area while affording the patient the greatest degree of modesty possible in this position.
7. The patient most likely will be unbalanced from the examination position.
8. To remove the lubricant used during the examination.
9. Explaining what happens next diminishes patient anxiety.

PROCEDURE: Assist patient in the knee-chest position

OSHA STANDARDS:

Terminal Performance Objective: Assist the adult patient into the proper position required for the examination of the rectal area within 1 minute, without any discomfort to the patient or breach of patient modesty.

EQUIPMENT: Examination table
Patient gown
Drape sheet
Wipes

PROCEDURE

1. Identify the patient and explain the procedure.

2. Assist the patient from a sitting or supine position into a kneeling position just before the physician is ready to examine the patient.

3. Instruct the patient to lay the head and chest on the table, placing the hands above the head, flexed at the elbow. Variation: Knee-elbow—patient may rest on the elbows if unable to lower the chest onto the table.

4. Place a small pillow under the head and chest.

5. Instruct the patient to bring the knees up to the chest as far as is comfortable. Stand by the patient to offer assistance.

6. Position the drape so that one corner covers the entire buttocks.

PRINCIPLE

1. To reduce the risk of error and provide assurance to anxious patients.

2. Gradual steps in positioning promote the patient's understanding and cooperation. Positioning too far in advance will result in patient discomfort.

3. This affords the greatest comfort and prevents the arms from getting in the way of the examination.

4. This affords more comfort.

5. This affords the greatest accessibility to the rectal area.

6. To afford privacy and comfort.

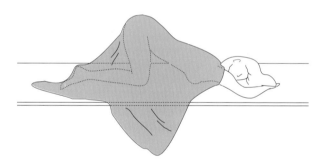

7. After the examination, assist the patient to a sitting position.

8. Hand the patient several wipes.

9. Let the patient know when you will return, and allow the patient time alone to dress.

7. This signals that the examination is completed and allows for greater patient comfort.

8. To remove lubricant used during the examination.

9. Explaining what happens next diminishes patient anxiety.

HIGHLIGHTS

The Paper Chase

Disposable gowns made of light-weight paper have been available for purchase for many years. During this time, we have witnessed an increased variety of styles and consistencies. What has not increased is the patient's comfort and satisfaction with the paper gown. As illustrated below, most patients would prefer to wear paper gowns over their clothes rather than next to their skin. Perhaps there is a more secure feeling in placing cloth as opposed to paper next to the skin.

If you participate in the selection of patient gowns, then you should consider the advantages and disadvantages of each type. The *advantages* of paper gowns are:
  - effective control of infection (the gown is disposed of immediately following patient use)
  - reduced cost (no laundering required)
  - easy storage (take up less room)

The *disadvantages* of paper gowns are:
  - tend to be extra large (for fitting all body sizes)
  - may tear, particularly when wet
  - difficulty conforming to body contour
  - patient may feel physically and psychologically uncomfortable
  - because the gowns may be rigid, slight movements tend to repeatedly alter its fit—oftentimes exposing body parts unintentionally
  - may convey an impersonal approach to the patient

Obviously, cloth gowns have contrasting advantages and disadvantages. When decisions are being made regarding the purchase of gowns, questions that should be asked are:

1. What are the intended objectives?
2. Who does this type of gown benefit? Benefit most?
3. Why? What are the reasons?
4. What patient reactions might be anticipated?
5. What are other factors which must be considered such as cost and storage?
6. Given the objectives, types of examinations to be performed, types and ages of patients, which type of gowning best meets the needs of this office practice?

Asking these questions may facilitate informed decision making to the benefit of the patient, physician, and staff.

CHAPTER OUTLINE

LEARNING OBJECTIVES

Upon completing this chapter, you will be able to:

1. List the purpose of and procedure for the general physical examination.
2. Describe how to prepare the examination room.
3. List the five basic methods the physician uses to examine the patient.
4. Simulate the preparation of the patient for examination.
5. List, arrange in appropriate order, and identify commonly used examination equipment.
6. Describe and demonstrate the care of the equipment used for the physical examination.

PERFORMANCE OBJECTIVE:

Upon completing this chapter, you will be able to:

1. Assist the physician to perform the general physical examination.

Chapter 19

General Physical Examination

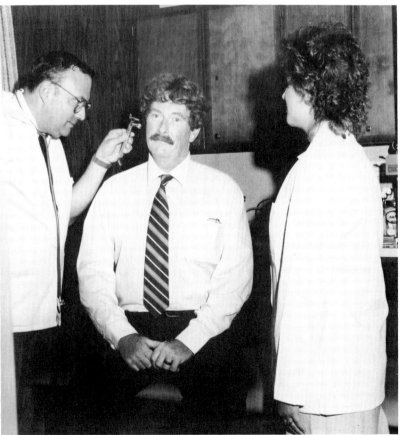

DACUM EDUCATIONAL COMPONENTS

1. Prepare examination and treatment area (4.5).
2. Prepare patients for examinations and diagnostic procedures (4.7).
3. Assist physician with examinations and treatments (4.8).
4. Obtain and record patient data (5.1).
5. Maintain and use aseptic techniques (4.1).

Glossary

Axilla: underarm area
Compliance: the extent to which a patient adheres to a prescribed health regimen
Diagnostic: pertaining to the identification of a disease or condition
Facilitator: an enabler of certain objectives achieved by another
Health maintenance: continued commitment to remaining healthy both mentally and physically
Hernia: protrusion or projection of an organ through the wall of the cavity in which it is normally contained
Symmetry: correspondence in the approximate shape, size, proportion, and position of body parts on opposite sides of the body
Visual acuity: visual clarity; being able to see precisely

Almost every patient who comes to the medical office receives a physical examination. The examination is either of *general* (complete) or *specific* (limited) nature. This chapter focuses on the general physical examination, sometimes referred to as the *comprehensive examination*. Specific examinations are discussed in the subsequent chapters.

Most physicians prefer to perform a general examination on new patients to assess their state of health and to establish some comparative base for future visits. Regular, or routine, examinations are performed at regular intervals as a preventive measure to ensure health maintenance. The major objective of the routine examination is early detection of disease itself or the signs that indicate the potential for disease. The evaluation of wellness and the diagnosis of certain diseases, however, depend on an assessment of *all* body parts and systems. In these instances, a general examination is performed.

The physical examination is the physician's primary diagnostic tool. As the physician's facilitator, the medical assistant not only must master the skills required to prepare the patient and to assist the physician, but must also comprehend the process of the physical examination—its purpose and methods. It is this combination of understanding and skill development that will enable the medical assistant to apply discretionary judgment to the diverse situations encountered when assisting with the general physical examination.

PURPOSE OF THE PHYSICAL EXAMINATION

The purpose of the general physical examination is to determine the patient's overall state of health. The entire body is examined, including all body *orifices* (open-

ings), all major organs, and all body systems. The physician interprets the findings of the examination and forms an initial judgment regarding the patient's present condition.

Laboratory and other diagnostic tests are used concurrently to supplement the physical findings. Laboratory testing is an essential component of the general physical examination, and of specific examinations as well. These laboratory tests and diagnostic testing procedures are described in later chapters.

DIAGNOSIS

The physical examination is the cornerstone of the diagnostic process on which all other nonphysical findings rest. Together, the patient history, physical examination findings, vital signs, laboratory and other diagnostic test results, the patients' expressed (*subjective*) symptoms, and the physician's general perceptions give shape and substance to the diagnostic puzzle. The physician studies and interprets these factors, forms a judgment, and concludes a diagnosis.

The physician may select from three basic categories of diagnoses to represent his or her own conclusions:

1. *Differential Diagnosis.* In this category, the physician attempts to rule out certain possibilities. The final diagnosis may emerge from these alternative diagnoses. A differential diagnosis is usually written in the following manner:

Differential Diagnosis:

1. Rule out (R/O) appendicitis
2. R/O gastroenteritis
3. R/O colitis

2. *Tentative Diagnosis (Impression).* At this stage, the physician has not yet reached a conclusion, and the diagnosis is therefore temporary and subject to change as the physician gains further insights from other diagnostic tools. These can include consultations with other physicians or further laboratory and other diagnostic studies. Sometimes, hospitalization is required. The tentative diagnosis is usually written in the following manner:

Diagnosis. Possible bowel obstruction

3. *Final Diagnosis.* The final diagnosis is the conclusion the physician reaches after the results of all diagnostic tools have been integrated and evaluated. The final diagnosis is written in the following manner:

Final Diagnosis. Gastritis

EXAMINATION METHODS

To establish a diagnosis, the physician uses four primary methods of physical examination: inspection, palpation, percussion, and auscultation. Frequently a fifth method, mensuration, is added. These methods are used collaboratively during the examination process, with attention being focused on uncovering abnormalities. A brief description of each of these methods follows.

INSPECTION During the process of examination, the physician visually inspects all body parts and exterior surfaces and, with illumination and the aid of instruments (some with magnifying capabilities), examines the eyes, ears, and throat and, in the female patient, may examine the cervix and vaginal wall. In certain patients, a sigmoidoscopic examination may also be performed. All body areas are inspected for the presence of any abnormality in size, color, continuity, shape, position, and symmetry (Fig. 19–1).

PALPATION Using different parts of the hand, the physician locates and feels all accessible body parts, including the major organs of the body and the lymph node pathways. During the process of examination, the physician palpates the chest, the abdomen, and the lymph nodes in the neck, *axillae* (underarms), and chest. The purpose of palpation is to detect any abnormality in characteristics of movement, size, shape, texture, temperature, and tenderness (Fig. 19–2).

PERCUSSION During the neurologic examination, the physician uses a percussion hammer to check the reflexes of certain body parts by tapping them. During the process of the general physical examination, the percussion hammer or fingers or knuckles are used to percuss the body parts. The chest wall and abdomen are percussed with parts of the hand by thumping, striking, or tapping the body surface. Through the use of percussion, the physician evaluates the normalcy of internal structures related to location, size, and density, and the presence or absence of fluid. These characteristics are determined by interpreting the vibrations and sounds caused by percussing (Fig. 19–3).

AUSCULTATION The physician listens to certain body sounds with a stethoscope. During the process of examination, the physician listens to the sounds made by the heart and respiratory system and for bowel sounds in the intestines (Fig. 19–4).

MENSURATION The physician uses calipers and measuring tape to evaluate the growth and development of specific body areas or to determine the size of abnormalities.

ROLE OF DIAGNOSTIC TESTS IN THE PHYSICAL EXAMINATION

Although not classified as a method of examination, diagnostic testing, including laboratory, x-ray, and

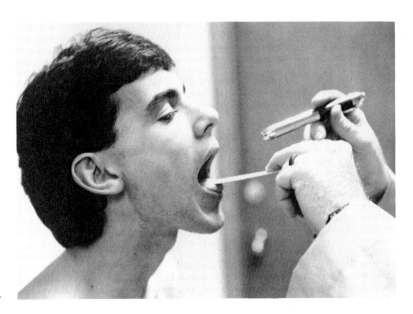

Figure 19–1. Inspection (looking).

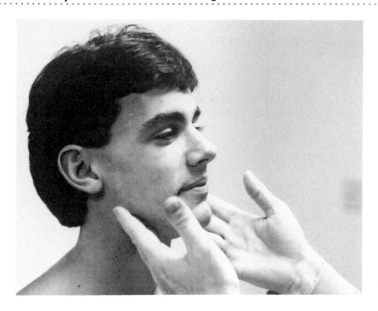

Figure 19–2. Palpation (feeling).

other measurements, is an integral part of the general, or comprehensive, physical examination. An examination of the blood and urine, a chest x-ray, and an electrocardiogram are commonly included in the diagnostic testing for evaluation of the general state of health. Usually the physician's own preferences and concerns would govern the choice of specific diagnostic tests for inclusion in the general physical examination.

EQUIPMENT USED IN THE PHYSICAL EXAMINATION

Special instruments are required for the physical examination. These instruments enable the physician to use the methods previously discussed to listen, inspect, visualize, and test the body parts. The instruments are readily accessible in a special tray or are stored permanently in each examination room.

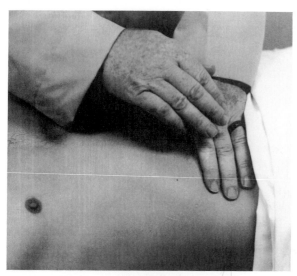

Figure 19–3. Percussion (tapping).

The instruments most commonly used for a complete physical examination are described below and illustrated in Figure 19–5.

1. *Ophthalmoscope*. This instrument is used to inspect the internal structures of the eye. The physician focuses light through the magnifying lens of the ophthalmoscope on the parts of the eye and checks for any abnormalities.
2. *Otoscope*. This instrument enables the physician to inspect the outer ear and tympanic membranes. Light is focused through a magnifying lens to view these structures. By changing the speculum, the physician can also inspect the nasal canals with the same instrument. Ear speculums are long and narrow and come in varying widths, whereas nasal speculums are short and wide.
3. *Pocket flashlight or headlight*. This light source supplies light during various phases of the examination.
4. *Ruler or flexible tape measure*. These measuring devices are used to determine the size of an abnormality (such as lesions). In infants, head circumference and body length are measured to assess developmental progress.
5. *Tongue depressors*. A tongue depressor is used to hold down the tongue to visualize the throat.
6. *Stethoscope*. This instrument is a listening device and is used to auscultate various parts of the body, specifically the heart, lungs, and abdomen.
7. *Gloves and lubricant*. Lubricated disposable examination gloves are used to protect the patient and physician from invading microorganisms while the physician palpates the inner structures of the vagina and rectum in the female, and the rectum in the male. The oral cavity is examined with a freshly gloved hand.
8. *Vaginal speculum*. This instrument is used by

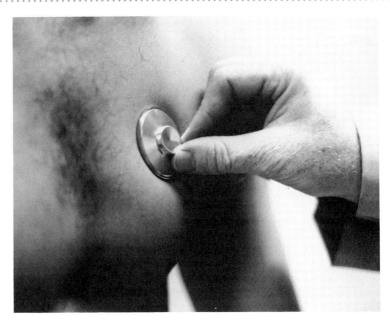

Figure 19–4. Auscultation (listening with a stethoscope).

the physician to expand the vaginal opening to facilitate examination of the vaginal wall and the cervix. An instrument called *uterine forceps*, which holds sponges (*gauze wipes*) that are used to clean the cervix or vaginal canal to facilitate visualization, is also usually included on the examination tray in preparation for complete physical examination of the female patient. For the patient's comfort, the vaginal speculum, since it is a clean rather than a sterile instrument, can be warmed by holding it under warm water just prior to examination.

9. *Reflex hammer.* Two types of hammers are available to test neurologic reflexes. The *reflex hammer* has a rubber, triangular-shaped head for testing neurologic reflexes such as in the tendons of the knee. The *neurologic hammer*, in addition to having a rubber tip on its head, also has a small insert that contains a brush and a needle for testing sensory functions.

10. *Tuning fork.* This instrument permits the physician to make judgments about patient's auditory (hearing) acuity. The vibration of the tuning fork produces a humming noise that is perceptible to the ears.

Certain supplies must also be available on the examination tray. These include cotton tipped applicators, Pap smear slides (when a Pap smear is anticipated), fixative, and wipes (4 × 4 gauze squares) or tissues. Specialty offices have specialized instruments that are used routinely, such as the fetoscope and Doppler, which are used in an obstetrician's office.

PROCEDURE FOR THE GENERAL PHYSICAL EXAMINATION

The physician may perform the physical examination aided by the medical assistant. The ability to effectively assist the physician is dependent on an understanding of how each physician proceeds through the examination. Equipped with this information, the medical assistant can better anticipate the needs of the patient and the physician. Table 19–1 compares the various areas for physical examination, listing the body parts, the corresponding positions of the patient, and the equipment needed for each.

Using the methods previously described, the physician assesses the general state of health of the body parts and systems. This assessment includes a general survey based on observation. As the physician interviews the patient, he or she notes signs of distress, skin color, stature, posture, motor activity and gait, grooming, presence of odors, facial expression, mood, body language, state of awareness, and speech. After the patient gowns and assumes the sitting position, the physician first proceeds to examine the head and the neck.

The patient's needs or the physician's preference, however, dictate the remaining sequence of the examination and what is included in it. The procedure for the comprehensive physical examination outlined below, although not absolute, is widely accepted and therefore serves as a useful guide. A detailed description of the procedure is provided at the end of this chapter.

SITTING POSITION

HEAD   The hair, scalp, skull, and face are examined using inspection and palpation.

EYES   A *visual acuity test* (eye chart examination) performed by the medical assistant before the physical examination may supplement the physician's initial ophthalmoscopic examination of the eyes.

EARS   The ear canals and eardrums are inspected with an otoscope. Auditory acuity is tested with a tuning fork.

NOSE AND SINUSES   With the use of an otoscope

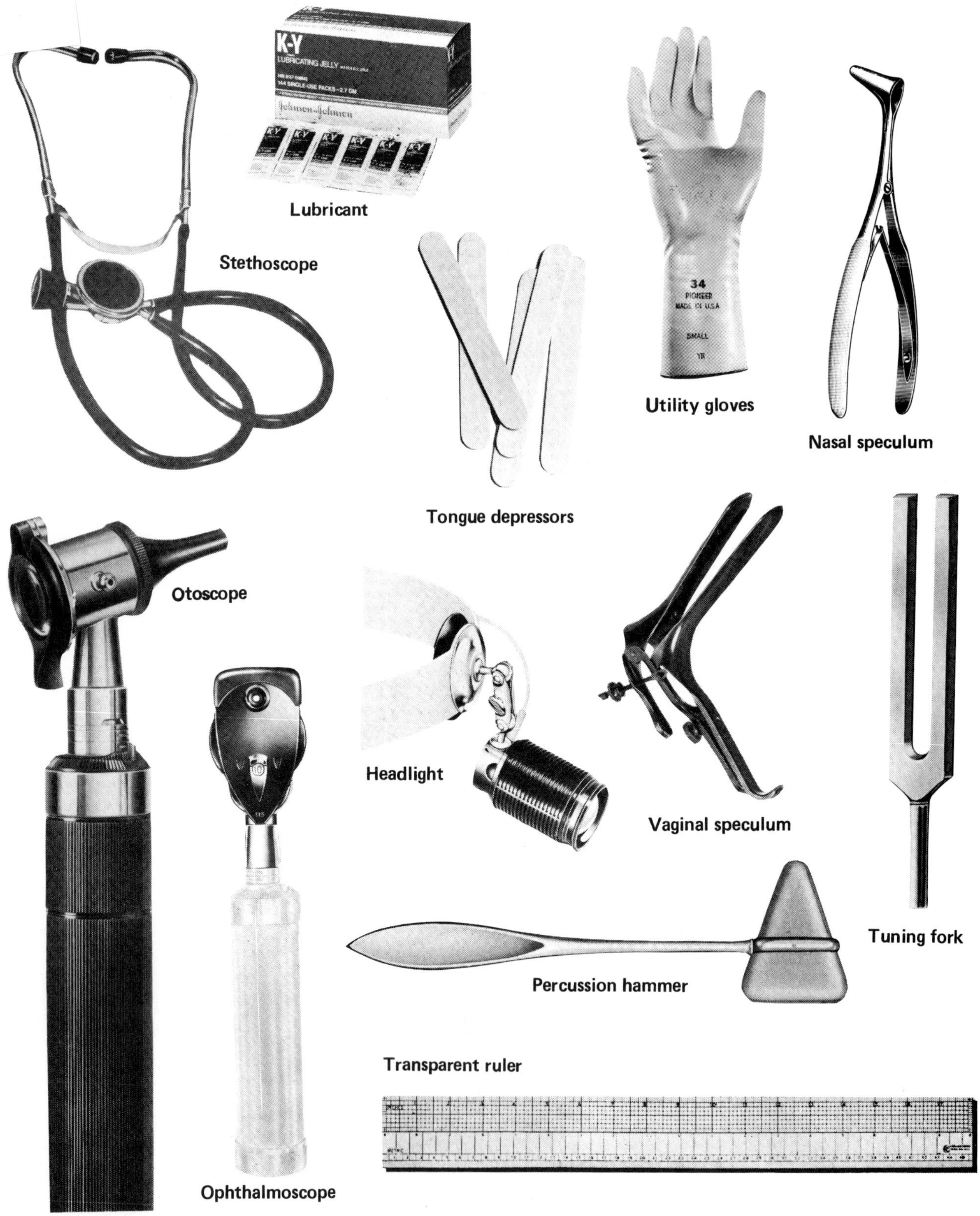

Lubricant

Stethoscope

Tongue depressors

Utility gloves

Nasal speculum

Otoscope

Headlight

Vaginal speculum

Tuning fork

Percussion hammer

Transparent ruler

Ophthalmoscope

Figure 19–5. Instruments commonly used in the general physical examination. (Courtesy of General Medical Corporation. Nasal speculum courtesy of Labtron Scientific Corporation and Villa Medical Supply.)

Table 19-1
AREAS FOR PHYSICAL EXAMINATION

Body Part	Position	Equipment Needed
Head and neck	Sitting	Ophthalmoscope, otoscope, nasal speculum, tuning fork, tongue blade, measuring tape
Chest (front and upper extremities)	Sitting	Stethoscope
Abdomen	Supine and dorsal recumbent (knees flexed)	Stethoscope
Genitalia and rectum	Sims', dorsal recumbent, or lithotomy positions	Glove, lubricant, vaginal speculum, slides, and curette stick (for Pap tests in women), sigmoidoscope—proctoscope
Lower extremities	Supine or sitting	None
Nervous system	Sitting	Reflex hammer

with a speculum attachment or a nasal speculum, which is specifically designed for the nasal examination, the nasal passages above and below the eyes (*frontal* and *maxillary*) are examined and palpated.

MOUTH AND PHARYNX (THROAT) The lips, interior mucosa, roof of the mouth, gums, teeth, tongue, and pharynx are inspected. The physician uses a light source and a tongue blade to visualize the pharynx. The mucosa of the mouth may also be palpated. If the medical assistant hands the physician a tongue blade, it is held in the center to allow the physician to grasp an end. A *laryngeal mirror* (a mirrored instrument used to visualize the larynx) is sometimes required for the examination or is included in the tray setup according to the physician's preference. When a laryngeal mirror is used, it is warmed first by momentarily placing the mirrored end under warm water. (Another technique is to warm the mirror by quickly passing it over the flame of an alcohol lamp). Fogging can be prevented by spraying the mirror with sprays specially formulated for this use.

NECK The *trachea* (windpipe) and the thyroid are inspected and palpated. The carotid artery is auscultated bilaterally, and the lymph nodes located on both sides of the neck (*cervical nodes*) are palpated.

BACK The spine and muscles of the back are palpated and inspected.

POSTERIOR THORAX (CHEST WALL) AND LUNGS The chest wall and the lungs are examined by inspection, palpation, percussion, and auscultation.

CHEST The chest is inspected for symmetry, the presence of masses or nipple discharge, and general appearance. The nodes in the axillary (underarm) region are palpated. A stethoscope is used to auscultate breath sounds. When these examination steps are concluded, the patient is assisted to assume the supine position for the continuation of the procedure.

SUPINE POSITION

BREASTS The breast examination is performed in the supine position using palpation. In this position,

female breast tissue spreads, facilitating examination of the outer layers of the breast.

ANTERIOR THORAX AND LUNGS All four methods of examination are used to examine the anterior chest and lungs. Some physicians initiate this examination while the patient is in the sitting position. A stethoscope is used for auscultation.

HEART Auscultation and inspection are the methods used to examine the heart. A stethoscope is used for auscultation to determine the heart's pumping sounds. Inspection focuses on external movements of the anterior chest to observe pumping action, which is observable only when the heart rate is fast and the pumping action is strong. Auscultation is also used to determine the apical pulse.

ABDOMEN All four methods are used to examine the abdomen. A stethoscope is used to auscultate bowel sounds and abdominal blood vessels. Inspection is used to determine the symmetry and contour of the abdomen. Percussion is used to outline the borders of organs within the abdomen and to outline the presence of air in the stomach or bowel. Palpation enables the physician to evaluate the abdominal wall, the abdominal aorta, and the abdominal organs for the presence of masses, pain, tenderness, or organ enlargement.

INGUINAL AREA The *inguinal area* (the flexion point between the hips and the legs) is examined using palpation for location of inguinal nodes and subsequent assessment of the normalcy of these nodes and detection of hernia. An *inguinal hernia* is the projection of a loop of intestine through an area of the abdominal wall. A *hernia* is the protrusion or projection of an organ through the wall of a cavity in which it is normally contained. Blood vessels in this region are auscultated.

GENITALIA AND RECTAL EXAMINATION IN MEN The penis, scrotal contents, prostate, anus, and rectum are inspected and palpated. A rectal examination is performed while the patient is in the Sims' (side-lying) position.

GENITAL EXAMINATION IN WOMEN The examination of the external genitalia, vagina, cervix, and rectum can be accomplished while the patient is in the modified-lithotomy position. First, a Pap smear is taken, and the cervix and vaginal lining is examined. Next, the physician palpates the internal structure of the vagina with the fingers of one gloved hand, which is inserted into the vagina, and then palpates the patient's abdomen to check the uterus, fallopian tubes, and ovaries with the other hand, which is ungloved (bimanual examination). A warmed vaginal speculum, headlight, gloves, lubricant, and wipes are needed. Pap test equipment is further described in Chapter 21.

LEGS The legs are inspected and palpated. Pulse sites are located and evaluated for irregularity and abnormality in volume. The patient then stands for further evaluation of the musculoskeletal and peripheral vascular systems.

STANDING POSITION

MUSCULOSKELETAL SYSTEM While standing, the range of motion and muscle strength are noted for both upper and lower extremities. Also noted is the alignment of the legs and feet and the arms and hands. The patient may be asked to walk so that the physician may observe the gait.

PERIPHERAL VASCULAR SYSTEM The legs are inspected for *varicosities* (varicose veins). The femoral, popliteal, and dorsalis pedis pulses are also assessed.

HERNIA In men, the inguinal area is again inspected and palpated this time in the standing position, because a hernia may become pronounced only when the patient is upright.

NEUROLOGIC EXAMINATION Assessment of the patient's gait, ability to do knee bends, to hop, to walk on toes and heels, and to perform other movements comprises the evaluation of the neurologic and musculoskeletal systems. The patient then assumes a sitting position for further neurologic testing of the knee reflex with a reflex hammer.

THE ROLE OF THE MEDICAL ASSISTANT

The medical assistant's role is to create a climate of comfort and security for the patient and efficiency and convenience for the physician.

ROOM READINESS

The medical assistant is responsible for readying the examination room. Inspection of the room for cleanliness is required. The patient should never be ushered into a "dirty room." The table sheet or disposable table cover should be fresh for each patient. Wastebasket contents, if odorous, sanguineous (bloody), or otherwise unpleasant, are removed. Contaminated instruments from previous procedures are removed for cleaning and sterilization. Countertops are cleaned, and instruments and equipment are arranged in an orderly manner. Equipment should be assembled and ready for use. Lighting should be adequate and, if movable, positioned appropriately. Prescription pads and other mate-

rials should be stored safely and be inaccessible to the patient or patient's family. The patient's record is usually placed outside the examination room door in a rack provided for this purpose. It is usually not left in the room with the patient because its contents may be misinterpreted by the patient or an individual accompanying the patient. However, when the patient asks to see the record, the physician is consulted.

PATIENT PREPARATION

Physical and psychological preparation are necessary to ready the patient for examination. Physical preparation of the patient includes the obtaining and recording of weight and height before the patient goes into the examination room. In addition, to facilitate the examination, the patient should empty his or her bladder and bowel. The medical assistant asks the patient to disrobe completely and to dress in a full gown, giving instructions as to how it is to be worn (opening in front or back), and then directs or assists the patient to sit on the examination table. A drape sheet is provided for the patient's legs.

Psychological preparation of the patient includes an assessment of the patient's level of anxiety. Some patients experience stress or uneasiness before examination. Explaining the procedure to the patient helps alleviate anxiety. Young children may also be anxious and restless and may require either the distraction provided by toys in the examination room or the comfort of sitting in their parent's lap rather than on the examination table while waiting for the physician. The medical assistant should observe the patient's facial expression before, during, and after the examination to detect signs of discomfort or anxiety.

The medical assistant may give special attention to pediatric, elderly, pregnant, or disabled individuals in preparing them for the physical examination. Pediatric patients should never be left alone in the room and will require an appropriate explanation of the examination procedure according to their age. (See also Chapter 21, the section titled the Pediatric Patient.) For instance, the medical assistant may show a preschool child the ophthalmoscope and explain that the examination will take place in the dark. The medical assistant can also show the child other instruments to promote cooperation and to prevent the child's becoming fearful. Elderly patients may, depending on their level of wellness, require the medical assistant's special assistance in preparing for the physical exam. In addition to offering empathetic support, the medical assistant may help the elderly or disabled patient obtain a specimen, sit on the examination table, or assume a comfortable position. Disabled individuals and pregnant women may require special accommodation in assuming a comfortable position or moving about the examination room or psychological preparation for the examination.

While interviewing the patient, the medical assistant has the opportunity to assess and respond to the patient's psychological needs. The patient often shares with the medical assistant valuable information related to the purpose of the visit and the severity of symptoms, as well as personal fears and anxieties. It is not uncommon for the medical assistant to spend more contact time than the physician with the patient. Needless to say, the medical assistant should relate all pertinent information to the physician.

The medical assistant may also prepare the patient for examination by interviewing him or her regarding symptoms, the time of onset of the illness, and the duration of the illness, as discussed in the chapter on patient interviewing. A history is also obtained during the first visit. The vital signs are taken. The physician, while examining the patient, may repeat the blood pressure procedure and will further interview the patient.

Certain diagnostic tests performed by the medical assistant are routine and are included as part of the general physical examination. These are typically the complete blood count, urinalysis, and electrocardiogram. For these and certain other studies which may require a referral, the proper laboratory order sheets for the physician's use can be readied.

In summary, as the liaison between the physician and the patient, the medical assistant prepares the patient for examination, sets the tone for the visit, makes general observations concerning the patient, attends to the patient's comfort, explains procedures, and answers questions.

ASSISTING THE PHYSICIAN

The medical assistant's role in assisting the physician with the examination is threefold: (1) handing instruments to the physician and obtaining other instruments and materials as directed; (2) assisting the patient to assume positions and exposing body areas for examination; and (3) offering the patient reassurance and providing comfort.

With the exception of obtaining vital signs, medical assistants do not perform the general physical examination; however, their presence and assistance are extremely valuable to the physician and the patient. When the physician is aided by the medical assistant, the examination can be performed in less time, with greater effectiveness, and with increased patient comfort. When male physicians examine female patients, the female medical assistant's presence is required for legal reasons.

The medical assistant may offer special assistance to pediatric, elderly, or disabled patients during the examination. For instance, the medical assistant may need to hold the young child's head immobile during otoscopic examination or instruct the parent to do so. Elderly and disabled patients may need help assuming and maintaining certain positions during examination to avoid

pain or discomfort. The procedure guide near the end of the chapter outlines in detail the medical assistant's role in the general physical examination of most adult patients.

PATIENT TEACHING CONSIDERATIONS

While preparing the patient for examination and following its completion, the medical assistant has the opportunity for patient teaching. This type of instruction should be adjusted to the patient's age and developmental level. One example is the differing set of instructions given to a parent versus a child regarding ear care and avoiding the placement of foreign bodies in the ear. This example illustrates that brief, purposeful information can help the patient improve or maintain general well-being.

Still another example of patient teaching is instruction of the female patient in the Breast Self-Examination. This self-examination procedure is described in Chapter 21. Women who consistently examine their breasts every month significantly increase their chances for early detection and successful treatment of breast cancer.

In the previous instances, the medical assistant is encouraging the patient to adopt positive health behaviors. Patient teaching methods and their application in time-constrained situations were discussed in Chapter 4, Patient Teaching.

RELATED ETHICAL AND LEGAL IMPLICATIONS

The medical assistant should recognize that beginning with the physician's first "laying of the hands" on the patient constitutes a contractual agreement between the physician and the patient, and the patient and the medical office staff. This implied contract begins with the first physical examination. For this reason, the physician must provide an acceptable standard of care using reasonable skill, experience, and knowledge. (Refer to Chapter 3, Medical Law and Ethics.)

SUMMARY

The medical assistant's role in assisting the physician with the general physical examination is to accommodate both the physician's and the patient's needs. To function effectively in this capacity, the medical assistant must possess a multitude of diverse skills, both clinical and interpersonal. The content of this chapter has been directed toward providing the information necessary to the development of these skills.

DISCUSSION QUESTIONS

1. During the process of the general physical examination, the physician tests the patient's reflexes. Identify the system being examined, what instruments the physician may need, and the patient's appropriate position.

2. A female patient being examined has very long hair. Assess what difficulty, if any, would be encountered during the examination. In what ways could the medical assistant facilitate the examination?
3. A patient is scheduled for a pelvic examination and a Pap smear. She is elderly and has arthritic knees. How would you position her for examination? What other assistance would you offer?
4. The physician is examining the patient's ears during the course of a general physical examination. The doctor hands the otoscope to you and pauses a moment. What would you anticipate to be the next step in the examination? Depending on your answer to the first question, what will you do with the otoscope?
5. The physician is about to perform a pelvic examination using a speculum. What other items are needed for this examination? How would you, as the medical assistant, function in this situation with regard to readying the room, preparing the patient, and assisting the physician?

BIBLIOGRAPHY

Anaveoli, C, et al.: Cecil Essentials of Medicine, 2nd ed. WB Saunders, Philadelphia, 1990.
Doenges, ME and Moorhouse, MF: Nurse's Pocket Guide: Nursing Diagnosis with Interventions, 3rd ed. FA Davis, Philadelphia, 1991.
Hogstel, M and Keen-Payne, R: Practical Guide to Health Assessment. FA Davis, Philadelphia, 1993.
Pottes, P: Physical Assessment. CV Mosby, St Louis, 1976.
Rakel, RE: Conn's Current Therapy, 1993. WB Saunders, Philadelphia, 1993.
Schwartz, MH: Textbook of Physical Diagnosis: History and Examination. WB Saunders, Philadelphia, 1989.
Stults, BM and Dere, WH: Practical Care of the Ambulatory Patient. WB Saunders, Philadelphia, 1989.
Talley, NJ and O'Connor, S: Examination Medicine: A Guide to Physician Training, 2nd ed. FA Davis, Philadelphia, 1991.

PROCEDURE: Assist with the general physical examination

OSHA STANDARDS:

Terminal Performance Objective: Assist the physician to perform the general physical examination without any discomfort to the patient or breach of patient modesty.

EQUIPMENT: General examination equipment (see Fig. 19–5)
Adjustable light source
Examination gloves (at least two pairs)
Patient gown and drape sheets
Wipes
Urine collection kit
Eye chart and cup
Scale
Vital signs equipment
Biohazard bags for disposal

PROCEDURE

1. Prepare the room by assembling the equipment and checking the cleanliness of the room, lighting, and temperature.
2. Identify the patient and escort from the waiting area.
3. Instruct the patient in the collection of a clean-catch midstream urine specimen if directed. Ask the patient to empty the bladder and bowel if necessary.
4. Measure and record visual acuity, if directed.

5. Escort the patient to the examination room after obtaining and recording the height and weight.

6. Obtain and chart the history and physical assessment, if directed.

7. Instruct the patient in disrobing and gowning and afford privacy.

8. If a urine specimen is obtained before the examination, label the specimen and deliver it to the laboratory.
9. Reenter the room and explain the anticipated procedure to the patient.
10. Obtain and record the vital signs.

11. Assist the patient onto the table by reaching under the patient's arms at the shoulder and helping to raise the patient onto the table. Cover the legs with a drape sheet.
12. Notify the physician that the patient is ready for the examination.

PRINCIPLE

1. To reduce the chance of transmitting microorganisms and to facilitate the efficiency of the examination.

2. To reduce the risk of error and to provide assurance to anxious patients.
3. An empty bladder and bowel facilitates palpation of the abdomen.

4. Visual acuity should be tested before disrobing. The patient should not be required to leave the examination room wearing a gown.
5. Depending on the location of the scale, the patient should not be required to leave the examination room wearing a gown. If the scale is in the examination room, this step can be completed with the vital signs.
6. This step saves the physician time and serves as a double-check system, as the physician will further interview the patient.
7. If the patient does not require assistance, then personal comfort is promoted by leaving the room while the patient disrobes.
8. Immediate labeling with the patient's name, date, time of collection, and the purpose prevents error.
9. An informed patient is less anxious and more cooperative.
10. This data is a necessary part of every physical examination, as it provides data to evaluate the patient's general state of health.
11. The physical examination begins with the patient in the sitting position. During the examination, the patient is assisted to lie down.

12. The physician usually relies on the medical assistant to announce that the patient is ready for the examination.

PROCEDURE	PRINCIPLE
13. As the physician proceeds with the examination, provide the appropriate instruments, assist the physician in exposing body areas, and maintain patient comfort and dignity by covering previously exposed areas.	13. The physician usually relies on the medical assistant to assist with the orderliness and efficiency of the examination. The more the medical assistant is able to anticipate the physician's procedures and to accommodate preferences, the more valuable a time-saving resource and quality-care provider the medical assistant becomes.
14. After the examination, assume follow-up duties such as administrating medication, performing further diagnostic tests, applying dressing, or performing other clinical procedures.	14. The physician usually relies on the medical assistant to carry out treatment plans.
15. Instruct the patient to dress, and assist if necessary. Allow opportunities for questions.	15. The physician usually relies on the medical assistant to share the responsibility for patient education. Allowing and encouraging questioning provides opportunities to instruct the patient regarding the treatment and ensures that the patient understands the treatment routine, thus increasing the probability of the patient's compliance.
16. When possible, escort the patient to the front desk, equipped with full instructions related to treatment and return visits.	16. Patient comfort depends on many variables. One of prime importance is the personal treatment provided by office personnel. In addition, since the medical assistant is usually the last person in the clinical area to come in contact with the patient, he or she should ensure that all the patient's questions are answered and the patient fully understands follow-up expectations.
17. Clean the equipment and the examination room.	17. To prevent the chance of transmitting microorganisms and to prepare the room for the next patient.
18. Chart the patient teaching session and remaining notes. Example: 12/20/93 10:30 AM ocular dexter (OD), 20/20, ocular sinister (OS), 20/15 with (w/) glasses; temperature (T) 36.5°C/98°F (o); pulse (P), 68; rate (R), 17; blood pressure (BP), 128/99 (right arm [r/a]); urinary specimen (US) sent to lab. Chief complaint (CC) and presenting illness (PI) none; CPE [complete physical examination] for college admission. Patient/instruction: Instructed patient on procedures for obtaining three hemoccult fecal samples over next week. Written instr and test kit given. Appointment: 12/27/93 (initials).	

HIGHLIGHTS
From Illness to Wellness

In our contemporary society, well-being is perceived to be every individual's right. Well-being is defined as the experience of an acceptable quality of life as determined by each individual. For most people, well-being includes a quality of life in which physical, spiritual, emotional, and social needs are met and the individual is regarded as "healthy." Implicit in the definition of well-being, then, are values associated with health.

The values (personal beliefs) which seem to be commonly associated with health are that health is a resource, a right and a personal responsibility. It is a resource because it is in limited supply for each individual and there is no substitute: "As long as you have your health, you have everything." It is a right equal to the rights to life, liberty and the pursuit of happiness . . . tenets established by our forefathers. It is a responsibility because effort is required for its maintenance and it is often personal choice to remain healthy. Today, further value is being placed on the state of one's health and new terms or terms with new meaning have been invented.

Many people today are attempting to achieve well-ness and high-level wellness. Wellness is more than absence of disease. It is the integration of physical, spiritual, emotional, and social needs indicative of a satisfying state of health. The term high-level wellness is further up on the illness-wellness continuum. High-level wellness refers to the individual functioning at his or her own highest or best level in relation to his or her own abilities and limitations. It differs from wellness in that it is beyond satisfactory. High-level wellness is an exemplary achievement in which all of the individual's lifestyle habits are connected together and directed toward the attainment of the highest end of the range of well-being. For example, an individual pursuing high-level wellness would keep abreast of the latest scientific medical information and accordingly determine his or her diet and exercise level. In addition, he or she would pursue the spiritual, social, and emotional paths leading to fullness of life, happiness, peace, and productivity. As health care practitioners, we must be aware of the values placed on health by contemporary society and understand the individualization of the definitions of wellness.

> The constitution of the human being is composed of a great number of organs, constructed upon the most beautiful chemical, physical, mechanical, and dynamic principles, and is governed by a system of organic laws, upon the proper observation of which the health of mankind depends.
>
> H. R. Burner, MD
> Lectures on How to Acquire
> and Preserve Health, 1874

CHAPTER OUTLINE

Chapter 20

Specific Phys
Examinations
Clinical Proce ___ es.
Part I

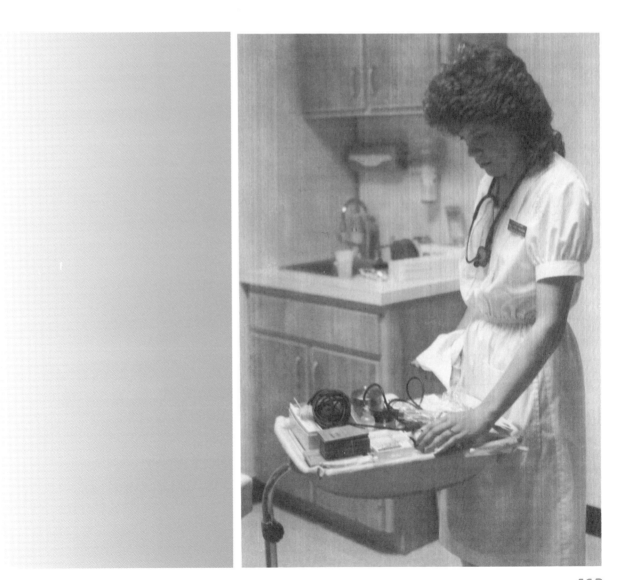

LEARNING OBJECTIVES

Upon completing this chapter, you will be able to:

1. Identify the body's symptomatic reaction to disease in each system discussed.
2. List and define diagnostic studies related to the systems and individual body parts discussed.
3. List the common diseases related to each system discussed.
4. Describe the process of specific physical examinations.
5. State the medical assistant's role in preparation of the room and the patient for the examinations, treatments, and procedures.
6. Provide instruction for the patient's office experiences and follow-up care.
7. Explain and discuss the principles of specific clinical procedures.

PERFORMANCE OBJECTIVES

Upon completing this chapter, you will be able to:

1. Test visual acuity (degrees of visual clarity) with the Snellen eye chart.
2. Using sterile technique, irrigate the eye to remove foreign particles, treat infections, or flush away harmful chemicals.
3. Using sterile technique, instill or apply medication to dilate or contract the pupil, relieve pain or discomfort, cleanse the eye, treat infection, or reduce inflammation.
4. Apply warm compresses to the eye to promote drainage or soothe inflammation and irritation.
5. Apply a sterile eye dressing to keep the eye at rest, protect the eye, absorb secretions, or reduce swelling.
6. Irrigate the external ear canal to remove discharge, cerumen, or foreign bodies.
7. Introduce medication directly into the ear canal or onto the ear drum to soften earwax or treat infection.
8. Using written instructions, instruct the patient in cast care at home to ensure safety and comfort and promote a positive outcome.

9. Using written instructions, instruct the patient to apply an ice bag to relieve pain or reduce swelling.
10. Using written instructions, instruct the patient to apply a cold compress to relieve inflammation, pain, swelling, or hematoma.
11. Using written instructions, instruct the patient to apply a hot water bag to relieve pain or reduce swelling.
12. Using written instructions, instruct the patient to apply a heating pad to relieve pain or reduce swelling.
13. Using written instructions, instruct the patient to apply warm soaks to relieve pain or reduce swelling.
14. Using written instructions, instruct the patient to apply warm compresses to relieve pain or reduce swelling.

DACUM EDUCATIONAL COMPONENTS

1. Prepare examination and treatment area (4.8).
2. Prepare patients for examinations and diagnostic procedures, and instruct patients in at-home care (4.7).
3. Assist physician with examinations and treatments (4.8).
4. Perform routine diagnostic tests (4.11).
5. Administer specified medications (4.13).
6. Maintain patient medication records and records of procedures (4.14).
7. Obtain and record patient data (5.1).
8. Maintain and use aseptic techniques (4.1).

Glossary

Ear: the organ of hearing and equilibrium
Endocrine system: deals with the internal secretions and their physiologic and pathologic relations
Eye: the organ of vision interacting with the nervous system
Homeostasis: the process of maintaining bodily equilibrium with respect to various functions and chemical compositions of the fluid and tissues

When a patient visits the office with specific symptoms, the physician may concentrate the examination on the system or body areas related to the patient's symptoms. To prepare for special procedures and assist the physician, the medical assistant must first have an understanding of the symptoms related to specific systems and the responses of these systems to disease.

Generally speaking, symptoms are subjective clues that indicate the presence of disease, whereas signs are objective, or observable, changes that indicate a disorder or response to disease. Symptoms, such as feelings of nausea or the sensation of pain, are usually what prompt the patient to seek medical treatment. Signs, on the other hand, although sometimes noticed by the patient, are usually observed or measured by the physician. These could include vital signs, skin color, and other visible abnormalities. The physician discusses these signs and symptoms with the patient and then performs an examination to identify physical findings that could connect them with a specific disorder. From the patient's symptoms, signs, and physical findings the physician formulates a diagnosis.

The medical assistant assists the patient in initiating effective communication with the physician. A basic description of common diseases, related diagnostic studies, and clinical procedures and their associated principles is presented in this chapter for the student's understanding, and to facilitate effective communication between patient and physician.

The next two chapters cover "general clinical medical assisting techniques." These include positive patient identification; preparation of the examination room and equipment; patient preparation and instruction regarding the examination; gowning and positioning; and assisting the physician by handing instruments, repositioning the patient, performing specified treatment, and providing specified supplemental instruction and teaching. This chapter focuses on the symptom-system relationship and examinations and treatment procedures specific to the nervous system, the eye, the ear, the endocrine system, the musculoskeletal system, and the integumentary system.

THE NERVOUS SYSTEM

SYMPTOMATIC REACTION TO DISEASE OR INJURY

The characteristics and symptoms of nervous system disease or injury encompass three major functions: mental status and cognitive abilities, sensory perception, and muscle activity. The body's response to disease or injury to any of these areas is an alteration in, or loss of, function. Symptoms related to mental status and cognitive abilities could include changes in level of consciousness; lack of orientation to time, place, or person; or inability to perform tasks that were once easy to perform. Changes in sensory perceptions affect the sensations of taste, hearing, smell, and pain or balance and positioning abilities. For example, a patient may burn himself and be unaware of the pain. Disturbances in muscle activity affect both gross and fine muscular strength and movement. Resulting symptoms include lack of muscle coordination (*ataxia*), partial or full paralysis (*plegia*), difficult swallowing (*dysphagia*), or uncontrolled shaking (*tremors*). There are many other symptoms associated with neurologic disease, but these are the major ones.

NEUROLOGIC EXAMINATION AND THE MEDICAL ASSISTANT'S ROLE

Table 20–1 describes the steps involved in a standard neurologic examination and the medical assistant's role and responsibilities. Figure 20–1 illustrates the instruments and other items required for the neurologic examination.

COMMON DIAGNOSTIC TESTS

These tests are performed at a radiology outpatient center or in a hospital. The medical assistant must obtain thorough patient instructions from the center

Table 20–1
THE NEUROLOGIC EXAMINATION

Body Part and Function	Method and Equipment	Medical Assistant's Role
Mental Status Survey Cognitive abilities	Inspection of body posture and general appearance. Interviewing with questions directed at measuring intelligence, memory, etc. Observe grooming, dress, hygiene, orientation to person, time, and place.	The medical assistant is usually not present for this portion of the examination as it might interfere with the relationship between the physician and the patient. The medical assistant, however, may provide input regarding mental status derived from time spent alone with the patient.
Face for Cranial Nerve Status Olfactory (smell)	Patient may be asked to identify common odors with eyes closed.	The medical assistant will be present and hand the physician the items required. Patient will be sitting.
Optic (sight)	Ophthalmoscope used to examine the eye. Visual acuity test may be performed to test vision capabilities.	The visual acuity test may be the responsibility of the medical assistant. See eye section in this chapter.
Pupil motor reaction	Flashlight inspection of the eyes. Palpation of the face. Patient clenches teeth and physician palpates muscles.	Lights out. Support unsteady patient on examining table.
Sensory	Patient closes eyes. Physician palpates the face. Safety pin may be used. Evaluate for light, touch, temperature, corneal reflex. Use sterile swab, tubes with warm and cold water.	The medical assistant may need to assemble various items that would assist the physician to test for pain or feeling sensation. Clean safety pins and cotton balls are most frequently used.
Facial motor ability	Inspection of the face as the patient is given directions such as to frown, smile, puff out cheeks, clench teeth. Observe symmetry and movement.	The medical assistant should note the degree of patient comfort. A complete examination tends to be lengthy. Rest periods are usually provided in which the physician leaves the room. The medical assistant can attend to the patient's comfort and remain for quiet conversation if time permits.
Voice	Evaluate for hoarseness/speech, tongue movements.	
Hearing	Physician may speak in various tones to test hearing capabilities. Weber's and Rinne tests.	Medical assistant may be asked to perform audiometry. See ear section in this chapter.

Continued

Table 20-1
THE NEUROLOGIC EXAMINATION—Continued

Body Part and Function	Method and Equipment	Medical Assistant's Role
Nerves of the Motor System Coordination and muscle strength; gait	Patient will be asked to walk, do knee bends, walk on toes, raise hands above head, flex extremities, and push and pull against examiner's hands. Finger-to-nose movements. Romberg test—balance.	Medical assistant should be close to patient if balance is lost to prevent patient's falling.
Nerves of the Sensory System Arms, trunk, legs	Inspection with pin and tuning fork, cotton balls.	The medical assistant assists the patient to assume a supine position. Patient may get very tired.
Reflexes All points of reflexes, such as knees, elbows, ankles	Reflex hammer.	The patient is assisted to a sitting position, then again to a supine position.

doing the test and set aside time during the patient's appointment to instruct the patient concerning the test procedures and any necessary restrictions. Understanding the procedure and what to expect will decrease the patient's anxiety, ensure completion of the test, and provide for accurate results.

Diagnostic tests of the nervous system are divided into two types: noninvasive and invasive. *Noninvasive procedures* do not require entering the body in any manner. Examples include skull radiography, computed tomography (CT) scan, electroencephalography (EEG), and magnetic resonance imaging. With the exception of the EEG these procedures are done by radiologists. *Invasive procedures* involve penetrating the nonsuperficial tissues of the body. Examples of invasive tests include catheterization, biopsy, injection of x-ray dyes, and so forth.

Electroencephalography is a test that records the electrical waves of the brain. When this test is done in the neurologist's office, the medical assistant will receive special training if responsible for electrode placement and running the test.

Invasive procedures are usually done in a hospital or imaging outpatient center and require the patient to sign a consent-to-procedure form after the radiologist has explained the procedure, its risks, and the alternatives. These radiology procedures include *cerebral angiography* (x-ray study of cerebral blood vessels), *myelography* (x-ray of the spaces around the brain and spinal cord), brain scan, and *pneumocephalography* (air injected into the brain ventricles).

Obtaining cerebrospinal fluid (CSF) samples requires the performance of another invasive procedure called *lumbar puncture.* With this procedure, CSF is obtained

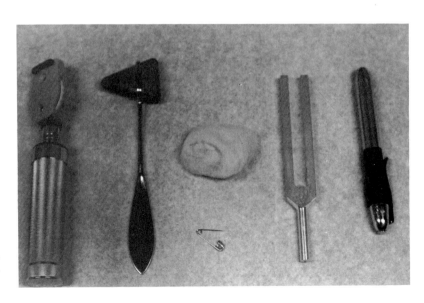

Figure 20-1. Instruments and equipment used for the neurologic examination.

by inserting a spinal needle between two lumbar vertebrae and into a space between the meninges. The fluid flows out through the needle and drips into test tubes. The CSF specimen(s) is sent to the laboratory for analysis.

COMMON DISEASES OF THE NERVOUS SYSTEM

A wide variety of diseases are associated with alterations in the nervous system. These include inflammatory conditions, pain-producing disorders, convulsive disorders, and demyelinating conditions. These conditions and others are listed in Table 20–2, along with their symptoms, treatment procedures, and the medical assistant's role.

Additional nervous system disorders associated with the aging process occur in the gerontologic patient. Symptoms include decreased hearing, decreased vision, alternations in strength, and reduced reflexes and muscle bulk.

Table 20–2

COMMON DISEASES OF THE NEUROLOGIC SYSTEM

Disease	Symptoms	Treatment	Medical Assistant's Role
Alzheimer's disease	Deterioration of intellectual capacity, extreme forgetfulness. Progressive mental and physical degeneration.	Frequent stimulation. Eventually requires total care.	This can be a devastating disease for family members and requires great empathy and support. Assist family in locating all available community services.
Encephalitis (inflammation of the brain caused by infection; may be transmitted by mosquito or tick; viruses are the most common cause)	Headache, drowsiness, convulsion.	Drug therapy is usually not effective. Therapy is supportive: rest, analgesics, fluids.	General clinical medical assisting procedures. The patient is usually hospitalized and seen in the office for initial diagnosis and follow-up. When there is suspicion of meningitis, aseptic precautions should be carefully followed to avoid contamination.
Epilepsy (abnormal discharge of nervous energy from the brain)	*Convulsions:* *Grand mal* seizures are characterized by longer-lasting loss of consciousness, and *petit mal* seizures are of short duration (5–30 sec). Two other classifications of seizures are commonly used to describe symptoms: *Jacksonian* seizures are characterized by jerking movements in one part of the body, and *psychomotor* seizures are characterized by brief, isolated, bizarre behaviors.	If symptoms are caused by a tumor, then surgery is performed. If not, the following measures are employed: drug therapy (anticonvulsants) and family psychotherapy if indicated.	General clinical medical assisting procedures. In addition, the medical assistant should be acutely aware of the needs of the patient and family, and can give significant input to the physician that will assist in making judgments relating to the emotional needs of the patient. Recommend support groups. Teach the family care during seizures. Encourage medication compliance.
Herpes zoster (shingles) (inflammation of skin or mucous membrane along the course of a nerve)	Pain usually along the course of the nerve. Skin eruption may form.	Drug therapy: analgesics. Warm soaks may also be applied. Cool compresses are also helpful. Advise patients to rest and decrease their stress level.	General clinical medical assisting procedures. The patient may be hospitalized or seen in the office for initial diagnosis and follow-up. Patient needs assistance with pain relief measures.

Continued

<u>Table 20-2</u>
COMMON DISEASES OF THE NEUROLOGIC SYSTEM—*Continued*

Disease	Symptoms	Treatment	Medical Assistant's Role
Meningitis (inflammation of the meninges caused by bacterial or viral invasion)	General symptoms of upper respiratory infection, usually accompanied by headache and stiff neck. Positive Brudzinski's and Kernig's sign. Photophobia.	Drug therapy: antibiotics and other drugs such as analgesics are used to relieve symptoms. Anti-inflammatory agents decrease edema. Anticonvulsants.	General clinical medical assisting procedures. The patient is hospitalized and seen in the office for initial diagnosis and follow-up. When there is suspicion of meningitis, isolation precautions should be carefully followed to avoid contamination.
Migraine (pain derived from dilation of blood vessels supplying the brain) Cluster headaches	Nausea and vomiting are the principal symptoms. Also, distorted vision, light auras, severe stabbing pain that is long lasting and localized.	Drug therapy: vasoconstrictors. Eliminate food triggers and nicotine. Avoid environmental triggers.	General clinical medical assisting procedures. The physician may suggest the application of an ice bag to the head on the area of the headache. The medical assistant should be certain the patient understands how, when, why, and for how long ice should be applied (described in this chapter).
Multiple sclerosis (demyelinating disease of white matter in brain and spinal cord)	Visual problems, numbness in extremities, tingling, weakness in legs, ataxia, urinary frequency and urgency.	Major therapy uses anti-inflammatory drugs during exacerbations. Avoid stress, infections, fatigue. Keep to an exercise program. Avoid food and environmental allergens.	The medical assistant can be very supportive. Tell family how to avoid infections. Provide balanced dietary information. Advise on support groups and contact with peers and positive attitude and behaviors.
Neuritis (inflammation of one or more nerves; different types have different causes)	Severe discomfort or pain; weakness and/or paralysis of the part affected.	Nonspecific. Drug therapy: analgesics for pain. Bedrest and physical therapy.	General clinical medical assisting procedures. The patient is usually hospitalized and seen in the office for initial diagnosis and follow-up. When there is suspicion of meningitis, aseptic precautions should be carefully followed to avoid contamination.
Parkinson's disease (degeneration of specialized brain neurons and decreased release of the neurotransmitter dopamine)	Slow, shuffling gait, rigid arms when walking, akinesia, masklike face, and tremors.	Aimed at relief of symptoms via drug therapy, physical therapy, and at times neurosurgery.	Patients and families need support. Reinforce the need for drugs. Help them to make schedules. Encourage activities and independence.
Sciatica (pain that follows the pathway of the sciatic nerve)	Pain (low back and radiates down the leg). Numbness, tingling of	Dependent on cause, e.g., inflammation, herniated nucleus pulposus,	General clinical medical assisting procedures. The medical assistant

Continued

Table 20–2
COMMON DISEASES OF THE NEUROLOGIC SYSTEM—*Continued*

Disease	Symptoms	Treatment	Medical Assistant's Role
	the part, may also be present.	trauma. Therapy involves rest, heat and cold, traction, surgery, or chemonucleolysis if disk involved.	should be aware that an intramuscular injection administered improperly can injure the sciatic nerve and cause sciatica (painful inflammation).
Trigeminal neuralgia (severe pain on one side of the face which follows the pathway of a nerve branch)	Severe, incapacitating pain.	Drug therapy; analgesics, sedatives, and other specialized drugs. Surgery may be required to sever nerve impulses and relieve pain.	General clinical medical assisting procedures, which include reassurance, since patient anxiety tends to be great.

SPECIFIC CLINICAL PROCEDURES

Although there are no specific clinical neurology procedures routinely performed by the medical assistant, the medical assistant's support and caring is important to the patient awaiting an examination, as neurologic symptoms are particularly frightening. It is possible, however, that a medical assistant could be instructed to perform procedures such as the EEG.

NERVOUS SYSTEM SPECIALTIES

The neurologist serves patients with suspected nervous system disorders. The neurosurgeon is trained in the microsurgical techniques required to treat disorders involving the brain and spinal cord, such as tumors, removal of blood clots (*hematomas*), or repair of injuries due to trauma.

There are additional surgical subspecialties that use microsurgical techniques, such as plastic or reconstructive surgery, ophthalmologic, ear, cardiovascular, musculoskeletal, and reproductive system surgery. Microsurgical techniques have applications to all systems.

THE EYE

The eye is an organ that has complex functions yet is a small and uncomplicated structure. Many consider the eye to be one of the most precious senses that an individual has. It is the principal organ of vision, and although it is not a part of the nervous system, it interacts with the nervous system. It is possible to look directly into the eye and observe its nerve and surrounding structures.

SYMPTOMATIC REACTION TO CONDITIONS AND DISEASES

Symptoms patients use to describe vision changes include blurred vision, changes in reading ability, loss of vision, blending of colors, and seeing spots. These impairments are called *visual defects.*

There are six major symptoms that bring the patient to the medical office. These include the visual defects just described, tearing, redness, itching, discharge, and pain. The terminology for describing visual defects correctable with glasses, along with their specific symptoms, is described in Table 20–3. Other common symptoms that may bring the patient to the office include:

Bulging eyeballs (*exophthalmos*)
Double vision (*diplopia*)
Drooping eyelids (*blepharoptosis*)
Lumps in eyelids
Light intolerance (*photophobia*)
Pain—mild to severe
Impaired eye movement
Constant tearing
Floating spots
Light flashes

COMMON DISEASES OR DISORDERS OF THE EYE

Disorders of the eye can occur in any of its structures. Visual defects correctable with glasses are by far the most common disorders.

There are a number of conditions that may require surgical correction. Among the more common are strabismus, blepharoptosis, *dacryocystitis* (inflammation of the tear sac), retinal detachment, and cataract. Common medical conditions include conjunctivitis, stye, corneal abrasion, and glaucoma. Table 20–4 provides a description of these conditions and the medical assistant's role. The role of the medical assistant in the treatment of eye disorders emphasizes patient reassurance and patient teaching.

The aging process alters both structure and function of the eye. The lens becomes more rigid and less capable of adjustment. Often, bifocal glasses are needed to correct vision. The supportive structures may atrophy and cause changes in placement and wrinkling of lids. Visual acuity decreases, and somewhere between the

Table 20-3
COMMON VISUAL DEFECTS CORRECTABLE WITH GLASSES

Condition	Definition
Myopia (nearsightedness)	Individual can see objects most accurately when close at hand. In myopia, the eyeball or the crystalline lens may be contoured defectively. Corrective lenses cause light to be focused directly on the retina and thus improve sight.
Hypermetropia (farsightedness)	Individual can see objects most accurately when they are at a distance. Again, the objective of the corrective lens is to allow the light to be focused on the retina.
Presbyopia	Individual can see only distant objects clearly, but the images cloud as they are drawn closer, thus resembling farsightedness. Again appears to be a common natural cause of presbyopia as the crystalline lens which is normally elastic becomes less accommodating. Corrective lenses can improve this condition.
Astigmatism	Individual cannot focus clearly; vision is blurred. The contour of either the cornea or the crystalline lens prevents light from being projected on the retina adequately. Corrective lenses can improve the condition.
Strabismus	Individual has difficulty directing both eyes toward the same objects. Muscle coordination in the eye is affected. Eyes may cross or turn outward. Corrective lenses and specific exercises or surgery may improve the condition.

Table 20-4
COMMON DISEASES OF THE EYE

Disease	Symptoms	Treatment	Medical Assistant's Role
Cataract (crystalline lens becomes clouded) Opacity of lens	Impaired vision: spots before the eyes. Blurred vision, halo around lights.	Surgical removal (phakolysis).	General clinical medical assisting procedures. Patient education is essential before surgery.
Conjunctivitis (inflammation of the conjunctiva)	Redness and swelling, pain, increased tearing (especially caused by allergy). Others are burning, itch, photophobia, and discharge.	Drug therapy: ophthalmic antibiotics, antiallergic drugs such as antihistamines. Instillation of antiseptic solutions. Eye irrigation. Warm compresses. Possible allergy testing, vasoconstrictors.	General medical assisting clinical procedures. Patient teaching includes instruction to prevent reinfection. Emphasis on reading and writing in good light with frequent rest periods is advised.
Galucoma (increased pressure within the eyeball with no known cause) Types: Open angle, chronic Closed angle, acute	Pain with gradual pressure and impairment of vision. Chronic pain, pressure inflammation, pupil dilation are acute symptoms.	Drug therapy. Surgery. Continuous monitoring.	Patient teaching includes emphasis on avoiding the lifting of heavy objects. Emotional stress should be avoided as this tends to increase ocular pressure. Stress drug compliance.
Stye (acute inflammation of the edge of the eyelid)	Stinging pain and the presence of a hordeolumn (swelling) are common.	Warm compresses. An incision may be made into the stye to allow drainage. Antibiotics may also be used.	Teach patient warm compresses 4 X daily to promote drainage. Prevent infection by cleanliness and no rubbing. Protect eye by decreasing reading, avoiding direct sun, increasing rest by closing eyes, and avoiding strain.

ages of 40 and 70 years a farsightedness called *presbyopia* develops. Cataracts are relatively common in the elderly. Cataracts are surgically corrected by removing the lens by a process called *phacolysis* and by inserting a lens implant. The risk of glaucoma increases greatly with age. Visual-field (extent of space visible) changes of glaucoma are permanent and may require patients to adapt their lifestyles and self-expectations. Patients need the encouragement to follow the physician's prescribed treatment while maintaining activities that promote maximum use of functions.

EYE EXAMINATION AND THE MEDICAL ASSISTANT'S ROLE

The interior of the eye can be examined with the ophthalmoscope (Fig. 20–2). This instrument allows for the direct visualization of the retina, including the optic nerve and the retinal blood vessels. Disease conditions may be diagnosed by the physician with the use of the ophthalmoscope. The medical assistant may ready the ophthalmoscope for the physician, and be responsible for checking its proper functioning.

COMMON DIAGNOSTIC TESTS

In addition to the ophthalmologic examination performed by the physician, the medical assistant may be responsible for testing the patient's visual acuity and color vision. *Visual acuity* is a term used to signify the degree of clarity or sharpness of vision. Normal visual acuity allows the individual to see without any impairment in details from short and longer distances. Color vision acuity tests the patient's ability to determine and differentiate between colors.

There are many types of tests for visual acuity. The test most commonly used in the medical office and performed by the medical assistant is the Snellen eye test (see description of the procedure at the end of this chapter). The Snellen eye chart (Fig. 20–3) features letters or images in rows of decreasing size to test the patient's ability to see at measured distances, both close and far away. There are charts available for non-

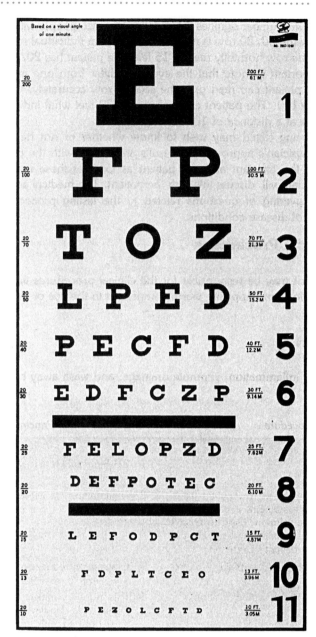

Figure 20–3. The Snellen eye chart.

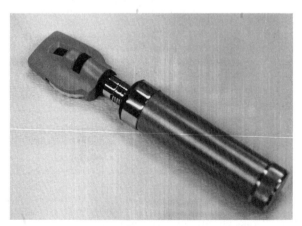

Figure 20–2. The ophthalmoscope.

English-speaking people, for preschoolers, and for English-speaking individuals who can read the alphabet. The chart for non-English-speaking individuals depicts the capital letter E in decreasing sizes and in various positions. The preschool chart illustrates certain common objects that children can readily identify. There is a greater margin of error, however, in the preschool test because a child may simply fail to recognize an object, while actually having no difficulty with visual acuity. The pattern of recognition of the objects must be carefully monitored. The child may also be tested for visual acuity by using cards with the letter E and instructing the child to point in the direction that corresponds to the middle line of the E. Comparing the E to a "table with three legs" is a more appealing concept to most children. The cards are then held in varying directions at the recommended distance. The charts are available as cardboard posters and as illuminated wall-mounted or portable units.

INTERPRETING THE RESULTS OF THE VISUAL ACUITY TEST

As mentioned, the Snellen visual acuity test consists of rows designated by numerals on the right and fractions on the left. There are 11 rows. Each row's fraction contains the top number 20, because the test is being conducted at a distance of 20 ft from the chart. The bottom number signifies the distance at which people with normal acuity can read the row. Below the 20/20 row is the 20/15 row. If an individual standing 20 ft from the chart can read the row normally read at 15 ft, the patient has 20/15 vision in the eye examined. It is important to note that each eye can differ in the degree of visual acuity. If the patient can read only the second row accurately with the left eye, the recording is oculus sinister, 20/100. The patient can only see at 20 ft what individuals with normal visual acuity can see at a distance of 100 ft.

The patient being treated may wish to know his or her visual acuity. With the physician's approval, the results can be shared with the patient. However, a discussion between the medical assistant and the patient regarding the implications of the results must be avoided. The physician will discuss these implications with the patient. The medical assistant's responsibility involves answering of questions related to the testing procedures only, and not the presence or degree of disease conditions.

SPECIFIC CLINICAL PROCEDURES

The medical assistant may be responsible for the clinical procedures of eye irrigation, eye instillation, application of warm compresses to the eye, and application of protective eye dressing, or for instruction of the patient in these techniques. (These procedures are described in detail at the end of this chapter.)

EYE SPECIALTIES

There are several medical specialties related to the care and treatment of the eyes. An *ophthalmologist* is a physician who diagnoses and treats disorders of the eyes. An ophthalmologist also tests visual acuity and interprets the results. An *optometrist* is a licensed practitioner (not a physician) whose expertise lies in testing visual acuity and the interpretation of results. An *optician* is a technician who prepares lenses according to prescription and fits them into frames of the patient's choice.

The medical assistant would most likely be employed in an ophthalmologist's office performing administrative or clinical functions, or both of these functions. In the specialist's office, the medical assistant will be trained, if required, to assist with examinations such as *tonometry* (measuring eyeball pressure), *gonioscopy* (measuring the angle of the anterior chamber), *slit-lamp examination* (magnified viewing of external eye structures), and color vision testing.

THE EAR

SYMPTOMATIC REACTION TO DISEASE OR DISORDER

The ear symptoms can indicate to the physician the location of the disease or disorder. The five major symptoms of ear disorder are ear discharge, pain, hearing loss, dizziness (*vertigo*), and ringing (*tinnitus*).

Acute ear disturbances commonly occur in children. Older patients frequently exhibit decreased hearing acuity. Hearing loss with age is known as *presbycusis* and usually begins with decreasing ability to hear high-pitched sounds. It is important that the medical assistant be aware of this change to effectively communicate with the older patient. When a patient has presbycusis, communication can be more effective if a lower vocal tone is used rather than higher tone.

EAR EXAMINATION AND THE MEDICAL ASSISTANT'S ROLE

The physician inspects the ear canal and eardrum with an otoscope. Although the illumination and magnification of the otoscope enable the physician to inspect these areas, much of the middle ear and inner ear are inaccessible to examination. The physician also tests for tenderness by grasping the tip of the ear and moving it back and forth and by pulling on the ear lobes.

To insert the otoscope in an adult's ear, the physician tilts the patient's head back, grasps the auricle gently, and pulls it upward and back, to permit complete visualization of the eardrum. A child's external canal is shorter and slants at an upward angle, so the auricle can be pulled slightly down and back. It is best to insert the otoscope slightly before moving the external ear as outer ear movement affects the shape.

The equipment for the ear examination includes an otoscope and a clean speculum, or cone-shaped attachment. Specula come in a variety of sizes, and several should be laid out for the physician's choice. Figure 20–4 shows examples of ear, nose, and throat instruments that may be used for examination and treatment. When the examination is complete, the equipment is cleaned, disinfected, and sterilized. It is important to remove all particles from the speculum with a small brush before soaking the instrument in disinfectant solution. Most facilities use disposable specula.

COMMON DIAGNOSTIC TESTS

The two diagnostic studies associated with the ear are *audiology* (for hearing loss) and *vestibular* tests (for disturbances in equilibrium).

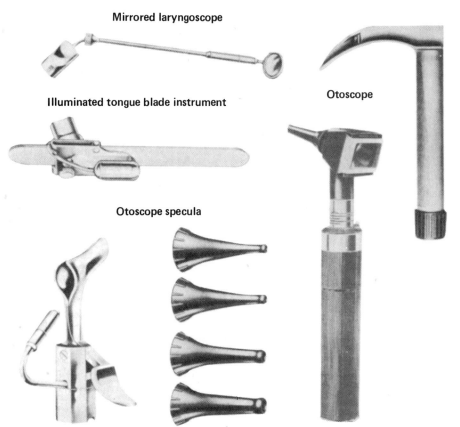

Mirrored laryngoscope

Illuminated tongue blade instrument

Otoscope specula

Otoscope

Figure 20–4. Instruments for ear, nose, and throat examination.

Audiology tests determine the presence of conduction defects or nerve impairment. The Weber and Rinne tests both use a tuning fork. The Weber test evaluates whether hearing is the same in both ears. The Rinne test compares bone and air conduction by placing the fork on the mastoid bone (behind the ear, Fig. 20–5), until the patient no longer feels the vibrations and then immediately placing the fork over the ear canal to see if any further sound can be heard. When the medical assistant is responsible for conducting these tests, the physician will provide instruction as to the exact procedures. *Audiometry tests* use an audiometer to detect very specific areas of hearing loss. This test can be performed by a medial assistant who has received the necessary technical training. A *tympanogram* evaluates middle ear function and is performed by an audiologist or physician.

Two types of vestibular tests evaluate balance and equilibrium: the falling and past pointing tests. These evaluations require the patient to make various motions with the eyes open and closed. Another vestibular test is electronystagmography, in which eye movements are recorded by electrodes placed around the eyes. The patient usually requires special preparation for this test, including abstinence from drugs and alcohol for 48 hours, and no tobacco, caffeine products, or heavy meals the day of examination. The medical assistant

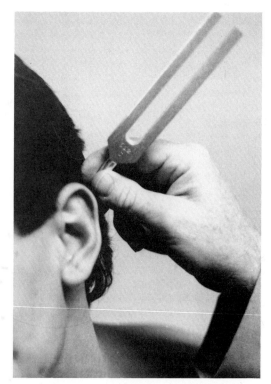

Figure 20–5. The tuning fork is used to test for certain audiologic defects.

performs the necessary patient education and instruction before the test.

COMMON DISEASES OR CONDITIONS OF THE EAR

There are two common conditions associated with each part of the ear. All of the conditions present with a variation in the symptoms discussed earlier. Foreign body obstruction and external otitis affect the outer ear. Obstructions can be removed manually or with irrigation. Any obstruction that can swell in size must not be irrigated. If the cause of the obstruction is excessive *cerumen* (earwax), oil base drops can be instilled before irrigation. An insect may enter the outer ear canal, creating irritation and uncomfortable noise. Insects may be removed by darkening the room and shining a light into the ear. The insect usually will migrate to the light and can be removed. One of the most common causes of external otitis is inadequately drying the ear canal. This is often called "swimmer's ear," although it is generally realized that improper cleaning, earphones, hairspray, and other irritants can also cause this condition. It is extremely painful and is usually treated with hot compresses, antibiotics, or fungicides depending on the causative organism, in addition to ear irrigation and debris removal.

Acute otitis media, *serous* (thin, water drainage) or *suppurative* (pus drainage), and *mastoiditis* (inflammation of the mastoid), are common inflammations of the middle ear. The major symptoms of serous otitis media are fullness of the ear, mild pain, and even hearing loss. If an accumulation of serous fluid is present, a *myringotomy* (surgical incision into the eardrum) may be performed to prevent rupture. In addition to a myringotomy, ventilatory tubes may be inserted into the eardrum to facilitate drainage and equalize pressure. Suppurative otitis, caused by pus-producing bacteria, is extremely painful for the patient and may include rupture of the eardrum with purulent drainage. Treatment includes antibiotic and decongestant therapy. Mastoiditis is an infection of the mastoid bone adjacent to the middle ear. It is usually due to chronically recurring otitis media in which the infection spreads to the bone tissue. The pain is located behind the ear and may be accompanied by a dull headache. Treatment requires that the patient be hospitalized and receive large doses of intravenous antibiotic. Myringotomy may be performed to allow for drainage or mastoidectomy to eliminate all sources of infection.

Inner ear disorders are extremely distressing to patients. Most of them are accompanied by both severe vertigo and tinnitus. Meniere's disease also involves hearing loss and violent acute symptomatic attacks of vertigo (dizziness) and tinnitis (ringing in the ear) lasting from a few minutes to hours. At times, epinephrine may be able to stop the attack. Patients are also advised to restrict sodium intake. If the disease becomes chronic, the only treatment is destruction of the labyrinth, which results in loss of hearing in that ear. *Labyrinthitis* (inflammation of the labyrinth) has a rapid onset and quickly incapacitates the patient with extreme vertigo, nausea, and vomiting, usually lasting 3 to 5 days. Symptoms disappear slowly over 3 to 6 weeks. Treatment includes bedrest, medication to control the symptoms, and antibiotics if the infection is caused by bacteria.

One has only to imagine being subjected to persistent attacks of dizziness, loss of balance, and ringing in the ears to understand the total disruption these conditions inflict on patients. These symptoms are extremely frightening and physically demanding on the patient.

SPECIFIC CLINICAL PROCEDURES

The medical assistant may be asked to perform clinical procedures to relieve patient discomfort. These treatment measures can include the instillation of ear medications and irrigation of the external canal. These procedures are described in a step-by-step fashion at the end of this chapter.

EAR SPECIALTIES

Several medical specialties are concerned with conditions affecting the ear. Among these are *otology*, which deals specifically with the ear and its anatomy, physiology, and pathology; *otoneurology*, which concentrates on the relationship of the ear to the nervous system; *otorhinology*, which deals with conditions of the nose and ear; and *otorhinolaryngology*, which treats diseases of the ear, nose, pharynx, and larynx.

THE ENDOCRINE SYSTEM

The endocrine system is composed of glands that are essential to the regulation and coordination of all body systems. The glands of this system secrete chemicals, called *hormones*, directly into the blood. Table 20–5 lists six important endocrine glands, the hormones that they produce, and the abbreviations for those hormones. Hormones may affect the entire body or act only on specific organs or tissues. Hormones affect body processes such as metabolism, growth, development, secretions of other glands, and reproductive and sexual functions. Hormonal balance is a complex process. The amount of a hormone contained in the blood is the regulating switch that turns hormone production on and off.

SYMPTOMATIC REACTION TO DISEASE OR DISORDER

The endocrine system, when in a state of malfunction, produces either too much or too little of a particular hormone. Symptoms are directly related to the functions controlled by these hormones. For instance, a disturbance of the pituitary gland in a child (Fig. 20–6) can cause overproduction of the pituitary hormone and result in gigantism, whereas inadequate production

Table 20-5

SIX MAJOR ENDOCRINE GLANDS, HORMONES PRODUCED, AND ABBREVIATIONS

Gland	Major Hormones	Abbreviation	Gland	Major Hormones	Abbreviation
Pituitary	Human growth hormone	hGH	Thyroid	Thyroxin	T_4
	Thyroid-stimulating hormone (somatotropin)	TSH		Triiodothyronine	T_3
			Parathyroid	Calcitonin	none
	Adrenocorticotropic hormone	ACTH	Adrenal	Parathyroid Hormone	PTH
				Aldosterone	none
	Follicle-stimulating hormone	FSH		Cortisol	none
	Lutenizing hormone	L.H.		Catecholamines	none
	Prolactin hormone	L.T.H.		Androgens	none
	Antidiuretic hormone (vasopressin)	ADH	Pancreas	Insulin	none
	Oxytocin	none	Reproductive	Estrogen	none
				Progesterone	none
				Testosterone	none

might result in dwarfism. Symptoms are related to the specific gland that is diseased and the aspect of body functioning influenced by the hormone's increased or decreased production. The glands are interdependent; that is, dysfunction of one gland tends to affect the normal functioning of other glands.

Symptoms associated with hormonal imbalance can be grouped into five major areas: complaints related to fatigue and weakness, weight changes, changes in ental status, sexual dysfunction or delayed maturity, and excessive urination and thirst. One or more of these symptoms is usually present with all conditions related to underproduction or overproduction of a hormone. The physician may find the patient complaining of many vague symptoms which will require extensive examination and testing before a definitive diagnosis can be reached. At other times, the symptoms may be so definitive as to allow for accuracy in diagnosis after objective examination.

ENDOCRINE SYSTEM EXAMINATION AND THE MEDICAL ASSISTANT'S ROLE

The endocrine examination may be general, or specific to the gland suspected of causing the symptoms. The medical assistant must be prepared to assist the physician with either of these examinations. The physician's preference should be confirmed before preparing the patient.

Diagnostic laboratory studies are often the most conclusive indicator of endocrine malfunction. Thus, the medical assistant must be prepared to draw blood if requested by the physician.

It is also important for the medical assistant to provide support for patients with endocrine malfunctions. The patient may not accurately understand his or her condition, and this can create anxiety. Often, endocrine conditions are chronic in nature and try patients' coping skill; consequently, patients may require constant supervision and care.

COMMON DIAGNOSTIC TESTS

Three major types of tests can aid the physician in diagnosing endocrine disease: blood serum tests, to measure directly levels of hormones in the blood; urine tests, to measure excreted hormones and metabolites, and procedures performed in a radiology facility, to measure gland function or structure.

Most hormones can be directly measured in blood serum. Refer to Table 20-5 to review the abbreviations commonly used in ordering tests.

Measurement of hormones and metabolites excreted in the urine is obtained by collecting a urine specimen for hormone analysis. Some tests require a 24-hour collection of urine. The method of collection is covered in Chapter 29. The medical assistant must thoroughly explain the procedure to the patient, so a complete urine collection can be obtained. In addition the medical assistant must become familiar with the names of all tests requested.

The major procedures performed in a radiology facility consist of radioactive iodine scans and ultrasound. Radioactive iodine is injected intravenously and x-rays are taken as it collects in the thyroid. This test assists in the diagnosis of thyroid malfunction. Ultrasound can be used to visualize structures and is an excellent tool for identification of growths and abnormalities of structure. The medical assistant must be able to prepare the patient for these procedures. Preparations for both of these procedures are explained in the chapter on radiology.

COMMON DISEASES OR DISORDERS OF THE ENDOCRINE SYSTEM

Tumors and inflammation are two causes of disorders affecting the glands of the endocrine system, but many causes of dysfunction are unknown. Table 20-6 lists the major endocrine disorders associated with each gland. Table 20-7 summarizes four common diseases that may be encountered.

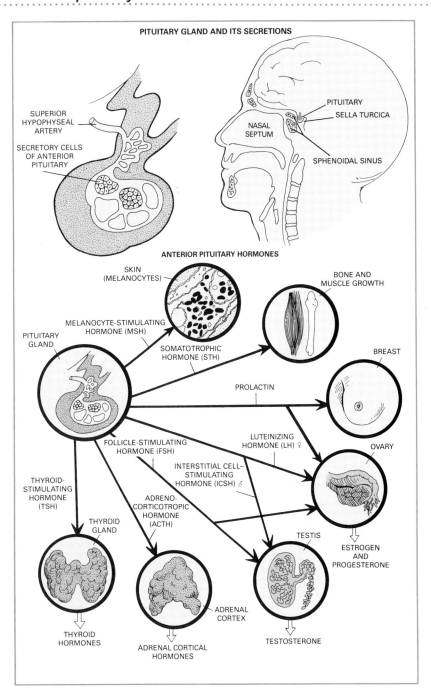

Figure 20-6. The pituitary gland is sometimes called the body's "master gland." (From Thomas, CL (ed): Taber's Cyclopedic Medical Dictionary, ed 17. FA Davis, Philadelphia, 1993, p 1515, with permission.)

Of these, the medical assistant needs to be especially familiar with diabetes, as it affects approximately 5% of the US population. Simply stated, *diabetes* is a persistent lack of insulin secretion which causes a disturbance of carbohydrate, fat, and protein metabolism and which results in extremely high blood sugar levels. Insulin is required to move sugar across the cell membrane. Once inside the cell, the sugar is used for cell metabolism. The cause of inadequate insulin is not understood. It is thought that predisposing factors include heredity, stress, pregnancy, and obesity. Some re-searchers are exploring the possibility that insulin is not produced because of an autoimmune response or viral infection. Another theory is that adequate amounts of insulin are produced, but for some unknown reason, the body produces antibodies that render it unusable.

The classic symptoms of diabetes are *polyuria* (excessive urination), *polydipsia* (excessive thirst), and *polyphagia* (excessive eating). The most common early symptom is fatigue. Progressive symptoms include sugar in the urine (*glycosuria*), weight loss, nausea, and vomiting.

Table 20–6
PRINCIPAL ENDOCRINE GLANDS AND THEIR DISORDERS

Name	Position	Function	Endocrine Disorders
Thyroid	Two lobes in anterior portion of neck.	Influences basal metabolic rate; indirectly influences growth and nutrition.	Hypofunction—Cretinism in young; myxedema in adult; goiter. Hyperfunction—Goiter; thyrotoxicosis.
Parathyroid	Four or more small glands near thyroid.	Calcium and phosphorus metabolism; indirectly affects muscular irritability.	Hypofunction—Tetany. Hyperfunction—Resorption of bone; renal calculi.
Adrenal cortex	One above each kidney.	Steroid hormones regulating carbohydrate metabolism and salt and water balance; some effects on sexual characteristics.	Hypofunction—Addison's disease. Hyperfunction—Adrenogenital syndrome; Cushing's syndrome.
Adrenal medulla	The inner portion of the adrenal gland. It is surrounded by the adrenal cortex.	Effects on sympathetic nervous system and carbohydrate metabolism.	Hypofunction—Almost unknown. Hyperfunction—Pheochromocytoma.
Anterior pituitary	Small gland at base of brain.	Influences growth, sexual development, skin pigmentation, thyroid function, adrenocortical function through effects on other endocrine glands (except for growth factor, which acts directly on cells).	Hypofunction—Dwarfism in child; decrease in all other endocrine gland functions except parathyroids. Hyperfunction—Acromegaly in adult; diabetes, gigantism in child.
Posterior pituitary	Attached to anterior pituitary.	Oxytocic factor influencing some aspects of uterine contraction. Antidiuretic factor influencing absorption of water by kidney tubule.	Unknown. Hypofunction—Diabetes insipidus.
Testes and ovaries	Testes—in the scrotum. Ovaries—in the pelvic cavity.	Development of secondary sex characteristics; some effect on metabolism.	Hypofunction—Lack of sex development or regression in adult. Hyperfunction—Abnormal sex development.
Pancreas (endocrine portion)	Abdominal cavity. Head adjacent to duodenum; tail close to spleen and kidney.	Secretes insulin and glucagon, which regulate carbohydrate metabolism.	Hypofunction—Diabetes mellitus. Hyperfunction—If a tumor produces excess insulin, hypoglycemia; if excess glucagon, diabetes mellitus.

Source: From Thomas, CL (ed): Taber's Cyclopedic Medical Dictionary, ed 17. FA Davis, Philadelphia, 1993, pp 641–2, with permission.

<u>Table 20–7</u>
COMMON DISEASES OF THE ENDOCRINE SYSTEM

Disease	Symptoms	Treatment	Medical Assistant's Role
Thyroiditis (inflammation of the thyroid)	Pain in the neck which may radiate to the upper arms and chest. General symptoms of inflammation may be present.	Nonspecific. Usually subsides without drug therapy.	General clinical medical assisting procedures.
Hyperthyroidism (Graves' disease) (activity of thyroid is increased with subsequent overproduction of thyroxine)	Weakness, increased appetite with weight loss, restlessness, insomnia, tremors, and anxiety. Palpitations and dyspnea may occur. Signs: exophthalmus (protruding eyes).	Alternatives: Radioactive iodine, antithyroid drugs, surgery. In addition, diet therapy is employed. A high-calorie diet is usually ordered.	General clinical medical assisting procedures.
Hypothyroidism (decreased activity of the thyroid gland with subsequent decreases in the production of thyroxine)	In children, cretinism (a lack of normal physical and mental development) may result. In adults, myxedema may result, which is a condition of dry skin and hair and sensitivity to cold. Slowed mental functions may be present. Signs: puffy facial appearance.	Therapy: thyroid supplement	General clinical medical assisting procedures.
Diabetes mellitus (inability of the body to metabolize carbohydrates adequately due to insufficient amount of insulin produced by the pancreas)	Major symptoms: polyuria (excessive urination), polydipsia (excessive thirst), polyphagia (excessive hunger). Major signs: increased amount of sugar in the blood, glycosuria (presence of sugar in the urine).	Combination of diet, exercise, and medication. Oral hypoglycemic agents or insulin by injection may be prescribed, depending on the severity of the disease. The diet usually recommended is balanced, with restricted carbohydrates. Diet therapy may be used without drug therapy depending on the individual disease profile.	General clinical medical assisting procedures. The medical assistant will also be responsible for patient teaching. Diet instructions, use of an exchange list, instruction in how to self-administer insulin, and the extreme importance of patient compliance with the regimen must be stressed. Instruct patient to wear medical ID (necklace or bracelet) and to carry a sugar source (e.g., hard candy) at all times.

Dietary regulation plays a major role in the treatment of both insulin-controlled and diet-controlled diabetes. The diabetic diet instruction is usually provided by the physician. Sample instructions are listed in Chapter 22, Nutrition and Diet Therapy. The American Diabetic Association provides sample diet information, and this organization is an excellent resource for other diabetic materials. Diet in combination with insulin therapy is essential in the treatment of insulin-dependent diabetics, whereas diet combined with exercise may be sufficient in other patients with less severe forms of the disease.

With diabetics, the medical assistant may be involved in patient teaching and reinforcing positive behaviors. Urine and blood testing can be done at home if prescribed, and the medical assistant must be able to ex-

Table 20–8
SYMPTOMS OF DIABETIC COMPLICATIONS

Ketoacidosis	Hypoglycemia
Weakness	Hunger
Thirst	Weakness
Headache	Nervousness
Loss of appetite	Tremors
Abdominal pain	Dizziness
Nausea	Profuse sweating
Vomiting	
Dry, flushed skin	

plain the procedures and the equipment used to the patient.

Diabetics should be provided with written instructions for their self-care and be given new instructions every time their self-care is changed. Juvenile onset diabetics (insulin-dependent diabetes mellitus) present special problems related to growth and development, coping with a chronic disease, and accepting the responsibility of self-care. Any medical assistant who consistently interacts with diabetics has an obligation to be well informed, knowledgeable, and current in diabetes care practices.

The medical assistant involved in screening patients for appointments must be alert to the patient's description of symptoms, as they may be indications of complications in patients who have diabetes (Table 20–8). In the insulin-dependent diabetic, for example, ketoacidosis can occur. *Ketoacidosis* is an excess accumulation of ketones in the blood caused by faulty metabolism due to inadequate insulin supply for energy conversion in the cell. The physician should consult immediately with the diabetic patient complaining of any of the symptoms of ketoacidosis or hypoglycemia. The skin provides important clues that can help the medical assistant decide whether the patient's condition is ketoacidosis or hypoglycemia. In ketoacidosis, the skin is warm and dry, whereas in hypoglycemia, profuse sweat is visible on the skin surface.

SPECIFIC CLINICAL PROCEDURES

The chief responsibilities of the medical assistant in relation to endocrine disorders are communication and patient teaching. In addition to stressing patient compliance with the physician's instructions, reinforcement of specific dietary regimens, the self-administration of specific medications, and the noting of potential and observed complications in the various endocrine diseases are all areas in which the medical assistant can greatly assist the patient.

ENDOCRINE SPECIALTIES

The physician specializing in disorders of the endocrine system is called an *endocrinologist.* The medical

assistant working in the office of this specialist would be expected to perform general medical assisting procedures with an emphasis on patient teaching and interaction. The endocrinologist in private practice receives patient referrals almost exclusively and is most often closely associated with a medical center or teaching facility. The field of endocrinology tends toward consultation and research.

THE MUSCULOSKELETAL SYSTEM

A close relationship exists between the muscular and skeletal systems; both have similar functions. The functions of these combined systems are protection, support, movement, *hematopoiesis* (manufacturing of blood cells), and storage of calcium.

SYMPTOMATIC REACTION TO DISEASE OR INJURY

The musculoskeletal systems reacts to disease or injury with four major symptoms: pain, swelling, immobility, or deformity. Injury to bone or joints causes pain, muscle strains, tears, sprains, swelling and stiffness, or immobility. Deformity is the result of broken bones and growths.

MUSCULOSKELETAL EXAMINATION AND THE MEDICAL ASSISTANT'S ROLE

During the musculoskeletal examination, the physician observes both structure and function of the skeleton and associated structures. See Table 20–9 for the medical assistant's role in this examination.

The physician directs the examination more specifically toward areas of abnormal functioning, such as decreased range of motion (ROM) (Fig. 20–7), swelling, tenderness, heat, decreased or unequal strength, deformities, or growths.

COMMON DIAGNOSTIC TESTS

X-ray is the most frequently used diagnostic tool for the skeletal system, usually for the diagnosis of broken bones (*fractures*). Other radiology tests include *myelography,* for diagnosis of intervertebral disk conditions; *arthrography,* for joint conditions; and *bone scans,* for analysis of bone age, density, and growth. All of these procedures are explained in the radiology chapter.

Three other tests are related to muscle strength, function, and structure. *Goniometry* is a measurement of joint function. The goniometer is an orthopedic protractor calibrated to measure the range of motion of the joint. *Electromyography* records muscular activity. *Muscle biopsy* is an invasive procedure in which a small piece of muscle tissue is obtained for microscopic examination. This procedure is often done to differentiate between *myopathic* (muscle disease) and *neurogenic*

Table 20–9
EXAMINATION OF THE MUSCULOSKELETAL SYSTEM

Body Part	Method and Equipment	Medical Assistant's Role
General systems	The physician usually instructs the patient to walk, sit, and assume various other positions and activities. Observations are noted relating to pain, swelling, mobility, and deformity.	The medical assistant should be aware that a detailed musculoskeletal examination is lengthy. Usually, only the parts related to the patient's symptomatology are examined. The medical assistant should be aware also that frequent position changes and maneuvers are required for the exam. For examination of the head and neck, the patient is sitting. The patient may be placed in the supine position for lower extremity exam.
Head and neck	Inspection and palpation. The physician may instruct the patient to rotate the neck and may give certain other directions to test the range of motion.	
Hands and wrists	Inspection and palpation. Evaluate ability to flex, extend, make a fist. Evaluate grip strength.	
Elbows	Inspection and palpation. Instructions to bend, straighten, flex, and turn the elbow.	
Shoulder	Inspection and palpation. Flexion, abduction, etc.	
Feet and ankles	Inspection and palpation. Range of motion (ROM), including inversion, eversion, plantar flexion, and dorsiflexion.	The medical assistant may be responsible for instructing the patient in ROM exercises according to the physician's prescription, but is never responsible for diagnostic evaluations.
Upper and lower legs	Inspection, palpation, resistance exercises, muscle strength.	The medical assistant may need to assist in leg raising and support, especially with the older patient.
Knees	Inspection and palpation. Maneuvers including flexion, extension, rotation, abduction, hyperextension.	The patient who has an existing joint disease or a deformity will have difficulty with some aspects of the testing and will be apprehensive. The medical assistant's role is to reassure the patient and offer the necessary assistance.
Spine	Inspection and palpation. Observing bending, rotation, pelvic height, curvatures, flexion, extension.	The patient is assisted to a standing position. The gown is opened completely at the back to allow visualization. Usually the assistant stands in front of the female patient, grasping the gown ties at each shoulder and holding the gown open for the physician. If the patient holds the gown herself, the anatomic and muscular structure may appear changed.

(nerve origin) disorders. At times, blood serum tests may be ordered to check levels of vitamins and minerals.

The physician also uses specific tests performed during the physical examination, such as ROM, straight leg raising, and muscle strength testing, along with inspection and palpation.

COMMON DISEASES OR DISORDERS OF THE MUSCULOSKELETAL SYSTEM

Musculoskeletal disorders are classified according to conditions of bones, joints and structures, and muscles and surrounding tissues. Musculoskeletal disorders are

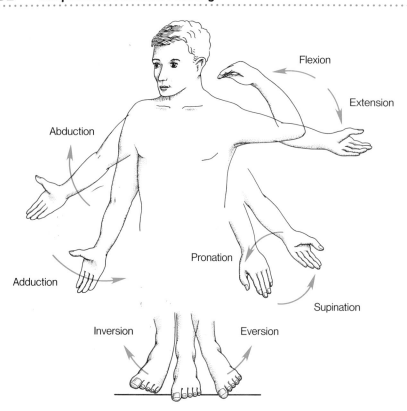

Figure 20–7. Movement of the body at the joints. (From Gylys BA and Wedding ME: Medical Terminology: A Systems Approach, ed 2. FA Davis, Philadelphia, 1988, p 208, with permission.)

common in the elderly, children, and the athletic. Table 20–10 describes common musculoskeletal disorders along with the medical assistant's role. One of the most common disorders is nonspecific back pain. Often, a physical therapist is brought into the treatment plan if back pain results from weakness and overuse. The physical therapist uses heat, cold, massage, exercise, and electrical stimulation as prescribed by the physician. It is important for the medical assistant to support the recommendations for physical therapy because it often provides pain relief.

The musculoskeletal system changes in adolescence and continues to change even after full growth is attained. Slow and subtle changes occur in the older patient that include thinning of intervertebral disks with decrease in height. These changes result in both a loss in muscle strength and a corresponding loss in muscle bulk, with decreased ROM. Loss of height, the most notable change, occurs because vertebral curves become exaggerated and the vertebral spaces narrow. Collagen tissue is not replaced, which results in loss of elasticity in subcutaneous tissues. In the female patient, more specific changes occur that are associated with hormonal changes and are discussed in the next chapter.

SPECIFIC CLINICAL PROCEDURES

The application of heat and cold are used frequently in treating disease and injury to the musculoskeletal system. The physician may refer the patient to the physical therapist for treatment. However, the medical

assistant may be responsible for applying or instructing the patient to apply various forms of heat and cold. For this reason, the medical assistant must understand the effects of heat and cold on the body.

Heat dilates blood vessels, increases the blood supply to the body part, and promotes healing. Heat also promotes drainage and is soothing, thereby increasing comfort.

Cold constricts blood vessels, decreases the blood supply to the body part, and reduces swelling. Cold is also used to relieve pain. Prolonged application of cold, however, has the reverse effect. Usually an application of not more than 30 minutes is recommended.

As you may recall from the discussion of temperature, the body's reaction to heat and cold is directed at maintaining normal body temperature. When heat is applied, the vessels dilate to rid the body of excess heat. When cold is applied, the vessels constrict to conserve heat.

MUSCULOSKELETAL SYSTEM SPECIALTY

Orthopedics focuses on the diagnosis and treatment of injury and disease of the musculoskeletal system. The responsibilities of the medical assistant associated with an orthopedic practice includes the performance of general duties, as well as assisting with casting procedures and possibly obtaining x-rays. Types of fractures occurring in the skeletal system are illustrated in Figure 20–8. Under the physician's supervision, the medical assistant may also be responsible for carrying out ROM exercises and providing assistance in other spe-

Table 20–10
COMMON DISEASES OF THE MUSCULOSKELETAL SYSTEM

Disorder or Disease	Symptom	Treatment	Medical Assistant's Role
Joints			
Arthritis (inflammation of the joints)	Two major types: Rheumatoid (most common): general symptoms of inflammation; joint stiffness and soreness, pain and swelling; deformities may develop. Degenerative (osteoarthritis): pain, stiffness, sensitivity to weather change; bones may become larger (hypertrophy) but deformity does not usually occur.	Related to severity. Alternatives: Drug therapy: anti-inflammatory agents such as salicylates (aspirin), ibuprofen, prednisone. Application of heat. Balanced diet and exercise. Rest, sometimes immobilization of joints. Occupational therapy. Physical therapy. Surgery: synovectomy (joint removal), arthroplasty (repair of joint using synthetic materials), arthrodesis (fusion of joint surfaces).	General clinical medical assisting procedures. The patient with arthritis can be elderly or very young. In either case the patient needs information regarding activities of daily living, medications, exercise, diet, heat treatments. Patient teaching is directed toward helping the patient to cope with the disease since it is chronic. Patience is of extreme importance when working with arthritic patients. Personality changes are not uncommon due to the frequent periods of pain and the anxiety associated with the disease.
Gout	Swollen, red, painful joint; usually distal joints, most commonly the great toe. May become chronic.	Aimed at lowering the serum uric acid levels. Drug therapy: analgesics, uricosurics, corticosteroids. Also bedrest, immobilization, heat or cold as ordered, and possible joint aspiration.	The medical assistant may need to give instruction in heat or cold application. Encourage the patient to rest, elevate extremity, drink at least 2 L of fluid, and follow diet as prescribed. Usually organ meats and alcohol are restricted.
Carpal tunnel syndrome (compression of median nerve by carpal ligament)	Pain, weakness, tingling, and numbness at wrist. Inability to clench fist.	Progressive from rest and splints, injection of corticosteroids, to surgical decompression of nerve.	The patient may be advised to change occupations and will need referral to occupational rehabilitation. Teach splint application. Range of motion after surgery when ordered.
Bones			
Fracture (broken bone usually caused by injury) Types: Simple (broken bone with skin intact) Oblique (line of break slanted) Transverse (break line straight across bone) Compound (break involves open wound)	Pain, swelling, deformity, bleeding if compound fracture has occurred. Inability to bear weight or use extremity.	Alternatives: immobilization, surgery, traction. Drug therapy: analgesics for pain; antibiotics if vulnerable to infection. Diet therapy: high-protein diet is usually ordered and may also be higher in calories, vitamins and minerals.	The patient with a fracture is usually not seen in the office but in the emergency facility of a hospital or medical center. However, follow-up visits are scheduled for the patient so that the physician may monitor progress. Patient

Continued

Table 20–10
COMMON DISEASES OF THE MUSCULOSKELETAL SYSTEM—*Continued*

Disorder or Disease	Symptom	Treatment	Medical Assistant's Role
Complete (break line extends completely through bone) Incomplete (break line extends only part way through bone) Greenstick (resembles a "green stick" break or a splintering) Comminuted (bone splintered into fragments) Impacted (bones are wedged together) (see Fig. 20–8)			teaching may involve explanation of the treatment alternative employed by the physician. Reinforce the need to prevent immobility complications with movement, fluids, range of motion, diet to prevent constipation. Instruct in cast care when applied in office.
Osteomyelitis (localized infection of the bone)	Pain is the major symptom.	Drug therapy (antibiotics and analgesics); surgery; casting. Diet therapy: high-protein diet usually recommended.	General clinical medical assisting procedures.
Scoliosis (lateral curvature of the spine)	Usually early onset is asymptomatic. Convex spine.	Exercises, brace (Milwaukee), surgical rod implantation.	The medical assistant should encourage all parents to bring adolescent children for screening either in office or at screening clinics. Adolescents need encouragement to wear brace as directed. Provide information about clubs or support groups. Inform physician of lack of compliance or negative attitude.
Herniated intervertebral disk (nucleus pulposus)	Severe low back pain, tenderness of spine and down sciatic nerve, inability to do straight leg raise because of pain.	Conservative: bedrest, traction, immobility, physical therapy, muscle relaxants. For acute severity: surgical laminectomy, possible spinal fusion, or chemonucleolysis	Medical assistant will need to use measures of support with patients with chronic pain. Encourage discussion of concerns with physician, need to take medications, and rest before pain onset. May need occupational rehabilitation.

Muscle and Connective Tissue

Disorder or Disease	Symptom	Treatment	Medical Assistant's Role
Bursitis (inflammation of the bursa) Tendinitis (inflammation of tendons and muscle attachments)	Pain, often severe, especially upon movement. Restricted motion, swelling.	Drug therapy such as cortisone. Aspiration of fluid that collects around the joint. Support with sling, heat therapy, physical therapy.	General clinical medical assisting procedures. Reinforce physician instructions for self-care. Written instructions may be supplied.

Continued

Table 20–10

COMMON DISEASES OF THE MUSCULOSKELETAL SYSTEM—*Continued*

Disorder or Disease	Symptom	Treatment	Medical Assistant's Role
Sprain (trauma to joint and ligament) Strain (trauma to tendon and muscle)	Joint swelling, tenderness, pain on motion, limited range of motion. Usually can tolerate some weight bearing.	Rest, elevate. Cold then heat per order. Analgesic. Support (Ace bandage or elastic support).	Before examination, elevate and support extremity with pillow. Stress rest, support, limited movement as ordered. Review instructions for applications of heat or cold.

cific orthopedic treatments. At the end of this chapter, some of the procedures performed by the medical assistant are described.

THE INTEGUMENTARY SYSTEM

The integumentary system consists of the skin. The total area and weight of the skin, or *integument,* make it the largest body organ. The skin has many functions. It protects from injury and infection, assists in the regulation of body temperature, secretes and excretes substances that lubricate the skin, and assists in the maintenance of fluid and electrolyte balance. Two other important functions include touch sensations and the synthesis of vitamin D during exposure to sunlight. In short, the skin is essential in maintaining homeostasis; thus, damage to large skin areas can be life-threatening.

The appendages of the skin are the hair and the nails. Both of these structures are keratin outgrowths from the skin. Their growth rate varies, and often they develop changes that reflect disease states.

One of the great abilities of the skin is its ability to repair itself after injury and often without any residual scarring. This is because epithelial tissues are capable of total regeneration.

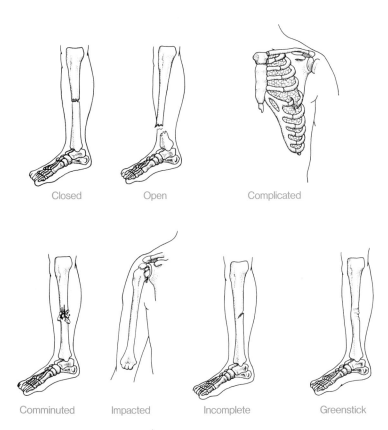

Figure 20–8. Types of fractures. (Adapted from Gylys BA and Wedding ME: *Medical Terminology: A Systems Approach,* ed 2. FA Davis, Philadelphia, 1988, p 218, with permission.)

Closed   Open   Complicated

Comminuted   Impacted   Incomplete   Greenstick

Symptomatic Reaction to Disease

Skin symptoms may be either local or systemic responses. Most responses relate to changes in texture, color, or temperature, or the development of rashes (*eruptions*). Texture changes include abnormal dryness or loss of elasticity (*turgor*); swollen, tight skin (*edema*); and excessive perspiration (*diaphoresis*). Color variations may include redness (*erythema*), blue tinges (*cyanosis*), paleness (*pallor*), purpleness, and yellowing (*jaundice*). Temperature changes manifest as sensations of excessive cold or heat, cold and clammy skin, and chills associated with fever (pyrexia).

Skin eruptions are classified in the following way (Fig. 20–9):

1. *Macular area:* discolored but not elevated (freckles)
2. *Papular area:* discolored, elevated, and small in size (pinpoint to pea size)
3. *Vesicular area:* elevated, fluid-filled (serous) blisters
4. *Pustular area:* elevated and pus filled

Because skin is the primary defense against entry of foreign bodies or agents, it is important for the medical assistant to know that certain injuries may be life-threatening, especially when related to hypersensitive (*allergic*) reactions. Any patient with hives (*urticaria*) that has developed over a large portion of the body or has swelling "all over" or is experiencing difficulty in breathing should be seen by the physician or should talk to the physician immediately.

Skin Examination and the Medical Assistant's Role

Depending on the patient's symptoms, the physician will determine whether to inspect all skin surfaces or confine the examination to local areas. The medical assistant must be able to anticipate the areas to be examined and position and drape the patient accordingly. Often, multiple lesions need to be examined, and the patient may require assistance in exposing areas for the physician's inspection.

Because the skin is the first line of defense, the medical assistant must ensure that at all times it is protected from harm by being careful when performing any procedures.

Common Diagnostic Tests

There are two commonly performed tests involving the integumentary system: the tuberculin skin test and allergy hypersensitivity testing. These skin tests are administered intradermally either by syringe (e.g., Mantoux) or by multipuncture methods (e.g., Tine, Aplitude, Mono-Vacc).

The tuberculin skin test screens for previous invasion by the tubercle bacillus. This test is routinely performed on all individuals having contact with children, those working in health care fields, and patients with a positive x-ray suggestive of infection. The tuberculin antigen can be introduced via the syringe; however, the four-pronged lancet (multipuncture method) is usually used for screening.

Testing to determine hypersensitivity to specific al-

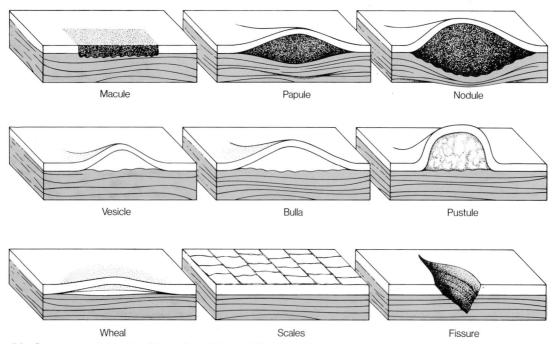

Figure 20–9. Lesions of the skin. (From Gylys BA and Wedding ME: *Medical Terminology: A Systems Approach*, ed 2. FA Davis, Philadelphia, 1988, p 71, with permission.)

lergens is frequently done. These tests include the patch and the scratch tests. Both tests evaluate the immune system's response to known allergens. Table 20–11 provides a further description of these tests and defines the medical assistant's role in each.

Occasionally, the medical assistant will assist the dermatologist in obtaining either scrapings of superficial skin or cultures of wounds and lesions for microscopic examination and identification of organisms. The procedures for these examinations are explained in the medical technology chapters of this book.

COMMON DISEASES OF THE SKIN

The types of diseases commonly associated with the skin include various forms of skin inflammation, acne, and burns. Table 20–12 summarizes these conditions and their symptoms, treatment approaches, and the medical assistant's role. The medical assistant should also learn the following terms:

Abscess: any local pus collection
Crust: dried serous fluid

Excoriation: abrasion of the epidermis
Fissure: crack in the skin
Furuncle: boil; acute deep inflammation that may involve hair follicle
Scale: flaking, dry epidermis
Ulcer: open sore
Urticaria: hives
Verruca: warts

SPECIFIC CLINICAL PROCEDURES

Specific clinical procedures related to the integument that are performed by the medical assistant include obtaining wound cultures and the application of sterile dressings after minor surgical procedures. Techniques for obtaining cultures are discussed in Chapters 28, 29, and 30.

The two most common minor surgical procedures are skin or lesion biopsy and wart removal. Biopsy requires a sterile tray and a small scalpel, curette, or a cutaneous biopsy punch, depending on the type of biopsy to be obtained. Wart removal is often performed with cryosurgery using liquid nitrogen–soaked sterile swabs.

Table 20–11
COMMON DIAGNOSTIC TESTS

Test	Description	Equipment	Medical Assistant's Role
Intradermal tuberculin skin test: Mantoux (syringe) Multipuncture: Tine, Aplitude, Mono-vacc	Antigen to which the patient may have been exposed is injected into the superficial skin with a needle and syringe or a four-pronged lancet. After a waiting period of 48 to 72 hr, the injected site is observed for a localized reaction.	Alcohol sponge, tuberculin syringe, vial of antigen diluent, antigen or antigen-containing multipuncture equipment.	Do not administer if acute inflammation or skin lesions are present. Explain the procedure and the possible reactions to the patient. Check for hypersensitivity to test antigen. If there is no hypersensitivity administer in the inner aspect of the forearm or other hairless area. Arrange to read in 48 hr or according to test directions.
Hypersensitivity allergy tests: Patch Scratch	Both tests evaluate immune system response to known allergens. The patch test antigens are applied to the skin and covered with gauze patches and tape. The tests are read after 24, 48, and at times 72 hr. The scratch test antigen is applied after the skin is scraped with a sterile lancet. The antigen is placed on the scraped area with an eyedropper and left in place for 30 to 40 min and then is read.	Patch test: "Patch" tray kit, patches, alcohol sponges, diluents, allergens, gauze, tape, millimeter ruler. Scratch test: Lancet to scratch skin, allergen, eyedropper, control solution, millimeter ruler.	Explain the procedure to the patient. Instruct the patient not to get patches wet. Apply antigen to normal hairless skin area. Do not administer if patient has an acute inflammatory condition or skin lesions. Read test areas at designated times. Positive readings include: erythema, papules, vesicles.

Table 20-12

COMMON SKIN DISEASES AND DERMATOLOGIC CONDITIONS

Disease	Symptoms	Treatment	Medical Assistant's Role
Acne vulgaris (inflammation of the sebaceous glands causing eruptions called "pimples" and "blackheads")	Skin eruptions: papules, pustules.	Drug therapy includes topical medications specific to the type of skin and cause of acne. Sunlamp treatments may also be ordered. Severe acne may be treated with systemic antibiotics.	General clinical medical assisting procedures. The medical assistant should be aware that the patient is most often an adolescent and embarrassed about his or her appearance. Patient teaching should include explanation of the need for meticulous cleansing. The patient should be cautioned against squeezing the pimples since in doing this permanent injury to the pore and/or spread of the inflammation may occur. Written care instructions should be given.
Burns (injury to the skin and body caused by heat or other agent)	Classification: *First-degree:* redness and pain present. *Second-degree:* redness and pain and blisters occur. *Third-degree:* skin destruction is irreparable. White in appearance and no pain. *Fourth-degree:* underlying tissue destroyed. No pain.	Depends on extent of area burned and doctor's preference for treatment.	General clinical medical assisting procedures. The medical assistant should be aware that the seriousness of burns depends on size, location, and degree. Usually, minor burns are self-treated and not seen in the office. Serious burns are usually an emergency situation. Dressing changes and application of ointment may be the assistant's responsibility when the burned patient does visit the office. Nothing is ever to be applied without a physician's order and examination.
Dermatitis (inflammation of the skin)	Redness and any or all forms of eruption: macules, papules, vesicles, pustules, and secondary lesions.	Dependent on type, usually ointment for specific treatment. May include skin testing for allergens, antibiotics for infections, corticosteroids for acute inflammation, scabicides for mite infestation.	General clinical medical assisting procedures. The medical assistant should be aware that dermatitis is a term that encompasses a broad spectrum of dermatologic conditions. Drugs, allergies, and prolonged sun exposure are examples of causes of dermatitis. Contact dermatitis is an allergic reaction to any of the poisonous plants such as ivy or oak or various chemicals such as in

Continued

Table 20-12

COMMON SKIN DISEASES AND DERMATOLOGIC CONDITIONS—*Continued*

Disease	Symptoms	Treatment	Medical Assistant's Role
			household cleaners. In persons susceptible to allergic reactions from poisonous plants, patient teaching would include instructing the patient to thoroughly wash following exposure to such plants to prevent the reaction.

The medical assistant maintains medical asepsis and uses sterile technique for treatments of lesions or wounds. Surgical procedures such as wound suturing, biopsy, or débridement require strict asepsis. Sterile dressings should be readily available for application to lesions and wounds. All soiled and contaminated material are removed, and the room should be cleansed in a manner that prevents any cross-contamination of infection or disease. This usually requires wiping the surfaces that were exposed to the patient with disinfectant.

The medical assistant also provides the patient with instructions for home care of the biopsy or wart removal site. The patient should be instructed to keep the site clean and dry until a scab forms or the wart falls off, usually in 1 to 2 days.

INTEGUMENTARY SPECIALTY

Dermatology is the medical specialty that studies and treats diseases and conditions of the skin. The medical assistant employed in the dermatologist's office, in addition to performing the general medical assisting responsibilities, may administer sun lamp treatments, apply topical medications, and assist with minor sterile dermatologic procedures. Often, growths are removed and sent for biopsy, or skin scrapings may be taken for examination under the microscope. (Refer to Chapter 23, Pharmacology and Drug Therapy, and the specific examination chapters for information on assisting with these procedures.) If the medical assistant works in a dermatologist's or allergist's office where skin testing is common, the procedures for patch and scratch testing will be taught by the physician.

PATIENT TEACHING CONSIDERATIONS

Throughout this chapter, the tables of the specialty examinations provide specific teaching information. Patients referred to the specialist's office require instruction and teaching in all phases of the examination, clinical testing and other procedures, and treatment. Anxiety levels are often high in a new setting, and teaching the patient what to expect, as well as what is expected of him or her, helps to provide a therapeutic environment conducive to the specific examination. The medical assistant can provide information reinforcing concepts regarding the structure and function of the involved system, explaining the rationale and procedures in diagnostic testing, and clarifying the preventive and therapeutic measures prescribed for home care. Use the principles of teaching discussed in Chapter 5 when preparing each patient teaching plan. It is important to use every available opportunity to teach patients who are seen in the specialist's office as the patients may have a limited number of visits. This requires that the medical assistant maximize the role as teacher during each patient visit.

RELATED ETHICAL AND LEGAL IMPLICATIONS

There are many facets of the specific physical examination that require the medical assistant's understanding of legal responsibilities. Patients must provide informed consent for the examination or procedure to be performed. The medical assistant needs to reinforce the physician's explanation of the examination. The explanation provides the patient or parent with an opportunity for implied or verbal consent, or the refusal of the examination or procedure. The procedures, treatments, and patient teaching must be performed after the physician has completed the explanation and has instructed the medical assistant to proceed.

The practice of providing patients with written materials for teaching self-care, drug administration, and other procedural preparations facilitates more accurate understanding and compliance. Again, patients who understand and are satisfied with their care are less likely to take legal action.

The medical assistant does not initiate, prescribe, or diagnose because these activities are outside the scope of medical assisting practice. The medical assistant who oversteps the bounds of "assistant," even at the physician's direction, puts both himself or herself and the physician in legal jeopardy.

SUMMARY

The role of the medical assistant in the specific physical examination is to facilitate the needs of both the physician and the patient. This results in a cooperative patient and a successful examination. The medical assistant must develop a number of diverse physical examination skills. The skills will aid the medical assistant in anticipating needs according to symptomatology, preparing the examination room for expected procedures, and providing patients with needed teaching and supplemental information. Patient information and education allays anxiety and increases patient compliance in the process of diagnosis, treatment, and follow-up care. This chapter has presented the necessary information to assist the medical assistant in the development of these skills.

DISCUSSION QUESTIONS

1. A man has just been told that he has multiple sclerosis. You see he is alone in the physician's office. What could you say to him?
2. A patient has been shown how to instill eye drops but states that she could never do it and has no help. What will you do?
3. The patient is afraid of the ear irrigation procedure. What would you do to allay the patient's fears?
4. A woman patient has lost weight, has protrusion of the eyeballs, and has enlargement of the thyroid gland. The physician orders a blood test for thyroid hormone. While you are performing venipuncture, she begins crying and states that she is afraid she has cancer. What will you say?
5. The patient is in the office for examination of a skin rash. You notice that he is breaking the pustules open while scratching. What do you do?
6. The patient is 73 years old and has been diagnosed for 1 month as being a diabetic. What would you discuss with the patient, and what would your approach be?
7. The patient has injured her ankle so badly that she can't walk or place any weight on it. She asks if it is broken. What do you say?
8. The patient asks to see his chart as you are placing it on the door rack. What would you do?

BIBLIOGRAPHY

Refer to Chapter 22 for a bibliography of works related to specific physical examinations and clinical procedures.

Barness LA: Manual of Pediatric Physical Diagnosis, ed 6. Mosby-Year Book, St. Louis, 1991.
Bates B: A Guide to Physical Examination and History Taking, ed 4. Lippincott, Philadelphia, 1987.
Magee DJ: Orthopedic Physical Assessment, ed 2. WB Saunders, Philadelphia, 1992.
Malasanas L: Health Assessment, ed 3. CV Mosby, St. Louis, 1986.
Seidel HM: Mosby's Guide to Physical Examination, ed 2. Mosby–Year Book, St. Louis, 1991.

PROCEDURE: Test visual acuity

OSHA STANDARDS:

Terminal Performance Objective: Test a patient's degree of visual acuity with the Snellen eye chart placed at a distance of 20 ft from the patient.

EQUIPMENT: Snellen eye chart mounted on a wall at eye level
Eye covering (eye spatula, paper cup, index card, etc.)
Floor marker positioned a distance of 20 ft from the chart

PROCEDURE

1. Prepare the room by assembling the equipment and checking the cleanliness of the room, lighting, and temperature.
2. Identify the patient and explain the procedure.

3. Ask the patient to continue wearing contact lenses or eyeglasses for distance, unless otherwise directed by the physician.
4. Instruct the patient to stand at the 20-ft marker and cover the right eye with the cup while keeping the right eye open.

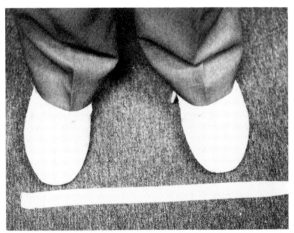

The distance marker is placed so that a person standing with toes on the far edge of the marker is 20 feet from the Snellen eye chart.

PRINCIPLE

1. To reduce procedure time and to facilitate the efficiency of the examination.

2. To reduce the risk of error and to provide assurance to anxious patients.
3. The test objective is to measure the patient's present visual acuity even with correction.

4. If the eye not being examined is closed, the visual acuity of the left eye is affected. Closing one eye causes squinting in the open eye, which temporarily increases visual acuity.

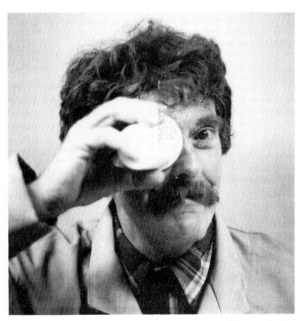

The patient uses the cup to cover the eye without closing it.

5. Stand by the chart and point to each row as the patient reads down the chart.
6. Ask the patient to verbally identify each letter in the row, beginning with row 3 (20/70). Continue down to the smallest row in which the patient can identify at least five letters accurately. (If the patient cannot read row 3, proceed up the chart to the row the patient can read.)

5. Pointing assists the patient to focus on one row at a time.
6. Skipping to row 3 saves time; however, the chart row order should be followed for both eyes to avoid error. If the patient cannot read row 1, move the patient closer to the chart until it can be read. Measure the distance to the chart with a tape measure.

PROCEDURE

7. Observe the patient for any reactions during the testing.

8. Repeat the procedure to test the other eye.

9. Record the results as two numbers. (Refer to the number on the left-hand side of the chart next to the smallest line that could be read most accurately.)
   Example: OD, 20/25
   OS, 20/20–2
   Note: Chart the use of contact lenses or eye glasses during the examination.
   Example: OD, 20/25 w/contacts
   OS, 20/20 w/contacts

10. Answer the patient's questions regarding the testing.

PRINCIPLE

7. Watering eyes, tilting of the head, or squinting are examples of symptoms that may indicate difficulty with visualization.

8. Both eyes are tested separately for the greatest accuracy. Visual acuity can be different in each eye.

9. The right eye is designated as OD (oculus dexter); the left eye, OS (oculus sinister). The numerator designates the number of feet from the chart (20 ft); the denominator, the distance at which a person with normal vision can read the row of letters. If the smallest line is read with errors, record the number of errors after a minus sign as part of the denominator.

10. The patient is usually interested in knowing the test results. While these results are usually shared with the patient, care should be taken to properly interpret the numeric results and not to make a diagnosis.

PROCEDURE: Irrigate the eye

OSHA STANDARDS:

Terminal Performance Objective: Irrigate the eye to remove foreign particles, treat infections, or flush harmful chemicals using sterile technique within a reasonable time standard.

EQUIPMENT: Curved basin
Towel
Sterile cotton balls
Sterile normal saline
Sterile eyedropper (for a small amount of solution)
Sterile bulb syringe (for a larger amount of solution)
Disposable irrigation set may be used
Sterile IV set (for copious use in chemical burns)
Order from the patient chart
Gloves (optional)*
Biohazard bag for disposal

PROCEDURE

1. Prepare the room by assembling the equipment and checking the cleanliness of the room, lighting, and temperature.
2. Identify the patient, and explain the procedure.

3. Assist the patient into the supine position.

4. Drape the toweling over the patient's neck and shoulder and under the head. Place the curved basin next to the affected eye to catch the solution.
5. Assist the patient to turn the head toward the side of the affected eye.
6. Instruct the patient to roll the eyes upward (look up) while pulling the lower conjunctival sac downward with gauze placed over the fingertips.

7. Pour the solution over the cotton ball. The solution should be at room temperature.
8. With a solution-dampened cotton ball, cleanse the eyelid and lashes, cleansing from the inner (near the nose) to the outer aspect of the lid *once*, and dispose of the cotton ball.

PRINCIPLE

1. To reduce procedure time and to facilitate the efficiency of the procedure.

2. To reduce the risk of error and to provide assurance to anxious patients.
3. To make the procedure more manageable, however, it can be performed in the sitting position.
4. To prevent the solution from soiling or wetting the patient's clothing.

5. To prevent the solution from running into the unaffected eye, thus preventing cross-contamination.
6. Looking upward prevents the chance of injuring the cornea with dropper and distracts the patient's attention from the dropper. The sac is pulled downward to catch the drops. The gauze prevents the finger from slipping and injuring the eye.
7. Placing the cotton ball in the solution would cause contamination of the solution.
8. Cleansing in one direction removes infectious material. If the step is to be repeated, a new solution-dampened cotton ball is used. Each wash is done with one sweep to prevent recontamination of the area.

*Tears are body fluids to which the CDC's universal precautions do not apply; however, CDC guidelines constitute minimum standards of practice. In institutions that have implemented universal precautions (applying them to *all* body fluids), it is acceptable to wear disposable gloves, especially for the patient at high risk for or with an infectious disease such as acquired immunodeficiency syndrome. Other barriers such as goggles, gown, and mask may also be worn depending on the extent of potential risk.

PROCEDURE

9. Pour the required amount of irrigating solution into a sterile container. Withdraw the solution into a bulb syringe by squeezing the bulb *before* inserting it into the solution, then releasing the bulb when the syringe tip is immersed in the solution.

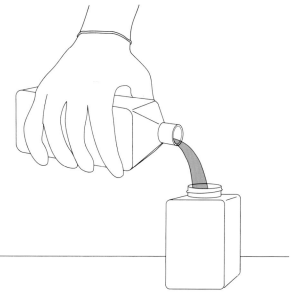

Pour the solution into the sterile container without touching the solution bottle to the container.

10. Separate the upper and lower eyelids with the index finger and thumb and hold in this position.

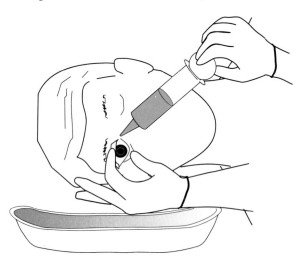

Use index finger and thumb to hold upper and lower lids apart while directing flow of solution toward the inner contour of the eye.

11. Squeeze the bulb, directing the solution toward the inner contour of the eye, allowing it to flow toward the outer corner slowly and steadily. Avoid touching the eye with the syringe. Repeat as required in the same manner.

12. Allow the eye to close immediately and instruct the patient to rotate the eyeball.

PRINCIPLE

9. To avoid injecting the contents of the syringe into the solution.

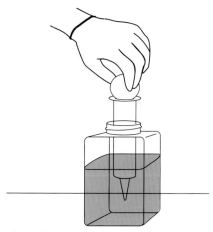

Squeeze the bulb, insert syringe tip into the solution, then release the bulb.

10. To dispose the conjunctiva and a greater area of the eye surface for irrigation.

11. The flow of solution is controlled to avoid eye injury. It is directed toward the inner contour so that it flows over the greatest surface without injuring the cornea.

12. Allows the upper and lower lids to meet, and may dislodge foreign material.

PROCEDURE

13. Pat dry the lid with a cotton ball from the inner to the outer corners of the eye.

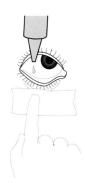

Dry the eyelid with a cotton ball, wiping from the inner to the outer corner of the eye.

14. Give follow-up instructions to the patient.
15. Record the date, time, procedure and solution, patient tolerance, patient instruction, and initial the record.
    Example: date, time: OD irrigation w/sterile normal saline (initials).
16. Clean the equipment and the examination room.

PRINCIPLE

13. To provide patient comfort and to reduce the chance of contamination.

14. To ensure proper continued care.
15. To ensure the quality of care and provide a point of future reference.

16. To prevent the chance of transmitting microorganisms and to prepare the room for the next patient.

PROCEDURE: Instill or apply eye medications

OSHA STANDARDS:

Terminal Performance Objective: Instill medication to dilate or contract the pupil, to relieve pain and discomfort, to cleanse, to treat infection, or to reduce inflammation using sterile technique within a reasonable time standard.

EQUIPMENT: Antiseptic solution or antibiotic ointment
2 × 2 sterile gauze squares
Sterile cotton balls
Sterile eyedropper
Medication order from the patient chart
Gloves (optional*)
Biohazard bag for disposal

PROCEDURE	PRINCIPLE
1. Prepare the room by assembling the equipment and checking the cleanliness of the room, lighting, and temperature.	1. To reduce procedure time and to facilitate the efficiency of the procedure.
2. Identify the patient and explain the procedure.	2. To reduce the risk of error and to provide assurance to anxious patients.
3. Assist the patient into the supine position without a pillow.	3. To make the procedure more manageable, however, it can be performed in the sitting position with the head tilted backward.
4. Double-check the medication container label and which eye is being treated with the physician's order.	4. To ensure that the correct medication is given. Accuracy cannot be overstressed.
5. Instruct the patient to roll the eyes upward (look up) while pulling the lower conjunctival sac downward with gauze placed over the fingertips.	5. Looking upward prevents the chance of injuring the cornea with dropper and distracts the patient's attention from the dropper. The sac is pulled downward to catch the drops. The gauze prevents the finger from slipping and injuring the eye.
6. For installation of eye drops: Instill the prescribed number of drops directly into the center of the lower conjunctival sac. Do not touch the eye with the dropper.	6. Eye medications are considered sterile. Placing the drops over the conjunctival sac prevents injury to the cornea.
7. Allow the eye to close without squeezing the eye shut and instruct the patient to rotate the eyeball. Remove the excess with care.	7. Rotating the eyeball ensures even distribution of medication. Squeezing would force out the medication.
8. For application of eye ointment: Holding the lower lid in place, squeeze a ribbon of ointment along the lower lid from the inner to the outer corners of the eye. Do not touch the tips of the tube to the eye.	8. Eye medications are considered sterile. Placing the drops over the conjunctival sac prevents injury to the cornea.
9. Allow the eye to close immediately and instruct the patient to rotate the eyeball. Remove excess with care.	9. Rotating the eyeball ensures even distribution of medication.
10. Give follow-up instructions to the patient.	10. To ensure proper continued care.
11. Record the date, time, procedure and solution, patient tolerance, patient instructions, and initial record. Example: 3/5/93 2 PM: Pilocarpine 1% gt i OD (initials).	11. To ensure quality of care and to provide a point of future reference.
12. Clean the equipment and the examination room.	12. To prevent the chance of transmitting microorganisms and to prepare the room for the next patient.

*Tears are body fluids to which the CDC's universal precautions do not apply; however, CDC guidelines constitute minimum standards of practice. In institutions that have implemented universal precautions (applying them to *all* body fluids), it is acceptable to wear disposable gloves, especially for the patient at high risk for or with an infectious disease such as acquired immunodeficiency syndrome. Other barriers such as goggles, gown, and mask may also be worn depending on the extent of potential risk.

PROCEDURE: Apply warm compresses to the eye

OSHA STANDARDS:

Terminal Performance Objective: Apply a warm water compress to the eye to promote drainage or soothe inflammation and irritation using sterile technique and within a reasonable time standard.

EQUIPMENT: Warm water or prescribed solution
4 × 4 sterile gauze squares
Sterile cotton balls
Order from the patient chart
Gloves (optional*)
Biohazard bags for disposal

PROCEDURE

1. Prepare the room by assembling the equipment and checking the cleanliness of the room, lighting, and temperature.
2. Obtain information from the physician as to how often and how long compresses should be applied and what, if any, special solution should be used.
3. Identify the patient and explain the procedure.

4. Assist the patient into the supine position.

5. Double-check the medication container label and which eye is being treated with the physician's order.
6. Inform the patient that gauze squares may be used, but a clean washcloth is satisfactory, provided the cloth is restricted to the infected eye and changed frequently.
7. Test the solution to ensure the temperature is 95°F to 105°F (35°C to 41°C) (warm on the inner wrist).
8. Teach the patient to soak the washcloth in warm water or in the solution prescribed, wring it out, and apply it to the eye for the duration recommended.
9. Give follow-up instructions to the patient.

10. Record the date, time, procedure and solution, teaching session, and initial the record. Example: 3/5/93 2:00 PM: Warm compresses applied OD 15 minutes. Patient instructed to apply warm compresses for 15 minutes OD 3 or 4 times per day for comfort for five days. Instructions given to patient (initials).
11. Clean the equipment and the examination room.

PRINCIPLE

1. To reduce procedure time and to facilitate the efficiency of the procedure.

2. Clear understanding of directions is necessary for solutions, and treatment times may vary with each patient.
3. To reduce the risk of error and to provide assurance to anxious patients.
4. To make the procedure more manageable, however, it can be performed in the sitting position.
5. To ensure that the correct medication is given. Accuracy cannot be overstressed.

6. Unless specified by the physician the use of gauze squares is costly and not necessary.

7. To prevent the patient from eye injury through burns from hot solutions.
8. Keeping instructions simple helps the patient to feel confident and to remember the information.

9. To ensure proper continued care, instructions should be in writing for the patient to take home.
10. To ensure quality of care and to provide a point of future reference.

11. To prevent the chance of transmitting microorganisms and to prepare the room for the next patient.

---

*Tears are body fluids to which the CDC's universal precautions do not apply; however, CDC guidelines constitute minimum standards of practice. For institutions that have implemented universal precautions (applying them to *all* body fluids), it is acceptable to wear disposable gloves, especially for the patient at high risk for or with an infectious disease such as acquired immunodeficiency disease. Other barriers such as goggles, gown, and mask may also be worn depending on extent of the potential risk.

PROCEDURE: Apply an eye dressing

OSHA STANDARDS:

Terminal Performance Objective: Apply a sterile eye dressing to keep the eye at rest, to protect the eye, to absorb secretions, or to reduce swelling within a reasonable time standard.

EQUIPMENT: Sterile solution or medication
Sterile eye dressing
Four to 10 adhesive tape strips (hypoallergenic type if the patient is allergic to tape)
Order from the patient chart
Gloves (optional*)
Biohazard bag for disposal

PROCEDURE	PRINCIPLE
1. Prepare the room by assembling the equipment and checking the cleanliness of the room, lighting, and temperature.	1. To reduce procedure time and to facilitate the efficiency of the procedure.
2. Obtain information from the physician as to how often and how long compresses should be applied and what, if any, special solution should be used.	2. Clear understanding of directions is necessary for solutions, and treatment times may vary with each patient.
3. Identify the patient and explain the procedure.	3. To reduce the risk of error and to provide assurance to anxious patients.
4. If a medication is ordered, place it in the eye before opening the eye dressing package. Double-check the medication container label with the physician's order.	4. To keep the dressing sterile. The need to check for accuracy cannot be overstressed.
5. Using aseptic technique, lift the dressing from the package by grasping the edge with the forefinger and thumb.	5. Only the tip of the oval dressing is touched. Touching the center of the dressing would contaminate the sterile inner area. Sterile gloves are not required.
6. Instruct the patient to close both eyes.	6. Closing only one eye is too difficult.
7. Lay the dressing over the eye lightly without touching the center of the eye dressing.	7. Only the tip of the dressing can be touched to prevent contamination of the dressing.
8. Secure the dressing corners with tape that is placed diagonally from the forehead over the unpatched eye across dressing to the cheek bone.	8. To apply a secure dressing that avoids putting pressure to the eye while permitting freedom of head movement.
9. Ask the patient to open the patched eye.	9. To ensure that the dressing is exerting enough pressure.
10. Give follow-up instructions to the patient.	10. To ensure proper continued care, instructions should be in writing for the patient to take home.
11. Record the date, time, procedure and medication, teaching session, and initial the record. Example: 3/5/93 2:00 PM: Antibiotic ointment OD and pressure dressing applied. Instructions given to patient (initials).	11. To ensure quality of care and provide a point of future reference.
12. Clean the equipment and the examination room.	12. To prevent the chance of transmitting microorganisms and to prepare the room for the next patient.

*Tears are body fluids to which the CDC's universal precautions do not apply; however, CDC guidelines constitute minimum standards of practice. In institutions that have implemented universal precautions (applying them to *all* body fluids), it is acceptable to wear disposable gloves, especially for the patient at high risk for or with an infectious disease such as acquired immunodeficiency disease. Other barriers such as goggles, gown, and mask may also be worn depending on the extent of potential risk.

PROCEDURE: Irrigate the external ear canal

OSHA STANDARDS:

Terminal Performance Objective: Irrigate the external ear canal to remove discharge, cerumen, or foreign bodies or to warm the tissues of the ear canal within a reasonable time standard.

ALERT: Ask the patient if there is any history of draining ears, eardrum perforation, or any complications from a previous irrigation. If so, notify the physician before continuing with the process. Do not proceed if the canal is swollen or the patient has a severe cold.

EQUIPMENT: 500 ml sodium chloride (normal saline) or distilled water
Wax softener or other medication ordered
50-ml Reiner's (metal) or bulb-type syringe
Ear or small emesis basin (for drainage)
Sterile large basin (for solution)
Towels and cotton balls
Order from the patient chart

PROCEDURE

1. Prepare the room by assembling the equipment and checking the cleanliness of the room, lighting, and temperature.
2. Identify the patient and explain the procedure.

3. Warm the solution to 95°F to 105°F (35°C to 41°C) or until it feels warm to the inner wrist.
4. Instruct the patient to assume a sitting position and to tilt head slightly forward and to the affected side.

5. Look at the ear canal and eardrum, if visible, with the otoscope.

PRINCIPLE

1. To reduce procedure time and to facilitate the efficiency of the procedure.

2. To reduce the risk of error and to provide assurance to anxious patients.

3. Cold solution may cause acute pain or symptoms of vertigo.

4. To allow the irrigation solution to continuously return to the ear basin. In the side-lying position, too much pressure would be exerted on the eardrum from the irrigation solution.

5. To provide a baseline comparison to determine when irrigation has been successful.

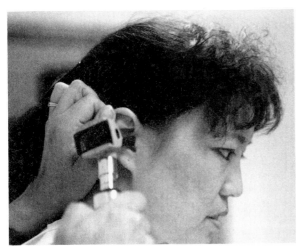

Use an otoscope to look into the ear canal and, if possible, at the eardrum.

6. If a wax softener is to be used, instill one or two drops in the affected ear.

6. Wax softener takes 15 minutes to have an effect.

PROCEDURE

7. Place a towel on the patient's shoulder on the side of the affected ear and fold up under the ear lobe. (Simulate a stand-up collar.)

8. Position the ear basin under the affected ear and instruct the patient to hold the basin in place.

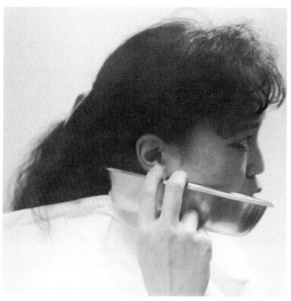

The patient holds the basin in place.

9. Cleanse the outer ear with a cotton ball dampened with the solution ordered (usually sterile normal saline).

10. Pour the warmed solution into the sterile basin, then withdraw the solution into the syringe.

11. Expel any air in the syringe.

12. Grasping the syringe with one hand, pull the auricle up and back with the other hand for adult patients and children older than 3 years of age.

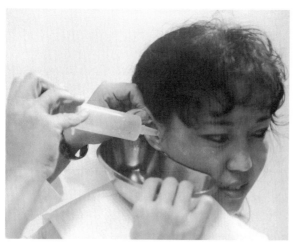

Ear irrigation.

PRINCIPLE

7. To prevent the solution from running down the neck, chest, and back.

8. The patient's assistance is required to free your hands for the procedure.

9. To prevent outer ear matter from being introduced inside the ear.

10. To prevent contamination, the solution should not be withdrawn from the original container.

11. A small amount of solution is expelled to prevent air from entering the ear. Air entering the ear under pressure causes discomfort.

12. To facilitate the flow of medication by straightening the ear canal.

PROCEDURE

13. For children younger than 3 years of age, pull the earlobe down and back.
14. Insert the tip of the filled syringe into the affected ear, pointing the tip slightly upward and posterior to direct the flow against the side of the canal.

15. Repeat the irrigation, removing the syringe tip periodically to enable the free flow of returning solution.

16. Dry the outer ear. Visualize the inner ear with the otoscope.
17. Call the physician to view the results.

18. Provide dry cotton or gauze if drainage continues.
19. Give follow-up instructions to the patient.

20. Record the date, time, procedure and medication if used, patient instructions, and initial the record. Example: 3/5/93 2:00 PM: Debrox and ear irrigation, right ear. Debrox instructions given to patient (initials).
21. Clean the equipment and the examination room.

PRINCIPLE

13. The direction of the ear canal differs in young children and infants.
14. This angle is more effective in dislodging cerumen than if the flow of solution were directed straight into the canal. If using a metal syringe, less pressure is exerted to avoid rupture of the eardrum.
15. Several irrigations are usually required to release the foreign body or cerumen. Perform each carefully to prevent discomfort, vertigo, or excessive tissue softening.
16. If matter is still present, irrigation is continued.

17. Once the ear canal is clean, the physician will want to examine the eardrum and the sides of the canal. Observation of the drained solution in the basin is also used as an evaluation tool.
18. To promote patient comfort and to protect clothing.
19. To ensure proper continued care, instructions should be in writing for the patient to take home.
20. To ensure quality of care and to provide a point of future reference.

21. To prevent the chance of transmitting microorganisms and to prepare the room for the next patient.

PROCEDURE: Instill medicated ear drops

OSHA STANDARDS:

Terminal Performance Objective: Introduce medication directly into the ear canal or onto the drum to soften earwax before irrigation or to apply antibiotic drops to treat infection within a reasonable time standard.

ALERT: Ask the patient if there is any history of draining ears, eardrum perforation, or complications from a previous irrigation. If so, notify the physician before continuing with the process.

EQUIPMENT: Medication
Cotton balls
Petroleum jelly (if ordered)
Towels
Medication order from the patient chart

PROCEDURE

1. Prepare the room by assembling the equipment and checking the cleanliness of the room, lighting, and temperature.
2. Identify the patient and explain the procedure.

3. Compare the medication to the written order.
4. Instruct the patient to assume a sitting position and to tilt head slightly forward and to the unaffected side.

5. Warm the medication and withdraw it into the dropper.
6. Hold the dropper in one hand, use the other hand to pull the auricle up and back (for adult patients and children older than 3 years of age) or down and back (for children younger than 3 years of age).
7. Instill the medication, and instruct the patient to remain in position for approximately 10 minutes.

8. If the physician has ordered this step, insert a cotton ball saturated with petroleum jelly.

9. Give follow-up instructions to the patient.

10. Record the date, time, procedure and medication (if used), patient instructions, and initial the record. Example: 3/5/93 2:00 PM: Penicillin gtt ii, right ear. Prescription instructions given to patient (initials).
11. Clean the equipment and the examination room.

PRINCIPLE

1. To reduce procedure time and to facilitate the efficiency of the procedure.

2. To reduce the risk of error and provide assurance to anxious patients.
3. To ensure accuracy of administration.
4. To allow the irrigation solution to continuously return to the ear basin. In the side-lying position, too much pressure would be exerted on the eardrum from the irrigating solution.
5. Cold medication may cause acute pain or symptoms of vertigo.
6. Pulling the auricle straightens the ear canal and makes it easier for the medication to flow. The direction of the ear canal differs in young children and infants.

7. To prevent the medication from draining out of the ear and to allow for medication retention in the external canal.
8. Improper insertion could cause damage to the canal. Petroleum jelly prevents the cotton ball from absorbing the medication.
9. To ensure proper continued care, instructions should be in writing for the patient to take home.
10. To ensure quality of care and provide a point of future reference.

11. To prevent the chance of transmitting microorganisms and to prepare the room for the next patient.

PROCEDURE: Instruct the patient in cast care

OSHA STANDARDS: Ⓘ

Terminal Performance Objective: Instruct the patient with written instructions in cast care at home, to ensure appropriate safety, comfort, and a positive outcome within a reasonable time standard.

EQUIPMENT: Written patient care instructions (see Chapter 5, Patient Teaching)

PROCEDURE

1. Prepare the room by assembling the equipment and checking the cleanliness, lighting, and temperature.
2. Identify the patient and explain the procedure.

   After the cast application, use a written teaching plan to instruct patients:
3. That the cast will feel warm for 24 hours after application.

4. Not to use palms when cast is wet to move extremity.

5. To elevate the cast above the heart and support with pillows.
6. To keep cast uncovered until completely dry.

7. To notify the physician of any of the following:
   a. Unusual sensations or tingling.
   b. Changes in skin color or temperature.
   c. Pain.
   d. Inability to move fingers or toes.
   e. Any drainage after surgery.
   f. Cracks in the cast.
8. After 24 hours, to follow physician's order for exercise and activity.
9. After 24 hours, to:
   a. Maintain body alignment.
   b. Exercise according to orders.
   c. Bear weight only if ordered.
   d. Wash and lubricate skin above and below the cast daily.
   e. Keep the cast dry.
   f. Report any previously listed symptoms.
   g. Report loose or moving cast.
   h. Put nothing inside the cast (back scratchers, rulers).
   i. Call with any questions.
10. Give follow-up instructions to the patient.

11. Record the date, time, procedure and medication (if used), patient instructions, and initial the record. Example: 3/5/93 2:00 PM: Long-arm cast applied. Cast care instructions given to patient (initials).
12. Clean the equipment and the examination room.

PRINCIPLE

1. To reduce procedure time and to facilitate the efficiency of the procedure.
2. To reduce the risk of error and provide assurance to anxious patients.

3. Plaster reaches its maximum temperature 5 to 15 minutes after it is applied and will then cool rapidly. Maximum plaster strength is obtained after the cast is dry (up to 48 hours for plaster casts; 30 minutes for synthetic casts).

4. Fingers dent and leave pressure areas which can lead to pressure sores.

5. To prevent or reduce swelling.

6. Circulating air increases the evaporation of water and dries the cast.

7. All are signs that the cast needs to be checked by the physician. The patient should not ignore any potential danger signs. The cast may have to be split or removed.

8. To prevent stiffness and contractures.

9.
   a. To prevent accidents.
   b. To maintain strength.
   c. To promote healing.
   d. To maintain cleanliness.

   e. To prevent breakdown of cast.
   f. To prevent injury from complications.
   g. Cast may need to be reapplied.
   h. To prevent skin abrasions and irritations.
   i. To ensure proper continued care.
10. To ensure proper continued care, instructions should be in writing for the patient to take home.
11. To ensure quality of care and provide a point of future reference.

12. To prevent the chance of transmitting microorganisms and to prepare the room for the next patient.

PROCEDURE: Instruct the patient in how to apply an ice bag

OSHA STANDARDS: Ⓘ

Terminal Performance Objective: Instruct the patient with written instructions in how to apply an ice bag to relieve pain, reduce swelling, and ensure safe and comfortable care within a reasonable time standard.

EQUIPMENT: Written patient care instructions (see Chapter 5, Patient Teaching)
Ice bag
Crushed ice
Towel

PROCEDURE

1. Prepare the room by assembling the equipment and checking the cleanliness of the room, lighting, and temperature.
2. Check the order from the physician regarding length of time the ice bag needs to be applied, how frequently it should be used, and the site to be treated.
3. Identify the patient and explain the procedure.

4. Instruct the patient to fill the bag one half to two thirds full with crushed ice.
5. Expel the air before capping by resting the bag on a flat surface so that the ice is level with the mouth of the bag.
6. Dry the bag and check for leakage.
7. Place a towel between the bag and body surface being treated.

8. Place the bag on the affected area for the proper duration (usually 20 to 30 minutes) for the first 24 hours.
9. Repeat the procedure the number of times indicated by the physician.
10. Instruct the patient to temporarily suspend the treatment if numbness occurs or pain increases.

11. Give written follow-up instructions to the patient.

12. Record the date, time, procedure and medication if used, patient instructions, and initial the record. Example: 3/5/93 2:00 PM: Patient instructed to apply ice bag to left calf 20 to 30 minutes at a time as many times as can be tolerated for 24 hours. Written instructions given to patient (initials).
13. Clean the equipment and the examination room.

PRINCIPLE

1. To reduce procedure time and to facilitate the efficiency of the procedure.

2. To ensure proper treatment at home and to write down the directions for the patient.

3. To reduce the risk of error and provide assurance to anxious patients. Writing down the information for the patient reinforces the instructions. Instruction forms with blanks to be filled in may be effective.
4. Overfilling the bag interferes with the bag's conformity to the part. Crushed ice conforms best.
5. Less air contains the cold and increases the flexibility of the bag.

6. To keep the patient dry.
7. Depending of the patient's sensitivity to cold, the towel can be used as a buffer and to keep the affected area dry.
8. To produce vasoconstriction, decrease edema, and reduce discomfort. After 24 hours, heat is usually the treatment of choice.
9. To fulfill the objectives of treatment.

10. Treatment should not cause the patient discomfort. Young children and the elderly tend to be more sensitive to cold.
11. To ensure proper continued care, instructions should be in writing for the patient to take home.
12. To ensure quality of care and to provide a point of future reference.

13. To prevent the chance of transmitting microorganisms and to prepare the room for the next patient.

PROCEDURE: Instruct the patient in the use of a cold compress

OSHA STANDARDS:

Terminal Performance Objective: Instruct the patient with written instructions in how to apply a cold compress to relieve symptoms of inflammation, pain, swelling, or hematoma and to ensure safe and comfortable care within a reasonable time standard.

EQUIPMENT: Written patient care instructions (see Chapter 5, Patient Teaching)
Clean washcloth or gauze
Ice water in a basin
Towel

PROCEDURE

1. Prepare the room by assembling the equipment and checking the cleanliness of the room, lighting, and temperature.
2. Check the order from the physician regarding length of time the compress needs to be applied, how frequently it should be used, and the site to be treated.
3. Identify the patient and explain the procedure using written instructions.

4. Instruct the patient to use gauze or washcloths that have been soaked in ice water and wrung out.
5. Apply to the affected body surface frequently resoaking the compress.
6. Repeat the procedure as directed and for the time specified (usually 15 to 20 minutes) for the first 24 hours.
7. Repeat the procedure the number of times indicated by the physician.
8. Give written follow-up instructions to the patient.

9. Record the date, time, procedure and medication (if used), instructions, and initial the record. Example: 3/5/93 2:00 PM: Patient instructed to apply cold compress to left calf 20 to 30 minutes at a time depending on tolerance for 24 hours. Written instructions given to patient (initials).
10. Clean the equipment and the examination room.

PRINCIPLE

1. To reduce procedure time and to facilitate the efficiency of the procedure.

2. To ensure proper treatment at home and to write down the directions for the patient.

3. To reduce the risk of error and provide rereassurance to anxious patients. Writing down the information for the patient reinforces the instructions. Instruction forms with blanks to be filled in may be effective.
4. Ice water ensures that the compresses will maintain the cold for a longer period of time.
5. The body tends to warm the compress in approximately 2 minutes.
6. To produce vasoconstriction, decrease edema, and reduce discomfort. After 24 hours, heat is usually the treatment of choice.
7. To fulfill the objectives of treatment.

8. To ensure proper continued care, instructions should be in writing for the patient to take home.
9. To ensure quality of care and to provide a point of future reference.

10. To prevent the chance of transmitting microorganisms and to prepare the room for the next patient.

PROCEDURE: Instruct the patient in the use of a hot water bag

OSHA STANDARDS:

Terminal Performance Objective: Instruct the patient with written instructions in how to apply a hot water bag to relieve pain or reduce swelling and to ensure safe and comfortable care within a reasonable time standard.

EQUIPMENT: Written patient care instructions (see Chapter 5, Patient Teaching)
Hot water bag
Warm water (115°F to 130°F [46°C to 54°C] maximum)
Towel

PROCEDURE

1. Prepare the room by assembling the equipment and checking the cleanliness of the room, lighting, and temperature.
2. Check the order from the physician regarding length of time the hot water bottle needs to be applied, how frequently it should be used, and the site to be treated.
3. Identify the patient and explain the procedure using written instructions.

4. Instruct the patient to fill the rubber bag approximately two thirds full with warm water (for adults, 130°F [54°C] maximum temperature; for children, 115°F [46°C] maximum temperature).
5. If water temperature cannot be measured, instruct the patient to adapt the temperature to body comfort.
6. Expel the air before capping by resting the bag on a flat surface so that the water is level with the mouth of the bag.
7. Dry the bag and check for leakage.
8. Place a towel between the bag and body surface being treated.

9. Repeat the procedure as directed and for the time specified (usually 15 to 20 minutes) four times a day.

10. Give written follow-up instructions to the patient.

11. Record the date, time, procedure and medication (if used), instructions, and initial the record. Example: 3/5/93 2:00 PM: Patient instructed to apply hot water bag to left calf for 15 to 20 minutes at a time four times a day. Written instructions given to patient (initials).
12. Clean the equipment and the examination room.

PRINCIPLE

1. To reduce procedure time and to facilitate the efficiency of the procedure.

2. To ensure proper treatment at home and to write down the directions for the patient.

3. To reduce the risk of error and to provide reassurance to anxious patients. Writing down the information for the patient reinforces the instructions. Instruction forms with blanks to be filled in may be effective.
4. Water temperature too high may burn the patient. Filling the bag two thirds full allows the bag to conform to body contour and is lighter in weight.

5. The bag should not feel hot, just warm. If redness occurs within the first 2 minutes, the water is too hot.
6. Less air contains the heat and increases the flexibility of the bag.

7. To keep the patient dry.
8. Depending on the patient's sensitivity to heat, the towel can be used as a buffer and to keep the affected area dry.
9. To promote circulation and absorption of the swelling. The effectiveness of heat application decreases after 20 minutes.
10. To ensure proper continued care, instructions should be in writing for the patient to take home.
11. To ensure quality of care and provide a point of future reference.

12. To prevent the chance of transmitting microorganisms and to prepare the room for the next patient.

PROCEDURE: Instruct the patient in the use of a heating pad

OSHA STANDARDS: (III)

Terminal Performance Objective: Instruct the patient with written instructions in how to apply a heating pad to relieve pain or reduce swelling and to ensure safe and comfortable care within a reasonable time standard.

EQUIPMENT: Written patient care instructions (see Chapter 5, Patient Teaching)
Heating pad
Heating pad cover

PROCEDURE

1. Prepare the room by assembling the equipment and checking the cleanliness of the room, lighting, and temperature.
2. Check the order from the physician regarding length of time the heating pad needs to be applied, how frequently it should be used, and the site to be treated.
3. Identify the patient and explain the procedure using written instructions.

4. Instruct the patient to use the appliance with great care.

5. Follow the product instructions carefully before applying.

6. Repeat the procedure as directed and for the time specified (usually 15 to 20 minutes) four times a day.
7. Give written follow-up instructions to the patient.

8. Record the date, time, procedure and medication (if used), instructions, and initial the record. Example: 3/5/93 2:00 PM: Patient instructed to apply heating pad to left calf for 15 to 20 minutes at a time four times a day. Written instructions given to patient (initials).
9. Clean the equipment and the examination room.

PRINCIPLE

1. To reduce procedure time and to facilitate the efficiency of the procedure.

2. To ensure proper treatment at home and to write down the directions for the patient.

3. To reduce the risk of error and provide assurance to anxious patients. Writing down the information for the patient reinforces the instructions. Instruction forms with blanks to be filled in may be effective.
4. Electric heating pads are capable of causing serious injury. The pad covering should be waterproof, dry, and well insulated.
5. Instructions should be read carefully to avoid body burns or electric shock. Do not go to bed for the night with a heating pad on; keep the affected area dry.
6. To promote circulation and absorption of the swelling.

7. To ensure proper continued care, instructions should be in writing for the patient to take home.
8. To ensure quality of care and provide a point of future reference.

9. To prevent the chance of transmitting microorganisms and to prepare the room for the next patient.

PROCEDURE: Instruct the patient in the use of warm soaks

OSHA STANDARDS: (III)

Terminal Performance Objective: Instruct the patient with written instructions in how to apply warm soaks to relieve pain or reduce swelling and to ensure safe and comfortable care within a reasonable time standard.

EQUIPMENT: Written patient care instructions (see Chapter 5, Patient Teaching)
Clean washcloth or gauze
Warm water (110°F [43°C]) or solution
Towel

PROCEDURE

1. Prepare the room by assembling the equipment and checking the cleanliness of the room, lighting, and temperature.
2. Check the order from the physician regarding length of time the warm soaks need to be applied, how frequently they should be used, and the site to be treated.
3. Identify the patient and explain the procedure using written instructions.

4. Instruct the patient to use the solution specified with tap water and heated to 110°F (43°C) maximum temperature.
5. If water temperature cannot be measured, instruct the patient to adapt the temperature to body comfort.
6. Soak the affected body part for 15 to 20 minutes by placing it in a basin with the water or solution.
7. Repeat the procedure as directed and for the time specified (usually 15 to 20 minutes) four times a day.

8. Caution the patient to maintain good body alignment so as not to cause further injury or discomfort.
9. Use towels or absorbent pads.

10. Give written follow-up instructions to the patient.

11. Record the date, time, procedure and medication (if used), instructions, and initial the record. Example: 3/5/93 2:00 PM: Patient instructed to apply warm soaks to left foot for 15 to 20 minutes at a time four times a day. Written instructions given to patient (initials).
12. Clean the equipment and the examination room.

PRINCIPLE

1. To reduce procedure time and to facilitate the efficiency of the procedure.

2. To ensure proper treatment at home and to write down the directions for the patient.

3. To reduce the risk of error and provide assurance to anxious patients. Writing down the information for the patient reinforces the instructions. Instruction forms with blanks to be filled in may be effective.
4. Water temperature too high may burn the patient. Excessive heat or burning is abnormal.

5. The water should not feel hot, just warm. If redness occurs within the first 2 minutes, the water is too hot.
6. Water will cool quickly. An even temperature is necessary to fulfill the treatment objective.
7. To promote circulation and absorption of the swelling. The effectiveness of heat application decreases after 20 minutes.
8. If body parts are twisted for the purpose of soaking, further discomfort will result.
9. To dry the affected part immediately following the soak.
10. To ensure proper continued care, instructions should be in writing for the patient to take home.
11. To ensure quality of care and to provide a point of future reference.

12. To prevent the chance of transmitting microorganisms and to prepare the room for the next patient.

PROCEDURE: Instruct the patient in the use of warm compresses

OSHA STANDARDS: (III)

Terminal Performance Objective: Instruct the patient with written instructions in how to apply warm compresses to relieve pain or reduce swelling and to ensure safe and comfortable care within a reasonable time standard.

EQUIPMENT: Written patient care instructions (see Chapter 5, Patient Teaching)
Clean washcloth or gauze
Warm water (110°F [43°C]) or solution
Towel

PROCEDURE

1. Prepare the room by assembling the equipment and checking the cleanliness of the room, lighting, and room temperature.
2. Check the order from the physician regarding length of time to be applied, how frequently it should be used, and the site to be treated.
3. Identify the patient and explain the procedure using written instructions.

4. Instruct the patient to use gauze or washcloths that have been soaked in water or the solution and wrung out.
5. Instruct the patient to use the solution specified with tap water and heated to 110°F (43°C) maximum temperature.
6. If water temperature cannot be measured, instruct the patient to adapt the temperature to body comfort.
7. Apply to the affected body surface frequently resoaking the compress.
8. Repeat the procedure the number of times indicated by the physician.
9. Repeat the procedure the number of times indicated by the physician.
10. Give written follow-up instructions to the patient.
11. Record the date, time, procedure and medication (if used), instructions, and initial the record. Example: 3/5/93 2:00 PM: Patient instructed to apply warm compresses to left calf 15 to 20 minutes at a time for four days. Written instructions given to patient (initials).
12. Clean the equipment and the examination room.

PRINCIPLE

1. To reduce procedure time and to facilitate the efficiency of the procedure.
2. To ensure proper treatment at home and to write down the directions for the patient.
3. To reduce the risk of error and provide assurance to anxious patients. Writing down the information for the patient reinforces the instructions. Instruction forms with blanks to be filled in may be effective.
4. Washcloths are the easiest, most accessible, and most comfortable form of compress.
5. Water temperature too high may burn the patient. Excessive heat or burning is abnormal.
6. The water should not feel hot, just warm. If redness occurs within the first 2 minutes, the water is too hot.
7. The body tends to cool the compress in approximately 2 minutes.
8. To promote circulation and absorption of swelling, discomfort. After 20 minutes, the maximum effectiveness of heat is reduced.
9. To fulfill the objectives of treatment.
10. To ensure proper continued care, instructions should be in writing for the patient to take home.
11. To ensure quality care and to provide a point of future reference.

12. To prevent the chance of transmitting microorganisms and to prepare the room for the next patient.

HIGHLIGHTS

Osteoporosis and Calcium Supplementation

Osteoporosis, a disease in which bone density diminishes, has been cited as the major cause of 70% of the fractures in persons 45 and older. Dr. A. Michael Parfitt, director of the Bone and Mineral Research Laboratory, Henry Ford Hospital, Detroit, Michigan, discussed the physiology of osteoporosis in April 1984, at the National Institutes of Health (NIH) Conference. He stated that while bone is continually being absorbed and formed, peak bone mass occurs at about 35 years of age. After 35, the balance begins to tip and age-related bone loss begins. Postmenopausal white women are at the highest risk. Women begin their lives with 30% less bone mass than men, and white people have 10% less than black people. Early menopause has been cited as the strongest prediction of osteoporosis. It is believed that low calcium intake may contribute to the problem. In 1984, panel members at the NIH Conference favored an increase in the recommended daily allowance of calcium from 800 mg to 1000–1500 mg (one glass of milk contains 275 mg of calcium). The panel cautioned against intake exceeding their recommendations because of the danger of developing renal calculi.

The recommendation of the NIH panel became public information. Along with this medical news came the onslaught of calcium products whose manufacturers promised prevention of osteoporosis with the regular intake of their own calcium supplements. Even food products, such as Total cereal, Citrus Hill orange juice, Breyer's yogurt, and Calcimilk, enjoyed the advertising promotions touting the high calcium content of their foods. Sales of calcium products soared from $18 million in 1980 to $240 million in 1986. Calcium fever continues to afflict Americans, particularly women. In the spring of 1987, the NIH became concerned about the commercial hype and reiterated its earlier counsel on daily intake. Dr. William Peck of Washington University cautioned that "calcium is not a panacea for osteoporosis. The ads promise more than calcium can deliver."

The fact remains that both the disease and the role of calcium are poorly understood. It is known that calcium cannot prevent osteoporosis after menopause. Extra calcium had little or no effect in slowing bone loss in menopausal women—even when the dosage was as high as 3000 mg per day. The most effective defense against osteoporosis in women, the NIH suggests, is estrogen replacement.

Regarding calcium supplement before menopause, researchers suggest that strong, healthy bone formation during youth is the strongest defense. Although calcium does help build bone and retain it, it is simply one factor in lifelong skeletal health. Exercise, such as walking, seems to be another significant factor in the prevention of osteoporosis.

In the final analysis, NIH continues to support its recommendations for the intake of calcium in the dosage previously advised but emphasizes that osteoporosis can be prevented in premenopausal women by total lifestyle modifications—not by overdosing on calcium.

*S*pecific Physical Examinations and Clinical Procedures: Part II

> Every vice, bad habit or indulgence, which weakens and debilitates the constitution, must be abandoned as inimical to recovery from consumption, such as the habitual use of tobacco, tea, coffee, etc.
>
> H. R. Burner, MD
> Lectures on How to Acquire
> and Preserve Health

CHAPTER OUTLINE

*S*pecific Physical Examinations and Clinical Procedures: Part II

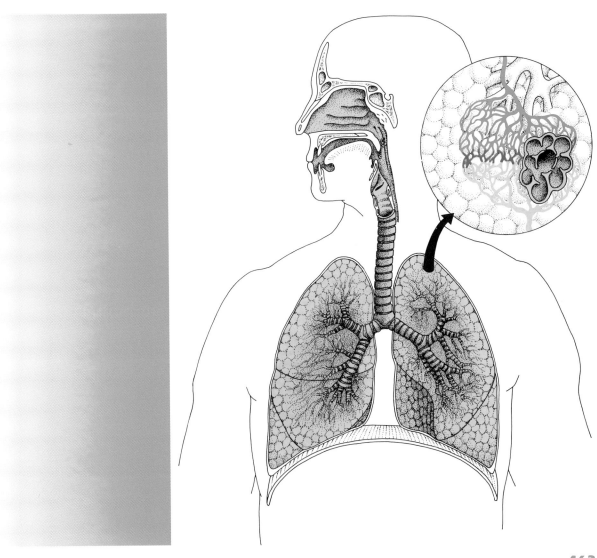

LEARNING OBJECTIVES

Upon completing this chapter, you will be able to:

1. Describe the basic structure and function of each anatomical system.
2. Identify the body's symptomatic reaction to disease in each specified system.
3. List and define diagnostic studies related to each system and individual body part specified.
4. List the common diseases related to each system.
5. Describe the process of each specific physical examination.
6. Describe the medical assistant's role in preparation of the room and the patient for the examinations, treatments, and procedures discussed in this chapter.
7. Provide instruction for the patient's office experiences and follow-up care.
8. Explain and discuss the principles of specific procedures.

PERFORMANCE OBJECTIVES

Upon completing this chapter, you will be able to:

1. Introduce medication directly into the nasal cavity to relieve pain, increase or decrease drainage, control nasal bleeding, or serve as an antiseptic application.
2. Irrigate the nasal cavity to relieve inflammation, increase drainage, or remove foreign bodies.
3. Instruct the patients to obtain a clear-catch urine specimen that will not be contaminated by bacteria.
4. Measure the head circumference of an infant or child.

DACUM EDUCATIONAL COMPONENTS

1. Prepare examination and treatment area (4.5).
2. Prepare patients for examinations and diagnostic procedures and instruct patients on at-home care (4.7).
3. Assist the physician with examinations and treatments (4.8).
4. Perform routine diagnostic tests (4.11).
5. Administer specified medications (4.13).
6. Maintain patient medication records, and prepare and maintain medical records (4.14).
7. Document accurately (5.1).
8. Maintain and use aseptic techniques (4.1).

Glossary

Alimentary canal: synonym for the digestive system
Alveolus (plural, alveoli): air cell of the lung
Body system: anatomically related structures that act in concert
Cilia: tiny specialized hairs in the nose that filter out foreign matter from the inhaled air
Congenital: present or existing at the time of birth
Dysmenorrhea: painful menstruation
Functional: affecting the function but not the structure of any part or organ
Functional disease: a disease affecting body function but having no known organic basis; self-originating; occurring without a known cause

Continued

Hematuria: urine containing blood
Normal flora: bacteria normally residing in an area
Organic disease: disease associated with a detectable organic lesion or change; due to or accompanied by structural changes in organs or tissues (as opposed to functional disease, see above)
Pacemaker: specialized cells in the heart that initiate cardiac activity
Perineal: pertaining to the area of pelvic outlet; obstetricians limit the term to the region between the anus and the vulva

This chapter continues the discussion of body systems and the medical assistant's role in assisting with special procedures begun in Chapter 20. The systems discussed are the respiratory system, the cardiovascular (CV) system, the gastrointestinal (GI) system, the urinary system, and the male and female reproductive systems. The final section of this chapter focuses on examination of the pediatric patient with emphasis on developmental stages and their behavioral characteristics. As in the previous chapter, the term *general clinical medical assisting techniques* refers to those techniques presented in Chapter 19.

THE RESPIRATORY SYSTEM

The function of the respiratory system is to exchange gases between the environment and body cells. The parts of the body involved in external respiration are the nose, pharynx, larynx, trachea, bronchi, and lung parenchyma (*alveoli*).

SYMPTOMATIC REACTION TO DISEASE

Inhaled air contains many microorganisms and allergy-producing particles. Specific organisms (*normal flora*) are present normally in the respiratory tree, but the invasion of disease-producing microorganisms leads to infection. Infection can easily spread throughout the respiratory system because of the numerous connecting structures. Common sites for upper respiratory infections are the nose, tonsils, adenoids, sinuses, and larynx.

Infections have both specific and general symptoms, depending on the causative organism. Most respiratory symptoms (Table 21–1) are associated with either poor gas exchange or obstruction. A simple cold can produce many symptoms of both. General symptoms of infection usually include both chills and fever, area redness, swelling, discharge, and pain. The patient describes these as nasal congestion, pain in the face or throat, difficulty in breathing, or difficult or painful swallowing. Yellow or greenish discharge usually dictates sinus infection; off-white discharge indicates the common cold; and clear discharge indicates allergy. Cough caused by excess drainage may be another symptom, as well as hoarseness resulting from laryngeal inflammation. As the infection progresses down the respiratory tree, the symptoms become more severe.

Table 21–1

COMMONLY SEEN SYMPTOMS IN PATIENTS WITH RESPIRATORY TRACT INFECTIONS

Fever (pyrexia)	Headache (cephalgia)
Shivering (chills)	Weakness, fatigue (malaise)
Pain—local or general	Rapid breathing (tachypnea)
Cough	Nosebleeds (epistaxis)
Discharge (catarrh)	Nasal congestion
Difficult breathing (dyspnea)	Watery eyes

Symptoms of noninfectious respiratory tract dysfunction occur because of structural or functional abnormalities or because of inflammatory processes. Older persons often show many of these symptoms. Because of decreased resistance, limited exercise, and inadequate diet, gerontologic patients often have an increased susceptibility to respiratory tract infections. Changes in the spinal curvature also can result in decreased lung capacity and poor lung expansion. The elderly are often easily overwhelmed by respiratory disease.

RESPIRATORY TRACT EXAMINATION AND THE MEDICAL ASSISTANT'S ROLE

The physician's examination of the respiratory tract usually begins with inspection of the face, nose, and throat and examination of the mucous membranes and visible respiratory system structures (Fig. 21–1). Although the ears are not a part of this system, they are usually examined because the eustachian tubes open into the pharynx. The medical assistant hands the otoscope with a short, wide nasal speculum, tongue depressor, penlight, and gauze sponges to the physician, and with the patient in a sitting position, the physician (with gloved hands) inspects the nose, sinuses, mouth, pharynx, salivary glands, and tonsils. The physician will request that the patient remove dentures to facilitate the examination. To examine ears and hearing, the physician will need an otoscope with earpieces (*specula*) that is a comfortable size for the patient and a tuning fork. The physician then inspects and palpates the neck muscles, cervical lymph nodes, thyroid, trachea, jugular veins, and carotid arteries. The medical assistant provides physical support as needed. The lymph nodes of the upper trunk are inspected. Breath sounds are auscultated with a stethoscope, and the skin, rib cage, and lungs are inspected, palpated, auscultated, and percussed. The medical assistant needs

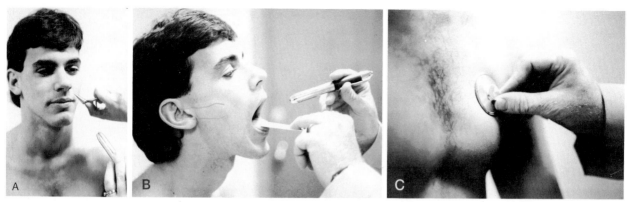

Figure 21–1. During a respiratory tract examination, the physician (**A**) inspects the sinuses and nasal passages, and (**B**) the throat, and (**C**) auscultates the lungs.

to drape the patient so only the area to be examined is exposed. The posterior chest and lungs are examined first, then the anterior chest and lungs. When the examination is over, the physician may discuss the findings in the examination room or may have the patient dress and go to another area. The medical assistant should assist the patient with dressing if necessary.

COMMON DIAGNOSTIC TESTS

The most commonly performed diagnostic test is the throat culture. Infections of the throat may be caused by viruses or bacteria. Most infections are viral, and these infections are not improved with antibiotic treatment. The throat culture can help determine if the infection is caused by one of several types of streptococci bacteria. Streptococcal infection, if not treated properly, can lead to such complications as rheumatic fever (arthritis and inflammation of the heart's inner lining) and nephritis (bleeding into the kidney and blood in the urine).

When the physician orders a throat culture, the medical assistant takes a specimen by swabbing the affected area of the patient's throat with a special applicator (Fig. 21–2). The specimen is sent to the medical laboratory for identification of any infectious organisms. The complete procedure for obtaining a throat culture is presented in Chapter 29.

The physician may request a sputum specimen to examine materials from the lung. To obtain a good specimen, it is important to have the patient cough deeply and expectorate the material from the lungs. Frequently, sputum specimens consist of saliva rather than lung expectorant. Unless the patient has a productive cough, a sputum specimen is difficult to obtain.

Radiography is used extensively to assist with diagnosis. The most commonly ordered studies are the chest x-ray and sinus x-ray. *Bronchography* involves the insertion of dye into the bronchi followed by x-ray.

Endoscopic procedures such as examination of the bronchi (*bronchoscopy*) and associated mediastinal examination (*mediastinography*) permit direct visualization. (The *mediastinum* is the mass of tissue and

organs, including the heart, that separates the two lungs.) Both procedures are done in an outpatient surgery facility. Bronchoscopy allows visualization of the entire respiratory tree using a flexible fiber-optic tube (*endoscope*) inserted through the mouth and windpipe into the bronchi. The procedure is done under local anesthesia. Mediastinography requires that a skin incision be made through which the endoscope is advanced into the mediastinum. Frequently, mediastinography requires a light general anesthesia. Both of these procedures are considered to be invasive and require that a written consent to treatment be signed by the patient.

Pulmonary function tests are noninvasive and are done using a spirometer. The *spirometer* is designed to measure and record inhalations and exhalations. The test results describe respiratory capacity and function. Patients with severe or chronic lung disease will often be referred to a pulmonary specialist for treatment.

The office manual should contain all the patient preparation instructions for all diagnostic tests ordered by the physician. Except for the sputum specimen and throat culture, the medical assistant is rarely required to collect other specimens.

COMMON DISEASES OF THE RESPIRATORY TRACT

Common respiratory tract diseases include sinusitis, tonsillitis, pharyngitis, laryngitis, otitis, bronchiolitis, tracheitis, pneumonitis, and pleuritis. Table 21–2 provides a comprehensive review of common diseases of the respiratory tract and the medical assistant's role. The medical assistant's role includes encouraging the patient to ask questions and providing the patient with teaching aids and community referrals as necessary.

SPECIFIC CLINICAL PROCEDURES

The medical assistant may be requested to perform nasal instillation, nasal irrigation, and the application of heat and cold. Irrigation of deeper structures such as the sinuses are always the physician's responsibility. The principles and procedures for nasal irrigation and

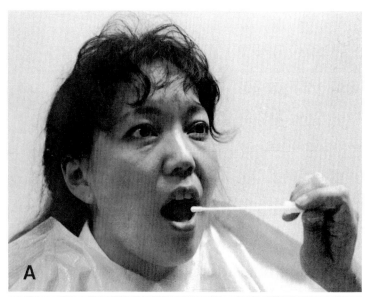

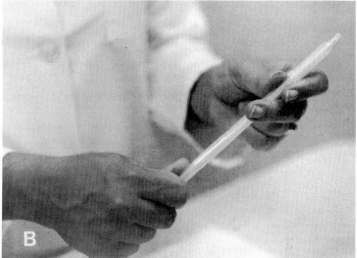

Figure 21-2. Obtaining a throat culture. (**A**) The medical assistant removes the culture stick from its sterile package and gently swabs the affected area of the patient's throat. (**B**) After swabbing, the medical assistant returns the culture stick to the sterile tube. Pressing firmly on the bottom of the tube releases a preservative that will keep microorganisms alive until the specimen reaches the laboratory.

instillation are delineated at the end of the chapter. Procedures and principles for the application of heat and cold are universal and are outlined in Chapter 20. If the treatment is to be continued at home, the medical assistant instructs the patient and provides the patient with written materials.

RESPIRATORY SYSTEM SPECIALTIES

The physician who has specialized education and training along with board certification in the diagnosis and treatment of respiratory disease may be referred to as a *pulmonologist* or *pulmonary specialist.* Surgeons specializing in the chest or lungs are called *thoracic surgeons.* Other respiratory specialists, referred to as *otorhinolaryngologists, otolaryngologists,* or ear, nose, and throat physicians, treat diseases of the ear, nose, and throat, but not the lungs. *Allergists* treat hypersensitivities manifested by respiratory or other symptoms.

The role of the medical assistant in the office of a respiratory specialist depends on the procedures done and equipment used. X-ray, audiometry, and spirometry equipment may be standard in the specialist's office. Medical assistants working in this type of office would build on and expand basic knowledge and specific skills required in clinical assisting.

THE CARDIOVASCULAR SYSTEM

The *CV system,* also called the *circulatory system,* transports oxygen and nutrients to the cells and carries away the cell waste products. The system consists of the heart and blood vessels.

The medical assistant must be able to visualize the position of the heart under the sternum and the ribs and know certain landmarks for electrocardiogram (ECG) lead placement and cardiopulmonary resuscitation. Additionally, the medical assistant takes and records a

Table 21-2
COMMON DISEASES OF THE RESPIRATORY TRACT

Disease	Symptoms	Treatment	Medical Assistant's Role
Acute rhinitis: inflammation of mucous membrane lining the nose that may be caused by viral infection (common cold) or by an allergic response (hay fever).	Sneezing, nasal discharge, tearing of eyes, headache.	Nonspecific treatment relieves symptoms rather than cures disease. Medication such as decongestants and analgesics (pain-relievers) may be ordered. Antibiotics cannot counteract virus. Antihistamines and desensitization if severe allergies.	Assist with examination; perform diagnostic tests if ordered; administer medication if ordered; patient teaching. Instruct patient to blow nose frequently but gently, keeping both nostrils open to prevent infected material from being blown into sinuses and eustachian tube, and into the middle ear. Patients with a common cold usually do not come to the office unless it has become chronic. When discharge is purulent (puslike) and yellowish or greenish in color, the patient should be instructed to be seen by the physician.
Sinusitis: inflammation of mucous membrane lining the sinuses (can become chronic).	Pain and tenderness over affected area. Facial headache with infection, fever, and malaise may be present.	Medication to relieve symptoms and antibiotics if bacterial infection is present. Local application of heat. Irrigation for increased drainage. Surgery is a last resort.	General clinical assisting procedures are performed. Nasal irrigation, instillation, or spray may be employed.
Pharyngitis (sore throat): inflammation of the throat caused by irritation or infection.	Pain, difficulty swallowing, red throat, fever.	Medication such as antibiotics, gargle, and analgesics.	General clinical assisting procedures are performed. In particular, obtain a throat culture if ordered.
Tonsillitis: inflammation of tonsils (adenoids may also be involved).	Symptoms same as pharyngitis, and exudate (pus) on tonsils.	Medication or surgery.	General clinical assisting procedures are performed. Patient teaching may be needed to prepare patient for surgery if indicated.
Laryngitis: inflammation of larynx (voice box) associated with infection or other disease, and vocal abuse.	Hoarseness, aphonia (loss of speech), cough, tightness in the throat, general symptoms of inflammation.	Inhalation of steam or medicated cool mist. Treatment differs depending on the cause. Antibiotics, warm mouth washes, voice rest.	General clinical assisting procedures. Patient teaching may include explanation of effects of steam or cool mist vaporizer. Patient should be instructed that the nozzle should be directed so the spray falls in a mist to be inhaled.

Continued

Table 21 – 2
COMMON DISEASES OF THE RESPIRATORY TRACT — *Continued*

Disease	Symptoms	Treatment	Medical Assistant's Role
Bronchitis: inflammation of the mucous membrane of the bronchi with increased mucus production (may become chronic).	Cough, usually worse in morning; general symptoms of inflammation.	Medication.	General clinical assisting procedures. In chronic bronchitis, prescription to stop smoking may be explained and progress managed by the medical assistant when indicated.
Pneumonia: infection localized in the lungs; can be bacterial or viral.	*Bacterial:* Symptoms of acute infection, fever, dyspnea (painful respirations), malaise, cough. *Viral:* Fever is usually present; dry hacking; cough initially less acute.	*Bacterial:* Antibiotics and other drugs to relieve symptoms. Hospitalization may be necessary. *Viral:* Nonspecific treatment, bedrest. Hospitalization may be necessary.	General clinical assisting procedures. Patient teaching includes instructing patient to cough into the tissue and dispose, to prevent the spread of disease. Obtain sputum for culture and sensitivity if ordered.
Emphysema: air spaces or alveoli become abnormally enlarged and less elastic.	Dyspnea, persistent cough, loss of weight.	Medication, postural drainage at outpatient facility, and physiotherapy (cannot be cured, only controlled). Respiratory therapist gives percussion and breathing treatments.	General clinical assisting procedures. Patient teaching includes explanation of need and procedure for mouth care as patient is usually a mouth breather. Dietary and exercise instructions should be given and fully explained. Give literature from the American Lung Association to help the patient stop smoking.

patient's pulse, which represents the rate of left ventricle contractions.

SYMPTOMATIC REACTION TO DISEASE

The five major symptoms associated with cardiovascular disease are chest pain, dyspnea, fatigue, irregular heartbeat, and peripheral circulation changes. Structural disturbances of the CV system include impairment of conduction of heart impulse, insufficiencies, insufficient blood circulation to the heart muscle or formations of blood clots in the coronary arteries, deterioration of the heart valves or chambers, interference with the movement of blood circulation, and inflammatory disease caused by bacteria. Functional diseases include a variety of congenital heart defects present at the time of birth.

Conditions related to heart disease produce symptoms of *dyspnea* (shortness of breath) on exertion, chest pain not relieved by medication, fatigue, irregular

heartbeat, and *edema* (swelling) in the extremities. Interference with blood circulation to heart muscle produces shortness of breath; chest pain that is substernal, crushing, and radiating to the left arm and jaw; *palpitations* (fluttering); irregular heartbeat; fatigue; and sometimes *cyanosis* (bluish tinge in nailbeds or around lips). In the adult, disease of the heart valves may produce dyspnea, fatigue, and occasionally palpitations. Chest pain is usually absent. Interferences with peripheral blood circulation present symptoms in the extremities, including aching pain, edema, ulcers that do not heal, pain that increases with walking and stops with rest (*claudication*), skin pigment changes, and the symptoms associated with inflammation (redness, swelling, and heat). Changes in peripheral veins, often caused by increased venous pressure, may produce dilated, twisted, and sclerosed veins called *varicose veins*. Table 21 – 3 lists symptoms and common diseases associated with the cardiovascular system and the medical assistant's role.

Table 21–3
COMMON DISEASES OF THE CARDIOVASCULAR SYSTEM

Disease	Symptoms	Treatment	Medical Assistant's Role
Hypertension (high blood pressure [BP]). Major cause of cerebrovascular accident, heart disease, left ventricular hypertrophy, renal failure.	Systolic blood pressure above 140, diastolic above 90. Headache, nervousness, vertigo (dizziness). (Usually no symptoms are present until vascular, kidney, and cerebral changes occur.)	Drug therapy, diet therapy. For essential hypertension without known cause: low-salt diet, weight loss, exercise, relaxation, antihypertensive drugs. For secondary hypertension, treat the cause.	General clinical medical assisting procedures. In patients with hypertension, patient teaching is extremely important. With the physician's approval, lifestyle patterns may need to be worked out with the patient. Stressing the importance of daily medication is essential as patients are reluctant to take medication when no symptoms are present. Diet instruction and planning per orders. Get a food list and handouts from the American Heart Association. Get lists of low-salt foods. Provide reading on relaxation techniques.
Varicose veins (dilated, knotted, and prominent veins).	Feeling of heaviness and weakness in lower legs; aching muscles of legs, especially after standing; edema.	Conservative measures such as avoiding sitting or standing for long periods may be recommended. Ace wraps, warm soaks. Surgery is another alternative.	General clinical medical assisting procedures. Patient teaching would include instructions such as how to wrap an Ace bandage, recommendation of elastic stockings, and other precautions as the physician dictates. No constrictive clothes. Elevate legs when possible.
Thrombophlebitis (blood clot in vein accompanied by inflammation). Phlebothrombosis (clot in vein without inflammation).	Pain, warmth, redness, swelling if superficial. Deep vein: severe pain, cyanosis, chills, fever, edema.	Drug therapy, surgery. Medical: bedrest, warm compresses, analgesics, antiembolism stockings, anticoagulants.	General clinical medical assisting procedures. Teach patient how to use warm compresses, how to measure extremities, leg elevation. Reinforce need for rest.
Buerger's disease. Thromboangitis obliterans. Inflammation and occlusion.	Intermittent claudication, blanching extremities; first cold then hot.	Exercise program, stay in temperate areas, lumbar sympathectomy, amputation.	Medical assistant must reinforce the need to reduce stress, stop smoking, and proper care of extremities.
Cerebral vascular accident: arteries of brain receive reduced blood supply (several causes).	Headaches, feeling of fullness in the head, vertigo. Could result in paralysis of part or side of body and coma. Short attacks of	Objective is restoration and rehabilitation after the acute phase is over. Involves physical, speech, occupational, and other therapies.	Medical assistant needs to be alerted to the possibility when screening patients over the phone with symptoms of severe

Continued

Table 21-3
COMMON DISEASES OF THE CARDIOVASCULAR SYSTEM—*Continued*

Disease	Symptoms	Treatment	Medical Assistant's Role
	blackouts, blocking of visual field.		headache, etc., that this may be an emergency condition.
Coronary artery disease. Arteriosclerosis (narrowing of arteries by lime deposits) or atherosclerosis (narrowing of arteries by fatty deposits).	Angina pectoris: pain under sternum (may spread down left shoulder). Pain can range from discomfort to severe squeezing pain. Results from decreased blood flow to myocardium.	Drug therapy includes sublingual or transdermal patches of nitroglycerin. Surgery may be angioplasty or bypass.	General clinical medical assisting procedures after the acute phase. Reinforce patient teaching regarding low-salt and low-fat diet, weight control, prescribed exercise program, decrease stressors, repeated visits for blood tests and evaluation, and drug compliance. Provide literature from American Heart Association for all patients.
Myocardial infarction (MI; heart attack): heart tissue death from inadequate blood supply; coronary artery is occluded.	Severe vise-like pain under sternum may radiate down left arm into jaw and shoulder. May start as anginal pain and accelerate. Patient presents with ashen face, diaphoresis, dyspnea, arms holding chest, increased pulse.	Drug therapy: treatment specific to individual condition and type and amount of tissue damage. The postacute phase is directed at rehabilitation.	Medical assistant must be alerted to all patients complaining of chest pain. Post-MI office visits require scheduling of examinations, electrocardiogram (ECG), stress testing, coronary follow-up care programs, promoting compliance with diet, drugs, exercise and other prescribed programs. The medical assistant should provide positive feedback and support.
Congestive heart failure: heart pump dysfunction; fluid collects in tissues and lungs.	Symptoms are dependent on which side of heart is affected. Left: fatigue, dyspnea, orthopnea. Right: peripheral edema, fatigue, neck vein distention.	Drug therapy, including cardiotonics, digoxin, and diuretics (Lasix). Bedrest, antiembolism stockings, low-salt diet.	General clinical medical assisting procedures for examination. Provide literature, assist patient by discussing methods of compliance with diet, potassium supplements and foods, low-salt foods, regular checkups. Put instructions and guidelines in writing.
Infection of the heart: endocarditis, myocarditis, pericarditis, rheumatic heart disease.	General and specific symptoms of inflammation. Nonspecific include, dyspnea, fatigue, palpitations, diffuse chest pain, joint pain.	Specific to location of infection. Bedrest, antibiotics, possible pericardial tap to remove fluid in hospital.	General clinical medical assisting procedures. Patients who are not hospitalized need encouragement and reassurance that help is available. Schedule them for frequent evaluation. Encourage questions.

Continued

Table 21–3
COMMON DISEASES OF THE CARDIOVASCULAR SYSTEM—*Continued*

Disease	Symptoms	Treatment	Medical Assistant's Role
Dysrhythmias: Inability of the heart to empty properly; can be life threatening.			
Sinus arrhythmia	Normally present in young children and infants. Pulse quickness at peak of inspiration, then decreases during expiration.	None	Dysrhythmias with pulse deficit must be reported immediately. Visits require scheduling of examination, ECG, BP, ambulatory ECG, coronary care follow-up programs, promoting compliance.
Sinus tachycardia	Rhythm regular, but rate 100+ beats/min caused by exercise, stress, stimulants, or heat abnormalities. Considered normal under 100 beats/min.	Digitalis preparations if the effect of the condition on cardiac output is negative; otherwise treatment is directed to the cause. With diet, drugs, exercise, and other prescribed programs.	The medical assistant should provide positive feedback and support.
Sinus bradycardia	Rhythm regular, but rate 40–60 beats/min. Common in athletes. May be caused by drug therapy.	Drug therapy: drugs that stimulate and accelerate heart rate. Pacemaker.	
Premature ventricular contractions	Rhythm irregular; caused by abnormal electrical conduction. It is the most common dysrhythmia accompanying other acute forms of heart disease and electrolyte instability.	Drug therapy: treatment specific to individual condition and type of acute care management. Postacute phase is directed to treatment of the initial cause.	

CARDIOVASCULAR EXAMINATION AND THE MEDICAL ASSISTANT'S ROLE

The physician usually begins the examination of the circulatory system by listening to the heart with a stethoscope, noting heart sounds, rate, and rhythm.

The physician also uses percussion, inspection, and palpation. Palpation of the heart and chest wall is performed to detect vibrations produced by *murmurs* (sounds other than normal heart sounds). Percussion, although more infrequently used, helps to detect areas of dullness outlining the heart and is helpful in the determination of cardiac enlargement.

The vessels in the extremities are also inspected, auscultated, and palpated, noting the symmetry of pulses as well as skin color and temperature and the presence of any edema.

The method for examination of the CV system is presented in Table 21–4. The medical assistant's role consists of maintaining a quiet environment for examination, draping the patient for examination of the heart,

providing physical support for painful extremities, and offering emotional support. The medical assistant should be prepared to assist with an ECG or *Doppler ultrasound* (a noninvasive ultrasound test used to detect blood flow). Patients with ulcers due to peripheral vascular disease that need dressings will require the medical assistant to prepare dressing materials necessary for sterile dressing application. Patients with possible heart problems have a great deal of anxiety about their conditions and the potential changes in their lifestyles. They need encouragement to ask questions and discuss fears.

COMMON DIAGNOSTIC TESTS

There are several diagnostic tests associated with the CV system. In addition to the electrocardiogram or Doppler ultrasound, x-ray, blood tests, *Holter monitoring* (ambulatory ECG monitoring), stress testing, echocardiography, nuclear scanning, arteriography, cardiac

Table 21-4

EXAMINATION OF THE CARDIOVASCULAR SYSTEM

Examination	Methods and Equipment	Medical A
Heart	Inspection, palpation, percussion, auscultation with stethoscope.	Position, c physicia
Arteries of trunk and head	Inspection, palpation of carotid arteries, venous pressure, auscultation with stethoscope, and blood pressure (BP) readings with BP apparatus and stethoscope.	Hand phy patient to change p... necessary. Take vital signs as requested by physician.
Peripheral vascular system (arteries which supply arms and legs, veins in the extremities and the lymphatic system)	Palpation of pulses in arms and legs; inspection of extremities; palpation of lymph nodes.	Place patient in supine position and assist in exposing extremities.
Presence of varicosities	Inspection of backs of calves; palpation.	Assist patient to standing position. Help patients reduce unnecessary exposure to ensure privacy. Redrape and assist to sitting position when examination is completed.

catheterization, angiography, and angiocardiography may be ordered. These and other tests are described in Table 21-5. The medical assistant should become familiar with these procedures and should include this information in the office procedure manual for future reference. Refer to the chapter on radiography for an explanation of radiologic examinations.

COMMON DISEASES OF THE CARDIOVASCULAR SYSTEM

The medical assistant should be familiar with the most common diseases associated with the CV system. These include hypertension, coronary artery disease, myocardial infarction, and congestive heart failure. These and other cardiovascular disorders, together with their symptoms and treatment, were presented in Table 21-3.

SPECIFIC CLINICAL PROCEDURES

The special clinical procedures related to cardiology for which the medical assistant assumes responsibility include obtaining the blood pressure and pulse measurements. (See Chapter 17.)

The medical assistant is also responsible for performing the ECG. This diagnostic study is discussed in Chapter 31.

CARDIOVASCULAR SPECIALTIES

The *cardiologist* is a physician trained in the treatment of heart diseases and dysfunctions. The cardiolo-

gist usually limits his or her practice to the examination, diagnosis, and medical treatment of the heart. Cardiac surgery is performed by a *cardiovascular surgeon* with special cardiac and vascular surgical training and board certification.

The medical assistant in the cardiologist's office may perform the ECG and assist with stress tests at the physician's direction. Patient teaching is an important responsibility as patients are often enrolled in postcoronary education programs. The medical assistant may answer questions in the areas of home management, medication scheduling, diet, exercise, and overall lifestyle. The medical assistant provides literature from the American Heart Association and encourages patients to become informed managers of their self-care program.

THE GASTROINTESTINAL SYSTEM

The *GI system*, also known as the *digestive system* or *alimentary canal*, is a long hollow tube with accessory organs and glands.

The organs of the system combine to perform the ingestion of food, mechanical digestion (moving the food through the system in wavelike contractions called *peristalsis*) and chemical digestion, the absorption of nutrients into the bloodstream, and the removal of waste materials. A more detailed assessment of the patient's nutritional status is discussed in Chapter 22.

SYMPTOMATIC REACTION TO DISEASE

The symptoms and reactions of the GI system to disease encompass variations of six major symptoms:

Table 21–5

COMMON DIAGNOSTIC STUDIES OF THE HEART

Test	Description
Electrocardiogram (ECG): (called a stress test when measured while the patient is actively exercised)	Graphic measurement of the electrical currents produced by contraction of heart muscles. Electrodes are placed in certain areas over the heart and vessels to detect abnormalities in heart function. The medical assistant can perform the ECG in the office. In the hospital, the ECG is performed by the ECG technician, and a computer often is available to assist with reading. Primary tool for cardiac evaluation.
X-ray and fluoroscopic examination	X-ray of the heart will present the heart's configuration. Fluoroscopic examination is x-ray of the heart as it is functioning. Reveals cardiac enlargement and aortic dilation.
Angiocardiography	An opaque dye is injected into a major blood vessel and an x-ray examination performed as the dye flows through the heart, lungs, and major vessels. This procedure is performed in the hospital, and special preparation of the patient is required.
Coronary arteriography	A long catheter (hollow plastic tube) is passed through an artery and into the heart. Opaque dye is injected through the catheter. Visualization through x-ray of the dye flowing through the coronary arteries is achieved. This procedure is performed in the hospital, and the patient requires special preparation.
Cardiac catheterization	A catheter is inserted into a vein in the arm and passed into the heart. Blood samples can be extracted for gas content analysis, and the amount of pressure in the heart's chambers is measured. This procedure is performed in the hospital, and the patient requires special preparation.
Aortography	X-ray study of the aorta. This study involves the same routine and particulars as those tests previously discussed.
Radiocardiography	Radioactive isotopes are injected into the bloodstream intravenously. Their course and the timing of their arrival at the heart are measured with a special counter. This procedure is performed in the hospital, and the patient requires special preparation.
Central venous pressure	A catheter is inserted into the vena cava or right atrium and is attached to a measuring device that detects the amount of pressure exerted by the blood in the catheter. This procedure is done only in the hospital.
Circulation time	A bitter substance is injected intravenously. The time it takes for this substance to be tasted is recorded. (Also called the "arm-to-tongue" test.)
Medical technology laboratory procedures	Blood serum tests, enzymes, and isoenzymes that indicate cardiac muscle damage. Examples are lactic dehydrogenase and creatine phosphokinase.
Echocardiography	Echoes obtained by ultrasound which are recorded on paper and used to evaluate the inner structures of the heart.
Phonocardiography	Graphically records the cardiac cycle sounds as heard through a stethoscope.

pain, nausea and vomiting, difficulty swallowing (*dysphagia*), constipation or diarrhea, fullness or bloating, and bleeding. In the upper tract, symptoms can include painful mouth sores, *indigestion* (burning sensation below the breast bone), belching (*eructation*), nausea and vomiting, and pain in the *epigastric* (upper and middle) region. Lower tract symptoms can be unlocalized pain, bloating, constipation, diarrhea, gas (*flatulence*), and bleeding. Bleeding can occur anywhere along the GI tract. Upper GI bleeding is expelled either in vomit or in stool, giving the stool a dark, tarry appearance. The lower the source of bleeding in the GI tract, the brighter the blood contained in the stool. Pain in the GI tract is either general and cannot be located or referred pain. *Referred pain* is pain the patient feels in an area different than its point of origin.

GASTROINTESTINAL TRACT EXAMINATION AND THE MEDICAL ASSISTANT'S ROLE

The GI examination includes direct examination of the abdomen and rectum. The physician examines the abdomen using standardized anatomic landmarks called *quadrants* (Fig. 21–3). The abdomen is generally divided into four main sections by imaginary lines that cross over the *umbilicus* (naval or belly button). These divisions are referred to as right upper quadrant, right lower quadrant, left upper quadrant, and left lower quadrant. Another descriptive approach divides the abdomen into nine regions (see Fig. 21–3). Any of these methods of description may be used by the medical assistant in charting the area of the patient's symptoms, the physician's findings, and procedures performed.

Other structures that are examined in a GI examination are the stomach, liver, pancreas, gallbladder, small and large intestines, and appendix. Major blood vessels that descend through the abdomen to the extremities may also be examined. The medical assistant's role in assisting with examination of the GI tract is explained in Table 21–6. The examination concludes with the rectal examination. The anus and perianal region is inspected for inflammation, lesions, ulcerations, or intestinal bulges. The internal anal canal and rectum are palpated with a gloved hand for masses, nodules, or tenderness. In men, the prostate gland is palpated. Any fecal material on the glove after the finger is withdrawn is tested for occult blood.

COMMON DIAGNOSTIC TESTS

The most common tests involving the GI system include analysis of gastric contents; examination of stool specimens for blood or parasites; radiologic examinations and procedures; and direct endoscopic visualization of the esophagus, stomach, colon, or rectum. The medical assistant should be familiar with the procedures that are explained in Table 21–7. Occasionally, the medical assistant may need to instruct the patient to bring a stool specimen from home.

COMMON DISEASES OF THE GASTROINTESTINAL SYSTEM

Although many diseases affect the GI system, the most common include stomatitis, peptic ulcer, gastritis, colitis, and hemorrhoids. These and other common conditions are discussed in Table 21–8, along with the medical assistant's role. Since many GI symptoms are similar to those produced by other systems, the medical assistant should be prepared to deviate from the expected GI examination.

SPECIFIC CLINICAL PROCEDURES

The most common GI procedures are the proctoscopy and sigmoidoscopy examination. These examinations provide for direct visualization of the rectal and sigmoid mucosa. Their purpose is to locate growths and identify tissue changes. Refer to Table 21–6 to review the medical assistant's role.

The medical assistant may teach the patient how to collect a stool specimen or may assist the patient while in the office.

Special clinical procedures done in the office of a proctologist require special instruments and equipment. For the proctologic examination, a table with jack-knife capability is required to raise the buttocks and lower the head for adequate visualization of the lower tract. The patient lies prone on the table and then adjusts his or her position to the jack-knife contour while the table is adjusted to accommodate this position. Figure 21–4 shows the proctologic table and some proctologic instruments.

GASTROINTESTINAL SPECIALTIES

A *gastroenterologist* is a physician who specializes in diseases of the entire GI tract, whereas a *proctologist* is a physician who concentrates only in disorders of the anus and rectum. Medical assistants in these offices are usually involved with the care of patients during postoperative visits. Patient teaching, preparing patients for surgery, and scheduling diagnostic studies are all routine activities.

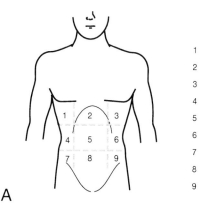

1	Right hypochondriac
2	Epigastric
3	Left hypochondriac
4	Right flank
5	Umbilical
6	Left flank
7	Right inguinal
8	Suprapubic
9	Left inguinal

A

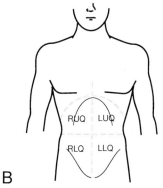

RUQ = right upper quadrant,
LUQ = left upper quadrant,
RLQ = right lower quadrant,
LLQ = left lower quadrant.

B

Figure 21–3. (**A**) Regions of the abdomen. (**B**) Quadrants of the abdomen.

Table 21-6

EXAMINATION OF THE GASTROINTESTINAL TRACT

Body Part	Method and Equipment	Medical Assistant's Role
Mouth, including the lips, oral cavity, and tongue.	Inspection for inflammation, infections, deformities that interfere with functions. Local swelling, redness, pain, loose teeth, ulcers of gum, tongue and mucous membrane, painful speech. Flashlight, tongue blade, culture and smear materials, clean rubber gloves.	General clinical medical assisting procedures. Prepare equipment and hand instruments as necessary. Provide instructions regarding mouth care with soft or liquid diet, mouth rinses. Reinforce physician's instructions.
All regions of the abdomen and lower thorax.	For all regions to be examined, the following methods are used: inspection, palpation, percussion, auscultation with stethoscope. Physician notes size, shape, contour, and appearance. Palpation notes rebound tenderness, guarding, masses, muscle tone, liver size, uterus. Auscultate for bowel sounds. Usually examines symptomatic quadrant last.	Instruct patient before examination to empty bladder. Assist patient to assume supine position and place a small pillow under his head for comfort. Instruct patient to fold arms across chest or preferably extended at side. For abdominal area, pull gown up to midriff and fold under the breast line. Pull drape sheet to suprapubic edge and fold over the pubic area. Hand physician stethoscope. Warming the diaphragm in the palm of the hands increases patient comfort. Flex knees to prevent abdominal tensing.
Rectum (In addition to the detection of abnormalities or disease of the rectum, general rectal examination can detect uterine displacement in the female, and prostatic enlargement and texture change in the male.)	Glove, lubricant, sponge forceps, sponges, rectal speculum or anoscope, applicator, culture material. The physician inserts a gloved, lubricated finger in the rectum. An anoscope or speculum may be used for visualization. Sponge forceps and sponges may be used to absorb bleeding or discharge. If a culture is required, the applicator is inserted to obtain a smear.	Instruct patient to put on a full gown. Drape and position properly. (Jack-knife or left side-lying position.) Remain with the patient during examination. Attend to patient's comfort by recommending relaxation breathing.
Rectum and lower sigmoid colon	Sigmoidoscope with obturator or proctoscope with obturator, transilluminators, rheostat, insufflator with bulb attachment, suction machine with suction tip, biopsy forceps (sterile), rubber gloves, rectal dressing forceps, gauze (4 × 4), lubricant, specimen materials.	Instruct patient to take the prescribed laxative the night before the examination and to have only liquids for breakfast on the morning of the test. Administer cleansing enemas immediately before the examination to rid the bowel of its contents and facilitate visualization. Position and drape the patient and attend to comfort needs. Remain with the patient during the examination. If a specimen is obtained, handle and process properly. (The physician may expect the medical assistant to attach the light source to the scope and hand the instruments. The medical assistant is also responsible for cleanup and instrument care.)

Table 21-7
DIAGNOSTIC TESTS OF THE GASTROINTESTINAL SYSTEM

Gastric analysis	Gastric contents are analyzed after being collected through a nasogastric tube. The tube is passed through the mouth and into the stomach by a nurse or physician in the hospital.
Stool specimen	Bowel movement sampling is collected by the medical assistant if the patient is in the office and then sent to the hospital laboratory for examination to detect the presence of blood. Provide dietary instructions before test for blood contained in stool.
Endoscopy (esophagoscopy and gastroscopy)	Visualization of an area of the upper gastrointestinal (GI) tract by passing a tube with a lighted instrument through the mouth and down into the stomach or area to be inspected. Specimens for microscopic study can also be obtained. Requires hospitalization and special patient preparation.
GI series	X-ray examination of the upper tract (barium swallow) and the lower tract (barium enema) employs a chalklike opaque substance introduced into the system for visualization of the tract outline. Performed in the hospital x-ray laboratory or special outpatient facility. (See Chapter 32.)
Anoscopy, proctoscopy, sigmoidoscopy	Special examination procedures performed by the physician to visualize the mucous membrane of the sigmoid, anus, and rectum. Special instruments are required.

Table 21-8
COMMON DISEASES OF THE GASTROINTESTINAL SYSTEM

Disease	Symptoms	Treatment	Medical Assistant's Role
Stomatitis, herpatic or aphthous (canker).	Sore gums and inner mucous membrane, burning, swelling, ulcers.	Mouth rinses, bland diet, topical anesthetic.	Assist with general examination. Enhance teachings related to decreasing stress, anxiety, fatigue, and irritating foods.
Gastroesophageal reflux: back flow of gastric juices into esophagus.	Initially no symptoms. Heartburn, may mimic angina, dysphagia.	Antacids, sit upright and positional eating, small meals. Rarely surgery required.	Teach patient to relieve by gravity, sleeping with head elevated. Take medications as ordered.
Hiatal hernia: diaphragm defect allows stomach to pass into thorax.	Initially no symptoms or as in reflux, a fullness in chest and dysphagia. Pain in severe nonreversing hernia.	Relieve symptoms with gravity, exercise, drug therapy, diet and eating pattern changes. Surgery a last resort.	Teach patient to avoid bending, coughing, straining; to modify diet to soft foods and small meals; not to eat 3 h before bedtime. No smoking, weight control, and medication compliance.
Peptic ulcer: eroded area of mucosa of upper gastrointestinal tract.	Painful, aching, burning, gnawing, or cramping sensations near to midline region under and to the left side of the sternum. Symptoms occur approximately 2 h after ingestion of food.	Drug therapy, diet therapy, surgery. Stress reduction techniques. Occasional recommendation for counseling. Stop smoking, decrease spicy and other irritating foods.	General clinical medical assisting procedures. The medical assistant should be alert to emergency conditions with any ulcer: perforation and hemorrhage. With perforation, there is sudden severe pain with nausea and vomiting. Hemorrhage will produce hematemesis (bloody vomitus), bloody stools, tarry stools, and symptoms of

Continued

Table 21–8
COMMON DISEASES OF THE GASTROINTESTINAL SYSTEM—*Continued*

Disease	Symptoms	Treatment	Medical Assistant's Role
			shock. Patient teaching in diet instruction and avoidance of stimulants may be required.
Gastritis: inflammation of the mucous membrane lining of the stomach.	Eructation, bloating, gastric discomfort.	Drug and diet therapies.	General clinical medical assisting. If requested, may need to assist with gastric lavage to obtain a sample of gastric juices (rare).
Appendicitis: inflammation of appendage attached to the colon. The appendix has no known physiologic use.	Generalized abdominal pain or localized in the lower quadrant, with fever, nausea, and vomiting.	Surgery (appendectomy).	Emergency scheduling of patient for surgery if seen in the office.
Colitis: inflammation of the colon; can be an ulceration (area of erosion).	Abdominal pain or cramping; frequent loose stools (diarrhea can contain pus, muscus, blood); malaise; weight loss; fever; recurrent bloody diarrhea.	Diet and drug therapy; psychotherapy if indicated. Surgery if indicated (ileostomy or colostomy).	General clinical medical assisting procedures. If patient passes stools during visit, instruct patient not to flush toilet so that stools may be inspected.
Spastic colitis	Alternating abdominal cramps and diarrhea with constipation.	Diet therapy to avoid food intolerances. Avoid stress. Relaxation necessary. Annual sigmoidoscopy.	Patient instruction to support diet restrictions, avoid caffeine, and literature for relaxation techniques.
Abdominal hernia: weakness in abdominal wall with outpouching.	Patient usually notices herniation, or it may be detected during routine examination.	Surgical repair.	General clinical medical assisting procedures. Medical assistant should be alert for severe inguinal or umbilical pain in area of hernia, which signals strangulated hernia (inadequate blood supply to part).
Hemorrhoids: dilatation of the veins in the anal canal or rectum; may protrude through the anus.	Anal itching; discomfort; bright red blood present upon defecation.	Diet therapy; surgery (hermorrhoidectomy).	General clinical medical assisting procedures. Explanation of preoperative and postoperative care.
Anal fissure: an ulcerated crevice in the anal wall. Fistula: an abnormal canal leading from the anus or rectum.	Pain and burning on defecation.	Nonspecific; surgery if indicated.	General clinical medical assisting procedures.

Proctologic table

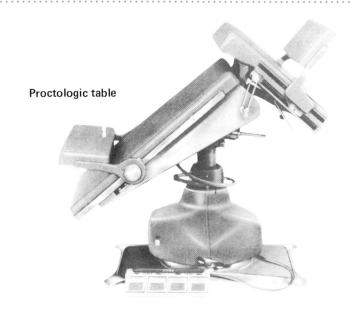

Proctoscope

Anoscope

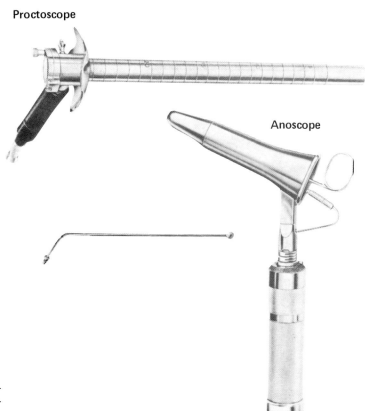

Figure 21–4. Proctologic table and instruments. (Courtesy of General Medical Corporation.)

THE URINARY SYSTEM

The urinary system helps regulate fluid and electrolyte balance and removes waste products of protein metabolism (*urea*) from the blood. All the body systems depend on the urinary system to maintain homeostasis.

SYMPTOMATIC REACTION TO DISEASE

Many of the genitourinary (GU) symptoms (Table 21–9) are similar and require testing to reach a definitive diagnosis. Inflammation may present symptoms such as burning while urinating, *nocturia* (voiding at night), polyuria (excessive urination), *dysuria* (painful

Table 21–9
SYMPTOMS ASSOCIATED WITH URINARY TRACT DISEASE

Output changes: polyuria, oliguria, nocturia.
Voiding pattern changes: frequency, urgency, nocturia.
Urine color changes: red, gray, black, green; diet and medications may cause expected color changes.
Pain: flank, lumbar, colic (spasm), burning, tenderness.

urination), *hematuria* (blood in urine), abnormal urine colors, and scanty urine (*oliguria*). Pain in the lumbar region or flank indicates that swelling is present.

EXAMINATION OF THE URINARY TRACT AND THE MEDICAL ASSISTANT'S ROLE

Since direct examination of the urinary tract is impossible without the use of invasive procedures, the physician's evaluation is based on the patient's symptoms and laboratory test results. If further data is needed, direct visualization of the urinary tract via cystoscopy or radiography is done.

The most common laboratory test performed as part of the physical examination is urinalysis. The medical assistant is responsible for obtaining the specimen. The physician may also order blood chemistry tests to obtain further data. The medical assistant must be prepared to perform venipuncture for specific tests as described in Chapter 28. The medical assistant should prepare patients for these office diagnostic tests by explaining the purpose and procedure. The physician uses all test results in conjunction with other collected data to form the diagnosis and initiate the treatment plan. When the physician requires even further data for making or confirming a diagnosis, the medical assistant will arrange for a patient appointment at other health care facilities, such as a radiology center or a specialist's office.

COMMON DIAGNOSTIC TESTS

Several different tests are associated with the urinary system, including urine tests (*urinalysis* and *urine culture*), x-ray tests (*pyelogram* and *cystoscopy*), x-ray studies of the kidneys, ureters, and bladder, blood tests, ultrasound studies, computed tomography of the kidney, and renal biopsy. The medical assistant should be familiar with each of these tests (Table 21–10). A complete list of diagnostic studies, along with comprehensive instructions for patient preparation and scheduling requirements, should be maintained in the office procedure manual.

COMMON DISEASES OF THE URINARY TRACT

The most commonly encountered diseases of the urinary system include infection of the bladder, inflamma-

tion of the kidney, and kidney stones. These are presented in Table 21–11, along with their symptoms, treatment procedures, and the medical assistant's role.

SPECIFIC CLINICAL PROCEDURES

The medical assistant must frequently teach patients procedures related to the collection of urine specimens. In the office setting, the patient may be instructed in how to obtain a specimen or how to bring the specimen from home. A commonly obtained specimen in the office is the *clean-catch urine specimen* (see procedure at end of chapter). Other types of urine specimens include:

1. *Spot.* Collected at any time of day in a clean container.

Table 21–10
COMMON DIAGNOSTIC STUDIES OF THE URINARY SYSTEM

Test	Description
Urinalysis	Laboratory analysis of urine, consisting of physical, chemical, and microscopic examination. Medical assistants can perform the test in the medical office if facilities and equipment are available.
Urine culture	Bacterial analysis. May also be performed in the office. Requires special training and equipment.
Pyelogram	X-ray examination using an opaque dye for visualization. Dye may be injected into the patient's vein (intravenous pyelogram), or the physician may insert a small catheter into the urethra through a cystoscope (retrograde pyelogram) and inject the dye through these catheters.
Cystoscopy	Examination of the bladder by visualization and inspection using a special instrument. The walls of the bladder and urethra can be examined. Special preparation and scheduling are necessary.
Kidney function	Various tests which determine normal kidney function: determination of waste removal capability in certain lengths of time. Special patient preparation and scheduling are necessary.
Blood chemistry studies	Medical technology study of blood substances that determines whether or not waste products are being removed from the blood stream.
Radiorenography	Dye injected as with pyelography but tagged with radioactive dye. Special patient preparation and scheduling are necessary.

Table 21–11

COMMON DISEASES OF THE URINARY TRACT

Disease	Symptoms	Treatment	Medical Assistant's Role
Cystitis: infection of the bladder.	Urgency and frequency of burning, painful urination (dysuria); bleeding may occur (hematuria); scant voiding (oliguria).	Drug therapy; antibiotics; increased fluid intake.	General clinical medical assisting procedures. Patient teaching. With almost all infections of the urinary tract, the importance must be stressed of drinking large amounts of fluid to dilute the bacterial concentration. In women, instruction may be necessary pertaining to cleansing of the perineum after voiding or defecating to avoid urethral contamination from the rectum. *The perineum should be wiped or cleansed from front to back.*
Pyelonephritis: inflammation of the kidney which can result in serious tissue damage.	General symptoms of inflammation, pain, and tenderness in the area of the kidney with frequent and painful voiding.	Drug therapy; antibiotics; increased fluid intake.	General clinical medical assisting procedures. Drink 2–3q of fluid daily. Provide information on diet. Instruct on collecting clean-catch urine specimen. Make reappointments.
Nephrolithiasis: kidney stones.	Characteristic pain in the region of the kidney; hematuria may occur.	Diet therapy, drug therapy, analgesics, muscle relaxants, application of heat, increased fluid intake. Surgical removal may be necessary: nephrolithotomy (incision into kidney for removal of stone) or ureterolithotomy (incision into ureter for removal of stone).	General clinical medical assisting procedures. If a specimen is obtained from the patient, it should be screened for the presence of stones. Instruct patient to strain urine at home and bring particles and stone in for analysis when obtained. Keep fluid intake at 2–3 L. Give list of low-calcium foods and foods to keep urine acid levels low.
Glomerulonephritis: inflammation of the kidney, especially the area composed of glomeruli. The disease may result in tissue damage. May be acute or chronic.	Oliguria, hematuria, weakness, headache, anorexia (loss of appetite), edema around eyes upon awaking, and edema of the feet in the evening. Hematuria and proteinuria first sign of acute.	Bedrest. Drug therapy; antibiotics, diet therapy—low sodium and moderate protein. Fluids restricted. If chronic, antihypertensive drugs are given.	General clinical medical assisting procedures. Each time the patient comes to the office (if not routine) weight is obtained to note fluid retention fluctuation. Patient teaching would involve stressing the importance of skin care. When skin is edematous (water-logged), it is more susceptible to injury and infection. Diet instruction.

2. *First Morning.* Collected immediately upon arising.
3. *Postprandial.* Collected immediately after meals.
4. *Timed.* Collected at a specific time during the day or for a specified period of time (most commonly, the 24-hour collection).
5. *Sterile Catheterized.* Collected by inserting a sterile catheter into the bladder. The specimen is stored in a sterile container. This type of specimen is most commonly collected in the hospital, outpatient facility, or the specialist's office.

URINARY TRACT SPECIALTIES

A physician whose practice is limited to diseases of the urinary tract and the male reproductive system is called a *urologist.* Urologists perform surgery on the urinary tract and employ a variety of nonsurgical treatments as well.

The medical assistant's responsibilities in the urologist's office include performing routine urinalysis, obtaining cultures, and assisting with postoperative procedures such as suture removal and dressing changes. The medical assistant must be knowledgeable about diseases of the urinary tract as well as diagnostic studies and related preparation and treatment procedures.

THE MALE REPRODUCTIVE SYSTEM

The male reproductive system consists of the testes; the vas, or ductus, deferens; the seminal vesicles; the prostate gland; the urethra; and the penis. The examination of the male genitalia includes inspection and palpation for hernias. A *hernia* is the protrusion of a portion of the intestine through an abdominal opening.

SYMPTOMATIC REACTION TO DISEASE

Male reproductive symptoms are usually related to five major areas: changes in voiding patterns, discharge from the urethra, tenderness or masses, impotence, and infertility. Voiding pattern changes may include frequency, urgency, hesitancy, and nocturia. Discharge can occur in many forms. Normally, the male has no discharge from the penis. Thus, any watery, thin, milky, thick, yellow, or blood-streaked discharge is abnormal. Tenderness may vary from local scrotal tenderness to low back pain or painful erection. Disturbances related to impotence may be associated with pain or decreased desire (*libido*). Infertility relates to either decreased sperm production or a lack of viable sperm.

As with other systems, there are normal changes that occur with aging. Testosterone levels may decrease, producing slower sexual initiation and recovery responses. Libido may slowly decrease. Prostatic enlargement is common and produces symptoms of difficulty in initiating and maintaining a forceful urinary stream.

MALE REPRODUCTIVE SYSTEM EXAMINATION AND THE MEDICAL ASSISTANT'S ROLE

During the physical examination, the physician examines the penis, scrotum, and inguinal regions for lesions; discharge; tenderness; and structural changes such as hernias, masses, or swelling. The examination of the male genitalia is best done with the patient standing. The patient's chest and abdomen remain draped for the sake of modesty, and only the groin and genitalia exposed. The physician wears gloves if any inflammatory lesions are present. The medical assistant may be asked to instruct the patient in performing regular testicular self-examinations. See Table 21–12 for a discussion of other aspects of the medical assistant's role during examination of the male reproductive system.

COMMON DIAGNOSTIC TESTS

Semen analysis requires the patient to obtain the specimen at home. The container, written instructions, and a laboratory slip are usually provided by the medical assistant at the physician's direction. This test evaluates fertility. Smears obtained from samples of discharges may be placed on glass slides for microscopic examination. Testicular biopsy, done in the hospital, involves obtaining a tissue sample for pathologic examination. Because this procedure is most frequently done when masses are palpated, the patient will be very anxious. The medical assistant should give hospital instructions carefully and slowly and provide a written copy of instructions. Another test frequently ordered involves hormone and metabolic evaluation of blood specimens. The medical assistant may be requested to draw the blood specimen and forward it to the laboratory or provide the patient with the completed laboratory request slip.

COMMON DISEASES OF THE MALE REPRODUCTIVE SYSTEM

Common diseases of the male reproductive system include hernias, inflammatory conditions, conditions created by structural change, and malignant disease. Sexually transmitted diseases (STDs) affect both males and females and are usually inflammatory in nature. Table 21–13 lists common diseases associated with the male reproductive system and discusses symptoms, treatment, and the medical assistant's role in patient management. Common sexually transmitted diseases are listed in Table 21–14 along with disease source, symptoms, diagnosis, treatment, and the medical assistant's role.

Sexually transmitted diseases are considered to be the leading communicable disease problem today. Anyone who is sexually active can contract these diseases and can transmit them to others, including offspring during childbirth. Since most cases of STDs are related to sexual activity, many patients avoid evaluation when

<u>Table 21–12</u>
EXAMINATION OF THE MALE REPRODUCTIVE SYSTEM

Body Part	Method and Equipment	Medical Assistant's Role
Penis	Inspection and palpation (gloves if lesion is present).	The patient is lying down with a drape sheet over the chest and abdomen. The medical assistant, if female, is usually not present during the examination of the male genitalia for purposes of avoiding embarrassment to the patient. However, since the presence of the medical assistant is ultimately at the discretion of the physician, basic knowledge of the examination process is required.
Scrotum	Inspection and palpation. Transillumination may be required. Examining room must be darkened and a penlight used.	
Inguinal hernia (examination of ridge between abdomen and thigh)	Inspection and palpation.	Patient stands.

the first symptoms of infection appear. The possible warning signs related to STD infection are unusual discharge from sex organs; sores, bumps, or blisters near the genitals or mouth; dysuria; and pelvic pain.

Because of the increasing incidence of STD, the medical assistant has the obligation to become well informed about these diseases.

MALE REPRODUCTIVE SYSTEM SPECIALTIES

The *urologist* specializes in male reproductive conditions. It is the urologist who usually performs the male sterilization procedure (*vasectomy*), as well as other surgical procedures, including hernia repairs and prostatectomies. Although the physician explains most procedures, the medical assistant may be asked to witness the signing of consent forms.

THE FEMALE REPRODUCTIVE SYSTEM

The female reproductive system has both internal and external organs. The internal organs of reproduction include two ovaries, two fallopian tubes, the uterus, and the vagina. The external organs (*genitalia*) are the mons veneris and the vulva. The mons veneris is the pad of fatty tissue over the pubic bone, covered by coarse skin that in adults is covered with hair. *Vulva* is the collective term for all the external genitalia below the mons veneris, including the labia majora, the labia minora, the clitoris, the vaginal vestibule, and the vaginal opening.

The perineum contains the body orifices of the female from the mons pubis (*pubic bone*) to the coccyx (*tail bone*) in this order; urinary meatus, vagina, rectal opening. The breasts, also referred to as the *mammary glands*, are included as reproductive system accessory organs.

SYMPTOMATIC REACTION TO DISEASE

An abnormality in one area of the female reproductive system can easily affect another area and may produce disorders with similar symptoms. The most common symptoms are associated with three categories of disease: inflammation and infection, benign lesions, and malignancy. Inflammatory symptoms include: (1) discharge, usually malodorous with amounts varying from slight to profuse and yellow-green in color; (2) pain on voiding, during intercourse, or persistent in the lower pelvic region; and (3) itching (*pruritus*) around the vulva and vagina.

Interestingly, it is the benign pelvic lesions that usually present with pain. Benign breast lesions are not usually painful. Lumps, masses, and ulcerations are the common presenting symptoms with benign lesions of the reproductive system, including the breast.

Malignancies present abnormalities in bleeding and occasionally pain. Breast malignancies may or may not have a palpable lump, and sometimes discharge from the nipples is a symptom.

Some disturbances in the menstrual cycle are caused by factors not solely related to disease. For instance, many women who are athletes in vigorous training may experience amenorrhea. Menopausal women also experience amenorrhea. The disturbances in menstruation have specific terminology:

1. *Amenorrhea.* The absence of menstruation. It normally occurs during pregnancy, lactation (breast-feeding), and menopause.
2. *Dysmenorrhea.* Abnormal painful menstruation.

<u>Table 21–13</u>
COMMON DISEASES OF THE MALE REPRODUCTIVE SYSTEM

Disease	Symptoms	Treatment	Medical Assistant's Role
Epididymitis (inflammation of the epididymis caused by bacterial infection).	Pain, swelling, tenderness in the scrotum, fever, and malaise.	Bedrest. Patient may be instructed to apply ice bag. Drug therapy: antibiotics, analgesics (pain-relievers). Surgery (vasectomy) for recurrent disease. Increase fluid intake.	If patient is instructed to apply ice bag for relief of pain and to reduce swelling, special instruction should be given regarding keeping the bag in place for a maximum of 15 min every hour to prevent tissue damage.
Orchitis (inflammation of the testes caused by bacterial infection or injury).	Pain, swelling, tenderness in scrotum, fever, malaise.	Bedrest. Patient may be instructed to apply ice bag. Drug therapy: antibiotics, analgesics. Surgery (vasectomy) for recurrent disease. Increase fluid intake.	Same as above.
Prostatitis (inflammation of the prostate usually caused by bacterial infection).	Dysuria (difficult and painful voiding), fever, and hematuria may occur.	Drug therapy: antibiotics, analgesics. Increase fluid intake.	Explain the treatment regimen and its purpose to the patient.
Hydrocele (collection of fluid in the scrotum which usually occurs in connection with infection of the epididymis or testes).	Scrotal enlargement without pain.	Fluid removal.	If procedure is performed in the office, the medical assistant will give the patient instructions to observe the dressing for signs of bleeding and to report this occurrence to the physician.
Varicocele (enlargement of spermatic veins).	Scrotum feels full, may be purplish color.	Suspensory. Surgery if persistent.	Same as above.
Benign prostatic hypertrophy.	Hesitancy, dribbling, stream flow decreases. Common in men over age 55.	Early treatment involves manual massage to temporarily relieve enlargement. Surgical: Usually transurethral resection of prostate.	General clinical assisting during examination. Provide privacy if requested. Surgery may result in impotence. Provide literature and encourage patient to ask questions.
Testicular cancer.	Mass felt in scrotum. Most common in men ages 20–40 y.	Immediate hospitalization with biopsy and possible unilateral or bilateral orchidectomy. Radiation. Chemotherapy.	Provide complete, written information for hospitalization. Be supportive.

3. *Menorrhagia.* Excessive amount of menstrual flow or a prolonged period of menstruation.
4. *Metrorrhagia.* Bleeding that occurs between menstrual periods. It may present as spotting between periods or frank, fresh bleeding.

From ages 40 to 55, as women enter menopause, many bodily changes occur. Although these changes are normal, some of them cause discomfort and may bring the patient to the physician for evaluation. With the decrease in hormone production, reproductive

Table 21–14
COMMON SEXUALLY TRANSMITTED DISEASES

Disease/Source	Symptom	Diagnosis/Treatment	Medical Assistant's Role
Gonorrhea. Bacteria. Sexual contact. "Clap" and "dose" are nicknames.	Men: milky white to yellow/green discharge, dysuria. Women: 80% no symptoms; vaginal itch, discharge, dysuria.	Obtain smear. Culture organism. Penicillin or other antibiotic. All sexual partners must return until cultures are negative.	Always provide privacy and confidentiality. Have glass slide and culture material. Provide medication. Reinforce need to tell sexual partners to report for tests and treatment.
Syphilis. Bacteria. Sexual contact. "Pox" and "stiff" are nicknames.	First stage: genital sore called chancre, hard, round; or oral sore. Lasts 1–5 wk. Second stage: flu-like symptoms with red rash over moist, fatty areas or whole body. Third stage: no symptoms. Damage to internal organs and brain.	Obtain serologic test (VDRL). Penicillin. Treat all contacts.	No sex until sores disappear. Teach patient to keep dry. Warm baths, loose cotton underwear.
Herpes. Viral. Sexual contact. Simplex I and simplex II can spread in both directions, oral to genital, and vice versa.	Fluid filled blisters on skin and mucous membrane of genital and oral area. Become shallow, painful ulcers.	Examination. Tissue culture. Smears/blood tests. No known cure. Drug: acyclovir treats outbreaks; antibacterials.	Refer to Herpes Resource Centers. Give literature on disease. Prepare medication. Provide handouts for safe sex.
Chlamydia. Microogranism. Sexual contact. Also called "nongonoccocal urethritis."	Women: itching and painful urination, cystitis, discharge, pelvic pain. Men: mucopurulent discharge, dysuria, swollen testes. May be asymptomatic.	Examination shows inflammation. Smear exam. Oral antibiotics. Vaginal cream.	Females no tampons. Abstain from sex until treatment is complete. Teach hygiene, condom use. Adequate fluids. Loose clothing.
Genital Warts. Viral. Skin-to-skin wart contact.	Small, painless, cauliflower-like bumps growing around genitals. Possible itch, dysuria.	Lesion examination. Local medication applied weekly as directed until falls off. Surgical: cold, laser, electric, or excision.	Without treatment, may spread. Use condom or abstain from sex. Return in 1 mo.
Acquired immunodeficiency syndrome. Virus—human immunodeficiency disease. Damages body's ability to fight disease. Sexual contact with semen, blood, vaginal secretions. Contaminated intravenous needle.	Unexplained chills, fever, night sweats; fatigue; weight loss; swollen glands; constant diarrhea; pink/purple skin blotches; pneumonia; repeated infections.	Physical examination. Serology for antibody. Treatment is palliative to reduce symptoms, relieve discomfort, avoid infection, treat specific secondary illness.	Patient may be weak and need help during examination. Casual contact does not put others at risk. Follow standard safety measures as with any communicable disease in handling blood, tissue, and semen.

organs may atrophy and secretion production decreases. Breasts lose firmness and become more pendulous. The vagina shortens, and intercourse may be painful and require the use of lubricating substances. The uterus and ovaries diminish in size.

FEMALE REPRODUCTIVE EXAMINATION AND THE MEDICAL ASSISTANT'S ROLE

Usually, the physician begins with the examination of the breast and axilla and proceeds to the pelvic examination (see Chapter 19). The medical assistant should instruct the patient to void before the examination and assist the physician in getting the patient to relax, so the pelvic examination can be performed with minimal discomfort to the patient. See Table 21–15 for a description of the medical assistant's role in these examinations. As the breast examination is performed, the physician often asks the patient questions regarding monthly breast self-examination and may ask the patient to demonstrate the procedure. The medical assistant should provide the new patient with written instructions and calendar reminders for breast self-examination. The most common resource for these materials is the local chapter of the American Cancer Society. There are many valid sample instructions available, and the instruction chosen should best meet the patient's needs. See Figure 21–5 for sample instructions.

COMMON DIAGNOSTIC TESTS

Common diagnostic tests to assess the female reproductive system may be performed in the medical office or may require hospital surgery or imaging services. The medical assistant prepares the equipment for the test or schedules an appointment for the patient at the appropriate facility and explains the procedures. See Table 21–16 for a description of the tests and studies used to diagnose pathology, infertility, and pregnancy.

Mammography, whether done by x-ray film or the Xerox technique (Xeroradiography), involves doses of low-level radiation to the breast. It is considered the best method to detect abnormal growths and lesions in their early stages. If the patient is symptom-free, a first (baseline) mammogram is recommended at about age 35 years; testing is then repeated every 1 to 2 years between the ages of 40 and 49 years and once a year for women aged 50 or older. The physician usually includes an annual breast examination on every patient after age 18 years or upon becoming sexual active.

Sonography uses high-frequency sound waves (*radar*). Echoes rebound differently from various internal structures, making it possible to distinguish between solid masses (such as *tumors*) and fluid-filled *cysts* (usually benign).

COMMON DISEASES OF THE FEMALE REPRODUCTIVE SYSTEM

The medical assistant needs to be familiar with the most common diseases of the reproductive system and

also with the complications associated with pregnancy. Both the reproductive organs and the breasts have common diseases related to: (1) inflammation, such as mastitis or vaginitis; (2) benign growths, such as fibrocystic disease and endometriosis; and (3) cancers, such as breast and cervical cancer. Table 21–17 covers these and other disorders.

SPECIFIC CLINICAL PROCEDURES

The medical assistant is responsible for instructing or reinforcing instruction in breast self-examination. This educational process enhances the detection of early breast cancer and successful treatment. Many physicians make use of breast models that contain simulated growths. The patient examines the model using the correct technique and discovers the growth. It is important to stress that breasts should be examined about the same date each month and not within a week of menstruation. Monthly examination allows the patient to become familiar with her body and therefore notice changes in the breast. As all breasts have irregularity in contour, it is often these changes that are the earliest sign of growths.

These steps offer a suggested teaching approach for breast self-examination.

1. Explain the purpose of the examination and what to feel for.
2. Assist the patient in attaining the lying and standing positions, and instruct the patient in the use of a large mirror to visualize the breasts during the procedure.
3. Demonstrate how to perform the small rotary motions with the flat pads of the fingers from the rim inward (including the armpit area) toward the nipple and how to inspect the nipples.
4. Ask the patient to practice the procedure.
5. Observe the patient's self-examination technique.
6. Suggest that the patient mark her calendar for a monthly reminder. Examination should be done 1 week after the onset of menses.
7. Give the patient a brochure on breast self-examination.

Clinical procedures involved with the reproductive organs are diagnostic and therefore are performed by the physician. Examples of such procedures are endometrial biopsy and culdoscopy. The medical assistant receives special training in assisting with these procedures. They are normally performed in the specialist's office.

FEMALE REPRODUCTIVE SPECIALTIES

The physician specializing in the female reproductive system is the *gynecologist*. When the physician has specialized training and cares for the pregnant woman, he or she practices *obstetrics* and is known as an *obste-*

Table 21–15

EXAMINATION OF THE FEMALE REPRODUCTIVE SYSTEM

Body Part	Method	Medical Assistant's Role
Breasts	Inspection. Note size, symmetry, color, veins, nipples, rashes, discharges.	Assist the patient to a sitting position and expose breasts (gown to waist). Instruct patient to keep arms at sides. The patient is then instructed by the physician to raise arms over head and then to lower arms and press hands against hips. The medical assistant may then, at the physician's request, grasp the patient's hands and extend the arms while the patient leans forward. While this procedure may cause embarrassment to the patient, it is an essential component of the examination. The procedure should be fully explained to the patient by the medical assistant before the examination to increase the patient's comfort and afford the opportunity for patient teaching.
	Palpation. Uses a rotary motion compressing tissue gently against chest wall. Note nodules, induration, tenderness, consistency.	Instruct and assist the patient to assume the supine position. Place a small pillow under patient's shoulder on the side to be examined. (This procedure distributes the breast more evenly on the chest wall.) The physician may instruct the patient to raise arms alternately above head. (Transfer the pillow to the side being examined.)
Axillae	Inspection and palpation. Note nodules, rashes, infection, increased pigment.	Instruct and assist the patient to assume sitting position and expose area.
External genitalia	Inspection.	
Cervix and vaginal wall (internal examination)	Inspection with head light or adequate overhead light, vaginal speculum, applicator or vaginal spatula, gloves, microscopic slides, fixative for Pap smear, normal saline and potassium hydroxide solution for wet mounts, lamp, drapes, laboratory slips.	The medical assistant, if female, should be in attendance and assist the physician with the examination, for purposes of efficiency and patient comfort. The patient should be prepared by the medical assistant for examination by instructing the patient to empty her bladder. The patient is then placed in the lithotomy position and draped properly with only the perineum exposed. The speculum should be warmed for patient comfort. The medical assistant may place lubricant on a gauze square or squeeze it on the physician's gloves when requested. The patient's facial expressions should be observed for signs of extreme discomfort and anxiety. After the Pap specimen is obtained, the medical assistant may be responsible for spraying the glass slide with fixative for later laboratory examination.
Cervix, rectum (bimanual examination)	Palpation with glove, lubricant. One gloved hand internally while the other palpates the lower abdominal wall.	Instruct the patient to breathe evenly and slowly through the mouth as an aid to relaxation.

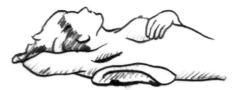

While lying down, place a towel or pillow under your right shoulder and put your right hand behind your head. Examine your right breast with your left hand.

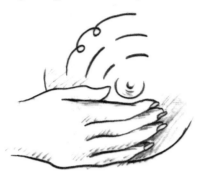

With your fingers flat, use sufficient pressure to press in small circles, starting at the outermost top edge of your breast and spiraling in toward the nipple. Examine every part of the breast. Repeat on the other side.

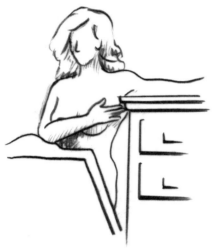

Now, rest your arm on a firm surface and use the same circular motion to examine the underarm area. This is breast tissue also.

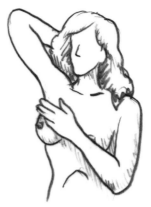

While in the shower, raise one arm. With fingers flat, touch every part of each breast using sufficient pressure to detect a lump or thickening. Use your right hand to examine the left breast and left hand to examine the right breast.

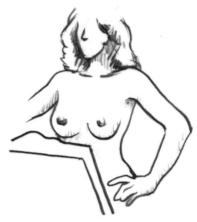

While in front of a mirror, look carefully for changes in the size, shape and contour of each breast first with arms at your sides then raised above your head. Look for puckering, dimpling or changes in skin texture.

Gently squeeze both nipples and check for discharge. Call your physician if you detect a lump, thickening or notice unusual changes in your breasts.

Figure 21–5. *Self-examination of the breast. The American Cancer Society recommends monthly self-examination.*

trician. There are also gynecology subspecialists who deal only with infertility and diminished ability to produce healthy, viable children. Larger medical centers have clinics involved with all aspects of maternal and fetal development, including genetic counseling.

The medical assistant employed in the office of the obstetrician and gynecologist assists with examinations, special laboratory procedures, such as pregnancy and reproductive system testing of blood and urine, colposcopy, ultrasonography, Pap and other bacterial smears, and patient teaching, such as the importance of prenatal care. The medical assistant also assists in minor surgical and sterile diagnostic procedures such as endometrial biopsies and amniocentesis. In the obstetricians' office, the medical assistant requires in-depth

knowledge about pregnancy, infertility, and newborn assessment to assist the physician and the patient.

Patients requiring breast procedures are usually referred to a general surgeon, a plastic surgeon specializing in breast disorder, or an oncology surgeon. Fine needle aspiration of the breast is a simple diagnostic procedure that may be performed in the office in a matter of minutes. The procedure is performed with a needle. The skin may be anesthetized (frozen) with a local injection. Since mammography is contraindicated in pregnant patients, fine needle aspiration is particularly useful during pregnancy for diagnosing breast masses.

Biopsy is the surgical removal of suspicious breast tissue for microscopic examination. It is the most accu-

Table 21-16
COMMON DIAGNOSTIC STUDIES OF THE FEMALE REPRODUCTIVE SYSTEM

Test	Description
Papanicolaou smear (Pap smear)	Smear is made on slide and fixative applied. To detect atypical cells. Specimen sent to laboratory.
Bacteriologic smear	Smear of discharge to detect causative agent. Wet smears in office identify most bacterial and fungal agents.
Biopsy (endometrial or vaginal)	Removal of tissue for examination and evaluation of abnormal bleeding, infertility, or hyperplasia.
Dilation and curettage	Surgical procedure that dilates cervix and scrapes uterus. Treats atypical bleeding. Also an abortion procedure.
Amniotic fluid analysis	Amniocentesis is performed under sterile procedure usually in operating room. Detects genetic, metabolic and other defects. Done at 14-16 wk gestation.
Radiology Exams: Hysterosalpingography Mammography Ultrasound	Evaluates patency of fallopian tubes and uterus size after instillation of dye or air. Detects breast growths. Nonradiation visualization of fetus or abnormal growths.

Table 21-17
COMMON DISEASES OF THE FEMALE REPRODUCTIVE SYSTEM

Disease	Symptoms	Treatment	Medical Assistant's Role
Inflammatory vaginitis (inflammation of the vagina usually caused by infection).	Itching, abnormal vaginal discharge: can be white (leukorrhea), yellow, frothy, or like cottage cheese. Discharge characteristics depend on the type of microbial invasion.	Drug therapy: antibiotics (systemic and/or local). Vaginal irrigations may also be recommended.	General clinical medical assisting procedures. Patient teaching may include instructions for using a vaginal cream or inserting a suppository. Special instructions should be given the patient regarding vaginal irrigation. Be sure type of solution and amount are specified as well as the length of time to continue treatment. Instruct the patient to move irrigation tip up and down and rotate it in the vagina so as to allow the solution to infiltrate the vaginal folds.
Cervicitis (inflammation of the cervix usually caused by infection).	Abnormal discharge may or may not be present.	Drug therapy: antiseptic, antibiotic (local and systemic). Vaginal irrigation or cauterization may be required. Cauterization destroys eroded tissue by electrical current. Eroded tissue can also be destroyed by chemical application. Removal of the tissue for laboratory examination is called biopsy.	In addition to general clinical medical assisting procedures, the medical assistant should explain cauterization to the patient if this procedure is to be performed.

Continued

Table 21–17
COMMON DISEASES OF THE FEMALE REPRODUCTIVE SYSTEM—*Continued*

Disease	Symptoms	Treatment	Medical Assistant's Role
Pelvic inflammatory disease (inflammation of several of the reproductive organs). May result from sexually transmitted disease.	General symptoms of infection. Large amounts of foul-smelling vaginal discharge may be present.	Drug therapy: antibiotics. Application of heat, vaginal irrigation. Surgery may be indicated. Venereal disease counseling if indicated.	The patient is usually hospitalized. During office visits, the medical assistant should offer patient teaching such as instructing the patient to change perineal pads frequently to avoid the spread of infection.
Mastitis: infection of the breast.	Swollen, painful breast and general symptoms of inflammation. Engorgement.	Drug therapy: hot or cold compress. Lactating females may have to stop breast feeding.	General clinical medical assisting procedures. May instruct patient in the use of compresses for relief of discomfort. Decrease caffeine, chocolate foods.
Benign lesions. Fibrocystic disease: irregular excessive growth of normal breast tissue which results in the formation of cysts (sacs containing fluid).	Patient feels small lumps in breast and axillae, tenderness and pain.	Conservative treatment is nonspecific. Surgery, however, may be performed to remove the cyst.	General clinical medical assisting procedures. Patient usually requires extensive reassurance of benign nature of disease. Dietary teaching avoiding caffeine, chocolate.
Benign tumor: abnormal growth of breast tissue (can occur in males). Adenofibroma.	Patient feels lump(s) in breast.	Biopsy performed. Surgical removal may be performed.	General clinical medical assisting procedures. Explanation of biopsy procedure and scheduling.
Endometriosis (particles of the mucous membrane lining present on the ovaries and/or throughout the pelvis).	Dysmenorrhea, pelvic pain, abnormal uterine bleeding, lower abdominal and/or back pain.	Drug therapy: hormones. Surgery may be required to remove the patches or cysts that form as a consequence of the displaced tissue.	General clinical medical assisting procedures. The medical assistant involved in the screening should be alert to certain symptoms in a patient diagnosed as having cervicitis. Symptoms that are similar to those of appendicitis would signal the occurrence of a complication such as cyst rupture.
Infections: *Monilia/Candida*.	White, cheesy discharge, dysuria, redness, itching.	Vaginal suppository.	For all vaginal infections, patients need to avoid stress, douching unless ordered, and sex without use of condom.
Trichomoniasis vaginalis.	Profuse, frothy, malodorous, yellow-green discharge, soreness, burning, dyspareunia.	Vaginal suppositories.	
Premenstrual syndrome.	Edema, bloating, weight gain, breast tenderness, headaches, mood shifts, palpitations, mild to	Symptomatic, including diuretics, tranquilizers, progesterone therapy before menses.	Reassure the patient. Restrict salt intake 10 d before menses. Avoid stimulants such as

Continued

Table 21–17
COMMON DISEASES OF THE FEMALE REPRODUCTIVE SYSTEM—*Continued*

Disease	Symptoms	Treatment	Medical Assistant's Role
	severe behavior changes.		alcohol and caffeine. Discuss reducing anxiety and life stressors.
Breast cancer: breast tissue malignancy (can occur in males).	Patient initially notices small hard lump in breast. Signs: dimpling ("orange peel"), depressed area, or puckering. Retraction of nipple, swelling.	Dependent on type and location of cancer. Alternatives: chemotherapy, radiation, surgery (mastectomy or lumpectomy).	Patient preparation, reassurance, explanation, and follow-up planning.
Endometrial cancer.	Abnormal spotting. Postmenopausal pain in later stages.	Includes any combination of the alternatives: surgery, chemotherapy, radiation.	Because of the difficulty in early treatment, it is essential to provide support for patients. Treatment may be complex and prognosis poor. Support for cancer patients demands sensitivity and education.
Carcinoma of the cervix.	None.	After detection: any of the cancer treatments, usually starting with surgery or radiation.	This cancer occurs most commonly in women 40–46 years. The need for annual Pap smear after age 40 must be encouraged in every female patient.

rate method of diagnosis. Biopsies are performed in a hospital outpatient setting or surgicenter with general sedation or anesthesia.

Mastectomy is the removal of all or part of the breast. Sometimes this procedure is performed in combination with radiation or chemotherapy (drug therapy). The *radical mastectomy* is performed to remove the breast, lymph nodes in the armpit, and underlying pectoral muscles. The *simple mastectomy* removes only the entire affected breast. The *partial mastectomy* is the resection of the tumor and some of the normal breast tissue surrounding the tumor. Radiation may be required after the surgery. The *lumpectomy*, which is increasingly being performed in situations where the tissue surrounding the tumor is not involved, removes the tumor and 1 to 2 cm of surrounding normal tissue. Frequently the lymph nodes in the armpit are also removed. Lumpectomy is followed by radiation therapy. Radiation therapy usually begins 2 weeks after surgery and continues for 5 to 6 weeks. After mastectomies, many women actively participate in rehabilitation programs, and for women who cannot adapt comfortably to their appearance without a breast, surgical reconstruction is available.

THE PEDIATRIC PATIENT

The pediatric patient warrants special consideration and discussion. Regardless of the type of practice, children are frequently encountered in the office setting. The age range of a pediatric patient usually falls between birth and 12 years. In some pediatric practices, the outside age limit may be 18 years.

Because of their particular stage of physiologic, psychological, and emotional development, children require special handling to provide the best possible atmosphere for patient comfort and the delivery of quality care. Young children frequently form judgments regarding medical personnel and medical care that influence their adult perceptions. Just as each adult is a unique individual, so too is each child.

In this section, the child is considered not in terms of physiologic structure, but rather in terms of age and behavioral expectations. The medical assistant who can relate effectively to children will be a valuable asset to the office team, facilitating the positive formation of the physician-patient relationship.

Although information regarding ages and stages at

which certain behaviors appear in children may differ somewhat according to the source, basic age-related behavior can be identified. The medical assistant can plan the optimal approach to the patient when a basic understanding of behavioral expectations in that patient's age range has been gained (Table 21–18).

SYMPTOMATIC REACTION TO DISEASE IN THE PEDIATRIC PATIENT

As with adults, symptomatic reaction to disease in children depends on the body system that is experiencing distress. The major concern in childhood disease is

Table 21–18
SUGGESTED APPROACHES TO THE PEDIATRIC PATIENT

Age Period	Behavior Expectations	Suggested Approach
Infancy (0–12 m)	Crying in the newborn period is expected, especially if the office visit takes place close to feeding time.	Since auscultation will be difficult when the baby is crying, encourage the mother to place the tip of her finger or pacifier in the baby's mouth when the stethoscope is being used to allow the chest sounds to be heard without distracting noises. The baby should not be fed during the examination as this would interfere with the sounds being analyzed when the stethoscope is in use. When the medical assistant is weighing the baby and performing other procedures, a gentle, quiet approach is recommended. Talking quietly and holding the baby securely are comforting.
	Infants have a short attention span and appear to be able to focus on only one stimulus at a time.	Distraction appears most successful to gain cooperation. Mobiles, body movements, a shining light, all can distract an infant. Experimentation is necessary since each child responds enthusiastically to different stimuli.
	Nudity is usually preferred. Keep child covered until physician is present.	In preparing the patient for the examination, all clothing is removed except the diaper.
	Infants need constant closeness to the mother.	The medical assistant or the mother may help position the baby during examination. With the physician's approval, the mother can hold the baby for most of the examination.
Early Childhood (1–5 y)	A child in this age group usually fears the office visit. The extent of the fear and behavior expressed are dependent on the patient's age and personality. However, vocal expressions of resistance such as crying, screaming, and physical struggle, and exasperated parents are common experiences. May need help in restraining very resistant child. Allow parent to help if able and willing.	The medical assistant is challenged to make the office visit a pleasant experience. Allowing the child to retain as much clothing as possible is comforting. Interesting toys and books in the waiting room and examining room help to reduce the child's discomfort. A gentle, quiet manner and conversation also help to gain the child's confidence. Truth is imperative. If a procedure will hurt, a brief, clear explanation of what is being done and why may be helpful, depending on age and personality. Complimentary remarks help to bridge the unfamiliarity the child feels in the presence of the office staff. If the physician prefers, the examination need not be performed on the examining table. The child may stand, or sit in the

Continued

Table 21–18

SUGGESTED APPROACHES TO THE PEDIATRIC PATIENT—Continued

Age Period	Behavior Expectations	Suggested Approach
		mother's, the medical assistant's, or the physician's lap. Demonstration of the procedure or explanation and demonstration of the examination on a doll is helpful. The medical assistant can allow the child to place the stethoscope in his ears and pretend to examine the doll or the medical assistant. Other equipment can be handled by the patient with supervision.
		First physical contacts set the stage for the child's reaction to the examination. For instance, the medical assistant may need to take a rectal temperature reading. The medical assistant should first touch the child in a gaming situation such as counting the fingers or toes. Injections are particularly unpleasant, and the child will resist. Unpleasant procedures should be performed quickly despite patient protest. Reassurance and explanation should take place following the procedure.
Childhood (5–12 y)	Usually, the school-age child is cooperative and curious, and wants to be treated as an adult. At this age, there is greater cooperation if children are allowed choices within ranges: i.e., which arm for injection, type of bandage, etc.	Questions should first be directed to the child. The parent can usually add to the response.
	Privacy needs are usually well established.	Preparation for the examination includes an awareness of this need. While gowning is usually necessary, the child should be left with his or her mother to undress. Underpants are usually not removed until required.
Preadolescence and adolescence	Rapid growth, awkward, self-conscious, involved in socialization tasks, very "I" oriented, sexual development and interests. Prefers to dress and be with physician alone.	Allow flexibility and choices. Encourage parent not to be present in examination room. Provide health teaching in private. Encourage nonjudgmental exchanges around common problem areas of sexuality, sexually transmitted disease, drug abuse, alcohol. Need to feel medical assistant is willing to listen, not condemn. Report suspected problems to physician.

that the symptoms of many diseases are quite similar. The general symptom of pain can be present in a child with pharyngitis (sore throat) and meningitis. The medical assistant responsible for patient screening in scheduling appointments must ask pertinent questions that will elicit clues about the severity and exact nature of the symptoms. The parents of small children are often alarmed when their children are ill because very young children cannot communicate the nature of their dis-

tress. Moreover, parents are often confused as to when a child should be brought to the physician.

Many pediatricians print pamphlets that provide helpful information in this regard. Some physicians, especially those in pediatrics, may schedule a telephone hour when parents can phone for advice. Often, the medical assistant assumes responsibility for initially receiving and referring the questions when necessary.

PEDIATRIC EXAMINATION AND THE MEDICAL ASSISTANT'S ROLE

The examination of the pediatric patient follows the same pattern as that for adults. Children, however, are growing and changing, and their anatomic and physiologic development must be closely monitored. To perform the comprehensive examination in children, the physician may alter the standard techniques and adapt certain other ones. The medical assistant's clinical responsibilities are also adapted. For instance, an infant's head measurement is taken to provide brain growth estimations (see procedure at end of chapter). Table 21–19 outlines the general pediatric examination and the medical assistant's role.

The medical assistant should be aware of the major problems affecting children in the various age groups. Because many pediatric conditions require corrective surgery or are of a chronic nature, it is important to develop skills in supporting parents as well as the children.

COMMON DISEASES OF CHILDREN

Children are susceptible to most adult diseases. Respiratory tract infections are common. There are a number of conditions and diseases common to various ages and stages of development. Many of the diseases are contagious but preventable with adequate immunizations. The suggested guidelines for immunization are

Table 21–19
THE PEDIATRIC EXAMINATION

Body Part or Function	Method and Equipment	Medical Assistant's Role
Vital signs	The medical assistant performs temperature, pulse, and respiration (TPR), height, weight, measures head and chest circumference. Blood pressure (BP) may be omitted, depending on physician preference. If performed, a small pediatric cuff is utilized. Use pediatric equipment that is the correct size for child.	The medical assistant usually takes the child's temperature. TPR is usually taken on every visit. The rectal temperature can be obtained by placing the young child over the lap or placing the child on the table. Spread the buttocks with one hand; with the other insert the lubricated thermometer approximately 1 inch. On insertion, hold the buttocks closed and the thermometer in place, as the child will have the urge to expel the thermometer. The medical assistant's arm should lie over the child's back with the body leaning forward to secure the child. The medical assistant's approach will greatly affect the ease in performing these procedures. Head and chest circumference are measured in the first 2 years. BP is usually obtained with a pediatric cuff at every visit when the child is over age 3. Before this time, if the BP is obtained, the physician usually performs the procedure.
Skin	Inspection	The medical assistant hands the physician the equipment and assists in positioning the patient.
Head and neck	Inspection. Palpation Transillumination of the skull with a flashlight.	The medical assistant can help the mother to position the child for ease in examination. Much of the examination of the infant can occur while the mother is sitting on the examination table, holding the child.
Eyes	Inspection with an ophthalmoscope.	The medical assistant will most likely be responsible for visual acuity tests in young children over 3 and in early school-age children. Some resistance to covering the eye may be experienced. Again, gaming may be helpful. For example, reference to a cover as a "pirate's patch" may be helpful.

Continued

Table 21–19

THE PEDIATRIC EXAMINATION — *Continued*

Body Part or Function	Method and Equipment	Medical Assistant's Role
Ears	Inspection with otoscope. Otoscope with pneumatic bulb (air-inflated) may be used.	The medical assistant must provide a small speculum for the pediatric patient. In very young children, or children offering resistance, the mother may be requested to lie across or hold down the child's legs while the medical assistant secures the patient's head. This is necessary to avoid injury to the ear.
Nose, mouth, throat	Inspection with light and tongue blade. Palpation.	Restraint of the young child may be necessary. Arms are held at sides. Head again immobile.
Thorax and lungs	Inspection. Palpation. Percussion. Auscultation with a stethoscope.	Keeping the child quiet during this part of the examination is extremely important for the physician's accuracy in judgment.
Heart	Auscultation with a stethoscope. Electrocardiogram may be done if congenital defects.	Keeping the child quiet during this part of the examination is important for accuracy in judgment.
Abdomen	Inspection. Palpation. Percussion.	The medical assistant will hold the child's legs flexed in order to relax the abdomen and facilitate the physician's examination.
Genitalia and rectum	Inspection. Palpation. Children 11–18 y may refuse.	The medical assistant helps the patient to maintain a supine position. May be deferred.
Musculoskeletal system	The physician puts the extremities and back through ranges of motion. The child who is able to walk is sometimes instructed to walk a short distance and is observed by the physician for abnormalities and deformities.	The medical assistant can be helpful in relaying to the physician any observation made while preparing the patient for examination.
Neurologic system: reflexes	Percussion using a hammer and specific hand movements and manipulations.	Assistance in positioning and handling instruments.

listed in Table 21–20. Contagious diseases are those that are easily transmitted from person to person. They are termed *communicable disease* because of the nature by which they are transmitted. These diseases become common as children become involved in social situations and their exposure to microorganisms increases. Common childhood infections and their incubation periods are listed in Table 21–21. Incubation period refers to the time between exposure to the disease-causing organism and the onset of symptoms.

The Centers for Disease Control and the American Academy of Pediatrics recommend immunizing all babies against hepatitis B. Mothers are routinely tested for hepatitis B during pregnancy. Babies born to mothers carrying the hepatitis B virus receive a first dose of vaccine *and* an injection of hepatitis immune globulin (rich in antibodies to hepatitis B) before leaving the hospital. Babies of mothers whose test results are negative are given the first dose of vaccine at the same time. There are two possible schedules for the three doses of vaccine:

	Schedule 1	Schedule 2
Dose 1	Newborn nursery	1 to 2 mo
Dose 2	1 to 2 mo	4 mo
Dose 3	6 to 18 mo	6 to 18 mo

There are two contagious diseases for which vaccines are not presently available: scarlet fever (*scarlatina*) and chickenpox (*varicella*). Scarlet fever is an acute bacterial infection producing a sore throat, red tongue, and finally a scarlet rash on the fatty fold areas of the

Table 21–20

GUIDE FOR USE OF SELECTED VACCINES AND TOXOIDS

This guide is intended to serve as a quick reference for commonly employed immunization procedures. It is based on recommendations made by the Public Health Service Advisory Committee on Immunization Practices and the Report of the Committee on Infectious Diseases 1982 (*Red book*) of the American Academy of Pediatrics. Reference should be made to the complete published reports of these two committees for more detailed information on general considerations and specific applications of accepted immunization practices.

Important: Avoid immunizing persons ill or febrile in preceding 24 hours. Carefully read the product description and directions supplied with each immunizing agent as potency (dosage) may vary with the manufacturer. In addition, agents may contain substances to which patients may be sensitive such as egg protein or antibiotics.

Disease	Immunizing Agent	Age Range	Administration (Intramuscular — IM) (Subcutaneous — SC)	Primary Immunization Intervals(s)	Booster Doses	Comments
Diphtheria, tetanus and pertussis (DTP)	Toxoids of diphtheria and tetanus, alum precipitated or adsorbed, combined with pertussis antigen (DTP)	For infants and children aged 6 wk through 6 y.	Three doses: 0.5 mL ea. IM. Fourth dose: 0.5 mL IM.	4–8 wk. 6–12 mo.	At age 4–6 y, preferably at time of school entrance. Dose: 0.5 mL, IM.	Do not use after seventh birthday.
Tetanus diphtheria (For adults)	Toxoids of tetanus and diphtheria; alum precipitated or adsorbed, combined. (Contains 1–2 Lf units diphtheria toxoid.)	7 y through adult	Two doses: 0.5 mL ea. IM. Third dose: 0.5 mL IM.	4–8 wk. 6–12 mo.	Every 10 y for life.	For severe wounds, it is unnecessary to use booster doses if the patient has completed a primary series and has had a booster dose within the preceding 5 y (within 10 y for clean minor wounds).
Influenza	Inactivated (killed) polyvalent, bivalent, or monovalent influenza virus vaccine. (Grown in chick embryo tissue.)	All ages, from 6 mo. Seasonally for high-risk groups such as the elderly and those with chronic illness.	May change from year to year. See instructions on manufacturer's package insert.	4 weeks or more, if 2 doses are needed.	Seasonally for high risk groups.	Does not protect after exposure. "Split," or "subunit" vaccine generally recommended for children.
Poliomyelitis	Inactivated (killed) trivalent poliovirus vaccine. Types 1, 2, 3, combined.	All ages, begin: 6 wk.	Three doses: 1.0 mL ea. IM. Fourth dose: 1.0 mL IM.	4–8 wk. 6–12 mo.	Booster dose every 5 y through age 17.	To be used in persons with altered immune states and in their households.
	Attenuated (live) trivalent oral	Begin: 6 wk. Routine use in persons	Three oral doses.	Between doses:	Preschool age (4–6 y) and when traveling	Can be given to pregnant women in

		Dose	Schedule	Contraindications/Comments
poliovirus vaccine. Types 1, 2, 3 combined.	age 18 and over in the United States is not needed.		1 & 2: 6–8 wk. 2 & 3: 6–12 mo. to endemic areas. Repeated "booster" doses are not needed.	outbreak situations. Avoid in persons with altered immune states.
Measles (Rubeola)* Attenuated (live) measles virus vaccine	Age 15 mo or older.	One dose: 0.5 mL SC.	One dose only. However, measles vaccine should be given again if there is a history of receiving (a) killed measles vaccine only, or live vaccine within 2 y of receiving killed vaccine; (b) vaccine before the first birthday; (c) live *further* attenuated vaccine with immune serum globulin or measles immune globulin.	Contraindications: Altered immune states such as leukemia, lymphoma, antimetabolite and radiation therapy, and generalized malignancy. As with any live virus vaccine, avoid during pregnancy.
Mumps* Attenuated (live) mumps virus vaccine	Age 15 mo or older.*	One dose: 0.5 mL SC.	One dose only.	As with any live virus vaccine, avoid during pregnancy and in persons with altered immune states.
Rubella* Attenuated (live) rubella virus vaccine	Susceptible infants age 12 mo or older*	One dose: 0.5 mL SC.	One dose only.	SHOULD NOT BE GIVEN DURING PREGNANCY. Women of childbearing age may be considered for immunization if advised of necessity to avoid pregnancy for 3 mo after vaccine administration. Avoid in persons with altered immune states.

SMALLPOX: As of 1980 there is no medical indication for smallpox vaccination in any part of the world except for persons handling variola and vaccinia-group viruses in research laboratories.
*Combined live attenuated vaccines are available for Measles-Mumps-Rubella; Measles-Rubella; and Mumps-Rubella. If combined vaccine including measles vaccine is used, give at age 15 mo or older.

Source: From State of California Department of Health Services, Infectious Disease Section, April 1983.

Table 21-21
COMMON INFECTIONS

Name	Incubation Period	Isolation of Patient
Acquired immunodeficiency syndrome	Unknown. Thought to be from a few months to years.	Blood and body fluid precautions. Private room if personal hygiene habits are poor.
Brucellosis	Highly variable. Usually 5–21 d; may be months.	None.
Chickenpox	2–3 wk.	1 wk after appearance of vesicles.
Cholera	A few hours to 5 d.	Enteric precautions.
Common cold	12 h–3 d.	None.
Diphtheria	Usually 2–5 d.	Until two cultures from nose and throat, taken at least 2 h apart, are negative. Cultures to be taken after cessation of antibiotic therapy.
Dysentery, amebic	From a few days to several months, commonly 2–4 wk.	None.
Dysentery, bacillary (shigellosis)	1–7 d.	As long as stool cultures remain positive.
Encephalitis, mosquito-borne	5–15 d.	None.
Giardiasis	Variable. Median, 7–10 d.	Enteric precautions.
Gonorrhea	2–7 d, may be longer.	No sexual contact until cured.
Hepatitis A	Variable, 15–50 d. Mean, about 30 d.	Enteric precaution until 1 wk after onset of jaundice.
Hepatitis B	Variable, usually 45–180 d. Mean, 60–90 d.	Blood and body fluid precautions until antibodies to virus disappear.
Hepatitis, non-A, non-B	15–64 d.	As for hepatitis A.
Influenza	1–3 d.	As practical.
Legionella	2–10 d.	None.
Malaria	12 d for *Plasmodium falciparum*; 14 d for *Plasmodium vivax*, Plasmodium ovale; 30 d for *Plasmodium malariae*.	Protected from mosquitoes.
Measles (rubeola)	8–13 d from exposure to onset of fever. 14 d until rash appears.	From diagnosis to 7 d after appearance of rash. Strict isolation from children under age 3 y.
Meningitis, meningococcal	2–10 d.	Until 24 h after start of chemotherapy.
Mononucleosis, infectious	4–6 wk.	None. Disinfect articles soiled with nose and throat discharges.
Mumps	2–3 wk.	Until the glands recede.
Paratyphoid fevers	1–3 wk for fever. 1 to 10 d for gastroenteritis.	Until cultures of three stool samples are negative.
Pneumonia, pneumococcal	Believed to be 1–3 d.	Until 24 h after administration of antibiotics.
Poliomyelitis	3 to possibly 35 d.	1 wk from onset.
Puerperal fever, streptococcal	1–3 d.	Transfer from maternity.
Rabies	Usually 2 to 8 wk. Occasionally only 10 d.	Strict for duration of illness danger to attendants.
Rubella (German measles)	16–18 d, with range of 23 d.	None, but avoid contact with nonimmune pregnant women.
Salmonellosis	6–72 h, usually 12–36 h.	Until stool cultures are salmonella-free on two consecutive specimens selected not less than 24 h apart.
Scabies	2–6 wk before onset of itching in patients without previous infections. 1–4 d after reexposed.	Excuse patient from school-work until day after treatment.
Scarlet fever	1–3 d.	7 d; may be terminated in 24 h.
Smallpox	8–17 d.	Strict; in screened hospital wards, until all scabs have disappeared.

Continued

Table 21-21
COMMON INFECTIONS—*Continued*

Name	Incubation Period	Isolation of Patient
Syphilis	10 d–10 wk, usually 3 wk.	In noncooperative patient, should be enforced until surface lesions are healed.
Tetanus	4 d–3 wk.	None.
Toxic shock syndrome	Unknown but may be as brief as several hours.	None.
Trachoma	5–12 d.	Until lesions disappear, but usually not practical.
Tuberculosis	4–12 wk to demonstrable primary lesion or significant tuberculin reaction.	Variable, depending on conversion of sputum to negative after specific therapy and on ability of patient to understand and carry out personal hygiene methods.
Tularemia	2–10 d.	None.
Typhoid fever	Usually 1–3 wk.	Until three cultures of fecal and urine are negative. These should be taken earlier than 1 mo after onset.
Typhus fever	7–14 d.	None.
Whooping cough	Usually 1 wk.	For 3 wk after onset of spasmodic cough.

Source: From Thomas, CL (ed): Taber's Cyclopedic Medical Dictionary, ed 16. FA Davis, Philadelphia, 1989, pp 903–904, with permission.

chest, trunk, and extremities. Very high temperature elevations (to 105°F [41°C]) are not uncommon. Administration of penicillin for 10 days is the course of treatment.

Chickenpox is caused by a virus. It presents with macules, papules, and finally vesicles, appearing on the trunk and spreading to the head and extremities. It may be accompanied by headache and fever. Children are contagious and should be isolated until the vesicles are completely dry and no new ones have developed.

PEDIATRIC SPECIALTIES

The physician specializing in the health needs of children is a *pediatrician*. The pediatrician diagnoses and treats diseases of childhood and, in addition, routinely monitors the normal growth and development of children. The medical assistant working in a pediatric office is responsible for recordkeeping, patient teaching, and preparation of patients for examination, as well as for assisting with treatment procedures and assuming other general office responsibilities.

There are other specialties pertaining to children, such as pediatric cardiology and pediatric neurology. In these specialties, the concentration is in the related systemic diseases of pediatric rather than adult patients.

PATIENT TEACHING CONSIDERATIONS

Throughout this chapter, specific teaching information has been presented in the charts and tables for the specialty examinations. The medical assistant must be aware that patients referred to the specialist's office require instruction and teaching in all phases of examination, clinical testing, and prescribed procedures and treatments. Anxiety levels are often high in a new setting, and teaching the patients what to expect and what is expected of them helps to provide a therapeutic environment that is conducive for examination.

The medical assistant can provide information reinforcing concepts regarding the structure and function of the involved system, explaining the rationale and procedures in diagnostic testing, and clarifying the preventive and therapeutic measures prescribed for home care. The principles of teaching discussed in Chapter 5 should be incorporated in each patient-teaching plan. As the patient encountered in the specialty office may have a limited number of visits, the medical assistant should make good use of every available opportunity for patient teaching.

RELATED ETHICAL AND LEGAL IMPLICATIONS

The specific physical examination has many facets that require the medical assistant's understanding regarding legal responsibilities. Patients must provide informed consent for the examination or procedure to be performed. The medical assistant needs to reinforce the physician's explanation of the examination. The explanation provides an opportunity for the patient or parent to give implied or verbal consent or to refuse the exami-

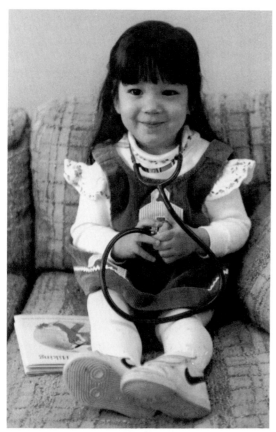

The young child is less fearful of the examination procedure when the equipment is familiar.

nation or procedure. The procedures, treatment, and patient teaching should be performed after the physician has completed the explanation and has instructed the medical assistant to proceed. Any patient who is infirm, disoriented, or confused should never be left alone in the examination room.

Patients being treated for STDs need informed, nonjudgmental information, encouragement to contact their sex partners so that they, too, can receive treatment instructions to avoid sexual contact until all medications and treatments are completed, and provisions for total confidentiality. Individual state laws provide for the reporting of certain communicable diseases, and STDs fall under such laws. The medical assistant must comply with the law while preserving confidentiality. Every office, including the pediatrician's office, should have information on STDs. The availability of information regarding AIDS is especially important, and the fact that this disease cannot be contracted by casual contact should be stressed during the office visit. AIDS counseling is mandatory before testing, and it is important that the medical assistant maintain absolute confidentiality as to the test results. In some states, the results of tests for the HIV antibody may not be released without the patient's written consent.

Special considerations apply to the care of children. As most children will answer to any name, the medical assistant should rely on the parent or accompanying adult for positive patient identification. Because children are unable to use abstract thinking, the medical assistant must always be alert to their safety. The medical assistant should be alert to possible environmental hazards such as slick floors, spilled liquids, electrical outlets, extension cords, and so forth. Children should never be left unattended on treatment tables, scales, and so forth. The assistance of the parent or accompanying adult can be enlisted to ensure the child's safety. Remember that children are inquisitive and want to explore their surroundings. Touch and taste are part of this exploration. The medical assistant should assess both the waiting area and treatment areas for potential hazards and take steps to correct them.

The patient has a right to privacy, comfort, and dignity. Medical assistants can meet these needs by remembering to shut doors, keep patients draped, provide pillows, talk in private areas, and teach self-care practices thoroughly.

The practice of providing patients with written materials for teaching self-care, drug administration, and other procedural preparations facilitates more accurate understanding and compliance. Patients who understand and are satisfied with their care are less likely to take legal action.

The medical assistant who is truly concerned about the patient will be careful not to make value judgments and will provide for the patient's basic needs, to prevent or minimize feelings of loss. Patient care should not be compromised by office personnel regardless of personal circumstances or beliefs.

The medical assistant does not initiate, prescribe, or diagnose, as all of these duties are outside the scope of practice. The medical assistant who oversteps the bounds of "assistant," even under the physician's direction, puts both himself or herself and the physician in legal jeopardy.

SUMMARY

The role of the medical assistant in the specific physical examination is to facilitate the needs of both the physician and the patient. This increases patient cooperation and contributes to a successful examination. The medical assistant must develop a number of diverse physical examination skills that will enable the medical assistant to anticipate needs according to patients' symptoms, prepare the examination room for expected procedures, and provide patients with needed teaching and supplemental information. Patient education and information allays anxiety and increases patient compliance in the processes of diagnosis, treatment, and home care. This chapter has presented the necessary information to assist the medical assistant in the development of these skills.

DISCUSSION QUESTIONS

Discuss possible solutions to the following situations.

1. The patient is coughing and not covering his mouth.
2. After the patient leaves the examining room, you notice that the doctor's written directions for a lung scan are in the trash container.
3. The patient has observed you carefully while you were taking her blood pressure. Now she asks if she has high blood pressure.
4. The patient asks you what kind of heart disease his palpitations indicate.
5. The patient vomits while gowning.
6. The patient asks why he is being referred to a proctologist after the physician has already explained this to him.
7. While you are preparing the patient for a vaginal examination, she informs you that she may have a sexually transmitted disease, but asks you not to tell the physician.
8. A 2-year-old child is scheduled for an ear examination. As you enter the room he begins to cry.
9. The mother of a 14-year-old has just been informed that her child has epilepsy. She is alone in the physician's office, and you've been asked to spend some time with her because she is upset.

BIBLIOGRAPHY

Please see the Bibliography for Chapter 20.

PROCEDURE: Instill medication drops into the nasal cavity

OSHA STANDARDS:

Terminal Performance Objective: Introduce medication directly into the nasal cavity to relieve pain, increase or decrease drainage, control nasal bleeding, or serve as an antiseptic application to irritated nostrils within a reasonable time standard.

EQUIPMENT: Medication with dropper
Tissue
Medication order from the patient chart

PROCEDURE

1. Prepare the room by assembling the equipment and checking the cleanliness of the room, lighting, and temperature.
2. Identify the patient and explain the procedure.

3. Compare the medication to the written order.
4. Instruct the patient to assume a semisitting (Fowler's) position and tilt the head over the pillow.
5. Grasping the filled dropper, hold the dropper over the affected nostril and expel the prescribed number of drops.
6. Instruct the patient to remain in position for a few seconds.

7. Instruct the patient to lean forward with the head tilted down for a minute or two.

8. Give follow-up instructions to the patient.

9. Record the date, time, procedure and medication (if used), patient instructions, and initial the record. Example: 3/5/93 2:00 PM: Neo-Synephrine 0.25% drops, right nostril. Prescription instructions given to patient (initials).
10. Clean the equipment and the examination room.

PRINCIPLE

1. To reduce procedure time and to facilitate the efficiency of the examination.

2. To reduce the risk of error and to provide assurance to anxious patients.
3. To ensure accuracy of the medication administration.
4. To allow the medication to flow onto the nose.

5. The dropper should not touch the nostril; otherwise it would contaminate the dropper and possibly cause the patient to sneeze.
6. To prevent the medication from draining out of the nose and to allow for medication retention in the nasal canal absorbing the medication.
7. To help spread the medication over the mucosa and to prevent the drug from running into the throat where it can be absorbed systemically. In contrast to nose drops, sprays are designed to be used with the head upright during administration.
8. To ensure proper continued care, instructions should be in writing for the patient to take home.
9. To ensure quality of care and to provide a point of future reference.

10. To prevent the chance of transmitting microorganisms and to prepare the room for the next patient.

PROCEDURE: Irrigate the nasal cavity

OSHA STANDARDS:

Terminal Performance Objective: Irrigate the nasal cavity to relieve inflammation, increase drainage, or remove foreign bodies within a reasonable time standard.

EQUIPMENT: 100 ml warmed normal saline
Bulb-type syringe
Ear or small emesis basin (for drainage)
Sterile large basin (for solution)
Towels
Medication order from the patient chart
Gloves (optional*)
Biohazard bag for disposal

PROCEDURE

1. Prepare the room by assembling the equipment and checking the cleanliness of the room, lighting, and temperature.
2. Identify the patient and explain the procedure.

3. Warm the solution in a basin of warm water or under warm running water.
4. Assist the patient into the Fowler's position with the head slightly forward.
5. Drape the toweling under the patient's neck and shoulders bib fashion. Instruct the patient to hold the basin below the affected nostril.

PRINCIPLE

1. To reduce procedure time and to facilitate the efficiency of the examination.

2. To reduce the risk of error and to provide assurance to anxious patients.
3. Warm solutions are more comfortable to the patient. Do not heat.
4. To allow the solution to run into a basin. Nasal drainage is promoted in the sitting position.
5. To prevent the solution from soiling or wetting the patient's clothing.

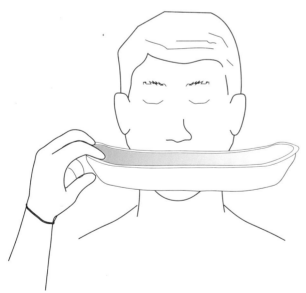

The patient holds the basin below the affected nostril.

*Nasal secretions are body fluids to which the Centers for Disease Control (CDC) universal precautions do not apply; however, CDC guidelines constitute a minimum standard of practice. In institutions that have implemented universal precautions (applying them to *all* body fluids), it is acceptable to wear disposable gloves, especially for the patient at high risk for or with an infectious disease such as AIDS. Other barriers such as goggles, gown, and mask may also be worn, depending on the potential for risk.

PROCEDURE

6. Pour the required amount of irrigating solution into a sterile basin or disposable container. Withdraw the solution into a bulb syringe by squeezing the bulb before insertion into the solution, then releasing the bulb when the bulb is immersed in the solution.

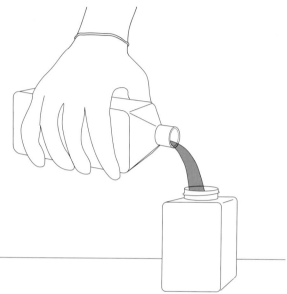

Pour the solution into a sterile container.

7. Instruct the patient to tilt the head slightly toward the affected nostril and insert the tip of the syringe into the unaffected nostril.

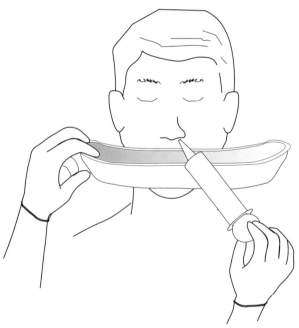

Insert the tip of the syringe into the *unaffected* nostril and squeeze the bulb gently, slowly, and evenly.

8. Squeeze the bulb gently, slowly, and evenly. Exert only slight pressure on the bulb.

PRINCIPLE

6. To avoid contaminating the entire contents of the solution.

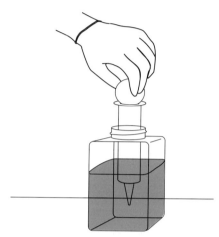

Squeeze the bulb before inserting the syringe into the solution; then fill the syringe by releasing the bulb.

7. The solution is inserted into the unaffected nostril to prevent the transfer of infectious material from the affected nostril into the unaffected side. Let the patient know why you are injecting into the unaffected side.

8. An excess of slight pressure may force the infectious material into the sinuses and eustachian tubes and into the ears. The solution should travel up into the nose, around the nasal septum that divides the nose, and out the opposite, or affected, nostril.

PROCEDURE

9. Repeat the irrigation several times or until the foreign body is removed or the discharge is clear (as instructed by the physician).

10. Stop the irrigation should the patient cough or choke and wait until the coughing ceases before beginning again.

11. Dry the patient's face.

12. Instruct the patient not to blow the nose for 5 to 10 minutes.

13. Give follow-up instructions to the patient.

14. Record the date, time, procedure and medication (if used), patient instructions, and initial the record. Example: 3/5/93 2:00 PM: nasal irrigation with 100 ml warm normal saline; no ill effects noted. Solution returned was green-tinged with a few flakes of dried blood. No active bleeding noted following the procedure. Patient stated his breathing was "easier" and his nose felt "opened up." Written follow-up instructions given (initials).

15. Clean the equipment and the examination room.

PRINCIPLE

9. To accomplish the purpose of the irrigation.

10. The solution has run down the patient's throat, obstructing breathing.

11. To provide patient comfort and to reduce the chance of contamination.

12. To prevent the remaining solution from being forced into the sinuses and ears.

13. To ensure proper continued care, instructions should be in writing for the patient to take home.

14. To ensure quality of care and to provide a point of future reference.

15. To prevent the chance of transmitting microorganisms and to prepare the room for the next patient.

PROCEDURE: Instruct the patient to collect a clean-catch urine specimen

OSHA STANDARDS:

Terminal Performance Objective: Instruct the patient using written instructions how to collect an uncontaminated urine specimen from the perineal area within a reasonable time standard.

EQUIPMENT: Written patient care instructions (see Chapter 5)
Six sterile gauze wipes (female patient)
Three sterile gauze wipes (male patient)
Antibacterial soap
Sterile rinse
Sterile specimen cup with lid and label
Gloves (optional*)
Biohazard bag for disposal
Note: A midstream clean-catch kit is also available for
medical office use.

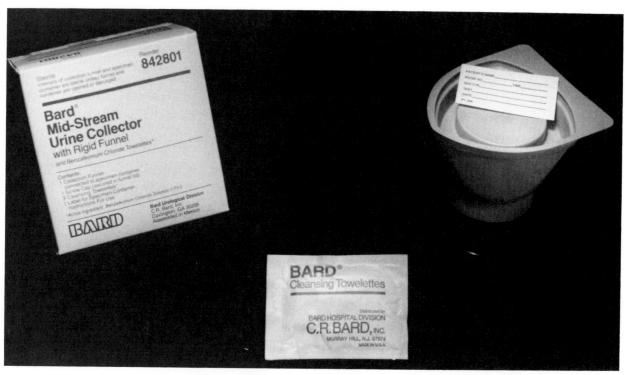

Midstream clean-catch kit.

---

*Urine not tinged or contaminated with blood is a body fluid to which the CDCs universal precautions do not apply; however, CDC guidelines constitute a minimum standard of practice. For institutions that have implemented universal precautions (applying them to *all* body fluids), it is acceptable to wear disposal gloves, especially for the patient at high risk for or with an infectious disease such as AIDS. Other barriers such as goggles, gown, and mask may also be worn, depending on the potential for risk.

PROCEDURE

1. Prepare the room by assembling the equipment and checking the cleanliness of the room, lighting, and temperature.
2. Identify the patient and explain the procedure.

3. Hand the patient the appropriate supplies.

4. Instruct the patient in self-cleansing technique in the following manner:
   a. Before voiding, wet the gauze pads and suds with the special soap.
   b. Female patients use one gauze pad to clean one side of the perineum, wiping from front to back. Dispose of wipe in biohazard bag.
   c. Using another wipe, cleanse the other side of the perineum from front to back. Dispose of wipe in biohazard bag.
   d. With the remaining wipe, cleanse the middle of the perineum from the front to back. Dispose of wipe in biohazard bag.
   e. Repeat same four steps using clean wet gauze wipes for rinsing off the soap.
   f. Male patients use a circular motion to wipe the penis starting at the center of the urethral opening to the exterior of the tip.
   g. Repeat the soap scrub a second time. If uncircumcised, retract the foreskin.
   h. Repeat the procedure with clean wet gauze to rinse off soap.
5. Instruct the patient to void as follows:
   a. Void briefly into the toilet.
   b. Void again and collect the urine in the sterile specimen cup.
   c. Remove the cup when the cup is not quite full and before voiding ceases.
   d. Place the lid on the cup and bring the specimen to you.
6. Label the container, not the lid, immediately with the patient's name, date, time, and contents.
7. Process the specimen according to the physician's orders or deliver the specimen to the laboratory area.
8. Give follow-up instructions to the patient.

9. Record the date, time, procedure, type of specimen, and disposition. Example: 3/5/93 2:00 PM: clean-catch specimen obtained 6/2/93 at 10:00 AM. Sent to laboratory (initials).
10. Clean the equipment and the examination room.

PRINCIPLE

1. To reduce procedure time and to facilitate the efficiency of the examination.

2. To reduce the risk of error and to provide assurance to anxious patients.
3. To use as visual confirmation while the procedure is explained.
4. Give a rationale for the steps to the patient to elicit compliance. Hairs of the perineum contain bacteria. Wiping from front to back avoids cross-contamination of the urethra from the other perineal orifices. Each wipe is used only once to prevent contamination.

5. Voiding a small amount of urine before collection washes away bacteria at the urinary meatus. The urine voided in midstream will be the "clean-catch." It is helpful to the patient if these instructions can be taped to the door in the bathroom for easy reference.

6. To reduce the chance of error, especially if the lid is misplaced during testing.
7. Urine specimens should be processed immediately or refrigerated.
8. To ensure proper continued care, instructions should be in writing for the patient to take home.
9. To ensure quality of care and to provide a point of future reference.

10. To prevent the chance of transmitting microorganisms and to prepare the room for the next patient.

PROCEDURE: Measure head circumference of children

OSHA STANDARDS: (III)

Terminal Performance Objective: Measure the head circumference (HC) of an infant or child within 1 minute.

EQUIPMENT: Measuring tape

PROCEDURE

1. Identify the patient and explain the procedure to the adult.
2. Place the child in the supine position.
3. Secure the measuring tape anteriorly over the lower forehead above the supraorbital ridge and posteriorly over the occipital bone (above the eyebrows) and over the greatest protrusion in the back of the head, usually midpoint to the ears.
4. Note and record the measurement immediately. Example: date, time HC 12.4 in (31 cm).

PRINCIPLE

1. To reduce the risk of error and to provide assurance to anxious parents.
2. To facilitate the measurement.
3. This area is the most reliable and perceptible as an indication of growth and development, especially brain growth. Small circumference may indicate underdevelopment; large circumference, congenital anomalies or hydrocephalus.
4. Normal HC at birth ranges from 12.4 in (31 cm) to 14.8 in (37 cm).

*N*utrition and Diet Therapy

> Let food be thy medicine.
>
> Hippocrates

CHAPTER OUTLINE

LEARNING OBJECTIVES

Upon completing this chapter, you will be able to:

1. List the functions and sources for each of the major nutrients.
2. List the daily requirements for each of the major nutrients.
3. Identify the food groups represented in the Food Group Pyramid, and state the number of servings per day for each.
4. List the modifications to the recommended daily allowances for pregnant and lactating women and for the elderly.
5. List and describe the relationship of body weight, lean body weight, and percentage of body fat to obesity and weight reduction or weight gain therapy.
6. Describe the standard diets commonly prescribed, the conditions for which they are used, and the characteristics of each.
7. State the factors accepted as contributing to obesity.
8. Describe the daily allowances usually prescribed for mild and moderate obesity and for the treatment of diabetes.
9. List four ways nutrients may adversely affect the patient on medication.

Chapter 22

*N*utrition and Diet Therapy

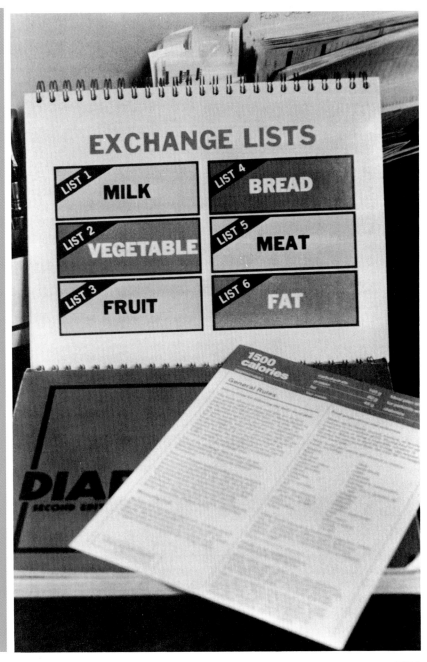

PERFORMANCE OBJECTIVES

Upon completing this chapter, you will be able to:

1. Interview the patient regarding nutritional status.
2. Calculate frame size, percentage of body fat, optimal percentage of body fat, ideal body weight, and weight loss or gain over time.
3. Measure and record skinfold thickness at four body sites.
4. Instruct the patient on how to apply a daily meal plan prescription to the food exchange list.

DACUM EDUCATIONAL COMPONENTS

1. Instruct patients with special needs (7.2).
2. Teach patients methods of health promotion and disease prevention (7.3).
3. Interview and take a patient history (4.6).
4. Perform selected tests that assist with diagnosis and treatment (4.11).

Glossary

Anabolism: the constructive phase of metabolism whereby simpler compounds derived from nutrients are converted into living, organized substances usable by the body cells

Appetite: the desire to eat

Basal metabolic rate: in physiology, pertaining to the lowest possible level; the minimal energy expended for the maintenance of vital body functions; about 25% of all energy from nutrients is used by the body to carry on its normal functions; the remainder becomes heat

Calorie: in nutrition, the energy content of foods, which is the "large calorie" or kilocalorie (1 kcal equals 1000 cal)

Catabolism: the breaking down phase of metabolism whereby compounds derived from nutrients are converted into simpler compounds, releasing energy

Energy: the capacity to be active that is derived from the consumption of food containing energy in chemical form; Carbohydrates, fats, and proteins are the three main sources of energy that, once in the cells, form chemical reactions that produce new forms of energy and yield by-products, such as waste and water

Hunger: the physiologic need to eat

Metabolism: the sum total of all the chemical reactions related to the body's processing of nutrients; there are two stages: anabolism and catabolism (see above)

Set point: the body's automatically regulated level of body weight; it is believed that elevation of the regulatory level or "set point" is responsible for obesity

Diet therapy is a treatment alternative the physician may select in providing comprehensive health care. Dietary requirements depend on age, sex, height, weight, activity, and percentage of body fat. The objective of a proper diet is to achieve and maintain the desired body weight and composition. In adults, body weight, in relation to height, gender, and percentage of body fat, is useful in assessing overall health. Diet therapy in medical practice is the primary method of treatment for patients who are undernourished or for the treatment of obesity. Permanently or temporarily altering the diet is also an important part of treatment plans for many diseases, after surgery, and during acute illnesses.

Diet therapy and the medical assistant's role in assisting with the implementation of diet prescriptions are discussed in this chapter. Although prescribing the diet is the physician's responsibility, the medical assistant is involved in interviewing the patient, taking specific anthropometric measurements, and aiding the patient in interpreting diet instructions. The medical assistant also serves often as a resource person to whom the patient directs questions and concerns related to the diet plan. Before the medical assistant can guide the patient in diet therapy, a basic background in normal nutrition is required. Normal nutrition is the foundation of diet therapy and of good health in general.

NUTRITION

Nutrition signifies the collective processes involved in the body's intake and utilization of food. Food is a physiologic requirement for growth, development, and maintenance of the body.

The importance of nutrition in clinical medicine is being increasingly acknowledged. The science of diet and nutrition involves the study of the body's need for, and utilization of, special food substances called *nutrients.* The patient's own dietary habits, conditions of food deprivation, or dependency on substances, such as alcohol or drugs, can interfere with the normal intake and utilization of the essential nutrients. When essential nutrients are lacking or are not supplied in sufficient quantities in the daily diet, a nutritional deficiency and disease results. The aim of therapy in this case is to increase the missing nutrients.

The excessive accumulation of body fat in obesity, on the other hand, also can cause serious nutrition-related complications, such as elevated cholesterol, hypertension, and diabetes. Therefore, the aim of all therapy for obesity is to eliminate harmful foods and to reduce the number of calories ingested below the number of calories expended as energy. By eliminating body fat, some diabetics actually can discontinue their medication, most people with hypertension can reduce their blood pressure, and obese patients can improve their health and lifestyle.

Normal physiologic states, such as pregnancy, lactation, infancy, and aging, and the practice of vegetarianism, can also change the body's need for specific nutrients. Disease and injury increase the body's need for certain nutrients, especially proteins, and can even interfere with the utilization of an otherwise healthy diet. Malnutrition frequently occurs during a prolonged illness and may accompany acute injury or complicated surgical or medical procedures. Many genetic disorders require special diets for their management, as do many degenerative diseases.

When the patient is undernourished, overnourished, or has a condition that responds to the increase or decrease of certain nutrients, diet therapy is used with specific food combinations, amounts, and dietary sources to return the patient to better health.

METABOLISM

Metabolism is the process of the physical and chemical changes related to the body's utilization of food. Body tissue is built up (through growth, repair, and maintenance) and broken down (through the manufacture of waste products) in the cyclic process of metabolism. The chapter on vital signs discusses how certain body states change metabolic activity. Metabolic activity produces heat and energy, and normal nutrition and diet therapy are concerned with the energy produced by the correct types and amounts of nutrients. About 25% of all energy from nutrients is used by the body to carry on its functions, and the rest becomes heat. The amount of energy required in the form of caloric intake for metabolic processes varies. In general, however, factors such as weight, percentage of body fat, age, activity, and a person's state of health all play a role in determining a person's metabolic rate and daily caloric requirement.

NUTRIENTS

Digestion is the term applied to the process whereby the body reduces food to usable "fuel," which the body "burns" inside the cells during chemical reactions. Chemical digestion is achieved by the actions of enzymes and digestive secretions that convert food into the specific molecular substances called *nutrients.*

There are six widely used classifications of nutrients: (1) proteins, (2) carbohydrates, (3) fats, (4) vitamins, (5) minerals, and (6) water. Each is described below according to its structure and sources. Table 22–1 describes the function, utilization, caloric requirement, and effects of deficiency for each.

PROTEINS

Amino acids are organic compounds occurring naturally in plant and animal tissues. These compounds form the chief constituents of protein. There are 20 amino acids necessary for body functioning. Eleven of these 20 can be synthesized by the human body; the other nine must be obtained from the diet. These nine, called *essential amino acids*, are absolutely essential in the diet because they supply human cells with needed protein.

Protein foods that provide a balance of the essential amino acids required by the body are called *complete proteins*. Complete proteins are found in animal sources, such as meat, eggs, fish, and milk. The World Health Organization (WHO) considers egg protein the perfect protein as it contains all the essential amino acids. Because it is the most complete and high-quality protein, it is used by the WHO as the reference to measure the quality of the proteins.

Complete protein is present in a variety of food substances. Daily sources include one egg or two egg whites, milk (low-fat or nonfat for adults), cooked lean and skinless meat or poultry, fish, and soybeans. Low-fat cooking methods should be used. Smoked or salt-cured meats contain substances linked to cancer of the stomach and esophagus; therefore, the amounts of these foods should be limited.

Plant proteins, with the exception of soybeans, do not contain all of the essential amino acids and are considered *incomplete proteins*, yet they are important in the daily diet. Plant protein sources such as nuts, dried beans, peas, and certain forms of wheat, although incomplete in essential amino acids, are low in fat and high in fiber. Incomplete protein sources can be combined in specific ways to provide all of the essential amino acids. Therefore, it is possible for a vegetarian who carefully selects vegetable proteins and includes milk products in the daily diet to be assured of adequate protein intake. More extreme vegetarians (those not including milk products in the diet) must plan more carefully to ensure a balanced protein diet.

Table 22–1
THE MAJOR NUTRIENTS

Nutrient	Functions	Utilization	Daily Requirement	Deficiency	Increased Levels
Proteins	1. Build and repair tissue. 2. Help to maintain water balance. 3. Antibody production and disease resistance. 4. Energy. 5. Maintain heat.	1. Completely absorbed. 2. Completely utilized. 3. Not stored. 4. Can provide quick energy in the abnormal absence of carbohydrates.	1 g = 4 cal Requirement: 1 g/kg adults; 2–3 g/kg children; 1–2 g/kg adolescents; (10%–20% of total caloric intake). Increased need in illness and body repair states.	1. Weight loss and fatigue. 2. Protein-calorie malnutrition. 3. Skin dryness and scaling. 4. Lowered resistance to infection. 5. Interference with normal healing, growth, and development.	1. Increased levels are found in liver disease, lead poisoning, phenylketouria, and folic acid deficiency.
Carbohydrates	1. Provide quick energy. 2. Source of heat. 3. Spare protein from being converted for energy uses. 4. Enable fat to be metabolized.	1. Quickest energy source. 2. Converted and used as glucose. 3. Stored in liver and muscle cells as glycogen. 4. Further excess of glucose converted into fat and stored as adipose tissue.	1 g = 4 cal Requirements: 50%–60% of total caloric intake.	1. Weight loss. 2. Protein loss. 3. Fatigue.	1. Increased body fat.
Fats	1. Most concentrated source of heat and energy. 2. Transportation of fat-soluble vitamins. 3. Feeling of satisfied hunger (more slowly digested). 4. Source of storage energy. 5. Insulation and protection for body organs (adipose tissue).	1. Digested more slowly than proteins or carbohydrates. 2. Stored as adipose tissue.	1 g = 4 cal Requirement: No more than 30% of total caloric intake, or 60–70 g/d.	1. Dry skin. 2. Disruption of vitamin utilization. 3. Fatigue.	1. Increased body fat. 2. Increased cholesterol levels. 3. Increased risk of heart and artery disease.

Continued

	Functions	Recommended Amount	Results
Fiber	1. Increase the bulk of stool. 2. Absorb organic wastes and toxins.	20–35 g Six or more servings of whole-grain products.	1. Increased risk of colon cancer and high blood cholesterol levels. 2. Increased blood glucose levels after eating.	1. Diarrhea. 2. Gastrointestinal disorders.
Vitamins	1. Essential to growth and development. 2. Infection resistance. 3. Specific functions to maintain body systems.	(See Table 22–3.)	(See Table 22–3.)
Minerals	1. Most absorbed directly into digestive tract. 2. Sunlight needed for vitamin D. 3. Water-soluble vitamins A, D, E, K not stored by body. 4. Fat-soluble vitamins stored by body.	(Most absorbed by the intestines.) (Most mineral excesses are eliminated.)	
	1. Bone, tooth formation. 2. Blood coagulation. 3. Heart and muscle contraction.	Calcium: 800–200 mg.	1. Bone fragility. 2. Osteoporosis in elderly.
	1. Bone, tooth formation acid-base balance. 2. Energy production.	Phosphorus: 800 mg.	1. Weakness. 2. Blood cell disorders.
	1. Hemoglobin. 2. Enzymes.	Iron: 10–18 mg.	1. Anemia, especially in women and during pregnancy.
	1. Thyroxin (T₄). 2. Triiodothyronine (T₃). 3. Energy control mechanisms.	Iodine: 100–150 mcg.	2. Hypothyroidism.
	1. Muscle activity. 2. Water retention. 3. Acid-base balance.	Potassium: 2–4 g.	1. Kypokalemia. 2. Paralysis. 3. Cardiac disturbances. 4. May be significant in persons taking diuretics (fluid or water pills).
	1. Acid-base balance. 2. pH of blood. 3. Osmotic pressure. 4. Muscle contraction.	Sodium: 1.1–3.3 g.	1. Hyponatremia.

Table 22–1
THE MAJOR NUTRIENTS—*Continued*

Nutrient	Functions	Utilization	Daily Requirement	Deficiency	Increased Levels
Water	1. Maintain fluid balance. 2. Lubricate moving parts. 3. Elimination of waste. 4. Transportation of nutrients and body secretions. 5. Solvent for chemicals. 6. Digestion and 7. Regulation of body temperature.	1. Continuous absorption, utilization, and excretion. 2. In healthy adults, input equals output.	Six to eight glasses per day.	1. Dry lips, mucous membranes. 2. Dehydration. 3. Hypovolemia.	1. Water intoxification (especially in babies). 2. Circulatory overload (vascular hypovolemia). 3. Edema.

CARBOHYDRATES

Carbohydrates are used by the body as an immediate source of energy. They are present in some amount in most foods, but the chief sources are sugars and starches. Carbohydrates are classified as monosaccharides, disaccharides, and polysaccharides.

Monosaccharides include *glucose*, also called *dextrose* and *grape sugar* (contained in fruits and vegetables); *fructose* (contained in fruits, vegetables, and honey); and *galactose* (derived from lactose found in milk). Disaccharides include *sucrose* (known as table sugar and found in syrups); *maltose* (found in malt products); and *lactose* (contained in the milk of animals and humans). Polysaccharides include *starches* (contained in grains and potatoes); *cellulose* (contained in fibrous vegetables, cereals, and fruits); and *glycogen* (stored in the muscles and liver).

All ripe fruits and many vegetables contain some natural sugars. The starches are present in breads, pastas, cereals, potatoes, and squash.

Carbohydrates may be stored in the body as glycogen for future use. If they are eaten in excess, however, the body changes them into fats and stores them in that form. The American Dietetic Association currently recommends natural sources loaded with complex carbohydrates, such as fruits and whole-grain breads and cereals. In addition to providing carbohydrates, fruits and vegetables provide fiber, vitamins, and minerals. They are also naturally low in fat. Bread and cereal carbohydrate sources are accompanied by B vitamins, iron, and protein and are naturally low in fat. Whole-grain products, such as whole wheat bread and brown rice, are also high in fiber.

Simple carbohydrates found in sugars such as table sugar, syrup, fructose, dextrose (found in many processed foods), and candy are sources of carbohydrates but provide few nutrients other than calories and thus are not considered to be of nutritional value.

Alcohol, like sugars, supplies calories with little or no nutrients. Alcohol is linked to many health problems, is the cause of many accidents, and can lead to addiction. If alcoholic beverages are consumed, a health guide is to limit consumption to two drinks a day for men and one drink per day for women and to abstain from drinking alcoholic beverages during pregnancy, during illness, and while taking medications. (One drink is equal to: $1\frac{1}{2}$ oz pure [80-proof] alcohol, 5 oz wine, or 12 oz of regular beer.)

DIETARY FIBER

Fiber is a special carbohydrate. It is composed of cellulose (which is the "skeleton" of most plant structures and plant cells), gums, lignin (obtained from wood or a woody plant), pectin (obtained from fruit rinds and skins), and other carbohydrates not digestible by humans. Fiber is necessary to increase the bulk of the stool and make it softer by taking up water as it passes through the colon. Fiber is also needed to absorb organic wastes and toxins and carry them out of the digestive tract. Dietary fiber is helpful in the treatment and prevention of uncomplicated constipation and hemorrhoids, diverticular disease, and irritable bowel syndrome.

Unable to be absorbed by the body, the bulk of fiber keeps the colon mildly distended, thus decreasing pressure pockets that cause spasm. Fiber hastens the passage of softer stools, which decreases the pressure exerted by stools against the intestinal walls. Fiber also has the capacity to unite with bile salts and cholesterol, thus preventing their absorption and hastening their elimination. Fiber slows the rate of carbohydrate breakdown and absorption from the intestinal tract and somewhat reduces the rise in blood glucose that occurs after eating. The American Cancer Society suggests a diet rich in fiber as a way to lower the incidence of some cancers, especially colorectal cancer.

For years, fiber-rich foods have been recommended because they are usually low in calories and promote regularity. Today, strong evidence links food high in fiber to a lowering of levels of blood cholesterol, a reduction in gallstone formation, and the ability to control diabetes mellitus and to decrease the risk of certain types of cancers. Scientists are uncertain, however, if fiber works alone or in combination with other substances to promote good health.

There are two major types of fiber: soluble and insoluble. Soluble fiber tends to swell when eaten and slows the absorption of food from the digestive tract. It also helps to control the blood sugar level of diabetics and lowers blood cholesterol levels. Sources of soluble fiber include oat bran, dried beans and peas, barley, and some fruits and vegetables.

Insoluble fiber promotes regularity and helps decrease the risk of colon cancer. Sources include wheat bran in whole wheat bread and brown rice. Fiber supplements do not contain all of the vitamins and minerals found in high-fiber food and are not recommended.

Excessive amounts of fiber can impair the absorption of essential minerals. Roughage in the intestinal tract can be harmful in bowel disease, where there is a narrowing of the bowel. Fiber intake must be increased gradually to prevent abdominal pain, gas, and diarrhea. More than six glasses of water per day are necessary because fiber needs water to work properly.

FATS

Fats, also known as *fatty acids*, are composed of the same basic elements as carbohydrates, but the proportions of the elements are different. Like carbohydrates, fats yield energy. In fact, more energy can be derived from a given amount of fat than from a similar amount of carbohydrate.

Fats are referred to as *lipids*. Lipids are fatty, greasy, oily, and waxy substances that are insoluble in water. They are soluble in ether or alcohol. About 95% of lipids are *simple lipids*, also called *triglycerides, neutral fats*, or *true fats*. They are an important source of fuel to the body and a much lighter form of energy storage than carbohydrates.

The other 5% of lipids are *compound lipids,* also known as *phospholipids* and *sterols.* Phospholipids include lecithin, the cephalins, and glycolipids. Lethicin is important in the transmission of nerve impulses. Cephalin is a substance needed for the clotting of blood.

All fatty acids are essential to the body. After digestion, fats are deposited and stored throughout the body (mostly in subcutaneous connective tissue) as a reserve source of energy. Fatty acids are also used to help form the membranes of all the body's cells. Too much fat storage, however, can complicate the functioning of the entire body system.

Fats are classified as *saturated* and *unsaturated,* and as *essential* and *false fatty acids.* Saturated fats, derived from animal sources, contain the highest concentration of hydrogen and are solid at room temperature. Butter and meat fat are examples of a saturated fat. Unsaturated fats are usually found in plant and nut oils. They are liquid at room temperature. An example is unsaturated vegetable oil. Highly unsaturated fats are referred to as *polyunsaturated fats.* Unsaturated fats can be hydrogenated; that is, additional hydrogen can be added through a special manufacturing process so that they are converted into solid fats for cooking. Thus hydrogenation process converts the unsaturated fat to a saturated form. Margarine is a prime example of the hydrogenation of unsaturated fatty acids into a solid substance.

Essential fatty acids are the fats found in butter, egg yolks, and milk. They are called essential fatty acids because they are necessary for growth and metabolism. False fats are those that have no nutritive value, such as mineral oil.

Some foods, such as meat, whole milk, and cheese, are naturally high in fat, whereas others, such as vegetables and fruits are almost fat-free. Animal sources of fat include meat, milk, eggs, and fish. Vegetable sources include corn, olives, cottonseed, safflower, soybeans, and nuts. All animal sources are saturated. Vegetable sources range from polyunsaturated (usually oils starting with the letter "S," such as sunflower or safflower oils) to saturated (coconut oil). Table 22–2 lists the sources of fats and oils.

As a rough guide, most people can eat 60 to 70 g of fat per day. About 10 g of fat are present in 3 slices of broiled bacon, 3 oz of roasted meat, 1½ oz cheese, 1¼ cups whole milk, and 1 tablespoon of margarine. On the low-fat side, however, it takes 18 oz of cooked fish, 25 cups of skim milk, 20 medium apples, or 100 cups of lettuce to provide the same amount of fat.

CHOLESTEROL

Associated with fatty acids is cholesterol. Cholesterol, however, is not a fat but a sterol, which means it is a steroid alcohol that combines with fatty acids to form an ester. In its free state, it aids in the functioning of hormones, vitamin D, and the formation of blood; but increased amounts of cholesterol as ester (combined with fatty acids) is associated with many diseases, including hypertension and atherosclerosis. Cholesterol

is a natural substance manufactured in the liver, but additional amounts are also derived from animal food sources and some plant sources.

VITAMINS

Vitamins are organic food substances that have been identified as essential elements for growth, development, and maintenance of body systems. They are more commonly assigned letters of the alphabet for reference with the exception of the B vitamin niacin.

Vitamins A, B, C, D, E, and K have been isolated and their functions established. Fat-soluble vitamins (those that dissolve in fat) are vitamins A, D, E, and K. Water-soluble vitamins (those that dissolve in water) consist of the B vitamins and vitamin C. Specific vitamins have specific sources, recommended allowances, functions, characteristics, and consequences from deficiencies or overdoses. These are listed in Table 22–3.

MINERALS

Minerals, not all of which are essential nutrients, are chemical compounds found in the body in differing quantities. Some minerals are found in such small proportions that they are called *trace minerals.* Other minerals are called *major minerals* because they are required by the body in greater proportion than trace minerals and because they compose a greater percentage of body weight. Calcium, phosphorus, iron, iodine, potassium, sodium, chlorine, and magnesium represent approximately 4% of body weight. All of these minerals, with the exception of iron, are major minerals. Iron, then, is a trace mineral. Both major and trace minerals perform essential functions; therefore a balanced diet must supply all the necessary minerals. The major sources of specified minerals are as follows:

Calcium. Milk and milk products; leafy green vegetables, such as kale, broccoli, spinach, and collard greens; tofu prepared with calcium; soft bones of sardines and salmon; oranges and calcium-fortified orange juice. In recent debates, physicians have disagreed over the value of milk as a source of calcium. Some studies show that there is no nutritional reason to drink milk, whereas others indicate that drinking milk lowers blood pressure in children aged 3 to 6 years. Still another study indicates that cow's milk may trigger juvenile diabetes. Despite seemingly contradictory evidence, most pediatricians still advise parents to include cow's milk in children's diets after a year of breast-feeding or formula feeding. The American Academy of Pediatrics recommends breast-feeding in the first year of life. A second choice is iron-fortified formula for the first 12 months of life, but absolutely no cow's milk should be given because of the risk of anemia. The American Academy of Pediatrics also recommends whole milk from ages 1 to 2 because fat is critically

Table 22-2
DIETARY SOURCES OF FATS AND OILS[a]

Animal Fats	Total Fat[b] (g)	Saturated Fat (g)	Polyunsaturated Fat (g)	Cholesterol (mg)
Beef fat	12.8	6.4	0.5	14
Chicken fat	12.8	3.8	2.7	11
Lard	12.8	5.0	1.4	12
Butter	11.5	7.2	0.4	31
Vegetable Oils				
Corn	13.6	1.7	8.0	0
Cottonseed	13.6	3.5	7.1	0
Peanut	13.5	2.3	4.3	0
Safflower	13.6	1.2	10.1	0
Soybean[c]	13.6	2.0	7.9	0
Mixed (mostly soybean and some cottonseed)[c]	13.6	2.4	6.5	0
Sunflower	13.6	1.4	8.9	0
Olive	13.5	1.8	1.1	0
Coconut[d]	13.6	11.8	0.2	0
Palm[d]	13.6	6.7	1.3	0
Margarine				
Hard (stick)	11.4	2.1	3.6	0
Soft (tub)	11.4	1.8	4.8	0
Vegetable shortening, hydrogenated	12.8	3.9	1.8	0
Salad Dressings				
Mayonnaise	11.0	1.6	5.7	8
Mayonnaise-type	4.9	0.7	2.6	4
Italian	7.1	1.0	4.1	0
Blue cheese	8.0	1.5	4.3	3
French	6.4	1.5	3.4	0
Thousand Island	5.6	0.9	3.1	4

[a]Amounts given are for 1 tablespoon.
[b]Total fat includes monounsaturated fat as well as the amounts of saturated and polyunsaturated fats shown in the two columns.
[c]Soybean oils and soybean oil mixtures are the vegetable oils most commonly available to consumers.
[d]Used in commercially prepared foods.

Table 22–3
SUMMARY OF VITAMINS SIGNIFICANT IN THE HUMAN DIET*

Vitamin	Chief Functions	Results of Deficiency	Characteristics	Good Sources	Recommended Daily Allowances
VITAMIN A Provitamin, carotene	Essential for maintaining the integrity of epithelial membranes. Helps maintain resistance to infections. Necessary for the formation of rhodopsin and prevention of night blindness.	*Mild:* Retarded growth. Increased susceptibility to infection. Abnormal function of gastrointestinal, genitourinary and respiratory tracts due to altered epithelial membranes. Skin dries, shrivels, thickens, sometimes pustule formation. Night blindness. *Severe:* Xerophthalmia, a characteristic eye disease, and other local infections.	Fat-soluble. Not destroyed by ordinary cooking temperatures. Is destroyed by high temperatures when oxygen is present. Marked capacity for storage in the liver. NOTE: Excessive intake of carotene from which vitamin A is formed may produce yellow discoloration of the skin (carotenemia).	Animal fats Butter Cheese Cream Egg yolk Whole milk. Fish liver oil. Liver. Vegetable 1. Green leafy, esp. escarole, kale, parsley 2. Yellow, esp. carrots. *Artificial:* Concentrates in several forms. Irradiated fish oils.	*Males (ages 11–51+y):* 1000 µg retinol equivalents. *Females (ages 11–51+ y):* 800 µg retinol equivalents. *In pregnancy:* 1000 µg retinol equivalents. *In lactation:* 1200 µg retinol equivalents. *Children:* 400–700 µg retinol equivalents. *Infants:* 400 µg retinol equivalents.
THIAMINE Vitamin B$_1$	Important role in carbohydrate metabolism. Essential for maintenance of normal digestion and appetite. Essential for normal functioning of nervous tissue.	*Mild:* Loss of appetite. Impaired digestion of starches and sugars. Colitis, constipation, or diarrhea. Emaciation. *Severe:* Nervous disorders of various types. Loss of coordinating power of muscles. Beriberi. Paralysis in humans.	Water-soluble. Not readily destroyed by ordinary cooking temperature. Destroyed by exposure to heat, alkali, or sulfites. Is not stored in body.	Widely distributed in plant and animal tissues but seldom occurs in high concentration, exception in brewer's yeast. Other good sources are: Whole-grain cereals Peas, Beans Peanuts Oranges Glandular— heart, liver, kidney Many vegetables and fruits	*Males (ages 11–51+ y):* 1.2–1.5 mg. *Females (ages 11–51+ y):* 1.0–1.1 mg. *In pregnancy:* 1.4–1.6 mg. *In lactation:* 1.5–1.7 mg. *Children:* 0.7–1.2 mg. *Infants:* 0.3–0.5 mg.

Continued

Table 22-3
SUMMARY OF VITAMINS SIGNIFICANT IN THE HUMAN DIET*—*Continued*

Vitamin	Chief Functions	Results of Deficiency	Characteristics	Good Sources	Daily Allowances Recommended
				Nuts. *Artificial:* Concentrates from yeast. Rice polishings. Wheat germ.	
RIBOFLAVIN Vitamin B$_2$	Important in formation of certain enzymes and in cellular oxidation. Normal growth. Prevention of cheilosis and glossitis. Participates in light adaptation.	Impaired growth. Lassitude and weakness. Cheilosis. Glossitis. Atrophy of skin. Anemia. Photophobia. Cataracts.	Water-soluble. Alcohol-soluble. Not destroyed by heat in cooking unless with alkali. Unstable in light, esp. in presence of alkali.	Eggs. Green vegetables. Liver. Kidney. Milk. Wheat germ. Yeast, dried. Enriched foods.	*Males (ages 11–51⁺ y):* 1.4–1.7 mg. *Females (ages 11–51⁺ y):* 1.2–1.3 mg. *In pregnancy:* 1.6 mg. *In lactation:* 1.8 mg. *Children:* 0.8–1.4 mg. *Infants:* 0.4–0.6 mg.
NIACIN Nicotinic acid Nicotinamide Antipellagra vitamin	As the component of two important enzymes, it is important in glycolysis, tissue respiration, and fat synthesis. Nicotinic acid but not nicotinamide causes vasodilation and flushing. Prevents pellagra.	Pellagra. Gastrointestinal disturbances. Mental disturbances.	Soluble in hot water and alcohol. Not destroyed by heat, light, air, or alkali. Not destroyed in ordinary cooking.	Yeast Lean meat Fish Legumes Whole-grain cereals and peanuts Enriched foods.	*Males (ages 11–51⁺ y):* 16–19 mg. *Females (11–51⁺ y):* 13–15 mg. *In pregnancy:* 17 mg. *In lactation:* 20 mg. *Children:* 9–16 mg. *Infants:* 6–8 mg.
VITAMIN B$_{12}$ Cyanoco-balamin	Produces remission in pernicious anemia. Essential for normal development of red blood cells.	Pernicious anemia.	Soluble in water or alcohol. Unstable in hot alkaline or acid solutions.	Liver. Kidney. Dairy products. Most of vitamin required by humans is synthesized by intestinal bacteria.	*Males and females (ages 11–51⁺ y):* 3.0 μg. *In pregnancy:* 4.0 μg. *In lactation:* 5.0 μg. *Children:* 2–5 μg. *Infants:* 1–2 μg.

Continued

Table 22–3
SUMMARY OF VITAMINS SIGNIFICANT IN THE HUMAN DIET*—*Continued*

Vitamin	Chief Functions	Results of Deficiency	Characteristics	Good Sources	Daily Allowances Recommended
VITAMIN C Ascorbic acid	Essential to formation of intracellular cement substances in a variety of tissues including skin, dentin, cartilage and bone matrix. Important in healing of wounds and fractures of bones. Prevents scurvy. Facilitates absorption of iron.	*Mild:* Lowered resistance to infections. Joint tenderness. Susceptibility to dental caries, pyorrhea, and bleeding gums. *Severe:* Hemorrhage. Anemia. Scurvy.	Soluble in water. Easily destroyed by oxidation; heat hastens the process. Lost in cooking, particularly if water in which food was cooked is discarded. Also loss is greater if cooked in iron or copper utensils. Quick frozen foods lose little of their vitamin C. Stored in the body to a limited extent.	Abundant in most fresh fruits and vegetables, esp. citrus fruit and juices, tomato and orange. *Artificial:* Ascorbic acid. Cevitamic acid.	*Males (ages 11–51+ y):* 50–60 mg. *Females (11–51+ y):* 50–60 mg. *In pregnancy:* 80 mg. *In lactation:* 100 mg. Children: 45 mg. *Infants:* 35 mg. The infant diet is likely to be deficient in vitamin C unless orange or tomato juice or other form is added.
VITAMIN D	Regulates absorption of calcium and phosphorus from the intestinal tract. Antirachitic.	*Mild:* Interferes with utilization of calcium and phosphorus in bone and teeth formation. Irritability. Weakness. *Severe:* Rickets, may be common in young children. Osteomalacia in adults.	Soluble in fats and organic solvents. Relatively stable under refrigeration. Stored in liver. Often associated with vitamin A.	Butter Egg yolk Fish liver oils Fish having fat distributed through the flesh, salmon, tuna fish, herring, sardines. Liver Oysters Yeast and foods irradiated with ultraviolet light. Formed in the skin by exposure to sunlight. Artificially prepared forms.	*Males and females (ages 11–51+ y):* 200–400 IU. After age 22, none except during pregnancy or lactation. *In pregnancy:* 400–600 IU. *In lactation:* 400–600 IU. Children: 400 IU. *Infants:* 400 IU.
VITAMIN E Alpha tocopherol	Normal reproduction in rats. Prevention of muscular dystrophy in rats.	Red blood cell resistance to rupture is decreased.	Fat-soluble. Stable to heat in absence of oxygen.	Lettuce and other green, leafy vegetables. Wheat germ oil. Margarine. Rice.	*Males (ages 11–51+ y):* 8–10 mg d-α-tocopherol. *Females 11–51+ y):*

Continued

Table 22–3
SUMMARY OF VITAMINS SIGNIFICANT IN THE HUMAN DIET* — *Continued*

Vitamin	Chief Functions	Results of Deficiency	Characteristics	Good Sources	Daily Allowances Recommended
					8 mg f-α-toco-pherol. *In pregnancy:* 10 mg d-α-toco-pherol. *In lactation:* 11 mg d-α-toco-pherol. *Children:* 10 to 15 IU. *Infants:* 5 IU.
VITAMIN B₆ Pyridoxine	Essential for metabolism of tryptophan. Needed for utilization of certain other amino acids.	Dermatitis around eyes and mouth. Neuritis. Anorexia, nausea, and vomiting.	Soluble in water and alcohol. Rapidly inactivated in presence of heat, sunlight, or air.	Blackstrap molasses. Meat. Cereal grains. Wheat germ.	*Males and females (11– 51+ y):* 1.8–2.2 mg. *In pregnancy:* 2.6 mg. *In lactation:* 2.5 mg. *Children:* 0.9–1.6 mg. *Infants:* 0.3–0.6 mg.
FOLACIN	Essential for normal functioning of hematopoi-etic system.	Anemia.	Slightly soluble in water. Easily destroyed by heat in presence of acid. Decreases when food is stored at room temperature. NOTE: A large dose may prevent appearance of anemia in a case of pernicious anemia but still permit neutrologic symptoms to develop.	Glandular meats. Yeast. Green, leafy vegetables.	*Males and females (ages 11–51+ y):* 400 μg. *In pregnancy:* 800 μg. *In lactation:* 500 μg. *Children:* 100–300 μg. *Infants:* 30–45 μg.

**Source:* From Thomas CL (ed): Taber's Cyclopedic Medical Dictionary, ed 15. FA Davis, Philadelphia 1985, pp 2054–2059, with permission.

needed during this time. Low-fat milk may be, or should be in some cases, used after the age of 2.

Phosphorus. Milk and milk products.

Iron. Liver and other meats, fish, poultry, and soybeans.

Iodine. Seafoods, iodized salt, and salt substitutes.

Potassium. Cereals; fruits including apricots, avocados, bananas, citrus fruits; dried fruits; and vegetables including artichokes, broccoli, potatoes, and tomatoes.

Sodium. Salt is the main source of sodium and is necessary for normal body functions. Most foods contain sodium, so care must be taken to select foods that do not contain excessive added amounts, for example, potato chips. When persons with high blood pressure decrease the amount of sodium they eat, their blood pressure usually decreases. Because there is currently no way to predict who will or will not develop high blood pressure, sodium intake should be limited by everyone, unless otherwise advised by the physician.

WATER

Like air, water is essential to the maintenance of normal body functioning and accounts for about 60% of the body weight. At least two thirds of this amount is intracellular, and most of the remainder functions extracellularly bathing the tissues, with approximately 5% present in the blood. Drinking water provides much of the body's need for water. Water is also contained in most foods.

Water and sodium are important in fluid balance because they are the components directly affecting the concentration of body fluids and, therefore, their distribution. There is a normal volume of fluid only as long as there is adequate *intake* and *output* of water. An accurate measuring of fluid intake and output can be a valuable aid in determining the amount of fluid replacement needed in disease and illness.

RECOMMENDED DIETARY ALLOWANCES

As a result of scientific investigation, the Food and Nutrition Board of the National Academy of Science publishes recommended dietary allowances (RDA), which are used as guidelines for planning and evaluating nutritional status (Table 22–4). Because of the safety margin in each recommended nutrient level (except calories), the suggested nutrient levels allow for the needs of most healthy individuals. Obviously, illness and injury would change these requirements.

THE FOOD GUIDE PYRAMID

The basic food groups represent the arrangement of nutrients in the daily diet. To provide the necessary nutrients for health and prevention of diseases, particularly cancer and heart disease, the United States Department of Agriculture (USDA) has developed the Food Guide Pyramid, a visual representation of a heavily researched nutritional guidance system (Fig. 22–1). The Food Guide Pyramid helps patients put the USDA's dietary guidelines into action.

Nutrition research has proved that many chronic diseases are linked to the foods we eat. Most nutrition experts agree that a high-fiber, low-fat diet is important in the prevention of heart disease and certain types of cancer. Many nutritionists also recommend that salt and sugar should be used only in moderation. In addition, staying active with regular exercise and maintaining proper weight and body fat proportions is an important part of nutritional awareness.

There are seven guidelines for a healthy diet for persons age 2 or older:

1. Eat a variety of foods.
2. Maintain a healthy weight and body fat proportion.
3. Choose foods low in fat, saturated fat, and cholesterol.
4. Include plenty of vegetables, fruits, and grain products.
5. Use sugars only in moderation.
6. Use salt and sodium only in moderation.
7. Drink alcoholic beverages in moderation, if at all.

The shape of the food pyramid provides a guide to the relative quantities of those foods that should be selected daily from each food group. A healthy diet includes choices from each group except the top group (fats, oils, and sweets). Each of the five lower food groups provides some of the nutrients needed each day. Foods in one group cannot replace those in another — all are needed for good health. A 29-page booklet on the Food Guide Pyramid is available for $1 from the Superintendent of Documents, Consumer Information Center, Pueblo, CO, 81009. The pamphlet details each section of the pyramid and provides information on serving sizes, calories, fat, cholesterol, sugar, salt, and sodium.

Although fat and oils are included in the preparation of many foods, the recommended allowance for fat is based on the number of calories eaten: fat should contribute no more than 30% of the total calories. As a rough guide, most people can eat 60 to 70 g of fat a day. Water, another nutrient not specifically identified in the Food Guide Pyramid, has a recommended allowance of 6 to 8 glasses daily. Although sweets provide energy, infrequent use is recommended because overconsumption tends to displace essential nutrients in the daily diet.

Generally, the pyramid emphasizes eating a variety of food from each food group and is inexact regarding carbohydrates, fat, and calories. The pyramid recommends *servings* of these foods rather than precise measurements in the form of a pyramid plan (2 to 3 servings each from the meat and milk groups; 3 to 5 servings

Table 22–4

RECOMMENDED DAILY DIETARY ALLOWANCES,ᵃ REVISED 1989

Category	Age (years) or Condition	Weight (kg)	Weight (lb)	Height (cm)	Height (in)	Protein (g)	Fat-Soluble Vitamins — Vitamin A (µg RE)ᶜ	Vitamin D (µg)ᵈ	Vitamin E (mg α-TE)ᵉ	Vitamin K (µg)	Water-Soluble Vitamins — Vitamin C (mg)	Thiamin (mg)	Riboflavin (mg)	Niacin (mg NE)ᵍ	Vitamin B₆ (mg)	Folate (µg)	Vitamin B₁₂ (µg)	Minerals — Calcium (mg)	Phosphorus (mg)	Magnesium (mg)	Iron (mg)	Zinc (mg)	Iodine (µg)	Selenium (µg)
Infants	0.0–0.5	6	13	60	24	13	375	7.5	3	5	30	0.3	0.4	5	0.3	25	0.3	400	300	40	6	5	40	10
	0.5–1.0	9	20	71	28	14	375	10	4	10	35	0.4	0.5	6	0.6	35	0.5	600	500	60	10	5	50	15
Children	1–3	13	29	90	35	16	400	10	6	15	40	0.7	0.8	9	1.0	50	0.7	800	800	80	10	10	70	20
	4–6	20	44	112	44	24	500	10	7	20	45	0.9	1.1	12	1.1	75	1.0	800	800	120	10	10	90	20
	7–10	28	62	132	52	28	700	10	7	30	45	1.0	1.2	13	1.4	100	1.4	800	800	170	10	10	120	30
Males	11–14	45	99	157	62	45	1000	10	10	45	50	1.3	1.5	17	1.7	150	2.0	1200	1200	270	12	15	150	40
	15–18	66	145	176	69	59	1000	10	10	65	60	1.5	1.8	20	2.0	200	2.0	1200	1200	400	12	15	150	50
	19–24	72	160	177	70	58	1000	10	10	70	60	1.5	1.7	19	2.0	200	2.0	1200	1200	350	10	15	150	70
	25–50	79	174	176	70	63	1000	5	10	80	60	1.5	1.7	19	2.0	200	2.0	800	800	350	10	15	150	70
	51+	77	170	173	68	63	1000	5	10	80	60	1.2	1.4	15	2.0	200	2.0	800	800	350	10	15	150	70
Females	11–14	46	101	157	62	46	800	10	8	45	50	1.1	1.3	15	1.4	150	2.0	1200	1200	280	15	12	150	45
	15–18	55	120	163	64	44	800	10	8	55	60	1.1	1.3	15	1.5	180	2.0	1200	1200	300	15	12	150	50
	19–24	58	128	164	65	46	800	10	8	60	60	1.1	1.3	15	1.6	180	2.0	1200	1200	280	15	12	150	55
	25–50	63	138	163	64	50	800	5	8	65	60	1.1	1.3	15	1.6	180	2.0	800	800	280	15	12	150	55
	51+	65	143	160	63	50	800	5	8	65	60	1.0	1.2	13	1.6	180	2.0	800	800	280	10	12	150	55
Pregnant						60	800	10	10	65	70	1.5	1.6	17	2.2	400	2.2	1200	1200	300	30	15	175	65
Lactating	First 6 mo					65	1300	10	12	65	95	1.6	1.8	20	2.1	280	2.6	1200	1200	355	15	19	200	75
	Second 6 mo					62	1200	10	11	65	90	1.6	1.7	20	2.1	260	2.6	1200	1200	340	15	16	200	75

ᵃThe allowances, expressed as average daily intakes over time, are intended to provide for individual variations among most normal persons as they live in the United States under usual environmental stresses. Diets should be based on a variety of common foods in order to provide other nutrients for which human requirements have been less well defined.

ᵇWeights and heights of Reference Adults are actual medians for the US population of the designated age, as reported by NHANES II (second National Health and Nutrition Examination Survey). The median weights and heights of those under 19 years of age were taken from Hamill et al (Physical Growth: National Center for Health Statistics percentiles. Am J Clin Nutr 32:607, 1979). The use of these figures does not imply that the height-to-weight ratios are ideal.

ᶜRetinol equivalents. 1 RE = 1 µg retinol or 6 µg β-carotene.

ᵈAs cholecalciferol. 10 µg cholecalciferol = 400 IU of vitamin D.

ᵉα-Tocopherol equivalents. 1 mg d-α tocopherol = 1 α-TE.

ᶠThose who smoke cigarettes regularly should take at least 100 mg of vitamin C daily.

ᵍ1 NE (niacin equivalent) = 1 mg of niacin or 60 mg of dietary tryptophan.

Source: National Research Council (Food and Nutrition Board): Recommended Dietary Allowances, ed 10. National Academy Press, Washington, DC, 1989.

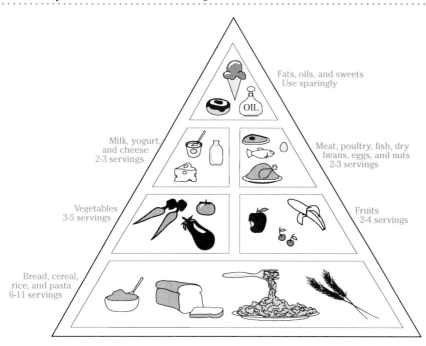

Figure 22–1. The Basic Food Guide Pyramid of the U.S. Department of Agriculture.

each from the fruit and vegetable groups; and 6 to 11 servings from the bread, cereal, rice, and pasta group). A pyramid guide for vegetarians consists of 2 to 3 servings of milk or milk products (or soybean milk fortified with vitamin B_{12}); 2 to 3 servings of protein-rich foods (beans or nuts); 6 to 11 servings of whole-grain foods; and 3 to 5 servings of fruit and vegetables. If a person is active, the upper level of daily servings should be followed. Less active people or persons who are watching their daily caloric intake should stay at the lower end of the range.

The pyramid presents eating guidelines that are quick and simple to use, but it does not guarantee nutritional adequacy because of nutrient variation in individual foods. Bread and cereal selections are one such example where nutritional values vary with respect to the choice of product. Further, the pyramid plan does not contain foods people may ordinarily eat, like soups and casseroles. Also, the nutrient content of foods can be greatly diluted by added fat, sugar, or water. However, a dietary regimen planned around the pyramid guide is more apt to be more nutritionally adequate than unstructured eating. The medical assistant should use the pyramid for teaching proper nutrition, keeping its limitations in mind.

PREGNANT AND LACTATING WOMEN

Assessing caloric needs and monitoring weight gain are major dietary concerns of the pregnant woman. Proper nutrition in pregnancy is essential for the normal development of the fetus as well as for maintaining the mother's good health. Although physicians may differ on the desired amount of weight gain, most usually recommend a 2- to 4.5-lb gain in the first trimester, with 0.8-lb gain per week thereafter. Total weight gain is then projected to be approximately 24 lb (20 to 27 lb

range), which accounts for the weight of the various components of the birth products such as the fetus, placenta, and the amniotic fluid. Weight gain is expected to occur steadily. Although some pregnant women gain considerably more weight (up to 60 lbs) without ill effects, excessive or sudden weight gain puts the pregnant woman at risk for serious complications. Specific dietary recommendations during pregnancy are as follows:

Increased Protein. An additional 30 g of protein should be consumed daily in the form of meat, poultry, fish, eggs, and dairy products.

Increased Calcium. The RDA for calcium during pregnancy is 12 mg. Some physicians recommend that pregnant women drink 1 qt of skim milk daily to ensure the recommended intake of calcium and high-quality protein. Skim milk is recommended because of its low-fat, lower-calorie content.

Normal Sodium Intake. Sodium should not be restricted. Normal consumption is recommended because of increased blood volume and fetal requirements.

Increased Folic Acid. The pregnant woman's need for folic acid doubles (800 μg) as compared with the need of the nonpregnant woman (400 μg).

Normal Nutrition. The pregnant woman is advised to avoid "empty" calories (nonnutritional foods) and to follow the USDA pyramid guidelines for the inclusion of the food groups in meal planning and food consumption. She should be cautioned that excess weight gain may complicate the pregnancy. In addition, she should be advised to drink six to eight glasses of water a day and to include fiber in the diet to help prevent constipation, a common side effect of pregnancy.

Caloric demands for the breast-feeding, or lactating, woman are greater than those for pregnancy, as the healthy infant will double its weight by the fifth month of life. The recommended dietary allowances for lactating women are as follows:

Caloric: additional 500 calories daily

Protein: additional 30 g daily

Folic Acid: 5500 μg daily

Calcium: 1200 mg daily

Iron: 30 to 60 mg daily

THE OLDER ADULT

Although exact nutrient requirements for older adults are unknown, certain physiologic events associated with aging, such as a decline in the metabolic rate, suggest certain dietary adjustments. The following dietary modifications are recommended:

Decreased Calories. The Food and Nutrition Board of the National Academy of Science recommends that the caloric intake of persons over 51 years of age should be reduced to 90% of that required by a young adult. Beyond age 75, a decrease to 75% to 80% of original caloric intake is suggested. Obviously, the level of physical fitness achieved by the elderly individual could greatly alter these percentages and allow for increased caloric intake.

Adequate Intake (RDA) of Vitamins and Minerals. Adequate intake of iron is necessary to prevent iron deficiency anemia; adequate intake (approximately 1500 mg daily) of calcium is necessary to prevent osteoporosis. Postmenstrual women actually require less iron than younger women because iron is no longer lost through menstruation. Supplements (tablets) may be required for adequate calcium, phosphorus, and magnesium intake for those patients unable to obtain recommended allowances from food sources.

Normal Nutrients. An adequate supply of nutrients in the diet is essential to good health. Consistency of foods may be modified depending on the presence of chewing difficulties. High-fiber foods and six to eight glasses of water a day should be included to compensate for decreasing muscle tone in the gastrointestinal tract.

Although protein needs are the same for the older and younger adult, the older adult must acquire protein from less food with fewer calories. Therefore, the individual must be instructed to choose high-quality protein foods, such as skim milk and meat products.

Twenty percent of the older individual's caloric intake should come from fat. Excesses should be avoided to help prevent atherosclerosis. Inadequate fat consumption should also be avoided to prevent poor absorption of the fat-soluble vitamins.

Special assistance may be required in planning meals that must be eaten alone or purchased with a small income, or in acquiring food from various community organizations.

NUTRITIONAL ASSESSMENT

Before diet therapy can be initiated, a thorough nutritional assessment is needed to determine the nutritional status of the patient. In addition to age, health status, height, weight, body frame type, and percentage of body fat, the patient's nutritional and exercise patterns should be known and certain anthropometric measurements should be obtained.

Questionnaries and interviewing are two convenient methods for determining a patient's eating habits. Factors that determine the patient's attitudes toward food include the following:

1. *Background information.* Cultural heritage, religious restrictions, family traditions, current socioeconomic status, effects of food fads and superstitions
2. *Food purchase and preparation.* Who purchases the food, types of food purchased, budgeting factors, where purchased and how often, foods served most often
3. *Relationship of food to lifestyle.* Food likes and dislikes, atmosphere of mealtimes, number of meals per day, food supplements, education about nutrition, frequency of meals eaten in restaurants, how much snacking
4. *Physical status.* Ability to eat, appetite, elimination (voiding and defecation), exercise and physical activity, mental status, and medications

Anthropometric measurements are necessary for assessment of nutritional status and diet planning. Anthropometric measurements include height, weight, body frame size, body circumference, and the skinfold (SF) test. These measurements are useful not only in determining overfatness or underfatness, but also for the early detection of protein-calorie malnutrition, sometimes called *protein-energy malnutrition.* These measurements must be evaluated together to determine the patient's total body weight (BW), frame size, percentage of body fat, and energy status.

DETERMINATION OF FRAME SIZE

Frame size can be determined by measuring the space between the two prominent bones of the elbow. Either a tape measure or skin caliper may be used. Using a tape measure, the prominences are measured with the elbow flexed at 90°. The fingers should be straight and the inside of the wrist toward the body. Measurements falling with the ranges listed on the frame size chart indicate a medium frame (Table 22–5). Lower measurements indicate a small frame; higher measurements, a large frame.

Table 22–5
FRAME SIZE CHART*

Height (in 1" heels)	Elbow Breadth*
Men	
5'2"–5'3"	$2\frac{1}{2}$"–$2\frac{7}{8}$"
5'4"–5'7"	$2\frac{5}{8}$"–$2\frac{7}{8}$"
5'8"–5'11"	$2\frac{3}{4}$"–3"
6'0"–6'3"	$2\frac{3}{4}$"–$3\frac{1}{8}$"
6'4"	$2\frac{7}{8}$"–$3\frac{1}{4}$"
Women	
4'10"–4'11"	$2\frac{1}{4}$"–$2\frac{1}{2}$"
5'0"–5'3"	$2\frac{1}{4}$"–$2\frac{1}{2}$"
5'4"–5'7"	$2\frac{3}{8}$"–$2\frac{5}{8}$"
5'8"–5'11"	$2\frac{3}{8}$"–$2\frac{5}{8}$"
6'0"	$2\frac{1}{2}$"–$2\frac{3}{4}$"

*This is the range of measurement indicating a medium range. Higher values indicate large frames; lower values indicate small frames.

DETERMINING BODY FAT AS A PERCENTAGE OF BODY WEIGHT

Although the human body is made up of many components, what is of most interest in health, nutrition, fitness, and longevity is body fat. However, simply weighing patients and comparing the results against normative measurements on height-weight charts cannot accurately measure their body fat or whether or not they are overfat or underfat. While height and weight charts are based on insurance statistics that relate overweightness to degenerative disease and death, they make no allowances for muscle development and frame size. They are based on body *weight* and not body *fat*. Unfortunately, this has lead to the general belief that overweight also means "overfat."

Recent studies suggest it is not how heavy a person is but rather how much fat a person carries or adds to body weight. Therefore, true obesity (excess fatness) rather than mere overweight must be assessed. The anthropometric measurement of subcutaneous fat from SFs is the most direct method to estimate leanness-fatness. From these measurements, the physician is able to evaluate nutritional status and to differentiate between overweight and obesity.

There are many reasons to monitor "percentage of body fat." For years, the SF test has been used in research to differentiate fat content between the sexes, age groups, sedentary and physically active workers, and athletes. In the physician's practice, percentage of body fat measurements can be used to (1) determine changes in muscle tissue over time, (2) diagnose patients who, although they may look fit, are overfat and undermuscled, (3) monitor the effects of diet and exercise on muscle tissue and fat, (4) evaluate patients,

particularly women, who are so lean that their lack of body fat may be harmful, and (5) determine whether the excess body weight of an athlete is due to increased fat or increased muscle mass and bone density. Whereas an athlete may be encouraged to diet in the first case, a diet could result in the loss of valuable muscle tissue in the second case.

BODY COMPOSITION

Body composition, which comprises the weight of an individual, can be divided into four components: fat, water, protein, and minerals, each expressed as a ratio to total BW. In some conditions (e.g., fluid accumulation) BW can increase due to an accumulation of water. Athletes, on the other hand, develop large muscles, and excess muscle mass can contribute substantially to total BW. In the normal person, however, fat tissue accounts largely for individual differences in body weight.

The most accepted body composition model divides the BW into lean body weight (LBW) and fat weight (FW). LBW represents the active energy-producing tissues. LBW contains the skeleton, the organs, and other tissues, but it is mostly made up of the muscles. Muscle mass alone accounts for approximately 40% to 50% of the LBW. FW, on the other hand, is the inactive storage of tissue that, although serving as a long-term energy pool, is considered excess baggage for most activities. The relative fat content, or "percentage of fat," is simply the ratio of FW to BW expressed as a percent (FW/BW = percentage of fat).

The most important use of percentage of body fat assessment is to monitor the changes in body fat and weight over time. The general trend of fat tissue in a person is attributable to age, activity, and appetite. The peaks of fatness are in early childhood and in later maturity. Therefore, the physician is faced with a prevalent problem of evaluating the onset of obesity in patients of many ages.

Although adult fat gain may be partly due to age and developmental factors, the main problem in obesity is an increased caloric intake accelerated by a decrease in energy expenditure. The excess of caloric intake over caloric expenditure leads to fat accumulation. With the increase of body fat, muscle tissue also can increase or decrease, depending on a person's diet, activities, exercise, and lifestyle. Lack of activity is probably the basis for the slow accumulation of excess fat in many sedentary middle-aged persons even though they do not change their eating patterns or increase their caloric intake. As a natural process, therefore, aging and decreased activity involves not only additive accumulation of body fat but most likely some replacement of muscle by fat. A patient can weigh the same at age 40 as she or he did at age 25 yet have far more fat at age 40 than at age 25.

SKINFOLD TEST

About one half of the total body fat is deposited in the subcutaneous tissues, which is loosely attached to the underlying tissue and can be pulled up between the thumb and forefinger into a fold. An *SF* is a pinch of skin plus the underlying fat taken at various sites over the body. An *SF caliper* provides a quantitative measurement of the amount of fat immediately below the skin. Because about 50% of the body fat is just below the skin and because the volume of subcutaneous fat is related to the volume of inner fat, the SF technique is a valid estimate of the total percentage of fat of an individual.

When measuring SF sites, the triceps and scapular sites are the best sites for this purpose. Other sites include points over the biceps muscle; above the iliac crest; and immediately under the costal margin, close to the umbilicus.

For the measurement to have meaning, the location of the site must be precise. Taking a SF measurement is simple, but acquiring proficiency requires practice. The proficient medical assistant can obtain the same measurement on different days and approximately the same value as another tester. The key to locating SF sites and getting accurate measurements is experience.

The triceps SF is made at the back of the upper arm (over the triceps), at the level midway between the tip of the acromial process of the scapula and the tip of the elbow. The scapular SF measurement is taken below the top of the right scapula with the right arm hanging free (see procedure at end of chapter for measurement at four different sites).

SKINFOLD CALIPERS

It is important to use a caliper with a built-in pressure mechanism (Fig. 22-2). The internal pressure mechanism enables the caliper to exert a constant pressure from reading to reading and over the range of SFs tested.

No caliper can give an accurate reading, however, unless the medical assistant picks up the SF in a standard manner. Several measurements should be taken at each site until they correspond within 2 mm. These values are then averaged.

Ideally, four or more sites should be used. If only one site is used, the triceps is the site of choice. If two sites are used, the triceps and scapular regions are used.

Example

Patient — 40-year-old woman, 5 ft 10 inches, 210 lb

	Triceps	Sub-scapular	Biceps	Supra-iliac
Measurement 1:	27	36	19	40
Measurement 2:	26	36	18	40
Measurement 3:	25	36	17	40
Site averages:	26	36	18	40

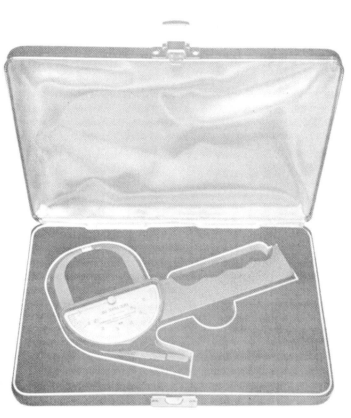

Figure 22-2. Skinfold caliper. Spring-loaded levers provide constant pressure. (Courtesy of Cambridge Scientific Industries, Cambridge, Maryland.)

26
36
18
40
120 = Sum of four sites = 42% body fat (see chart, Fig. 22–3)

The averages at each site are added together, and the sum is compared with chart measurements to determine the patient's percentage of body fat (Table 22–6). Charts with ideal range measurements have been developed for adult men and women and for male and female children. Some physicians use computation tables that eliminate the need for charts.

CALCULATING IDEAL PERCENTAGE OF BODY FAT

Every person has an optimal or ideal body weight (IBW), based not on height or body frame but on being at an optimal percentage of body fat. The weight of the skin plus subcutaneous tissue accounts for approximately 17% of BW in the adult men. Of this 17%, the skin in "normal" men accounts for 6% of body weight, and the fat, for 11%. The optimal range of body fat for men younger than 50 years is 10% to 14%, and for men age 50 and older, 12% to 19%.

In "normal" adult women, the percentage of skin is the same as that of normal men, 6%, but the subcutaneous tissue can account for 14% to 23% of a woman's BW. The optimal percentage of body fat for women younger than 50 years is, therefore, 14% to 23%, and for women age 50 and older, 16% to 25%.

Men are considered obese if the triceps measurement is greater than 15 mm. In men 6 ft, 2 inches or taller, 18 to 20 mm is the lower limit of normal. Women are considered obese if the triceps measurement is greater than 25 mm.

The patient's current BW and percentage of body fat, determined from the percentage of body fat chart, can now be used to calculate the patient's LBW and FW.

$$\text{Percentage of body fat} \times BW = FW$$
$$BW - FW = LBW$$

Example (from above)

$$42\% \times 210 \text{ lb} = 88 \text{ lb FW}$$
$$210 \text{ lb} - 88 \text{ lb} = 122 \text{ lb LBW}$$

As stated previously, the optimal percentage of body fat for women younger than 50 years is 14 to 23%, and for women aged 50 and older, 16 to 25%. Since this woman is 5 ft 10 inches with a large body frame, the upper limit of 23% can be used as her desired percentage of body fat. If the patient's weight and percentage of body fat are known, it is possible to calculate what the patient's ideal weight should be for any desired percentage of body fat, which in this case is 23%. To find the IBW for a desired percentage of body fat, subtract the *current* percentage of body fat from 100 and divide the answer by 100 minus the desired percentage of body fat:

$$\frac{100 - \text{Percentage of body fat}}{100 - \text{Percentage of desired body fat}}$$
$$\times \text{Current weight} = IBW \text{ for percentage of body fat}$$

Example (from above)

$$\frac{100 - 42}{100 - 23} = \frac{58}{77} = 0.75 \times 210 \text{ lb} = 157.5 \text{ lb IBW}$$

$$\begin{array}{r} 210.0 \text{ BW} \\ -157.5 \text{ IBW} \\ \hline 52.5 \text{ FW} \end{array}$$

52.5 lbs of body fat must be lost to reach the IBW of 157.5 lb and the desired 23% body fat.

If the IBW is less than the BW, the difference is the amount of weight the patient must lose to reach his or her optimal weight.

It is important to note that no matter how much weight is to be lost, the loss must be gradual. If the patient loses no more than 2 lb per week until the IBW is reached, his or her nutritional status is not jeopardized and he or she is more likely to stay at the IBW.

Both diet restriction and exercise should be prescribed, and because weight loss usually does not remain constant, the patient should be reevaluated periodically for progress. With exercise, usually only FW is lost, provided the patient maintains the same dietary pattern. Extreme exercise may actually increase the lean BW, and even if there is a decrease in fat weight, the patient may either gain BW or show no change in BW. In either case, however, the decrease in the body fat-to-total weight ratio is what is important.

As stated earlier, the measurement of muscle loss or gain compared with amount of fat loss or gain is one of the most important uses for body fat measurements. After the patient has been on a diet and exercise program, the measurements are repeated. Any change up or down represents the patient's progress.

Example (from above)

Two months later: BW: 195, SF: 38% body fat

$$\text{Percentage of body fat} \times BW = FW$$
$$BW - FW = LBW$$
$$38\% \times 195 \text{ lb} = 74 \text{ lb FW}$$
$$195 \text{ lb} - 74 \text{ lb} = 121 \text{ lb LBW}$$

Difference in LBW between first and second visits:
$$\begin{array}{r} 122 \text{ lb} \\ -121 \text{ lb} \\ \hline 1 \text{ lb} \end{array} \qquad BW: \begin{array}{r} 210 \\ -195 \\ \hline 15 \text{ lb} \end{array}$$

Result: This patient has lost a total of 15 lb. What is most important is that of the 15 lb lost, 14 lb is FW and only 1 lb is muscle. The patient is doing extremely well on her diet and exercise program.

The ideal *weight loss* program is moderate exercise

Table 22–6

BODY FAT AND SKINFOLDS MEASUREMENTS

The equivalent fat content, as a percentage of body weight, for a range of values for the sum of four skinfolds (biceps, triceps, subscapular, and suprailiac) of males and females of different ages.

	Males					Females			
Skinfolds (mm)	Ages 17–29	30–39	40–49	50+	Skinfolds (mm)	Ages 16–29	30–39	40–49	50+
15	4.8	—	—	—	15	10.5	—	—	—
20	8.1	12.2	12.2	12.6	20	14.1	17.0	19.8	21.4
25	10.5	14.2	15.0	15.6	25	16.8	19.4	22.2	24.0
30	12.9	16.2	17.7	18.6	30	19.5	21.8	24.5	26.6
35	14.7	17.7	19.6	20.8	35	21.5	23.7	26.4	28.5
40	16.4	19.2	21.4	22.9	40	23.4	25.5	28.2	30.3
45	17.7	20.4	23.0	24.7	45	25.0	26.9	29.6	31.9
50	19.0	21.5	24.6	26.5	50	26.5	28.2	31.0	33.4
55	20.1	22.5	25.9	27.9	55	27.8	29.4	32.1	34.6
60	21.2	23.5	27.1	29.2	60	29.1	30.6	33.2	35.7
65	22.2	24.3	28.2	30.4	65	30.2	31.6	34.1	36.7
70	23.1	25.1	29.3	31.6	70	31.2	32.5	35.0	37.7
75	24.0	25.9	30.3	32.7	75	32.2	33.4	35.9	38.7
80	24.8	26.6	31.2	33.8	80	33.1	34.3	36.7	39.6
85	25.5	27.2	32.1	34.8	85	34.0	35.1	37.5	40.4
90	26.2	27.8	33.0	35.8	90	34.8	35.8	38.3	41.2
95	26.9	28.4	33.7	36.6	95	35.6	36.5	39.0	41.9
100	27.6	29.0	34.4	37.4	100	36.4	37.2	39.7	42.6
105	28.2	29.6	35.1	38.2	105	37.1	37.9	40.4	43.3
110	28.8	30.1	35.8	39.0	110	37.8	38.6	41.0	43.9
115	29.4	30.6	36.4	39.7	115	38.4	39.1	41.5	44.5
120	30.0	31.1	37.0	40.4	120	39.0	39.6	42.0	45.1
125	30.5	31.5	37.6	41.1	125	39.6	40.1	42.5	45.7
130	31.0	31.9	38.2	41.8	130	40.2	40.6	43.0	46.2
135	31.5	32.3	38.7	42.4	135	40.8	41.1	43.5	46.7
140	32.0	32.7	39.2	43.0	140	41.3	41.6	44.0	47.2
145	32.5	33.1	39.7	43.6	145	41.8	42.1	44.5	47.7
150	32.9	33.5	40.2	44.1	150	42.3	42.6	45.0	48.2
155	33.3	33.9	40.7	44.6	155	42.8	43.1	45.4	48.7
160	33.7	34.3	41.2	45.1	160	43.3	43.6	45.8	49.2
165	34.1	34.6	41.6	45.6	165	43.7	44.0	46.2	49.6
170	34.5	34.8	42.0	46.1	170	44.1	44.4	46.6	50.0
175	34.9	—	—	—	175	—	44.8	47.0	50.4
180	35.3	—	—	—	180	—	45.2	47.4	50.8
185	35.6	—	—	—	185	—	45.6	47.8	51.2
190	35.9	—	—	—	190	—	45.9	48.2	51.6
195	—	—	—	—	195	—	46.2	48.5	52.0
200	—	—	—	—	200	—	46.5	48.8	52.4
205	—	—	—	—	205	—	—	49.1	52.7
210	—	—	—	—	210	—	—	49.4	53.0

In two thirds of the instances, the error was within ± 3.5% of the body weight as fat for the women and ± 5% for the men.

Source: Adapted from Durnin JVGA and Womersley J: Body fat assessed from total body density and its estimation from skinfold thickness. Measurements on 481 men and women aged from 16 to 72 years. Br J Nutr 32:77–97, 1974.

and limited dietary restriction. The best exercises for high caloric expenditures are jogging, swimming, cross-country skiing, and rope jumping. For patients who wish to *increase* BW, the best program is weight training or calisthenics, which tends to increase LBW while leaving the FW relatively unaffected.

Patients *below* optimal 5% body fat may not wish to gain BW, especially when the gain would be mostly FW, and may choose not to exercise during an increased caloric diet plan. For the patient who does want to gain BW, vigorous exercise will increase LBW for those below average in LBW for their age while leaving their FW relatively unchanged.

Although the SF measurement has a long research history, physicians use this tool more often as a simple and direct measurement of fatness, which might otherwise be obscured by reference to height-weight charts alone. Body composition and fitness is essential to good health. With as much as 40% of the school-age population classified as obese, it is vital to the health of the nation that patients be made aware of ways body composition can be modified. Rather than referring to vague ideals of body frame or weight, skinfold measurement can be used to show a patient that his or her total BW is unneeded and a detriment to good health.

DIET THERAPY

The arrangement of foods in the daily diet is significant in the prevention and treatment of disease. Much is still unknown concerning the interaction of nutrients and health. However, the medical profession has become increasingly aware of the relationship between patterns of food consumption, exercise, and the incidence of disease, and physicians are increasingly using diet therapy as a treatment measure.

Diet therapy signifies the design and prescription of a diet to prevent or treat disease. The normal diet is adjusted to meet the individual physiologic needs of the patient. These adjustments are based on the physician's understanding of the need for and effect of certain types of foods and nutrients as relates to the patient's condition.

In some disease states, such as diabetes, and in some disease prevention plans, such as the prevention of atherosclerosis, diet therapy may be the only treatment employed. Usually, however, diet therapy is used in combination with other treatment alternatives. The normal diet is most often modified in one or more of the following ways:

1. Adjusting the calorie allowance
2. Changing the consistency or texture of foods
3. Avoiding or restricting certain foods
4. Changing the number of meals or feedings
5. Emphasizing certain foods
6. Increasing or decreasing certain nutrient levels

The physician may prescribe a standard diet plan that increases the intake of certain nutrients. For example,

the physician may order a high-protein diet for a patient with a fracture. When the body's metabolism is increased (during certain growth states and illness) energy requirements are also increased and more calories are needed. Because protein is necessary for tissue growth and repair, protein intake needs to be increased as well.

Certain food excesses are linked to disease. For example, overconsumption of saturated fats and sodium is associated with heart disease. The physician, in this case, would prescribe a diet that is low in fat and low in sodium. Certain food consistencies and flavors are irritating to the mucous membrane lining the gastrointestinal tract when inflammation is present in diseases such as gastritis and ulcer. In this case, a patient may be prescribed a bland diet; that is, one that is free from any irritating or stimulating foods, or a low-fiber diet if the patient is suffering from severe diarrhea.

Much of diet therapy is based on the interrelationships between the chemical and physical properties of food and body physiology. Table 22–7 outlines the dietary modifications applied to specific diseases and conditions frequently encountered in the medical office. Specific concepts underlying diet therapy can be detected on reviewing this table.

PATIENT TEACHING

Certain general principles of effective patient teaching are applicable to diet therapy. The objectives are to gain the patient's cooperation and to assist the patient to understand the diet prescription. The medical assistant's role is to offer reassurance, give accurate nutrition information, help the patient plan the diet, and reinforce the physician's explanations. In many instances, the medical assistant may consult with, or at the physician's direction, refer the patient to a professional nutritionist who can offer expert and elaborate instruction.

When the medical assistant is responsible for patient teaching related to diet, a few factors should be considered before providing instruction. The medical assistant must fully understand the diet prescription, the foods to be included and avoided, and the specific goals of the diet. In addition, a nutritional assessment regarding the patient's normal eating habits and dietary difficulties must be obtained first. The diet plan cannot be successful if the patient's own eating patterns and habits are unknown or excluded. Third, the patient's reaction to the diet prescription must be considered, whether the diet plan is short term or long term, so that the medical assistant can provide further explanation and reassurance. Since the patient does not always verbalize concerns, the medical assistant must be alert for nonverbal signs. The ethnic and economic condition of the patient's dietary habits must also be considered. Finally, care should be taken to provide diet instruction within the boundaries of the medical assistant's professional responsibility. Remember, the medical assistant does not design the prescription but provides supplemental information and reinforcement.

Table 22-7
DIETARY MODIFICATIONS APPLIED TO SPECIFIC DISEASES AND CONDITIONS

Diet Prescription	Conditions for Use	Characteristics
High-calorie/ High-protein	Infection, fever, burns, surgery	A. Calorie intake increased to 3000–5000 daily. B. Increased carbohydrate and slightly increased fat food sources. C. Avoidance of large servings of low-calorie foods such as lettuce.
Low-calorie	Obesity	A. Calories are restricted but usually do not fall below 1000 calorie allowance per day. B. Carbohydrates and fats are restricted; protein is maintained. C. Foods emphasized include fruits, vegetables, lean meats, and whole grains. Foods avoided include desserts, snack foods, creams, sauces, starchy foods, and refined sugars.
High-carbohydrate	Liver and gallbladder disease	A. Increased carbohydrate intake by emphasis on whole-grain breads and cereals, fruits, vegetables with high-carbohydrate content, natural sugars, and starches.
Restricted or modified carbohydrate	Diabetes	A. Carbohydrate restrictions correspond to the physician's use of drug therapy. Carbohydrate intake must be managed by the drug prescribed to control the diabetes. B. Food exchange list is most frequently used to assist the patient in maintaining normal nutrition.
Low-protein	Kidney disease, such as nephritis; cardiac conditions	A. Protein allowances are maintained at a low-normal level. B. Foods that are high-protein sources are restricted. Fruits, vegetables and whole grains are stressed.
Low-fat	Obesity; gallbladder disease; digestive disturbances	A. Fats that are more easily digested are emphasized, such as lean meat, skim milk, and cottage cheese. B. Fats are restricted to include only the low-fat sources. C. Avoidance of sauces, gravies, and fatty or tough meats is encouraged.
High-fiber	Severe or continued constipation	A. Fiber content is increased. B. Raw fruits and vegetables are stressed, along with whole-grain cereals and leafy green vegetables. C. Refined foods are avoided. D. Increase fluids.
Low-fiber	Severe diarrhea, ulcerative colitis, and other gastrointestinal (GI) disorders; diverticulitis	A. Rests the GI tract but can only be used for a brief period, because of inadequacies in vitamins and minerals. B. Lean meats, fruit juice, gelatins, milk-free beverages, and fat-free soups are stressed.

Continued

Table 22–7

DIETARY MODIFICATIONS APPLIED TO SPECIFIC DISEASES AND CONDITIONS — *Continued*

Diet Prescription	Conditions for Use	Characteristics
		C. Whole grains, milk, cheese, raw fruits, vegetables, and spicy foods are avoided.
High-iron	Certain anemias	A. High-iron food sources are stressed, such as liver, egg yolk, beans, and whole-grain cereals.
Liberal bland	Peptic ulcers	A. Eliminate irritating foods according to personal tolerances. B. Avoid caffeine, (cola, cocoa, decaffeinated and caffeinated coffee, tea), alcohol, nicotine, peppers and chili powder. C. Eat frequently. D. Avoid stress (relax) between and during meals.
Soft diet	Chewing difficulties	Strong flavors and spices are permitted, but foods must be pureed.
Clear-liquid diet	Acute diarrhea	A. Used for short periods of time because of nutritional inadequacies. B. Tea, fat-free broth, noncitrus juices, carbonated beverages, Popsicles, and gelatin are included.
Full-liquid diet	Recovering diarrhea	A. Foods allowed include strained cooked cereals, plain ice cream, sherbet, pudding, strained soups.
Low- or restricted-sodium diet	Cardiovascular, liver, pancreas and gallbladder disease	A. Avoid cooking or table use of salt. B. Avoid highly salted snacks, including potato chips, corn chips, salted popcorn and pretzels. C. Avoid salty condiments, including barbeque sauce, catsup, mustard, soy and worchestershire sauce. D. Avoid salted commercially prepared foods, including pickles and olives, bacon, luncheon meats, salad dressing, beverages, and baking mixes. E. Read labels of all foods to keep within prescribed limits.
Low-tyramine diet	Migraine headaches; patients taking MAO inhibitors	A. Avoid foods containing tyramine: aged cheeses, red wine, beer, cream, chocolate, yeast.

OBESITY

Much controversy surrounds the reasons for overeating. Obesity has recently been classified as being one of three types: mild (20% to 40% overweight); moderate (41% to 100% overweight); and severe (greater than 100% overweight). The cause of obesity is unknown, but the mechanism is simple — consuming more calories than the calories expended. At least seven factors are accepted as contributing to obesity. These are as follows:

SOCIAL FACTORS Obesity is far more prevalent among lower-class than upper-class children, with significant differences apparent by the age of 6. Economic and other social factors, such as ethnic and religious backgrounds, are closely linked to obesity. Differences in lifestyle, dietary, and exercise patterns also play a major role.

ENDOCRINE AND METABOLIC FACTORS Usually endocrine and metabolic factors are the result of obesity rather than the cause of it. One exception is hyperadrenocorticism (Cushing's syndrome). In this case, there is overactivity of the adrenal cortex, which leads to a greater demand for insulin and in turn stimulates the transformation of nonfat food materials into fat.

PSYCHOLOGICAL FACTORS The influence of psychological factors is still obscure. Psychological factors may be suspected especially in young women of upper and middle socioeconomic classes who have been obese since early childhood. In this group, disordered eating patterns may lead to a poor body image, which in turn results in self-consciousness and impaired social functioning. What is not understood, however, is why some people overeat when emotionally upset and gain weight, and others do not.

Two extreme eating patterns thought to be caused by stress and emotional disturbance may also contribute to the obesity of some individuals. *Bulimia* is the compulsive eating of large amounts of food in a short time, followed by self-condemnation and, usually, self-induced vomiting. The *night-eating syndrome* is characterized by self-starvation (*anorexia*) in the morning, then evening overeating (*binging*) and insomnia.

GENETIC FACTORS A genetic predisposition to obesity gains strong support from family studies as well as studies of twins and adopted children. Evidence from family studies has shown that 80% of the children of two obese parents are obese, indicating that obesity runs in families. Twin studies and adoption studies are also beginning to provide convincing evidence that genetics plays a role in obesity. There is evidence of a higher incidence of obesity in twin populations (even when separated at birth), and in adoptee populations born to obese parents and their birth siblings.

DEVELOPMENTAL FACTORS Fat tissue may begin to develop in adulthood and be characterized by an increase in the size (*hypertrophy*) of fat cells with no increase in number; or fat tissue may begin to develop in childhood and be characterized by an increase in the number of fat cells (*hyperplasia*) or in both the number and size of fat cells (*hyperplastic-hypertrophic obesity*). In hyperplastic-hypertrophic obesity, individuals may have up to 5 times as many fat cells as people of normal body fat or as those who are just hypertrophically obese. Such a condition may set a biologic limit to weight reduction. This anatomic change associated with lifelong obesity is a strong reason for preventing obesity in children. With aging, there is also the tendency to accumulate body fat. Statistics show that the occurrence of obesity doubles from ages 20 to 50.

PHYSICAL ACTIVITY Although food intake increases with increased physical activity, food intake may not decrease proportionately with decreased physical activity past a certain level. Therefore, a sedentary lifestyle or restricting physical activity may contribute to obesity and may actually increase food consumption in some individuals.

BRAIN DAMAGE Although very rare, damage or disease of the hypothalamus may lead to obesity.

WEIGHT REDUCTION DIETS

If untreated, obesity tends to progress. Treatment may consist of diet therapy alone or in combination with behavior modification or medication. Patients with disease-linked reasons for reducing their weight tend to be more successful in achieving weight loss, because their motivations may be greater when the cause is more focused. Attempts to lose weight for the obese patient, however, more often cause complications and anxiety or depression. Although much progress has been made in recent years, treatment for obesity is only modestly effective.

In weight reduction diets, the physician prescribes the caloric allowance and the distribution of the nutrients. The medical assistant's responsibility is to guide the patient in understanding and accepting the dietary restrictions. To achieve these objectives, the medical assistant must be aware of the patient's true motivation, support systems, and understanding of basic principles of nutrition.

Treatment

For mild obesity (the most common weight disorder), physicians usually recommend a total daily allowance of about 1200 cal for women and 1500 cal for men, as these levels can still provide adequate nutrition. Allowances below 1000 cal are very restrictive and usually appropriate only for the moderately or severely obese. Treatment is combined with behavior modification that involves a gradual change in eating patterns to increase the intake of complex carbohydrates (fruits, vegetables, and cereals) and decrease the intake of fats and nonnutritional carbohydrates. In mild obesity, behavior modification does not require medical monitoring, unless it is complicated by other disease, such as high cholesterol, diabetes, or high blood pressure.

In moderate obesity, the primary goal of treatment is to prescribe the largest caloric deficit that can be safely and comfortably tolerated by the patient. The same levels recommended for mild obesity (1200 to 1500 cal) can be prescribed but may not produce a fast enough weight loss. A very low calorie diet, called the *protein-sparing modified fast*, may be prescribed. This diet usually provides between 400 and 700 cal per day and consists largely or entirely of protein, either as formula or natural foods, such as fish, poultry, or lean meat. This diet is safe when administered under medical supervision for up to 3 months. It should not be confused with "liquid-protein" diets, which have been associated with a number of deaths.

Motivation

The greatest problem in moderate and severe obesity is maintenance of weight loss. Behavior modification must first focus on eating habits, then on lifestyle patterns that precede food intake. Techniques include patient recordkeeping and plans to modify behavior, monitoring, nutrition education, increased exercise to decrease appetite and food intake, and counseling to develop self-esteem and positive attitudes towards weight reduction.

The medical assistant must recognize the importance of self-motivation to the success of the weight reduction diet and choose an approach that will help the patient to become motivated. Allowing the patient the opportunity to discuss personal feelings and providing positive reinforcement can help to encourage the patient to follow the dietary regimen.

Support

The medical assistant needs to be empathetic and appreciative of the personal and emotional obstacles the patient encounters in overcoming the habit of overeating. The patient following a weight reduction diet requires support. The medical assistant should draw the family into the supportive network formed by the physician and the medical office staff. Family members should be included in discussions of the patient's diet plan. This is especially important if the individual will not be preparing his or her own meals.

Fad Diets

Before effective patient instruction can begin, the medical assistant must possess accurate information concerning weight reduction. A vast amount of misinformation clouds and distorts the issue of weight reduction.

The medical assistant should caution the patient not to abandon the diet regimen for a "quick weight loss" diet. There are no magic formulas for losing weight. Calories not expended become fat tissue. When more energy is expended than the number of calories ingested, weight reduction results. A person will gain or lose weight most successfully by keeping to a daily diet with a calorie count above or below the daily requirement. Fad diets, on the other hand, may lead to vitamin, mineral, and protein depletion; dehydration; toxicity; cardiac, renal, and metabolic disorders; and even death.

The special arrangement of nutrients is important in weight loss diets to meet nutritional needs and to maintain body functions; therefore, daily recommended percentages of nutrient must be maintained. Special exercise and activities are also an important part of the plan to ensure that the weight lost is FW and not muscle tissue. A successful weight reduction plan will be long-term, well-balanced, and provide adequate nutrition while reducing the number of calories.

Weight Loss Groups

The physician may recommend a more comprehensive approach to weight loss by encouraging the patient to participate in an organized weight reduction group. Participation in such a group may help the patient to remain motivated and learn practical dietary suggestions as well as to receive understanding and support. Such groups are numerous, and the patient may need guidance in selecting a group appropriate for his or her own needs and circumstances.

Because maintenance of the weight loss is perhaps the single most difficult aspect of weight reduction, patients may need encouragement to remain in the group and continue with the specialized instruction of the medical office staff after achieving weight loss.

Medical offices may themselves provide group partici-

pation for their patients by designing, organizing, and staffing their own weight reduction support groups.

DIET THERAPY FOR THE DIABETIC PATIENT

The patient with diabetes requires special attention and consideration in providing dietary instruction because of the crucial relationship between diet, medication, and the disease. Because the diabetic diet is continued for a lifetime, the patient needs to become an expert in all aspects of the diet and the disease. Food intake is carefully measured against the body's capability to metabolize carbohydrates and other nutrients.

The foods in a diabetic diet are often weighed to ensure proper portions. The medical assistant may be responsible for instructing the patient in the use of the weighting scale if required, the intimate relationship between diet and insulin therapy, and the food exchange list.

The food exchange list is a standard diet model designed specifically for the diabetic patient and frequently used by patients on weight reduction diets. The physician specifies the calories, number of meals per day (usually four), and the amount of nutrients, with particular emphasis on carbohydrate allowance. A daily meal plan could be as follows:

Plan:	Total calories per day:	1200 cal
	Number of meals per day:	4
	Total daily carbohydrates:	150 g
	Total daily protein:	65 g
	Total daily fat:	**40 g

Figure 22–3 shows a typical daily meal plan.

The patient then uses the daily plan guide in conjunction with the food exchange list (Table 22–8). The food exchange list provides a convenient and practical reference for the patient in determining an accurate intake of specified calories, carbohydrates, proteins, and fats. Another advantage of the food exchange list is that it allows the patient to measure rather than weigh food. The food exchange program is divided into six exchange lists: milk, vegetables, fruit, bread, meat, and fat. Items in each exchange list (in the quantities stated) provide approximately the same amounts of carbohydrate, protein, and fat. Foods on the same list are interchangeable.

The patient is instructed to make substitutions, or "exchanges," within the allowable ranges of food groups on each list. For each food listed, specified portions are given together with their equivalents both in calories and in grams. For instance, the fruit group included listings for half of a banana and one small orange and one small apple. These and all the other fruits listed each contain approximately 10 g of carbohydrates and 40 cal. When the meal plan calls for one fruit exchange, any food listed under the fruit exchange may be used in the amount stated. If two exchanges

DAILY FOOD ALLOWANCES

Breakfast

2 fruit exchanges	fruit list
1 bread exchange	bread list
1 medium fat meat exchange	meat list
1 fat exchange	fat list
1 milk exchange (no fat)	milk list

Lunch

2 lean meat exchanges	meat list
2 bread exchanges	bread list
1 vegetable exchange	vegetable list
1 fruit exchange	fruit list
1 fat exchange	fat list

Dinner

2 lean meat exchanges	meat list
1 bread exchange	bread list
1 vegetable	vegetable list
vegetable(s) as desired	vegetable list, Grp A
1 fruit exchange	fruit list
2 fat exchanges	fat list
1/2 milk exchange (no fat)	milk list

Bedtime snack

1 bread exchange	bread list
1/2 milk exchange (no fat)	milk list

Figure 22–3. A sample daily meal plan for a diabetic patient.

Table 22–8
FOOD EXCHANGE LISTS

Vegetable Exchange

Group A: These vegetables contain very small amounts of carbohydrate, fat, and protein. Because there are so few calories, unlimited amounts of the raw vegetable are permitted. If vegetable is cooked, limit the serving to 1 cup.

Asparagus	Cabbage
Broccoli	Cauliflower
Brussels sprouts	Celery
Chicory	Turnip
Cucumber	Lettuce
Eggplant	Mushrooms
Escarole	Okra
Greens	Pepper, green
Beet	Radishes
Chard	Sauerkraut
Collard	String beans
Dandelion	Summer squash
Kale	Tomato
Mustard	Watercress
Spinach	

Continued

Table 22–8
FOOD EXCHANGE LISTS — *Continued*

Vegetable Exchange

Group B: Each serving of these vegetables contains 7 g of carbohydrate and 2 g of protein, which equals 36 cal. Each ½ cup serving equals one exchange.

Beets	Pumpkin
Carrots	Rutabaga
Onions	Squash, winter
Peas, green	Turnips

Fruit Exchange

Each serving contains 10 grams of carbohydrate and 40 calories.

Apple	1 (2-in diameter)
Applesauce	½ cup
Apricots	2 medium
Apricots, dried	4 halves
Banana	½ small
Blackberries	1 cup
Blueberries	⅔ cup
Cantaloupe	¼ (6-in diameter)
Cherries	10 large
Dates	2
Figs	
Dried	1 small
Fresh	2 large
Grapefruit	½ small
Grapefruit juice	½ cup
Grapes	12
Grape juice	¼ cup
Honeydew melon	⅛ (7-in diameter)
Mango	½ small
Nectarine	1 medium
Orange	1 small
Orange juice	½ cup
Papaya	⅓ medium
Peach	1 medium
Pear	1 small
Pineapple	½ cup
Pineapple juice	⅓ cup
Plums	2 medium
Prunes	2
Raisins	2 tablespoons
Raspberries	1 cup
Strawberries	1 cup
Tangerine	1 large
Watermelon	1 cup

Bread Exchange

Each serving contains 15 g of carbohydrate, 2 g of protein, and 68 cal.

Bread	1 slice
Biscuit, roll	1 (2-in diameter)
Cornbread	1 (1½-in cube)
Muffin	1 (2-in diameter)

Continued

Table 22–8
FOOD EXCHANGE LISTS — *Continued*

Bread Exchange

Cereal
Cooked	½ cup
Dry (flakes, puffed, etc.)	¾ cup

Crackers
Graham	2
Oyster	20
Saltine	5
Soda	3
Round	6–8
Flour	2½ tablespoons
Ice cream (omit 2 fat exchanges)	½ cup
Rice or grits, cooked	½ cup
Spaghetti, noodles, etc.	½ cup
Sponge cake, plain	½-in cube

Vegetables
Baked beans, no pork	¼ cup
Beans (dry, cooked)	½ cup
Corn	⅓ cup
Parsnips	⅔ cup
Peas (dry, cooked)	½ cup

Potatoes
Sweet	¼ cup
White, baked or boiled	1 (2-in diameter)
White, mashed	½ cup

Meat Exchange

Each serving contains 7 g of protein, 5 g of fat, and 73 cal. Remove bone and other wastes when measuring.

Cheese
Cheddar, American	1 ounce slice
Cottage	1 cup
Codfish, mackerel, haddock Halibut, etc.	1 ounce slice
Cold cuts	1½ ounces
Egg	1
Frankfurter	1
Meat and poultry (beef, lamb, pork, chicken)	1 ounce slice
Oysters, shrimp, clams	5 small
Peanut butter (limit to one exchange per day unless carbohydrate is allowed)	2 tablespoons
Salmon, tuna, crab, lobster	¼ cup
Sardines	3 medium

Fat Exchange

Each serving contains 5 grams of fat and 45 calories.

Avocado	⅛ (4-in diameter)
Bacon, crisp	1 slice
Butter or margarine	1 teaspoon

Cream
Heavy	1 tablespoon
Light	2 tablespoons
Cream cheese	1 tablespoon

Continued

Table 22–8
FOOD EXCHANGE LISTS — *Continued*

Fat Exchange

French dressing	1 tablespoon
Mayonnaise	1 teaspoon
Nuts	6 small
Oil or cooking fat	1 teaspoon
Olives	5 small

Milk Exchange

Each serving contains 12 g of carbohydrate, 8 g of protein, 10 g of fat, and 170 cal.

Buttermilk	1 cup
Evaporated milk	½ cup
Powdered milk	¼ cup
Skim milk (add 2 fat exchanges)	1 cup
Whole milk	1 cup

are allowed, a single selection may be doubled or two selections may be made. The exchange list provided in Table 22–8 is based on the recommendations of the American Diabetes Association and the American Dietetic Association.

The diabetic patient should be instructed to eat only those foods that are allowed on the exchange list, to never skip a meal, and to eat all of the specified portion. The exchange list enables the diabetic patient to experience the greatest freedom of choice reflective of normal living while remaining within the dietary restrictions necessary for disease control.

NUTRIENT-DRUG INTERACTIONS

In recent years, the topic of nutrition as it relates to drug therapy has gained the attention of health professionals. It is now well documented that drugs affect nutritional status and that nutritional status affects the efficiency of drug metabolism. The purpose of this section is to introduce the medical assistant to the general concept of the interrelationship between food and drugs.

Information regarding nutrient-drug interactions can be found in the *Physician's Desk Reference*, the *Compendium of Drug Therapy*, and the printed material accompanying drugs. Factors that influence adverse nutrient deficiencies as a result of drug therapy are as follows:

1. Long-term drug administration
2. Multiple drug prescriptions
3. Poor nutritional status at the time drug treatment is initiated

The elderly and people with high nutritional requirements are more likely to be affected by the food-drug interaction. Nutrients and drugs may interact in several ways:

1. Food intake may be altered.
2. Absorption of the nutrient or the drug may be altered.
3. Interference with the intended action of the drug may occur.
4. Metabolism and excretion of the nutrient or the drug may be altered.

While some drug-nutrient interactions may be intended, most are not. Most unintended reactions are of a gastrointestinal nature. Certain classifications of drugs, such as amphetamines, laxatives, and cardiac glycosides, depress the appetite. Previously, amphetamines were commonly prescribed specifically for appetite depression, but they are used less today for appetite depression than in the past. However, amphetamines are still used to treat hyperactive children and, in these patients, cause appetite depression as an unintended side effect. Drugs such as antihistamines, alcohol, insulin, thyroid hormones, tranquilizers, and corticosteroids can stimulate the appetite. Other drugs, such as analgesics, antibiotics, and anti-inflammatory drugs, can cause nausea or vomiting. Still other drugs, such as penicillamine, amphetamines, and anesthetics, can alter taste sensitivity.

The absorption of drugs can also be positively or negatively affected by the presence of particular nutrients in the gastrointestinal tract. Absorption of drugs can likewise be affected by the presence of certain food. Foods can affect a drug by delaying, enhancing, or decreasing absorption. Calcium in milk, for example, can bind with and diminish the absorption of tetracycline, and tetracycline, in turn, can decrease protein metabolism. Drugs can also alter digestive secretions and gastrointestinal motility. In addition, drugs can alter nutrient excretion. These potential drug-nutrient interactions should be investigated by the medical assistant involved in diet instruction. More information about this topic is covered in Chapter 23.

PATIENT TEACHING CONSIDERATIONS

Healthy, life-long eating habits affect BW, body fat, and basic health. During early life, the amount and kinds of food we eat depend on others; in adulthood, food choices become almost unlimited until the older years, when they once again become limited for economic or medical reasons, or because of restricted mobility. Aside from voluntary dieting, other factors that may decrease choice and therefore body weight include surgery, infections, malnutrition, and such diseases as diabetes, cancer, high blood pressure, and diseases of the heart and kidney. Understanding the emotional issues related to food choice and intake decisions is important as the medical assistant approaches the patient to explore the patient's feelings about food choices and diets.

In addition to choice, patients have a wide range of nutritional *needs*. Nutritional requirements depend on a variety of factors, including developmental, physical, economic, and emotional needs. During the various stages of human development, specific consideration must be given to children: parents depend on the physician and medical assistant for growth and childhood nutritional information and for diets to treat children with special needs. Even before birth, expectant couples need instructions for proper nutrition during pregnancy and breast-feeding.

Nutritional deficiencies represent an entire spectrum of causes and needs. Deficiencies may be temporary or chronic and dependent on economic factors, or they can be the result of negative emotions about one's self or food intake. In some cases, a deficiency may be fulfilling an unhealthy "need" of the patient or it can stem from a lack of nutritional information or access to better nutrition. In illness, intake needs are adjusted to specifically treat diarrhea, infections and fever, and disease, or when medications may interfere with nutrients (or vice versa).

Nutrition is considered an integral part of medical care. Adequate food intake is necessary to maintain a healthy nutritional state or to improve a poor one. For many, adequate food intake alone is all that is required to restore the body to good health, whereas for others, it may be one of several methods used.

Although the medical assistant is not a nutritionist or a professional diet therapist, his or her role often encompasses providing dietary information as well as reinforcing the importance of carrying out diet prescriptions ordered by the physician. The wise medical assistant understands that the ultimate purpose of presenting nutritional information is to allow patients to evaluate their own dietary practices and to make their own dietary decisions. To strengthen the impact of educational activities, the medical assistant must guide patients through particular nutrition-related decisions with careful instructions, repetition of concepts, soliciting the patient's direct participation, and a sincere concern for the patient's well-being.

Few medical personnel come into contact with as many patients as the medical assistant. The medical assistant has unlimited teaching opportunities to promote better nutrition, positive attitudes toward food and nutrition, and healthy dietary habits.

RELATED ETHICAL AND LEGAL IMPLICATIONS

Nutritional information is constantly and rapidly changing. Some topics are debated by nutrition experts, and many new research claims have not yet been proved scientifically. The medical assistant must be able to critically evaluate new nutritional information as it becomes available through the scientific literature and the media.

The medical assistant must respect all local social customs and be sensitive to personal issues regarding diet. At the same time, the medical assistant must have an appreciation for the right kinds and amounts of food and the scientific principles of normal diets, hospital diets, and therapeutic diets. Equipped with this knowledge, the medical assistant can combat misinformation about food forced on patients by food faddists, quacks, and self-appointed untrained food specialists. Fad reducing diets may be fast and easy, but they cannot keep off weight. These diets usually are monotonous and detrimental because they decrease self-esteem and are self-defeating and hard on the body. Medical assistants must be careful to follow the science of nutrition and the principles of nutrition and diet therapy. The following diet programs are considered "fad diets" by nutritionists and the medical profession:

"Fabulous" form diet

Elimination diet

Banana and skim milk diet

Egg and leafy vegetable diet

Various 7- or 9-day "wonder" diets

Low-protein diet

High-protein diet

Reducing pills, candies, etc.

"Eat all you want" diet

"Air Force" diet (not connected with the Air Force)

Grapefruit diet

Grapejuice diet

Starvation diet

Mayo diet (not connected with the Mayo Clinic)

When helping the patient to understand the physician's dietary instructions, the medical assistant must remain within the parameters of the professional medical assistant role. The medical assistant should have a clear understanding of the diet prescription, its purpose, and how it fits into the overall treatment regimen before attempting to instruct the patient. While the patient's own dietary habits and food likes and dislikes often are taken into consideration in formulating the actual diet plan, harmful departures from the prescription must be avoided. For example, the medical assistant should never tell a diabetic patient who is taking insulin and insisting on not eating lunch that it is okay to skip this meal when the diet prescription calls for three meals and two snacks. In this and similar instances, the medical assistant must use discretion based on the correct principles of disease and diet therapy. When in doubt, the physician should be consulted and clarification obtained. This approach is not only helpful in promoting the patient's wellness, but it serves as legal protection for both the medical assistant and the physician.

SUMMARY

The role of the medical assistant in diet therapy is of great importance and value to physicians in the management of their own time. Medical assistants who understand the concepts of basic nutrition and diet therapy and who can successfully apply these concepts in patient teaching enable physicians to use their office time more effectively. Although the medical assistant is not a nutritionist or a professional diet therapist, the role of the medical assistant is to provide information and to support the patient in carrying out the diet prescription ordered by the physician.

DISCUSSION QUESTIONS

1. Can a vegetarian diet be nutritionally sound? Why or why not? Defend your answer.
2. Choose five currently popular "fad" weight loss diets. Are any of these nutritionally adequate? Why or why not?
3. What services exist in your area that are designed to assist the older adult in planning or obtaining nutritious meals? Do these appear adequate?
4. Several new insights regarding the weight gain and loss cycle are related to research on the body's *set point*. Consult nutrition journals and texts (see Bibliography at the end of the chapter) for discussions on set point. Discuss the research findings and their relationship to the problems of weight reduction.

BIBLIOGRAPHY

AAHPERD Lifetime Health Related Physical Fitness Test Manual, The American Alliance for Health, Physical Education, Recreation and Dance, Reston, VA, 1980.

American College of Sports Medicine: Guidelines for Exercise Testing and Prescription, ed 4. American College of Sports Medicine, 1991.

Chernoff R: Geriatric Nutrition: The Health Professional Handbook. Aspen, Gaithersburg, MD, 1991.

Cooper KH: The Aerobic Way. M Evans and Co, New York, 1977.

Donoghue WC: How to Measure Your % Bodyfat, ed 3. Creative Health Products, Plymouth, MI, 1992.

Frankle RT and Yang M-U: Obesity and Weight Control: The Health Professional's Guide to Understanding and Treatment. Aspen, Gaithersburg, MD, 1988.

Kretchmer N: Frontiers in Clinical Nutrition. Aspen, Gaithersburg, MD, 1986.

Perkin J: Food Allergies and Adverse Reactions. Aspen, Gaithersburg, MD, 1991.

Powers MA: Handbook of Diabetes Nutritional Management. Aspen, Gaithersburg, MD, 1987.

Reiff DW and Reiff KKL: Eating Disorders: Nutrition Therapy in the Recovery Process. Aspen, Gaithersburg, MD, 1992.

Simko MD, Cowell C, and Hreha MS: Practical Nutrition: A Quick Reference for the Health Care Practitioner. Aspen, Gaithersburg, MD, 1989.

PROCEDURE: Measure skinfold thicknesses and the circumference of the adult arm

OSHA STANDARDS:

Terminal Performance Objective: Measure patient's skinfold thicknesses at four sites and arm circumference (AC), and calculate percentage of body fat and arm muscle circumference (AMC) within a reasonable time.

EQUIPMENT: Lange skinfold calipers (adipometer)
Percentage of body fat charts (see Table 22–6)
Measuring tape
The following formulas:
a. Percentage of body fat × body weight (BW) = Fat weight (FW)
b. BW − FW = Lean body weight (LBW)
c. $\dfrac{100 - \text{Percentage of body fat}}{100 - \text{Percentage desired}} = \text{IBW}$
d. AC (mm) − [thickness of skinfold (TSF; mm) × 3.14] = AMC

PROCEDURE

1. Identify the patient and explain the procedure.

2. Remove clothing at the skinfold test sites on the right side of the body.

3. If only one location is used, use the triceps site. If two sites are used, use the triceps and subscapular sites. Separate charts are available for the triceps site and the triceps-subscapular sites.

Triceps Measurement

1. Choose the site at the right deltoid triceps behind the upper arm midway between the tip of the elbow and the shoulder.

2. Take the fold in a vertical direction directly at the center of the back of the arm while the patient's arm is flexed at a 90° angle.

3. With a grease pencil, mark the point.

4. Ask the patient to extend the arm, then grasp the skinfolds making both sides of the fold parallel.

PRINCIPLE

1. To reduce the risk of error and to provide assurance to anxious patients.

2. Skinfold measurements must be taken directly on the skin and, unless otherwise ordered, on the right side of the body.

1. This site is the most accessible in both men and women. Because the thickness of subcutaneous fat from elbow to shoulder is not uniform, the location of the site must be precise.

2. The level is located with the forearm flexed at a 90° angle. (The triceps muscle is relaxed in this position.)

3. Until experienced, marking the site should not be eliminated.

4. The skinfold is lifted parallel to the long axis of the arm and the measurement is taken with the arm hanging free.

PROCEDURE

5. With the thumb and forefinger far enough apart, pinch up a full fold firmly and cleanly from the underlying tissue $\frac{1}{4}$ inch above the grease mark. (See figures, below.)

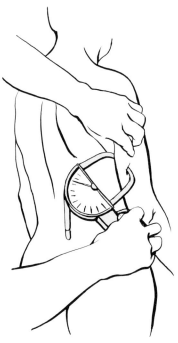

Skinfold measurement over the triceps muscle of the upper arm; maintain the original pinch grasp of the nondominant hand to ensure proper measurement.

6. If it feels that you have grasped underlying muscle, ask the patient to contract the muscle.

7. Apply the caliper jaws (parallel to one another) to the skinfold so that the grease mark is midway between the jaws.

8. Do not release the fingers of the nondominant hand during the measurement.

9. Release the thumb from the caliper handle, so that the tips of the caliper have full exertion on the skinfold.

10. Completely release the trigger of the caliper.

11. Take the reading immediately after the first rapid fall.

12. Read three different measurements at the site and record each reading.

13. Average the three readings.

14. Repeat the procedure for the four locations. The order makes no difference.

PRINCIPLE

5. Calipers will be applied $\frac{1}{4}$ inch below the fingers grasping the skin. The amount of skinfold must be proportionate to the site: grasp more fat on heavier patients; less on thin patients.

6. If there is muscle in the skinfold, the fold withdraws from the pinch. It is rare that muscle is included in the pinch.

7. The fold must be held firmly between the fingers while the jaws of the caliper are applied in the middle of the pinch. This allows the pressure at the point measured to be exerted by the caliper jaws and not the fingers.

8. To ensure the calipers measure just the thickness of the fold and not any of the forces required to keep it folded.

9. Skinfold calipers have springs that exert a certain pressure on the skinfold and a scale which measures the thickness in millimeters.

10. To allow the entire force of the jaws to close onto the skinfold. The patient will not be uncomfortable.

11. The calipers will register a lower reading at the instant they are released, then settle on the correct reading.

12. Rounding to within $\frac{1}{2}$ mm is sufficient. Readings should agree within 2 mm. Skinfold values may appear to diminish with subsequent measurement because area fluid has been squeezed out of the tissue, especially on larger patients.

13. The mean of three readings is gathered to create a single reading from each of the four sites.

14. The mean reading from the triceps, biceps, subscapular, and suprailiac sites are added together.

PROCEDURE

Subscapular Measurement

1. Pick up the skinfold just under the right shoulder blade, following the natural fold of the skin.

2. With a grease pencil, mark the midway point of the fold.
3. While holding the skinfold approximately 1 inch from the mark, take the measurements. **Note:** Measure this site holding the calipers at a 45° angle.

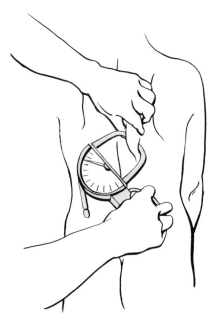
Subscapular skinfold measurement.

Biceps Measurement

1. With a grease pencil, mark the midpoint of the muscle belly on the flexed right biceps muscle.
2. Following the natural fold, pick up the skinfold with the thumb and forefinger of the nondominant hand.
3. Pinch the fold in a vertical direction directly at the center of the front of the upper arm (Fig. below).
4. Take three readings from the site and average the three to obtain the skinfold measurement at this site.

Suprailiac Measurement

1. Pick up the skinfold, following the natural horizontal fold of the skin.
2. With a grease pencil, mark midway on the fold.

PRINCIPLE

1. The skinfold below the tip of the scapular provides a good characterization of overall fatness. The thickness of subcutaneous tissue in this area is fairly uniform. Precise localization of this site is less critical than in the triceps area.

PROCEDURE

3. While holding the skinfold approximately 1 inch from the mark, take the measurements. **Note:** Measure this site holding the calipers horizontally.

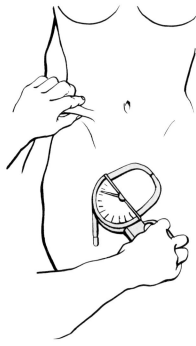

Suprailiac skinfold measurement.

Calculating Percentage of Body Fat

1. Add up the four site readings and determine the percentage of body fat by age group on the "Sum of Four Sites" male or female chart.

2. Record the percentage of body fat from the chart and calculate the LBW and FW:
   a. Percentage of body fat $\times$ BW = FW
   b. BW $-$ FW = LBW
3. Calculate the IBW:
   $$\frac{100 - \text{Percentage of body fat}}{100 - \text{Percentage desired}} \times BW = IBW$$
4. Calculate the amount of weight to be lost or gained:
   a. BW $-$ IBW = Amount to lose
   b. IBW $-$ BW = Amount to gain

Measure Arm Circumference and Arm Muscle Circumference

1. Place the measuring tape around the nondominant arm at the midpoint between the elbow and shoulder.
2. Measure with the measuring tape taut but not compressing the muscle.
3. Record the measurement to the nearest ¼ inch.

4. Convert inches to centimeters, then convert centimeters to millimeters.
5. Use the AC in millimeters to calculate the AMC:
   AMC (mm) = AC (mm) $-$ [TSF (mm) $\times$ 3.14]
6. Briefly explain the results to the patient.

PRINCIPLE

1. Separate charts are available depending on the number of sites measured. If only one location is measured, use the triceps only charts. If two sites are measured, use the triceps-subscapular charts.
2. See text for calculation examples.

3. See text for calculation examples.

4. See text for calculation examples.

1. Arm muscle circumference in conjunction with TSF is used to estimate the protein-calorie status.
2. To obtain an accurate measurement of the muscle at rest.
3. The average AC for adult men is 11.6 inches (29.3 cm); for adult women, 11.4 inches (28.5 cm).
4. 1 inch = 2.5 cm = 25 mm
   ¼ inch = 0.625 cm = 6.25 mm
5. In severely underweight patients, a small AMC may be an early indication of protein-calorie malnutrition.
6. Increased TSF is an indicator of the degree of obesity. Small AC may indicate inadequate protein and caloric intake.

HIGHLIGHTS
Eating Disorders

Our society's emphasis on thinness is at least one contributing factor in the incidence of eating disorders such as anorexia nervosa and bulimia. According to a 1985 statistic, anorexia nervosa, or self-induced starvation, affects about 0.5% (1 out of every 200) of American females typically 12 to 18 years of age. Bulimia, a cycle of food binges followed by purging (e.g., vomiting or laxative or diuretic abuse) appears to be more prevalent. It is estimated that bulimia affects 5% of adolescent and young adult females. The reported evidence of these eating disorders among males is much less than among females.

The American Psychiatric Association has published specific criteria for the diagnosis of these disorders. Anorexics and bulimics share the desire to become and remain thin, but can be differentiated according to their specific characteristics.

ANOREXIA NERVOSA

Reportedly, there are three common characteristics related to the diagnosis of anorexia nervosa in females: (1) self-induced starvation, (2) fear that fatness will result from loss of control of eating, and (3) amenorrhea. These features represent a behavioral, psychological, and physiologic dimension.

The typical anorexic is a white adolescent female described as "perfect": obedient, highly motivated, and successful socially and academically. Frequently, anorexics are members of families that are overly involved or enmeshed with each other, are highly controlling, and highly value achievement, perfection, and physical appearance. Psychologists theorize that the afflicted female, seemingly in pursuit of thinness, is actually struggling to exert some control in her life. Afflicted males, however, tend to be underachievers and have been chastised in their approach to life.

While the specific cause(s) of anorexia nervosa remains unknown, the metabolic and chemical changes resulting from starvation are predictable. Among these changes are decreased metabolic rate, lowered heart rate (bradycardia), hypotension, hypothermia, leukopenia, hypoplasia of bone marrow, low erythrocyte sedimentation rates and fibrinogen levels, electrolyte imbalance, increased blood levels of cholesterol and carotene, and decreased blood glucose concentration. The anorexic patient may also experience symptoms such as abdominal pain, constipation, dry skin, brittle hair and nails, and peripheral edema.

Treatment of anorexia nervosa is based on the understanding that it is a multidetermined disorder. Therefore, treatment measures are used in combination and include nutritional rehabilitation, individual and family psychotherapy, behavior modification, and medications. A treatment of choice has not yet emerged.

The prognosis regarding anorexia nervosa is controversial due to the sample number, length of study, and criteria used to define recovery (such as restoring the patient's body weight to about 95% of the ideal weight). The general consensus, however, is that a poor recovery can be expected in patients with late age of onset, long illness, distorted family background, and delayed treatment. A significant proportion of patients continue to demonstrate some disordered eating patterns after treatment, and 6% of patients treated die because of complications. Unfortunately, a great deal is still unknown about the cause, criteria for diagnosis, and effective treatment of anorexia nervosa.

BULIMIA

Bulimia is defined as the recurrent, rapid, and uncontrollable ingestion of large quantities of food in a short period of time followed by purging. Purging may be accomplished by vomiting and using laxatives or diuretics. Paradoxically, for the bulimic patient, these episodes are an attempt to bring control to their lives and their weight.

According to the American Psychiatric Association, bulimia is diagnosed on the basis of the following criteria:

1. Recurrent episodes of binge eating
2. Awareness that the eating disorder is abnormal and fear of not being able to stop voluntarily
3. Depression
4. Self-deprecating thoughts after the episodes

The typical bulimic is a white, college-educated female of normal weight for height who seeks treatment in her early twenties, but has a history of a 4- to 6-year manifestation of bulimic behavior. Ten to 13 percent of bulimic patients are male. It is interesting to note that 30% to 50% of anorexics develop bulimic behavior. In all patients, purging occurs with some regularity, ranging from vomiting after every meal to vomiting daily or once or twice weekly.

Behavioral characteristics of bulimic patient include problems with impulse control, chronic depression, intolerance to frustration, exaggerated sense of guilt, and recurring anxiety. Typically, bulimics are overdependent on the approval of others and have low self-esteem, difficulties expressing certain emotions, such as anger, and tend to be extraverted and volatile.

Precipitating factors culminating in the binge-purge cycle are emotional stress, boredom, or loneliness. Bulimics often feel panicked concerning the binge—afraid the weight will be gained (a sign of lack of

Continued

self-control)—and they vomit to retaliate and exert their "control."

While consistencies in the psychological profile of bulimics can be noted, the actual cause remains unknown. Consistencies in the medical and physical changes can also be recognized. Among these are enlarged parotid glands, facial puffiness, sore throat, menstrual irregularities, dental problems, and electrolyte disturbances. Serious complications arising from prolonged and severe bulimia are urinary infections, renal failure, and cardiac arrhythmias.

Treatment goals for bulimics are similar to those for the anorexic in that they draw on the collaboration of medical specialities (behavioral and cognitive therapy and medication) and are supportive rather than curative.

Much remains unknown regarding the treatment of bulimia. However, according to recent studies, the outcome appears more favorable for normal-weight bulimics than for anorexics who binge and purge or bulimics who abuse alcohol or drugs or whose disorder is severe or who experience suicidal feelings. As in the case of anorexics, proven means of preventing this disorder are unknown. It is the hope of health professionals, however, that teaching children and young adults the importance of nutrition and effective methods of weight control and the risks associated with eating disorders will decrease the incidence of these dangerous eating disorders.

CHAPTER OUTLINE

LEARNING OBJECTIVES

Upon completing this chapter, you will be able to:

1. Describe the role of the federal government and state and local agencies in the regulation of drugs.
2. Define terms related to drug interactions and classifications.
3. Discuss the general uses and actions of the specific drug categories.

Chapter 23

*P*harmacology and Drug Therapy

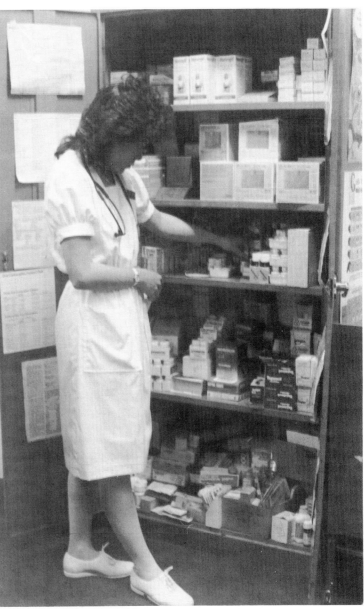

4. List the variables in individuals that could result in expected or unexpected drug responses.
5. Define the terms related to drug side effects.
6. List the major pharmacologic reference books for drug information.
7. Define and give examples of nonprescription, prescription, and controlled drugs.
8. List the seven parts of a complete prescription.
9. Name the seven rights and three checkpoints for preparing and administering medication.

PERFORMANCE OBJECTIVES

Upon completing this chapter, you will be able to:

1. Interpret a medication order and calculate drug dosages.
2. Prepare the patient for medication administration.
3. Administer oral medication in liquid or tablet form, or instruct a patient to administer an oral medication safely and accurately.
4. Administer a sublingual or buccal medication in tablet form, or instruct the patient to self-administer the medication safely and accurately.
5. Instruct a patient to deliver a topical medication to the respiratory tract safely and accurately.
6. Insert a rectal suppository, vaginal suppository, or vaginal cream, and instruct the patient to self-administer rectal and vaginal medications safely and accurately.
7. Instruct a patient to safely apply and remove a transdermal infusion unit.
8. Prepare a sterile injectable solution.
9. Administer a parenteral subcutaneous (or intramuscular) injection safely and accurately.
10. Perform an intradermal skin test to assess a patient's sensitivity to drugs or other antigens.

DACUM EDUCATIONAL COMPONENTS

1. Apply principles of aseptic technique and infection control (4.1).
2. Recognize emergencies (4.3).
3. Prepare and maintain examination and treatment area (4.5).
4. Prepare patients for procedures (4.7).
5. Prepare and administer medications as directed by the physician (4.13).
6. Maintain medication records (4.14).
7. Document accurately (5.1).
8. Dispose of controlled substances in compliance with governmental regulations (5.5).
9. Instruct patients with special needs (7.2).

Glossary

Ampule: glass or plastic container holding medication in either liquid or powdered form *one dose*

Controlled substance: classification of drugs regulated by the Food and Drug Administration because of the potential for abuse or misuse

Formulary: a listing of medical preparations including their chemical formulas

Hypersensitivity: abnormal or unusual response to a drug occurring after the body has been previously exposed (and sensitized) to the same drug, occurring in some patients but not others; drug allergy

Hypodermic: beneath the skin; an injection

Idiosyncrasy: abnormal or unusual response to a drug in patients who are abnormally sensitive to a small dose the first time it is administered, usually due to hereditary defects

Isotonic: a solution having the same osmotic pressure as body fluids

Over-the-counter drug: medication that can be purchased without a prescription

Parenteral: occurring outside the alimentary canal; an injection

Potentiation: process where one inactive drug nevertheless increases the action of another drug

Synergism: process of one drug producing the same effect as a second drug, with their combined action resulting in an increased intensity or prolonged affect of one or both drugs

Vial: a sterile, vacuum-sealed container of injectable medication available in multidose and single-dose sizes

Viscosity: resistance to flow; thick, not easily flowing

Wheal: a localized area of edema on the body surface

Drug therapy is used in the treatment and prevention of diseases or conditions. Many patients' conditions require treatment with one or more prescription medications. Many individuals also use nonprescription, over-the-counter (OTC) drugs, which may be purchased in drug stores and supermarkets.

In modern society, the use of drugs is often taken quite casually. This attitude, however, must be avoided by health care personnel. Although the use of drugs in patient care plans is prevalent, chemical intervention in human body processes always includes some element of risk. Medical assistants must acquire an appreciation for the serious responsibility they assume in the administration of drugs. This clinical function carries with it a greater potential for error than all other clinical functions within the scope of medical assisting. To reduce the risk of error, medical assistants need to acquire an understanding of basic pharmacology concepts and drug therapy applications.

The assistant's responsibility in drug therapy includes not only the administration of drugs, but also the awareness of side effects, the interpretation of the prescription for the patient, and the reinforcement of the physician's instructions. To remain current and provide accurate information to the patient, the medical assistant must learn to use the various drug reference books described later in this chapter.

LEGAL STANDARDS AND REGULATIONS

Federal, state, and local regulations govern the manufacturing, distribution, dispensing, and sale of drugs. With the passage of the Pure Food and Drug Act in 1906, the federal government established the first standards for the manufacturing of drugs.

The Food, Drug, and Cosmetic Act of 1938 established additional federal regulations governing the manufacture, sale, distribution, and clinical use of all drugs. This act is amended periodically and enforced by the federal Food and Drug Administration (FDA), a branch of the Department of Health and Human Services.

A specific category of drugs (those with abuse or addictive potential) is regulated by the Controlled Substances Act of 1970. The importation, manufacture, transportation, distribution, sale, prescription, and administration of controlled substances is federally monitored by the Drug Enforcement Agency (DEA), a branch of the Department of Justice. Drugs that fall within the domain of this law are categorized into five schedules (Fig. 23–1). The schedules are labeled with the Roman numerals I through V. Schedule I drugs have the highest potential for addiction and possible abuse and are not approved for medical use. Schedule V drugs have the least potential for addiction or abuse but still must be controlled. A complete list of scheduled drugs may be obtained from the regional offices of the DEA.

State and local agencies also play a role in the regulation of drugs. Individual states may add drugs to the schedules or change the classifications of some controlled substances, especially schedule II drugs, depending on whether state or federal regulation prevails. The state health department also mandates how drugs are stored and dispensed in public facilities (e.g., outpatient facilities). State registration and licensing boards have regulations specifically outlining who may dispense medications and under what circumstances. Various pieces of state or local legislation can regulate the intrastate transport of drugs, and interstate commerce laws are concerned with out-of-state drug transportation.

DRUG ENFORCEMENT AGENCY REGISTRATION AND DRUG SECURITY

To ensure compliance with legal standards for dispensing drugs, the medical assistant's responsibilities include the following:

1. Monitoring the currency of the physician's DEA federal and state registrations
2. Maintaining legally designated records and inventories
3. Providing security for all drugs, controlled substances, and prescription pads
4. Destroying drugs when expired

Physician registration is administered by the DEA. The initial physician application may be obtained through a regional office or by directly applying to the DEA Registration Section, PO Box 28083, Central Station, Washington, DC 20038-8083. A registration is issued to each licensed physician and must be renewed every 3 years. The DEA will send an application renewal form (Form 226) to the physician about 60 days before renewal is due. The medical assistant should make a note in the management calendar 45 days before the renewal date. A request for the renewal form must be made to the Washington address if the form has not been received by this time. Some states require separate state registration for controlled substances every 1 or 2 years. When state registration is required, the DEA will not reissue a federal certificate unless the state registration is current and valid.

Special recordkeeping is required of all physicians who administer or dispense scheduled drugs to their patients. The records must always be available for inspection and must account for all drugs administered and dispensed. The records must be kept for a minimum of 2 years and include the following information: the patient's name and address; date of administration; medication name, dosage, and route; method of dispensing; and indication for the drug. This specific recordkeeping is required *only* when the physician administers or dispenses a scheduled drug in the office.

When the physician prescribes a scheduled drug by giving the patient a completed prescription for a pharmacy to fill, keeping this detailed record is not required.

Schedule I: This schedule lists drugs of high potential for abuse and that have no current accepted medical use. Schedule I drugs will be used by physicians only for purposes of research, approved by the Food and Drug Administration and the DEA, and only after a separate DEA registration as a researcher is obtained. The manufacture, importation and sale of these drugs is prohibited. However, some states have enacted legislation to permit the use and possession of marijuana for certain medical patients.

Examples: heroin, marijuana, and LSD.

Schedule II: These drugs have current accepted medical use in the United States, but with severe restrictions. There is with these drugs a high potential of abuse that may lead to severe psychological or physical dependence.

Examples: *Narcotics:* morphine, codeine, Percodan.
Non-narcotics: amphetamines, Ritalin, Nembutal, and Quaalude.

When Schedule I and II drugs are ordered, the physician must use a special order form (DEA Form 222) that is preprinted with the physician's name and address. The form is issued in triplicate. One copy is kept in the physician's file while the remaining copies are forwarded to the supplier who, after filling the order, keeps a copy and forwards the third copy to the nearest DEA office.

Prescription orders for Schedule II drugs must be written and signed by the physician. Some states, by law, require special prescription blanks with more than one copy. The physician's registration number must appear on the blank. The order may not be telephoned in to the pharmacy except in an emergency, as defined by the DEA. A prescription for Schedule II drugs may not be refilled.

Schedule III: These drugs have less potential for abuse than substances in Schedule I and II. They have accepted medical use for treatment in the United States, but abuse may lead to moderate or low physical dependence or high psychological dependence.

Examples: *Narcotics:* various drug combinations containing codeine and paregoric.
Non-narcotics: amphetamine-like compounds and butabarbital.

Schedule IV: These drugs have a lower potential for abuse than those in Schedule III and have accepted medical use in the United States, but their abuse still may lead to limited physical or psychological dependence.

Examples: Chloral hydrate, meprobamate, Librium, Valium, and Darvon.

Schedule III and IV drugs require either a written or oral prescription by the prescribing physician. If authorized by the physician on the initial prescription the patient may have the prescription refilled up to the number of refills authorized, which may not exceed five times or beyond six months from the date that the prescription was issued.

Schedule V: These drugs have less potential for abuse than drugs in Schedule IV, and their abuse may be limited to physical or psychological dependence. Refills are the same as for drugs in Schedules III and IV.

Examples: This schedule includes cough medications containing codeine and antidiarrheals such as Lomotil.

According to the law, the only person authorized to issue prescriptions is the registrant. A prescription issued by the physician may be communicated to the pharmacist by the medical office employees. This regulation may be less restrictive for medications *not* in the Controlled Substances Act.

If your state requires triplicate prescription blanks, they will be used for prescribing drugs. These are not to be confused with the Form DEA 222 described earlier for the ordering of Schedule I and II drugs. The triplicate blanks will be furnished by the state, and the regulations should be followed.

All prescriptions for controlled substances must be dated and signed on the day issued, bearing full name and address of the patient and the name, address, and DEA registration number of the physician. The prescription must be written in ink or typewritten and must be signed by hand by the physician.

Physicians must know the laws of their state on controlled substances. The state regulations may be more strict than Federal regulations and may require a separate state registration.

Narcotics laws should be studied carefully by any physician who opens an office. *The Code of Federal Regulations, Title 21,* should be obtained from the nearest Federal government bookstore and studied carefully before handling of controlled substances in the medical office.

Figure 23–1. Schedule (listing) of drug categories as mandated by the Controlled Substances Act of 1970.

The physician records all prescribed drugs in the patient record. A record of all prescription renewals also must be recorded in the patient record.

Inventory regulations require that a completed inventory record form for Schedule II drugs be submitted every 2 years to the DEA at the time of registration. To be complete, this record requires an accounting of the "on-hand" inventory, the patients receiving the drug, and a reconciliation with the amount remaining. All inventory records require the physician's name, address, DEA registration number, date of inventory, and the signature of the person taken the inventory.

Controlled substances must be stored separately from other drugs in a locked cabinet. Federal regulations define the storage "container" as "adequately constructed." However, some state divisions of licensing and certification specify double locks for "narcotics" (Schedule II drugs). Prescription forms also must be secured because of the potential for unauthorized or illegal use. Forms should be kept out of patient and public areas and should not be used for note pads. It is wise to keep the forms in the locked safe or cabinet, but the physician can keep one form with him or her for ready use. The DEA Registration Form 222 and the state triplicate form should also be kept in the locked safe or cabinet. Many offices are choosing not to keep any controlled drugs on the premises because of the increased incidents of armed robbery. Any loss of drugs must be reported to the regional DEA office and local law enforcement agencies immediately after its discovery.

All medications must be removed from the shelf and destroyed when the expiration date has been reached. Under no circumstances is a drug to be administered or given to a patient as a prescription after its expiration date. To dispose of outdated medications, liquids and ointments may be rinsed down the sink drain to be further destroyed in the sewage system. Powders should be mixed with liquid (usually water or alcohol) and poured down the drain. Pills and capsules should either be dissolved in water and poured down the drain or they may be flushed down the toilet. For liquids in vials and ampules, the vial is to be opened or the ampule broken and the liquid disposed of by pouring it down the drain. The local DEA office must be contacted for disposal instructions and the required paperwork for controlled substances.

DRUG INTERACTIONS AND CLASSIFICATIONS

According to the Food, Drug, and Cosmetic Act, the term *drug* refers to any article or substance other than food that is intended to affect the structure or any function of the body and that is recognized and approved by the FDA. Generally, a drug has three names: a trade name (trademark), a generic name (nonproprietary name), and a chemical name (describes the chemical configuration of the drug).

The *trade name* is patented by a pharmaceutical company. This means that no other company can manufacture exactly the same compound until the patent expires. However, other companies can produce a similar compound with similar action. A single drug may be manufactured by several companies each having a different trade name, but all have only one official name. For example, Advil, Nuprin, and Motrin are all trade names of a drug whose official name is Ibuprofen USP. The official name is published in a volume titled the *United States Pharmacopoeia*, or *USP*. All drugs marketed by their official names have the letters "USP" after their names.

The *generic name* is also the *official name* of the drug and usually refers to its active ingredient. The advantage of a generic drug is that the generic drug costs less to purchase. The quality of a generically manufactured drug may or may not be considered the same as a trade name drug. Many states permit the pharmacist to substitute a generic drug anytime a prescription requests a drug by the trade name as long as the physician and patient approve of the substitution. A physician may include the words "medically necessary" on a prescription. In this case, the pharmacy cannot substitute a generic product for a trade name product.

The *chemical name* indicates the chemical makeup or molecular structure. Generally, it is only used by chemists and occasionally pharmacists who must compound a drug. The chemical name assists physicians and pharmacists in anticipating drug-drug interactions in specific situations. For example, a drug may be given to bind or bond with a previously administered drug either for potentiation or inactivation. *Potentiation* occurs when one drug intensifies the action of a second drug. *Inactivation* occurs when one drug cancels out the effects of another drug.

VARIABLES AFFECTING DRUG ACTION

Certain variables can alter a patient's response to a drug:

1. *Potency.* All drug containers are stamped with an expiration date. If a drug is used after the expiration date, its composition may be altered or decomposed, possibly causing the drug to become toxic or inactive. Environmental factors such as excessive cold or heat or exposure to light may also cause chemical alterations or decomposition. For example, unusual but reversible impaired kidney function has been traced to tetracycline products that were outdated or degraded as a result of improper storage.

2. *Route of administration.* Drug actions depend on the appropriate administration route. If routes other than those specified are used to administer the drug, the desired action may not occur at all or not occur at the desired rate.

3. *Physiologic variances.* The usual effects of a drug can be altered by the presence of food in the stomach, the individual's rate of drug ab-

sorption, reduced or increased peristaltic activity, reduced responsiveness to a drug (tolerance), and so forth. Individual patient variations influence drug distribution in the body. Less body weight, particularly in pediatric and geriatric patients, can increase the effect of a drug. Metabolism and drug elimination vary with each person and decreased elimination may produce increased drug concentrations from the accumulation of a drug on the body. Age, gender, diurnal rhythm, pathology, genetics, environmental, and emotional factors can all alter a patient's expected response to a drug.

4. *Drug-drug interactions.* The presence of specific foods or other drugs in the stomach or in the body may alter the usual effects of a drug. This is termed a *drug-food interaction* when a food, not a drug, affects the drug response. The result may be an increased or decreased response to a drug. Sometimes a drug can be prescribed to combine with and increase the effects of another drug. Two drugs that work together to produce effects greater than the sum of their individual effects are called *synergistic.* Codeine, for example, can be given with aspirin to relieve pain more effectively. *Potentiation* is the term used when drugs having dissimilar individual actions give a greater total effect when they are combined. When drugs taken together counteract the effects of each other, the result is known as *antagonism.* Drug-drug interactions may be desirable or therapeutic, or they may be seriously harmful. A drug that is absorbed faster than it is excreted has a cumulative effect. This may be due to physiologic variances, dosage, or the continuous use of the drug.

SIDE EFFECTS OF DRUGS

Drugs are prescribed to achieve desired therapeutic effects, but at the same time, all drugs have side effects. These side effects are results that are not specifically intended but are normal physiologic accompaniments to the desired effects of the drug. Not all side effects are undesirable; some side effects are harmless and even useful. An example of a drug with some positive side effects is aspirin. One side effect of aspirin (a pain-reliever) is mild sedation. A person taking aspirin for pain will also experience a state of mild relaxation. Although sedation is not the purpose of the prescription, it is usually beneficial to the patient.

An untoward effect is a side effect that is undesirable. An unexpected or unusual reaction to a drug the first time it is administered is termed *idiosyncrasy.* An abnormal reaction that occurs repeatedly after the first administration is termed an *allergic reaction.* Other unintended effects of drug administration may be related to factors such as strong emotions or psychological responses such as hope, fear, and belief.

Certain drugs, when used for prolonged periods, can become ineffectual in their action. The patient builds up a tolerance to the drug, and dosages must be steadily increased to achieve the same desired results. *Cross-tolerance* can occur when one drug increases the body's resistance to the effects and actions of other similar drugs. Occasionally, *physical dependence* on a drug occurs; in this case, the cells are unable to function without high levels of the drug circulating through the bloodstream. *Addiction* is the physiologic need for a drug, whereas *habituation* is the psychological need.

A drug may also produce certain effects that warrant special warning. These effects are called *contraindications.* This term applies to certain conditions under which the drug should not be administered.

Precautions are those measures taken to avoid contraindications. An example of a contraindication would be the warning "do not take this drug with other medication" or "do not administer to patient with hypertension." An example of a precaution would be a directive to "take the medication with milk" or a statement that "alcohol will complicate the effects of this medication."

DRUG CLASSIFICATION

Drugs can be classified either according to their effects and actions on certain body systems or in terms of their general therapeutic function. In Table 23-1, drugs in various classes are categorized according to their actions and uses. These classifications include the drugs commonly used in medical office practice. Please note that the table does not include all classifications or all possible uses and examples for the drug groups listed.

Placebos have not been included. Placebos, in fact, are not categorized as drugs at all, because they have no specific physiologic effects or actions. They are prescribed but rather are selectively (rarely) for psychological purposes only. Although usually simple sugar pills, placebos can also take the form of sterile water or saline injections. The desired effect is to make patients feel better in the assurance of receiving and taking "medication." The use of placebos is uncommon in modern medical office practice and has long been a controversial issue.

The study of pharmacology is an ongoing process. Each day, new drugs and new uses for old drugs are discovered. As part of a general commitment to continuing professional education, practical office pharmacology must be studied and understood by the medical assistant.

REFERENCES FOR DRUG INFORMATION

As a member of the health care team involved in administering drugs, it is important to keep current with pharmacologic advances. Drug information can be obtained from several reference publications. Medical Economics Company publishes the *Physicians' Desk Reference* (*PDR*) annually and supplements it with semiannual updates. The reference contains nine sections:

Table 23-1
CLASSIFICATION OF DRUGS

Class	Effects and Actions	Common Use	Examples
Adrenergics	Affect heart muscle, increasing the rate and strength of contractions. Act as vasoconstrictors, dilate pupils, and relax the muscular walls of gastrointestinal and urinary tracts. Dilate bronchi.	Treatment of bronchitis, asthma, allergic conditions, and nasal congestion. Used in the treatment of shock to increase blood pressure.	Isuprel Sudafed Neo-Synephrine Visine Epinephrine Alupent Intropin Brethine
Adrenergic blocking agents	Accomplish vasodilation, increase peripheral circulation, decrease blood pressure, and increase the tone of the muscle walls of the gastrointestinal tract.	Treatment of hypertension, migraine headache, peripheral disease.	Aldomet Ergotrate Inderal
Analgesics	Relieve pain and lower blood pressure. Vasodilation results. Decrease peristalsis; may cause constipation, nausea, and vomiting.	Narcotic and nonnarcotic analgesics are used to relieve varying intensities of pain.	Aspirin Talwin Tylenol Darvon Demerol Morphine
Anesthetics	Block nerve impulses to the brain to achieve loss of consciousness. Dilate pupils, decrease respiration, pulse, and blood pressure.	Can be used for general or local anesthesia in minor or major surgery. In local anesthesia there is loss of pain sensation without loss of consciousness. In general anesthesia, loss of consciousness also results.	Pentothal (general) Xylocaine (local)
Antacids	Neutralize the hydrochloric acid in the stomach.	Treatment of hyperacidity (indigestion) and peptic ulcers.	Aluminum hydroxide Sodium bicarbonate Riopan Maalox
Antihelminthics	Rid the body of parasitic worms by paralyzing or killing action or inhibiting growth.	Treatment of roundworm, tapeworm, and other infestations.	Povan Vermox
Antiarrhythmics	Act in various ways to regulate the heartbeat.	Treatment of cardiac arrhythmias.	Digoxin Dilantin

Antibiotics	Kill microorganisms, or inhibit or prevent their growth.	Treatment of diseases caused by bacteria (gram positive or negative), spirochetes, and rickettsiae. Used prophylactically in viral infections to reduce vulnerability to bacterial infection. Antibiotics, however, cannot kill viruses.	Penicillin
			Tetracycline
			Erythrocin
			Bacitracin (topical)
			Keflex
			Mefoxin
			Ceclor
			Sulfonamides
			  Bactrim
			  Septra
			  Azo Gantrisin

Anticholinergics	Increase heart rate, relax smooth muscle, reduce peristalsis, decrease glandular secretions, and dilate pupils.	Used to reduce muscle spasm (antispasmotic), to treat bronchial asthma, peptic ulcers, and hypermobility of the gastrointestinal tract.	Bentyl Banthine Pro-Banthine Atropine Sulfate Cogentin

Continued

Table 23–1
CLASSIFICATION OF DRUGS — *Continued*

Class	Effects and Actions	Common Use	Examples
Anticoagulants	Inhibit blood coagulation (blood clotting).	Treatment of thrombophlebitis, other specialized usages.	Dicoumaril Coumadin Heparin
Anticonvulsants	Prevent seizures or convulsions by depressing the brain's motor center or by stimulating the seizure threshold of the central nervous system.	Treatment of epilepsy and other neurologic disorders.	Dilantin Valium Phenobarbital Luminal
Antidepressants	Mood elevators.	Treatment of psychotic and neurotic types of depression and anxiety.	Elavil Nardil Tofranil Sinequan
Antidiarrhetics	Inhibit diarrhea and hypermobility of the gastrointestinal tract by affecting the tract's musculature.	Treatment of diarrhea, flatulence, and GI disorders.	Kaopectate Lomotil Donnagel
Antiemetics	Prevent vomiting and reduce nausea by acting on the medulla of the brain or reducing vertigo by acting on the vestibular mechanism of the ear.	Treatment or prevention of nausea, vomiting, vertigo, and motion sickness.	Compazine Dramamine Tigan
Antiflatulents	Relief of gastric or intestinal distention by changing the surface tension of gas and causing air bubbles to coalesce (usually used in combination with antacids).	Treatment of abdominal distention.	Oil of peppermint Simethicone Ilopan
Antifungals	Kill or check the growth of fungus.	Treatment of diseases caused by fungi.	Mycostatin Nystatin Fulvicin
Antihistamines	Counteract the production of an abnormal amount of histamine produced in the body.	Treatment of symptoms of allergies and coryza (common cold).	Dimetane Phenergan Benadryl
Antihypertensives	Reduce blood pressure by lessening resistance to blood flow, through relaxation of vasoconstricted peripheral vessels.	Treatment of hypertension, migraine, headache, arterioclerosis, and angina pectoris.	Reserpine Aldomet Apresoline Papaverine Capoten Catapres Tenormin
Anti-inflammatory agents	Act to diminish inflammation.	Treatment of arthritis, gout, and other inflammatory conditions.	Aspirin Indocin Butazolidin Ibuprofen Clinoril Corticosteroids Prednisone
Antipruritics	Relieve itching.	Treatment of skin disorders or allergies which cause itching.	Calamine lotion Temaril Hydrocortisone ointment

Continued

<u>Table 23–1</u>
CLASSIFICATION OF DRUGS — *Continued*

Class	Effects and Actions	Common Use	Examples
Antipyretics	Reduce body temperature in a febrile state. Dilate peripheral vascular system and increase heat loss, thus returning body temperature to normal.	Treatment of pyrexia (fever).	Aspirin Tylenol Ibuprofen
Antiseptics	Applied to living tissue to prevent growth of microorganisms. Disinfectants have some action on nonliving tissue.	For skin irritations and cleansing.	Cepacol pHisoHex Boric acid Furacin Hydrogen peroxide Mercurochrome
Antitoxins Vaccines	Antitoxins contain specific antibodies that provide short-term passive immunity to disease. Serum is obtained from animal blood in which the diseased animal produces the antibodies to fight the disease. (Sometimes human blood is the origin of the antibodies.) Vaccines are composed of certain "antigens" which are usually live disease-causing agents. For vaccination they are weakened or partially detoxified and cause the body to manufacture its own antibodies.	Given to prevent disease or make it less severe in an individual who has been exposed to the disease.	Sabine vaccine Diphtheria and tetanus toxoids Diphtheria, pertussis, and tetanus vaccine Measles and mumps virus vaccines Measles, mumps, rubella vaccine Measles and rubella vaccine Trivalent polio Tetanus toxoid Botulism antitoxin Diphtheria antitoxin
Antitussives	Protect mucous membranes from irritation by coating the membrane to prevent the cough reflex by depressing the medulla.	Cough suppressant in allergies or respiratory infections.	Hycodan Tuss-Ornade Romilar Sucrets (lozenges)
Astringents	Change the surface tension of cells. Reduce oiliness of skin and excessive perspiration. Stop bleeding from minor cuts.	Treatment of conditions and forms of dermatitis. Stop bleeding of cuts from shaving, etc.	Zinc oxide Calamine Witch hazel Aluminum acetate solution Aluminum hydroxide gel Tannic acid Styptic pencil
Cardiotonics	Increase strength of myocardial contraction. Pulse strengthens and slows.	Treatment of congestive heart failure.	Digoxin Digitoxin
Cathartics Laxatives	Cause the bowel to evacuate its contents. Several types of cathartics with different actions are available: fecal softener stimulants (stimulate smooth muscle of the bowel), bulk cathartics (increase fecal matter by adding nonabsorbable substance), saline cathartics. Water is retained in intestine, which promotes peristalsis.	Treatment of constipation. Used also as a preparatory drug for certain diagnostic tests.	Fleet enema Milk of magnesia Ex-Lax Metamucil Dulcolax Docusate sodium (Colace) Senokot

Continued

Table 23-1
CLASSIFICATION OF DRUGS—*Continued*

Class	Effects and Actions	Common Use	Examples

Antineoplastics	Poisonous to both normal and cancerous cells. Interfere with cell reproduction.	Used in chemotherapy in treatment of cancer.	L-asparaginase
			Alkylating:
			  Cytoxan
			  Leukeran
			Antimetabolites:
			  5-Fluorouracil
			  Cytarabine
			Antibiotic:
			  Adriamycin

Demulcents Emollients Protectives	*Demulcents* protect and coat the mucous membrane. *Emollients* soften, coat, and protect the skin, and can also relieve pain and itching. *Protectives* form a film on the skin to cover raw areas.	Treatment of throat irritations, cough, ulcerations, and cracked, dry skin.	Cold cream Glycerine Tincture of benzoin
Diuretics	Increase the production of urine by their action on renal tubules in the kidney.	Control of edema in cardiac disease such as hypertension. Also control premenstrual retention of fluid.	Diuril Lasix Aldactone (Spironolactone)
Emetics	Cause vomiting by irritating the mucous membrane of the GI tract.	To induce vomiting when a toxic substance has been ingested.	Ipecac
Expectorants	Assist removal of mucus by liquifying tenacious mucus.	Treatment of bronchitis and other respiratory conditions.	Robitussin Terpin hydrate Eucalyptus oil
Hematinics	Stimulate production of blood cells and increase amount of hemoglobin in the blood.	Treatment of anemias.	Ferrous sulfate Imferon
Hemostatics (coagulants)	Stop and control bleeding or hemorrhage.	Treatment of hemophilia (condition of defective clotting). Also used in surgical procedures to stop or control bleeding.	Gelfoam Fibrinogen Surgicel Thrombin

Hormones	Used to replace specific hormonal deficiencies in the body.	Treatment of hypothyroidism and diabetes. Other selected uses. Major constituent of oral contraceptives.	Thyroxine
			Insulin
			Ovarian hormones
			Pituitary hormones
			  Corticotropin
			  Somatotropin
			  Vasopressin
			Calcitonin

Hypnotics Sedatives	Act on the central nervous system and interfere with nerve impulse transmission to the cerebral cortex. Heart rate and respiration are depressed. Depending on the specific drug and dosage, drowsiness, sleep, decreased awareness, loss of muscle coordination, and other changes can occur.	Treatment of convulsions and insomnia. Selected use in specific conditions.	Nembutal Seconal Doriden Placidyl Dalmane Halcion

Continued

<u>Table 23–1</u>
CLASSIFICATION OF DRUGS — *Continued*

Class	Effects and Actions	Common Use	Examples
	The difference between sedative and hypnotic effects is the dosage. Hypnotics produce sleep; sedatives facilitate a feeling of restfulness.		
Tranquilizers	Act as central nervous system depressants. Reduce anxiety and tension. Some also act as smooth muscle relaxants.	Treatment of tension and anxiety. Treats symptoms of neuroses and psychoses. Some are also used in treatment of muscle spasms.	Librium Equanil Thorazine Valium
Stimulants	Stimulate the operations of the central nervous system and increase the activity of the vasomotor and respiratory centers of the medulla. Act to elevate mood and to suppress fatigue and appetite.	Treatment of obesity, exhaustion, and specific abnormal patterns of behavior.	Benzedrine Dexedrine Tenuate Caffeine
Sulfonamides	Interfere with the growth of specific bacteria.	Treatment of certain infectious disorders, especially those affecting the urinary and respiratory tracts, the vagina, and the eye.	Gantrisin Sulfa Sultrin Septra Sulfisoxazole Bactrim
Vasodilators	Dilate peripheral blood vessels in the heart, skeletal muscles, and various organs. Increase circulation and blood flow to the extremities.	Specific drugs have specific actions and may be used for peripheral vascular disease, dysmenorrhea, angina, and hypertension.	Nitroglycerin Vasodilan Isordil Cardilate

1. Manufacturers' index (white)
2. Product name index and discontinued products (pink)
3. Product category index (blue)
4. Generic and chemical name index (yellow)
5. Product identification section
6. Product information section (white)
7. Diagnostic product information (green)
8. Poison control centers
9. Guide to management of drug overdoses

The advantages of using the *PDR* is the ease in obtaining needed information. However, data for all drugs are not included. Older drugs, such as digoxin, may be listed but include no drug information.

Another source of drug information is the package insert in the drug container. The information is usually very similar to that contained in the *PDR*.

Two other official sources of information are the *USP* and the *National Formulary* (*NF*). Both are published every 5 years. The drugs listed in the *USP* have met specific standards related to purity, strength, shelf life, usage, and dosage, and they bear the initials *USP* after their names. The back of the *USP* also contains a thorough listing of the Controlled Substances Act regulations. The *NF*, published by the American Pharmaceutical Association, contains many drugs that are not commonly used or published in the *USP*. Other useful works include the *Desk Reference for Nonprescription Drugs* and the *Compendium of Drug Therapy*, with separate volumes published for family practice and certain specialties.

DRUG ADMINISTRATION

Physician, medical assistants, and Pharmacists use a well-defined universal system of abbreviations and terminology to exchange drug information. Most of these traditional abbreviations and terms have Latin or Greek roots.

Drug administration begins with the physician's order for treatment with drugs. The physician writes a medication order on a prescription that is given to the patient, telephones the prescription information verbally to the pharmacist, or gives the medical assistant instructions for administering a medication in the office. The patient's record should include all medications dispensed to the patient from the office supply, administered to the patient while in the office, or given as prescriptions to the patient.

Drugs administered in the medical office are usually *stat* orders. Stat means immediately. The stat drug is given to the patient in a single dose at the time of the visit. Although the medication order should always be placed in writing, there are times when the medical assistant must administer the drug on the verbal rather than on the written order of the physician. When this occurs, the medical assistant should always repeat the medication order back to the physician for accuracy verification, and as soon as possible, the physician must write down the order previously given verbally. When a medication is administered on a verbal order, the medical assistant writes the order on the patient's record as ordered by the physician, signs the physician's name, writes "verbal order" in the appropriate space, and countersigns the notation. When recording the procedure, medical assistants write "VO" before their signature.

The patient's record and the prescription form must include the following:

1. Date that the order was written
2. Name of the drug (either the generic or the trade name)
3. Dosage specified
4. Route of administration
5. Specific instruction regarding how frequently the drug is to be taken
6. Physician's signature

Depending on individual state requirements, special prescription forms are necessary for prescribing controlled substances. Some states require single-carbon or duplicate forms, whereas others require triplicate forms. Physicians may purchase "Trip-scripts" from the DEA. These are serialized (numbered) prescription pads. The medical assistant files one copy in the patient's medical record, and the patient is given the original copy and the second copy to give to the pharmacist. The pharmacist then sends the second copy to the state's health department.

There are seven components to a valid prescription:

1. Date, patient's name and address
2. Superscription: the symbol Rx (meaning "take thou" from the Latin "recipe")
3. Inscription: name of the drug or ingredients and the quantity(ies)
4. Subscription: directions to the pharmacist specifying how to compound the drug(s), if the drug is not already premanufactured
5. Signature (sig): instructions to the patient on when and how to take the medication (from the Latin "signetur" meaning "write on label")
6. Physician's signature, address, registry number, and when prescribing controlled substances, the DEA number
7. Number of times a prescription may be refilled, generic approvals, and instructions for labeling the container
8. Medical assistant's signature

State laws specify which members of the health care team are permitted to administer medications. Only a physician or pharmacist may dispense medications. In some states, nurse practitioners, nurse clinicians, and physician's assistants are permitted to prescribe medications. These prescription privileges are mandated by licensing agencies in individual states. The medical assistant practices under the direct supervision of the physician and may only administer drugs as prescribed by the physician. It is important for the medical assistant to be informed of individual state laws if persons other than physicians are prescribing medications in an office.

PRESCRIPTIONS

A prescription is a written order giving instructions to a pharmacist for the purpose of supplying a patient with a specific drug prepared and dispensed according to specific directions. It is a legal document. The prescription contains all the essential components of the medication order with special directions written specifically for the pharmacist's interpretation. Although medical assistants do not prescribe, they must know how to interpret the information on prescriptions to administer medications, transcribe medical records, and answer any questions either patients or pharmacists may have. This requires knowledge of prescription format, abbreviations, and terms. Table 23–2 lists commonly used abbreviations.

Figure 23–2 is an example of a prescription.

DRUG THERAPY AND THE ROLE OF THE MEDICAL ASSISTANT

Drug therapy is the use of natural or chemical substances in the treatment of the patient to relieve symptoms, replace body substances, or arrest or eliminate a condition or disease. Ordering and prescribing drugs is a treatment modality every physician uses. The physician, although well-grounded in general concepts of pharmacology, derives much knowledge concerning new drugs from journals and pharmaceutical representatives. This statement does not imply that the physician is deficient in pharmacologic knowledge, but rather that the physician must continually learn and be aware of new developments. The medical assistant's

Table 23-2

COMMONLY USED PRESCRIPTION ABBREVIATIONS

ABBREVIATION	MEANING	ABBREVIATION	MEANING
a	Before	os	Mouth
aa	Of each	oz	Ounce
ac	Before meals	p	After
ad	Up to	pc	After meals
ad lib	As desired	per	By
am, AM	Morning	po	By mouth
amt	amount	prn	when necessary
aq	Water	pt	Pint
bid	Twice a day	pulv	Powder
c̄	With	q	Every
caps	Capsules	qam	Every morning
cc	Cubic centimeter	qd	Every day
d	Day	q 2 h	Every 2 hours
dc	Discontinue	qid	Four times a day
dil	Dilute	qn	Every night
disp	Dispense	qod	Every other day
dr	Dram	qs	Quantity sufficient
elix	Elixir	®	Right
ext	Extract	R	Rectal
fl	Fluid	Rx	To take
g	Gram	Tx	Treatment or therapy
gr	Grain	s̄	Without
gt, gtt	Drop, drops	sat	Saturated
h, hr	hour	SC or subcut	Subcutaneous
(H)	Hypodermic	Sig	Write on label
hs	Hour of sleep	sol	Solution
ID	Intradermal	sos	Once if necessary
IM	Intramuscular	sp	Spirits
IV	Intravenous	ss	One half
kg	Kilogram	stat	Immediately
L	Liter	syr	Syrup
Ⓛ	Left	tab	Tablet
lb	pound	tbsp	Tablespoon
μ	Microgram	tid	Three times a day
mEq	Milliequivalent	tinct or tr	Tincture
m̜	minim	TO	Telephone order
mL	Milliliter	tsp	Teaspoon
MOM	Milk of magnesia	TX	Treatment
NPO	Nothing by mouth	U	Unit
N/S	Normal saline	UD	As directed
pt	Pint	ung	Unguent
OD	Right eye	VO	Verbal order
OS	Left eye	x	Times
otic	Ear	#	Number (of tablets to disperse)
ophthal	Eye		

Source: Adapted from Lane K: Medications: A Guide for the Health Professions. FA Davis, Philadelphia, 1992, p 2.

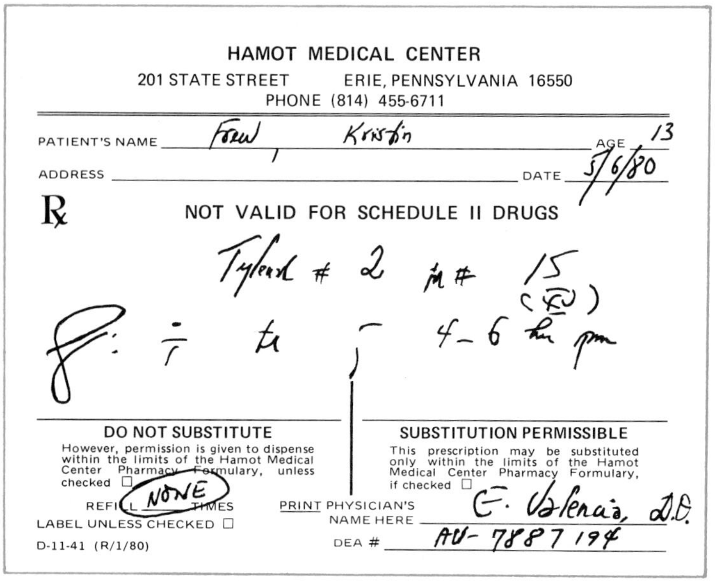

Figure 23–2. A typical prescription from a medical center.

role in drug therapy is to assist the physician to meet the objectives of the treatment. The medical assistant should not only prepare and administer the drug accurately, but also should share with the physician the responsibility of acquiring new knowledge and preventing errors in administration. Medical assistants enhance the physician's credibility whenever they check a reference source when concerns arise related to dosage or any other aspect of drug administration. The physician determines which drug will be prescribed and how it will be administered. The medical assistant checks the *PDR* or the specific literature on the drug to confirm the methods for preparation, safe handling, and administration.

No medication should be administered by the medical assistant unless sufficient information about the drug is first understood. Although the physician has prescribed the drug, the amount, and the route, errors are possible. By referring to the *PDR*, the medical assistant may save the patient from a drug overdose or promote optimal drug effects by providing specific instruction or by following certain procedures in administration.

Obviously, individual physicians acquire certain drug preferences. As medical assistants become more familiar with the drugs used, they will gain confidence in their own knowledge of dose preparation, how various drugs should be administered, and the normal dosage ranges.

GENERAL RULES OF DRUG ADMINISTRATION

There are "seven rights" to be observed when preparing and administering medications. They are as follows:

1. Right patient
2. Right drug
3. Right dosage
4. Right route
5. Right time

6. Right technique
7. Right documentation

The medical assistant must also observe the following rules to ensure the accurate handling and administration of medications:

Storage

1. Maintain original labels on all drugs kept in the office.
2. Store drugs in locked areas inaccessible to patients.
3. Remove and safely discard illegibly labeled and outdated drugs.
4. Contact a local pharmacist or the manufacturer for any questions regarding drugs that cannot be answered by the physician or a drug reference source.

Preparation

1. Wash hands before preparing medications.
2. Avoid distractions by preparing the medication in a quiet, well-lighted area.
3. Read the medication label three times:

   ❑ When removing the medication from the storage area
   ❑ When preparing (measuring) the medication
   ❑ When returning the container to storage or disposing of an empty container

4. Have calculations rechecked by the physician when unsure or when there is a particularly complicated order.
5. Never leave medications unattended.

Administration

1. Give only medications ordered by the physician. To avoid errors, the order should be written.

2. Never administer medication that has been prepared by someone else. The person administering the medication is responsible for any errors made. The physician may request that a medication be prepared for him or her to administer.

3. Identify the patient by asking him or her to state his or her name.

4. Determine the presence of any allergies and their possible relationship to the medication about to be given.

5. Observe the patient after administration for any untoward reactions.

6. Provide the patient with full medication instructions if necessary.

7. As soon as possible, record on the patient's chart the date, time, drug name, amount given, route of administration, and your signature. (Follow the rules for charting presented in Chapter 16.)

8. Record any controlled substances administered in the controlled substance inventory record.

When the seven rights and the above principles are scrupulously observed, the medical assistant can be assured of safe, error-free administration of medications.

SYSTEMS OF MEASUREMENT

To calculate dosages in pharmacology, two systems of weight and measurement are used: metric and apothecary (Table 23–3). The metric system is a decimal system, which means that all the units of measurement are derived by dividing or multiplying by powers of 10. Liters (L) refer to volume, grams (g) to weight, and meters (m) to length. In the metric system, doses are written as a decimal, and the unit of measurement follows the Arabic numerals. For example, one and one-half milliliters is written 1.5 mL. Other metric rules include:

1. When dividing to make subunits smaller than the basic units, Latin prefixes are used to denote the subunit: deci equals 0.1 (1/10); centi equals 0.01 (1/100); milli equals 0.001 (1/1000).

2. When multiplying to increase the number of basic units, Greek prefixes are used: deka equals 10 × unit; hecto equals 100 × unit; kilo equals 1000 × unit.

The apothecary system is the oldest system of measurement. Prescriptions written using this system may have either Roman or Arabic numerals written as whole numbers or fractions preceded by the weight symbol or abbreviation.

In the apothecary system, the basic units of weight are grain (gr), gram (g), dram (ʒ), ounce (℥), and pound (lb). Fluid measurements are represented as minims (mn), fluid drams (f/ʒ), fluid ounces (f/℥), pints (pt), quarts (qt), and gallons (c). Units of measure in the form of symbols are combined with Roman numerals to indicate the number of units; for example, 3 drams would be represented as ʒ iii, and 2 grains would be represented as gr ii. For apothecary orders, fractions are used; for example, one fourth of a grain would be represented as gr ¼.

Although drug dosages are now written in the metric system, some physicians still use the apothecary system. For this reason, a knowledge of both systems is necessary.

Although household measurements (teaspoon, table-

Table 23–3
COMMONLY USED APPROXIMATE EQUIVALENTS

Weight		Volume	
Apothecaries'	**Metric**	**Apothecaries'**	**Metric**
⅟₆₀, ⅟₆₄, or ⅟₆₅ grain (gr)	1 mg or 1000 μg	1 minim (m̥)	0.06–0.07 mL
1 gr	0.06, 0.064, or 0.065 g	4 m̥	0.25 mL
1 gr	60, 64, or 65 mg	8 m̥	0.5 mL
1 gr	60,000, 64,000, or 65,000 μg	15 or 16 m̥	1 mL or 1 cubic centimeter (cm³)
5 gr	0.3 or 0.33 g	1 fluid dram (flʒ) or 60 or 64 m̥	4 mL
10 gr	0.6 or 0.67 g	1 flʒ or 8 flʒ	30 or 32 mL
15 or 16 gr	1 g	1 pt or 16 flʒ	480 or 500 mL
1 dram ʒ	4 g		
1 oz ℥	30 or 32 g	1 qt or 32 flʒ	960 or 1000 mL or 1 L
1 lb (avoirdupois)	450 g		
1 lb	0.4536 kg		

Source: Adapted from Cornett EF and Blume DM: *Dosages and Solutions: A Programmed Approach to Meds and Math,* ed 5. FA Davis, Philadelphia, 1991, p 229.

spoon, dropper full) are not conventional medical units, these measurements are most practical when instructing patients in dosage amounts for fluids. Table 23–4 lists the common metric weights and the approximate corresponding apothecary and household equivalents.

CONVERSION TABLES

The medical assistant needs to know how to calculate dosages because a drug sometimes will not be remeasured or it will be ordered in one system but labeled in the other. When weights and measurements are not in the same system, conversion is necessary before measurement or calculations can be performed. See Table 23–3 for the commonly used approximate equivalents.

To accurately measure or calculate dosage, the medical assistant must first check whether both the order and the drug label have been expressed in the same system of measurement. If not, the conversion table is used to convert to the same system as that used on the manufacturer's label. A table for conversion from one system to another, such as the one listed above, should be available at all times for quick reference.

If an equivalent is not listed on a conversion table, a hand calculation must be used. Conversions are calculated by division and multiplication.

One simple way to tackle conversion is to *divide something by itself to get 1.* For example, to determine the milliliter equivalent of 4 oz, the total number of ounces must be changed into milliliters:

$$4 \text{ oz} = ? \text{ milliliters}$$

Using the conversion table (see Table 23–3), find how many milliliters equal 1 oz. The answer is:

$$30 \text{ mL} = 1 \text{ oz}$$

Now, a fraction is used to represent division with the *known unit* of measurement always as the *denominator* (bottom of the fraction). Since 30 mL is the same as 1 oz, when 30 milliliters is divided by 1 oz, the answer is 1:

$$\text{(known units)} \ \frac{30 \text{ mL}}{1 \text{ oz}} = 1$$

When something is divided by itself, the answer is always 1.

Next, the known measurement is used to multiply the fraction

$$\frac{30 \text{ mL}}{1 \text{ oz}} \text{ (or, the value of 1):}$$

$$4 \text{ oz} = \frac{4}{1} \times \frac{30 \text{ mL}}{1} = \frac{4 \times 30 \text{ mL}}{1}$$

$$= \frac{120 \text{ mL}}{1 \text{ mL}} = 120 \text{ mL}$$

Therefore:

$$4 \text{ oz} = 120 \text{ mL}$$

Table 23–4
APPROXIMATE HOUSEHOLD EQUIVALENTS

Household	Household
60 drops	1 tsp
2 tsp	1 dessertspoon
2 dessertspoons (4 tsp)	1 tbsp
2 tbsp	1 fl oz
6 fl oz	1 teacup
8 fl oz	1 glassful or 1 measuring cup

Household	Apothecaries'	Metric
1 drop	1 minim	0.06 mL
1 tsp	1 fluid dram (fl℥)	4 or 5 mL
1 tbsp	4 fl℥	15 or 16 mL
2 tbsp	1 fluid ounce (fl℥)	30 or 32 mL
1 teacup	6 fl℥	180 or 192 mL
1 glass or 1 measuring cup	8 fl℥ or ½ pt	240 or 250 mL
2 glasses or 2 measuring cups	16 fl℥ or 1 pt	480 or 500 mL
4 glasses or 4 measuring cups	1 qt	960 or 1000 mL

Source: Adapted from Cornett EF and Blume DM: Dosages and Solutions: A Programmed Approach to Meds and Math, ed 5. FA Davis, Philadelphia, 1991, pp 35–36.

As another example, reverse the process and convert the other way:

$$120 \text{ mL} = ? \text{ oz}$$

$$\text{(known units)} \frac{1 \text{ oz}}{30 \text{ mL}} = 1$$

$$120 \text{ mL} = \frac{120}{1} \times \frac{1 \text{ oz}}{30} = \frac{120 \times 1 \text{ oz}}{30}$$

$$= \frac{120 \text{ oz}}{30} = \frac{4 \text{ oz}}{1} = 4 \text{ oz}$$

Therefore:

$$120 \text{ mL} = 4 \text{ oz}$$

The same process is used to convert grains to milligrams and vice versa. For example: How many milligrams are there in ½ gr?

$$\frac{1}{2} \text{ gr} = ? \text{ mg}$$

$$\text{(known units)} \frac{60 \text{ mg}}{1 \text{ gr}} = 1$$

$$\frac{1}{2} \text{gr} = \frac{2}{1} \times \frac{60 \text{ mg}}{1} = \frac{2 \times 60 \text{ mg}}{1} = \frac{30 \text{ mg}}{1}$$

$$= 30 \text{ mg}$$

Therefore:

$$\text{½ gr} = 30 \text{ mg}$$

As another example, reverse the process: How many grains are there in 30 mg?

$$30 \text{ mg} = ? \text{ gr}$$

$$\text{(known units)} \frac{1 \text{ gr}}{60 \text{ mg}}$$

$$30\text{mg} = \frac{30}{1} \times \frac{1 \text{ gr}}{60} = \frac{30 \times 1 \text{ gr}}{60} = \frac{30 \text{ gr}}{60} = \frac{1}{2} \text{ gr}$$

Therefore:

$$30 \text{ mg} = \frac{1}{2} \text{ gr}$$

RULES OF CALCULATIONS

Once the drug order and the drug label are expressed in the same system and unit, a ratio and proportion equation is used to calculate the dosage, where:

DS equals desired strength.
AS equals available strength (on hand).
DA equals amount to give or ?, the unknown.

AA equals available amount (usually tablet or diluent amount on the label).

These abbreviations are used in the proportion:

$$\frac{DS}{AS} = \frac{? \text{ (DA)}}{AA}$$

The equal sign between two fractions designates *cross-multiplication*:

$$\frac{DS}{AS} \quad \frac{? \text{ (DA)}}{AA}$$

Using the algebraic function to get the unknown (?) alone on one side of the equation, the formula becomes:

$$? \text{ (DA)} \times AS = DS \times AA$$

$$? \text{ (DA)} = \frac{DS \times AA}{AS}$$

The following example uses this formula: The physician wants Ms. Jones to receive aspirin 300 mg po stat. The aspirin on hand is in a bottle: ASA 5 gr/tablet.

To calculate the dosage, first convert the order to the unit of measurement on the label. Then calculate the exact dosage using the proportion formula and cross-multiplication.

Step 1

$$5 \text{ gr} = ? \text{ mg}$$

$$\text{(known units)} \frac{1 \text{ gr}}{60 \text{ mg}} = 1$$

$$5 \text{ gr} = \frac{5 \text{ gr}}{1} \times \frac{60 \text{ mg}}{1 \text{ gr}} = \frac{5 \times 60 \text{ mg}}{1}$$

$$= \frac{300 \text{ mg}}{1} = 300 \text{ mg}$$

Therefore:

$$5 \text{ gr} = 300 \text{ mg}$$

Step 2

$$\frac{DS}{AS} = \frac{? \text{ (DA)}}{AA}$$

$$\frac{300 \text{ mg}}{300 \text{ mg}} = \frac{1 \text{ (DA)}}{1 \text{ tablet}}$$

$$? \times 300 = 300 \times 1 \text{ tablet}$$

$$? = \frac{300 \times 1 \text{ tablet}}{300} = \frac{1 \times 1 \text{ tablet}}{1} = \frac{1}{1} = 1 \text{ tablet}$$

Therefore, Ms. Jones would be given 1 tablet.

DRUG ROUTES AND FORMS

Medication can be administered by various routes and in a variety of forms. The drug *route* refers to how the drug will be introduced into the body. The drug *form* refers to how the drug is manufactured.

The choice of a drug route is based on several considerations. The first is the drug's action on the body. One drug may act on the body systemically, and another may act locally. A drug may have a slow or rapid onset of action as a result of whether the drug's rate of absorption is slow or rapid. Drugs administered intravenously, for example, reach the bloodstream and become effective most rapidly. Drugs absorbed through the mucous membranes are administered by injection and are also rapidly absorbed. Oral medications, on the other hand, usually take a longer time to reach the bloodstream, with a slower onset of action. There are exceptions, of course, to these rules for each of the routes. A drug may also have a long or short duration. Some injectable drugs—for example, those in repository forms—are designed for slow absorption and therefore remain in the body longer. In general, rapid-acting drugs usually have a short duration, whereas slower-acting drugs have a longer duration or therapeutic effect.

Another consideration in selecting the drug route is the patient's physical and emotional state. Although a drug may be available in a variety of forms, the route selected will ultimately be affected by the patient's level of consciousness, physical limitations, and emotional difficulties.

A third consideration is the characteristics of the drug. For example, before choosing a drug route, the relationship between the desired dosage and the route must be considered in terms of safety. The cost and availability of the drug in the desired form may or may not determine the route chosen.

The form of a drug is determined in manufacturing by (1) the nature and properties of the drug, (2) the intended purpose, and (3) the ability of the drug to be absorbed safely and effectively by a particular route. For example, bitter-tasting substances may be best packaged in capsule form or in a liquid with flavoring. If the medication is to be inhaled, it will be manufactured in liquid form and contained in an appropriate inhaling device. Logically, medications to be administered intramuscularly must be in a sterile liquid form, and those to be applied topically can be in liquid, cream, gel, ointment, or paste form.

ORAL DRUGS

The oral route is perhaps the most widely used method of administering and prescribing medication because it is convenient and does not require special equipment and because it is safest (see procedures at the end of this chapter).

Oral medications are those that can be swallowed or otherwise absorbed by the mucous membranes in the mouth when they are placed inside the cheek or under the tongue. Drugs placed inside the cheek are termed *buccal* and are absorbed through the capillaries in the mucous membrane lining the cheek. Drugs placed under the tongue are termed *sublingual* and are rapidly absorbed through the capillary network under the tongue.

Several forms of drugs are available for oral administration.

1. *Tablets.* Powdered or granulated substances molded into a particular shape (round, oval, and so forth). Tablets can be uncoated, which allows the medication to dissolve rapidly, or enteric coated, which protects the drug from destruction by acidic secretions in the stomach and provides a longer shelf-life for the drug. Enteric-coated tablets can also be layered in such a way as to release periodic doses. Certain drugs, such as vitamins, are flavored and manufactured in chewable form.
2. *Capsules.* Drugs placed in a gelatinous container. Hard capsules consist of two halves and contain powdered substances; soft capsules contain liquid substances. Capsules sometimes contain tiny pellets that are released over a span of time.
3. *Troches (lozenges).* Drugs mixed with mucilage and sugar and molded into desired shapes. The drug is slowly released as the lozenge dissolves in the mouth.
4. *Solutions.* Drugs contained in a homogenous mixture with a liquid (solute and solvent). Several types of solutions are available: (a) saturated solutions, which are concentrated; (b) aromatic solutions, which usually contain a volatile oil to disguise the taste of the drug substance; (c) liquors, which contain nonvolatile material (alcohol) as the vehicle; and (d) syrups, which are flavored sugar solutions used to carry the drug in a palatable form. Some syrups are also available in a sugar-free form.
5. *Alcohol solutions.* A drug (solute) mixed with alcohol (solvent) to enhance the drug's properties and act as a vehicle for drug delivery. Several types of alcohol solutions are available: (a) elixir, which is a solution containing the drug substance, sugar, alcohol, water, and flavoring; (b) spirit, which is a solute consisting of volatile materials; (c) fluid extract, which is a concentrated plant preparation of 100% strength in solution; (d) extract, which is a concentrated syrup-like fluid; and (e) tincture, which is a drug dissolved in alcohol and available in 10 to 20% strength.

INHALATION DRUGS

Gases, or vapors, of a drug are inhaled and passed into the circulation through the capillaries in the mucous membrane lining of the nose and lungs. Usually, the drug action is specific to the respiratory tract. Medication can be administered by inhalation in various forms (see the procedure at the end of this chapter).

1. *Nebulizer.* A hand-held atomizer that produces a fine mist
2. *Vaporizer.* A device that produces a fine, moist mist, either warm or cool
3. *Inhaler.* A device with an open tip to insert into the nostrils for inhalation of medication
4. *Spray bottle.* A bottle held upright and squeezed to release mist
5. *Aerosol.* A forceful spray operated by depressing a valve on the container
6. *Ampule.* A small bottle that is serrated and when broken releases vapors

Special instruction needs to be given to the patient who will self-administer inhalants. The patient should hold the inhalant in the dominant hand, with the index finger on the top and the thumb underneath and synchronize the actions of depressing the adapter and inhalating to maximize dosage. Some inhalant-type cartridges contain special instructions on the package insert. The adapter tip should be washed with soap and lukewarm water and allowed to dry. To prevent overdose, the patient should record the date, time, and effect of inhalants that are taken to relieve respiratory distress.

TOPICAL DRUGS

Drugs administered topically to the outer or external body surface may have a local or systemic action. Topical drug forms include:

1. *Creams.* Drugs contained in semisolid preparations applied to the skin in long strokes following the direction of hair growth. This prevents medication from entering the hair follicle and causing infection.
2. *Lotions.* Medicated liquid suspension applied to the skin in long smooth strokes.
3. *Ointments.* Drugs usually contained in an oily base that liquifies on contact with the skin. Ointment excess should be removed before reapplication of the next dose. This prevents skin irritation.
4. *Transdermal drugs.* A measured dosage of medication applied with an adhesive disk or ointment that releases a controlled dose of medication into surface capillaries and directly into the bloodstream for longer systemic effects. Although these drugs are administered via the topical route, the resulting action is systemic (see the procedure at the end of this chapter).

VAGINAL DRUGS

Drugs administered vaginally (inserted into the vaginal canal) primarily have a local action. Vaginal drug forms most frequently include tablets (compressed powder), suppositories (compressed gel), creams (thick, semisolid liquids), and solutions (liquids instilled through a douching procedure). See the end-of-chapter procedure for a detailed description of this process.

URETHRAL DRUGS

Drugs can also be inserted into the urethra (the canal that leads to the bladder), but these are seldom administered in office practice because of specialized application and patient discomfort.

RECTAL DRUGS

Drugs administered rectally may have a local or systemic action and are usually available in the form of suppositories or solutions instilled via enema. Antiemetics (drugs for control of nausea and vomiting) and local analgesics (pain-relievers) are commonly administered by this route. See the end-of-chapter procedure for a detailed description of this process.

PARENTERAL DRUGS

Parenteral indicates administration of medication by injection. There are two main advantages to the introduction of medication by the parenteral route: (1) rapid drug action can be produced, and (2) the route offers a necessary alternative when drugs cannot be taken orally because they cannot be absorbed through the digestive process or because of the patient's condition.

Although injection is a required or desired route for certain medications and for administering medications in certain conditions, it carries the greatest risk. When a drug is injected, the rate of absorption cannot be altered. When an oral medication is administered, the drug usually can be retrieved or diluted with food and water and absorption slowed if untoward effects develop. In addition, penetration of the skin carries with it the potential hazard of introducing bacteria, as well as traumatizing the tissue if the procedure is performed incorrectly. The procedures for performing injections and intradermal skin tests are given in detail at the end of this chapter.

There are several routes (*tissue depths*) available for depositing drugs by injection (Fig. 23–3).

INTRADERMAL INJECTION An intradermal (ID) injection is the introduction of a small amount of drug substance into the dermis, the layer just beneath the skin. Absorption is very slow, and the intended drug action is local rather than systemic. The site of choice for ID injections is the forearm, although the hairless areas of the upper back may be used.

The diagnostic skin test for allergy diagnosis is the most widely used ID procedure. Allergic extract is introduced under the epidermis by scratch, puncture, prick, or ID injection. Within 15 to 20 minutes, a wheal and reaction develops in sensitive individuals, and a diagnosis can be made.

Small amts.

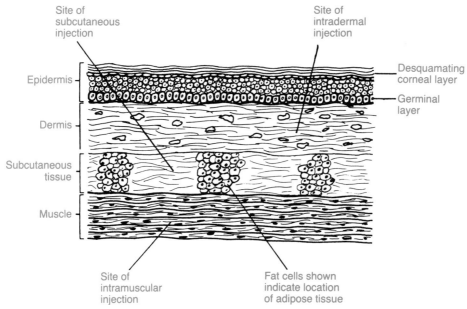

Figure 23–3. Cross-section of skin showing subcutaneous, intradermal, and intramuscular injection sites. (From Saperstein AB and Frazier MA: Introduction to Nursing Practice. FA Davis, Philadelphia, 1980, p 612, with permission.)

Another use of the ID injection in allergy is the challenge test. Before a patient can begin receiving drug immunotherapy ("allergy shots") for the treatment of allergic rhinitis, a minute dose (0.02 mL) of the allergy serum is administered as an ID skin challenge test or vial test. Depending on the reaction at the site of injection, the vial of serum is determined as safe to administer subcutaneously or the serum must be diluted before administering the initial dose.

One method used to test for skin sensitivity to tuberculin is the Mantoux test. This is a single ID injection of 0.1 mL of tuberculin purified protein derivation. The production of a 10-mm or greater wheal within 48 to 72 hours is usually interpreted as a positive indicator of past or present infection with the *Mycobacterium tuberculosis* organism.

SUBCUTANEOUS INJECTION   Any injection into the fatty tissue beneath the skin (the subcutaneous layer) is termed a *subcutaneous (SC) injection* (Fig. 23–4). The sites used are the deltoid regions of the upper arms, the anterior thigh, the scapular region of the back, and the abdomen.

When the patient must self-administer daily doses of a drug, such as insulin for diabetes, or must come to the office for frequent SC injections, a system injection-site rotation must be established (Fig. 23–5). By rotating the sites used, the patient can help to avoid the discomfort and tissue damage that could occur from repeated use of a single site.

A maximum of 2 mL of an easily absorbable solution can be given to an adult in this manner. For children, no more than 0.5 mL should be administered. Drugs given subcutaneously should be isotonic, nonirritating, and water-soluble. This route is used when a slower rate of absorption is desired. Drugs commonly administered

by the SC route include the MMR (measles, mumps, rubella) vaccine and some other vaccines (depending on each manufacturer's recommendation), heparin, insulin, vitamin B_{12}, and some narcotics.

INTRAMUSCULAR INJECTION   The intramuscular (IM) route of injection is preferred for larger amounts of medication or when a faster rate of absorption is desired. The safest sites are the muscle tissue of the deltoid area of the arm (Fig. 23–6), the vastus lateralis muscle of the thigh (recommended for infants and children) by the American Academy of Pediatrics (Fig. 23–7), and the ventrogluteal area of the buttocks (Fig. 23–8). The dorsogluteal (gluteus maximus) (Fig. 23–9) site is no longer considered a safe site for children because of poor circulation in the area and the large number of reported injuries to the sciatic nerve.

Long-acting, insoluble medications that would be irritating to SC tissues are most often administered into muscle mass. Since not as many nerve endings are distributed in muscle as in fatty tissue, IM injections are less painful than SC ones; therefore, thick medications are usually given intramuscularly. The maximal recommended doses are 2 mL in the deltoid area and 5 mL in the vastus lateralis and gluteal regions.

The deltoid site is used to administer IM vaccines, narcotics, vitamins, and sedatives. The vastus lateralis is used in children to deliver larger amounts of medication, such as an antibiotic, and to administer drugs via the Z-tract method. The ventrogluteal site is an alternative site for the vastus lateralis and for medications that may discolor the skin.

The Z-tract method of IM injection is frequently used for those solutions that may irritate the SC tissues or discolor the skin if the drug leaks along the track of the needle during insertion or removal. The Z-tract method

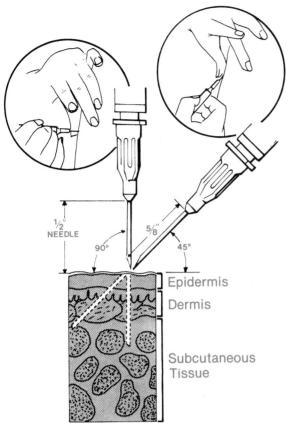

Figure 23–4. Subcutaneous and deep subcutaneous injections. The ⅝-inch needle is inserted at a 45-degree angle to the skin, and the ½-inch needle at a 90-degree angle. Both needles are short enough to remain within the subcutaneous tissue layer. (From Saperstein AB and Frazier MA: Introduction to Nursing Practice. FA Davis, Philadelphia, 1980, p 637, with permission.)

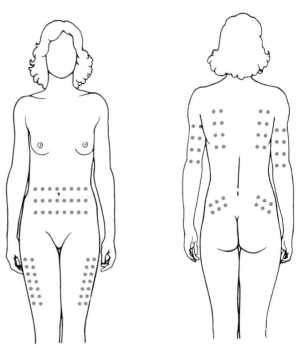

Figure 23–5. Sites for subcutaneous injections. (From Deglin JH and Vallerand AH: Davis's Drug Guide for Nurses, ed 3. FA Davis, Philadelphia, 1993, p 1237, with permission.)

also may prevent skin lesions and reduce pain. This procedure varies from the IM procedure in that the skin is retracted and held to one side. After the medication is completely injected and the needle is withdrawn, the skin is released (Fig. 23–10). The site is not massaged after using this technique, unless otherwise directed by the physician or the manufacturer of the drug. Encouraging reports of research on this method have led some authorities to recommend the Z-track method for all IM injections.

INTRAVENOUS INJECTION An intravenous (IV) route deposits the medication directly into the vein for the most rapid absorption of the drug. It is, therefore, the most dangerous method of injection. The method is seldom employed in the physician's office and is not performed by the medical assistant.

Special precautions must be observed at the site of any injection:

1. Avoid injecting into any abnormal skin area (scar, edema, inflammation, or reduced circulation) or areas in close proximity to major nerves, blood vessels, or bony prominences.

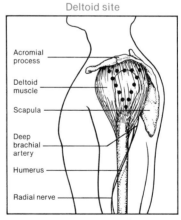

Figure 23–6. Mid-deltoid site for IM injection. The recommended area is a small rectangle bounded on the top by the lower edge of the acromion and on the bottom by a line parallel to the armpit. The side boundaries of the recommended area are parallel lines one third and two thirds of the way around the outer lateral aspect of the arm. This is a small area and cannot tolerate repeated or large doses. (From Deglin JH and Vallerand AH: Davis's Drug Guide for Nurses, ed 3. FA Davis, Philadelphia, 1993, p 1238, with permission.)

Vastus lateralis site

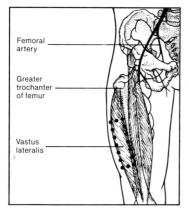

Figure 23–7. Vastus lateralis site for IM injection. This recommended area extends from the middle of the anterior (front) thigh to the middle of the lateral thigh; the top of the area is one handsbreadth below the greater trochanter and the bottom is one handsbreadth above the knee. The patient should be supine or sitting. (From Deglin JH and Vallerand AH: Davis's Drug Guide for Nurses, ed 3. FA Davis, Philadelphia, 1993, p 1238, with permission.)

2. Palpate the site before cleansing to ensure that a site is not tender or becomes firm when grasped.

INJECTION EQUIPMENT

Medication to be administered by injection is usually dissolved in an aqueous (water) solution or suspended in oil. The medication to be administered may be pack-

Dorsogluteal site

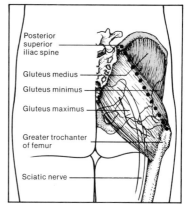

Figure 23–9. Dorsogluteal site for IM injection. To avoid the sciatic nerve, the recommended site is above and lateral to a line drawn from the greater trochanter to the posterior superior iliac spine. (From Deglin JH and Vallerand AH: Davis's Drug Guide for Nurses, ed 3. FA Davis, Philadelphia, 1993, p 1238, with permission.)

aged as (1) a solution in a single- or multiple-dose vial, (2) a powder in a vial which must be reconstituted with sterile isotonic saline or sterile water labeled "for injection," (3) a solution in an ampule, or (4) a solution in a prefilled cartridge-needle syringe unit. Figure 23–11 depicts these methods of packaging. Table 23–5 lists some of the commonly used drugs in the medical office.

Vials are most commonly used for packaging injectable medications. When a medication is in powder form, specific directions for reconstituting the medication are enclosed with the drug package and must be followed exactly.

Ventrogluteal site

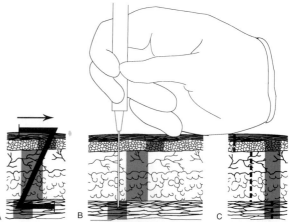

Figure 23–8. Ventrogluteal site for IM injection. When injecting into the left side of the patient, place the palm of the right hand on the greater trochanter and the index finger on the anterior superior iliac spine. Spread the middle finger posteriorly away from the index finger as far as possible along the iliac crest. Make the injection in the center of the V formed by the index and middle fingers, with the needle directed slightly upward toward the crest of the ilium. (From Deglin JH and Vallerand AH: Davis's Drug Guide for Nurses, ed 3. FA Davis, Philadelphia, 1993, p 1238, with permission.)

Figure 23–10. Z-track method of IM injection. (**A**) Pulling the skin at the injection site to one side before inserting the needle causes the epidermis, dermis, and subcutaneous layer to slide over the underlying muscle tissue. (**B**) The needle is inserted at a 90-degree angle, straight through the displaced layers into the muscle. (**C**) Releasing the tension on the skin *while withdrawing the needle* allows the tissue planes to slide back into their normal position, sealing the track of the needle and preventing the backflow of medication.

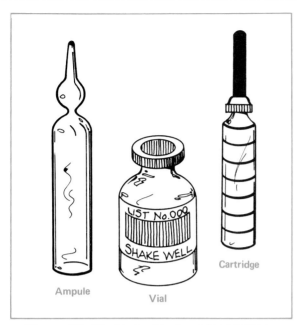

Figure 23-11. Medication forms for injection.

The equipment needed to administer a parenteral medication is determined by the viscosity of the medication, the patient's body size, the route, and the site of injection.

SYRINGES A syringe is a barrel-shaped, calibrated container with a plunger (Fig. 23-12). Medication is withdrawn into the syringe in the required amount. Syringes are available in 1-mL, 2.5-mL, 3-mL, 5-mL, 6-mL, 10-mL, 12-mL, 20-mL, 30-mL, and 60-mL capacities. The 3-mL size is the most commonly used and is calibrated both in tenths of a milliliter and minims. One-half and 1-milliliter tuberculin syringes are calibrated in one hundredths ($\frac{1}{100}$) of a milliliter and minims, and are used for minute doses such as those injected in tuberculin skin testing. Insulin syringes are available in 1-mL capacity and calibrated in a scale of 100 U, or in low-dosage sizes with either 0.3-mL (30-U) or 0.5-mL (50-U) capacities. Some insulin and tuberculin syringes have permanently attached needles.

NEEDLES Different needle lengths allow needles to penetrate to the various layers of tissue. The patient's size (amount of fatty tissue) must also be taken into consideration. Needles are available in lengths of $\frac{3}{8}$, $\frac{1}{2}$, $\frac{5}{8}$, $\frac{3}{4}$, 1 inch, and $1\frac{1}{4}$, $1\frac{1}{2}$, and 2 inches. For a SC injection, lengths between $\frac{1}{2}$ and $\frac{3}{4}$ inch are usually sufficient. An ID injection usually requires a needle length of $\frac{3}{8}$ or $\frac{1}{2}$ inch. Insulin needles are usually $\frac{1}{2}$ or $\frac{5}{8}$ inch and permanently attached to the needle to minimize "bubble" problems and the loss of insulin owing to needle "dead space" (insulin remaining in the needle after the insulin is injected).

The *gauge* of the needle refers to its inside diameter. At its tip, the inside diameter, or lumen, of the needle opens into a beveled edge (tip). Beveling a needle point gives the needle a sloped, minute cutting edge that allows the needle to penetrate the skin with less trauma. The choice of needle gauge is based on the thickness or viscosity of the medication to be administered. The numbers assigned to identify the diameter sizes are in descending order. Needle gauges range from 30 (thinnest) to 16 (thickest). The average gauges for IM injections range from 23 to 21. For SC, the usual gauges are 26 and 25. ID injections require 27- to 25-gauge needles. Hypodermic needles also are available in regular bevel, regular bevel–thin wall, short bevel, short bevel–thin wall, and intermediate bevel.

Disposable syringe-needle units and disposable needles are color-coded to the needle gauge. Syringe-needle units may be purchased in peel-away packages or encased in rigid plastic tubes. Insulin syringes are color-coded to standard insulin strengths.

OSHA BLOODBORNE PATHOGEN STANDARDS

The medical assistant must be protected from injury when disposing of used needles. Accidental sticking of oneself with a contaminated needle is a source of disease transmission, especially via bloodborne pathogens. Disposable needles and syringes are discarded intact in a rigid, puncture-proof, sharps collector. Medical offices are now required by law to have a rigid, plastic collector that is self-sealing with a lock-tight cap and a safety neck, which prevents the contents from being extracted. When the needle container is $\frac{3}{4}$ full, it is sealed and labeled with the bright red international biohazard caution sticker, which alerts all personnel that the container holds dangerous and contaminated materials, and properly disposed of by incineration or autoclaving. In addition to the OSHA regulations, the Environmental Protection Agency (EPA) lists specific regulations for the disposal of contaminated needles and sharp items.

If the medical assistant is accidentally stuck with a contaminated needle, the physician must be notified of the incident immediately so appropriate treatment can be given. OSHA's bloodborne pathogens standard includes provisions for medical follow-up for workers who have a puncture exposure incident. (For detailed OSHA standards, see the Highlights at the end of this chapter.)

PATIENT TEACHING CONSIDERATIONS

Patient preparation is essential to the safe and accurate administration of medication. Ideally, the patient should be informed by the physician that medication is to be administered. Occasionally, the patient is informed of the procedure as the medical assistant walks into the room with the medication. The patient should also know what medication he or she is receiving and why and should be given any special instructions. Before administering the medication, the medical assistant should identify the patient by name, even when familiarity exists, to avoid error and should ask the patient whether he or she is allergic to any drugs, and specifically to the drug in question, to prevent a drug reaction.

Table 23–5

INJECTABLE DRUGS COMMONLY PURCHASED FOR THE MEDICAL OFFICE

Generic Name	Trade Name	Strength	Unit Size	Route	Indication	Classification
Amitriptyline HCl	Elavil	10 mg/mL	10 mL	IM	Depression	Antidepressant
Bropheniramine maleate	Dimetane	10 mg/mL	10-mL vial, 1-mL ampule	SC, IM	Allergies	Antihistamine
Chlorpheniramine maleate	Chlor-Trimeton	10 mg/mL	1-mL ampule	SC, IM	Allergy	Antihistamine
Chlorpromazine HCl	Thorazine	25 mg/mL	1-mL ampule; 10-mL vial	IM	Psychotic disorders	Antipsychotic
Dexamethasone maleate, aqueous suspension	Decadron-LA suspension	8 mg/mL	5-mL vial	IM	Drug hypersen-sitivity reactions, endocrine and rheumatic disorders	Cortiosteroid hormone
Diazepam	Valium	5 mg/mL	2-mL ampule; 2-mL prefilled syringe; 10-mL vial	IM	Anxiety	Antianxiety
Dicyclomine HCl	Bentyl	10 mg/mL	2-mL ampule; 2-mL prefilled syringe; 10-mL vial	IM	Irritable bowel syndrome	Antispasmodic
Dimenhydrinate	Dramamine Injection	50 mg/mL	1-mL ampule; 5-mL vial	IM	Motion sickness	Antinauseant/ antiemetic
Diphenhydramine HCl	Benadryl	10 mg/mL; 50 mg/mL	1-mL ampule; 1-mL prefilled syringe; 10, 30-mL vials	IM	Allergic reactions	Antihistamine
Diphtheria and tetanus toxoids adsorbed, USP (Pediatric)	Same	—	0.5-mL cartridge-needle unit; 5-mL vial	IM (deeply)	Immunization	Vaccine, active
Estradiol cypoinate	Depo-Estradiol	1 mg/mL; 5 mg/mL	5-, 10-mL vials	IM	Menopausal vasomotor symptoms	Estrogen hormone
Furosemide	Lasix	10 mg/mL	10-mL vial	IM	Edema associated with congestive heart failure	Loop diuretic
Gentamicin sulfate	Garamycin	40 mg/mL (10 mg pediatric)	2-mL ampule, prefilled syringe, vial; 20-mL vial	IM	Serious infection	Antibacterial

Generic name	Trade name	Strength	How supplied	Route	Use	Classification
Heparin sodium	Heparin Sodium	1,000, 5,000, 10,000, 20,000, 40,000 USP Units	1-mL ampule; 1-mL cartridge-needle units; 1-, 2-, 4-, 5-, 10-, 30-mL vial	SC	Prevention of clotting	Anticoagulant
Hydromorphone HCl	Dilaudid	1,2,4 mg/mL	1-mL ampule; 20-mL vial	SC or IM	Moderate to severe pain	Controlled substance analgesic
Lidocaine HCL	Xylocaine 1%; 2%	10 mg/mL; 20 mg/mL	50 mL	Local injection	Minor surgery	Local anesthetic
Prednisolone tebutate	Hydeltra-TBA	20 mg/mL	1.5-mL single-dose vial	Local injection into joints	Joint inflammation	Corticosteroid hormone
Prochlorperazine	Compazine	5 mg/mL	2-, 10-mL vial	IM (deeply)	Psychotic episodes	Antipsychotic
Promethazine HCl	Phenergan Injection	25 mg/mL; 50 mg/mL	1-mL ampule, 1-mL cartridge-needle unit; 10-mL vial	IM	Immediate-type allergic reactions; nausea and vomiting	Antinauseant/antiemetic
Sodium chloride injection with benzyl alcohol 0.9%	Sodium Chloride, Bacteriostatic	—	30 mg	—	Diluent for injection	Normal (isotonic) saline
Sodium thiosalicylate	Sodium Thiosalicylate	50 mg/mL	30-mL vial	IM	Pain or fever	Nonnarcotic Analgesic/antipyretic
Tetanus and diphtheria toxoids adsorbed, USP (adult)	Same	—	0.5-mL cartridge-needle unit; 5-mL vial	IM (deeply)	Immunization	Vaccine, active
Tetanus antitoxin purified (equine)	Same	—	15,000-U vial; 20,000-U vial	IM	Prophylaxis	Vaccine, passive
Tetanus immune globulin	Hyper-Tet	—	250-U vial or prefilled disposable syringe	IM	Prophylaxis	Vaccine, passive
Tetanus toxoid adsorbed, USP	Same	—	0.5-mL cartridge-needle unit; 5-mL vial	IM (deeply)	Immunization	Vaccine, active
Tuberculin purified protein derivative	Tine Test	5 tuberculin units	10 tests/vial; 50 tests/box	ID	Tuberculin testing	Diagnostic
Vitamin B$_{12}$	Cyanocobalamin	100 μg; 1000 μg	10-, 30-mL vial	IM, SC	Vitamin B$_{12}$ deficiency; pernicious anemia	Antianemic
Water for injection with benzyl alcohol 0.9%	Water for Injection, Bacteriostatic	—	10, 30 mL	—	Diluent for injection	Sterile water

HCL = hydrochloride; ID = intradermal; IM = intramuscular; SC, subcutaneous.

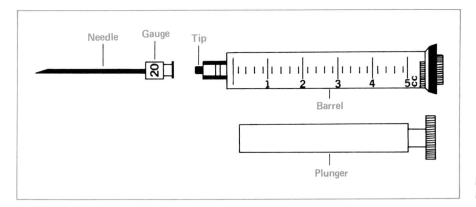

Figure 23–12. A syringe and its parts.

When oral medication is administered in the medical office, the medical assistant must witness the patient consume the drug to ensure that the drug has been taken.

If the patient is to self-administer medication, it is extremely important to instruct the patient about the name and type of medication, proper dosage, as well as any precautions, contraindications, and side effects. If the patient does not understand the directions or the need for carrying them out, the medication may be taken incorrectly, possibly resulting in ineffective treatment. For example, a patient should not drink water after a dose of cough syrup, as water will dilute the syrupy coating intended to relieve the mucous membrane of the throat. Patients given medication that can induce drowsiness should be warned of the dangers of driving or operating machinery while taking the medication.

The patient should also be instructed to take all of the drug dispensed with the prescription. Some drugs do not reach their full effects for days or even weeks. For example, antibiotics need a full 5, 7, or 10 days to adequately eliminate bacteria-causing infection. Accurate spacing between doses is also imperative to successful treatment with many drugs. Thus, the patient's taking the drug exactly as ordered helps to maintain adequate levels of the drug circulating in the bloodstream.

Misinformation is a frequent reason for lack of patient compliance with drug therapy. Patients must be educated about their responsibilities as they pertain to prescription drugs. The medical assistant must remember that the more the patient understands about how to take the medication and why it is being prescribed, the greater the possibility of successful treatment.

RELATED ETHICAL AND LEGAL IMPLICATIONS

The medical assistant must be extremely careful and knowledgeable when administering medications in the medical office. Medication should only be administered after the physician has given a written or verbal order to the medical assistant. All verbal orders must be signed by both the medical assistant and the physician. This completes the communication cycle and allows for no chance of error in interpreting the order. If doubt remains about any part of the order, the medical assistant should reconfirm the order with the physician.

The medical assistant's principal legal responsibility in drug therapy is the prevention of error by scrupulously observing safe practice in both drug preparation and subsequent administration. Observing the three checkpoints and the "seven rights" outlined in this chapter can help to reduce error. The medical assistant must further protect the patient by observing for side effects or untoward effects of the medication. This requires knowledge about the actions of the drugs to be administered and their potentially serious complications. Use of drug references is essential to this process. Finally, the medical assistant must assure compliance with all laws governing controlled substances and their administration and maintain drug and prescription pads in a secure place.

Ethical considerations in drug administration center on the disposal of contaminated substances and error-free dosing. The medical assistant cannot risk giving contaminated medications to a patient. If a break in procedure occurs, the medical assistant must be honest enough to discard the medication and begin again. If an incorrect amount of medication or the wrong medication is given, the medical assistant should immediately report the error to the physician. The physician will have to provide time for patient observation or intervention. Although it is very difficult to admit that a mistake of this seriousness has taken place, it is absolutely necessary.

In a pediatric office, the medical assistant should double-check the calculations for drug administration with a coworker or the physician. Errors in dosage with young children are extremely dangerous.

The administration of medications not only requires safe, legal practice, but also involves ethical principles that always put the patient first.

SUMMARY

The medical assistant who administers drugs in the physician's office must clearly understand the basic concepts of drug administration. The responsibility of participating in this treatment alternative is perhaps the most demanding of the clinical medical assistant's functions, because error could be lethal.

The medical assistant should not be fearful of drug administration, but rather should acquire respect for the process and respond to the challenge to continue to maintain high standards of practice.

DISCUSSION QUESTIONS

Discuss solutions to the following situations:

1. You are about to administer an injection to Mrs. Gordon. She refuses to cooperate.
2. After administering medication, you realize that you gave too small of a dose.
3. As you walk into the examining room, the medication spills onto the floor.
4. You are giving an injection, and when you withdraw the plunger you aspirate blood.
5. You notice that the prescription pad is missing from the examination room.
6. You are newly employed and when about to administer a drug you notice that its expiration date has passed.
7. Mrs. Jones is swallowing the medication and begins to cough. Some of the drug is spit out.
8. Mrs. Smith calls the office and states that she is feeling flushed and dizzy. She was in the office 3 days before and was placed on medication.

BIBLIOGRAPHY

Blume D and Cornett F: Dosages and Solutions, ed 3. FA Davis, Philadelphia, 1991.
Lane K: Medications: A Guide for the Health Professions. FA Davis, Philadelphia, 1992.
Lewis MA and Warden CD: Law and Ethics in the Medical Office. FA Davis, Philadelphia, 1983.
OSHA: Occupational Exposure to Bloodborne Pathogens; Final Rule. 29 CFS Part 1910, 1030, 1991.
Physician's Desk Reference. Medical Economics, Oradell, NJ, published annually.
Thomas CL (ed): Taber's Cyclopedic Medical Dictionary, ed. 17. FA Davis, Philadelphia, 1993.

PROCEDURE: Administer an oral medication

OSHA STANDARDS:

Terminal Performance Objective: Administer an oral medication in liquid or tablet form or instruct the patient to administer an oral medication safely and accurately and within a reasonable time.

EQUIPMENT: Oral medication (tablet or liquid)
Calibrated medicine cup
Paper cup
Glass of water (when appropriate)
Straw (when appropriate)
Medication order from the patient chart
Patient instruction sheet

PROCEDURE

1. Prepare the room by assembling the equipment and checking the cleanliness of the room, lighting, and temperature.
2. Select the proper medication and check the label against the medication order. Discard any questionable preparations.

3. If the drug is unfamiliar, read the package insert or other drug reference or consult with the physician.
4. Correctly calculate the dosage if necessary.
5. Select the correctly calibrated medicine cup and place the cup on a flat surface.

6. Shake the liquid first if required.

7. Check the label again.
8. Uncap and place the cap inside up on the counter.

9. Hold the bottle with the label in the palm of the hand.

PRINCIPLE

1. To reduce procedure time and to facilitate the efficiency of the procedure.

2. Proper checking includes confirming the drug's expiration date, verifying the name and strength of the drug, and inspecting the drug for color and appearance.
3. Obtaining proper information ensures safe, effective administration.
4. Not all drugs are immediately measurable.
5. The type of calibrations on the cup and the amount of medication to be administered determine the correct container to use.
6. Liquid medications that contain undissolved substances dispersed in a liquid vehicle must be mixed before dispensing.
7. Checking and rechecking prevents error.
8. The inside of the cap is considered sterile and should not come into contact with surfaces.
9. Facing the label up in the palm of the hand prevents the liquid from running down the surface of the label. Keeping the label clean ensures that the label will be intact and legible.

PROCEDURE

10. a. Pour the liquid drug into the cup on a flat surface and at eye level.
    b. If the drug is in tablet form, shake the number of tablets ordered into the bottle cop and then into a paper cup.

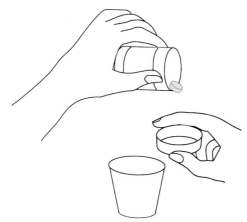

Do not touch tablets or capsules when dispensing them.

11. Do not pour back excess liquids. Discard excess liquids into the sink.
12. Check the dosage measured against the medication order.
13. Replace the cap and read the label when returning the drug to the shelf.
14. Prepare a cup of water. Use a straw if necessary.

15. Identify the patient and explain the procedure.

16. Ask the patient if he or she has any allergies.

17. Remain until the patient has swallowed the drug.

18. Give written follow-up instructions to the patient.

19. Record the date, time, procedure and medication, patient instructions, and sign the record. Example: 3/5/93 2:00 PM: Benadryl liquid, 25 mg orally. Written instructions given to patient (signature).
20. Dispose of the medication equipment and clean the examination room.

PRINCIPLE

10. A flat surface and an eye-level reading ensures a measurement taken at the bottom of the meniscus.
    This technique allows excess tablets in the cap to be returned to the bottle. The correct number of tablets can then be transferred to a cup without touching them.

11. Returning medications to their original containers would contaminate the original contents.
12. To be certain the dosage measured is exactly the dosage ordered.
13. Checking and rechecking prevents error.

14. With the exception of cough syrups, medications can be taken with water. Acids and iron preparations are given through a straw to avoid staining and injury to the teeth.
15. To reduce the risk of error and to provide assurance to anxious patients.
16. The patient could be allergic to any of the component parts of the medication.
17. To ensure the patient's safety and that the physician's orders are followed.
18. Patient education facilitates cooperation and compliance with the physician's orders. Instructions should be in writing for the patient to take home.
19. To ensure the patient's safety and that the physician's orders are followed.

20. To prevent transmitting microorganisms or patient access to medications and to prepare the room for the next patient.

PROCEDURE: Administer a sublingual or buccal medication

Terminal Performance Objective: Administer a sublingual or buccal medication in tablet form or instruct the patient to self-administer the medication safely and accurately within a reasonable time.

EQUIPMENT: Sublingual or buccal medication
Paper cup
Medication order from the patient chart
Patient instruction sheet

PROCEDURE

1. Prepare the room by assembling the equipment and checking the cleanliness of the room, lighting, and temperature.
2. Select the proper medication and check the label against the medication order. Discard any questionable preparations.
3. If the drug is unfamiliar, read the package insert or other drug reference or consult with the physician.
4. Correctly calculate the dosage if necessary.
5. Check the label again.
6. Shake the tablet ordered into the bottle cap and then into a paper cup.
7. Check the dosage measured against the medication order.
8. Replace the cap and read the label when returning the drug to the shelf.
9. Identify the patient and explain the procedure.
10. Ask the patient if he or she has any allergies.
11. For sublingual: Instruct the patient not to swallow but place it under the tongue until dissolved.
For buccal: Instruct the patient not to swallow but place it between the cheek and gum.

PRINCIPLE

1. To reduce procedure time and to facilitate the efficiency of the procedure.
2. Proper checking includes confirming the drug's expiration date, verifying the name and strength of the drug, and inspecting the drug for color and appearance.
3. Obtaining proper information ensures safe, effective administration.
4. Not all drugs are immediately measurable.
5. Checking and rechecking prevents error.
6. This technique allows excess tablets in the cap to be returned to the bottle. The tablet can then be transferred to a cup without touching it.
7. To be certain the dosage measured is exactly the dosage ordered.
8. Checking and rechecking prevents error.
9. To reduce the risk of error and to provide assurance to anxious patients.
10. The patient could be allergic to any of the component parts of the medication.
11. Absorption is rapid under the tongue because of the vast capillary network close to the surface in the area. Mucous membranes have rich blood supplies that facilitate rapid drug absorption.

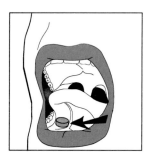
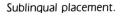   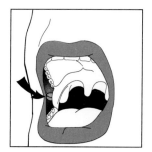

Sublingual placement.   Buccal placement.

12. Instruct the patient not to swallow any fluids until the table is dissolved.
13. Remain with the patient until the tablet has dissolved.
14. Give written follow-up instructions to the patient.

12. Fluids would wash away the medication and eliminate its effectiveness.
13. To ensure the patient's safety and that the physician's orders are followed.
14. Patient education facilitates cooperation and compliance with the physician's orders. Instructions should be in writing for the patient to take home.

PROCEDURE

15. Record the date, time, procedure and medication, patient instructions, and sign the record. Example: 3/5/93 2:00 PM: nitroglycerin 1 tablet sublingually. Patient instructed in administration and care of drug. Written instructions and precautions given to patient. To call and report progress at 5:00 PM today (signature).

16. Dispose of the medication equipment and clean the examination room.

PRINCIPLE

15. To ensure the patient's safety and that the physician's orders are followed.

16. To prevent transmitting microorganisms or patient access to medications and to prepare the room for the next patient.

PROCEDURE: Instruct the patient in the use of a nasal inhaler

OSHA STANDARDS:

Terminal Performance Objective: Instruct the patient to deliver a topical medication to the respiratory tract accurately and safely for a local or systemic effect within a reasonable time.

EQUIPMENT: Medication
Inhaler device
Tissue
Medication order from the patient chart
Patient instruction sheet
Biohazard disposal bag

PROCEDURE

1. Prepare the room by assembling the equipment and checking the cleanliness of the room, lighting, and temperature.
2. Select the proper medication and check the label against the medication order. Discard any questionable preparations.

3. Identify the patient and explain the procedure.

4. Review the medication insert with the patient.

5. Instruct the patient to blow nose.
6. Have patient tip head back and place inhaler tip into one nostril.
7. Instruct patient to use opposite hand to occlude the open nostril.
8. Instruct the patient to inhale while pressing inhaler.
9. Have the patient remove the inhaler tip and exhale slowly through the mouth.
10. Instruct patient to shake the cartridge and repeat steps 6 through 9 in the other nostril.
11. Remain with the patient to determine effectiveness of the intended action of the drug.
12. Give written follow-up instructions to the patient.

13. Record the date, time, procedure and medication, patient instructions, and sign the record. Example: 3/5/93 2:00 PM: Patient instructed to safely and accurately use a nasal inhaler. Written care instructions given to patient (signature).

PRINCIPLE

1. To reduce procedure time and to facilitate the efficiency of the procedure.

2. Proper checking includes confirming the drug's expiration date, verifying the name and strength of the drug, and inspecting the drug for color and appearance.
3. To reduce the risk of error and to provide assurance to anxious patients.
4. Understanding the procedure allows the patient to perform accurately and teaches the patient to check medication labels and directions.
5. Clears the nostrils for inhalation.
6. Proper position increases medication disbursement.

7. Provides maximum inhalation through the nostril.

8. Releases premeasured dose.
9. Rapid exhalation may expel some medication.

10. Complete the dosage and distribution through the respiratory system.
11. To ensure the patient's safety and to allow the patient to ask questions about the treatment.
12. Patient education facilitates cooperation and compliance with the physician's orders. Instructions should be in writing for the patient to take home.
13. To ensure the patient's safety and that the physician's orders are followed.

PROCEDURE: Insert a rectal or vaginal suppository or vaginal cream

OSHA STANDARDS:

Terminal Performance Objective: Insert a rectal suppository, vaginal suppository, or vaginal cream safely and accurately and instruct the patient to self-administer rectal or vaginal medications within a reasonable time.

EQUIPMENT: **Rectal Application**
Rectal suppository
Nonsterile glove(s)
4 × 4 gauze squares
Warm water

Vaginal Application
Vaginal suppository or vaginal cream and applicator
Sterile gloves
Warm water
Sanitary napkin
Medication order
Patient instruction
Two biohazard waste bags

PROCEDURE

1. Prepare the area by assembling the equipment and checking the cleanliness of the room, lighting, and temperature.
2. Select the proper suppository and check the label against the medication order. Discard any questionable preparations.

3. If the drug is unfamiliar, read the package insert or other drug reference or consult with the physician.
4. Identify the patient and explain the procedure.

5. Review the medication insert with the patient.

6. Ask the patient to remove underclothing from the waist down.

For Rectal Suppositories:

7. Assist the patient into the side-lying position and drape.
8. Peel open the suppository and drop it onto a 4 × 4 gauze field.

9. Put on one nonsterile glove.

10. Moisten the suppository.
11. If the patient prefers to insert the suppository, proceed with instructions at this step.
12. Ask the patient to breath slowly through the mouth.

13. With the ungloved hand, separate the buttocks. With the other gloved hand, pick up the suppository and insert, pushing it about 1 to 1½ inches until it passes through the internal sphincter.

PRINCIPLE

1. To reduce procedure time and to facilitate the efficiency of the procedure.

2. Proper checking includes confirming the drug's expiration date, verifying the name and strength of the drug, and inspecting the drug for color and appearance.

3. Obtaining proper information ensures safe, effective administration.

4. To reduce the risk of error and to provide assurance to anxious patients.

5. Understanding the procedure allows the patient to perform accurately and teaches the patient to check medication labels and directions.

6. Outer clothing can be positioned out of the way without further undressing.

7. Proper positioning exposes the rectal area.

8. Prevents contamination of the suppository and reduces the chance of introducing harmful microorganisms.

9. To protect yourself from contamination of fecal contents.

10. To lubricate it for easier insertion.
11. Patients who are able should b encouraged in self-care activities.

12. Mouth breathing helps to relax the anus and anal sphincter, providing a more comfortable entry of the suppository.

13. The suppository should rest along the wall of the rectum to promote more rapid absorption.

PROCEDURE

14. Hold the buttocks closed with the ungloved hand. Instruct the patient not to bear down.
15. Wipe dry the anal area with gauze then dispose.
16. Instruct the patient to remain in position for approximately 15 to 20 minutes.

For Vaginal Suppositories

17. Assist the patient into the dorsal recumbent position with legs wide apart and drape properly.
18. Peel back the wrapper of the sterile glove pack, but leave the gloves in place on the inside panel of the wrapper.
19. Peel open the suppository and drop it onto the sterile field created by the glove wrapper's inside panel. If an applicator is involved, drop it onto the sterile field next to the suppository.
20. Use sterile technique to glove.

21. If an applicator is filled with creams or gels, open the tube of medication with ungloved hands first, then glove one hand and hold the applicator with the gloved hand while the tube is squeezed with the ungloved hand. Set down the medication and place the filled applicator on the sterile field. Glove the remaining hand.
22. If the patient prefers to insert the suppository, proceed with instructions at this step.
23. With one gloved hand, separate the labia minora. With the other gloved hand, pick up the suppository and insert, pushing it one finger length into the vagina.
24. If using an applicator, gently insert it with a slight downward pressure angled toward the coccyx and deposit all of the medication.

PRINCIPLE

14. This aids in absorption of the suppository.

15. Drying the area provides comfort.
16. To allow the suppository time to dissolve and to prevent expulsion.

17. Proper positioning exposes the vaginal orifice.

18. The glove pack will serve as a sterile field for the suppository; otherwise the open suppository cannot be placed on a work surface.
19. Prevents contamination of the suppository and reduces the chance of introducing harmful microorganisms.
20. See sterile gloving technique described in Chapter 24. Although gloves are not necessary if the patient is being instructed to self-administer the suppository, gloving at this point enables intervention and assistance if the patient has difficulty completing the procedure.
21. The tube of medication is not considered sterile and would contaminate a gloved hand. The second glove cannot be put on until the applicator and suppository are ready for use. Another assistant can present the tube of medication if both hands are gloved.

22. Patients who are should be encouraged in self-care activities.
23. The folds of the labia minora must be separated to visualize the vaginal opening.

24. An applicator allows for easier insertion and medication may be placed deeper and alongside the lateral wall of the vagina.

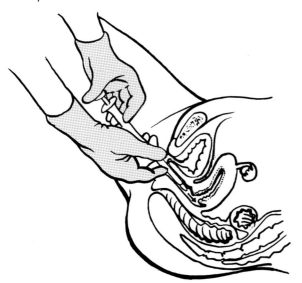

Use gentle, steady pressure on the plunger of the applicator.

PROCEDURE

25. After depositing the medication, remove the applicator and place it on the glove wrapper.
26. Instruct the patient to remain in position for approximately 10 minutes.

27. Place all used materials in a biohazard bag with the gloved hand.
28. Remove glove(s) by grasping cuff and pulling inside out. Hold the bag with the used materials in the gloved hand while removing the glove.
29. Provide a sanitary napkin.

30. Remain with the patient to determine the effectiveness of the intended action of the drug.
31. Give written follow-up instructions.

32. Record the date, time, procedure and medication, patient instructions, and sign the record.
Example for RECTAL suppository: 3/5/93 2:00 PM: Anusol-HC suppository with hydrocortisone. Patient instructed to safely and accurately insert a rectal suppository. Written care instructions given to patient (signature).
Example for VAGINAL suppository: 3/5/93 2:00 PM: Monistat,3, 200 mg vaginal. Patient instructed to safely and accurately insert a vaginal suppository. Written care instructions given to patient (signature).

PRINCIPLE

25. To prevent contaminating work surfaces.

26. To allow time for the medication to dissolve and to prevent expulsion. This is why inserting vaginal medications is best at bedtime.
27. To prevent cross-contamination of microorganisms, materials are disposed of while still wearing gloves.
28. As the glove is removed inside out, it is pulled over the biohazard bag thus sealing the bag in the glove. Dispose of all materials inside of a 2nd biohazard bag.
29. The sanitary napkin prevents soiling of patient's clothing upon ambulation.
30. To ensure the patient's safety and to allow the patient to ask questions about the treatment.
31. Patient education facilitates cooperation and compliance with the physician's orders. Instructions should be in writing for the patient to take home.
32. To ensure quality care, provide a point of future reference, and maintain legal standards.

PROCEDURE: Apply a transdermal infusion unit

OSHA STANDARDS:

Terminal Performance Objective: Instruct a patient to apply and remove transdermal infusion units accurately and safely within a reasonable time.

EQUIPMENT: Transdermal infusion unit
Medication order from the patient chart
Patient instructions
Waste receptacle

PROCEDURE	PRINCIPLE
1. Prepare the room by assembling the equipment and checking the cleanliness of the room, lighting, and temperature.	1. To reduce procedure time and to facilitate the efficiency of the procedure.
2. Select the proper medication and check the label against the medication order. Discard any questionable preparations.	2. Proper checking includes confirming the drug's expiration date, verifying the name and strength of the drug, and inspecting the drug for color and appearance.
3. If the drug is unfamiliar, read the package insert or other drug reference or consult with the physician.	3. Obtaining proper information ensures safe, effective administration.
4. Identify the patient by name and explain the procedure.	4. To reduce the risk of error and to provide assurance to anxious patients.
5. Review the medication insert with the patient.	5. Understanding the procedure allows the patient to perform accurately and teaches the patient to check medication labels and directions.
6. Ask the patient to expose any reasonably hair-free site on the chest or upper arms. Inspect the site.	6. Avoid areas below the knees or elbows, skinfolds, scar tissue, and burned or irritated areas. Body hair interferes with skin adherence. The patient can shower and swim while wearing the unit.
7. Instruct the patient to use a different site every day.	7. To prevent irritation from overusing one site.
8. Tear open the pouch, starting at the slit corner. Lift out the unit with the manufacturer's backing facing the patient in an up-and-down position.	8. Prevents contamination of the hands during application. Any skin surface will absorb the medication on contact.
9. Bend the sides away then toward the patient to hear a "snap."	9. The patient can hear when the backing is opened.
10. Peel off one side of the plastic backing and using the other half of the backing as a handle apply and press down the sticky side of the patch to the skin.	10. Prevents contamination of the hands during application. Any skin surface will absorb the medication on contact.

PROCEDURE

PRINCIPLE

11. Grasp the edge of the plastic applicator by the stripe and pull the backing off the patch. Smooth down the edges of the patch.

11. A tight seal is important to provide maximum absorption of the drug and to make the patch waterproof.

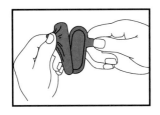

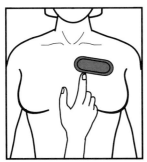

Plastic backing is peeled off on one side. The other half is used to apply the patch to the skin. Immediately following application, the edges are smoothed down to secure the patch.

12. Instruct the patient to apply the transdermal unit at the time of day and for the number of hours instructed by the physician.

12. Transdermal infusion works by releasing drugs through the skin into the bloodstream at a controlled rate. Application is usually prescribed at the same time each day and for a particular length of time. For patients wearing unit around the clock, a new unit is usually applied 30 minutes before removing the old one.

13. Have the patient wash hands thoroughly after each application.

13. To clear the hands of any medication.

14. Instruct the patient how to remove the patch: Press down the center of the unit with the finger, raising the outer edge away from the skin. Grasp the edge and slowly peel away from the skin.

14. Prevents the medication from coming into contact with the patient's hands.

15. Instruct the patient to dispose of the unit in a lined container. Wash hands.

15. Units can be dangerous if they come in contact with others, especially children and including pets.

16. Remain with the patient to determine the effectiveness of the intended action of the drug.

16. To ensure the patient's safety and to allow the patient to ask questions about the treatment.

17. Give written follow-up instructions to the patient.

17. Patient education facilitates cooperation and compliance with the physician's orders. Instructions should be in writing for the patient to take home.

18. Record the date, time, procedure and medication, patient instructions, and sign the record. Example: 3/5/93 2:00 PM: Nitro-dur II, 5 mg/24 h transdermal infusion system. Patient instructed to safely and accurately apply and remove patches. Written care instructions given to patient (signature).

18. To ensure the patient's safety and that the physician's orders are followed.

PROCEDURE: Draw a medication into a syringe for injection

Terminal Performance Objective: Prepare a sterile injectable solution within a reasonable time.

EQUIPMENT: Disposable regular syringe with a needle gauge of 25 and
          a needle length of ⅝ inch
      Alcohol swab
      Vial of medication to be administered
      Medication order from the patient chart
      Biohazard sharps collector

PROCEDURE

1. Prepare the area by assembling the equipment and checking the cleanliness of the room, lighting, and temperature.

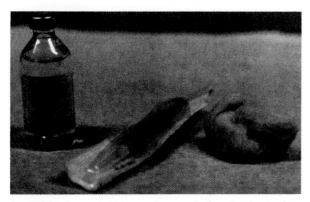

Assemble the necessary equipment before beginning the procedure.

2. Select the proper medication and check the label against the medication order. Discard any questionable preparations.

3. If the drug is unfamiliar, read the package insert or other drug reference or consult with the physician.
4. Correctly calculate the dosage if necessary.
5. Select the correct syringe and needle gauge and length.

6. Shake the vial if required.

PRINCIPLE

1. To reduce procedure time and to facilitate the efficiency of the procedure.

2. Proper checking includes confirming the drug's expiration date, verifying the name and strength of the drug, and inspecting the drug for color and appearance.

3. Obtaining proper information ensures safe, effective administration.
4. Not all drugs are immediately measurable.
5. The amount of medication determines syringe size; the route, injection site, patient size, and viscosity of the medication determine the needle length and gauge.

6. Liquid medications that contain undissolved substances dispersed in a liquid vehicle must be mixed.

PROCEDURE

PRINCIPLE

7. Cleanse the top of the vial with an alcohol swab and allow the alcohol to dry.

7. Antiseptic reduces contamination of the medication as the needle passes through the stopper. Allowing the alcohol to dry prevents "dragging" liquid on the stopper into the vial.

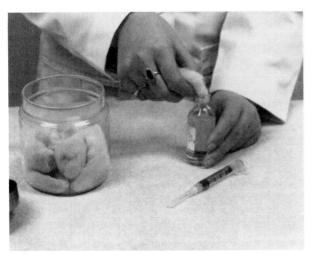

Clean the top of the vial with an alcohol swab.

8. Check the label again. Place the vial on the counter.

9. While holding the syringe at eye level, pull back the plunger to withdraw an amount of air in the syringe equal to the amount of medication to be withdrawn.

8. Checking and rechecking prevents error. Check before inserting the syringe into the vial.

9. Before withdrawing medication from the vial, air is inserted into the vial to make it easier to withdraw the medication.

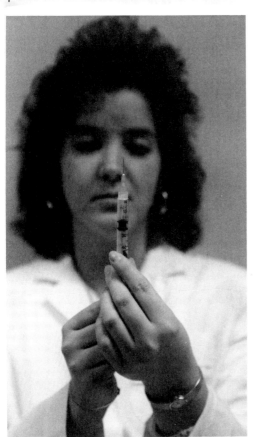

Hold the syringe at eye level to accurately withdraw the appropriate amount of air into the plunger.

PROCEDURE

10. Remove the cap from the syringe and hold the cap end between two fingers or the little finger cupped against the palm.
11. With the vial firmly on the work surface, insert the needle into the vial, just above the solution line, and release the air into the vial by pushing the plunger.
12. Lift up the connected vial-syringe to eye level with the vial label facing up in the palm of one hand and the syringe calibrations facing up in the other hand.
13. With the thumb and forefinger of the hand holding the syringe, grasp the plunger and slowly withdraw an amount of medication that is slightly more than the amount ordered.

14. Hold the syringe-vial in an absolute vertical line and tap the syringe to dislodge any air bubbles formed. The bubbles should float to the top and gather as a single one air bubble in the tip (hub) of the syringe.
15. Eject the bubble, then inject any excess medication back into the vial, until the plunger is positioned on the exact calibration ordered.
16. Add 0.2 mL of air to accurate dosage, when appropriate, according to office policy and the drug manufacturer's recommendation.*

17. Withdraw the syringe by pulling on the barrel and recap the needle.
18. Check the drug label with the order for a third time before replacing the vial in storage. The physician may request the medication be left out with the filled syringe as a double check, if someone else is administering the medication.

PRINCIPLE

10. The inside of the cap is considered sterile and should not come into contact with surfaces. The cap opening should not be contaminated by the hand.
11. If air is inserted into the solution, bubbles will form and make removal of the medication more difficult.

12. Keep the label face up to check for the correct medication and the calibrations at eye level to ensure the correct amount is withdrawn.
13. Withdrawing the medication too quickly causes a "fizzing" effect, which results in air bubbles forming in the syringe. The excess eliminates having to draw up more medication after the air bubbles have been released and assures that medication, not air, has cleared the needle.
14. Air bubbles displace medication and reduce the amount of medication actually in the syringe. The vertical position allows the bubbles to pass into the tip of the syringe.
15. If the air bubble in the top of the syringe were injected, absorption of medication would be impaired.

16. To clear the medication from the needle shaft and the syringe tip (known as dead space) and to prevent seepage of irritating drugs into the subcutaneous tissues during injection.
17. Capping keeps the needle sterile while the syringe is being transported to the patient.
18. Checking and rechecking avoids errors in medication preparation.

---

*In most situations, the dead space (usually 0.002 to 0.3 mL, depending on the size of the needle) is not important. The amount of extra medication in the needle shaft and syringe tip after withdrawal from the vial is offset by the same amount of medication remaining in the shaft and tip after the plunger has injected the medication. When the air-bubble method is used, the dead space volume of medication is cleared and added to the medication in the syringe. The use of an air bubble is *not recommended* for injections with infants or in small dosages of less than 1.0 mL. In both cases the ratio of dead space to total medication can be significant and result in overdosage. More appropriate alternatives to withdrawing additional air into the syringe include the use of the Z-tract injection technique for irritating medications and the use of the smallest calibrated syringe for small doses, especially with infants and children.

PROCEDURE: Administer a parenteral (subcutaneous or intramuscular) injection

OSHA STANDARDS:

Terminal Performance Objective: Administer a subcutaneous (SC) or an intramuscular (IM) injection safely and accurately and within a reasonable time.

EQUIPMENT: Subcutaneous Injection
Disposable 2.5-mL syringe
25g, ⅝-inch needle
Intramuscular Injection
Disposable 3-mL syringe
22g, 1½-inch needle
Alcohol swab
Dry cotton balls
Nonsterile gloves
Vial of medication to be administered
Medical order from the patient chart
Biohazard waste disposal bag
Biohazard sharps collector

PROCEDURE

First, follow the procedure on pages 586–588 for withdrawing medication into a syringe.

1. Prepare the room by assembling the equipment and checking the cleanliness of the room, appropriate lighting, and temperature.
2. Select the proper medication and check the label against the medication order.
3. Check the amount measured in the syringe against the medication order.
4. Identify the patient and explain the procedure.

5. Ask the patient if he or she has any allergies.

6. Position the patient to reduce strain on the part to be used.

7. Help the patient expose the part to be injected.

8. Apply nonsterile gloves, if it is facility policy.

9. Inspect and palpate the site.

10. Locate the anatomic landmarks and the specific point for injection.
11. Cleanse the site with an alcohol swab using a circular motion moving from the site downward.

For Subcutaneous Injection

12A. ⟍Pick up and hold the skin tissue surrounding the site in a pinching and cushioning fashion.

For Intramuscular Injection

12B. ⟍Stretch the tissue. For thin patients and children, firmly grasp a muscle bundle and squeeze while the needle is inserted.

PRINCIPLE

1. To reduce procedure time and to facilitate the efficiency of the procedure.

2. Checking and rechecking prevents error.

3. To be certain the dosage measured is exactly the dosage ordered.

4. To reduce the risk of error and to provide assurance to anxious patients.

5. The patient could be allergic to any of the component parts of the medication.

6. Tense muscles make the injection more painful and difficult. Correct positioning is important for identifying landmarks.

7. The site must be free of constrictions and inspected before injecting.

8. Since an injection is an invasive procedure, there is the possibility of exposure to blood.

9. To ensure that a site is not tender or becomes firm when grasped. Drugs should never be injected into an inflamed area, scar tissue, or into an area with reduced circulation.

10. Marking off landmarks for proper positioning of the needle prevents nerve damage.
11. To prepare the skin for the injection.

12A. Cushioning the SC tissue helps ensure that the needle will penetrate only the SC tissue.

12B. "Bundling" a small muscle mass helps ensure that the needle will not penetrate deeper than the muscle layer. Stretching the skin allows the needle to penetrate the skin more easily.

PROCEDURE	PRINCIPLE

PROCEDURE

13. Place a dry cotton swab between the fingers holding the skin for later use. Remove the needle cap with the same fingers holding the skin.

14A. Hold the needle in a dartlike fashion with the dominant hand and insert the needle with one swift movement, keeping the beveled opening upward and leaving ⅛ inch of the needle shaft above the skin.

For Subcutaneous Injection

14B. Insert at a 45° to 90° angle.

For Intramuscular Injection

14C. Insert at a 90° angle.

15. Immediately bring the fingers and thumb of the other hand to grasp the hub of the needle. Leave enough of the hub visible for signs of discoloration during aspiration.

16. Aspirate (withdraw) the plunger for 2–3 seconds and watch the hub for any signs of discoloration.

17. If blood appears, the syringe must be withdrawn and a new syringe prepared.

18. If no blood is present, slowly push the plunger and inject the medication.

19. Keep the needle motionless while injecting.

20. Hold the cotton swab next to the hub and withdraw the needle quickly.

21. Dispose of the intact syringe unit into a disposable sharps container. Do not recap the needle. Do not sit the needle on any surface.

22. At the same time the needle is withdrawn and disposed of with one hand, use the cotton to apply pressure and gentle massage with the other.

23. Remain with the patient until patient is able to dress and leave the examination room.

24. Give written follow-up instructions to the patient.

25. Record the date, time, procedure and medication, patient instructions, and sign the record. SC Example: 3/5/93 2:00 PM: measles, mumps, rubella II, 0.5 mL SC right arm (R/A). No egg allergy, pregnancy test negative. Nothing in past history contraindicates immunization. Written instructions and precautions given to patient (signature). IM Example: 3/5/93 2:00 PM: Hepatavax-B, 1.0 mL IM R/A. Patient instructed to return for second immunization in 1 month. Written instructions and precautions given to patient (signature).

26. Dispose of the gloves and the cotton materials in a biohazard bag, and clean the examination room.

PRINCIPLE

13. The other hand must be left free to inject the medication.

14A. Inserting the needle swiftly reduces pain. Should a needle break off at the hub, it can be retrieved by the shaft exposed above the skin.

B. Deep SC injections are administered at a 90° angle and are used for solutions exceeding 2.5 mL.

C. The 90° angle is necessary to penetrate the deeper muscle layers.

15. To anchor the syringe in place while the plunger is withdrawn.

16. Waiting allows time for blood to travel up the needle and into the syringe. **Note:** Do not aspirate for SC heparin and insulin injections.

17. If blood appears, then a blood vessel has been penetrated. A new medication must be prepared because the medication is contaminated with blood. Blood must not be injected free into the tissues.

18. Slow, steady pressure allows the tissue to adjust to the volume of drug being deposited. Too forceful a flow will cause tissue tearing and pain.

19. Movement could cause the needle to enter a blood vessel after checking by aspiration.

20. The cotton will absorb any blood that appears as the needle is withdrawn.

21. A rigid sharps container should be accessible in every area used for administrating injections. The container should be in easy reach while still attending to the patient. Older methods of recapping the needle have been discontinued according to OSHA Guidelines.

22. Massage helps to increase circulation and decrease pain. SUBCUTANEOUS INJECTION: DO NOT massage after heparin or insulin injections. INTRAMUSCULAR INJECTION: Check the manufacturer's recommendations for massage after injecting long-acting IM drugs or when using the Z-track technique.

23. To ensure the patient's safety.

24. Patient education facilitates cooperation and compliance with the physician's orders. Instructions should be in writing for the patient to take home.

25. To ensure quality of care, provide a point of future reference, and maintain legal standards.

26. To prevent transmitting microorganisms or patient access to medications and to prepare the room for the next patient.

PROCEDURE: Perform an intradermal skin test

OSHA STANDARDS:

Terminal Performance Objective: Perform an intradermal skin test safely and accurately to assess a patient's sensitivity to drugs or other antigens within a reasonable time.

EQUIPMENT: Disposable 1-mL tuberculin syringe
26 or 27 g, ⅜- to ⅝-inch needle
Acetone swab
Dry cotton balls
Nonsterile gloves
Vial of antigen to be tested
Testing order from the patient chart
Patient instructions
Biohazard disposal bag
Biohazard sharps collector

PROCEDURE

First, follow the procedure on pages 586–588 for withdrawing medication into a syringe.

1. Prepare the room by assembling the equipment and checking the cleanliness of the room, lighting, and temperature.
2. Select the proper medication and check the label against the medication order.
3. Check the amount measured in the syringe against the medication order.
4. If the test is unfamiliar, read the package insert or other drug reference or consult with physician.
5. Identify the patient and explain the procedure.

6. Inspect and palpate the site.

7. Locate the anatomic landmarks and the specific point for injection.

8. Apply nonsterile gloves, if it is facility policy.

9. Position the patient's forearm in the palm of your hand and pull the skin tightly across the patient's forearm by wrapping your fingers around the arm and grasping the skin.
10. Cleanse the site with an acetone swab using a circular motion moving from the site outward.

11. Place a dry cotton ball between the fingers holding the skin for later use. Remove the needle cap with the same fingers holding the skin.

PRINCIPLE

1. To reduce procedure time and to facilitate the efficiency of the procedure.

2. Checking and rechecking prevents error.

3. To be certain the dosage measured is exactly the dosage ordered.

4. Obtaining proper information ensures safe, effective testing.

5. To reduce the risk of error and to provide assurance to anxious patients.

6. To ensure that site is not tender or becomes firm when grasped. Drugs should never be injected into an inflamed area, scar tissue, or into an area with reduced circulation.

7. Marking off landmarks for proper positioning of the needle ensures injection into the volar surface of the forearm.

8. Since an injection is an invasive procedure, there is the possibility of exposure to blood.

9. Taut skin helps ensure the needle penetrates only the epidermis. Holding the arm in this manner minimizes patient arm movement.

10. To prepare the skin for the injection. Acetone is preferred because it is quick drying and removes the oil from the skin.

11. The other hand must be left free to inject the medication.

PROCEDURE	PRINCIPLE

PROCEDURE

12. Hold the needle, bevel up, parallel to the skin surface and slide the needle into the dermis just past the beveled opening.

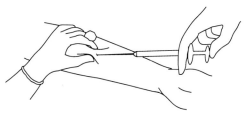

Hold needle level side up while injecting medication.

13. Do not aspirate.
14. Keep the needle motionless while slowly injecting the medication.

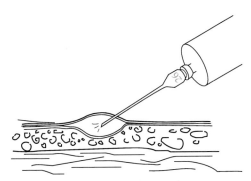

The medication is deposited under the outer layer of epidermis.

15. Hold the cotton ball next to the hub and withdraw the needle quickly.
16. Dispose of the intact syringe unit into a disposable sharps container. Do not recap the needle. Do not sit the needle on any surface.

17. At the same time the needle is withdrawn and disposed of with one hand, use the cotton to blot the area dry. Do not massage.
18. Remain with the patient to determine the presence of the intended action of the drug.
19. Give written follow-up instructions for allergy testing or tuberculin testing follow-up.

20. Record the date, time, test, patient instructions and sign the record. Example: 3/5/83 2:00 PM: Mantoux test: 0.1-mL tuberculin purified protein derivative into right forearm. Patient to return for reading in 48 hours. Written care instructions given to patient (signature).
21. Dispose of the medication equipment and clean the examination room.

PRINCIPLE

12. The needle is embedded only far enough to be under the epidermis.

13. There are no blood vessels in the epidermis.
14. Movement could cause the needle to break through the skin. Slowly injecting the material allows a wheal to form, too forceful a flow could force the medication out through the skin. A small raised wheal should form at the site.

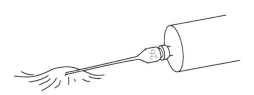

Properly formed, the intradermal injection causes a wheal, or raised circle, on the skin.

15. The cotton will absorb any blood that appears as the needle is withdrawn.
16. A rigid sharps container should be accessible in every area used for administrating injections. The container should be in easy reach while still attending to the patient. Older methods of recapping the needle have been discontinued according to Universal Precaution Guidelines.
17. Massage may alter the response to the drug when used for allergy testing. Massage may break the wheal that was formed with the injection.
18. To ensure the patient's safety. A local reaction may or may not be expected.
19. Skin testing includes interpreting the size of the skin reaction, in 15 to 20 minutes for allergy testing and 24 to 48 hours later for both allergy and tuberculin testing.
20. To ensure quality of care, provide a future point of reference, and maintain legal standards.

21. To prevent transmitting microorganisms or patient access to medications and to prepare the room for the next patient.

Highlights

Reporting Incidents of Possible Exposure to Bloodborne Pathogens

Occupational Safety and Health Administration's (OSHA's) new bloodborne pathogens standard includes provisions for medical follow-up for workers who have an exposure incident. The most obvious exposure incident is a needlestick. But any specific eye, mouth, other mucous membrane, nonintact skin, or parenteral contact with blood or other potentially infectious materials is considered an exposure incident and should be reported to the employer.

Exposure incidents can lead to infection from hepatitis B virus (HBV) or human immunodeficiency virus (HIV) which causes acquired immunodeficiency syndrome (AIDS). Although few cases of AIDS are directly traceable to workplace exposure, every year about 8700 health care workers contract hepatitis B from occupational exposures. Approximately 200 will die from this bloodborne infection. Some will become carriers, passing the infection on to others.

Why Report?

Reporting an exposure incident right away permits immediate medical follow-up. Early action is crucial. Immediate intervention can forestall the development of hepatitis B or enable the affected worker to track potential HIV infection. Prompt reporting also can help the worker avoid spreading bloodborne infection to others. Further, it enables the employer to evaluate the circumstances surrounding the exposure incident to try to find ways to prevent such a situation from occurring again.

Reporting is also important because part of the follow-up includes testing the blood of the source individual to determine HBV and HIV infectivity if this is unknown and if permission for testing can be obtained. The exposed employee must be informed of the results of these tests.

Employers must test their employees to ensure that they know what to do if an incident occurs.

Medical Evaluation and Follow-up

Employers must provide free medical evaluation and treatment to employees who experience an exposure incident. They are to refer exposed employees to a licensed health care provider who will counsel the individual about what happened and how to prevent further spread of any potential infection. He or she will prescribe appropriate treatment in line with cur-

rent US Public Health Service recommendations. The licensed health care provider also will evaluate any reported illness to determine if the symptoms may be related to HIV or HBV development.

The first step is to test the blood of the exposed employee. Any employee who wants to participate in the medical evaluation program must agree to have blood drawn. However, the employee has the option to give the blood sample but refuse permission for HIV testing at that time. The employer must maintain the employee's blood sample for 90 days in case the employee changes his or her mind about testing—should symptoms develop that might be related to HIV or HBV infection.

The health care provider will counsel the employee based on the test results. If the source individual was HBV positive or in a high-risk category, the exposed employee may be given hepatitis B immune globulin vaccination, as necessary. If there is no information on the source individual or the test is negative, and the employee has not been vaccinated or does not have immunity based on his or her test, he or she may receive the vaccine. Further, the health care provider will discuss any other findings from the tests.

The standard requires that the employer make the hepatitis B vaccine available, at no cost to the employee, to all employees who have occupational exposure to blood and other potentially infectious materials. This requirement is in addition to postexposure testing and treatment responsibilities.

Written Opinion

In addition to counseling the employee, the health care provider must give a written report to the employer. This report simply identifies whether hepatitis B vaccination was recommended for the exposed employee and whether or not the employee received vaccination. The health care provider also must note that the employee has been informed of the results of the evaluation or treatment. Any added findings must be kept confidential.

Confidentiality

Medical records must remain confidential. They are not available to the employer. The employee must give specific written consent for anyone to see the records. Records must be maintained for the duration of employment plus 30 years in accordance with OSHA's standard on access to employee exposure and medical records.

Source: From US Department of Labor, Occupational Safety and Health Administration.

CHAPTER OUTLINE

LEARNING OBJECTIVES

Upon completing this chapter, you will be able to:

1. Recognize and define terms related to disinfection, sterilization, and asepsis.
2. Describe the steps of cleaning instruments either manually or with the use of a ultrasonic cleaner.
3. Describe the use of various cleaning agents and disinfectants.
4. Differentiate between chemical disinfection and cold sterilization.
5. List the different methods of wrapping articles for sterilization.

Chapter 24

Sterilization Procedures, Asepsis, and Surgery: Part I

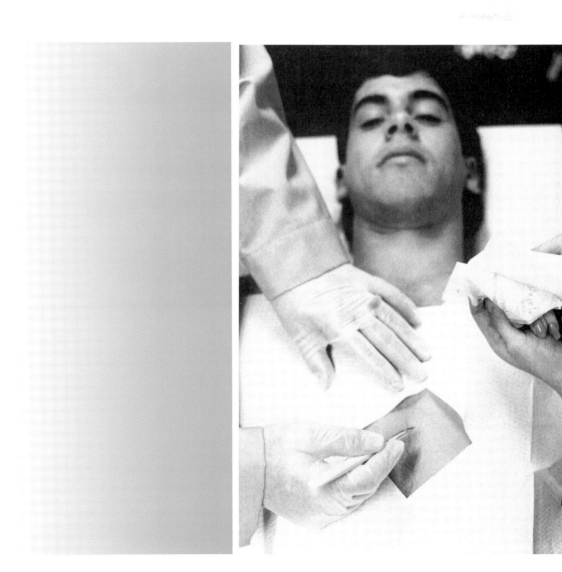

6. Discuss the need for sterility indicators, control monitors, and shelf-life monitoring.
7. Describe how steam sterilization destroys microorganisms.
8. Explain the correlations among temperature, pressure, and time during steam sterilization.
9. Explain "wet packs" and why the autoclave is loaded in a prescribed manner.
10. Recognize the different types of instruments by category and describe how to care for them properly.
11. Identify the various suture materials.
12. Differentiate between medical asepsis (clean technique) and surgical asepsis (sterile technique).
13. Explain the rules for the aseptic handling of instruments and supplies.

PERFORMANCE OBJECTIVES

Upon completing this chapter, you will be able to:

1. Wash hands to remove transient bacteria and to reduce the number of resident bacteria.
2. Scrub hands to remove transient bacteria, reduce and retard the growth of resident bacteria.
3. Put on sterile gloves for use of hands on a sterile field.
4. Clean and shave the patient's skin to eliminate as much as possible the transference of microorganisms.
5. Move sterile objects on or to a sterile field or into the hand of a gloved person.
6. Pour a sterile solution into a sterile basin situated on a sterile field.
7. Open a sterile pack of instruments, towels, or sponges.

DACUM EDUCATION COMPONENTS

1. Apply principles of aseptic technique and infection control (4.1).
2. Prepare and maintain examination and treatment area (4.5).
3. Prepare patients for procedures (4.7).
4. Maintain the physical plant (6.1).
5. Operate and maintain facilities and equipment safely (6.2).

Glossary

Antiseptic: a chemical substance that inhibits the growth of bacteria in contrast to a germicide, which kills bacteria; antiseptics may be used to clean the skin before surgery and to treat wounds and infections

Asepsis: free from pathogenic microorganisms

Clean technique: maintaining a process or area that is pathogen-free

Cold sterilization: the use of chemical solutions to render instruments sterile (10 hours) or clean (10 minutes); a complete germicide

Disinfect: to immerse instruments in chemical disinfectants for 10 to 20 minutes and render the instruments "clean"; to scrub work surfaces with chemical disinfectants

Disinfectant: agent that renders instruments clean but does not sterilize them

Germicide: a chemical substance that kills bacteria and is used to disinfect inanimate objects and work surfaces; the types and numbers of organisms killed depends on the type of germicide

Neutral pH: referring to a solution that is neither acidic nor alkaline

Resident bacteria: bacteria found under the fingernails, in hair follicles, and in the sebaceous glands; resident bacteria come to the surface with perspiration, which is why sterile gloves are worn and the patient's operative site is draped with sterile towels

Sterilant: an Environmental Protection Agency–approved chemical agent that renders instruments sterile after 10 hours of immersion; a germicide that destroys all microorganisms and their spores

Sterile technique: an absolute term that means no living organisms survive

Transient bacteria: skin bacteria that remains for a short time and can easily be removed

In surgery, patient protection is of the utmost importance. When a procedure breaks the skin barrier or invades the sterile, internal organs, the danger of infection always exist for the patient. The medical assistant must be constantly on the lookout for situations that might be harmful to the patient. Two areas that are strongly affected by an awareness of patient safety are sterilization procedures and aseptic technique. The medical assistant must acquire accurate skills in both of these areas before being able to prepare the patient for surgery and to assist the physician with surgical routines.

Environmental protection in the form of sterile conditions is essential to patient care. Disease-producing bacteria have certain environmental requirements necessary for their transmission and growth. Infection control is necessary to prevent disease transmission and is the responsibility of all who work with patients. Because surgical instruments and equipment must be sterile, the medical assistant must be able to distinguish the process of sterilization from other processes that do not achieve sterility.

A second method of protection is through aseptic technique. Certain instrument movements and body movements are required to keep areas in a state of sterility. Sterility is an absolute term; an object is sterile only when it is free from all microorganisms. An object cannot be partially sterile. Incomplete sterilization or a break in sterility could lead to serious wound contamination and infection.

As the medical assistant works around sterile fields, such as trays or the patient, sterility awareness is important. A break in sterile technique could lead to infection in the patient, the physician, or the medical assistant. The practice of sterile technique is the responsibility of every team member during a surgical procedure. Breaks in technique must be reported immediately, even if reporting the break means a delay in the procedure or embarrassment to the medical assistant or another team member. Honesty, integrity, attention, and self-confidence are necessary to exercise good judgment regarding patient safety.

This chapter and Chapter 25 together are for the medical assistant who will assist in those procedures that require the use of sterile equipment and technique. This chapter describes the processes of sterilization, instrumentation, and the sterile techniques necessary as antecedents to sterile procedures performed on patients. Chapter 25 focuses on specific surgical routines and patient care during the preoperative, intraoperative, and postoperative phases.

STERILIZATION AND MAINTENANCE OF EQUIPMENT

Instruments and surgical materials require special care and handling. After each procedure, reusable instruments must be cleaned and sterilized in preparation for the next procedure. After cleaning and before sterilization, instruments must be inspected to ensure good condition and functioning. After sterilization, instruments for nonsterile procedures are stored in covered containers, and sterile instrument packs are stored in a clean, dry, dust-free area, ready for use with the next sterile procedure.

CLEANING INSTRUMENTS

Immediately after surgery, instruments are rinsed under warm (not hot) running water to remove blood, body fluids, and tissue. If the instruments are not cleaned immediately, they should be submerged in water and a neutral pH detergent. A neutral pH detergent is used because it does not cause stains and corrosion if it is properly rinsed off the instruments. High pH detergents cause surface deposits of brown stain; low pH detergents break down stainless protective surfaces and cause black staining. In addition to having a neutral pH, a detergent chosen for instrument cleaning should be nonetching to glass, low sudsing, and an effective blood solvent.

Most instrument manufacturers recommend ultrasonic cleaning for surgical instruments, especially those with hinges and other moving parts. In addition to loosening debris, ultrasonic cleaning helps to reduce the risk of injury when cleaning sharp instruments. Ultrasonic cleaners use sound waves (above 20,000 cycles/sec) beyond the audible range. The sound waves cause the solution to vibrate which, in turn, breaks up the debris attached to the instruments. Instruments are processed according to the manufacturer's instructions, usually for 5 to 10 minutes.

Hinged instruments are placed in the ultrasound solution in the open position. Sharp instruments should be cleaned separately to avoid injury to other instruments. Dissimilar metals (stainless, copper, chrome plated, etc.) should not be placed together in the same cleaning cycle as the ultrasonic vibrations could cause the alloys in the different metals to disintegrate and fuse with one another. After cleaning, the instruments are rinsed under running water to remove the ultrasonic cleaning solution. Ultrasonic solutions should be changed frequently according to the manufacturer's instructions.

If instruments are washed by hand, utility gloves must be worn to protect against accidental skin puncture or contamination. Instruments should be cleaned with plastic brushes, never steel wool or wire brushes. Delicate instruments are washed separately from general instruments. Sharp instruments should be cleaned separately and singly in a washing tray or basin.

After thorough cleaning, instruments should be visibly clean and free from stains and tissue. After scrubbing, each instrument is rinsed thoroughly under running water. Once the instruments are cleaned, they should be checked for proper functioning and condition. Table 24–1 is a checklist for inspecting instruments.

Table 24-1
CHECKLIST FOR INSPECTING INSTRUMENTS

Instrument	Working Order	Test
Scissors	Smooth, gliding blades; not loose in the closed position; shanks straight; no chips along blades.	Cut into thin gauze. The blades should cut from three fourths the length from tip to tip and not "hand up."
Forceps	Properly aligned tips; tips closely parallel to one another.	
Hemostats and needle holders	No visible light between the jaws; lock and unlock easily; joints not loose.	Close and lock ratchets, then rap the edge of the finger ring gently on a firm surface. An instrument that is "sprung" will pop open.
Suction tubes	Clean inside.	
Scalpels	Sharp blades with no nicks or chips.	
Nonmovable instruments	In correct shape to function properly.	

STERILE PACKS

Instruments and supplies to be stored in a sterile condition require special wrapping or protective covering to prevent contamination after the autoclave procedure and during handling and storage (Table 24-2). Wrapping of instruments is performed after the cleaning and drying procedure. Wrapping materials include clean muslin, cotton, paper sheets, disposable paper bags, and plastic-like pouches. Linen materials require laundering. They spread lint, which can act as a carrier of airborne bacteria. Since linen is not waterproof, strikethrough contamination (wetness) can occur at any time. The advantage of linen wrappers is that they are supple and fall nicely into folds. Paper wrappers are somewhat stiff and are more likely to be contaminated by personnel brushing against edges that do not lie flat after folding and sterilizing.

Several principles apply to packaging instruments for sterilization:

Table 24-2
WRAPPING AND PACKAGING MATERIALS FOR ARTICLES TO BE STERILIZED

Material	Grade or Thickness	Suitable for		
		Steam	Dry Heat	Ethylene Oxide Gas
Textile				
Muslin	140 Thread count	Yes	Yes	Yes
Broad cloth	200 Thread count	Yes	No	Yes
Canvas	—	No	No	No
Paper				
Kraft-Brown	30-40 lb	Yes	No	Yes*
Kraft-White	30-40 lb	Yes	No	Yes*
Glassine†	30 lb	Yes	No	Yes
Parchment	Patapar 27-2 T	Yes	No	Yes
Crepe	Dennison Wrap	Yes	No	Yes
Cellulose Film				
Cellophane	Weck Sterilizable	Yes	No	Yes
Plastic				
Polyamide	1-2 mils	‡	No	Yes
Polyethylene	1-3 mils Low-density	No	No	Yes
Polypropylene	1-3 mils	‡	No	Yes
Polyvinylchloride	1-3 mils	No	No	No
Nylon	1-2 mils	‡	No	No
Foil				
Aluminum	1-2 mils	No	Yes	No

*Papers with chlorine formulations should not be used.
†Glassine is a coated paper; it may adhere to hard objects when dry and may tear.
‡Difficult to eliminate air from package.
Source: American Sterilizer Company.

I. Wrapping Sets
   A. Hinged instruments are packaged open (un-hinged) to allow steam to penetrate all surfaces. Heavy instruments are placed on the bottom of a set if two layers of instruments are required.
   B. Items to be envelope-wrapped using linen or paper sheets are placed in the center of the square wrap diagonal to the wrapper. Two layers or sheets are always used. The bottom corner of the wrap is placed over the object, with a small corner tab turned back to allow grasping the corner without contaminating the instruments underneath. The two sides are then folded over, then the top of the wrap is folded down to form the outside flap of the envelope. The flap is secured with sterilizer tape. Labeling tape is used to identify and date the contents of the pack.
   C. Flat instrument trays without lids may also be placed under the instruments in a wrapped set to form a solid sterile field when the pack is opened for use.
   D. The label of every set should include the date the set is sterilized, the name of the set (e.g., suture removal) or the instruments contained (e.g., forceps and suture scissors) and the wrapper's initials.

II. Open instruments
   A. Instruments for immediate use or that are stored unwrapped can be sterilized in instrument trays. The lid of the instrument tray is sterilized beside its open tray of instruments.
   B. After the sterilization procedure, the sterile lid is carefully placed over the instruments in the tray, and the instruments are ready for immediate use or short-term storage.
   C. Usually a plastic-type wrap or muslin toweling is placed in the tray under the instruments to absorb excess moisture during autoclaving.

III. Sterilization Pouches and Bags
   A. Sterilization pouches and bags are ideal for storing individual instruments. They are available in a variety of lengths and widths. Their disadvantage is that they may rupture during sterilization and are easily punctured by sharp instruments or handling.
   B. Only small lightweight items should be wrapped in pouches or bags.
   C. Wide pouches should be used for instruments with ratchet locks so the instrument can be sterilized in an open position.
   D. Pouches and bags are available with sterilization indicators both inside and outside the package.

STERILITY INDICATORS AND CONTROL MONITORS

Biologic monitors are the most reliable way to assure the sterility of an instrument or to verify that the sterilization process did actually render the instruments free from all microorganisms. A biologic monitor consists of spores in a test pack. The pack goes through a normal sterilization cycle and then is sent to a medical laboratory to see if the spore survived or was killed. Positive cultures indicate problems with the sterilization equipment or operator technique. Biologic indicators should be run at least weekly. Many facilities test daily.

Chemical indicator strips are placed in the center of the pack to indicate that the physical conditions required to sterilize instruments in a pack have been reached in that portion of the pack. The physical conditions are: 1) temperature reached; 2) length of time at optimal temperature; and 3) for autoclaving, moisture. Chemical indicator strips are especially important when packages of varying thicknesses are autoclaved. When all required conditions have been reached, a color change from white to black occurs along the entire length of the strip, which provides visible proof of uniform sterilization.

Chemical indicator tape is used to secure the outside of the package. It also turns black when exposed to the sterilization process. Indicator tape serves only as an indication of exposure to a sterilization process. It cannot guarantee that sterilization has taken place deep within the package.

CHEMICAL DISINFECTION AND COLD STERILIZATION

Instruments may be submerged in chemical agents for varying lengths of time to accomplish either chemical disinfection or cold sterilization.

Nonsurgical instruments (e.g., thermometers) that come in contact with the skin or that are inserted into nonsterile body orifices are usually disinfected rather than sterilized after use, because these body surfaces are not considered sterile. The exception to this is when an instrument in or on a nonsterile area comes into contact with surface blood or any blood-tinged body fluid or tissue. In this case, the instrument must be sterilized, regardless of the requisites for its use, to protect against future blood-borne pathogen contamination.

For instruments that do not need to be sterilized, chemical disinfection for 10 minutes will safely disinfect them. It must be remembered, however, that disinfection is never a substitute for sterilization. Cold sterilization solutions, designated as Environmental Protection Agency (EPA)–approved sterilants, can effectively sterilize instruments *only* after a 10-hour immersion. This prolonged chemical process can be more harmful to some instruments than the usual 20-minute autoclave cycle; therefore, care should be taken to read the instrument manufacturer's recommendation for each type of instrument considered for cold sterilization. Table 24–3 lists the specific trade names of commonly used disinfectants and antiseptics. (Antiseptics are used on human tissues. Although the term *antiseptic* includes disinfectants, disinfectants are too strong to be applied to human tissues.)

Table 24-3

COMMONLY USED DISINFECTANTS AND ANTISEPTICS

Common Name	Disinfectant Trade Name	Antiseptic Trade Name	Sterilant Trade Name	Disinfectant Use	Sterilant Use	Shelf-Life	Corrosive	Inactivated by Blood, Serum, Mucous, or Soap
Glutaraldehyde (2%)	Cidex Cidex 7 long-life Cidexplus	Not for antiseptic use	Cidex Cidex 7 long-life Cidexplus	Yes 10–30 min	Yes 10 h	14–28 d	No	No
Chlorine compounds	Chlorinated lime Bleach (10%)	Not for antiseptic use	None None	Yes Yes	No No	N/A N/A	Yes Yes	Yes Yes
Phenolic detergents (0.1%–0.03%)	Cresolyne Hydrasol Phenolor Amphyl O-Syl Staphene	Gamophen pHisoHex Surgi-Cen Surofene	None	Yes	No	N/A	Yes	Yes
Quaternary ammonium compounds (2%)	Benasept Germacin Roccal Zephiran chloride (17%) Hyamine 3500	Not for antiseptic use Zephiran chloride (1:750)	None	Yes	No	N/A	No; Yes to tungsten carbide instruments	Yes
Iodine compounds (0.045%) Iodophors (Iodine mixed with detergent)	Hi-Sine Wescodyne	Prepodyne Betadine Isodine	None	Yes	No	N/A	Yes	Yes
Alcohol (70%–90%)	None	Isopropyl (70%)	None	Limited value	No	When dry	Yes	Yes
Formaldehyde (10%)	Formalin	Not for antiseptic use	None	Yes	No	N/A	Yes	No

N/A = not available.

Instructions for solution strength and the time required to accomplish disinfection by chemical agents are usually listed on the container label. The chemicals described in this chapter do not represent a complete list, but rather are those in common use. Only those chemicals that are EPA-approved sterilants should be used to sterilize instruments.

HEAT STERILIZATION

Sterilization is required for surgical instruments that come in contact with the internal tissues or sterile body cavities, such as the bladder. In addition to cold sterilization using chemicals, there are two *physical methods* of sterilization commonly used: moist heat (steam) and dry heat.

USING THE AUTOCLAVE

Principles

Moist heat sterilization in the medical office is done in the autoclave (Fig. 24–1). An *autoclave* is a specially designed sterilizer that provides steam under pressure. Steam under pressure is the simplest and

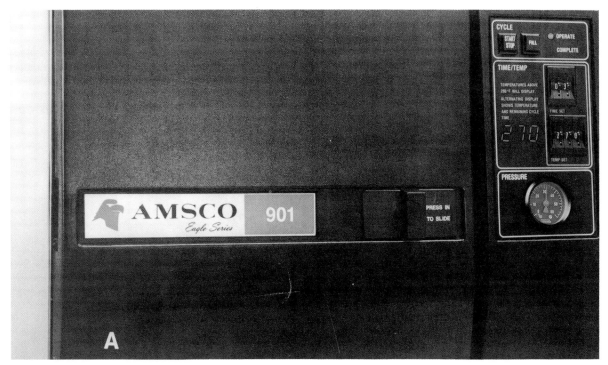

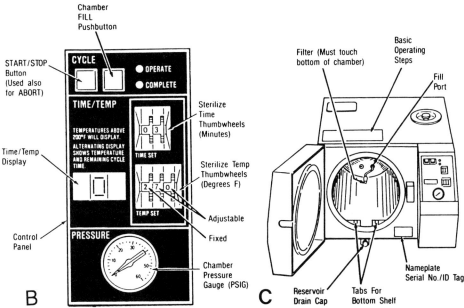

Figure 24–1. Moist (steam) sterilization of medical office instruments and materials is done in the autoclave. (**A**) A typical countertop autoclave. (**B**) The control panel. (**C**) A diagram of the interior. (Courtesy AMSCO.)

most reliable method available for sterilizing surgical items. Effective sterilization requires the presence of *saturated steam* at a proper *temperature* for a proper amount of *time.*

It is not the heat produced in steam sterilization but the steam condensing on the items that kills microorganisms. Heat is transferred to the items on which the steam condenses, and it is this heat that kills all microorganisms present and their spores. Air pockets in the wrapped packages hinder steam penetration and protect the microorganisms from moisture in steam; therefore a pump removes air from the inside of the autoclave to begin the cycle. Once the air is removed, temperature and pressure build up and change the water in the autoclave chamber into hot, pressurized steam that circulates throughout the autoclave.

The temperature and pressure gauges must be monitored during each cycle. There is a set correlation between specific temperature and pressure and the ability of the steam to saturate what is in the chamber. The medical assistant's responsibility during the autoclave cycle is to verify usually that the temperature and pressure gauges reach the desired *temperature-pressure*

combination. When these two gauges reach the readings recommended for the load, the medical assistant begins to time the cycle. The exposure time required for each load is also governed by specific *time-temperature combinations.* The time-temperature combinations listed by each manufacturer are minimum recommendations and should be strictly followed. Never decrease the time-temperature combinations recommended by the manufacturer. Table 24–4 lists the temperature-pressure and time-temperature combinations.

Procedure

Instruments may be autoclaved individually or in wrapped sets. Unwrapped instruments and supplies usually require 15 minutes of exposure at 270°F (132°C) and 27 lb pressure or 30 minutes at 250°F (121°C) and 15 lb of pressure to achieve sterilization. Other materials vary in the length of time needed. The composition of the objects being autoclaved, the positioning of the objects in the autoclave, and the size of the load are factors that influence the time required for sterilization. Special instructions for operating an auto-

Table 24–4

CLEANING AND STERILIZATION RECOMMENDATIONS*

Sterilization or Cleaning Method	Load	Exposure Time	Temperature F(C)	Pressure (psig)	Dry Time
Ultrasound		5–10 min	—	—	Rinse immediately
Steam gravity	Fabric packs	30 min	250(121)	15	30
	Wrapped instrument sets	15 min	270(132)	27	45
(Flash)	Unwrapped metal instruments (without lumens); trays and other empty, nonporous containers	3 min	270(132)	27	0
Steam prevacuum	Fabric packs	4 min	270(132)	30	20
	Wrapped instrument sets	4 min	270(132)	30	30
(Flash)	Unwrapped metal instruments (without lumens); trays and other empty, nonporous containers	3 min	270(132)	30	0
Dry heat	Metal instruments; glassware	1 h 2 h 6 h 9 h	340(170) 320(170) 270(132) 250(121)		
Chemical vapor	Paper-wrapped packs	20 min	270(132)	20–40	
Ethylene oxide		2–3 h	120(49)		
Chemical sterilant (cold sterilization)	Open metal instruments; delicate rubber, plastic, fiber optic instruments	10 h	—	—	To use immediately: Rinse-sterile water To store: Rinse with running water and dry

*Consult device manufacturer's and sterilizer manufacturer's recommendations.
Source: American Sterilizer Company.

clave are provided by each manufacturer and should be carefully followed.

All items should be placed in the autoclave tray so that steam can surround each pack. Fabric and hard goods packs should be placed on edge to aid air removal and steam penetration (Fig. 24–2).

Distilled water is preferred over tap water to prevent the build up of lime deposits inside the autoclave chamber. Commercial cleaning products are available to clean grease and grime from autoclaves and retard scale (lime) deposits.

Improperly loading or overloading the autoclave interferes with complete sterilization during the autoclave cycle. Improper placement of articles may form air pockets that do not allow the penetration of steam. Instruments and utensils should be spaced so as not to touch one another. When possible, utensils, treatment trays, and glassware should be inverted with their lids or caps removed and autoclaved sterile side down.

A major factor governing the sterility of supplies is a state of dryness. Wet materials transmit bacteria; therefore, a state of wetness (strikethrough contamination) could compromise the sterility of a just-processed pack or instrument. No single factor stands out as the primary cause of "wet packs," but rather several factors cause wet pack conditions.

To prevent wet packs, make sure that proper pack preparation and sterilizer loading techniques have been followed. A towel placed on the bottom of the autoclave tray to absorb excess moisture reduces the chance of wet packs. (Make sure the towels have been laundered in a neutral pH detergent and do not contain bleach.) If towels are not used, the autoclave tray should have a perforated bottom (Fig. 24–3). When processing mixed loads of fabric and hard goods, place the hard goods on the lower tray or rack. This prevents wetting of the fabric packs due to condensate dripping from the hard goods during the drying cycle.

At the end of the autoclave cycle but before the drying cycle, open the autoclave door about ¾ of an inch (1.9 cm) (no more). Then run the dry cycle for the time recommended by the manufacturer. If the autoclave door is fully opened before the drying cycle, the colder air in the room will rush into the autoclave

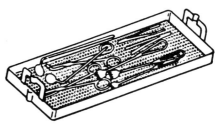

Figure 24–3. The bottom of the autoclave tray is perforated to prevent accumulation of condensation and subsequent "wet-through" of wrapped packs. When sterilizing a mixed load of hard goods and soft packs, place the hard goods on the lower tray, so that condensation dropping of the instruments or hard-good packs does not drop onto fabric packs.

chamber, causing too much condensation on the instruments and packs. This condensation will cause not only wet packs but stains on instruments.

When removing articles from the autoclave, inspect each pack and instrument for moisture. The following are unacceptable conditions in which the articles must be considered *not* sterile:

1. The presence of external droplets or visible moisture on the exterior of the pack or on the tape (unless the wrap is completely impermeable to water, e.g., plastic wrap).
2. The presence of water droplets on the interior of a wrap or on the items within the pack.
3. A pack that is damp or wet when ready to store or opened for use. A general guideline is that autoclaved articles should be completely dry when removed from the autoclave and *remain* completely dry for a minimum of 1 hour after their removal from the autoclave.

Shelf-Life

Wrapped articles and articles stored in the open may be removed from the autoclave with clean, dry hands. Sterile transfer forceps or gloved hands are required to remove unwrapped sterile objects for immediate use under sterile conditions.

Autoclaved articles are stored in a clean and dry storage area. The area should be closed to prevent dust accumulation. Generally the shelf-life of wrapped goods is 21 days, but shelf-life is dependent on the type of wrapper or pouch material used. Each product manufacturer provides shelf-life information. Storage beyond the shelf-life expiration date on the package necessitates recleaning and resterilization. Articles may not be reautoclaved in the same package or without first washing, rinsing, drying, and rewrapping.

DRY HEAT

Dry ovens are used to provide sufficient heat to destroy microbial life and its spores. Dry ovens are useful for supplies that would be damaged by moisture. They

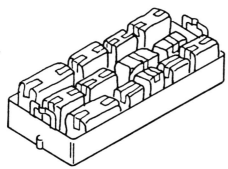

Figure 24–2. Packs of wrapped instruments and other hard goods should be placed standing on edge in the autoclave tray, with sufficient space around each pack so that steam can circulate throughout.

are also useful for home sterilization in emergency situations where sterile towels or linens are needed. The disadvantage of dry heat is the time required for complete sterilization. At a temperature of 270°F (132°C), steam sterilization occurs in 15 minutes, whereas the dry heat method requires 6 hours. Dry ovens require strict adherence to the manufacturers' instructions listed on each sterilizer.

INSTRUMENTATION

Surgical instruments are precision instruments designed for use in operative procedures. Instruments are named according to their use and manufacturer.

The medical assistant should be able to identify a variety of surgical instruments, know their function, and be able to select the correct instruments to be used for specific procedures. The usual minor surgical setup consists of several different instruments. Some instruments are multipurpose, whereas others are specific for only one procedure.

CUTTING AND DISSECTING INSTRUMENTS

Scalpels are knives used to make incisions. They are available either as disposable or reusable instruments. Several shapes and sizes of blades and handles are designed for making specific types of incisions. Figure 24–4 illustrates the most commonly used blades and handles.

Surgical scissors (Fig. 24–5) are used primarily to cut tissue and sutures. Scissor blades touch precisely at the tips and are either curved or straight to meet various needs. Blade points are either sharp or blunt, and both can be combined in one pair. The probe at the end of the tip of the scissors is used to slide under bandages

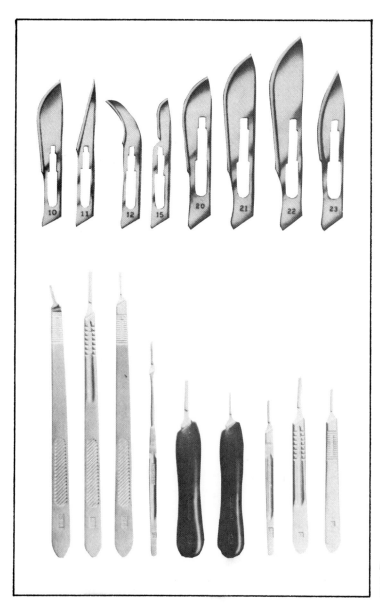

Figure 24–4. A selection of commonly used scalpel blades and handles. (Courtesy of General Medical Corporation.)

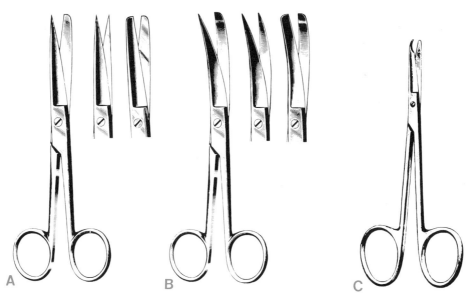

Figure 24–5. Surgical scissors (**A**) straight; (**B**) curved; (**C**) Spencer stitch scissors. (Courtesy Herwig Surgical Instrument Company.)

for cutting the dressing without injuring the skin. Stitch scissors are designed with a hook or beak to get under and sever the suture.

GRASPING AND CLAMPING INSTRUMENTS

Forceps (Fig. 24–6) are instruments designed to grasp objects or tissue. There are several types. *Hemostatic forceps*, or "hemostats," when applied to a blood vessel, grasp tightly enough to stop the flow of blood. This is an important instrument that holds "bleeder" vessels until they can be sutured. Forceps tips are either straight or curved with a variety of types of serrations or teeth and different lengths and sizes to meet special needs. The handle clamps together to prevent slipping and serves to hold the hemostat closed without using the hands.

Tissue forceps are used specifically to grasp tissue. *Thumb forceps* are used to grasp tissue, dressings, and other sterile objects. In surgery, they are primarily used to grasp and apply dressings. Thumb forceps are available in lengths up to 12 inches, with serrations varying from coarse to fine.

Lucae bayonet forceps are used primarily to remove foreign bodies from the ear and nose. They are curved in such a fashion as to permit the entry of scopes for visualization. Lengths up to 8½ inches (21.3 cm) are available. *Splinter forceps* are designed to grasp foreign

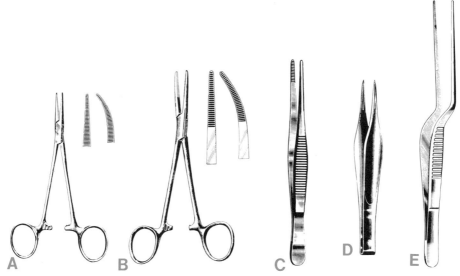

Figure 24–6. Forceps: (**A**) Halstead-Mosquito; (**B**) Kelly-Murphy; (**C**) Dressing forceps; (**D**) Feilchenfeld splinter forceps; (**E**) Lucae ear forceps. (Courtesy of Herwig Surgical Instrument Company.)

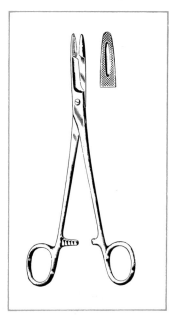

Figure 24–7. Olsen-Hegar needle holder. (Courtesy of Herwig Surgical Instrument Company.)

bodies imbedded in the skin or under the nails. The tips are usually fine and pointed. *Sterilizer forceps* are used to remove sterile objects from containers and sterilizers. Objects such as syringes, metal instruments, and dressing packs can be grasped by the jaws of these forceps.

Figure 24–7 is an example of a *needle holder*, used to grasp the needle during a suturing procedure. The curved needle fits into the special slot inside the tip. The handle clamp prevents slipping. A variety of lengths and jaw sizes are available for holding various sizes of needles.

Figure 24–8 illustrates *towel clamps* for grasping a sterile drape or toweling and holding it in place. Drapes are used to create a sterile field around the surgical site. The drape can be secured to the incision flaps with a towel clamp as the sharp points can pierce tissue. The handle clasp holds the clamp in place, freeing the physician's hands during surgery.

DILATING AND PROBING INSTRUMENTS

This group of instruments is used to enter body cavities for various purposes in both surgical and nonsurgical procedures. Such instruments are often used in surgery of the ear, nose, or rectum (Fig. 24–9).

A *scope* is an instrument used to visualize the interior of a body orifice. It is usually equipped with a light source. A scope differs from a *speculum* in that a speculum has movable parts to widen the orifice and is not usually lighted. An example of a scope is the sigmoidoscope; an example of a speculum is the vaginal speculum.

An *obturator* is an instrument that fits inside a scope and protrudes forward to guide the scope into the canal or body cavity. Some obturators also puncture tissue for insertion.

An *applicator* is a long-handled instrument used to apply medication by twisting cotton at the top. These can usually be inserted through the scope.

A *director* is an instrument, often grooved, used to guide the direction and depth of a surgical incision.

Probes are instruments used to explore cavities, wounds, or foreign bodies. The ends may be straight or curved to facilitate conformity to the shape of the canal or cavity.

A *fingernail drill* (Fig. 24–10) is used to perforate the injured nail when a blood clot or infection makes drainage and pressure release necessary.

Extractors are used to remove substances (such as

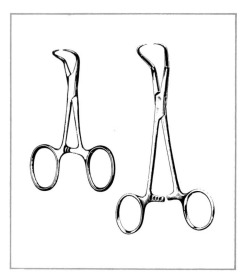

Figure 24–8. Backhaus towel clamps. (Courtesy of Herwig Surgical Instrument Company.)

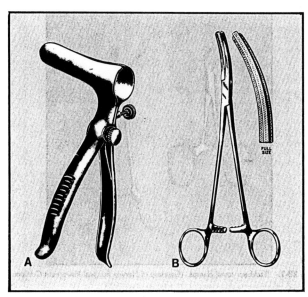

Figure 24–9. Instruments for rectal surgery: (**A**) Bodenhammer rectal speculum; (**B**) Buie pile clamp. (Courtesy of Herwig Surgical Instrument Company.)

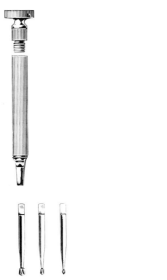

Figure 24–10. Fingernail drill. (Courtesy of Herwig Surgical Instrument Company.)

comedones, or blackheads) from the superficial layer of skin (Fig. 24–11).

Biopsy instruments are used for the removal of tissue for examination, usually for the detection of cancer cells. Biopsies are rarely performed in the medical office. If a biopsy is performed in the office, it is usually of the cervix, uterus, or the rectal region and is accomplished by inserting a *biopsy punch* through a scope.

EAR, NOSE, AND THROAT INSTRUMENTS

Various ear, nose, and throat instruments are pictured in Figure 24–12. *Snares* have a sharp cutting wire used to remove polyps. They are used in nose or ear surgery.

"Alligator" forceps are so termed because of the appearance of their jaw closure. These forceps are inserted through a speculum in the ear or nose to remove foreign bodies. The *Wieder tongue depressor* is a metal strip that holds the tongue in place during a procedure or prolonged examination. *Ear curettes* are used to scrape accumulated or impacted cerumen from the ear canal. A *eustachian catheter* is a tube through which air can be blown into the eustachian canal and into the middle ear cavity. It is often used to clear an obstruction or to test the patency of the canal. *Retractors* are used to separate incisions for expanded visualization. A *trocar* is a set of instruments used to drain fluid from a cavity by piercing the site. The set consists of a *cannula* (outer tube) and a *stylette* (sharp, pointed instrument).

GYNECOLOGIC INSTRUMENTS

Various gynecologic instruments are pictured in Figure 24–13. The *curette* (not pictured) is an example of an instrument used to scrape cells from the cervix for a Pap test, to remove minor polyps, and to obtain secretion samples for testing.

The *vaginal speculum* is an instrument for opening and exposing the interior of the vaginal canal for proper visualization.

Dressing forceps are used to hold a dressing in place to absorb discharge or to apply medication to the cervix and vaginal walls. Other gynecologic forceps include the *vulsellum forceps* and the *tenaculum forceps* (not pictured), which are used to grasp cervical or vaginal tissue.

The *pelvimeter* is an instrument used to measure the female pelvis to determine the adequacy of the pelvic basin for pregnancy and delivery.

SUTURE MATERIALS

Minor surgical procedures disrupt the integrity of the skin. The resulting "wound" may require the use of suture materials to stitch the edges together. Use of these materials promotes more rapid healing and minimizes scarring.

Sutures are available in various materials and thicknesses (gauges). Choice of material and gauge depends on the wound size and location and the type of tissue to be repaired. A rule of thumb is that the suture should be as strong as the tissue it approximates. Sizes are registered in gauge numbers from the smallest (6-0) through the largest (0). For instance, preferences for use of eyelid sutures range for 6-0 to 4-0. Sutures used in skin over the movable joint such as the knee may be as thick as 2-0. Table 24–5 summarizes suture types and sizes. Both absorbable and nonabsorbable sutures are commonly used in the medical office. Table 24–6 compares these two suture types.

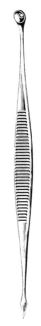

Figure 24–11. Saafield comedone extractor. (Courtesy of Herwig Surgical Instrument Company.)

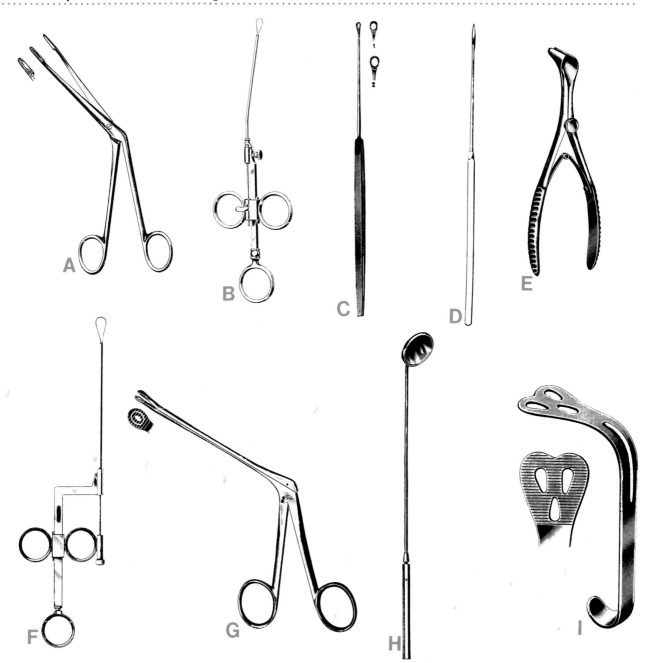

Figure 24–12. Ear, nose, and throat instruments; (**A**) Hartman ear dressing forceps; (**B**) Krause ear snare; (**C**) Shapleigh ear curette; (**D**) myringotome knife; (**E**) Vienna speculum; (**F**) Wilde (Bruening) nasal snare; (**G**) Ferris-Smith alligator forceps; (**H**) laryngeal mirror; (**I**) Weider tongue depressor. (Courtesy of Herwig Surgical Instrument Company.)

Materials other than sutures are available for wound closure. *Sterile tapes* are adhesive and serve to approximate skin edges in the same manner as the suture. They are available in sizes from ⅛ inch (0.312 cm) to 2 inches (5 cm) in width. One popular brand of sterile tape is the Steri-strip. Sterile tapes, although easy to use, must be placed by the physician, as wound closure is considered a surgical procedure that must be performed by licensed personnel.

Tissue approximation also can be performed with *stainless steel staples* that secure the wound edge in a "B" shape. Staples are placed with a surgical cartridge-stapler. Some stapling units are intended for single use and are disposable. As with suture thread, stainless steel staples are available in a variety of sizes to suit the surgical site and the physician's preference.

SURGICAL NEEDLES

Surgical needles are precision-made instruments that are classified according to shape and the type of point, shaft, and eye. The most common needles are curved.

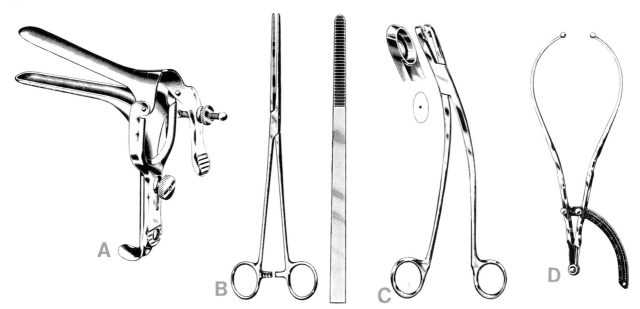

Figure 24-13. Gynecologic instruments: (**A**) Pederson vaginal speculum; (**B**) Bozeman uterine dressing forceps; (**C**) Gellhorn cervical biopsy forceps; (**D**) Martin pelvimeter. (Courtesy of Herwig Surgical Instrument Company.)

The curvature allows the physician to dip beneath the surface of the tissue and retrieve the point as it emerges. The deeper the tissue, the greater the need for a sharper curvature. Fully curved needles are used with needle holders. Straight needles are used without needle holders. The straight needle is hand-held and usually limited to the skin surfaces.

Needle points can be taper, cutting, or reverse cutting. *Taper needles* are similar to the point on a sewing needle and are used on delicate tissues. *Cutting needles* have a triangular cutting tip and are used to lacerate the tissue as they pass through. Cutting needles are used to cut through skin and connective tissues. *Reverse cutting needles* are used to cut through tougher tissues such as the fascia and certain skin areas.

Needles may be manufactured without suture thread. A *sutureless needle* contains an eye and must be threaded with suture packaged on spools or as strands of varying lengths. Eyeless needles are called *atraumatic needles* because they cause the least amount of tissue damage. They are manufactured with the suture material already inserted into the head of the needle.

MEDICAL AND SURGICAL ASEPTIC TECHNIQUES

A primary objective in any surgical procedure is the prevention of infection. Even minor surgery performed in the medical office carries the risk of infection. Aseptic techniques must be observed to control contamination and to prevent surgical complications.

Asepsis is a term applied to the control and elimination of all disease-producing organisms by either clean or sterile techniques. Asepsis interferes with the components necessary to promote infectious growth. These components include the *agent,* which is a factor that

can cause disease; the *host,* which is the vulnerable recipient of the agent; and the *environment,* which is the arrangement of conditions that support microbial life. Aseptic techniques impose changes in one or all of the components.

There are two categories of asepsis: *medical asepsis*

Table 24-5
RECOMMENDED SUTURE USES AND SIZES

Use	Type of Material	Recommended Gauges
Blood vessels/ ligation	Chromic gut	3-0 to 0
	Cotton	3-0
	Silk	3-0 to 0
	Polyester	5-0 to 0
Eyelid	Silk	6-0 to 4-0
	Polyester	6-0, 5-0
Fascia	Chromic gut	2-0 to 0
	Silk	2-0 to 0
	Stainless steel	4-0 to 3-0
	Polyester	2-0 to 0
	Cotton	2-0 to 0
Lip	Chromic gut	5-0
	Plain gut	5-0
Muscle	Plain gut	3-0 to 0
	Chromic gut	3-0 to 0
	Cotton	3-0 to 0
	Silk	3-0 to 0
	Polyester	3-0 to 0
Skin	Nylon	6-0 to 2-0
	Polyethylene	5-0 to 3-0
	Silk	6-0 to 2-0
	Polyester	6-0 to 3-0
	Stainless steel	5-0 to 2-0

Table 24-6

SUTURE COMPARISON

	Absorbable	Non-absorbable
Use	Deeper wounds.	Superficial laceration.
Healing	Difficult or occurs more slowly. Wound needs additional support.	Occurs rapidly. Tissue support not required.
Removal	Not needed; have varying absorption rates.	When adequate closure has occurred and no longer requires support.
Infection Risk	Very low.	Higher.
Types Used	Catgut, plain and chromic, synthetics.	Silk, cotton, synthetics (nylon).

(clean technique) and *surgical asepsis* (sterile technique). Table 24-7 compares the two categories. The major objectives in medical asepsis are to reduce the number of pathogens (disease-producing organisms) and to inhibit their transmission. The techniques of medical asepsis are referred to as "clean techniques." Handwashing before performing clinical procedures is an example of medical asepsis. Removing a lid from a container that houses clean or sterile equipment and placing it upside down on the countertop is an example of medical asepsis; placing it face down would contaminate the inner lid. Pouring oral medication into the bottle cap or a cup rather than into the hand is another example of medical asepsis.

The major objective in surgical asepsis is to free the surgical site of all microbial life and its spores. The techniques of surgical asepsis are referred to as *sterile techniques*. Wearing sterile gloves to apply a sterile dressing is an example of surgical asepsis. Using sterilized instruments in a surgical procedure also is an example of surgical asepsis. Administering an injection requires surgical asepsis. For all surgical and sterile procedures, therefore, sterile techniques are observed.

Important rules to remember in applying aseptic techniques are that

1. Clean must always go against clean.
2. Unclean must always go against unclean (soiled dressings in waste disposal).
3. Sterile must always go against sterile (sterile gloves for holding sterile instruments).
4. Nonsterile must always go against nonsterile (in urinary catheterization, for example, the nonsterile gloved hand retracts the labia for insertion of the sterile catheter by the sterile gloved hand).

MEDICAL ASEPTIC HANDWASHING

Proper handwashing removes soil and acquired microorganisms from skin surfaces. Frequent handwashing is essential because in the course of the day the skin continually acquires microorganisms that, under the right conditions, can become pathogenic (disease causing). Medical office personnel should *always* wash hands before and after seeing each patient, before handling clean or sterile supplies, after handling contaminated items, before any procedure, and at other times as needed or indicated. There are three main components to effective handwashing: (1) running water, (2) friction, and (3) soap or cleansing agent. (See procedure at the end of this chapter.)

SURGICAL SCRUB

Medical aseptic handwashing becomes a surgical scrub by including the adaptations described in the procedure at the end of this chapter. Although sterilizing the skin is impossible, it can be rendered "clean" and prepared surgically by following the steps listed in the procedures at the end of this chapter. Surgical scrub reduces the number of microorganisms because the causal relationship triangle (host, agent, and environment) has been interrupted.

STERILE GLOVES

Sterile gloves are used whenever the patient needs to be protected from all microorganisms or whenever the

Table 24-7

DIFFERENCES BETWEEN MEDICAL AND SURGICAL ASEPSIS

Medical Asepsis	Surgical Asepsis
Absence of pathogens	Absence of microorganisms
Uses "clean' technique	Uses "sterile" technique
Prevents cross-contamination	Prevents organism introduction
Requires thorough handwashing	Requires surgical scrub
Uses clean supplies and equipment	Uses sterile supplies and equipment

medical assistant is required to handle sterile equipment and supplies while maintaining their sterility. In these instances, the use of sterile forces would be inadequate or inefficient. (See the procedure at the end of this chapter.)

SKIN PREPARATION

It is important to remember that skin cannot be sterilized. Some resident microorganisms remain on the skin surface even after thorough cleaning. The objective of presurgical skin preparation is to remove as many transient microorganisms as possible so as to reduce the likelihood of introducing microorganisms into the open surgical area. Preparatory techniques ready the skin for surgery.

The area may be shaved, because bacteria cling to hair. A wet rather than dry shave is preferred to reduce cuts and scrapes. The hair should be shaved in the direction of growth for less irritating removal. (See the procedure at the end of this chapter.)

ASEPTIC HANDLING OF INSTRUMENTS AND SUPPLIES

There are applications for surgical asepsis in the handling of instruments and supplies. The objective is to keep the instruments and supplies free from contamination. Again, remembering the simple precept — clean against clean, sterile against sterile — is helpful. Nothing can be "almost sterile"; it is either sterile or nonsterile. An awareness of these principles, coupled with skillful handling of equipment, will result in effective surgical asepsis.

The following techniques are required to maintain asepsis:

1. Transfer forceps are used to handle sterile instruments and supplies when sterile gloves are not worn. Often the physician is performing a sterile procedure and requests an instrument or other item. Putting on gloves to hand the physician the instrument takes too much time. Therefore, transfer forceps are usually kept standing in a container on the counter in the examination room for ready use. The handle of the forceps is nonsterile; the tips are sterile. (See procedure at end of chapter.)

2. Lids removed from containers housing sterile instruments and supplies always face up when placed on the counter surface. The outside of the lid is nonsterile; the inside is sterile. Lids removed from containers housing sterile instruments and supplies that are not placed on the counter surface are held face down to avoid breathing into the inside of the lid.

3. Pouring sterile solution from a bottle requires opening the lid carefully to avoid touching the inside and pouring the solution at a height above the receptacle to avoid touching the rim

of the sterile receptacle with the bottle. Solution must not splash on the sterile field. (See the procedure at end of chapter.)

4. Commercially packaged sterile instruments and supplies are opened by using the flaps provided on the package. The package is opened in one movement by pulling the flaps apart. The contents can be pulled out by an individual wearing sterile gloves, or the contents may be gently slid onto the sterile field while holding the package above the field. Commercial packs available include towel packs, drape packs, skin preparation packs, shave preparation packs, irrigation sets, drainage tube sets, suture sets, suture removal sets, catheterization sets, and biopsy sets. (See the procedures for sterile packets and envelope-wrapped packs at end of chapter.)

5. Opening sterile wrapped instruments and supplies requires placing the package on a flat surface. Grasp and open the corners with the fingertips, the farthest flaps first and then the nearest. Do not reach over the sterile field. The area inside the package becomes the sterile field. The area approximately 1 inch (2.5 cm) around the edge of the wrap is considered contaminated. If equipment in the package has to be handed to a gloved individual or dropped onto a sterile field, it is best to move the package contents with the transfer forceps. (See the procedures for sterile packets and envelope-wrapped packs at end of chapter.)

6. Ointments must be placed on a sterile gauze pad with a sterile cotton-tipped swab or tongue blade.

7. A sterile tray must be covered with a sterile towel if it is not to be used immediately.

8. When there is any *break* in these techniques, the entire field is contaminated and must be set up again.

The following are important basic rules of asepsis:

1. Sterile team members should keep within the surgical area. Members should not wander around the room or leave the room for any reason.

2. Movement around the sterile field is kept to a minimum, as movement stirs up dust and air currents.

3. Talking releases droplets into the air and should be kept to a minimum.

4. Nonsterile persons may not reach over sterile surfaces (tables, trays, supplies, the patient).

5. Team members face each other and the sterile field. The back is never turned on a sterile field. When sterile team members pass one another, they do so back to back.

6. Nonsterile persons should never pass between two sterile persons or a sterile person and a sterile field.

7. If the sterility of an item is in question, it is considered contaminated.

8. Sterile fields are only sterile at table height; the height of the work surface must not be changed after the procedure is begun.

9. Gowns are considered sterile only in front, from the armpits to the waist, and from the sleeves to 3 inches (7.5 cm) above the elbow. Hands must be kept within this sterile boundary of the gown.

10. The edge of any container is considered not sterile.

11. Handling of sterile goods should be kept to a minimum.

12. Moisture carries bacteria from nonsterile surfaces to sterile surfaces in what is called *strike-through contamination.*

13. Certain areas of the patient cannot be considered sterile. These areas include the patient's nose, mouth, perineal region. Aseptic technique is still observed to prevent gross contamination to the sterile field.

DISCUSSION QUESTIONS

See end of Chapter 25.

BIBLIOGRAPHY

Centers for Disease Control. Update: Universal precautions for prevention of transmission of human immunodeficiency virus, hepatitis B virus, and other bloodborne pathogens in health-care setting. MMWR 37(24):377–382, 387–388, 1988.

Fuller JR: Surgical Technology, ed 3. WB Saunders, Philadelphia, 1992.

Lane K (ed): The Saunders Manual of Medical Assisting Practice. WB Saunders, Philadelphia, 1993.

Reichert, M and Young, JH: Sterilization Technology in the Health Care Facility. Aspen, Gaithersburg, MD, 1993.

PROCEDURE: Perform a medical aseptic handwash

Terminal Performance Objective: Wash hands to remove transient bacteria and to reduce the number of resident bacteria on the hands and wrists within the time designated by office policy.

EQUIPMENT: Dispenser soap
Two to three paper towels
Hand lotion

PROCEDURE

1. Remove jewelry.
2. Ready all materials.

3. Stand away from the sink and keep hands and arms above the waist.

4. Turn on the faucet and regulate the water temperature to tepid.

5. Wet hands and wrists while keeping them in a *downward* position.

6. Apply the cleansing agent from a soap dispenser (not bar soap).

7. Wash hands and wrists vigorously soaping and washing in the crevices between fingers and around fingernails for approximately 2 minutes.

8. Rinse hands thoroughly.

9. Pat hands dry with paper toweling, working from the wrists to the fingertips.
10. Turn off the faucet with a new dry paper towel.

11. Apply hand lotion.
12. Replace jewelry if cleansed.

PRINCIPLE

1. Microorganisms accumulate on inanimate objects.
2. Assembling equipment will prevent recontamination by contact with unclean areas.
3. The sink harbors microorganisms that can be transferred to clothing or skin. All areas below the waist are considered contaminated.
4. Running water is one of the key factors in aseptic cleansing. Water that is too hot or too cold chaps the skin. Dry, cracked skin can be a source of cross-infection.
5. In an upward position, water would run from raised wet hands to uncleaned portions of the arms and then back down, thus recontaminating just-cleaned hands.
6. Surgical soaps contain antibacterial and oil-removing agents that remove transient (surface) bacteria and oils from the skin. Bar soap harbors bacteria.
7. Friction and the cleansing agent are the other two key factors that reduce the activity of microorganisms. Friction is perhaps the most effect because the motion dislodges much of the transient bacteria.
8. Running water rinses away the dislodged transient bacteria.
9. Rubbing would cause chapping. Patting motions should be limited only to the area cleansed.
10. The faucet is unclean. A dry towel prevents contact and recontamination through moisture.
11. Hand lotion helps to prevent chapped hands.
12. Plain bands such as wedding rings and other keepsakes can be worn if they have been scrubbed and placed in disinfectant solution. It is preferable to avoid wearing hand jewelry when you are coming into contact with patients.

PROCEDURE: Perform a surgical hand scrub

Terminal Performance Objective: Scrub hands to remove transient bacteria, reduce the number of resident bacteria, and retard the growth of resident bacteria on the hands, wrists, and lower arms for the time standard designated by policy.

EQUIPMENT: Dispenser soap
Sterile scrub brush
Sterile towel pack, opened to expose two towels (or two to
    three paper towels)
Glove pack

PROCEDURE

1. Remove jewelry.
2. Ready all materials.

3. Stand away from the sink and keep hands and arms above the waist.

4. Turn on the faucet and regulate the water temperature to tepid.

5. Wet hands from the fingertips to the elbows while keeping the hands directed *upward*.

6. Apply the cleansing agent from a dispenser (not bar soap).

7. Wash hands and wrists vigorously with a scrub bush, working toward the elbow and being careful not to abrade the skin. Allow 5 minutes for each hand.*

8. Raise the hands, bending the arms at the elbows, and pass under running water to rinse.

9. Pat hands dry with a sterile towel or paper towel, working from the fingertips to the wrists. Ideally, sterile toweling should be used for drying, if available.

10. Turn off the faucet with a new sterile towel or new dry paper towel. Ideally a foot or forearm lever should be used, if available.

11. Glove immediately. Keep hands folded together and above the waist.

PRINCIPLE

1. Microorganisms accumulate on inanimate objects.
2. Assembling equipment will prevent recontamination by contact with unclean areas.

3. The sink harbors microorganisms than can be transferred to clothing or skin. All areas below the waist are considered contaminated.

4. Running water is one of the key elements in aseptic cleansing. Water that is too hot or too cold will chap the skin. Dry, cracked skin can be a source of cross-infection.

5. In a downward position, water would run down from unscrubbed portions of the arm and back down, thus recontaminating just-cleaned hands.

6. Surgical soaps contain antibacterial and oil-removing agents that remove transient (surface) bacteria and oils from the skin. Bar soap harbors bacteria.

7. Friction and the cleansing agent are the other two key factors that reduce the activity of microorganisms. The brush adds further friction, and longer wash time interrupts the growth of microorganisms.

8. The hands are elevated and elbows flexed to prevent water flowing from unclean (upper arm) to clean (elbows and the lower arms).

9. Rubbing would cause chapping. Patting motions should be limited only to the area cleansed.

10. The faucet is unclean. A dry towel prevents contact and recontamination through moisture.

11. Resident bacteria in the deeper skin layers come to the surface with perspiration. If the gloves are torn during a procedure, the surgical hand scrub minimizes contamination of the patient.

---

*Although some recommend surgical hand scrubbing for a number of minutes, others count the number of scrub strokes. Follow the guidelines of the facility.

PROCEDURE: Glove from a double-wrapped glove pack

OSHA STANDARDS:

Terminal Performance Objective: Put on sterile gloves for the use of hands on a sterile field without a break in sterile technique.

EQUIPMENT: Double-wrapped sterile glove pack

> **NOTE:** It is assumed that this procedure follows a properly performed surgical hand scrub.

PROCEDURE

1. Assemble the equipment and check the tape, date, and condition of the package.

2. Place the package on a flat surface at waist height with the envelope tip pointed toward you.
3. Peel open the outer wrapper and discard or leave in place as a sterile field.
4. Open the inner wrapper by grasping the folded edges and pulling outward to the right and left.

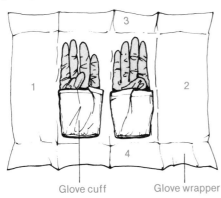

Glove cuff   Glove wrapper

Open the inner wrapper without reaching over package or touching inside of the wrapper. Some manufacturers specify a numbered sequence for opening the flaps.

5. Glove the dominant hand first, then glove the non-dominant hand.

PRINCIPLE

1. Sterility is not guaranteed if the package is old, damaged, or exposed to moisture during storage. If the sterility of an item is in question, consider the item contaminated.
2. Any item below your waist must be considered contaminated. Sterile items are sterile only at table height.
3. If packs are double-wrapped, the outer wrapping can be left underneath as the sterile table field.
4. Nonsterile persons do not reach over a sterile field.

5. The second gloving requires more skill. It is more skillfully accomplished using the dominant hand.

PROCEDURE

PRINCIPLE

6. Keep the gloves above the waist and well away from the body and objects.

6. Sterile items are considered sterile only above waist or table height.

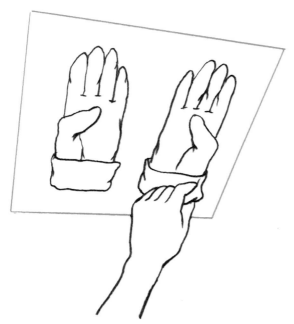

Be sure to touch only the folded cuff of the first glove (for the dominant hand) with only the thumb and fingers of the nondominant hand.

7. Lift the first glove up and off the sterile field by holding the end of the glove cuff between your thumb and fingers and "dangle" the glove fingers downward.

7. The inside of the cuff will be next to your skin and may be touched by a nonsterile person.

8. Note the position of the glove thumb and slide the hand to be gloved down into the glove. (**Note:** If fingers or thumb fail to insert into the matching glove fingers, do not adjust until the second glove in on.)

8. Adjustments must be made later to prevent touching the sterile outside surface with your bare hand.

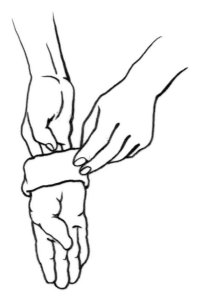

Keep the thumb of the gloved hand tucked against the palm while donning the second glove.

PROCEDURE

9. Slide the gloved fingers *under* the cuff of the second glove. Keep the thumb of the gloved hand tucked against the palm.

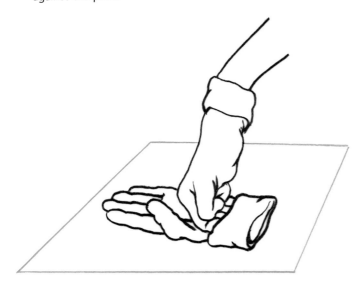

10. With a slightly cupped hand position, lift the second glove straight up and off the field without touching the inside glove surface.
11. Slide the second hand into the glove, then unroll the cuff by pulling the cupped fingers up and out. Keep the gloved hand away from your bare arm. Gently release the cuff (do not snap it) while unrolling it over the wrist.

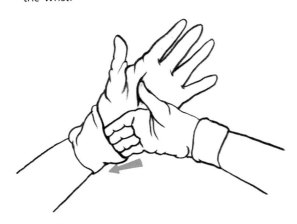

12. Unroll the cuff of the first gloved hand in the same manner.
13. Adjust the fingers in the glove, if necessary, keeping hands above waist level and out in front of the body.
14. Remove first glove by grasping the edge of the glove, then unroll the glove over the hand and discard.
15. With the bare hand, grasp the remaining glove cuff on the inside surface and remove by inverting it over the hand, then discard.

PRINCIPLE

9. Sterile surfaces may only touch sterile surfaces. A free thumb is often the cause of contamination.

10. Sterile items are considered sterile only above waist or table height. The inside glove surface will be considered contaminated when the cuff is unrolled.
11. Cuffs must be eliminated before contact with the patient. If you are gowned, the cuff is rolled over the sleeve of the gown to secure a sealed extremity.

12. Sterile surfaces may only touch sterile surfaces.

13. The glove must form a snug fit with the contours on the fingers.
14. Turning the glove inside out seals in blood and body fluids.
15. Turning inside out by the inside surface prevents bare handed contact with blood and body fluids.

PROCEDURE: Prepare the patient's skin for surgical procedures

OSHA STANDARDS:

Terminal Performance Objective: Prepare the patient's skin to eliminate, as much as possible, the transfer of microorganisms to the incision site or wound. Shave the site per order.

EQUIPMENT: Mayo tray or side tray
Antiseptic soap
Sterile saline
Antiseptic
Waste receptacle
Sterile cotton applicators (eight)
Biohazard bags

Sterile Packs
Sterile gloves
Towel pack (four towels)
Patient drape (with window) pack
Sterile basin pack (three)
4 × 4 sponge pack (12 to 24 sponges)
Shave preparation pack

Note: It is assumed that this procedure follows a properly performed surgical hand scrub.

PROCEDURE

1. Prepare the room, open and set up equipment on a side stand or table, and adjust the lighting.

2. Reinforce the physician's explanation of the procedure. Have the patient sign a consent form.
3. Instruct the patient on clothing removal and gowning. Position and drape the patient to provide exposure and availability to the operative site.

4. Pour germicidal skin detergent in one basin, sterile saline in the second, and the antiseptic in the third.

5. Wash hands and put on gloves.
6. Drape the site with two towels 3 to 6 inches (7.5 to 15 cm) above and below the surgical site.

7. Dip the first sterile gauze into the soapy solution and prepare the patient's skin by cleansing in a circular motion, working from the site outward and passing over each area only once.

8. Use a new sponge for each pass. Repeat the process until the site is completely cleansed.

9. Immediately discard each sponge into the waste receptacle.

10. Rinse with the sterile saline and clean gauze, then pat dry with dry gauze, staying within the area just cleaned.

11. Resoap in the same manner, then using the razor, shave the area in the direction in which the hair grows.
12. Rinse with the saline solution and pat dry.

PRINCIPLE

1. A clean room diminishes the chance of infection. Equipment readiness is essential to save time and to ensure procedural safety.
2. Facilitates patient understanding and relieves anxiety and reduces the risk of liability.
3. To ensure patient comfort and safety during the procedure. Enough clothing must be removed to fully expose the operative site.

4. Once you are gloved, you cannot pour liquids.

5. To prevent the transfer of resident bacteria.
6. The area cleansed should be 3 to 6 inches (7.5 to 15 cm) larger than the window drape opening.

7. To prevent dragging microorganisms back over the cleansed area, always work from clean to unclean.

8. With each sweep, the sponge becomes contaminated with the debris on the skin.

9. To keep soiled materials clear of the sterile working areas.

10. The first scrub debris should be wiped away before the area is shaved. Shaving may inadvertently cause a skin abrasion and break the natural protective barrier of the skin.

11. Enables a close shave yet is not as irritating to the skin as shaving against the direction of hair growth.

12. Rubbing could cause skin abrasion and potential injury to natural skin barriers.

PROCEDURE

13. Moisten a new gauze with the soapy solution and begin the skin preparation as described above. Repeat the process for 5 minutes or for the length of time dictated by office policy. Rinse using the same single-pass, circular motion.

14. Dry the area with the third sterile towel by patting dry. Check to ensure there is no pooling of solutions under the patient.

15. Paint on the antiseptic using the cotton applicators in the same circular technique, using one applicator per sweep.

16. Cover the site with the fourth sterile towel.

17. Dispose of soiled materials and gloves in a biohazard plastic bag:
    a. Remove one glove inside out.
    b. Put the bare hand into a plastic bag.
    c. Through the bag, remove the second glove.
    d. Pick up all soiled materials and hold them through the bag; use the other hand to grasp the top edge of the bag and pull it down over the hand and dressings.

PRINCIPLE

13. The skin prep does not begin until the area is first shaved.

14. A moist site would contaminate the window draping. Antiseptics could irritate or burn the skin.

15. The antiseptic is the last skin protectant and is applied to retard the growth of bacteria during the procedure.

16. The site must be protected from air currents carrying bacteria.

17. All soiled materials must be in a plastic bag before disposing for incineration or other disposal.

PROCEDURE: Transfer sterile objects using transfer forceps

OSHA STANDARDS:

Terminal Performance Objective: Move sterile objects on or to a sterile field or into the hand of a gloved person with transfer forceps.

EQUIPMENT: Sterile transfer forceps
Forceps container filled with sterilant, such as Cidex
Sterile 4 × 4 package, opened
Mayo stand with sterile field of instruments

PROCEDURE

1. Grasp the forceps handles and keep them together.

2. Slowly lift the forceps in a vertical position.

3. Lift the forceps above the solution line without touching the sides of the container.

4. Gently open and close the forceps handles to "tap" excess solution from the forceps tips or dry the tips by touching them, tip downward, to a dry, sterile 4 × 4 gauze.

5. Use the forceps to transport sterile materials, keeping the forceps pointed downward and without touching the sterile field.

6. Securely grasp instruments midshank.

7. Place items on a sterile field inside an imaginary 1-inch (2.5 cm) perimeter.

8. Replace forceps in container, not touching the sides of the container.

9. Clean and autoclave the forceps and the container, then fill the container with fresh solution at least weekly.

PRINCIPLE

1. Open forceps could touch the side of the container, which is contaminated.

2. Tilting the forceps into a horizontal position would allow the solution to travel up the forceps onto the surfaces not soaking in the solution. The solution would then run from the nonsterile part of the forceps to the sterile part, dragging down bacteria and thus contaminating the forceps.

3. The sides of containers are considered not sterile.

4. Excess solution could wet the sterile field. A sterile field remains sterile only as long as it is dry.

5. A drop of moisture results in the contamination of a sterile field. Spills contaminate a sterile field.

6. Grasping the tips of instruments could damage the instrument; grasping the handles would make the instrument transfer too difficult.

7. A 1-inch (2.5 cm) perimeter around the entire sterile field is considered contaminated because the edges are in contact with the work surfaces.

8. Forceps may not rest on a sterile surface as the handles are contaminated; they must be replaced in solution immediately after use.

9. Specific "Shelf-lives after activation" vary according to manufacturer's recommendations. Solutions lose their effectiveness due to evaporation.

PROCEDURE: Transfer sterile solutions to a sterile field

OSHA STANDARDS:

Terminal Performance Objective: Pour a sterile solution into a sterile basin situated on a sterile field without spilling the liquid onto the sterile field or contaminating the solution.

EQUIPMENT: Sterile saline or hydrogen peroxide
Sterile basin
Mayo stand with sterile field and basin

PROCEDURE

1. Assemble the equipment and check the expiration date of the solution.
2. Remove the cap by touching only the outside of the cap and place it on a surface, inside facing up. If the cap is held in the hand during the pouring, hold the cap inside facing downward.
3. Hold the bottle with the label against the palm of one hand and approximately 6 inches above the sterile container, which is located in the sterile field.

4. Remove the bottle from over the sterile field and immediately replace the lid.

PRINCIPLE

1. The effectiveness against microbial activity is diminished if the solution is old.
2. To prevent contamination of the sterile inside of the cap and subsequent contamination of the solution. If the cap is held in the hand, keeping the inside downward prevents contamination from air currents.
3. Holding the bottle in this manner prevents the solution from dripping on the label while pouring. Holding the bottle too high would cause the solution to splash onto the sterile field, whereas holding the bottle too low might result in touching the lip of the bottle to the sterile container.
4. Motions over a sterile field must be kept to a minimum.

PROCEDURE: Open a sterile packet

OSHA STANDARDS:

Terminal Performance Objective: Place sterile items onto a sterile field or into the hand of a gloved person without a break in sterile technique.

EQUIPMENT: Sterile syringe and needle package
Sterile, double-wrapped package containing nonabsorbable suture material and needle

PROCEDURE

1. Assemble the equipment and check the expiration date and condition of the package.

2. Locate the unsealed extended edges.

3. Grasp each edge with the thumb and forefinger of each hand and pull apart evenly.

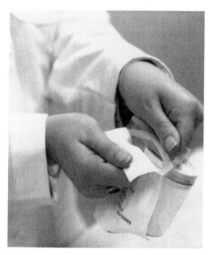

4. Secure the package by forming a fist with the last three fingers against the packet and peel apart the package flaps.

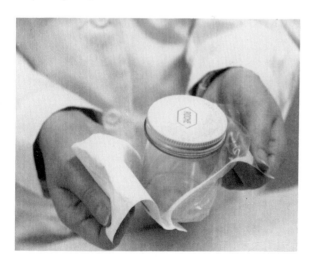

PRINCIPLE

1. Sterility is not guaranteed if the package is old, damaged, or exposed to moisture during storage. If the sterility of an item is questionable, consider the package contaminated.

2. The edges indicate where the package is to be opened and are usually marked by the word "open" printed on the package.

3. Tearing the package exposes the contents to the outside wrapper, which is not considered sterile.

4. Peeling the package back fully exposes the contents. Sterile items must not come in contact with the wrapper edges. The wrapper edges, packs, and towels are not considered sterile.

PROCEDURE

PRINCIPLE

5. Hold the contents 8 to 12 inches (20 to 30 cm) from the field and drop the contents inside the sterile field. In some situations, instead of dropping the item onto a sterile field, you will present the item to the physician, with the item sticking straight out between the peeled back sides of the package.

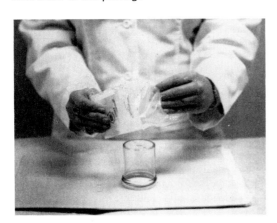

5. Nonsterile persons do not reach over a sterile field. A 1-inch (2.5-cm) perimeter around the sterile field is set up as an imaginary barrier and is considered contaminated at all times.

PROCEDURE: Open a sterile envelope-wrapped pack

OSHA STANDARDS:

Terminal Performance Objective: Open a sterile pack of instruments, towels, or sponges without a break in sterile technique and within a reasonable time frame.

EQUIPMENT: Autoclaved instrument pack
Autoclaved towel pack
Autoclaved pack of 4 X 4 sponges

PROCEDURE

1. Assemble the equipment and check the tape, date, and condition of the package.

2. Place the package on a flat surface at waist height with the envelope tip pointed toward you.

3. Unfold the first triangular corner away from you, touching only the folded back tab.

4. Unfold the right and left corners.

5. Unfold the last corner by pulling its tab toward you, uncovering the contents of the package.

6. If the contents are not to be used immediately, leave the last corner covering the materials.

PRINCIPLE

1. Sterility is not guaranteed if the package is old, damaged or exposed to moisture during storage. If the sterility of an item is in question, consider the item contaminated.

2. Any item below your waist must be considered contaminated. Sterile items are sterile only at table height.

3. Beginning in this fashion will prevent you from having to reach over the sterile contents later.

4. Each tab acts as a touchable barrier to the sterile inside surface and becomes part of the 1-inch (2.5-cm) barrier around the field not considered to be sterile.

5. Although the last flap of the wrap is considered sterile, the tab allows you to lift the pack without coming into contact with the sterile contents.

6. Never turn your back or wander from an exposed sterile field. If you lose a sterile field from your line of vision, you can no longer assume it is sterile. Air currents carry bacteria, so exposure to air should be kept to a minimum.

HIGHLIGHTS

The Evaluation of Surgical Risk

The term *surgical risk* refers to the probability of death from surgery. Certainly, in minor surgical procedures performed in the medical office, death is not a conceivable outcome. However, it is likely that medical assistants will come into contact with this term at some point during their careers.

Anesthesiologists categorize surgical risk according to a rating scale:

Class I   Normal and healthy
Class II   Mild systemic disease
Class III   Severe systemic disease that is not incapacitating
Class IV   Incapacitating systemic disease that is a threat to life
Class V   Not expected to live with or without surgery

Specifically, the degree of surgical risk depends on the nature, duration, and location of the condition, magnitude and urgency of the surgical procedure, the mental attitude of the person toward surgery, and the caliber of the professional staff and health care facility.

Nature of condition: Is it benign or malignant? (Malignancy increases risk.)
Location of condition: The importance of the organ and its function (heart and brain conditions cause an increase in surgical risk).
Magnitude and urgency of surgical procedure: Is surgery extensive or limited? Emergency surgery and surgery that is very extensive, such as colon resection, carries an increased surgical risk.
Mental attitude of the person: Fear and stress increase surgical risk. Confidence and patience decrease risk.
Caliber of staff and facility: Competent staff and a well-equipped facility decrease surgical risk. It is also likely that the behavior of physicians and staff influence risk. Poor bedside manner affects the patient adversely.

In patient teaching and helping to prepare patients for major or minor surgery, the medical assistant must be cognisant of his or her attitude and the attitude of the patient toward the surgical procedure.

> The fact that an operation is technically minor does not mean that a person experiences it as "minor" and is free from fear.
>
> Joan Luckman and
> Karen C. Sorenson,
> *Medical-Surgical Nursing*

CHAPTER OUTLINE

LEARNING OBJECTIVES

Upon completing this chapter, you will be able to:

1. Recognize and define terms related to surgery.
2. List the presurgical routines the patient goes through and why each is performed.
3. Identify the various routes and types of conduction anesthesia.
4. Describe the steps of terminal disinfection either manually or with the use of a sterilizer-washer and ultrasonic cleaner.
5. List the materials and human substances that are considered hazardous medical wastes.
6. Compare the various wound types and classifications of healing.
7. List the purpose of bandaging.

Chapter 25

*S*terilization Procedures, Asepsis, and Surgery: Part II

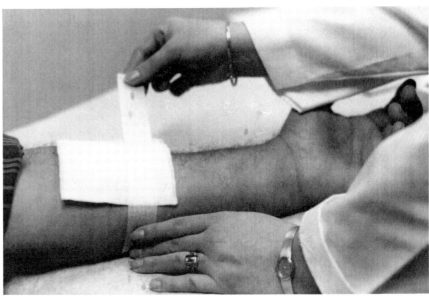

PERFORMANCE OBJECTIVES

Upon completing this chapter, you will be able to:

1. Ensure that all materials and equipment are accounted for, ready to use, and prepared with sterile technique during a surgical routine.
2. Assist in the repair of an incision or a laceration.
3. Assist in the removal of an ingrown nail under local or topical anesthesia.
4. Assist with an incision of an abscess and the drainage of accumulated infectious materials.
5. Assist with the excision of a benign sebaceous cyst.
6. Apply a sterile dressing after the completion of minor surgery and instruct the patient in wound and dressing care.
7. Care for healing wounds and apply a new dressing.
8. Remove dermal sutures from a closed incision.

DACUM EDUCATIONAL COMPONENTS

1. Apply principles of aseptic technique and infection control (4.1).
2. Prepare and maintain examination and treatment area (4.5).
3. Prepare patients for procedures (4.7).
4. Assist physician with examinations and treatments (4.8).
5. Maintain the physical plant (6.1).
6. Operate and maintain facilities and equipment safely (6.2).
7. Instruct patients with special needs (7.2).

Glossary

Approximate: in surgery, to close together wound edges
Cauterize: to destroy tissue with a caustic agent, hot instrument, electric current, or laser beam
Débridement: the removal of foreign material or contaminated tissues until only healthy tissues remain: drainage or excision
Electrosurgery: using an electrocoagulation "pencil" to cauterize blood vessels and excise tissue with electrical current
Fiberoptics: the transmission of an image along flexible bundles of glass or plastic fibers
Infiltration anesthesia: local or regional anesthesia introduced directly into the tissues; anesthesia deposited directly into the wound or wound edges
Laser: acronym for light amplification by stimulated emission of radiation; using thermal lasers to heat tissues at a microscopic level, causing vaporization and coagulation of the target tissue
Laceration: a wound in which tissue is torn

Ambulatory surgery (office surgery, outpatient surgery, day surgery, in-out surgery, surgicenter surgery) is now more prevalent than ever. This increase is due to many reasons, mostly economic. Hospital stays for minor procedures are very costly and most often unnecessary. New managed care limitations on the patient's length of hospital stay and insurance coverage limitations on procedures considered medically unnecessary have contributed greatly to the development of outpatient surgical facilities as a separate department of the hospital or in the private setting.

There are many advantages to outpatient surgery. Perhaps the greatest advantage is the reduced cost to the patient and to insuring and governmental agencies. Not requiring hospitalization for surgery also reduces the psychological stress to the patient and the time lost from work and the family. The major disadvantage of outpatient surgery is that it provides less time to assess and evaluate the patient and decreases the face-to-face opportunity to care for the patient preoperatively and postoperatively. This lack of in-person care often reduces the rapport between the patient and the surgical staff.

Usually outpatient surgery is limited to procedures that can be completed in 15 to 60 minutes. Candidates for outpatient surgery usually have noninfected conditions that require procedures where the risk of postoperative complications are low. Except in emergency suturing of minor wounds, conditions that involve infection or a risk of infection or other postoperative complications are usually performed in the hospital on an inpatient basis.

Surgery is classified as optional, elective, required, urgent, or emergency. *Optional surgery* is scheduled completely at the discretion of the patient. It is considered not medically necessary. Cosmetic surgery is an example of optional surgery. Most insurance companies will not reimburse the patient who has optional surgery. *Elective surgery* is surgery that is considered medically necessary, but only at the convenience of the patient. Failure to have surgery would not result in harm to the patient. Removal of a cyst is an example of elective surgery.

If a surgery is deemed medically necessary within a few weeks, it is considered required surgery. One example of required surgery is removal of cataracts. Surgical problems that require attention in 1 to 2 days are considered *urgent* (e.g., cancer), and problems that require intervention without delay are *emergency* procedures (e.g., fractures, lacerations). Most outpatient surgery performed is of the elective type or for minor emergencies. Frequently preformed elective surgeries include excision of skin lesions, oral surgery, myringotomy, dilation and curettage, tubal ligation, vasectomy, cystoscopy, and diagnostic laparoscopy. Frequently performed emergency surgeries include wound repair, incision and drainage for abscesses, and toenail resection. Surgical conditions requiring electrosurgery (electrocoagulation) and laser surgery are also frequently performed on an outpatient basis.

PRESURGICAL PROCEDURES

With so many procedures being performed outside the hospital, the medical assistant plays a key role in preoperative and postoperative processes. The medical assistant must understand the general principles of surgical procedures and become competent in the skills necessary to assist the patient in preparing for surgery.

INFORMED CONSENT (OPERATIVE PERMIT)

Informed consent is when the patient understands and consents to the procedure being performed. The responsibility for obtaining the patient's consent is explained in detail in Chapter 3, Medical Law and Ethics.

Any procedure where scalpel, scissors, suture, hemostats, or electrocoagulation may be used requires the patient's permission to perform surgery. Other procedures requiring patient permission include entering a body cavity (bronchoscopy, cystoscopy), local infiltration anesthesia, and regional block anesthesia.

The medical assistant is often responsible for having the patient sign a consent form. The patient's signature provides documentation that the risks and probable outcome have been disclosed to the patient. The medical assistant usually witnesses that the patient affixed his or her signature to the form.

PREOPERATIVE INSTRUCTIONS

Some surgical procedures may require the patient to complete specific preparations before the procedure is done. These preoperative instructions are presented in written form to facilitate preoperative teaching. Booklets, brochures, videotapes, and models are all helpful instructional tools. Patient education may include the family and significant others. During patient instruction, the medical assistant should encourage questions and provide needed clarifications. Patient education increases the patient's understanding of the procedure and ensures greater compliance with presurgical preparations.

Preoperative education includes explaining what preoperative laboratory tests, if any, are needed. Other subjects include cleansing enemas, bathing, restrictions on food intake (discontinuing food and fluids the midnight previous to the day of surgery), and bedtime sedatives. Patients also need to be instructed to notify the office should they contract a cold, have a fever, or have any illness just before surgery. Patients also should be told to arrive at a specific time and to have someone with them who can drive them home. Most facilities have preprinted instructions for each surgical procedure performed on site or (for a surgical practice) in the hospital.

ASSISTING WITH SURGICAL PROCEDURES

With orientation to office protocol and with experience, the medical assistant will learn the steps and equipment necessary for specific procedures. But even the novice medical assistant will be able to apply general principles of assisting with minor surgery. For example, if an incision is required, a local anesthetic, suture material, sponges, scalpel, and scissors will be needed (Fig. 25–1). In addition, preparing the site by prepping and cleansing will also be necessary. As more experience is acquired, it will be easier to anticipate specifically what is needed. At the end of this chapter, step-by-step descriptions of common surgical procedures are provided, including assisting with minor surgery, suturing, incision and drainage, and removal of a cyst; and performing the application of a sterile dressing and postsurgical routines, changing dressings, and removal of sutures from a healed incision.

POSITIONING AND DRAPING

The general principles of positioning and draping as described in Chapter 18 apply to surgical procedures. All clothing and jewelry in the vicinity of the surgical site must be removed. A properly prepped and draped surgical site both enhances visibility for the physician and provides a sterile field from which to work.

Steps should be taken to make the patient as comfortable as possible because the length of the procedure or required position can cause the patient physical and

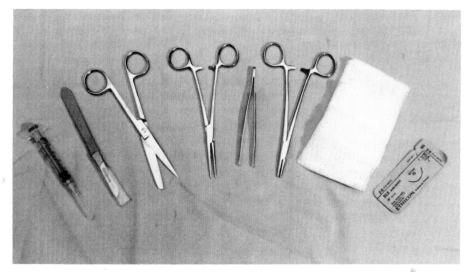

Figure 25–1. General surgical tray set-up.

psychological discomfort. Patient privacy should be maintained to the extent possible.

ANESTHESIA

Anesthesia is the partial or complete loss of sensation. It is used to allow the performance of surgery or other painful procedures. Anesthesia acts to block sensation to pain, to achieve muscle relaxation, to calm fear and anxiety, and to produce amnesia or sleep during surgery.

Anesthetics are classified as general or conduction depending on whether or not they produce unconsciousness. A *general anesthetic* produces unconsciousness by systemic central nervous system (CNS) depression. This type of anesthesia is usually introduced by inhalation or intravenous injection, although it can be administered intramuscularly, rectally, or via the gastrointestinal tract.

Inhalation agents are gases or volatile liquids. For surgical anesthesia, inhalants are usually used in combination with other preanesthetic medications such as sedatives or opiates to relieve pain before and after surgery and tranquilizers to relieve anxiety. Preanesthetic medications may be administered intramuscularly before surgery or intravenously just before the introduction of intravenous anesthetics.

Intravenous anesthetics are sedative-hypnotic drugs that can produce general anesthesia if given in large enough doses. Sodium pentothal is a popular short-acting barbiturate. It can be used alone for procedures of short duration or in combination with inhalation anesthetics for longer procedures.

General anesthesia must be administered on an empty stomach to prevent vomiting and aspiration. General anesthesia causes psychomotor impairment for at least 24 hours after surgery. Patients must be cautioned not to drive or engage in any activity that involves alertness that otherwise could result in harm to the patient. Patients should not consume alcohol or depressant drugs 3 days before and 1 day after anesthesia to avoid the accumulation of CNS depression, or liver damage.

Local anesthetics produce limited and brief effects by decreasing sensation only in the area of injection, freezing, or application. The patient remains conscious. Local anesthetics work by blocking the conduction of nerve transmissions that relate to sensation and pain; therefore they are called *conduction,* or *local anesthetics.*

Agents used for conduction anesthesia act on nerve endings (topical, local infiltration), a single nerve (nerve block), or a group of nerves (regional block, epidural, spinal, saddle block, etc.). Anesthesia by injection is termed *local infiltration anesthesia* and is injected directly into the tissues that will be incised, probed, or sutured. When an agent is injected into and around nerves not at the immediate surgical site, it is termed a *nerve block.* Nerve blocks are commonly used for procedures performed on the fingers and toes. *Topical anesthetics* are applied to the skin; they act by numbing nerve endings. Topical anesthetics may be sprayed, swabbed, or applied in drops, as for eye procedures. Examples of topical anesthetics include benzocaine (Solarcaine) and bucaine (Nupercainal). Ethyl chloride is a spray anesthetic that is used to temporarily "freeze" the skin. Topical anesthetics also are useful in inhibiting cough and gag reflexes during procedures such as bronchoscopy. Patients who have had their gag and cough reflexes anesthetically depressed should not be allowed to eat or drink until the effects of the anesthesia wears off.

Some local anesthetics contain epinephrine. Epinephrine helps to minimize systemic absorption of the anesthesia and prolongs the effects of the anesthesia. When highly vascular areas are anesthetized, epinephrine causes vasoconstriction, which holds the anesthetic in the tissue and helps to minimize local bleeding. There are two conditions in which epinephrine should not be used, however. Because epinephrine can increase cardiac irritability, the drug should not be used with patients who have heart conditions or who are taking certain cardiac medications. Epinephrine also may not be desired in delicate facial surgery where prolonged localization, and therefore prolonged swelling of the tissues, could result in imperfect approximation of the skin edges and a lesser cosmetic result. Plain anesthesia and anesthesia with epinephrine should be stored separately so that the one type is never confused with the other.

Local anesthesia occurs in a few minutes. The physician assesses the patient's feeling before and a few minutes after administration. Procedures are not initiated until the physician is satisfied that the anesthesia has taken effect. Local anesthetics are injected with a 25-, 16-, or 30-gauge, ½- or ⅝-inch (0.125 or 1.6 cm) needle.

High levels of local anesthesia are toxic and should not be used for extensive surgery. Local anesthesia may produce severe allergic reactions or anaphylactic shock. An emergency tray should be on hand whenever a local anesthesia is used.

Topical anesthetics are often used by patients for the temporary relief of minor skin or mucous membrane irritations. The patient should be instructed to avoid contact of the anesthesia with the eyes and to discontinue the medication if a rash or irritation develops at the site.

The first conduction anesthesia was cocaine. Although local anesthesia is commonly referred to as *Novacaine* (procaine), Novacaine is rarely used today. The names of local anesthetics all end in *-caine*. The most common local anesthetics are listed in Table 25–1.

TYPES OF PROCEDURES

In practices that are not surgical specialties, the most frequent surgical procedures are for injuries and conditions of the integument and subcutaneous tissues. These include:

LACERATION REPAIR   Often, a patient will come to the office rather than go to an emergency facility for surgical repair or suturing of a laceration. The wound site is first cleansed and anesthetized, then the wound edges are approximated (closed) with suture, staples, or Steri-strips. Wounds containing debris, such as dirt or glass, must be débrided before skin closure.

TOENAIL RESECTION   A paronychia is an acute bacterial inflammation of the nail bed. If a pocket of purulent material develops under the nail, an incision with a scalpel can be performed under local anesthetic to promote drainage and healing. If the infection is widespread or difficult to heal, removal of the nail may be necessary.

ABSCESS DRAINAGE   An abscess is the accumulation of infectious materials (pus) contained in an area of deteriorated tissue. An abscess is commonly referred to as a "boil." Abscesses can occur anywhere on the body and are painful. Usually, they are surgically incised and drained. The wound is thoroughly cleaned and left unsutured for healing to occur from the innermost region

Table 25–1

LOCAL ANESTHETIC AGENTS

Compound	Dosage (% solution)*	Duration (hours)	Use	Comments
Procaine	0.5, 1.0, 2.0, 4.0	0.3–0.7	Infiltration only, nerve block, spinal (max. 5%)	Ineffective topically, widely used for infiltration
Chloroprocaine	1.0, 2.0, 3.0	0.2–0.5	Infiltration only, nerve block, epidural	Ineffective topically, short duration with epidural
Tetracaine	0.25–2.0	6	Infiltration or topical (1%–2%), nerve block, spinal (max. 0.5%)	Slow in onset and long duration, about 10 times more toxic than procaine after systemic injection
Benzocaine	10.0	>10	Topical only (10%)	Insoluble
Cocaine	1.0–10.0	1–2	Topical only (4%–10%) (respiratory tract)	Central nervous system stimulant, cardiac depressant, vasoconstrictor, drug of abuse
Lidocaine	0.5–4.0	1–2	Infiltration or topical (2%–4%), spinal (max. 5%), epidural	Widely used for infiltration
Mepivacaine	1.0, 1.5, 2.0, 3.0	1–2.5	Infiltration nerve block (1%–3%), spinal	Similar in pharmacologic properties to lidocaine, more rapid onset and longer duration
Etidocaine	0.5, 1.0	3–6	Infiltration or topical, epidural	Two to three times longer acting than lidocaine

Source: Adapted from Conn PM and Gebhart GF: Essentials of Pharmacology. FA Davis, Philadelphia, 1989, pp 179–80.
*Epinephrine or other vasoconstrictor agents are often added to solutions of local anesthetic agents. Addition of a vasoconstrictor will prolong the duration of action, and it is often possible to reduce the amount of local anesthetic agent used.

of the wound outward. Occasionally, a drain or gauze packing is inserted into the wound to prevent premature closing of the skin, which would disrupt the drainage that is necessary for the wound to heal.

CYST REMOVAL A sebaceous cyst is a benign capsule containing a fatty substance secreted by the oil glands. Ordinarily, cysts are attached only to the skin and move freely over the underlying tissue. Sebaceous cysts may occur in any sebaceous gland in the body, but are most common on the scalp, face, ears, neck, and back. Because they are frequently a source of irritation and pain, they are removed. If a cyst becomes infected, the usual procedure is to drain it first with a needle aspiration, then remove it surgically after the infection subsides.

DECONTAMINATION AFTER SURGERY

Once the patient has left the room after a surgical procedure, the medical assistant decontaminates the room. This process is called *terminal decontamination.* Both unused and soiled instruments are gathered and decontaminated, all linen is placed in appropriate bags or hampers, and disposable items are placed in appropriate biohazard bags or disposable sharps collectors. Large equipment and the room itself also must be cleaned.

The safest method for decontaminating instruments is to place the instruments opened in a *washer-sterilizer,* which may be available in the larger facilities that perform a large amount of outpatient surgery. The washer-sterilizer works in the same way as the autoclave. The washer sends cold then hot soapy water over the instruments; then a steam-sterilizing cycle occurs at the end of the wash cycle. The washer-sterilizer removes about 60% of all debris on instruments. After the instruments have been processed in the washer-sterilizer, they are placed in an ultrasound cleaner, which removes the remaining debris from the instruments. After the ultrasonic cycle the instruments are thoroughly rinsed and prepared for sterilization.

If a washer-sterilizer is not available, both unused and soiled instruments are gathered and decontaminated in warm water and detergent and then processed open on trays in the autoclave to render the instruments free of microorganisms that might pose a health hazard to personnel handling the equipment. The medical assistant must wear utility gloves when handling instruments before they are sterilized. Items should be soaked long and well enough to remove all visible debris so that bits of blood and tissues are not "cooked" onto the surface of instruments during the autoclave cycle. The instruments should not be cleaned with a brush before autoclaving to prevent droplets of contaminated moisture from being released into the air. After sterilizing, the instruments are cleaned in the ultrasonic cleaner or by hand using a new pair of utility gloves.

All used and unused linen is placed in a hamper that is color-coded orange-red or labeled with the universal biohazard sign. Large equipment used during surgery is wiped with disinfectant before removal from the room or placing in storage. If spills have occurred on the floor, the floor is disinfected. Any stationary equipment (examination table, electrosurgical power unit) is wiped clean with disinfectant. Any other surfaces showing visible signs of blood or tissue are washed with disinfectant. During all of these procedures, the medical assistant must wear utility gloves and place used cleaning materials in plastic biohazard containers. Please refer to Chapter 24 for further information regarding disinfection.

Removal of medical wastes is regulated by Occupational Safety and Health (OSHA) regulations. Most offices employ an Environmental Protection Agency–approved, licensed waste management service. Each waste hauler provides specific directions for the preparation of items to be removed from the office. For linens, only a laundry service that abides by all OSHA laundering regulations should be used.

Information about the disposal of any chemicals used during surgery is included on the Material Safety Data Sheet provided by the manufacturer. Flushable chemicals can be washed down the sink with large quantities of water. Nonflushable chemicals must be sealed in glass or metal containers and labeled for the waste hauler to properly dispose of the material. Liquid wastes safe for sanitary sewage may be flushed in the toilet. If virulent organisms are suspected or known to be present, they should be autoclaved before the waste is transported. Some facilities prefer to have two autoclaves: one autoclave is used for terminal decontamination and disposal; the other, to sterilize equipment for contact with the patient.

The medical facility is responsible for the handling and disposal of hazardous medical wastes from the time wastes are created. Hazardous medical wastes to which OSHA management regulations apply include the following:

- ❏ Blood products
- ❏ Body fluids
- ❏ Human tissues
- ❏ Human cultures and inoculating loops
- ❏ Vaccines, live and attenuated
- ❏ Sharps
- ❏ Table paper, linen, towels, and gauze with body fluids on them
- ❏ Gloves
- ❏ Disposable instruments and specula
- ❏ Cotton swabs and disposable applicators

POSTOPERATIVE PATIENT CARE

After the office surgical procedure, patient care may include cleansing of the wound, applying dressings to prevent infection and absorb drainage, and patient instructions for preventing complications.

WOUND TYPES

A *wound* is any interruption in the continuity of internal or external soft tissues. A *closed wound* is an injury that occurs without a break in the skin. For example, a closed wound occurs in trauma when a blunt object causes internal bruising (*contusion*) or bleeding (*hematoma*) but does not cause a break in the skin. An open wound involves a break in the skin or mucous membranes.

Wounds are also classified according to the depth of injury. A *superficial wound* does not extend beyond the subcutaneous layer. Examples are abrasion (scraping away of the skin by trauma, heat, or chemicals), second-degree burns, and surface lacerations (tear in the skin). *Deep wounds* are those that extend beyond the subcutaneous layer. A puncture wound is a hole made with a thin, sharp instrument and is an example of a deep wound.

THE HEALING PROCESS

Wound repair is classified according to the way the healing process occurs. Classification depends on (1) the nature of the wound, (2) the amount of tissue lost or removed, and (3) the potential for infection.

When wounds such as sutured surgical incisions heal, there is minimal tissue damage and scarring. This type of healing is called *first intention* (*primary union* or *closure*). *Second intention* wound healing, also known as *granulation* or *indirect union*, occurs when the wound edges are not sutured or approximated. Examples are deep ulcerations, abscesses, and gaping or torn wounds. The body's repair of these wounds is slower and produces more scarring. Repair by *third intention* results when a surgical wound becomes infected and requires reopening of the initial wound. As in secondary intention, these wounds take longer to heal and produce much scar tissue.

The body's ability to heal after surgery or trauma depends on several factors:

1. Adequate circulation and normal clotting time
2. Good general health
3. Proper intake of essential nutrients

Specific cleansing procedures are determined by the physician. As with surgical procedures, there are three general principles in all types of wound cleansing:

1. In using an antiseptic solution, proceed from a clean to a contaminated area.
2. Use one swab or gauze pad per stroke when circular motions cannot be used.
3. If a drain is present, clean around it after the suture is cleansed.

When necessary, the patient, with proper instruction, can perform all these procedures at home.

APPLYING DRESSINGS AND BANDAGES

A dressing is a sterile cover for a wound. Dressings protect the wound from contamination and further injury, help control bleeding, absorb blood or other wound secretions, and help hold the edges of the wound together.

Dressings can be made of many kinds of material; there are several commercially available dressings already lubricated or impregnated with antiseptic. In the medical office, the most commonly used dressing is 4 X 4 inch gauze.

Bandages differ from dressings in that they are nonsterile long strips ranging from 1 to 6 or more inches (2.5 to 15 cm or more) in width. The purposes of a bandage are to:

1. Splint or protect an injured tissue
2. Maintain pressure over an area
3. Aid in circulation of an extremity
4. Hold a sterile dressing in place

The correct procedure for applying a bandage (Fig. 25-2) is as follows: starting at the distal end of the body part and progressing proximally, roll the gauze without stretching or pulling. A bandage applied too tightly can impair circulation and neurologic function. Therefore, it is important to keep the distal body part accessible to visual inspection. At the first sign of cyanosis of the extremity or a complaint of numbness, the bandage must be removed immediately.

PATIENT INSTRUCTION

After the surgical procedure, patients must be informed of the care to be self-administered and the precautions to be observed. While specific instructions depend on the nature of the surgery, some general principles apply. The patient should be instructed to immediately report (1) excessive bleeding; (2) fever; (3) swelling, redness, or streaking around the surgical site; or (4) a dislodged drain.

The patient should be instructed to keep all dressings clean and dry. If the patient is to change the dressing at home, instructions should be given regarding where dressing materials can be purchased, how to proceed, and how often dressing change is required. The physician will usually request a follow-up patient visit to remove sutures, if necessary, and to check the healing process.

SUTURE REMOVAL

After the fifth or sixth day, sutures cease to be effective. If allowed to remain in place too long, they can irritate the skin and act as wicks, carrying bacteria below the skin and into the subcutaneous tissues. The timing of suture removal for nonabsorbable sutures depends on the location of the wound.

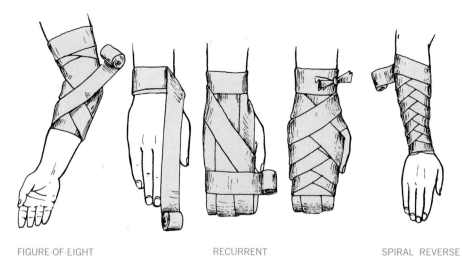

FIGURE-OF-EIGHT RECURRENT SPIRAL REVERSE

Figure 25–2. Types of bandages. (From Thomas CL: Taber's Cyclopedic Medical Dictionary, ed 17. FA Davis, Philadelphia, 1993, p. 190, with permission.)

- ❏ Sutures in the head and neck generally remain in place for 3 to 5 days.
- ❏ In the chest and abdomen, 5 to 7 days.
- ❏ In the lower extremities and over large joints, 7 to 10 days.
- ❏ In delicate facial surgery, sutures may be removed after 24 to 48 hours, to minimize scarring.

To remove sutures, the medical assistant first removes the surgical dressing. If the dressing sticks to the sutures, wet the dressing with hydrogen peroxide or sterile saline and after a moment gently pull it away from the skin. When the moistening agent is allowed to saturate the dressing for a few moments, the dressing usually is easily loosened.

PATIENT TEACHING CONSIDERATIONS

The medical assistant must become actively involved in patient teaching in an office where minor surgery is performed. During the process of obtaining written consent, the medical assistant can reinforce the physician's explanation of the procedure and thereby allay patient anxiety. Simple concepts of asepsis can be introduced so the patient can use the necessary techniques in home care. Sterile and nonsterile techniques may be easily demonstrated when applying a dressing to the wound.

One of the most rewarding moments of medical assisting occurs when the patient's physical and psychological needs have been met. This can be accomplished when the medical assistant, rather than asking "Do you have any questions?," proceeds to verify that the patient has sufficient information to be comfortable before, during, and after a procedure.

RELATED ETHICAL AND LEGAL IMPLICATIONS

The surgical procedures in the medical office require an awareness of legal responsibilities for all related duties. The medical assistant must know that the physician has explained the procedure to the patient before obtaining the patient's signature on the consent form. Many offices have short consent forms for all minor surgical procedures. When preparation at home is necessary, the preoperative instructions are usually given in writing at the physician's direction. The possibility of legal action occurs when complications result from a failure to follow surgical asepsis procedures. For instance, any nicks accidentally made in the skin must be reported immediately to the physician and treated. The physician may even decide it is necessary to cancel the procedure because of the skin break.

When sterilization procedures for birth control are performed in the office, in addition to obtaining written consent, it is essential to have spouse conferences if necessary and wait the required time before the procedure is performed. In many states, the spouse is also required to sign the consent form.

The medical assistant must assure confidentiality for all procedures and surgeries performed in the medical office. The medical assistant must keep confidential any information that is obtained in the course of daily responsibilities. Caution should be exercised to ensure that patient information cannot be overheard by others in the office. Care should be taken during telephone conversations, and patient medical records should never be placed in a public area, such as on a waiting room table. The medical assistant must always be aware of the responsibility to protect the patient's privacy and right to confidentiality.

Insurance billing must accurately reflect the procedure performed. A laceration repair of a ⅕-inch (0.5-cm) wound must state the *exact* size of the wound. Insurance reimbursement is determined by the size or length of a laceration and the number of sutures placed. Patients may receive insufficient reimbursement if billing is incorrect. Intentional failure to report and bill the exact procedures is fraud.

SUMMARY

Strict adherence to aseptic technique is mandatory when assisting with medical office surgery. A possible break in technique should never be disguised. Contamination can and does occur, and the medical assistant should be prepared with additional supplies for immediate correction. Preventing infection must be the ultimate goal of all actions.

The medical assistant who skillfully and knowledgeably handles sterile supplies and equipment enhances the physician's practice and minimizes the patient's risk of infection.

The medical assistant who ensures that the patient understands not only home-care procedure but also the reasons these procedures make a significant contribution toward ensuring the patient's compliance.

DISCUSSION QUESTIONS

1. While putting on sterile gloves, you accidentally touch the little finger of the left-hand glove to your uniform. Dr. Adams is involved in a procedure needing your immediate assistance. What is your response?
2. While removing sterilized instruments from the autoclave, you notice an instrument with a small particle resembling blood that has been baked on. What is your response?
3. You notice that another assistant is removing sterile gauze from a container without sterile gloves or forceps. What is your response?
4. While shaving Mr. Jones in preparation for surgery, you notice that he has been cut slightly. What is your response?

BIBLIOGRAPHY

Centers for Disease Control: Update: Universal precautions for prevention of transmission of human immunodeficiency virus, hepatitis B virus, and other bloodborne pathogens in health-care setting. MMWR 37(24):377–382, 387–388, 1988.
Cohen IK: Wound Healing. WB Saunders, Philadelphia, 1990.
Fuller JR: Surgical Technology, ed 3. WB Saunders, Philadelphia, 1992.
Goldman MA: Pocket Guide to the Operating Room. FA Davis, Philadelphia, 1988.
Hill G: Outpatient Surgery, ed 3. WB Saunders, Philadelphia, 1988.
Lane K (ed): The Saunders Manual of Medical Assisting Practice. WB Saunders, Philadelphia, 1993.
Ripley J: Focus on . . . Physician Office Laboratories Pamphlet "Office Disposal of Hazardous Wastes." College of American Pathologists, Northfield, IL, April 1990.
Roggow PA, Berg DK, and Lewis MD: The Home Rehabilitation Program Guide. Slack, Thorofare, NJ, 1990.
Stoddard CJ and Smith JAR: Complications of Minor Surgery. WB Saunders, Philadelphia, 1986.

PROCEDURE: Prepare equipment and assist during a minor surgical procedure

OSHA STANDARDS:

Terminal Performance Objective: Ensure that all materials and equipment are accounted for, ready to use, and prepared with sterile technique during a surgical routine.

EQUIPMENT:
Mayo stand
Transfer forceps
Anesthesia
Topical hemostatic agent
Waste receptacle
Specimen container
Side stand
Biohazard bags
Sharps collectors

Sterile Packs
Sterile gloves (two pairs)
Towel pack
4 × 4 sponge pack
Patient drape (with window) pack
Needle and syringe pack
Instrument pack
Nonabsorbable suture pack
Absorbable suture pack
Sterile basin pack (two)

PROCEDURE

1. Open the sterile tray packs on the Mayo stand and side surfaces, using the wrappers as the sterile fields, or open a sterile towel package and transfer sterile instruments and supplies to towels from peel-away packages or with transfer forceps.
2. Arrange the articles on the sterile field with transfer forceps.
3. Open sterile needle and syringe unit and "snap" it onto the sterile field.
4. Open a pair of sterile gloves for the physician.
5. Open a sterile window drape package, an adhesive-backed drape package, or a package containing four sterile towels and four towel clamps.
6. Open a sterile towel package, pick up the towel by the two corner ends, and place it slowly over the sterile field starting at the side nearest you (if the procedure is not to begin immediately). **Note:** Once supplies are opened, an assistant should stay in the room.

Operative Procedure

7. Swab the vial of anesthesia and hold upside-down in the palm of your hand at the physician's eye level. Hold the vial firmly with the label facing the physician while the physician withdraws the medication from the vial.

PRINCIPLE

1. Procedure materials, such as antiseptics, anesthetics, instruments, glove sizes, syringe and needle sizes, suture sizes, and dressings, are set up in advance of the physician's arrival.
2. Instruments and supplies are neatly arranged in the sequence of the procedure or in groups of like instruments for safe and efficient location during the procedure.
3. The sterile syringe will be handled by the gloved physician to administer the local anesthetic.
4. A nonsterile assistant opens sterile supplies before and during the procedure.
5. Disposable drapes mark the boundary of the operative site and create a sterile field that separates the work area from the resident bacteria on the patient's skin.
6. Towels should not be fanned to prevent airborne contamination. Starting this procedure at the far side of the tray would pass the arms directly over the field and contaminate it. After gloving, the physician first sets up the surgical site with the fenestrated drape.

7. A nonsterile assistant handles the nonsterile vial of anesthesia during the procedure. If the medical assistant is to wear gloves, the surgical hand scrub is performed while the physician is waiting for the local anesthesia to take effect.

PROCEDURE

8. Assist as required and anticipate the physician's needs.
   a. Uncover the sterile tray.
   b. Adjust lighting as needed.
   c. Restrain patients or limbs.
   d. Hold basin for receipt of soiled sponges (gauze).
   e. Hold specimen container for receipt of specimens.
   f. Hand instruments and supplies (if gloved).
   g. Keep sterile field neat and orderly (if gloved).
   h. Retract tissue (if gloved).
   i. Sponge blood from site (if gloved).
   j. Cut sutures (if gloved).
9. Reassure the patient and offer support as needed. Stay with the patient and assist the patient throughout the recovery period.

PRINCIPLE

8. A nonsterile assistant provides the physician with another set of hands for obtaining additional instruments or assisting. This cooperative effort ensures the quality of patient care and asepsis. During the procedure, a gloved assistant touches only sterile items, cares for the open sterile field, and passes instruments and supplies to the physician. If the assistant is to glove, the gloves are put on while the physician is draping the operative site and administering the anesthesia.

9. Physicians often must rely on the medical assistant to provide patient support since their attention is necessarily focused on the surgical procedure. Patients may become dizzy or disoriented after minor surgery and should be protected from accidental injury.

PROCEDURE: Assist with suturing

OSHA STANDARDS:

Terminal Performance Objective: Assist in the repair of an incision or a laceration without a break in sterile technique.

EQUIPMENT: Mayo stand
Transfer forceps
Anesthesia
Topical hemostatic agent
Sterile saline
Side stand
Biohazard bags
Waste receptacle
Sharps collectors

Sterile Packs
Sterile gloves (two pairs)
Towel pack (four towels)
4 X 4 sponge pack (24 to 36)
Patient drape (with window) pack
Needle and syringe pack
Nonabsorbable suture and needle pack
Absorbable suture and needle pack
Sterile basin pack (two)
Scalpel blade packs (No. 11 or 15)
Suture pack: needle holder, No. 3 scalpel handle, two
scissors, three hemostats, thumb dressing forceps, two
Allis tissue forceps or skin hooks

PROCEDURE

1. Glove yourself.

2. Position yourself across from the physician.
3. Place two sponges next to the wound site.

4. Pick up additional sponges and mop the wound when directed by the physician.
5. If skin edges are to be trimmed, hold surgical scissors halfway down its shaft and pass it with a firm and purposeful motion until the handles "snap" in the physician's palm. Do not let go of the instrument until you feel the physician grasp it.
6. If the laceration needs to be incised, grasp the scalpel blade with a hemostat and mount the blade onto the scalpel handle. Keep the blade visible and pass the scalpel to the physician blade edge down.
7. Dispose of soiled sponges in a waste receptacle (previously placed nearby) and place two dry sponges next to the wound.
8. Pick up additional sponges and mop the wound when directed by the physician or hand to the physician as needed.

PRINCIPLE

1. During the procedure the scrub (gloved) assistant must protect the sterile field from contamination, notify the physician if there is a break in sterile technique, pass instruments, assist in the suturing, and keep the operative site free from blood.
2. Sterile team members face each other.
3. The physician will use the sponges to mop up blood and drainage during inspection of the wound.
4. The assistant is responsible for keeping the site free from blood.
5. The physician will not have to look up to take the instrument. Letting go too soon may cause the instrument to drop to the floor or onto the patient.

6. Safe handling of sharp instruments protects the physician from injury. Blades should never be held in the bare hand.

7. Additional bleeding will occur during the incision. Sponges should be used only once, then discarded.

8. The assistant is responsible for keeping the site free from blood.

PROCEDURE

9. If a hemostat is requested, pass it to the physician.

10. If the laceration needs to be grasped, pass toothed forceps to the physician.

11. Hold the suture needle point up 4 to 5 inches (10 to 12.5 cm) over the sterile field.

12. Pick up the needle holder and clamp the needle at the upper third of the needle.

13. With your nondominant hand, hold the suture thread up and off the sterile field.

14. With your dominant hand, hold the needle holder halfway down its shaft with the suture needle pointed up and pass it to the physician. Let go of the thread only when you are sure the physician sees it.

15. Pick up the surgical scissors with your dominant hand and two sponges with your nondominant hand.

16. After the physician has tied a suture and holds the threads taut, with the scissors parallel to the wound site cut both strands together above the knot, at the length requested. (Tails are usually ⅛ to ¼ inch [0.312 to 0.625 cm].)

17. Mop the closure gently once with the sponge and discard the sponge.

18. Repeat the process as each suture is placed.

19. Receive used instruments and place them back on the field or in a basin and continue to mop up blood from the surgical site.

20. Instruct the patient in postoperative care:
    a. Follow-up appointment for the removal of sutures or explanation of suture absorption process if absorbable sutures were used
    b. Reporting signs of infection or other complications
    c. Keeping dressing dry and intact and technique for reapplying if patient is to change it
    d. Skin care and recognition and care of wound drainage
    e. Application of cold dry compresses
    f. Medications prescribed for pain

PRINCIPLES

9. If there is sudden hemorrhage from a blood vessel, the vessel must be clamped.

10. Toothed forceps will grasp the tissue when the needle is passed through.

11. Keeping the suture needle and thread unit close to the field prevents the thread from contact with a nonsterile area.

12. Clamping too near the point may damage the needle, clamping in the middle bends the metal, and clamping too near the thread may cut the thread. **Note:** straight needles are held by the hand not in a needle holder.

13. To prevent the thread from contact with a nonsterile area.

14. Pointing the needle upward keeps the needle visible and protects the physician from injury.

15. To prepare for the suture cutting and to mop up additional bleeding that may occur as the needle is passed through the tissues.

16. Too short a strand may loosen the knot; too long a strand may cause serious irritation to the patient during the healing process. Holding the scissors parallel provides control when cutting and prevents cutting the tissue.

17. Friction may damage the newly created wound edge. Once a sponge has been used, it must be discarded.

18. The continuous suture technique requires only one cut. The interrupted technique requires several cuts. In the interrupted technique, the physician places the first suture midpoint of the wound, dividing the wound in half. The next sutures are placed midpoint between the first suture and the wound ends, thus dividing the wound into fourths, then so on until the physician is satisfied that enough sutures are spaced evenly. The tissues need only be approximated.

19. The physician will not have to look away from the surgical site.

20. Thorough patient instruction ensures continuity of care and minimizes potential problems.

PROCEDURE: Assist with an incision and drainage

OSHA STANDARDS: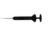

Terminal Performance Objective: Assist with an incision of an abscess and the drainage of accumulated infectious materials without a break in sterile technique.

EQUIPMENT:
Mayo stand
Transfer forceps
Anesthesia
Gauze packing or penrose drain
Specimen container
Side stand
Waste receptacle
Biohazard bags
Sharp collectors

Sterile Packs
Sterile gloves (two pairs)
Towel pack (four towels)
4 × 4 sponge pack (24 to 36)
Patient drape (with window) pack
Sterile basin pack (two)
Scalpel blade packs (No. 11 and 15)
Irrigation and drainage pack: No. 3 scalpel handle,
  two pairs of scissors, Mosquito hemostat,
  thumb dressing, probe, abscess needle

PROCEDURE

1. Glove yourself.

2. Position yourself across from the physician.
3. Place two sponges next to the abscess site.

4. Pick up additional sponges to mop the drainage when directed by the physician.
5. At the time of the incision, grasp the scalpel blade with a hemostat and mount the blade onto the scalpel handle. Keep the blade visible and pass the scalpel to the physician blade edge down.
6. Hold the scalpel halfway down the shaft and pass it with a firm and purposeful motion until the handle "snaps" in the physician's palm. Do not let go of the instrument until you feel the physician grasp it.
7. Dispose of soiled sponges in a waste receptacle (previously placed nearby) and place two dry sponges next to the abscess.
8. Pick up additional sponges and mop the abscess when directed by the physician or hand to the physician as needed.
9. Receive used instruments and place them back on the field or in a basin and continue to mop up blood and drainage from the surgical site.
10. If a drain is to be inserted, pass a rubber penrose drainage tube or a gauze wick.

PRINCIPLE

1. During the procedure the scrub (gloved) assistant must protect the sterile field from contamination, notify the physician if there is a break in sterile technique, pass instruments, assist in the suturing, and keep the operative site free from blood.
2. Sterile team members face each other.
3. The physician will use the sponges during the inspection of the abscess.
4. The assistant is responsible for keeping the site free from blood and drainage.
5. Safe handling of sharp instruments protects the physician from injury. Blades should never be held in the bare hand.

6. The physician will not have to look up to take the instrument. Letting go too soon may cause the instrument to drop to the floor or onto the patient.

7. Additional bleeding will occur during the incision. Sponges should be used only once, then discarded.

8. The assistant is responsible for keeping the site free from blood.

9. The physician will not have to look away from the surgical site.

10. To keep the edges of the tissues spread apart, which facilitates drainage.

PROCEDURE

PRINCIPLES

Postoperative Procedure

11. Apply a sterile or nonsterile bandage and tape to the dressing.

12. Instruct the patient in postoperative care:
    a. Follow-up appointment and when to return to usual routines
    b. Reporting signs of infection or other complications
    c. Daily dressing changes in the presence of copious drainage
    d. Skin care and recognition and care of wound drainage
    e. Application of warm, moist compresses
    f. Medications prescribed and their purposes

11. Pressure dressings protect the abscess from injury or contamination, maintain constant pressure, hold the abscess edges together, and control bleeding.

12. Thorough patient instruction ensures continuity of care and minimizes potential problems.

PROCEDURE: Assist with the removal of a cyst

OSHA STANDARDS:

Terminal Performance Objective: Assist with the excision of a benign sebaceous cyst without a break in sterile technique.

EQUIPMENT: Mayo stand
Transfer forceps
Anesthesia
Topical hemostatic agent
Sterile saline
Side stand
Biohazard bags
Waste receptacle
Sharps collectors

Sterile Packs
Sterile gloves (two pairs)
Towel pack (four towels)
4 × 4 sponge pack (24 to 36)
Patient drape (with window) pack
Needle and syringe pack
Nonabsorbable suture pack
Absorbable suture pack
Sterile basin pack (two)
Scalpel blade packs (No. 11 or 15)
Suture Pack: needle holder, No. 3 scalpel handle, two
    scissors, three Kelly hemostats, thumb dressing for-
    ceps, two Allis tissue forceps, dissector, skin hook

PROCEDURE

1. Glove yourself.

2. Position yourself across from the physician.
3. Place two sponges next to the surgical site.

4. Pick up additional sponges and mop the incision when directed by the physician.
5. Grasp the scalpel blade with a hemostat and mount the blade onto the scalpel handle. Keep the blade visible and pass the scalpel to the physician blade edge down.
6. Pass grasping forceps to the physician. Hold the forceps halfway down its shaft and pass it with a firm and purposeful motion until the handles "snap" in the physician's palm. Do not let go of the instrument until you feel the physician grasp it.
7. Dispose of soiled sponges in a waste receptacle (previously placed nearby) and place two dry sponges next to the wound.
8. Pick up additional sponges and mop the wound when directed by the physician or hand to the physician as needed.

PRINCIPLE

1. During the procedure the scrub (gloved) assistant must protect the sterile field from contamination, notify the physician if there is a break in sterile technique, pass instruments, assist in the suturing, and keep the operative site free from blood.
2. Sterile team members face each other.
3. The physician will use the sponge to mop up blood during the first incision.
4. The assistant is responsible for keeping the site free from blood.
5. Safe handling of sharp instruments protects the physician from injury. Blades should never be held in the bare hands.

6. The physician will not have to look up to take the instrument. Letting go too soon may cause the instrument to drop to the floor or onto the patient. The forceps will hold the ellipse of skin as the physician makes an elliptical incision.
7. Additional bleeding will occur during the incision. Sponges should be used only once, then discarded.

8. The assistant is responsible for keeping the site free from blood.

PROCEDURE

9. Pass surgical scissors to the physician. Hold surgical scissors halfway down its shaft and pass it with a firm and purposeful motion until the handles "snap" in the physician's palm. Do not let go of the instrument until you feel the physician grasp it.
10. If the incision needs to be retracted, pass Allis tissue forceps to the physician or retract the ellipse of the skin with the Allis forceps.
11. If a vessel begins to bleed, or if a hemostat is requested, pass it to the physician. If bleeding points must be controlled by sutures, prepare fine catgut ligatures (sutures). The skin is closed with nonabsorbable sutures.

12. Hold the suture needle point up 4 to 5 inches (10 cm to 12.5 cm) over the sterile field.

13. Pick up the needle holder and clamp the needle at the upper third of the needle.

14. With your nondominant hand, hold the suture thread up and off the sterile field.
15. With your dominant hand, hold the needle holder halfway down its shaft with the suture needle pointed up and pass it to the physician. Let go of the thread only when you are sure the physician sees it.
16. Pick up the surgical scissors with your dominant hand and two sponges with your nondominant hand.

17. After the physician has tied a suture and holds the threads taut, place the scissors parallel to the wound site and cut both strands together between the knot and the physician to the length requested. (Tails are usually ⅛ to ¼ inch [0.312 to 0.625 cm].)
18. Mop the closure gently once with the sponge and discard the sponge.
19. Repeat the process as each suture is placed.

20. Receive used instruments and place them back on the field or in a basin and continue to mop up blood from the surgical site.

Postoperative Procedure

21. Instruct the patient in postoperative care:
    a. Follow-up appointment for the removal of sutures or explanation of sutures absorption process if absorbable sutures were used
    b. Reporting signs of infection or other complications
    c. Keeping dressing dry and intact and technique for reapplying if patient is to change it
    d. Skin care and recognition and care of wound drainage
    e. Application of cold dry compresses
    f. Medications prescribed for pain

PRINCIPLE

9. The physician will not have to look up to take the instrument. Letting go too soon may cause the instrument to drop to the floor or onto the patient. The physician will use the scissors to remove the cyst intact, if possible.
10. Toothed forceps will grasp the tissue and expose the cyst to be removed.
11. If there is sudden hemorrhage from a blood vessel, the vessel must be clamped or ligated.

12. Keeping the suture needle and thread unit close to the field prevents the thread from contact with a nonsterile area.
13. Clamping too near the point may damage the needle, clamping in the middle bends the metal, and clamping too near the thread may cut the thread. **Note:** straight needles are held by the hand not in a needle holder.
14. To prevent the thread from contact with a nonsterile area.
15. Pointing the needle upward keeps the needle visible and protects the physician from injury.

16. To prepare for the suture cutting and to mop up additional bleeding that may occur as the needle is passed through the tissues.
17. Too short a strand may loosen the knot; too long a strand may cause serious irritation to the patient during the healing process. Holding the scissors parallel provides control when cutting and prevents cutting the tissue.
18. Friction may damage the newly created wound edge. Once a sponge has been used, it must be discarded.
19. The continuous suture technique requires only one cut. The interrupted technique requires several cuts. In the interrupted technique, the physician places the first suture midpoint of the wound, dividing the wound in half. The next suture is placed midpoint between the first suture and the wound ends, thus dividing the wound into fourths, and so on until the physician is satisfied that enough sutures are spaced evenly. The tissues need only be approximated.
20. The physician will not have to look away from the surgical site.

21. Thorough patient instruction ensures continuity of care and minimizes potential problems.

PROCEDURE: Apply a sterile dressing and complete postsurgical routines

OSHA STANDARDS:

Terminal Performance Objective: Apply a sterile dressing after the completion of minor surgery, instruct the patient in wound and dressing care, and clean the operatory in preparation for the next patient.

EQUIPMENT: Mayo stand
Topical hemostatic agent
Sterile saline
Side stand
Adhesive tape
Biohazard bags
Waste receptacle

Sterile Packs
Sterile gloves (two pairs)
Patient drape (with window) pack
Dressings
Bandage
Sterile basin pack
4 × 4 sponge pack (6 to 10)

PROCEDURE

1. Obtain the dressing and bandage materials, then cut the lengths of adhesive tape needed.
2. Open the dressing packages and create a sterile field.
3. Put on gloves.
4. Cleanse the operative site with wet and dry sponges. Place a dry sponge on the sutures and gently clean the surrounding area with saline dampened gauze.
5. Apply a sterile dressing without touching the wound or the patient's skin.
6. Lift the sterile window drape off the field with minimal movement.
7. Apply the bandage as ordered, either as a circular bandage or additional dressings and tape.

8. Secure the bandage with tape to hold the bandage in place. The bandage should conform to the contour of the body part being bandaged.
9. Instruct the patient in postoperative care:
   a. Follow-up appointment and when to return to usual routines
   b. Reporting signs of infection or other complications
   c. Keeping dressing dry and intact and technique for reapplying if patient is to change it
   d. Skin care and recognition and care of wound drainage
   e. Application of cold or warm, moist compresses
   f. Medications prescribed and their purposes
10. Give written follow-up instructions.

11. Break down the Mayo tray and sterile field after the patient has left the room.

PRINCIPLE

1. Equipment readiness is essential to save time and ensure procedural safety.
2. Routines are performed in a sterile field.
3. Postsurgical dressings are sterile.
4. The dry sponge protects the wound edges during cleaning.

5. The patient's skin would contaminate the sterile gloves.
6. The sterile field should not be removed until the wound is covered and ready for bandaging.
7. To apply pressure to control bleeding; to protect a wound from contamination; to hold medication or a dressing in place; or to protect, support, or immobilize an injured part of the body.
8. To seal the wound and stay in place.

9. Thorough patient instruction ensures continuity of care and minimizes potential problems.

10. Patient education facilitates cooperation and compliance with the physician's orders. Instructions should be in writing for the patient to take home.
11. If there is an unexpected contamination of the operative site, more materials may be needed from the sterile field.

12. Provide for the safe removal of needles and sharp instruments.
    a. Glove with disposable gloves.
    b. Place syringe-needle units, disposable scalpel blades, and suture needles into a sharps container at the site.
    c. Carefully place sharp instruments into a basin to be rinsed off immediately in cold running water.
13. Dispose of soiled materials and gloves in a plastic bag:
    a. Remove one glove inside out.
    b. Put the bare hand into a plastic bag.
    c. Through the bag, remove the second glove.
    d. Pick up all soiled materials and hold them through the bag; use the other hand to grasp the top edge of the bag and pull it down over the hand and dressings.
14. Clean the room and dispose of contaminated objects in appropriate waste containers.
15. Chart the procedure and patient instructions. Label the specimen container and complete a laboratory request form. Chart the specimen disposition. Chart the next appointment.

12. Prevents accidental punctures through the use of universal blood and body fluid precautions.

13. All soiled materials must be in a plastic bag before disposing for incineration or other disposal.

14. Prevents the spread of infectious materials and possible cross-contamination to the next patient.
15. To protect against legal action in the event the patient fails to follow instructions or causes injury to the operative site.

PROCEDURE: Change a dressing

OSHA STANDARDS:

Terminal Performance Objective: Care for healing wounds and apply a new dressing using sterile technique and without injury to the approximated skin edges within a reasonable time standard.

EQUIPMENT: Mayo stand
Sterile saline or hydrogen peroxide
Antiseptic solution
Waste receptacle
Adhesive tape
Bandage scissors
Baby oil
Plastic biohazard bag

Sterile Packs
Sterile gloves
Sterile towel pack
4 × 4 sponge pack (6 to 10)
Dressing and bandage

PROCEDURE

1. Prepare the room, assemble and set up equipment on a side stand or table, and adjust the lighting.

2. Instruct the patient on clothing removal and gowning. Position and drape the patient to provide exposure and availability to the wound site.

3. Position and support the bandaged part. Place dry toweling underneath the area.

4. Inspect the bandage and ask the patient to point to the wound.

5. Put on disposable gloves.

6. Slowly peel back the tape edges along the longitudinal axis of the wound by holding the skin taut and pushing the skin away from the tape.

7. Use baby oil if the tape does not release easily.

8. If the dressing is wrapped with roller gauze, cut through the bandage on the side opposite the wound and lift the bandage by the ends toward the wound. Leave the dressing in place.

9. Examine the bandage and place in a plastic bag.

10. Loosen the dressing by lifting one corner toward the wound site. Check that the dressing is not adhering to the wound.

11. Release the first corner, then lift the opposite corner toward the wound and off.

12. If the dressing adheres to the wound, soak a clean 4 × 4 gauze in hydrogen peroxide or sterile saline solution. Place the soaked 4 × 4 on the dressing and allow it to set for a few seconds.

13. Place the dressing in a waste receptacle skin side facing up.

14. If the wound must be cleaned, hold a dry 4 × 4 gauze sponge over the wound and gently scrub the surrounding area with 4 × 4 sponge soaked in hydrogen peroxide, sterile saline solution, or surgical soap.

PRINCIPLE

1. A clean room diminishes the chance of infection. Equipment readiness is essential to save time and ensure procedural safety.

2. To ensure patient comfort and safety during the procedure. Enough clothing must be removed to fully expose the bandaged part.

3. To keep the part to be examined immobilized and to set up a work field.

4. Verifies the location of the wound and ensures safety in removal of the bandage.

5. Dressings should not be handled by ungloved hands.

6. Removing tape in the same plane is less painful.

7. Oil is soothing and works as well as the more irritating adhesive solvents.

8. To avoid injuring the wound with the scissors.

9. To enclose soiled materials.

10. Pulling a dressing away from the wound may tear some of the newly formed tissues.

11. Pulling away from the wound may tear some of the newly formed tissues.

12. Moisture will loosen the tissues from the dressing.

13. The physician will examine the dressing for amount of bleeding or drainage.

14. In the process of liberating oxygen, peroxide will loosen dried blood and exudate. For suture removal, skin surfaces must be as clean as possible.

15. Rinse with sterile water or sterile saline using a new 4 × 4 sponge or a syringe and pour antiseptic solution over the wound.

15. To remove the soap and debris.

16. Cover the area with sterile gauze and ask the physician to examine the wound.

16. The physician will observe the skin and wound site and order suture removal, redressing, or leaving the area exposed.

17. Dispose of dressing and gloves in a plastic bag:
    a. Remove one glove inside out.
    b. Put the bare hand into a plastic bag.
    c. Through the bag, remove the second glove.
    d. Pick up all soiled materials and hold them through the bag; use the other hand to grasp the top edge of the bag and pull it down over the hand and dressings.

17. All soiled materials must be in a plastic bag before disposing via incineration or some other form of disposal.

18. Document the condition of the wound on the patient chart. Include drainage; if present; color; smoothness, inflammation; or signs of irritation.

18. To protect against legal action in the event the patient fails to follow instructions or causes injury to the wound.

PROCEDURE: Remove sutures from a healed incision

OSHA STANDARDS: —

Terminal Performance Objective: Remove dermal sutures from a closed incision with sterile technique and without injury to the approximated skin edges.

EQUIPMENT: Mayo stand
Sterile saline
Biohazard bags
Waste receptacle
Sharps collectors

Sterile Packs
Sterile gloves
Sterile towel pack
4 × 4 sponge pack (6 to 10)
Suture removal pack: suture
removal scissors, thumb
dressing forceps

PROCEDURE

1. Follow the steps for removing a dressing.
2. Wash hands after removing the dressing and cleaning the site.
3. Open the suture removal pack.
4. Glove with clean or sterile disposable gloves.

5. Place one 4 × 4 gauze sponge on a clean towel next to the patient.
6. Using the forceps, grasp the knot and gently pull upwards.
7. Cut the shorter end of the suture as close to the skin as possible. Pull the suture out by the knot.

8. For continuous suture removal, cut the suture at each skin puncture site on one side only and remove the suture through the opposite side.
9. Pat the site with antiseptic. If there is oozing, apply a small dressing.

10. Instruct the patient to avoid injury to the tender and newly healed skin.
11. Document the condition of the wound on the patient chart. Include drainage, if present; color; smoothness; inflammation; or signs of irritation.

PRINCIPLE

1. To ensure appropriate handling of dressing materials.
2. To prevent the transfer of microorganisms.

3. Sterile instruments and gauze are used.
4. Gloves that have handled soiled dressings should not be used for a sterile procedure.
5. The sutures will be deposited on the gauze for a suture count.
6. To pull the suture away from the skin.

7. To allow the suture to be pulled free so that only the part of the suture which is under the skin touches underlying tissue. No segment of the suture above the skin should be drawn below the skin. Drawing the suture under the skin would drag surface bacteria into the underlying tissues.
8. To avoid dragging suture material and bacteria under the skin.

9. The small suture punctures are a potential site for infection. Do not overmoisten the incision area with too much antiseptic.
10. Thorough patient instruction ensures continuity of care and minimizes potential problems.
11. To protect against legal action in the event the patient fails to follow instructions or causes injury to the wound.

HIGHLIGHTS
Protect Yourself When Handling Sharps

A needlestick or a cut from a contaminated scalpel can lead to infection from hepatitis B virus (HBV) or human immunodeficiency virus (HIV) which causes acquired immunodeficiency syndrome (AIDS). Although few cases of AIDS have been documented from occupational exposure, approximately 8700 health care workers each year contract hepatitis B. About 200 will die as a result. The new Occupational Health and Safety Administration standard covering blood-borne pathogens specifies measures to reduce these risks of infection.

PROMPT DISPOSAL

The best way to prevent cuts and sticks is to minimize contact with sharps. That means disposing of them immediately after use. Puncture-resistant containers must be available nearby to hold contaminated sharps—either for disposal or, for reusable sharps, later decontamination for reuse. When reprocessing contaminated reusable sharps, employees must not reach by hand into the holding container. Contaminated sharps must never be sheared or broken.

Recapping, bending, or removing needles is only permissible if there is no feasible alternative or if required for a specific medical procedure such as blood gas analysis. If recapping, bending, or removal is necessary, workers must use either a mechanical device or a one-handed technique. If recapping is essential—for example, between multiple injections for the same patient—employees must avoid using both hands to recap. Employees might recap with a one-handed "scoop" technique, using the needle itself to pick up the cap, pushing cap and sharp together against a

hard surface to ensure a tight fit. Or they might hold the cap with tongs or forceps to place it on the needle.

SHARPS CONTAINERS

Containers for used sharps must be puncture-resistant. The sides and the bottom must be leakproof. They must be labeled or color coded red to ensure that everyone knows the contents are hazardous. Containers for disposable sharps must have a lid, and they must be maintained upright to keep liquids and the sharps inside.

Employees must never reach by hand into containers of contaminated sharps. Containers for reusable sharps could be equipped with wire basket liners for easy removal during reprocessing, or employees could use tongs or forceps to withdraw the contents. Reusable sharps disposal containers may not be opened, emptied, or cleaned manually.

Containers need to be located as near to as feasible the area of use. In some cases, they may be placed on carts to prevent access to mentally disturbed or pediatric patients. Containers also should be available wherever sharps may be found, such as in laundries. The containers must be replaced routinely and not be overfilled, which can increase the risk of needlesticks or cuts.

HANDLING CONTAINERS

When employees are ready to discard containers, they should first close the lids. If there is a chance of leakage from the primary container, the employees should use a secondary container that is closable, labeled, or color coded and leak resistant.

Careful handling of sharps can prevent injury and reduce the risk of infection. By following these work practices, employees can decrease their chances of contracting bloodborne illness.

Source: US Department of Labor, Occupational Safety and Health Administration.

> In the past, it was expected that the physician would assume absolute responsibility for the diagnosis and treatment of the patient. No longer can this view be upheld. Physicians must now rely on the competence of co-workers not trained as medical practitioners, but whose specialized knowledge is of vital importance to the diagnosis and treatment of patients.
>
> John Walters, MD
> Principles of Disease

CHAPTER OUTLINE

Chapter 26

*R*ehabilitation Medicine

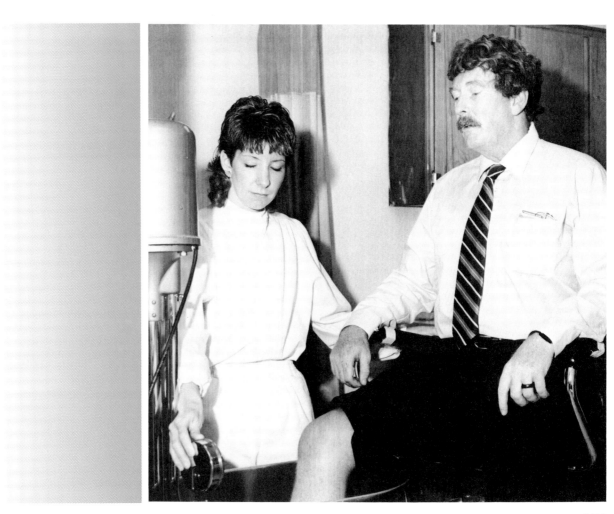

PATIENT TEACHING CONSIDERATIONS

RELATED ETHICAL AND LEGAL IMPLICATIONS

SUMMARY

DISCUSSION QUESTIONS

BIBLIOGRAPHY

HIGHLIGHTS
Exercise and Health

LEARNING OBJECTIVES

Upon completing this chapter, you will be able to:

1. List the objectives of physical therapy.
2. Define and describe the various types of exercises.
3. Describe the various devices for assisting the patient in mobility and how to assist patients in learning to use crutches.
4. Describe the procedures and precautions necessary when treating the patient with deep heat.
5. List the objectives of sports medicine.
6. List the objectives of occupational therapy.
7. Describe the role of psychotherapy in comprehensive patient care.
8. List some of the services performed in podiatry.

DACUM EDUCATIONAL COMPONENTS

1. Serve as a liaison between the physician and others (2.5).
2. Schedule and monitor appointments (3.2).
3. Locate resources and information for patients and employers (3.6).
4. Operate and maintain facilities and equipment safely (6.2).

Glossary

Cerebral vascular accident: a disorder of the blood vessels supplying the cerebrum, due to an impaired blood supply to, and ischemia in, parts of the brain; commonly called a "stroke"

Contractures: abnormal shortening of muscle tissue which can lead to permanent disability

Débridement: to revitalize a wound or the tissue surrounding a wound by removing devitalized tissue until only healthy tissue is exposed

Edema: the abnormal accumulation of fluid in the intercellular tissues of the body

Fitness: to be in overall good physical condition, including cardiovascular strength, muscular strength, and flexibility

Isometric contraction: muscle contraction without any appreciable shortening of the muscle, produced by either isometric exercise or electronic muscle stimulation

Isometric exercise: active exercise performed against a stable resistance with no appreciable change in the length of the muscle

Isotonic exercise: active exercise performed by moving weights or pulleys, with shortening of the muscle

Physiatry: the field of medicine using physical therapy

Reeducation: muscle training taught to the patient who has lost some control over a major skeletal muscle

Sprain: twisting of a joint with partial rupture of the ligaments and possible damage to muscle, tendons, blood vessels, and nerves; a sprain is much more serious than a strain

Strain: the overstretching of a muscle without swelling from overexercising

Comprehensive health care is a creative process. Physicians rely on a team of health care professionals to work together and contribute specialized services for the good of the patient. When does the family physician recommend that a patient see a psychologist, for example? Many times it will be for basic psychological problems or psychological reactions to a disability. The parameters for referral at first may be unclear or may appear not to require the specialist's expertise. In some instances, the general practitioner will perform the basic procedures used by specialists in these disciplines. Although the highest levels of physical, mental, social, emotional, educational, and vocational rehabilitation will be applied by trained therapists, medical assistants should be prepared to offer assistance and information to the patient regarding the rehabilitation concepts presented in this chapter, while respecting the skill parameters of their profession.

There are three reasons for presenting the materials in this chapter. First, as the field of rehabilitation has grown in both sophistication and complexity, many subspecialties have emerged that have greatly enhanced the potential for comprehensive patient care. In the field of sports medicine, for example, enormous strides have been made in the rehabilitation of athletic injuries. These advances are no longer the private domain of a privileged few professional athletes. In fact, the benefits of advances in sports medicine have been passed along to the family physician and have resulted in the development of a new awareness about sports injuries as well as the introduction of new treatment techniques in the primary care physician's office. Medical assistants must be aware of the nature of these specialties and of their own roles as pertains to them, so that they can provide appropriate assistance when the generalist prescribes treatments related to physical therapy, psychotherapy, or other disciplines.

A second important reason for medical assistants to familiarize themselves with these professions is to enable them to participate in patient teaching. Often, when a patient is instructed to visit a specialist, such as a physical therapist, the patient (or the family) will have questions and concerns regarding the referral. The medical assistant should be prepared to respond appropriately to these questions and concerns and to help the patient feel more positive about visiting a new member of the health care team. If the patient's basic queries are met with uncertainty by the medical assistant, the proposed treatment will seem even more mysterious and threatening and thus will undermine the patient's confidence in the prescribed therapy.

A third compelling reason for discussing these allied disciplines is related to their increasing interaction and overlap with other areas of medicine. Therefore, they represent attractive additions to the potential employment opportunities for medical assistants. Although the scope of medical assisting practice may be somewhat limited because of the nature of the work performed in these offices, the medical assistant may function appropriately and according to the skill parameters of the medical assisting profession in a number of capacities. For instance, medical assistants may assume office management responsibilities in these disciplines and may, within well-defined guidelines, offer assistance in aspects of running the clinical practice.

Although there are arguably more disciplines than those represented here, the five listed were chosen because of the frequency with which physicians refer patients to specialists in these areas.

Physical therapy. The process of using exercise or manipulation of body parts to facilitate or assist the restoration of an injured body part to normal functioning

Sports medicine. The use of a number of different modalities that enable the patient to recover quickly and return to high levels of activity with minimal loss of the desired fitness level

Occupational therapy. Preparation and training that enable the patient to return to work or to obtain employment after a medical problem

Psychotherapy. The attempt to improve psychological functioning via personality, behavioral, and interpersonal analysis

Podiatry. The treatment of medical problems of the foot

PHYSICAL THERAPY

The *physical therapist* is an allied health professional who has completed at least a 4-year baccalaureate training program in physical therapy and has received state licensure. A physician who specializes in physical medicine and rehabilitation is called a *physiatrist.* Physical therapists deal primarily with movement dysfunction and work with body parts that have been damaged or injured due to disease, accident, or amputation. The physical therapist may use physical and mechanical agents such as massage, active or passive exercise, hot or cold application, electricity, or diathermy to diagnose, treat, and prevent disease. In some instances, although more infrequently today, the physician will present a program of physical therapy for a patient and then expect the physical therapist to implement the mechanics of the program. Usually the physician refers the patient and completely relies on the physical therapist's judgment relative to program development and implementation. The approach taken depends on the physician, the physician's specialty, the patient, the nature of the physical problem, and the relationship between the physician and the therapist. The objectives of physical therapy are usually to relieve pain; to increase or improve circulation; to increase or restore muscular function; or to improve strength, range of motion, or joint mobility. In addition to the use of exercise and physical agents, physical therapists teach patients how to exercise and new ways of locomotion, transportation, and daily activities. In situations where the physician prescribes an elementary physical routine and the expertise of the therapist is not required, the medical assistant may be used to instruct the patient.

Physical medicine is an enormously broad field, and although subtopics listed below do not represent a summary of its methods, they have been chosen for discussion because they represent the majority of practical applications in the primary care physician's office.

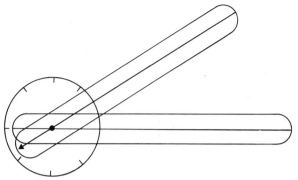

Figure 26-1. A universal goniometer.

RANGE OF MOTION

Almost every joint in the body allows some sort of movement of the bones that make up the joint. The amount of movement that the joint allows, expressed in degrees, is called the *range of motion* (*ROM*). See Figure 20-7 for examples of the normal movements of the body at the joints. The measurement of joint motion, referred to as *goniometry*, is critical to the work of physical therapy. It allows the physician and therapist to determine if range of motion is normal or has been limited because of disease or injury, thus helping to monitor the success of treatment or the progress of disease. The traditional instrument for measuring joint motion is the goniometer (Fig. 26-1), which is a simple 360° protractor with a movable pointer arm. Once the correct measurement has been obtained, the physical therapist compares this against a *list of standards for that particular joint*. For example, the average person who lies flat on his back can move his elbow from 30° to 180°, as recorded on the goniometer (Fig. 26-2).

Because many physicians obtain joint motion measurements, the medical assistant may be required to assist with, or be instructed to assume the responsibility for, joint mobility testing. In assisting the physician with goniometry, it is important to understand the terminology used (Table 26-1).

MUSCLE TESTING

Many physicians employ manual muscle testing for the same reasons that joint mobility is measured. The general purpose is to evaluate the strength of muscle groups so that patients can be assisted in the process of regaining function after injury or disease. Muscle testing usually includes the following components:

1. *Range of motion tests.* Testing that is focused on muscle flexibility and resilience
2. *Strength tests.* Testing whose purpose is to establish the force with which a muscle or muscle group can act
3. *Task skill tests.* Testing the person's capacity to carry out certain important activities

Many other tests are designed to test the condition of the musculature, but only the basic evaluations used most frequently in the medical office have been listed.

EXERCISE THERAPY

Exercise therapy is the use of body motion to prevent deterioration of ROM or to achieve an improvement of a particular function in one or more of the specific parts of the body. For the trained athlete, exercise may be used to attain high levels of performance in an activity such as running or jumping. In physical therapy, however, exercise is substantially more than a tool for improved athletic strength and endurance. Exercise is a therapeutic technique for helping patients to prevent deformities, regain body movement, improve muscle

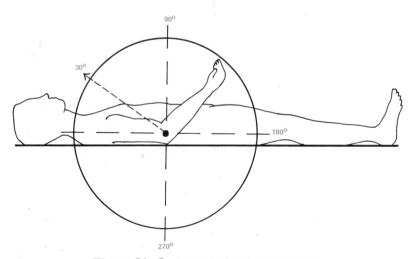

Figure 26-2. A standard goniometric test.

Table 26 – 1
GONIOMETRIC TERMS

Term	Description
Flexion	Motion toward closing the joint or bringing two body parts together
Extension	Motion toward opening the joint or spreading two body parts apart
Abduction	Motion away from midline of body or axis of limb.
Adduction	Motion toward midline or axis of body or limb
Circumduction	Circular rotation of a body part
Pronation	Lifting up or down of the palm at the wrist point
Supination	Twisting of the palm at the wrist joint
Inversion	Inward bending of foot at the ankle
Dorsiflexion	Upward flexing of foot
Plantar Flexion	Downward flexing of foot

strength, stimulate circulation, and retrain for neuromuscular coordination and resuming normal daily activities.

In addition to being of benefit in the management of primary disabilities such as arthritis, fractures, and pulmonary disorders, exercise therapy provides both preventative and therapeutic benefits in the management disabilities due to inactivity, such as those commonly found in postoperative patients, the elderly, stroke patients, burn victims, and amputees. For instance, a 70-year-old patient may perform certain exercises in order to regain walking ability.

Exercise is a very powerful tool. It involves the function of muscles, nerves, bones, and joints as well as the cardiovascular and respiratory systems. It may have as great an effect as medication or other treatment alternatives. Thus it is important that the practitioner be knowledgeable of the types of exercises and their specific effects on the body. Therapeutic exercises are prescribed by the physician or therapist after a thorough evaluation of the physical problem.

The role of the medical assistant in exercise therapy is clearly to function as a resource person. Medical assistants must understand the goals and objectives to be achieved for the exercises prescribed. They should encourage and support the patient as he or she moves toward completion of the program.

Exercise programs may employ one or more of the following forms of exercise:

1. *Active-voluntary mobility.* Self-directed exercises accomplished by the patient without assistance, usually to increase muscle strength and function
2. *Passive-involuntary mobility.* Body parts are moved by the therapist without assistance by the patient, usually to retain as much range of motion as possible or to improve circulation

3. *Aided mobility.* Voluntary mobility with conducive aids, such as a therapy pool
4. *Active resistance.* Active exercise with counterpressure produced either manually or by mechanical means, usually to increase muscle power
5. *Isometric.* Active contracting and relaxing of muscles while keeping a body part in a fixed position to maintain muscle strength when a joint is temporarily or permanently immobilized

Because the process of exercise therapy is dynamic, the dosage (repetition frequency) must constantly be adjusted as the patient get stronger. Exercises are individually planned, since there is a wide variation in body builds, age capabilities, and the degrees of motion physically possible.

RANGE OF MOTION EXERCISES

In some cases, the medical assistant may be asked to assist with exercises that are designed to maintain patient joint mobility. These exercises may be *active* (performed by the patient) or *passive* (performed by another person for the patient). Although ROM exercises do not promote muscle tone, they do help to maintain joint mobility. The medical assistant may be asked to demonstrate these exercises for the patient and to give instruction regarding their application (Fig. 26 – 3).

MASSAGE

Massage, the manipulation of external body tissues, is one of the oldest known methods to promote healing. Various massage techniques appear to be almost instinctive in both humans and lower animals. In cases of strains, bruises, muscle soreness, lower back pain, dislocations, and other problems in which muscle relaxation or increased circulation is desired, the physical therapist may prescribe therapeutic massage.

There are basically three approaches to massage, and the therapist may choose one or all of them for a particular patient.

1. *Stroking.* The systematic movement of the hand across the skin (this is the most common massage modality used in the medical office)
2. *Compression.* The squeezing, pressing, or kneading of soft tissues
3. *Percussion.* The alternating thumping of the skin with various parts of the hand

Most persons regard massage as an art that is based on scientific understanding of the body and its injury. Often, the physical therapist or physician will demonstrate a massage technique and ask that the patient or a family member carry out massage on a systematic basis.

The medical assistant should understand the basic principles of massage therapy to prepare the patient for the procedures. These are listed and explained below.

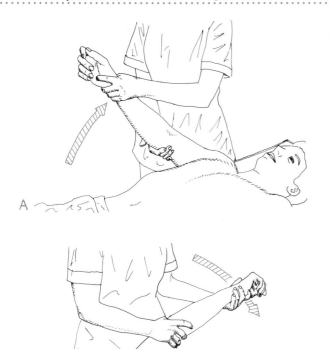

Figure 26–3. The medical assistant may be asked to demonstrate passive range of motion exercises to the patient's family member, who will perform them on the patient at home. (**A**) Beginning and (**B**) ending positions for passive shoulder flexion. (From Kisner C and Colby LA: Therapeutic Exercise: Foundations and Techniques, ed 2. FA Davis, Philadelphia, 1990, p. 24, with permission.)

Principal Guidelines for Massage

THE PATIENT MUST BE RELAXED. For massage to be effective, all muscles should be completely relaxed. Relaxation techniques such as breathing exercises can be employed. Thus, the first step is to calm the patient. Have him or her wear comfortable clothing, lie down, and expose only the area to be massaged.

A LUBRICATING CREAM OR OIL SHOULD BE USED. Skin surface friction is reduced with the use of these substances and the patient is helped to relax.

PRESSURE IS TRANSMITTED THROUGH RELAXED MUSCLES. TENSE MUSCLES IMPAIR EFFECTIVE MASSAGE. A relaxed muscle has the characteristics of a liquid so that pressure is transmitted. A tense muscle will resist pressure and cause discomfort during massage.

TRACTION

Traction, the act of pulling or stretching applied to the musculoskeletal system, is sometimes employed by the physician to ensure proper alignment of bones after injury or disease, to correct or prevent deformities, and to achieve other specific treatment objectives. The physical therapist applies traction according to a variety of different methods. Traction can be accomplished manually (using the hand to exert a pull), or by means of appliances, weights, or weighted pads applied to the sides of limbs. Skeletal traction may be effected by surgical insertion of pins, wires, or tongs.

CONDITIONS REQUIRING PHYSICAL THERAPY

A major role of physical therapy is the care of the amputee. Unless working for a physical therapist or an orthopedic specialist, the medical assistant will probably not be involved in the care of an amputee. However, contact with patients who use some kind of prosthesis is inevitable. A *prosthesis* is an artificial replacement for a missing part of the body.

Many persons are erroneously convinced that amputations are followed by the fitting of an artificial limb and that after a brief training program, all problems are resolved and the patient adapts. For most amputees, the truth is far from this common assumption. The prosthesis requires constant attention; it may wear out, cause pain, become obsolete, or in other ways cause difficulties. Meanwhile, the patient almost always faces the major psychological and emotional adjustment problems of realistic hopefulness and acceptance. While technological science is continuously offering new improvements in prosthesis design and function, the loss of a limb has lifetime repercussions for the affected individual. The medical assistant must develop empathy for these problems, offer the patient reassurance, and reinforce the physician's or therapist's prescription. Information concerning prosthetic appliances can be obtained from the American Orthotic and Prosthetic Association, 717 Pendleton Street, Alexandria, VA 22314.

In addition to deformities and complications resulting from amputation, physical therapy procedures are often recommended for the following conditions commonly encountered in the medical office:

1. *Arthritis.* To increase circulation or restore muscle strength, and to prevent flexion contractures through early passive exercise and then active exercise as inflammation subsides
2. *Cardiovascular disease.* To restore strength and increase circulation through change of positioning, exercise, and elastic stockings
3. *Pulmonary disorders.* To promote postural drainage through clapping and vibration and deep breathing exercises
4. *Cerebral vascular accidents.* To restore function and strength to affected limbs; to achieve proficiency in eating, dressing, and toilet functions; to retrain with hearing aids and walking frames and, occasionally, speech therapy
5. *Low back pain.* To relieve discomfort and maintain mobility through orthopedic corsets, muscle-strengthening exercises, and deep heat

6. *Muscle spasm.* To relax the musculature and relieve pain through resistance exercise and massage modalities and deep heat

7. *Muscle diseases and injuries.* To maintain mobility and prevent deformity and atrophy using ROM exercises, whirlpool baths, heat, and passive and active exercises

8. *Pressure sores (decubitus ulcers, bedsores) and infections.* To promote healing and kill microorganisms through changes of position, teaching patients to raise themselves and to use devices to support specific areas of the body

9. *Skin disorders.* To promote healing, reduce inflammation, and kill microorganisms with the use of infrared and ultraviolet therapy

10. *Burns.* To preserve function and appearance as burn wounds heal with positioning, exercising, and pressure garments; to prevent contractures and joint function with splints and positioning; and to preserve function through active and passive ROM exercises

MOBILITY-ASSISTING DEVICES

Quite often, patients find that they require the use of a mobility-assisting device. The medical assistant should be knowledgeable in the use of these supports in order to respond to the patient's questions and concerns.

WHEELCHAIRS

There are several criteria that should be considered by a patient who requires a wheelchair.

1. *Term of use.* Perhaps the most important issue is whether the patient will require the chair for an indefinite or limited time. For instance, when the period of use will be brief, the patient may be best served by a rental unit and may be able to live with standard models that have not been specifically adjusted to his or her needs.

2. *Size.* Wheelchairs are available in a wide range of sizes. it is essential that the chair fit properly to offer adequate support.

3. *Patient disorder.* Many design options are available, depending on the special needs of the patient. Neck braces, specialized foot braces, and different transfer systems can be combined to facilitate the needs of individual patients.

4. *Lifestyle.* Wheelchair models can also be purchased that fold or are, by design, compatible with outdoor use and are available with a number of other modifications that serve the special needs of particular patients.

The patient who faces long-term use of a wheelchair is usually referred to a medical supply house that can provide a precise chair prescription. In the long run, a used or borrowed "bargain" chair does not facilitate the patient's physical or psychological needs, since the fit may be improper or the mobility hampered by the type of model. Figure 26–4 is an illustration of a standard wheelchair.

WALKING WITH CRUTCHES

Patients for whom crutches have been prescribed should be assisted in understanding how to use them effectively. Under the physician's or therapist's supervision, the medical assistant may assume this responsibility. For the young or healthy patient with one "good" leg, the task of crutch training is uncomplicated. Most persons who spend a few moments with a pair of crutches will quickly learn how to manipulate them. Special instructions may be required in the following cases:

1. *Stairs.* Place both crutches under one arm and balance the body between the pair of crutches and the handrail (Fig. 26–5). Care should be taken so that the patient does not "jackknife" and fall.

2. *Obstructions.* Obstructions such as curbs or steps without handrails can be approached by placing the lead crutch either up (ascending) or down (descending) and then twisting and elevating (or lowering) the body simultaneously (Fig. 26–6).

3. *Single crutch.* Patients for whom one crutch is prescribed should be advised to carry the crutch on the side of the "good" leg, not the "bad"

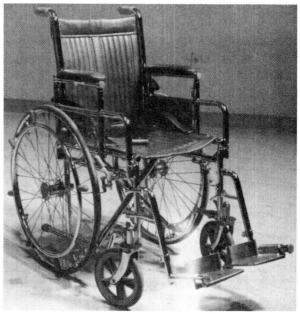

Figure 26–4. A standard wheelchair. (From Palmer ML and Toms JE: *Manual for Functional Training,* ed 3. FA Davis, Philadelphia, 1992, p. 112, with permission.)

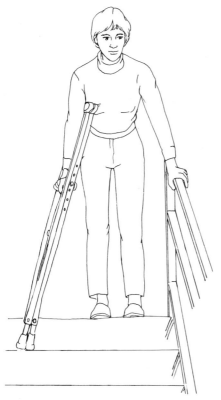

Figure 26–5. Descending stairs using crutches and a handrail. (From Palmer ML and Toms JE: Manual for Functional Training, ed 3. FA Davis, Philadelphia, 1992, p. 234, with permission.)

leg. Most patients intuitively take the reverse approach.

4. *Crutch gaits.* The approach to instructing a patient in a particular walking technique will depend on the patient and the injury. The physician may prescribe a two-, three-, or four-point gait.

Four-point gait:

   a. Right crutch
   b. Left foot
   c. Left crutch
   d. Right foot
   e. Repeat steps a through d

Three-point gait:

   a. Two crutches and weak leg
   b. Strong leg
   c. Repeat steps a and b

Two-point gait:

   a. Right crutch and left foot
   b. Left crutch and right foot
   c. Repeat steps a and b

There are two major types of crutches (Fig. 26–7): the *axillary crutch* and the *Lofstrand (Canadian) crutch,* which offers wrist support.

CANES AND WALKERS

The needs of patients are best served by one of a variety of available types of canes or walkers designed for specific purposes. A few of these are illustrated in Figures 26–8 and 26–9.

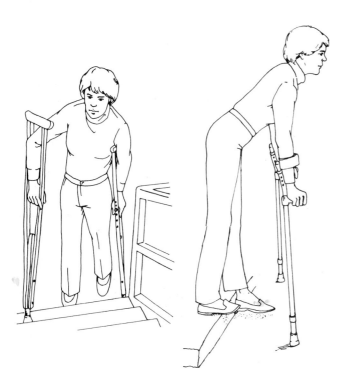

Figure 26–6. (*Left*) Ascending stairs without a handrail. (*Right*) Descending curbs. (From Palmer ML and Toms JE: Manual for Functional Training, ed 3. FA Davis, Philadelphia, 1992, pp. 239 and 238, with permission.)

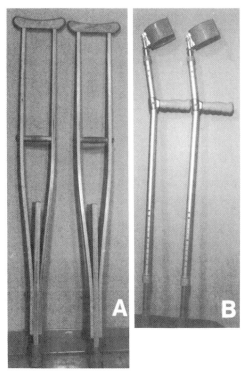

Figure 26-7. (**A**) Axillary crutch. (**B**) Lofstrand or Canadian crutch. (From Palmer ML and Toms JE: Manual for Functional Training, ed 3. FA Davis, Philadelphia, 1992, pp. 120 and 121, with permission.)

ORTHOTIC DEVICES

An orthosis is an orthopedic appliance that provides support and alignment to correct or prevent deformities and improve body function. There are many different types of splints and braces available, and a detailed

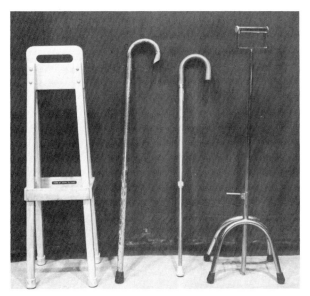

Figure 26-8. Types of canes. (From Saperstein AB and Frazier MA: Introduction to Nursing Practice. FA Davis, Philadelphia, 1980, p. 511, with permission.)

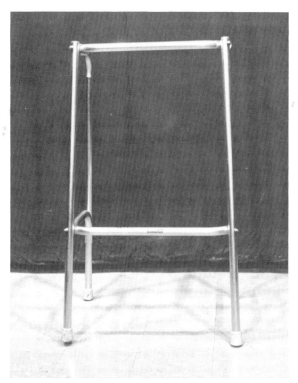

Figure 26-9. A Type of walker.

discussion of these is not possible in this chapter. When a patient is in need of a brace, the medical assistant who may be collaborating with the physician or therapist should make a special effort to prepare for patient teaching by learning as much as possible from the salesperson or manufacturer. It is not uncommon for special representatives of brace companies to give detailed instructions to the patient.

SPECIFIC THERAPEUTIC PROCEDURES

Physicians commonly prescribe heating (*thermotherapy*) or cooling (*cryotherapy*) or both for treatment of problems such as sprains or muscle spasms. The application of cold is accomplished by immersion in cold water, the use of ice packs, or cold bath. Cold acts primarily by constricting blood vessels and contracting the involuntary muscles of the skin. These two actions result in a reduced blood supply to the skin and may be used to control bleeding or check an inflammatory process. Although cold can prevent bleeding and swelling, it will not reduce edema that is already present in the tissues. The secondary effects of cold are the opposite of its primary action. Thus, observing the time limits of the prescription is essential with the use of cold applications, since prolonged application may result in tissue damage. Specific procedures related to the application of topical heat and cold are discussed in Chapter 20.

There are several ways of applying dry heat, including heating pads, hot water bottles, and heat lamps using ultraviolet, infrared, or in candescent bulbs in a heat cradle. Moist heat methods include heat packs, immersion, hydrocollator, soaks, and compresses. Methods used for the deeper penetration of heat into tissue includes shortwave, ultrasound, and microwave diathermy. The general precautions outlined below contain guidelines for heat therapy. It should be noted that generally heat is applied to facilitate drainage from an infected area by hastening the inflammatory process and to relieve congestion and swelling by dilating blood vessels in an injured area. This causes circulation to increase and improves repair of injured tissues by increasing local metabolism. Specific time intervals and the length of treatment are individually prescribed for each patient. Overtreatment may increase skin secretions, resulting in softened skin and lowered resistance. Extreme heat may constrict blood vessels or localize infection and swelling. Patients who already suffer from chronic edema may not be able to tolerate the application of heat.

INFRARED THERAPY

Infrared therapy, as a dry heat form, is administered by a heat lamp. Surface heat is transmitted that penetrates the skin to a depth of 5 to 10 mm. Placing the heat lamp a distance of 2 to 4 feet from the area is generally recommended to avoid burning the skin. Exposure time is usually 15 to 20 minutes. In addition, there are some general precautions to be followed in the application of heat. See Precautions for the Application of Heat, on the next page. In recent years, physicians and physical therapists have abandoned the use of infrared heat in favor of newer, and more effective therapies.

DIATHERMY

Diathermy is a form of heat therapy in which the area to be treated requires deep (internal), rather than superficial, heat penetration. Diathermy works by creating a high frequency in the tissue that is capable of creating moderate heat, thus heating the tissue and increasing circulation. Diathermy penetrates deep into muscle tissue with negligible heating of the fatty layer or bone. Beneficial effects include decreased joint stiffness, increased vasodilation, muscle spasm relief, and reduced pain from ligamentous sprains and strains. There are three basic approaches to diathermy:

1. *Microwave.* Radar waves capable of converting energy into heat in the tissues. Use of this method as clinically safe was questioned in 1980 by the FDA and is presently not prescribed in many physical therapy facilities.
2. *Shortwave.* Radio waves travel through the body between two condenser plates and are converted into heat.
3. *Ultrasound.* High-frequency acoustic vibrations are directed to the tissues and converted into heat.

Each of these forms of therapy requires the use of specific equipment. Microwave diathermy uses the highest frequency and is generally the least complicated. It requires aiming a beam of heat toward the affected area. Shortwave diathermy usually requires the manipulation of a somewhat complex control panel, and sometimes the use of rather cumbersome and specialized appliances for application. Microwaves cannot be used in high dosages on edematous (swollen) tissue. It is never used over wet dressings or near metal implants in the body because of the danger of burns. Shortwaves and microwaves are never used on persons with implanted electronic cardiac pacemakers.

Ultrasound energy is administered with a transducer treatment head held against the skin. The skin is covered with a transmission lotion or gel, or the body part may be under water. Ultrasound can cause bone damage and should not be used over areas where bones are near the surface of the skin.

Since equipment technology changes quite rapidly and varies from manufacturer to manufacturer, the medical assistant must be specifically trained to operate such equipment by the physician or the sales representative. Because of the enormous heat that is generated in the diathermy process, it is vitally important to adhere to recommended dosage and time allowances. Treatments are usually ordered for 15- to 20-minute periods. The manufacturers' stepwise instructions and corresponding principles for these procedures are listed for each therapy unit.

ULTRAVIOLET THERAPY

Many skin problems are treated with *ultraviolet therapy*, which is the use of ultraviolet lamps on the skin. Generally speaking, the lamp is one of three types: a hot quartz lamp, a cold quartz lamp, or a sunlamp. Each of these is a complex electrical unit that has distinct characteristics. The physician determines the type to be used and the medical assistant implements the physician's prescription. The appliance may be fixed or portable; in either case, the distance between patient and lamp is as critical as the exposure time. Exposure time, distance and angle depend on the reason for use. Ultraviolet is highly bactericidal and produces skin erythema (redness) quickly. Common medical office uses include treatment for acne, psoriasis, and superficial infection. The patient's sensitivity to ultraviolet light must be tested before lamp application of full dosage. Different areas of the body are exposed to different dosages of ultraviolet light, according to the physician's instructions and then compared for changes in coloration. Although some light redness is expected, deeper red color would indicate increased sensitivity. The physician usually prescribes the time and distance that achieved the desired coloration. The physician may order the exposure time to be increased after repeated applications are achieved without ill effects. During the procedure, protective goggles are worn by the medical assistant and the patient to protect the eyes from harmful rays.

HYDROTHERAPY

Hydrotherapy is the use of external water applications for therapeutic purposes. Physicians are likely to prescribe whirlpool baths, contrast baths, or underwater exercise in particular applications. The patient is usually referred to the physical therapy department of a medical center for hydrotherapy treatments. A description of the most commonly prescribed forms of hydrotherapy follows.

1. *Whirlpools.* These provide the heat that is also available in immersion along with a gentle massage action. There are a number of different kinds of whirlpools available, including wheelchair stalls, total body immersion baths, and smaller tubs for specific body parts.
2. *Contrast Baths.* The baths employ two different containers of water: one hot and the other cold. The patient is required to move the affected body part quickly from the hot to the cold and then back to the hot bath.
3. *Underwater Exercise.* This is often prescribed in cases of joint injuries, burns, or arthritis. In some instances when the instruction is minimal, this therapy can be carried out by the patient in any swimming pool.

These three modalities provide varying degrees of relaxation, increased or improved circulation, and improved mobility. For patients with burns, hydrotherapy may be prescribed for débridement (removal of devitalized tissue).

PARAFFIN WAX BATH

A *paraffin wax bath* involves melting and heating wax and dipping the patient's body part (usually an extremity) into the substance. Paraffin wax baths are often used for patients who have arthritis to relieve pain caused by chronic joint inflammation and to relax stiffness and relieve muscle spasm. The wax is usually melted and heated anywhere from 26°F to 130°F (−3.3°C to 54°C) and mixed with mineral oil in a proportionate amount (usually 7 : 1). The dry body part is immersed in the wax and quickly lifted out. The paraffin coating is often used for at-home treatment. The medical assistant may be responsible for explaining the procedure and instructing the patient in the technique.

PRECAUTIONS FOR THE APPLICATION OF HEAT

EXTREME CAUTION SHOULD BE USED IN APPLYING HEAT ON AFFECTED BODY PARTS OF VERY YOUNG CHILDREN TO AVOID BURNING. Infants and young children have increased sensitivity to heat because they are not sufficiently matured to have acquired a normal heat tolerance and may develop adverse heat reactions or burns.

ELDERLY PATIENTS SHOULD BE OBSERVED CAREFULLY FOR LOW TOLERANCE TO HEAT AND SUBSEQUENT BURNING. Older people may find that localized heat applications challenge cardiovascular reserves, thus reducing heat tolerance.

PATIENTS SHOULD BE FOREWARNED OF THE DANGERS OF HEATING PADS. In addition to the danger of electric shock, heating pads can also produce excessive heat and cause adverse reactions.

DOSAGES OF INFRARED RAYS SHOULD BE CAREFULLY OBSERVED. An insufficient heat penetration does not achieve the required effect; overly sufficient dosages can lead to skin damage.

SOAKING OR IMMERSION SHOULD OCCUR IN WATER TEMPERATURES BETWEEN 104°F AND 113°F (40°C AND 45°C). Temperatures of 116°F (47°C) or above can cause burning.

ELECTRONIC MUSCLE STIMULATION

One of the more powerful and complex forms of therapy available to the physical therapist is the use of electrical frequencies for neuromuscular stimulation. Muscle stimulation works by using a mild electric current to stimulate a muscle contraction in the same way a natural nerve impulse would contract a muscle. Muscle stimulation is used for orthopedic or neurologic rehabilitation in two specific ways. The first is to control pain and relax muscle spasm due to damaged peripheral nerves. The second important function is to isolate and passively exercise a specific muscle or muscle group to prevent muscle atrophy from disease, to increase local circulation, and to assist in muscle reeducation. This is accomplished when the muscle stimulator is used to enhance range of motion movements electronically.

Medical assistants should not be involved in electrical diagnosis or therapy since these procedures are not within the parameters of their expertise. They should, however, possess an understanding of why and how the procedures are performed to prepare patients.

SPORTS MEDICINE

In recent years, a rather sudden and unexpected increase has occurred in physical activities pursued by men and women of all ages. Jogging, tennis, and weekend athletic activities are becoming increasingly popular. The result of this trend is an ever-growing interest in the treatment and prevention of athletic injury.

The proper treatment of the athlete must be approached from a special perspective. The sedentary person with a sprained ankle is interested only in having the pain reduced. The tennis player with a sprained ankle wants pain relief and, in addition, wants to know when he or she can play tennis again and how the process can be accelerated.

Athletes are typically willing to invest a great deal of energy in pursuing therapeutic programs that will speed their recovery. Often, zeal motivates them to try to return to activity too soon, thus risking aggravation of the injury. Substitute activities are usually suggested to reduce the athlete's temptation to resume full activity prematurely. The jogger with tendinitis of the knee, for example, might be encouraged to temporarily substitute a swimming program until the knee is healed. Generally, then, when working with injured athletes, the role of the medical assistant is to reinforce and clarify the physician's orders.

Sports medicine is currently one of the fastest growing areas of medicine in the United States. It has been estimated that by the year 2000, every major hospital will have its own sports medicine department and that many of these will be freestanding facilities that will be located close to concentrations of exercisers, rather than in proximity to hospital facilities themselves. A number of large hospitals, for example, have purchased or built exercise complexes featuring Nautilus-type equipment, running tracks, and swimming pools, and either have included their sports medicine departments or satellite offices of those departments within the exercise facility. This allows the sports medicine staff to closely supervise exercise therapy and, at the same time, serves the community by providing an exercise club. In addition, hospitals are finding these innovations financially advantageous.

The major purpose of sports medicine is to treat the patient in terms of overall athletic and conditioning objectives. For example, for the sports medicine practitioner to cure a sprained ankle but let the athlete lose his or her conditioning and thus miss an important contest is inadequate and unacceptable health care.

In addition to the treatment of sports injuries, sports medicine practitioners are also interested in the promotion of fitness and the prevention of athletic trauma. For this reason, most sports medicine facilities offer consulting and other services to athletic teams or to the general public in the form of seminars and workshops. This aspect of sports medicine includes the design of training programs for both the formal, or professional, athlete and the informal, or amateur, athlete.

SPORTS MEDICINE PRACTITIONERS

Many of the persons who staff the typical sports medicine facility are either the same types of professionals or, in some cases, the same individuals who staff other areas of the hospital or medical center. The services of orthopedists, for example, are needed in the departments of sports medicine and orthopedic surgery. As the field of sports medicine expands, sports medicine orthopedists will most likely only practice sports medicine and not be required to offer their services to other departments. For the next few years, however, and in smaller and newer facilities, the health care consumer will continue to be confused by the variety and overlap of the professionals assuming multiple responsibilities.

In addition, there may be an overlap between sports medicine and physical therapy. Since much of the rehabilitative process in this field involves exercise as a therapy, it is common for the sports medicine department to own or share a cadre of physical therapy specialists with the hospital.

There are other kinds of specialists within the sports medicine function as well. The services of nurses and x-ray and laboratory technicians are necessary in order to provide complete care in the sports medicine arena.

ATHLETIC INJURIES

The most common complaints in sports medicine are related to the legs, arms, and neck, all of which are in motion during most sports activities. In particular, the joints are prone to injury and are difficult to rehabilitate. The knee, ankle, elbow, wrist, foot, hand, shoulder, and neck seem to demand the most attention from sports medicine therapists. The frequency of injury to a particular body part is also related to the athletic event in question. Football seems to cause knee injuries; running has been linked to foot and knee injuries; and tennis players are prone to elbow and shoulder problems. In general, however, the injuries frequently fall into the following categories:

Bursitis. Inflammation of the linking of a joint such as the shoulder; a common baseball injury

Hyperextension. Injury caused by moving a joint beyond its straight position

Sprain. An injury in which ligaments are ruptured but not severed along with attendant muscles, nerves, and tendons

Strain. Overextension or overstretching of a muscle or group of muscles

Tendinitis. Inflammation of a tendon such as the Achilles tendon or the elbow in tennis elbow

The medical assistant's role within a sports medicine facility or his or her involvement in helping patients who have been referred to a sports medicine facility by a family physician is largely the same as that suggested in the physical therapy section of this chapter.

OCCUPATIONAL THERAPY

Occupational therapists (OTs) are health professionals who have obtained a bachelor's degree or beyond in occupational therapy. As professionals, they are concerned with the reentry or, in some cases, the initial entry, of persons into the home or workplace. The basic premise of occupational therapy is that all persons need to develop mastery of self and the environment to be involved in meaningful, productive activity.

Although there is a broad range of clients for whom the OT offers important services, the most frequently encountered clients include:

1. Skilled workers who have lost their jobs because of an illness or accident

2. Amputees who find that they are unable to continue with their previous occupations
3. Stroke victims who must readapt basic skills to their jobs
4. Learning disabled teenagers who need to move from the special education environment to the work world
5. Young persons with birth defects who must begin to prepare for jobs
6. Emotionally disturbed persons who are trying to seek employment
7. Persons who are stricken with arthritis or other crippling diseases

Occupational therapists view their functions macroscopically. The task is not only one of helping persons to acquire skills and training, but also one of helping them adapt to home or work roles. *Occupational therapy* has been defined as:

> "the art and science of directing man's participation in selected tasks to promote and maintain health, to restore, reinforce, and to enhance everyday performance, and to diminish or correct pathology caused by illness."*

In the area of rehabilitation, there is a range of problems that arise in the typical medical practice from the minor (advising) problems to the major dilemmas that require the expertise of an OT.

Many physicians make an effort to understand the delicate relationship between work and health and may counsel patients regarding the interaction between medical problems and occupation. The role of the medical assistant is to support the advice of the physician and to serve as an additional facilitator for the patient. It is imperative that the patient understand the clear link between occupational satisfaction and personal health and the ways in which an OT may be able to help the patient effect a more satisfactory adjustment. In addition to the OT, social workers and vocational counselors may be consulted to determine the patient's socioeconomic status, interests, and attitudes for a more successful adjustment to home or work environments.

Among the disease-related uses of occupational therapy for which the physician may refer the patient to an occupational therapist are the following:

1. *Cerebral vascular accidents and spinal cord injuries.* To assist the patient in maximizing function. Self-dressing and self-feeding techniques may be stressed for patients with paralysis. Applications of splints to extend usefulness of body parts may also be necessary. Adaptation of automobiles and work and home environments may be necessary to restore the individual to independent functioning.

2. *Arthritis.* To assist the patient experiencing debilitation to maintain or restore self-care.
3. *Cerebral palsy.* To provide self-care instructions to encourage independence and maximization of functional ability.
4. *Psychiatric disorders.* To supplement psychotherapy objectives.

PSYCHOTHERAPY

A great many therapeutic activities fall within the general classification of psychological treatment. As in the case of physical therapy and occupational therapy, there are many levels of psychological function and dysfunction. They range from minor adjustment or adaptation problems, which the general or family physician might encounter and treat, to extreme problems, such as helplessness and total or near total disruption of occupational performance, that may require specific medications, referrals for extensive therapy, or institutionalization.

There are many resources in the psychotherapy treatment system: state and national health care planning and services; health services in the community; organization- and institution-based programs, which include school programs and support groups; comprehensive interdisciplinary group treatment plans; occupational and activity therapy groups; directive group therapy (which is a specialized form of group therapy designed to meet the needs of acutely ill, minimally functioning patients); and individual treatment by a psychiatrist or a psychologist. Among the many participating professionals in the general area of the psychological helping professions are the following major groups:

1. *Psychiatrists.* Physicians who specialize in the study, treatment, and prevention of mental disorders; can employ drug therapy when needed
2. *Psychologists.* Persons who are trained (usually at the doctoral level) in methods of psychological analysis, therapy, and research; cannot employ drug therapy because they are not physicians
3. *Counselors.* Trained persons (usually having master's degrees) who generally specialize in a particular problem area, such as marriage counseling, drug rehabilitation, or mental health counseling

As in the other areas, general physicians will typically be drawn into psychological counseling in administering to the needs of the patient until the nature of the problem transcends the physician's expertise. The patient is then referred to a specialist or therapist.

Again, the role of the medical assistant is supportive in nature. When a patient is referred to a psychotherapeutic specialist, the medical assistant must encourage the patient to follow through and help him or her to feel comfortable and confident with such therapy.

---

*Abott M and Franciscus ML: Opportunities in Occupational Therapy. VMG Career Horizons Books, New York, 1979, p 1.

THERAPEUTIC APPROACHES

There are a number of very different methods for pursuing therapy. The approach used depends on the patient and his or her beliefs, the problem encountered, and the therapist's training. Most of the problems encountered by the family physician involve adaptation difficulties in the areas of marriage, employment, or family relationships. Sometimes these issues lead to the identification of a more serious emotional or mental illness. Often, the patient's problems can be linked to external circumstances that require the assistance of a skilled and interested listener. Initially the physician may attempt to assist with these difficulties without recommending an outside referral. When the problem persists or an underlying psychological difficulty is suspected, however, the physician will refer the patient to a therapist. One of several approaches may be recommended:

Psychotherapy. An investigation of the root causes of a patient's emotional or psychological difficulties. This is usually attempted only by a psychologist or psychiatrist.

Group therapy. The use of a directed group of persons with similar difficulties to support each other in the solution of a problem. Weight Watchers and Alcoholics Anonymous are examples of this approach.

Specialized counseling. Marriage, parenting, cancer, career, and other forms of counseling are often prescribed by physicians whose patients are having specific problems.

TOWARD OPTIMAL MENTAL HEALTH

Health care practitioners are beginning to understand the importance of happiness and satisfaction in the attainment of optimal wellness and are therefore placing emphasis on ministering to the needs of the whole multidimensional person. Although the medical assistant will not be expected to function as a counselor, he or she must be aware of, and concerned about, the problems and difficulties of each patient. The development of this concern requires that the medical assistant become a careful listener and be alert to signals in conversation with the patient or family that may potentially indicate the need for counseling. When such needs are suspected, the medical assistant should share his or her observations with the physician and cooperate with other members of the health care team in providing comprehensive patient care.

PODIATRY

Podiatrists are persons who complete a specialized form of training beyond the baccalaureate degree and receive a doctorate in podiatric medicine. They are licensed to perform medical procedures on feet.

Podiatry has been brought to the forefront of medicine in recent years because of the fitness movement. For instance, podiatrists have taken a special interest in foot mechanics and the technical aspects of running. Many running magazines have advocated consultation with podiatrists for individuals who are either interested in improving their running skills or who are experiencing foot problems related to use or overuse. Some physicians recommend podiatrists or sports podiatrists to their patients with foot problems related to activity. Others prefer the use of orthopedic physicians and physical therapists.

Among the services performed by podiatrists are treatments for skin problems such as fungus or warts, corrective foot surgery, the design of special appliances (orthotics) to correct foot mechanics, and the treatment of injuries. Podiatrists also treat many diabetic patients with foot or circulatory complications from their disease. They also see many elderly patients for bunions, corns, and other conditions.

PATIENT TEACHING CONSIDERATIONS

In most cases, physicians are not acting as special therapists when they offer advice such as "you should do some stretching exercises for your stiff back," or "you've been working too hard," or "you should try to spend more time talking with your wife." Instead, they are viewing the problems of the patient in an expanded light — one that perceives the relatedness of specific symptoms to lifestyle behaviors. It is common practice for the physician to make inquiries regarding problems related to employment or family relationships when a patient complains of certain symptoms, such as a persistent headache. This approach is characteristic of *holistic* medicine, which recognizes, accepts, and treats the total, integrated person.

It is crucial that the medical assistant support the suggestions of the physician and help the patient to understand and follow them. The medical assistant's role is to reinforce the physician's advice by emphasizing and restating it to convince the patient that the physician's suggestion, if followed, will be effective and is as important to recovery as any other type of treatment. Medical assistants should also apprise the physician of their observations when a patient is resisting advice or not assigning it due importance.

Occasionally, patients may presume that since there is no explicit organic problem suggesting the need for drug or surgical intervention, they will recover automatically. To counter this common reaction, the medical assistant should emphasize the need for the patient to take an active role in his or her treatment. The patient must grasp the fact that some medical problems do not lend themselves to specific drug or surgical procedures, but that these problems must still be treated by following the practical suggestions made by the physician.

It is also important that medical assistants understand their role as a liaison between patient and physician. The medical assistant should ensure that the patient clearly understands the physician's recommendation and does not confuse a serious recommendation, such as "you ought to slow down and take time off from work," with a more casual comment, such as "take it easy."

Two basic questions that medical assistants can ask themselves to evaluate the patient's potential for compliance are: Did the patient understand the purpose of the suggestion and how to integrate the recommendation into his or her lifestyle? Has the patient taken the advice seriously?

RELATED ETHICAL AND LEGAL IMPLICATIONS

Practicing within the parameters of one's own profession is both an ethical and a legal issue. Medical assistants must be extremely cautious in assuming the basic responsibilities and performing basic tasks associated with other health care fields. Legislation in each state sets specific guidelines and defines the parameters of practice for all health professions. Medical assistants, to afford themselves legal protection, need to become aware of these regulations in their own state. For instance, many states do not allow supportive personnel (anyone other than physical therapists) to perform diathermy, ultrasound, or shortwave procedures.

In addition, when using the machinery described in this chapter, the medical assistant must take care to precisely follow manufacturer's directions for use and physician's orders to avoid injury to the patient and potential litigation. Also, to provide legal protection for the physician, the medical assistant, and the patient, all procedures should be recorded in the patient record, identifying the date, time, procedure, patient's response (when appropriate), and the health professional's signature.

SUMMARY

The medical assistant who has a working understanding of the various components of the health care delivery system, including fields such as physical therapy, psychotherapy, and sports medicine, is a valuable asset to the physician's office staff. Patient preparation and patient teaching are facilitated by the medical assistant's awareness of the role of each of the medical services available. In addition, a broad understanding of the practical dimensions of the allied health care fields enhances his or her potential for professional employment and contribution.

DISCUSSION QUESTIONS

1. In what types of situations would patients be referred to a physical therapist as opposed to receiving treatment in the medical office?
2. For what types of situations would patients most likely be referred to a sports medicine treatment center?
3. How can either cold or heat therapy be mishandled? What would be the danger to patients?
4. What psychological or emotional problems may accompany the use of mobility-assisting devices?

BIBLIOGRAPHY

Aspen Reference Group: Geriatric Patient Education Resource Manual. Aspen, Gaithersburg, MD, 1993.
Bisbee CC: Educating Patients and Families About Mental Illness: A Practical Guide. Aspen, Gaithersburg, MD, 1991.
Brown M: Therapeutic Recreation and Exercise. Slack, Thorofare, NJ, 1990.
Davis CM: Patient Practitioner Interaction. Slack, Thorofare, NJ, 1989.
DiDomenico RL and Ziegler WZ: Practical Rehabilitation Techniques for Geriatric Aides. Aspen, Gaithersburg, MD, 1989.
Dossey BM: Holistic Health Promotion: A Guide for Practice. Aspen, Gaithersburg, MD, 1989.
Grana WA and Kalenak A: Sports Medicine. WB Saunders, Philadelphia, 1991.
Kaplan K: Directive Group Therapy. Slack, Thorofare, NJ
Keilhofner G: Conceptual Foundations of Occupational Therapy. FA Davis, Philadelphia, 1992.
Lewis CB and McNerney T: Exercise Handouts for Rehabilitation. Aspen, Gaithersburg, MD, 1993.
May BJ: Home Health and Rehabilitation: Concepts of Care. FA Davis, Philadelphia, 1993.
Mayall J and Desharnois G: Positioning in a Wheelchair. Slack, Thorofare, NJ, 1988.
Mueller FO (ed): Prevention of Athletic Injuries: The Role of the Sports Medicine Team. FA Davis, Philadelphia, 1991.
Palmer ML and Toms JE: Manual for Functional Training, ed 3. FA Davis, Philadelphia, 1992.
Pheasant S: Ergonomics, Work and Health. Aspen, Gaithersburg, MD, 1991.
Reed KL: Quick Reference to Occupational Therapy. Aspen, Gaithersburg, MD, 1991.

HIGHLIGHTS

Exercise and Health

During the past decade, our country has experienced an exercise and fitness revolution. The sedentary society that John F. Kennedy admonished in the early 1960s has become a nation of joggers, tennis players, and bike riders. No one knows exactly how this transition came about or the extent to which we can expect it to be permanent. There is no doubt, however, that the fitness revolution has brought about dramatic changes in our lifestyles.

It is inevitable that a change of such proportions would have an impact on medical practice in a number of ways. More patients are involved in fitness programs and are expecting physicians to treat injuries incurred. The athlete's concern, however, is not limited to the healing of the injury. Perhaps an even greater concern is being able to immediately return to the activity that most probably caused the injury. Also, more individuals are beginning to feel that they have an insight into these common—and often serious—medical problems and are seeking self-treatments or advice from "friends" in lieu of early medical care. Often, the consequence of this mind-set is that physicians encounter aggressive patients who are likely to rush their recoveries and patients who may have procrastinated seeking treatment for a serious or chronic injury. In addition, many individuals involved in fitness regimens overtrain, and by so doing, are more vulnerable to athletic injury.

The problems cited represent the negative side of the fitness revolution. Health care practitioners must become alerted to the tendency for many fitness-oriented individuals to carry their programs to extremes. While the focus for health professionals has been to promote the movement toward fitness on the basis of the positive outcomes of exercise, they must not be—or allow their patients to become—oblivious to the fact that exercise can be overdone. As previously mentioned, orthopedic injury is more likely to occur in individuals who train excessively. However, these injuries are not the only detrimental outcomes of an overzealous, perhaps obsessive, pursuit of fitness. Exercise can become negatively addictive and can have an impact on the individual both physically and psychologically. Recently, researchers have been reporting a syndrome that is similar to anorexia nervosa (the eating disorder). Individuals become somehow addicted to the training process and begin to expand the number of hours spent in exercise beyond reasonable limits. This syndrome appears to be more prevalent in males and in runners. The persons affected may begin by becoming psychologically addicted to the positive feelings that are associated with training. After some time, it appears that the addiction may take on a physiological component as well.

Researchers have also observed changes in hormonal chemistry in the overtrained athlete. Adrenal gland stimulation has been noted, which in turn affects the central nervous system. While the changes can be observed, the long-term effects of altered activity in the central nervous system are unknown. The overtrained runner, for instance, is in effect wasting his or her training time. By spending dozens of extra hours in training, he or she may make only a minuscule gain in athletic ability. Often, the overtrained person has reduced capacity to energetically and productively complete his or her daily tasks. Meanwhile, the individual may suffer from imbalance in his or her life since the job, the family, and other concerns are placed in a position of secondary importance. Withdrawal, compulsiveness, and rigidity may characterize all of his or her life systems. Further complications and resultant depression may arise from a permanent or chronic injury sustained in overtraining.

Recent studies have indicated that a running regimen that is in excess of 20 to 25 miles per week is potentially dangerous and adds little to what might be characterized as a reasonable level of fitness for most individuals. Fitness experts have also suggested that an exercise routine that includes several different kinds of activities (running, walking, biking, and swimming, for example) minimizes the specific risks to joints and muscle groups.

In light of these findings, the physician and his or her staff should be prepared to set limits on, and suggest moderation in, exercise. Certainly, exercise should be encouraged since the benefits to both health and well-being have been documented. However, health care professionals must become involved in counseling fitness-oriented individuals and must present both the positive aspects of exercise and the negative aspects of overtraining. The objective for all exercise programs is always wellness—in body, in mind, in spirit. Health professionals need to assume the responsibility for guidance as well as treatment of those attempting to achieve fitness.

*M*edical Office Emergencies

> Injury or sudden illness becomes an emergency when life is threatened, suffering occurs or problems develop that endanger physical or psychological well-being.
>
> ———————
>
> Guy Parcil
> Basic Emergency Care

CHAPTER OUTLINE

LEARNING OBJECTIVES

Upon completing this chapter, you will be able to:

1. Define the concepts of emergency care and first aid.
2. Describe the medical assistant's role in medical office emergencies.
3. List the five general procedures for emergency care.
4. List and describe the 10 components of general patient assessment in emergency situations.
5. In the context of problem-solving simulations, identify emergency situations.

Chapter 27

*M*edical Office Emergencies

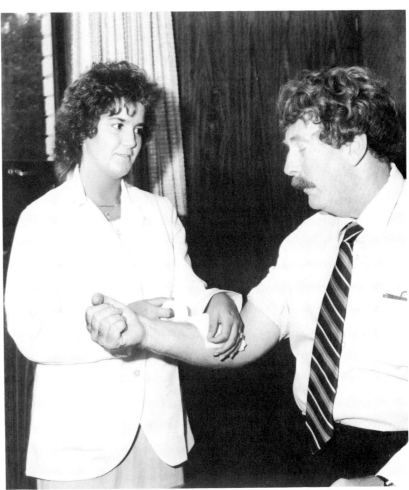

PERFORMANCE OBJECTIVES

Upon completing this chapter, you will be able to:

1. Simulate the administration of first aid for sudden illness (fainting, epileptic seizure, allergic reaction to drugs, chest pain, diabetes-related problems, nosebleed) wounds, shock, bleeding, burns, heat and cold exposure, and poisoning.
2. Describe how to assemble and maintain emergency supplies.
3. Define the relationship of a "safety mentality" to medical office emergencies.

DACUM EDUCATIONAL COMPONENTS

1. Recognize emergencies (4.3).
2. Perform first aid and cardiopulmonary resuscitation (4.4).

Glossary

Aura: a subjective sensation preceding a convulsive attack
Blister: a collection of fluid below the epidermis
Cyanosis: discoloration of the skin due to abnormal reduction of hemoglobin in the blood
Emergency: sudden, urgent, unforeseen occurrence requiring immediate attention
Noxious: smell irritating to nasal mucosa
Patent: open, not unobstructed, or not closed.
Syncope: temporary loss of consciousness due to inadequate blood supply to the brain; fainting

---

Occasionally, the medical assistant is required to respond to emergency situations in the office. If the physician is not present, the medical assistant is responsible for the management of the emergency situation and for the administration of first aid. If the physician is present, the medical assistant is responsible for aiding the physician in managing the situation and caring for the patient.

Although the emergency situations presented in this chapter are particularly relevant to medical office practice, the principles of first aid discussed are applicable to situations outside the office as well. As a health professional, the medical assistant is expected to have expertise in managing emergency situations knowledgeably and skillfully, regardless of the setting in which they occur.

THE MEDICAL ASSISTANT'S ROLE IN OFFICE EMERGENCIES

An emergency situation implies that a crisis has arisen that requires an immediate response. The medical assistant's role is to manage the crisis effectively by ordering priorities and demonstrating competency. He or she must make decisions that affect the physical and mental well-being of all persons involved. Each situation must be assessed apart from preconceived assumptions or past experiences. In addition, the medical assistant must promote an atmosphere of calm control while administering first aid. Sensitivity and awareness

are needed to prevent expanding or intensifying a crisis situation.

The medical assistant will encounter emergencies in the medical office involving staff members, the physician, patients and their families, and visitors. The anticipation of potential causes of accidental injury will help to reduce the incidence of emergency situations in the medical office.

FIRST AID PRINCIPLES APPLIED TO OFFICE EMERGENCIES

DEFINITION AND PURPOSE

First aid is the immediate care given to a person who has suddenly become injured or ill. First aid encompasses life support measures that are temporary resolutions to a crisis.

PRIORITY ASSESSMENT

The urgency of a situation must be determined before the type of care to be administered can be decided. Immediate attention must be given to the following cases:

1. Respiratory or circulatory collapse (cardiopulmonary arrest) or choking (obstructed airway)
2. Severe bleeding

3. Poisoning or severe allergic reactions (anaphylaxis)
4. Shock or burns

Other situations may also warrant urgent attention. The objective in assessing priorities is to establish the urgency of the illness or injuries regardless of the number of persons involved. Take, for example, the case of a patient who, while awaiting the physician, falls to the floor of the examination room and hits his head on the table. He is bleeding from a head laceration and clutching his chest. An appropriate assessment of priorities would require that the patient's condition be generally assessed to determine which injury is most serious or life-threatening. In the example given, the laceration may be of secondary concern if the person is having cardiac or respiratory distress. In other cases it may be necessary to treat life-threatening bleeding first and then to treat shock or wounds. Therefore, general assessment enables the medical assistant to determine priorities.

GENERAL PROCEDURES FOR EMERGENCY CARE

There are five general procedures that must be followed to provide competent emergency care regardless of the type of emergency situation. Because each emergency is an unpredictable event that challenges the knowledge and skills of the care provider, standardized and organized procedures must be followed to prevent oversights and errors, further injury to the patient, and a further deterioration of a crisis environment. These procedures are as follows:

1. Assess the situation.
2. Assess the patient.
3. Administer appropriate first aid.
4. Transport to an emergency care facility if necessary and notify appropriate medical personnel and family.
5. Obtain follow-up care.

ASSESSING THE SITUATION

When emergencies occur in the medical office or elsewhere, assessing the situation requires that the medical assistant make immediate general observations to pinpoint clues as to the nature of the emergency. A quick response is necessary for questions such as:

1. What person or persons are involved?
2. What factors produced the emergency?
3. What immediate dangers and concerns exist?

For instance, in the medical office waiting room, a sick child in his or her mother's arms may begin to have breathing difficulties, and the mother may become emotionally upset. The medical assistant, in assessing this situation, immediately recognizes who is involved, the potential hindrances to maintaining control of the situation, and who will require attention first. The observation provides the medical assistant with the information needed to plan for appropriate action. In this instance, assuming the physician is present, the medical assistant would immediately notify the physician and bring the mother and child to the examination room. While the physician attends the child, the medical assistant offers necessary assistance and administers to the mother's needs as well. Appropriate action is selected on the basis of individual situations and inherent observations.

ASSESSING THE PATIENT

The following patient assessment guidelines should be observed in all emergency situations:

1. Determine the level of consciousness by talking to or questioning the patient.
2. Obtain a description of the incident and the physical condition from the afflicted individual, if possible, or a bystander. When appropriate, ask "Are you okay?" "Where does it hurt?" "How does it feel?" "When does it hurt?" "How long does it hurt?"
3. If the individual's medical history is unknown, check for medical identification, such as a bracelet or card, that identifies a chronic condition.
4. If you are unable to obtain information as to the exact nature of the illness or injury, then the individual must be assessed for injury by palpating the body parts and loosening or removing clothing. Check for vital life signs (patent airway, breathing, circulation), severe bleeding, internal poisoning, shock, sudden illness, and nontraumatic problems. The examination of the patient begins with evaluating the vital signs and then proceeds from the most serious to the least serious to detect the nature of the emergency. Be alert to corresponding symptoms. Never expose the individual without cause.
5. Observe the individual's general appearance and color, especially the inner surface of the lips, the mouth, eyelids, and nail beds. The colors white or blue warrant concern because they may indicate a lack of oxygenated blood supply.
6. Check the pulse for regularity and strength of beat (radial and carotid pulses are most frequently used). In the unconscious individual, check for head injury by noting the contour of the face for signs of drooping or abnormal contortion.
7. Observe the eyes, especially the size and reactive qualities of the pupils. (Pupils should constrict equally in size then light is flashed and dilate equally when the light is eliminated.)
8. In suspected poisoning, check the mouth for stains or burns.

9. Keep the individual warm to prevent excessive loss of body heat and chilling, which could indicate further complications such as shock.
10. The individual must not be moved if there is a suspected neck or back injury. Otherwise, if possible, the individual should be allowed to remain in, or be assisted to, a supine position. A change of position may cause further injury, and the supine position facilitates assessment.

ADMINISTERING FIRST AID

The selection of appropriate first aid procedures depends on the interpretation of data collected in assessing the situation and the patient. Cardiopulmonary arrest and severe bleeding are the highest priorities. Internal injuries and severe shock are also high priorities.

Next in terms of assigning priority are life-threatening medical emergencies that require immediate medical intervention. These include coma, heart attack, heat stroke, cardiovascular accident, and surgical emergencies such as appendicitis and difficult or complicated childbirth.

Once life-threatening conditions are resolved, assessment of the patient proceeds to uncover lesser conditions or injuries. Appropriate intervention related to specific conditions and injuries (with special application to the medical office setting) is discussed later in this chapter.

Administering life-support measures and preventing further injury or worsening of the condition do not include diagnosis. Assessment differs from diagnosis. Assessment pinpoints the symptomatic nature of the illness or injury, whereas diagnosis refers to qualitative judgments regarding the physiologic state, cause, and treatment decisions related to patient care.

ARRANGING TRANSPORTATION AND NOTIFYING APPROPRIATE INSTITUTIONS

By definition, first aid refers to care provided that is immediate and temporary and does not imply that the emergency care provider will assume complete responsibility for the resolution of the emergency. Both medical and legal responsibility for the patient's emergency care is transferred to the physician or transport paramedics.

Decisions regarding who should be notified and when depend on the nature of the emergency. In most instances, because of the availability of emergency equipment it is better to rely on professional rather than on private transportation when arranging for emergency transport.

When providing information for transport, include the following:

1. Your name, phone number, and location
2. Nature of the emergency
3. Summary of the treatment given
4. Directions for locating the site, if necessary

Be calm, talk clearly, and provide an opportunity for the person being notified to ask questions.

FOLLOW-UP CARE

Follow-up care refers to those procedures that are necessary to support, supplement, and follow first aid.

1. Make the person comfortable by maintaining appropriate body temperature and by providing support for limbs and body parts.
2. Provide emotional support and reassurance.
3. Complete arrangements for hospital admission when ordered by the physician, or encourage the person to obtain follow-up care for minor injuries or less serious illness.

Although the medical assistant may not be involved in follow-up care, these procedures should be considered when the circumstance is appropriate. Perhaps the key concept underlying first aid treatment in emergency situations is to *act with purpose and with regard to consequences* and to work within the parameters of expertise defined by the medical assisting profession.

COMMON MEDICAL OFFICE EMERGENCIES

The medical office is not a setting free of accidents. Patients, family members, office staff, and visitors may develop a sudden illness. The structure and activities of the medical office setting create an environment where certain types of illnesses and injuries are more likely to occur than elsewhere. For example, many of the patients visiting the office are already acutely ill, and their conditions are subject to sudden change. The equipment found in the office can cause injury. Patients could fall off examination tables. Patients or staff walking on wet floors from spilled solutions or discharges could slip and fall. It is easy to imagine numerous other situations conducive to accident or illness in the medical office. The medical assistant must, therefore, be prepared to manage and handle the emergency effectively.

SUDDEN ILLNESS

Fainting

Fainting, or syncope, is caused by a temporarily diminished supply of blood to the brain. The individual may suddenly collapse, but recovery almost always occurs within minutes if a reclining position is assumed. To prevent fainting when symptoms of weakness and dizziness occur, the head should be brought to the level of the knees with the individual in a sitting position. The usual symptoms of an impending fainting attack include paleness; perspiration; clammy, cold skin; dizziness; nausea; a numbness and tingling of the hands and feet; and spots before the eyes or tunnel vision.

After a fainting attack, the individual should assume a reclining position to promote circulation, and the clothing should be loosened for comfort. If vomiting occurs, the individual should be rolled on his or her side to prevent aspiration and choking. Sips of water should be given only if the victim is fully revived. If a fall was sustained, examination for injury should be made.

Fainting can occur as a result of certain diseases, such as diabetes, in which hypoglycemia may be experienced. Emotional pain or distress can also cause fainting.

Consequently, when the individual is a patient in the office, he or she should be brought to the examination room as soon as possible. Regardless of where the incident took place, the individual should be examined by a physician if underlying disease is even remotely suspected.

Epileptic Seizure

Epilepsy is a disease characterized by convulsions of a variety of types. The individual may have a history of epilepsy known to office staff or may carry identification in the form of a card or bracelet. He or she may be aware of the onset of the seizure (aura) and lie down suddenly. People around the afflicted person may recognize certain behaviors as forerunners of the seizure. Warning signs may include sudden paleness or disorientation.

The major objective in first aid treatment of an epileptic person experiencing a grand mal seizure is to keep the airway patent. Grand mal seizures may be observable as either localized or general body movement accompanied by loss of consciousness, followed by a gradual period of awakening. During the seizure, the tongue may fall back across the trachea, obstructing the airway. The patient is rolled to one side, and the head is held to the same side to facilitate the tongue falling to one side and opening the airway. The patient is held in this position but not restrained from convulsing.

If airway obstruction has occurred and difficulty in breathing is apparent, mouth-to-nose ventilation is initiated when convulsions cease. Mouth-to-nose ventilation requires the rescuer to place his or her mouth over the individual's nose and breathe into the nostrils at an even rate, allowing a pause for exhalation or keeping the mouth apart to facilitate exhalation.

Basic first aid for a grand mal epileptic episode consists of the following measures:

1. Remove any objects from the surroundings that may cause injury.
2. Roll the individual to a side-lying position, with the head turned and held to one side.
3. Loosen clothing after the convulsion to make the individual comfortable.
4. Maintain the individual in a side-lying position to provide rest. If the seizure occurs in the office waiting room, wait until the seizure ends and, with assistance, move the individual to the examination room.
5. If the individual vomits, maintain the side-lying position to avoid aspiration of vomitus.
6. If breathing is obstructed, perform mouth-to-nose respiration when the seizure has ceased.
7. Allow the individual to rest after a seizure.
8. If the individual is a patient, record the incident on the patient's record. If the individual is not a patient, appropriate individuals should be notified, and as a precautionary measure, the physician's insurance company should receive a written report of the incident.

A petit mal epileptic seizure can go unnoticed and may be evidenced only by lip smacking, disorientation, and staring. Regardless of the severity of the attack, first aid measures should be administered and subsequent examination performed by the physician.

Allergic Reaction to Drugs

Occasionally after receiving medication in the office (especially injections), a patient develops an anaphylactic reaction, which is an extreme allergic response. Breathing and swallowing may become difficult. Without immediate aid, the victim could die of an impaired airway. As a precaution, most physicians require the patient to remain in the office for 20 to 30 minutes after receiving an injection of certain drugs. Various degrees of allergic response may also occur outside the office setting when the patient has ingested or come in contact with an allergy-causing substance. The same principles of first aid apply when anaphylaxis is suspected, regardless of the setting: check for a patent airway and ascertain breathing and pulse beat. In the medical office, oxygen and the drug epinephrine (adrenaline) will be on hand to be administered on the physician's order.

A sitting or reclining position is usually more comfortable for a patient experiencing breathing difficulties. An airway can be inserted only by the physician or trained emergency medical technician. Transportation to a medical center may be necessary.

Chest Pain

Severe chest pain can be indicative of a heart attack and is treated as a heart-related emergency until a diagnosis can be established.

Signs and symptoms of a heart attack include (1) ashen skin coloring; (2) profuse perspiration; (3) cyanosis of the nail beds and lips; (4) severe, crushing pain in the midchest region (pain may also radiate to the neck and jaw or the left shoulder and down the left arm); (5) pulse usually rapid and weak; and (6) nausea.

First aid measures in a heart-related emergency are as follows:

1. Keep the patient in a comfortable position. Usually a reclining position is preferred. If the attack occurs in the waiting room, move the patient to the examination room. A wheelchair or a desk chair with rollers can be used for transport.
2. If the physician is present, call him or her imme-

diately. Prepare the medication per the physician's request.

3. Administer oxygen, if instructed by the physician.
4. If the physician is not present, call an ambulance or rescue team. Ask the patient if he has a medication that he takes for chest pain, such as nitroglycerin. Administer this medication if the reply is affirmative.
5. If the patient becomes unconscious and breathing has ceased (no air flow is heard or felt) and the pulse in the carotid artery is absent for 5 to 10 seconds, begin cardiopulmonary resuscitation (CPR). If a pulse is present, omit chest compressions and work to restore breathing by mouth-to-mouth artificial respiration.

When cardiac arrest is apparent (as evidenced by the absence of a pulse), CPR is required. This procedure is described at the end of this chapter, as is the procedure for mouth-to-mouth resuscitation, but they should be learned in first aid and CPR classes. The medical assistant is required to attend classes in first aid and CPR and to obtain CPR certification.

Diabetes-Related Problems

Diabetic Coma

Diabetic coma occurs as a result of an insufficient supply of insulin circulating in the bloodstream (hyperglycemia). Symptoms of diabetic coma include (1) rapid, deep, gulping respirations; (2) flushed face; (3) dry and reddened skin; (4) apparent confusion or disorientation; and (5) "acetone breath," which has the odor of fruit or nail polish remover. Diabetic coma requires immediate hospitalization. If the physician is present in the office, he or she should be alerted and an ambulance called.

Insulin Shock

Insulin shock occurs as a result of an excess of insulin and an insufficient amount of sugar circulating through the bloodstream (hypoglycemia). The symptoms of insulin shock include (1) weak, rapid pulse; (2) profuse perspiration; (3) cold, clammy skin; (4) convulsions or tremors; and (5) restlessness, confusion, and fainting.

Immediate relief can be obtained by offering the patient sugar in some available form. In the medical office, packets of sugar or soft drinks may be on hand. However, if the patient has fainted, nothing should be forced into the mouth because the patient may aspirate. When in the office, the physician should be alerted immediately. When the physician is absent, arrange immediate transportation to the hospital. When symptoms of diabetic coma and insulin shock are not discernible, it is advisable, when possible, to give the patient a packet of sugar to ingest before transport. The rationale is that if the patient is experiencing insulin shock, the patient's life will be saved; if the patient is experiencing ketosis, the effects can be reversed.

Epistaxis (Nosebleed)

Nosebleed may occur for a variety of reasons ranging from blowing the nose forcefully to hypertension. Although the experience can be frightening, nosebleeds rarely cause severe blood loss. Nose bleeds are very common among children, especially at night. Repeated small bleeds over a long period of time could be caused by a more serious blood disorder, such as low platelets, leukemia, or hemophilia. Repeated nosebleeds could also lead to anemia.

Nosebleeds can be caused by local irritation from dryness or sneezing, from a cold or allergy, from foreign bodies in the nose (usually associated with a disagreeable odor and discharge of pus) or from injury, nose blowing or picking, and nasal infections. Basic first aid procedures include the following:

1. Elevate the patient's head by placing the patient in a semi-Fowler position.
2. Pinch the nostrils closed for approximately 2 to 5 minutes while the patient leans forward over a basin. If bleeding restarts, place a cotton ball coated with petroleum jelly in the affected nostril and pinch the nostrils again. Pinch for a longer period of time.
3. Apply a cold compress over the bridge of the nose, and use it to pinch the nostrils closed for 3 to 5 minutes.
4. Alert the physician when a nosebleed occurs in the medical office. Advise patients to apply a small amount of vaseline inside each nostril for a week to prevent crust formation. Humidification during the heating season often helps to eliminate nosebleeds.

Since HIV may be transmitted through mucous membrane or open wound contact with a carrier, gloves should be worn to prevent direct or indirect contact with potentially infected blood or secretions, or items contaminated with such blood or secretions. Masks and gowns are needed if splatter or soiling with blood or body fluids is likely. Hands should be washed immediately if contaminated with blood or body fluids, and needle-stick injuries should be carefully avoided. Contaminated articles should be discarded or bagged and decontaminated before reuse. Blood spills should be cleaned up immediately with 5.25% sodium hyperchlorite (bleach) diluted 1:10 with water.

Hemorrhage

Hemorrhage is profuse bleeding. Hemorrhage can be internal or external. In addition, hemorrhage from a wound can occur from arterial or venous bleeding. Bright red spurting blood indicates arterial bleeding, whereas a continuous flow of dark red blood indicates venous bleeding. Although venous bleeding can be life-threatening, arterial bleeding is usually more serious and necessitates immediate control, as there is greater pressure in the arteries than in the veins. Loss of 2 to

10 pt of blood in the average adult can cause shock and ultimately death.

The first objective of wound treatment, therefore, is to stop the bleeding. Further assessment includes: (1) establishing the need for repair or sutures; (2) noting any damage to adjacent structures, such as the eye or internal structures; (3) ascertaining the risk of infection (clean or dirty wound); and (4) determining the risk of tetanus and immunization status.

To control the bleeding, apply gentle pressure directly on the wound (minor bleeding), or for more serious bleeding, apply firm pressure at the arterial pressure point distal to the wound on the blood vessel feeding the hemorrhage. Figure 27–1 shows the arterial pressure points. Tourniquet application is usually avoided and is used only as a last resort when there is the threat of loss of life and when the bleeding cannot be controlled by any other means; using a tourniquet involves risking a limb to save a life. Once a tourniquet is applied, care by a physician is imperative. The tourniquet should only be loosened by the physician.

If there are multiple wounds with uncontrollable bleeding (bleeding does not subside after 10 minutes of direct pressure), the patient should be transported to the emergency room immediately.

Please refer to the preceding page, Epistaxis (Nosebleed) for a discussion of relevant OSHA universal precautions.

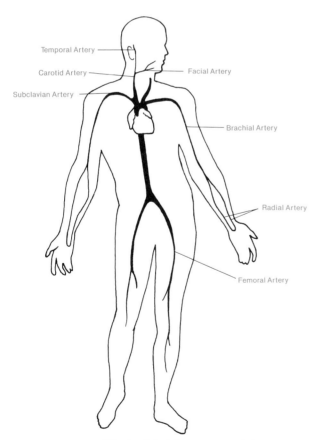

Figure 27–1. Arterial pressure points.

INJURY

Eye Injuries

Eye injuries include foreign objects in the eye, lacerations, and burns, all of which can occur to either medical office patients or personnel.

A foreign object can be removed from the eye by following these steps: (1) clasping the upper lash between the thumb and forefinger; (2) folding the lash over an applicator swab at the midline of the upper lid; (3) instructing the patient to look down to expose the upper surface of the eye; and (4) irrigating the eye with sterile water (see Chapter 24), or, if the object can be located and identified, removing it with the corner of a clean handkerchief. When the physician is present in the office, he or she, and not the medical assistant, attempts removal of the foreign object in the patient's eye. A foreign object that cannot be removed by the medical assistant or the physician in the office must be removed in a medical center or hospital facility. First aid measures include covering the eye, or preferably both eyes, with a light patch and bandage to avoid further injury and to prevent eye movement.

Lacerations of the eyelid require a sterile pressure dressing to stop bleeding and transportation to a medical center. Laceration of the eye itself requires application of a loose dressing and transportation to a medical center.

Burns of the eye require emergency treatment to prevent permanent damage. Chemicals splashed into the eye should be flushed with water to dilute the strength of the chemical. The Occupational Health Safety Administration (OSHA) Hazardous and Toxic Substances Act requires flushing the eye(s) with constant water flow for a minimum of 15 minutes when on-the-job injuries occur. Devices that attach to a water faucet and regulate the water flow for eye irrigation are now available commercially. The medical assistant can help the victim by holding the eyelid open so that water can make contact with the eye. Do not use an eye cup. Notify the physician immediately, while the eye is still being washed. If the victim is lying down, turn the head to the side of the infected eye and pour water from the inner canthus of the eye outward (see Chapter 20, irrigating the eye). Make sure that the chemical does not wash into the other eye. Cover the eye with a dry, sterile, noncotton dressing and bandage in place. With heat burns of the eye, both eyes are covered with a loose, moist dressing until the physician arrives.

Head Injuries

Injuries to the skull include concussions, fractures, and scalp hematoma. The most serious head injury results in an injury to the brain, in which case unconsciousness may occur. The most common injury to the brain is a concussion. A *concussion* is a closed head injury in which there is a transient loss of consciousness, followed by disorientation, then gradual recovery. Not all patients lose consciousness. Some patients experience temporary loss of vision, pallor, listlessness, memory loss, or vomiting. Symptoms may disappear almost immediately or last several hours. Skull x-rays are of no help in diagnosing concussions.

More severe head injuries such as contusion, bleeding into the brain (subdural or epidural hematoma), and skull fractures are extremely serious. The symptoms are similar to those associated with concussion but more profound. In these cases, immediate hospitalization is required.

A bump, bruise, or "goose-egg" on the head after injury is caused by bleeding into the skin (hematoma). When this type of injury occurs on the forehead, there is usually a color change from purple to yellow. Bruising sometimes spreads to the spaces around the eyes. Bruising most often resolves in 7 to 10 days. Repeated traumas of this type in children may indicate child abuse.

Symptoms of severe head injury include (1) skull deformity; (2) unequal or poorly reacting pupils; (3) blood or clear liquid in, or flowing from, the eyes, ears, or nose; (4) paralysis; (5) vomiting; (6) convulsions; and (7) respiratory arrest or distress.

First aid measures in cases of head injury involve (1) maintaining an open airway, (2) covering open wounds, (3) administering oxygen with the physician's consent, (4) minimizing movement by immobilizing the head and neck, and (5) telephoning for an ambulance.

Bone Injuries

Fractures are the primary type of bone injury. Falls often are the cause of fractures sustained in the medical office. Fractures can be confirmed only by x-ray.

Signs and symptoms of bone injury may include (1) exposed bone ends (not present in every fracture), (2) deformity, (3) pain and tenderness, (4) swelling and discoloration, and (5) restriction or loss of movement.

First aid measures involve (1) stopping the bleeding and applying a dressing to open wounds, if present, (2) immobilizing the affected body part, and (3) alerting the physician.

There are several types of fractures (see Fig. 20–8). Common types are reviewed below:

Comminuted fractures involve crushing or splintering of the bone.

Greenstick fractures have a break on one side of a bent bone. Greenstick fractures are so named because they resemble the breaking of a young tree limb.

Impacted fractures involve fragmented bone ends pushed forcibly into one another.

Oblique fractures occur at an angle or slant in the bone shaft.

Spiral fractures include a twisting apart of the bone shaft.

Transverse fractures are a straight-line break across the bone shaft.

Fractures can also be open or closed. An *open fracture* is one in which there is visible soft tissue injury and a protruding bone. A *closed fracture* is one in which the skin has not been broken and the fractured bone is contained in the surrounding tissue. Fractures most commonly occur in the extremities.

Immobilization of a fracture in an emergency may require temporary makeshift splinting until a more appropriate splint can be applied. Splinting will relieve pain, support the break, improve circulation, and prevent tissue damage caused by movement. Medical offices use a variety of slings and splints specific to the injury and available from various manufacturers.

Wounds

Wounds appear in many forms, each requiring specific emergency care. Table 27–1 considers the basic types of wounds, including their history, pathology, symptoms, identifying characteristics, treatment, and complications. The types of wounds most frequently sustained in the office by patients and staff are lacerations from falls or objects, contusions, and punctures.

Wounds of the forehead, mouth, and tongue are sometimes misleading as these areas have a rich blood vessel supply. Wounds around the genitalia of minors should raise suspicion of child abuse. Tetanus can infect any laceration or puncture wound, especially if the injury occurred outside. Tetanus is not a concern if the patient's tetanus immunizations are up to date or if the injury is just an abrasion.

Puncture wounds and minor cuts should be washed thoroughly with soap and then flushed with cool tap water. Foreign material that projects from a wound should be removed. Foreign material that is embedded in the wound should be removed by flushing the wound with tap water or sterile water in a syringe. Serious lacerations should be immediately covered with a clean compress, and pressure should be applied to control the bleeding. Gloves should be worn when treating any open wound.

Puncture wounds and abrasions should be blotted dry and inspected when all bleeding has stopped. An antiseptic, such as betadine, 3% hydrogen peroxide, or mercurochrome should be applied. The wound should be covered with a Band-Aid or sterile gauze if the cut is in an area that is likely to get dirty. Telfa nonstick dressings should be used if the injury is a large abrasion.

Shock

Any injury can stimulate the physiologic reaction of shock, in which blood vessels dilate and blood volume is reduced because the heart provides inadequate circulation. Central nervous system dysfunction triggers inadequate circulation.

Symptoms and signs of shock include (1) cool, clammy skin; (2) ashen color; (3) dilated pupils; (4) rapid, thready, weak pulse; (5) rapid, shallow respirations; and (6) decreased blood pressure.

First aid measures are intended to restore oxygena-

Table 27–1

CLASSIFICATION OF WOUNDS

Type	History	Pathology	Symptoms and Color	Points of Identification	Treatment	Transportation	Complications
Bite (human, animal, or insect)	Bite of a reptile or rabid human or animal. Sting or bite of poisonous insect.	Tissue degeneration at site of wound. Muscular paralysis. Venom has a drastic effect on respiratory nerve centers.	Type of wound: Snake—two fang wound. Human—shape of denture. Dog—laceration. Patient shows rabid disposition. Insect—elevated wheal with pain and itching or burning sensation, or single or double red dot.	Shape of wound; odor of colon bacillus about the wound in human bite; presence of stinger.	Dog bite: Observe victim and dog for signs of rabies for 2 weeks. Snake bite: Apply tourniquet just tight enough to prevent venous return. Use ice packs to prevent absorption of venom. Incision and suction as swelling rises. Sting: Neutralize with alkalies. Treat for shock. Respiratory stimulants for snake or insect venom. Specific antivenins are available for certain snake bites.	Keep patient quiet; avert apprehension; keep muscles of the area elevated and at rest.	Infection introduced by pathogenic organisms. Venom of toxic nature depresses victim. Death if delay in treatment.
Brush Burns or Abrasions	Friction of body against rough surface.	Surface effaced with nicks and dotted with small drops of blood.	Skin discolored. Surface peeled off with fine beadlike dots of blood. Skin may be permeated with foreign material.	Surface of the skin is brushed completely away, or remains very lightly attached to the area.	Carefully brush away loose dirt. Cleanse the wound with soap and water. Use antiseptic solutions, ointment, and apply dressings. Tetanus toxoid or antitoxin as required.	Use loose applications of sterile dressings held in place by loose-fitting triangle.	Infection. May retain rough, unsightly scars.

Continued

Table 27–1

CLASSIFICATION OF WOUNDS—Continued

Type	History	Pathology	Symptoms and Color	Points of Identification	Treatment	Transportation	Complications
Contusions	Blow or fall.	A bruise (hematoma) or petechial area with underlying injury.	Skin surface is rough; the area includes a large or small hematoma (depending upon the extent of injury).	Skin is not broken. Underlying tissues may be slightly or markedly crushed.	Apply cold to area for 24–48 h.	Keep part well elevated. If there is additional abrasion, cover with loose-fitting bandage.	Destruction of underlying tissue if hematoma is not aspirated early. Infection if skin is punctured or probed.
Gun Shot	Accident in care of a gun. Victim of deliberate gunfire.	Wound of single outer puncture site with deep injury consisting of twisting and tearing of tissue.	Aperture is small. Powder burns are occasionally found.	Puncture site. Deep wound shows characteristic twisting of the deeper tissues.	Cleanse and irrigate. Débridement when necessary. Wet antiseptic dressings. Tetanus toxoid or antitoxin as required.	Keep patient very quiet; head slightly lower than body. Treat for shock. Watch TPR and blood pressure if blood has been lost or patient is in shock.	Shock; internal hemorrhage; tetanus bacillus infection.
Lacerations	Accident wherein sharp instruments have cut and torn an area of the body.	Jagged or torn and roughened edges of tissues. May include avulsion of certain parts.	Injury has produced area of two raw or bleeding edges of the skin. Blood may be oozing or spurting from the wound.	Wound edges are jagged and irregular. Wound may contain amount of debris or dirt and usually is infected.	Remove the large debris and dirt. Clean the wound by water dripping from sterile cloth, or use soap and warm water; mild antiseptics and sterile dressings.	Edges of wound may be united with flamed strip of adhesive tape. Cover the area with loose dressings held by triangle or cravat bandage. Tetanus toxoid or antitoxin as required.	Infection and septicemia. Wound usually heals with very unsightly scar if not properly sutured.

Puncture	Accidental or intentional piercing of body with a pointed object.	Tissues are pierced. Small opening through the tissues providing an excellent course or inlet for infection.	Area usually manifests no bleeding. Trauma of tissues usually evident.	Puncture site is very small. Object usually withdrawn with fair amount of ease.	Probe the wound very carefully to enlarge bore for irrigation with antiseptic solutions. Tetanus toxoid or antitoxin as required. Treatment for prevention of gas gangrene may be required.	Cover the area with sterile dressings and triangle or cravat bandage.	Infection of the anaerobic type (tetanus bacillus) and septicemia.
Stab	Injury by a blunt or pointed object, incurred during a fight or acquired by a fall or push.	Size of hole in the tissues varies with the size of the instrument. Foreign material and pathogenic bacteria of anaerobic nature are usually introduced.	Evidence of the instrument that was used, such as knife, ice pick, etc. Victim shows pallor, syncope, and later collapse.	Large, very deep puncture site. Instrument may still be in wound. Victim may be pinned to an object by the force of the blow.	Cleanse and irrigate the wound when possible. Irrigation and inclusion of antiseptic drain or wet dressings. Early use of antitetanic sera. Tetanus toxoid or antitoxin as required.	Keep patient very quiet with head and chest slightly elevated. Treat for shock. If chest is involved, watch TPR and blood pressure.	Internal hemorrhage from, or damage to, organs underlying site of wound, such as puncture and collapse of lung, abdominal visceral injury, or severance of a nerve. Pulmonary hemorrhage. Infection of body by anaerobic organisms.

Source: From Thomas CL (ed): Taber's Cyclopedic Medical Dictionary, ed 15. FA Davis, Philadelphia, 1985, pp 2119–2121, with permission.

TPR = temperature, pulse, and respiration.

tion to the brain and include the following: (1) the physician is alerted to manage the patient; (2) the patient's feet are elevated if the procedure does not interfere with the management of the injury; (3) the patient's body is kept warm to reduce metabolic activity; and (4) the medical assistant may administer medication as ordered by the physician.

Choking

Remember that coughing and choking are two different things. Choking emergencies occur as a result of the inability to completely or successfully swallow a substance. The substance becomes lodged in the trachea or pharynx and prevents the flow of air to the lungs.

The act of choking sometimes may be masked by signs of cyanosis, protruding eyes, the waving of the arms, and frantic motions. However, the choking victim cannot talk; therefore, when possible, ask the person if he or she can talk before beginning first aid.

First aid measures consist of performing the *Heimlich maneuver*, illustrated in Figure 27–2. This procedure includes the following steps:

1. Wrap your arms around the patient's waist from behind (patient is standing or sitting).
2. With one hand, make a fist and place the thumb side of the fist against the victim's abdomen in the midline slightly above the navel and well below the tip of the xiphoid process.
3. With your free hand, grasp the fist and press the fist into the abdomen with a quick, forceful, upward thrust. (Each thrust should be a distinct movement.)
4. Repeat the procedure until the bolus is expelled and choking subsides.

Note that the Heimlich maneuver can be applied to the unconscious patient placed in the supine position with the face up. The rescuer uses the same technique with the exception of kneeling astride the victim's thighs.

In the markedly obese or a victim in the advanced stages of pregnancy who is conscious, a chest thrust technique can be applied. The rescuer stands behind the victim and places his or her arms directly under the victim's armpits and encircles the chest. The thumb side of the fist is placed on the middle of the breastbone while avoiding the xiphoid process and the margins of the rib cage. The other hand is placed over the fist and backward thrusts are applied.

The pediatric victim requires some modification of technique. Hold an infant or small child in your lap. With your index and middle fingers of both hands above the navel and below the rib cage, press into the abdomen with a quick upward thrust. An alternative method is to place the infant face up on a firm surface and perform the procedure directly overhead.

To avoid causing injury in both the adult and pediatric victim, *do not*:

1. Slap the back.
2. Compress the chest.
3. Perform the procedure while kneeling alongside a supine victim.
4. Turn the supine victim's head to the side while performing the maneuver.

Burns

Burns occur as a result of contact with heat, chemicals, or electricity. Burns differ in extent of injury and degree of severity.

Degrees of Burns

A *first-degree burn* is a superficial injury involving the epidermis. The outer layer of skin becomes red-

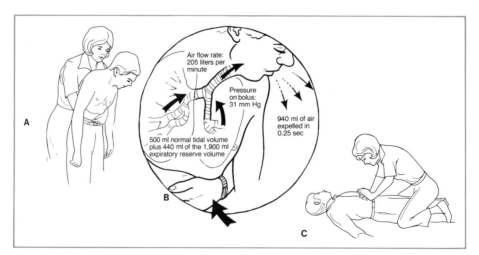

Figure 27–2. (**A**) The Heimlich maneuver with a standing choking victim. (**B**) Physiologic mechanism of the Heimlich maneuver. (**C**) Application of the Heimlich maneuver to a victim in the supine position. (Adapted from Saperstein, AB and Frazier, MA: Introduction to Nursing Practice. FA Davis, Philadelphia, 1980, p 73.)

dened and painful. A sunburn or scalding with hot water are examples of first-degree burns.

A *second-degree burn* is an injury that involves the epidermis, the dermis, and the capillaries within the dermis. It is a deeper burn, causing redness and blister formation and is quite painful. Blisters form as a result of plasma seeping into the tissue and raising the top layer of skin. A second-degree burn does not cause permanent damage to the tissue, although the patient sustaining the burn may become quite ill depending on the total body area involved. A burn that blisters can become secondarily infected. If a burn develops a discharge or the patient runs a fever, the burn should be rechecked.

A *third-degree burn* involves the epidermis, the dermis, and the subcutaneous tissue and is therefore the deepest burn. Third-degree burns often appear charred but are not as painful as second-degree burns because the nerves of the skin are destroyed. Muscle and bone could also be involved. These burns are often called *full-thickness burns* because of the depth of the injury. Third-degree burns cause permanent tissue damage and require surgical treatment. Burns involving subcutaneous tissue and muscle are referred to by some medical practitioners as fourth-degree burns.

First Aid for Burns

First aid measures for burns depend on the type of agent causing the burn.

Heat burns are treated by (1) flushing with cold running water (or ice water) for 5 to 10 minutes to reduce pain and to prevent further tissue damage, (2) applying wet dressing of 2 tablespoons of sodium bicarbonate in 1 quart of warm water, (3) covering burns with a sterile or clean dressing, and (4) treating for shock if apparent. In third-degree burns where the skin is burned off *do not* use ointment or grease.

Chemical burns are treated by (1) flooding the body areas affected with large amounts of running tap water; and (2) when the chemicals have been washed from the skin, covering with a sterile dressing. There are certain exceptions. Chemical burns can be a problem because the substance being flushed can splash and scatter to other areas, including the face and eyes.

Acid burns caused by phenol (carbolic acid) should be washed with ethyl alcohol before flooding with water, since phenol is not water-soluble.

Electrical burns are treated by: (1) covering with a sterile dressing, and (2) administering CPR if required. Electrical burns resulting from children playing with or biting into live wires can cause extensive damage to the tissues of the mouth and tongue.

Topical anesthetics such as Solarcane are not recommended for sunburns that have peeled or that blister as they can irritate broken skin or cause allergic reaction. Sunburns that have peeled or blistered can be relieved with cool tap water and application of vaseline. Sunburned skin usually peels in 5 to 7 days.

Any burn around the genitals or buttocks in minors should raise the suspicion of child abuse.

EMERGENCIES OUTSIDE THE MEDICAL OFFICE

The emergencies previously discussed can occur in the medical office or clinical setting, as well as outside the office. Those emergencies occurring from exposure to environmental heat or cold, poisoning or stress do not usually take place in the office setting. Nevertheless, the medical assistant needs to be aware of first aid measures applicable to these situations.

COLD EXPOSURE

Emergencies due to exposure to cold are usually local injuries that can cause permanent tissue damage in severe cases. The symptoms occurring from prolonged exposure to below-freezing temperatures may be delayed several hours after exposure or may appear within minutes. The conduction of heat and the presence of force of wind are major influential factors.

Emergencies from cold exposure are of two types: general cooling of the entire body surface, and local cooling of a body part.

The symptoms of general cooling include (1) shivering, (2) listlessness and apathy, (3) glassy stare, and (4) slowed pulse and respirations. First aid measures include (1) removing wet clothing; (2) applying warm clothing and blankets; and (3) using hot baths, hot liquids, and hot-water bottles.

Local cooling emergencies are usually referred to as *frostbite*. The symptoms of frostbite include (1) reddened skin that becomes gray and blotchy, and (2) numbness. The skin becomes white when actually frozen, and no pain is felt since the nerve endings are deadened. First aid measures in cases of frostbite include the following:

1. Warm the part immediately by placing it in contact with warmed areas of the victim's body, such as underarms and between the legs.
2. Immerse the part in warm water.
3. Do not put pressure on the frostbitten part.
4. Administer other comfort measures. Coffee or tea is beneficial in treating frostbite because it is a stimulant and causes dilation of peripheral blood vessels. Tobacco, however, should be avoided because it constricts blood vessels. Remember that with the application of cold, the vessels are already constricted.

HEAT EXPOSURE

It is important for the medical assistant to be able to identify and differentiate heatstroke and heat exhaustion, as these two conditions are frequently encountered, especially in the summer months and in warmer climates. Table 27–2 presents a concise comparison of common heatstroke and heat exhaustion.

Table 27–2

COMPARISON OF HEATSTROKE AND HEAT EXHAUSTION

Heatstroke. Definition: A condition or derangement of the heat-control centers due to exposure to the rays of the sun or very high temperatures. Loss of heat is inadequate or absent.	**Heat Exhaustion.** Definition: A state of very definite weakness produced by the excess loss of normal fluids and sodium chloride in the form of sweat.
History: Exposure to sun's rays or extreme heat.	History: Exposure to heat, usually indoors.
Differential Symptoms:	Differential Symptoms:
Face: Red, dry, and hot.	*Face:* Pale, cool, and moist.
Skin: Hot, dry, and no sweating.	*Skin:* Cool, clammy, with profuse diaphoresis.
Temperature: High, 106° to 110°F (41.1° to 43.3°C).	*Temperature:* Subnormal.
Pulse: Full, strong, bounding.	*Pulse:* Weak, thready, and rapid.
Respirations: Dyspneic and sonorous.	*Respirations:* Shallow and quiet.
Muscles: Tense and possible convulsions.	*Muscles:* Tense and contracted.
Eyes: Pupils are dilated but equal.	*Eyes:* Pupils are normal, eyeballs may be soft.
Treatment: Absolute rest with head elevated; cool by any means available until hospitalized, but do not use alcohol applied to skin. Take temperature every 10 minutes, and do not allow it to fall below 101°F (38.5°C).	Treatment: Keep patient quiet; head should be lowered; keep body warm to prevent onset of shock.
Drugs: Allow no stimulants; give infusions of normal saline (to force fluids).	*Drugs:* Salty fluids and fruit juices should be given frequently in small amounts. Intravenous isotonic saline will be required if patient is unconscious.

Source: From Thomas CL (ed): Taber's Cyclopedic Medical Dictionary, ed 17. FA Davis, Philadelphia, 1993, p 862, with permission.

POISONING

Poisoning can occur from inhalation of substances such as cleaning fluids and sprays, from ingestion of toxic substances, from absorption of substances such as insecticides, and from injection of drugs, or by means of bites. Table 27–3 presents emergency measures and supportive and follow-up treatment in cases of poisoning. Procedures such as lavage and the administration of medication are not performed by the medical assistant because they are outside the scope of medical as-

sisting. However, they are included in this chapter to alert the medical assistant to what action will be required in managing the poisoning victim and to facilitate the medical assistant's role in preparing, assisting in, or obtaining care.

Carbon monoxide is the most frequently inhaled poison. Symptoms of carbon monoxide poisoning include (1) headache, (2) dizziness, and (3) an unmistakable cherry-red skin color. First aid measures in cases of inhaled poisons consist of pulmonary resuscitation and immediate transportation to a medical center.

The first order of importance in emergencies involving ingested poisons is to ascertain what and how much was ingested (Table 27–4). The main objective of treatment is usually to rid the stomach of its contents by inducing vomiting. However, certain chemicals and other substances cause further injury, if vomited. These substances include strong acids or alkalines and petroleum products. In cases where immediate elimination of the poison by vomiting can be accomplished, apply one of the following first aid measures:

1. Administer 1 tablespoon of ipecac syrup followed by several glasses of warm water.
2. Administer warm water in large quantities with table salt or mustard added.
3. Tickle the back of the throat to produce a reflexive action of vomiting.

Poisons absorbed through the skin must be flooded with water and the patient observed for shock and other symptoms.

Always obtain expert advice on the handling of poison emergencies. Contact the poison control center in your area. The telephone number of the center should be placed in an accessible location. Report the following information to the center: time the incident occurred, the name of the poison, the amount, the age and weight of the victim, and any signs and symptoms noted. This should be the first course of action, as the poison control center can tell you whether it would be dangerous to induce vomiting with that particular poison.

Drug abuse accounts for a large number of cases of emergencies due to poisoning (Table 27–5). For example, cocaine use is a national epidemic and health professionals should be alert to signs and symptoms of cocaine use and should participate in patient teaching directed at educating the public regarding the dangers of cocaine use.

Recognition of the patient's symptoms is important in determining the proper first aid measures for any case of poisoning.

PSYCHOLOGICAL EMERGENCIES

Psychological emergencies encountered in the medical office are usually panic episodes of stress. Office staff members or patients may experience these attacks, which are characterized by an increase in blood pressure; clammy, moist skin; and increased pulse and respi-

Text continues on p. 689.

Table 27–3
POISONS AND POISONING

Toxic Substance	Probable Lethal Dose for Adult Humans (mg/kg body weight)	Symptoms of Poisoning	Emergency Measures	Supportive and Follow-up Treatment	Pathology
Acetaminophen		Early: may be asymptomatic. Nausea and vomiting, pallor, diaphoresis, early signs of liver damage. Late: In 24–48 h nausea and vomiting, jaundice, blood coagulation defects, hypoglycemia, hepatic and renal failure.	Emesis, gastric lavage; N-acetylcysteine should be given as soon as possible with the first dose being 140 mg/kg and then 70 mg/kg every 4 h for 3 d.	If liver and renal failure develop, treat accordingly.	Liver and kidney damage.
Acids	Variable.	Immediate pain and corrosion of mucous membranes of mouth, throat, and esophagus; difficulty in swallowing; stomach pain; nausea; coffee-ground vomitus; thirst, shock syndrome with death in circulatory collapse.	Give orally, magnesium oxide, milk of magnesia, lime water, or aluminum hydroxide gel. Avoid carbonates as neutralizers. Give large amounts of water. Demulcents and morphine for pain.	Correct shock with fluids, plasma, or whole blood. Tracheotomy or gastrectomy may become necessary.	Asphyxia from glottic edema, gastric and pyloric strictures, and stenosis or perforation.
Ammonia	Variable. Even a small amount may kill.	Irritation of eyes and respiratory tract (sometimes pulmonary edema, glottic spasm, or laryngeal edema). Other symptoms are like lye poisoning (see Lye in table).	Give large amounts of diluted vinegar, lemon juice, or orange juice. Demulcents and morphine for pain. Oxygen under pressure to help prevent pulmonary edema.	Treat for shock. Tracheotomy may be needed. **Note:** Do not give drugs such as narcotics which would depress respiration.	Corrosive esophagitis and gastritis, laryngeal edema, pulmonary edema.
Antihistamines	5–50 mg.	Drowsiness; lethargy; fatigue; ataxia; dryness of	Lavage or induce emesis. Cautious sedation if excited. Oxygen	Ice packs and alcohol sponges for hyperpyrexia.	Mechanism of death not precisely known.

Continued

Table 27–3
POISONS AND POISONING—*Continued*

Toxic Substance	Probable Lethal Dose for Adult Humans (mg/kg body weight)	Symptoms of Poisoning	Emergency Measures	Supportive and Follow-up Treatment	Pathology
		mouth; fixed dilated pupils; coma. Sometimes however, only excitement is seen with tremors, anxiety, delirium, convulsions, hyperpyrexia, nausea, vomiting, diarrhea, death in cardiovascular collapse or respiratory arrest.	and artificial respiration.		Cerebral edema is described.
Aspirin	50–500 mg.	Stimulation of the CNS including the respiratory center. The resulting hyperpnea leads to CO_2 loss. Respiratory alkalosis, hyperthermia, convulsions and shock, hypokalemia, and dehydration.	Gastric lavage with several liters of warm tap water with activated charcoal added.	The patient may be in acidosis or alkalosis; thus determine acid-base status and treat accordingly. Dehydration requires vigorous therapy.	Disturbed acid-base balance. Children often exhibit metaboic acidosis while adults more commonly show respiratory alkalosis. Intense CNS stimulation followed by depression.
Caffeine	50–500 mg.	Restlessness; excitement alternating with drowsiness; ringing in ears; fast pulse; nausea; vomiting; fever; diuresis; dehydration; thirst; tremor; delirium; convulsions; coma; death in cardiovascular and respiratory collapse.	Lavage, induce emesis with saline cathartic unless vomiting and purging have already begun. Treat CNS excitation with appropriate barbiturate therapy.	Oxygen and artificial respiration. Maintain fluid and electrolyte balance.	CNS stimulation and gastric ulceration.

Continued

Table 27-3
POISONS AND POISONING—*Continued*

Toxic Substance	Probable Lethal Dose for Adult Humans (mg/kg body weight)	Symptoms of Poisoning	Emergency Measures	Supportive and Follow-up Treatment	Pathology
Camphor	50–500 mg.	Nausea; vomiting; feeling of warmth; headache; confusion; vertigo; excitement; restlessness; delirium; hallucinations; tremor; convulsions; depression; coma; death from respiratory failure.	Short-acting intravenous barbiturates to prevent or stop convulsions. Be very careful not to overdose. Gastric lavage with tap water.	Protect the patient from all possible sensory stimuli. Oxygen and artificial respiration as needed. Avoid fats, oils, alcohol, and opiates.	Intense CNS excitation.
Carbon monoxide	1.5% concentration in the air causes unconsciousness in a few minutes. Continued exposure will cause death. Young children are more susceptible than adults.	Mild headache; breathlessness on moderate exertion; irritability; fatigue; nausea; vomiting; confusion; ataxia; syncope with period of convulsions; incontinence of urine and feces; death from respiratory arrest.	Artifical respiration and oxygen. Give 100% oxygen in a pressure chamber if possible. Glucose, 50% solution, IV for cerebral edema.	Keep patient warm. Use antibiotics at the first sign of infection. Give whole blood transfusions or washed red blood cells.	High concentrations of carboxyhemoglobin in circulating erythrocytes lead to an asphyxial death.
Carbon tetrachloride	5–10 ml total dose.	Nausea; vomiting; intense abdominal pain; headache; confusion; drowsiness; CNS depression; coma; late kidney and/or liver injury with possible acute renal failure. Death from respiratory	If swallowed: Gastric lavage or emetic. If inhaled: Artificial respiration, oxygen, stimulants but avoid alcohol. Remove clothes contaminated with carbon tetrachloride.	No specific therapy but be prepared to treat renal and hepatic failure.	CNS depression, hepatic central lobular necrosis, necrosis of renal tubular epithelium.

Continued

Table 27–3

POISONS AND POISONING—*Continued*

Toxic Substance	Probable Lethal Dose for Adult Humans (mg/kg body weight)	Symptoms of Poisoning	Emergency Measures	Supportive and Follow-up Treatment	Pathology
		arrest, circulatory collapse, or ventricular fibrillation.			
Iodine	5–50 mg.	Burning pain in mouth, throat, and stomach; lips and mouth are stained brown; thirst; vomiting (blue vomitus if stomach contained starches); bloody diarrhea; anuria or strangury, urine containing albumin or blood. Death from circulatory collapse, asphyxia from glottic edema or aspiration pneumonia.	Immediately give orally cornstarch or flour solution, 15 g in 500 ml (2 cups) water. Lavage with starch solution or 2% sodium thiosulfate. Morphine for pain and mild stimulants as indicated. Epinephrine, diphenhydramine (Benadryl) or hydrocortisone for anaphylaxis.	Give fluids and electrolytes, supportive therapy for circulatory collapse, antibiotics for secondary infections, prepare for emergency tracheotomy.	Irritation and swelling within throat (glottic edema), esophagus, and stomach. Shock secondary to fluid and electrolyte loss. More rarely, late esophageal stenosis.
Ipecac syrup or fluid-extract	Variable 1–2 oz of fluid extract (14 times more concentrated than the syrup).	Nausea: vomiting; diarrhea; albuminuria; abdominal cramps; bloody vomitus and feces; dehydration; myocarditis; myocardial infarction; cardiac arrest or shock secondary to cardiac depression and fluid loss.	Lavage or induce emesis if spontaneous vomiting has not occurred. Do not give additional emetic agents. Saline cathartic if purging has not occurred. Once toxin has been removed vomiting may respond to intravenous chlorpromazine.	General supportive and symptomatic measures for impending shock.	Intractable vomiting and diarrhea due to intense irritation of entire gastrointestinal tract leading to shock. Direct, specific cardiac damage.
Isopropyl alcohol	500–5000 mg.	Dizziness; incoordination; headache; confusion; stupor; and coma.	Lavage with tap water; oxygen and artificial respiration; mild stimulants.	Intravenous glucose and saline. Anticipate liver or kidney injury.	Acetonuria without glycosuria is pathognomonic. Severe CNS

Continued

Table 27-3
POISONS AND POISONING—*Continued*

Toxic Substance	Probable Lethal Dose for Adult Humans (mg/kg body weight)	Symptoms of Poisoning	Emergency Measures	Supportive and Follow-up Treatment	Pathology
		Symptoms closely resemble ethyl alcohol intoxication. Death from circulatory collapse or respiratory failure.			depression. Aspiration pneumonitis.
Kerosene (coal oil)	500–5000 mg if retained in stomach. If aspirated, a few can be lethal.	Burning sensation in mouth, throat, and stomach; nausea with vomiting and diarrhea; drowsiness; restlessness; disorientation; coma. Signs of pulmonary involvement indicate grave prognosis of impending fulminating hemorrhagic broncho-pneumonia.	If risks of lavage are undertaken, an endotracheal tube with inflatable cuff should be employed. Diluted sodium bicarbonate is satisfactory lavage fluid; follow with the instillation of olive oil and saline cathartic.	Antibiotics for secondary infection and positive pressure oxygen. Corticosteroids for pulmonary edema.	Severe chemical pneumonitis.
Lead	0.5 g of absorbed lead. (Chronic poisoning is much more common than acute.)	Metallic taste in mouth; burning pain in stomach and abdomen; constipation followed by diarrhea; convulsions; muscular weakness; paralysis of extremities; skin cold and cyanotic; delayed severe anemia; death is due to peripheral vascular collapse or encephalo-pathy.	Gastric lavage with magnesium or sodium sulfate. Analgesics for pain. Diazepam IV for convulsions. Intravenous calcium disodium edetate in accordance with supplier's directions. Dimercaprol is also used.	Keep patient quiet. Maintain fluid and electrolyte balance. Long-term therapy (1–2 mo for adults and 3–6 mo for children) with penicillamine to decrease the blood lead level to 60 mg/dL.	Gastrointestinal inflammation, liver and kidney injury when sufficient lead has been absorbed. Encephalopathy is frequent in children.

Continued

Table 27-3
POISONS AND POISONING—*Continued*

Toxic Substance	Probable Lethal Dose for Adult Humans (mg/kg body weight)	Symptoms of Poisoning	Emergency Measures	Supportive and Follow-up Treatment	Pathology
Lye	Total dose of 10 g may be fatal.	Severe pain in mouth and difficulty in swallowing; gastrointestinal pain and purging; weak and rapid pulse; death in shock or asphyxia from glottic edema.	Large amounts of water by mouth; diluted vinegar or lemon juice; avoid emetics and lavage. Olive oil by mouth or milk and egg whites. Mild stimulants to prevent shock. Tracheotomy may be required.	Morphine for pain; fluids and electrolytes; cortisone. Use of bougies to prevent esophageal stricture. Broad-spectrum antibiotics.	Laryngeal or glottic edema; corrosion and possible perforation of upper gastrointestinal tract; late esophageal stenosis.
Nicotine	Less than 5 mg.	Burning sensation in mouth and throat; salivation; vomiting; diarrhea; headache; sweating; dizziness; weakness; pupils contracted at first then dilated; pulse slow at first then rapid; respirations deep and rapid at first then dyspneic; death from paralysis of respiratory musculature.	Slurry of activated charcoal as lavage fluid with additional portion left in stomach. Artificial respiration and oxygen.	Control convulsions with small doses of intravenous barbiturates. Relief for visceral symptoms is obtained with atropine or phenoxy-benzamine (Dibenzyline).	Transient stimulation then depression of CNS, all autonomic ganglia and nerve endings in skeletal muscle.
Turpentine	500 mg to 5 g.	Sensation of warmth or pain in mouth, throat, and stomach followed by abdominal pain, vomiting and diarrhea. Aspiration into lungs may cause pneumonitis. Excitement,	Gastric lavage with weak bicarbonate solution, followed by demulcents and saline cathartic.	Morphine sulfate for intense pain and a short-acting barbiturate for excitement. Mild stimulation if indicated, e.g., caffeine sodium benzoate. Force fluids.	Irritation of kidneys; hematuria, albuminuria, and sometimes complete urinary suppression. Kidney symptoms appear to be related to composition of the turpentine,

Continued

Table 27–3
POISONS AND POISONING— *Continued*

Toxic Substance	Probable Lethal Dose for Adult Humans (mg/kg body weight)	Symptoms of Poisoning	Emergency Measures	Supportive and Follow-up Treatment	Pathology
		ataxia, delirium, and stupor, followed by convulsions, coma, and death from respiratory failure.			and often never appear.

Source: Adapted from Thomas CL (ed): Taber's Cyclopedic Medical Dictionary, ed 15. FA Davis, Philadelphia, 1985, pp 2088–2109, with permission. Most of the probable lethal dose values from data in Gleason MN, Gosselin RE, Hodge HC, and Smith RP: Clinical Toxicology of Commercial Products, ed 3. Williams & Wilkins, Baltimore, 1969.

ration rates caused by a surge of body chemicals such as epinephrine (adrenaline).

When a patient experiences panic, supportive measures should be provided. The patient should be instructed to take even breathes while sitting with the eyes closed. It is sometimes useful to help the individual put the situation in perspective by asking, "What's the worst thing that could happen?" and then helping the patient to consider alternatives and to select a practical solution. Sometimes, touching the patient or offering emotional support by silent presence is successful in calming the patient. Hyperventilation can occur during these episodes, and the medical assistant should be alert for potential signs (inability to catch breath, gasping). Providing the individual with privacy is, of course, essential.

Table 27–4
DOSE EQUIVALENT EXPRESSED IN HOUSEHOLD MEASURES

Less than 5 mg/kg	A taste; less then 7 drops
5–50 mg/kg	Between 7 drops and 1 tsp
50–500 mg/kg	Between 1 tsp and 1 oz
500–5000 mg/kg (0.5 to 5 g)	Between 1 oz and 1 pt
5000–15,000 mg/kg (5 to 15 g)	Between 1 pt and 1 qt
Greater than 15,000 mg/kg (15 g)	Greater than 1 qt

Source: From Thomas CL (ed): Taber's Cyclopedic Medical Dictionary, ed 15. FA Davis, Philadelphia, 1985, p 2109, with permission. Adapted from data in Gleason MN, Gosselin RE, Hodge HC, and Smith RP: Clinical Toxicology of Commercial Products, ed 3. Williams & Wilkins, Baltimore, 1969.

PREVENTION OF EMERGENCIES

In the medical office, safety precautions must be followed carefully. Because of the nature of medical practice, many potential situations exist that can easily develop into emergency situations. The medical assistant must be aware of possible hazards in the office and work toward their removal. For example, hurried performance of procedures increases the potential for accidents. Every individual in the office should consciously develop a "safety mentality." Instruments and equipment should be well maintained and handled with great care and proper technique. The floor should be kept free of obstructions such as rugs, electrical cords, and equipment. Patients with questionable orientation states or conditions should not be left unattended. Drugs should be kept in a locked cabinet. Being safety conscious also requires that the staff have plans for evacuation in case of fire or other disaster.

EMERGENCY READINESS

In the medical office, supplies are readily available for most emergencies. Nevertheless, there should be an area especially designated for emergency medications and special equipment. The medications should be checked weekly for expiration dates, and the equipment should be checked for proper functioning.

Table 27–6 provides a list of emergency medical supplies that should be preassembled.

DOCUMENTING EMERGENCY SITUATIONS

When an emergency arises in the medical office involving a patient, the event and the care given should

Table 27 – 5

TOXIC EMERGENCIES PRODUCED BY ABUSED SUBSTANCES

	CNS Excitation-Confusion	CNS Depression	Vital Signs*	Withdrawal Reaction
CNS Stimulants				
Amphetamines	Irritability, confusion, agitation, delirium, paranoia; sympathomimetic effects prominent	Exhaustion or collapse only from prolonged excitation	↑	"Crashes" after long excitation, otherwise mild depression
Methylphenidate and phenmetrazine	Stimulation, possibly convulsions		↑	No specific syndrome
Strychnine	Spinal convulsions, rigidity, trismus, hyperacusis	Postictal or exhaustion	↑ (↓)	None
Cocaine	Excitement, emotional instability to convulsions, sympathomimetic effects	Muscle paralysis, coma, CV or respiratory failure	↑ (↓)	None
Hallucinogens				
Substituted indoles		Coma with high overdose	↑ or ↓	None

LSD
  Harmines
  Ibogaine
  DMT (bufotenine), DET, DPT
	Anxiety, panic hallucinations; rare convulsions or catatonia			

Morning glory derivatives	Mild LSD-like			
Psilocybin Psilocyn	LSD-like plus fever and convulsions; rarely in children with high doses			
Mescaline (peyote)	LSD-like, plus nausea, vomiting, sweating		↑	None
Ditran and analogues	Resembles anticholinergics			None
Psychotomimetic amphetamines DOM (STP), DOET, DOP MDA, myristicin (nutmeg), PMA	Similar to LSD and amphetamines (hallucinogenic with strong sympathomimetic effects); panic reactions greater than with LSD	Coma with high overdose	↑	None
Phencyclidine (PCP), derivatives, ketamine	Convulsions in most severe (early) excitation, hallucinations, rigidity, paranoia at lower than depressant doses, hyperacusis	Coma followed by excitation and confusion, rarely respiratory depression	↑ (↓)	None
Cannabis (marijuana, THC, hashish)	Perceptual and body image distortions, rarely hallucinations	Mild hypotension occasionally		None

Anticholinergics
  Datura
  Belladonnas
  Antihistamines
  (Nonbarbiturate sedatives)
	Disorientation, hallucinations, excitement, sympathomimetic effects; fixed, dilated pupils Pathognomonic	Coma with extreme doses, collapse after prolonged excitation	↑ (↓)	None

Methysergide amantadine	Probably LSD-like			None

Continued

Table 27–5

TOXIC EMERGENCIES PRODUCED BY ABUSED SUBSTANCES—*Continued*

	CNS Excitation-Confusion	CNS Depression	Vital Signs*	Withdrawal Reaction
Inhalants				
Solvents	Delirium, psychosis, hallucinations, rarely sudden death	Coma, cardiorespiratory arrest with extreme exposure, suffocation not uncommon	↑ or ↓	None
Vasodilator-hypoxic agents, amyl and butyl nitrite	Drunken sensorium, disorientation, headache	Coma, hypotension, methemoglobinemia, coronary insufficiency on exertion	↓ (resp. ↑)	None
Opiates and Opioids				
Morphine, codeine, heroin, and derivatives meperidine, methadone, propoxyphene	Convulsions rarely, especially with codeine, propoxyphene, meperidine; otherwise confusional state most likely a sign of withdrawal; pinpoint pupils (except terminally) with all except meperidine	Coma, respiratory depression, hypothermia, CV collapse	↓	Restlessness, nausea, vomiting, diarrhea, muscle aches and spasms, weakness, chills, gooseflesh, yawning, accentuated vital signs
Pentazocine	Like other opiates, plus delirium			May precipitate withdrawal from another opioid
Sedative-Hypnotics				
Barbiturates Meprobamate Glutethimide Methyprylon	Some confusional manifestations from depressant effect; no excitatory state	CNS depression to coma, hypotension, respiratory depression, hyporeflexia, CV collapse or respiratory failure	↓	Tremulousness, insomnia, fever, agitation, delirium, psychosis; seizures not uncommon; death is possible
Benzodiazepines	Same as barbiturates	Rarely, severe depression with cardiorespiratory insufficiency	(↓)	Anxiety, restlessness, rarely convulsions
Chloral hydrate	Resembles barbiturate poisoning	Resembles barbiturate poisoning	↓	Resembles mild DTs
Alcohol	Inebriation, inhibition loss, disorientation	Coma, hypotension, hypothermia, respiratory or circulatory failure	↓	DTs, hallucinations, possible convulsions
Methaqualone	From muscle spasticity and hyperactivity to convulsions; hyperacusis, vomiting, bronchial hypersecretions	Coma, respiratory failure, rarely delayed CV collapse		Headache, cramps, anorexia, nausea, rarely convulsions, not fatal

*Vital signs ↑ = accentuated; ↓ = decreased; sign in parenthesis is less common, usually seen only in especially severe cases or as a postexcitatory depressive effect.

CV = cardiovascular; DMT = dimethyltryptamine; DET = diethyltryptamine; DOM = dimethoxymethylamphetamine (or STP = serenity, tranquility, and peace); DOET = dimethoxygethylamphetamine; DOP = dimethoxypropylamphetamine; DPT = dipropyltryptamine; DTs = delirium tremens; LSD = lysergic acid diethylamide; MDA = methylenedioxyamphetamine; PMA = paramethoxyamphetamine

From Thomas CL (ed): Taber's Cyclopedic Medical Dictionary, ed 15. FA Davis, Philadelphia, 1985, pp 2110–2113, with permission. From Emergency Medicine: March 15, 1980, with permission. Prepared by Alan K. Done, MD.

Table 27-6
EMERGENCY MEDICAL SUPPLIES

1. Airways of various sizes
2. Endotracheal tube
3. Emergency medications including:*
   Injectable epinephrine (adrenaline)
   Injectable phenobarbital
   Nitroglycerin tablets—sublingual†
   Injectable diphenhydramine HCl (Benadryl)
   Injectable diazepam (Valium)
   Syrup of ipecac
   Injectable isoproterenol (Isuprel)
   Injectable lidocaine
   Injectable sodium bicarbonate
   Sterile water for injection
   IV dextrose in saline (D5/NS)
   IV dextrose in water
   IV tubing/needles
4. Needles/syringes for injection
5. Thoracentesis needle (4 inch [10 cm], 18-gauge bevel with stylet)
6. Dressing supplies:
   Adhesive tape
   Alcohol wipes
   Angiocaths or butterflies
   Bandage strips
   Roller bandage (gauze and elastic)
   Sterile gauze pads
   Bandage scissors
7. Padded tongue blade
8. Tourniquet
9. Small paper bag (for hyperventilation)
10. Intact ice bag
11. Aromatic spirits of ammonia
12. Sugar packets (for diabetics)
13. Ambu bag
14. Oxygen tank‡

*While all emergency supplies should be included according to the physician's preference, the inventory of emergency medications, in particular, requires the physician's special attention. The physician may prefer to omit drugs from the above list or include others. In addition, he or she is responsible for ordering dosages to be kept on hand.

†Nitroglycerin tablets must be exchanged for a fresh supply every 3 months.

‡The oxygen tank should be checked for proper functioning and full content periodically according to a designated schedule. Face masks of adult and pediatric sizes should be kept with the tank, along with tubing that appropriately fits the Ambu bag.

be documented in the patient's medical record, both for legal protection and medical reference.

The procedures manual should contain guidelines for handling the specific emergencies and their documentation. An incident report form may be used to record the event and should be filed in the medical record. A staff member should be predesignated to make notations of medications and procedures on the patient's chart during an emergency. Obviously, the physician will record the event after its resolution. Emergency incidents involving staff must also be reported according to pre-

determined guidelines. Physicians are now subject to recordkeeping requirements for all recordable occupational injuries and illnesses. OSHA requires that a log, known as OSHA Form 200, be maintained and retained for 5 years. Figure 27-3 is an example of the form. Regardless of who experienced the emergency, seeking the advice of the physician's insurance carrier or observing OSHA guidelines will ensure proper documentation and processing.

PATIENT TEACHING CONSIDERATIONS

Patients should be taught both by example and actual instruction to adhere to safety measures in the medical office and at home. Patients can be instructed in home safety through the use of brochures available in the office.

If toys are available for children's play in the waiting room, signs should instruct the parents to keep toys within a particular area. No smoking signs should also be posted to prevent fire as well as to promote respiratory health.

In the examination room, parents may be reminded not to allow their children to touch instruments, as these could cause injury. While positioning patients on the examination table, give clear, concise directions to prevent their falling. As the medical assistant becomes alert to potential emergency-causing hazards, he or she can better assist patients in developing safety consciousness as well.

RELATED ETHICAL AND LEGAL IMPLICATIONS

Medical emergencies present particular legal concerns. It is helpful for the medical assistant to understand the legal responsibilities and rights of the caregiver. Regardless of the ethical and moral considerations, a physician or other health care professional is not legally obligated to stop at the scene of an accident and render emergency care. The Good Samaritan statutes provide protection for physicians (and nurses in some states) administering medical first aid at the scene of a sudden injury or accident. Legal liability is limited to gross neglect of or willfully causing further injury to the victim. The caregiver is required to act as a reasonable person and cannot be held liable for personal injury resulting from an act or its omission. The statute provides for discretionary evaluation of the caregiver's judgment.

An individual never trained in CPR cannot be expected to perform the procedure. However, in many states, a health care professional possessing the skills and training would be declared negligent if an accident occurred and the health professional present at the scene did not administer CPR.

The victim's consent for care is implied by virtue of his or her immediate need. If the victim is conscious or relatives are present, verbal consent can be obtained.

Bureau of Labor Statistics
Log and Summary of Occupational
Injuries and Illnesses

| NOTE: | This form is required by Public Law 91-596 and must be kept in the establishment for 5 years. Failure to maintain and post can result in the issuance of citations and assessment of penalties. (See posting requirements on the other side of form.) | RECORDABLE CASES: You are required to record information about every occupational death; every nonfatal occupational illness; and those nonfatal occupational injuries which involve one or more of the following: loss of consciousness, restriction of work or motion, transfer to another job, or medical treatment (other than first aid). (See definitions on the other side of form.) |

Case or File Number	Date of Injury or Onset of Illness	Employee's Name	Occupation	Department	Description of Injury or Illness
Enter a nonduplicating number which will facilitate comparisons with supplementary records.	Enter Mo./day.	Enter first name or initial, middle initial, last name.	Enter regular job title, not activity employee was performing when injured or at onset of illness. In the absence of a formal title, enter a brief description of the employee's duties.	Enter department in which the employee is regularly employed or a description of normal workplace to which employee is assigned, even though temporarily working in another department at the time of injury or illness.	Enter a brief description of the injury or illness and indicate the part or parts of body affected. Typical entries for this column might be: Amputation of 1st joint right forefinger; Strain of lower back; Contact dermatitis on both hands; Electrocution—body.
(A)	(B)	(C)	(D)	(E)	(F)

PREVIOUS PAGE TOTALS ➞

TOTALS (Instructions on other side of form.) ➞

OSHA No. 200   ☆U.S. GOVERNMENT PRINTING OFFICE: 1989 241-374/08097

Figure 27–3. OSHA form No. 299, Log and Summary of Occupational Injuries and Illnesses.

SUMMARY

Medical office emergencies present yet another challenge to medical assistants. They must possess the knowledge and skills to meet their responsibilities in emergency situations. Becoming certified in first aid and CPR is essential to the development of these skills. The information presented in this chapter serves as a basic foundation and reference for identifying and responding to medical office emergencies. Obviously, the role of the medical assistant in the management of emergency situations is determined by the presence or absence of more qualified medical personnel. However, the medical assistant's responsibility to check and replace office emergency supplies and equipment routinely and to initiate and monitor safety measures for accident prevention remains constant.

For Calendar Year 19 _____   Page ___of___

Company Name		Form Approved
Establishment Name		O.M.B. No. 1220-0029
Establishment Address		See OMB Disclosure Statement on reverse.

Extent of and Outcome of INJURY | **Type, Extent of, and Outcome of ILLNESS**

Fatalities	Nonfatal Injuries					Type of Illness							Fatalities	Nonfatal Illnesses				
Injury Related	Injuries With Lost Workdays				Injuries Without Lost Workdays	CHECK Only One Column for Each Illness *(See other side of form for terminations or permanent transfers.)*							Illness Related	Illnesses With Lost Workdays				Illnesses Without Lost Workdays
Enter **DATE** of death. Mo./day/yr.	Enter a **CHECK** if injury involves days away from work, or days of restricted work activity, or both.	Enter a **CHECK** if injury involves days away from work.	Enter number of **DAYS** away from work.	Enter number of **DAYS** of restricted work activity.	Enter a **CHECK** if no entry was made in columns 1 or 2 but the injury is recordable as defined above.	Occupational skin diseases or disorders	Dust diseases of the lungs	Respiratory conditions due to toxic agents	Poisoning (systemic effects of toxic materials)	Disorders due to physical agents	Disorders associated with repeated trauma	All other occupational illnesses	Enter **DATE** of death. Mo./day/yr.	Enter a **CHECK** if illness involves days away from work, or days of restricted work activity, or both.	Enter a **CHECK** if illness involves days away from work.	Enter number of **DAYS** away from work.	Enter number of **DAYS** of restricted work activity.	Enter a **CHECK** if no entry was made in columns 8 or 9.
(1)	(2)	(3)	(4)	(5)	(6)	(7)							(8)	(9)	(10)	(11)	(12)	(13)
						(a)	(b)	(c)	(d)	(e)	(f)	(g)						

INJURIES *ILLNESSES*

Certification of Annual Summary Totals By _____Title_____ Date _____

OSHA No. 200   POST ONLY THIS PORTION OF THE LAST PAGE NO LATER THAN FEBRUARY 1.

Figure 27–3. Continued.

DISCUSSION QUESTIONS

1. What is the definition of an emergency?
2. What are the five general procedures for providing emergency care?
3. What are the legal implications of the medical assistant administering emergency care?
4. What is the appropriate method of documentation for patients and employees injured in the medical office?
5. What is the meaning of "safety mentality"?

BIBLIOGRAPHY

Banks C: Learn CPR and save a life. The Professional Medical Assistant, Sept/Oct, 1986.

Conner K: Emergency! Are you prepared? The Professional Medical Assistant, Sept/Oct, 1986, p 7.

Frew, DR and Breening, N: Coping with emergencies: When stress becomes panic. The Professional Medical Assistant, Sept/Oct, 1986.

Luckmann J and Sorensen K. Medical-Surgical Nursing, ed 3. WB Saunders, Philadelphia, 1987.

Standards and Guidelines for Cardiopulmonary Resuscitation and Emergency Cardiac Care. American Heart Association: Textbook of Advanced Cardiac Life Support, ed 2. 1990.

PROCEDURE: Perform mouth-to-mouth resuscitation

OSHA STANDARDS:

Terminal Performance Objective: Using a training manikin, demonstrate and explain the steps to take in establishing an open airway. (NOTE: This procedure is to be demonstrated only by students who have successfully completed a certified CPR course.)

EQUIPMENT: Mouth-to-mouth resuscitation mask
Training manikin
Nonsterile gloves
Gauze squares
Bleach (household) for cleaning the manikin and equipment
Biohazard bag

PROCEDURE

1. Don gloves.

2. Shake patient. Shout "Are you OK?"
3. Wipe any foreign material from the victim's mouth. (This may be done with the gloved finger or a gauze square.)
4. Tilt the victim's head back so that the chin is pointing up and pull the jaw outward.

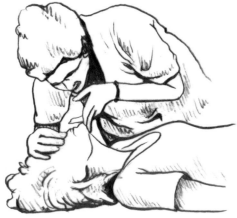

Head tilt/chin lift.

5. Look for any foreign body.
6. Establish breathlessness.

7. Following manufacturer's instructions, place the resuscitation mask on the victim's mouth.

PRINCIPLE

1. Although CDC Guidelines do not classify CPR as a Category I exposure unless blood is visible, gloves should be used as personal protective equipment when training to perform CPR as well as responding to an actual emergency resuscitation (if at all possible).
2. Establish unresponsiveness.
3. To provide a clean, unobstructed area to apply mask.

4. To establish a patent airway and to prevent the tongue from obstructing the airway.

5. An obstructive air passage prevents air exchange.
6. Respiratory movements or sounds preclude mouth to mouth resuscitation. If breathing is present, keep the victim safe until help arrives.
7. No transmission of HBV or HIV during mouth-to-mouth resuscitation has been documented, but because of the risk of salivary transmission of other infectious diseases and the theoretical risk of HBV/HIV transmission, OSHA recommends the use of disposable airway equipment or resuscitation bags during emergency artificial ventilation.

PROCEDURE

8. If the mask does not cover the victim's nostrils, close the nostrils by pinching them together with the fingers.

9. Blow two forceful breaths into the victim's mouth, taking care a good seal prevents air from escaping from the victim's mouth or nose. (Take a deep breath between ventilations.) Observe for spontaneous, non-assisted breathing.

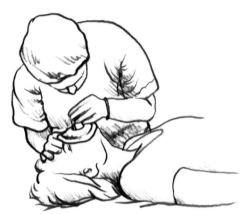

Begin resuscitation with two long breaths.

10. Check the carotid pulse for at least 5 seconds. If there is no pulse, initiate CPR. Otherwise, continue resuscitation.

11. After each breath blown into the mouth, turn your head to one side and listen and feel for the return rush of air.

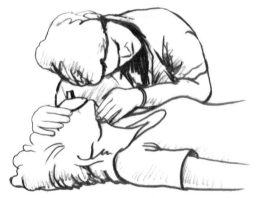

After each breath, turn your head to listen and feel for the rush of air out of the chest.

12. Repeat the blowing procedure with approximately 12 breaths a minute for adults and 20 for children.

13. Continue ventilation and checking for pulselessness until breathing is restored or other medical personnel are available to care for the victim.

PRINCIPLE

8. To prevent air from escaping through the nose.

9. To force air into the lungs for the exchange of O_2 and CO_2. Two ventilations (1 to 1½ seconds per breath) allow adequate chest expansion. A spontaneous return of breathing eliminates further need of ventilatory assistance.

10. To determine pulselessness. If the heart is not beating, circulation must be accomplished through manual compression of the chest. If pulse is present, it will be more readily apparent at the carotid artery.

11. The return flow of air signals lung deflation.

12. The number of breaths administered corresponds to the average number of breaths per minutes normally required to sustain life.

13. The presence of breathing and pulse determine whether assistance can be discontinued or cardiopulmonary resuscitation required.

PROCEDURE: Administer adult cardiopulmonary resuscitation

OSHA STANDARDS:

Terminal Performance Objective: Using a training manikin, demonstrate and explain the steps to take in providing cardiopulmonary resuscitation. (NOTE: This procedure is to be demonstrated only by students who have successfully completed a certified CPR course.)

EQUIPMENT: Mouth-to-mouth resuscitation mask
Training manikin
Nonsterile gloves
Gauze squares
Bleach (household) for cleaning the manikin and equipment
Biohazard bag

PROCEDURE

1. Don gloves.

2. Shake patient. Shout "Are you OK?"
3. Wipe any foreign material from the victim's mouth. (This may be done with the gloved finger or a gauze square.)
4. Tilt the victim's head back so that the chin is pointing up and pull the jaw outward.
5. Look for any foreign body.
6. Establish breathlessness.

7. Following manufacturer's instructions, place the resuscitation mask on the victim's mouth.

8. If the mask does not cover the victim's nostrils, close the nostrils by pinching them together with the fingers.
9. Blow two forceful breaths into the victim's mouth, taking care a good seal prevents air from escaping from the victim's mouth or nose. (Take a deep breath between ventilations.) Observe for spontaneous, non-assisted breathing.

PRINCIPLE

1. Although CDC Guidelines do not classify CPR as a Category I exposure unless blood is visible, gloves should be used as a personal protective equipment when training to perform CPR as well as responding to an actual emergency resuscitation (if at all possible).
2. Establish unresponsiveness.
3. To provide a clean, unobstructed area to apply mask.

4. To establish a patent airway and to prevent the tongue from obstructing the airway.
5. An obstructive air passage prevents air exchange.
6. Respiratory movements or sounds preclude mouth to mouth resuscitation. If breathing is present, keep the victim safe until help arrives.
7. No transmission of HBV or HIV during mouth-to-mouth resuscitation has been documented, but because of the risk of salivary transmission of other infectious diseases and the theoretical risk of HBV/HIV transmission, OSHA recommends the use of disposable airway equipment or resuscitation bags during emergency artificial ventilation.
8. To prevent air from escaping through the nose.

9. To force air into the lungs for the exchange of O_2 and CO_2. Two ventilations (1 to 1½ seconds per breath) allow adequate chest expansion. A spontaneous return of breathing eliminates further need of ventilatory assistance.

PROCEDURE

10. Check the carotid pulse for at least 5 seconds. If there is no pulse, initiate CPR. Otherwise, continue resuscitation.

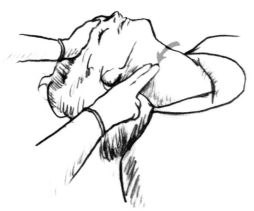

Feel for a carotid pulse.

11. Locate the lower half of the sternum. If you are kneeling on the patient's right side, run the index and middle fingers of your right hand up the lower margin of the victim's rib cage and locate the sternal notch with your middle finger.

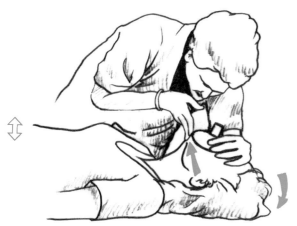

Begin resuscitation with two long breaths.

PRINCIPLE

10. To determine pulselessness. If the heart is not beating, circulation must be accomplished through manual compression of the chest. If pulse is present, it will be more readily apparent at the carotid artery.

11. The heel of the hand closest to the victim's head is the one to place on the compression point, with the other hand on top of that one.

PROCEDURE

PRINCIPLE

12. Place your right index finger on the sternal notch. Place the heel of your left hand on the sternum next to, but not covering, your index finger. Place your right hand on top of the left hand.

12. Correct placement is essential to avoid injury and for successful CPR.

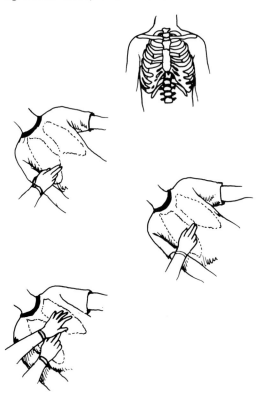

It is important to find the correct compression point.

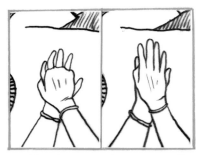

Place the second hand over the first; you can, if you prefer, lace the fingers of the second between those of the first.

13. Apply pressure straight down to depress the sternum 1½ to 2 inches, using all of your upper body weight. Hold for approximately three-quarter second (15 compressions each 10–11 seconds), then release.

14. Release each compression quickly. Release time should equal compression time.

15. Alternate heart compressions with lung ventilation at the rate of 15 compressions to 2 breaths.

16. Check for a pulse after every 4 ventilation-compression cycles.

13. To sufficiently compress the chest, and force blood circulation at a rate of 80–100 compressions per minute.

14. To create suction as the chest rebounds, which helps draw blood from the veins into the heart.

15. Successful CPR replaces the activity of the lungs (by ventilation) and the heart (by chest compression/release).

16. It is necessary to regularly reevaluate the pulse to determine whether the victim has resumed spontaneous heart contraction (pulse) and respiration.

PROCEDURE

17. If there is no pulse, resume CPR. If there is a pulse but no breathing, continue with only mouth-to-mouth resuscitation. Continue until normal heart-lung action is restored or qualified medical personnel take over management of the victim.

PRINCIPLE

17. Circulation and ventilation continues as long as the procedure is continued.

NOTE: For infants and small children:
  Ventilations: 40–60 per minute.
  Compressions: 120 per minute.
  Place both thumbs on the lower third of the sternum (or use two fingers—the ring and middle). Take care not to compress the xiphoid portion of the sternum. Compress the sternum by only ½"–¾".
  In the small infant or neonate, when using the thumbs for compression, encircle the torso and support the back with your fingers. Use the two-finger compression method for larger infants.
  Keep Pediatric CPR Resource Cards, which are charts of the appropriate ventilation/compression rates, readily available and visible in the medical office.

HIGHLIGHTS

A Question of Protection: The Good Samaritan Laws

Prior to the passing of the Good Samaritan acts, health care professionals were reluctant to render emergency assistance at the scene of an accidental injury occurring outside the medical setting for fear they could be held liable for malpractice. The health care professional presently is offered immunity under the Good Samaritan laws. However, the law still holds an individual responsible for his or her own actions. Immunity offers protection only when the individual acts appropriately and does not intentionally or recklessly cause the patient harm. Obviously, *appropriately* is a matter of discernment. Generally, to act appropriately is interpreted as acting reasonably (as any reasonable person would act) and rendering care according to an expected level of medical expertise (the expectations for a particular profession).

The Good Samaritan acts do not apply to medical office emergencies but only to accidents occurring outside the health care setting. The reason for special applications of these acts is based on the interpretation of several components of the law:

1. **Duty:** The health professional does not have a legal duty to assist the accident victim. If the health professional is the only one at the scene or if he or she has initiated care, care must be administered or continued until someone of similar or more extensive training arrives, or police or other officials assume responsibility for the patient.

2. **Injury:** It is understood that the Good Samaritan is helping an already injured individual in an emergency situation. The health professional is not expected to make the patient well or to perform specific procedures but to offer supportive care according to the standard of care for the individual's profession. Liability for the injury can only result when the health professional *causes* the victim's condition to worsen considerably.

3. **Relationship:** No contractual relationship exists between the victim and the health professional. However, a temporary relationship does exist with the victim once care is initiated and until more appropriate care can be provided. In the medical office setting, the medical assistant does have a legal duty to, and a legal relationship with the patient. Specific care measures are expected and quality determined by standard-of-care for medical assistants.

Unit 5

Laboratory and Diagnostic Procedures

This unit focuses on the role of the medical assistant in laboratory and other diagnostic tests. The medical assistant responsible for office laboratory testing must understand the basic concepts of laboratory medicine. This unit introduces the medical assistant to the various components of laboratory medicine, electrocardiography (ECG), and diagnostic imaging.

One of the most frequently used diagnostic tools is laboratory testing of body substances. Most medical office laboratories are fairly limited in the scope of tests performed. However, it is routine in most medical office settings to order and in some cases to perform certain blood and urine tests and to take specimens for the isolation, culture, and microscopic examination of microorganisms from selected body substances. This requires the medical assistant to be knowledgeable and skillful in obtaining the specimens and performing the appropriate procedures.

The ECG is also a valuable diagnostic tool, indispensable in the diagnosis and treatment of heart disease. The ECG procedure requires precise skill and knowledge, and the medical assistant who is competent in performing this procedure is an asset to the medical office practice. This unit also provides an overview of the relationship of diagnostic imaging, including radiology, ultrasound, and nuclear medicine procedures, to medical office practice. The medical assistant must be knowledgeable about this changing technology despite limited responsibility.

Unit Objectives

Upon completing this unit, you will be able to:

1. Perform medical office tests using quality controls.
2. Explain medical office laboratory tests to patients and their families.
3. Refer the patient to outside laboratory testing facilities and schedule appointments.
4. Prepare the patient for and explain the ECG procedure.
5. Perform an electrocardiogram.
6. Perform certain radiologic testing procedures, when appropriate.
7. Position the patient and explain the radiologic procedure before performing it.
8. Describe the ethical and legal issues associated with these procedures.
9. Understand the need for and follow CLIA regulations and OSHA standards when performing diagnostic and laboratory procedures.

> *O*ffice laboratory testing is a challenging opportunity to work with the physician to improve and promote health care.
>
> Margaret Watkins

CHAPTER OUTLINE

TYPES OF LABORATORY TESTS
  Clinical Laboratory Tests
  Profile Laboratory Tests

THE CLINICAL LABORATORY IMPROVEMENT
    AMENDMENTS: REGULATIONS AND
    REQUIREMENTS
  Quality Assurance
  Quality Control
  Recordkeeping

REGULATIONS CONCERNING HAZARDOUS AND
    TOXIC SUBSTANCES
  Material Safety Data Sheets
  Hazard Labels

OCCUPATIONAL EXPOSURE TO BLOODBORNE
    PATHOGENS
  Standard Operating Procedures
  Personnel Training and Evaluation

SPECIMEN COLLECTION
  Preparation and Collection
  Transport
  Chain of Custody
  Specimen Waste

PHLEBOTOMY
  Patient Teaching Considerations
  Venipuncture
  Specimen Tubes
  Site Selection
  Syringe Method
  Withdrawing a Blood Sample for Culturing
  Serum Separation
  Hemolysis

Capillary Puncture
Automatic Sample Collecting Devices

BASIC LABORATORY EQUIPMENT
  Pipettes
  Centrifuge
  Spectrophotometer

THE MICROSCOPE
  Microscope Components
  Magnification
  Care and Maintenance

GENERAL RULES OF SAFETY
  Housekeeping
  Emergency Precautions
  Protection from Aerosols
  Pipetting Safeguards

RELATED ETHICAL AND LEGAL IMPLICATIONS

SUMMARY

DISCUSSION QUESTIONS

BIBLIOGRAPHY

PROCEDURES
  Withdraw a Venous Blood Sample Using
    the Evacuated Blood Collecting System
    or a Syringe
  Perform a Capillary Puncture on a Finger
    or Heel
  Focus and Care for the Microscope

HIGHLIGHTS
  Personal Protective Equipment Cuts Risk

Chapter 28

*T*he Physician's Office Laboratory: Part I

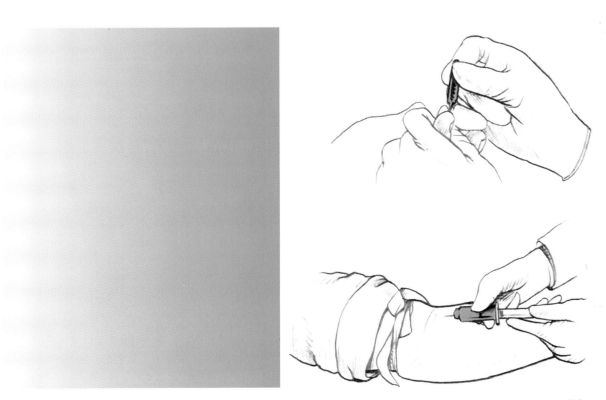

LEARNING OBJECTIVES

Upon completing this chapter, you will be able to:

1. List the waiver tests established by the Clinical Laboratory Improvement Amendment of 1988.
2. Describe each component necessary to implement complete laboratory quality assurance and quality control programs.
3. Define and describe the proper use of instrument calibration, reagents, controls, and standards.
4. Identify four types of quality control records.
5. Identify three federal laws that regulate safety in the physician's office laboratory.
6. List the information that should be included on the Materials Safety Data Sheet for at least five hazardous substances found in the office laboratory.
7. Classify specimen collection tasks according to the three exposure categories developed by the Occupational Health and Safety Administration.
8. List five basic criteria for a properly collected specimen.
9. List the precautions necessary for labeling, packaging, transporting, and disposing of specimens and in the chain of specimen custody.
10. Describe four types of blood specimens obtained by venipuncture and the color-coded rubber stoppers indicated for each type.
11. List the order of tubes used when multiple blood tests are performed.
12. List the causes of hemolysis.
13. List the general safety rules for the office laboratory.

PERFORMANCE OBJECTIVES

Upon completing this chapter, you will be able to:

1. Obtain a single sample or multiple blood samples for diagnostic testing and prepare blood specimens for transport.
2. Obtain a small volume of capillary blood for diagnostic testing and prepare the specimen for transport.
3. Demonstrate focusing and the proper care of the microscope.

DACUM EDUCATIONAL COMPONENTS

1. Apply procedures of aseptic technique and infection control (4.1).
2. Use quality control (4.9).
3. Collect and process specimens (4.10).
4. Document accurately (5.1).
5. Operate and maintain facilities and equipment safely (6.2).

Glossary

Absorbance: in spectrophotometry, the amount of light absorbed by a solution is directly proportionate to the concentration of the solution

Additives: usually anticoagulants added to blood during the collection process

Anticoagulants: a substance in the body or testing container that suppresses, delays, or prevents the coagulation of blood

Blank solution: solution containing all the components, including solvents and solutes, except the specimen to be measured

Bloodborne: carried by the blood

Calibration: means by which a piece of equipment or glassware is checked with a known substance to ensure that it will measure or deliver exact amounts

Capillarity: the action by which the surface of a liquid is elevated or depressed when it comes into contact with a solid, such as in a capillary tube

Control specimen: material or solution with known values; used for quality control where the control results must be within certain limits for the unknown specimen values run in the same "batch" to be considered reportable

Continued

Decantation: the pouring of a clear supernatant liquid from a sediment

g: abbreviation for gravity; the unit of force exerted upon a body during acceleration and deceleration

Hemolysis: rupture of the red blood cell membrane and release of hemoglobin into the plasma; the plasma appears reddish; used as an indicator of an antigen-antibody reaction

Numerical aperture (NA): measurement of the resolving power of a microscope or lens

Qualitative analysis: to identify and characterize one or more constituents of a specimen; to identify the components of a specimen as to kind and amount

Quantitative analysis: determining the proportionate quantities of the constituents of a specimen or mixture

Reference laboratory: a central laboratory setting where special or complex tests or tests requiring special technology are performed

Relative centrifugal force: the method of comparing the forces generated by various centrifuges by measuring the speed of rotation and the radius from the center of the rotation

Resolution: magnification limitations; tells how small and how close objects can still be recognized

Standard solution: solution of fixed and known composition of the specimen being tested

Laboratory medicine is a broad subject, too broad to completely cover in a book such as this. This chapter and the two following chapters do not, therefore, attempt to discuss all laboratory testing methods and equipment. Rather, these chapters introduce the medical assistant to the basic concepts and techniques of laboratory medicine.

Laboratory testing performed in the physician's office laboratory (POL) offers a convenience for both the patient and the physician. The patient's anxiety can be relieved when a diagnosis is confirmed or ruled out by a laboratory test result without waiting. When an immediate diagnosis is important for treatment, the physician can immediately initiate treatment after on-site testing.

The type of laboratory testing performed in the office varies depending on the physician's specialty and state or federal standards. The individual physician decides which tests are cost effective when done in the office, based on the complexity of the tests, the cost of the equipment, and the type of personnel required by law for the overall operations of the laboratory. Tests that are too costly or too complex are performed by independent, outside medical laboratories, called *reference laboratories.* Patients may be referred to a laboratory or their specimens are collected by the medical assistant and sent to the laboratory for testing.

This chapter describes the role of the medical assistant in specimen collection and clinical laboratory testing. Discussion of the importance of clinical tests as a diagnostic tool includes an introduction to the issues of quality assurance (QA) and quality control (QC).

In the role of phlebotomist, the medical assistant follows the basic criteria for the collection of laboratory specimens. The technical aspects of obtaining a blood sample by venipuncture or capillary puncture are presented along with communication skills that can help to reduce patient anxiety during the drawing of blood. A general understanding of laboratory medicine and diagnostic testing, along with the ability to perform a phlebotomy skillfully, is necessary to assist the physician effectively and to provide patient instruction and reassurance.

Basic laboratory equipment frequently used in the POL is described. Information about the microscope is presented in detail, as it has widespread use in the office setting. The chapter concludes with rules of laboratory safety to protect the medical assistant from biologic hazards while collecting specimens and doing laboratory testing.

TYPES OF LABORATORY TESTS

CLINICAL LABORATORY TESTS

The laboratory test is a valuable diagnostic tool. Specific laboratory tests can often be used to diagnose a particular disease; for example, an abnormal glucose level may indicate diabetes mellitus. Laboratory tests are also used to monitor a patient's therapeutic drug level. Many physicians include a blood profile and a urinalysis as a part of a complete physical examination. This utilization of laboratory tests acts as a preventive medicine measure. Test results that deviate from normal values can be indicative of a particular disease state or health problem. Table 28–1 lists several laboratory tests and their related diseases or conditions.

PROFILE LABORATORY TESTS

Although laboratory tests are indications of the body's state of health at the time a specimen is obtained, not all laboratory results can be correlated with disease states. For this reason, the patient's overall physical condition must be assessed by the physician in conjunction with the laboratory data. Many physicians routinely order a profile or panel of laboratory tests that can be performed by using a single blood sample (Table 28–2). A profile can be designed to screen several of the body's 12 systems or one particular function, such as liver function tests. If any test result is abnormal, the physician can further investigate the abnormal result.

Table 28-1

COMMON LABORATORY TESTS AND DISEASE STATES OR CONDITIONS

Test	Disease or Condition
Acetone	Metabolic acidosis
Acid phosphatase	Prostatic cancer
Alanine aminotransferase (ALT); formerly serum glutamic-pyruvic transaminase (SGPT)	Liver disease
Amylase and lipase	Acute pancreatitis
Antistreptolysin-O titer (ASOT) and erythrocyte sedimentation rate (ESR)	Rheumatic fever and other streptococcal infections
Aspartate aminotransferase (AST); formerly serum glutamicoxaloacetic transaminase (SGOT)	Heart or liver disease
Bence-Jones protein (BJP)	Multiple myeloma
Bilirubin and alkaline phosphatase	Liver function
Cholesterol/triglycerides	Atherosclerosis
Calcium and phosphorus	Parathyroid function
Carbon dioxide (CO_2), chloride (Cl), blood pH, PO_2, PCO_2	Acid-base balance, respiratory function
Cold agglutination test	Primary atypical pneumonia
Creatine kinase (PK); formerly creatine phosphokinase (CPK)	Heart disease, myocardial infarction
Eosinophil count	Allergic state, parasitic infection
Erythrocyte sedimentation rate (ESR) and C-reative protein (CRP)	Inflammatory process
Febrile agglutinins	Typhoid fever, brucellosis, Rocky Mountain spotted fever, tularemia, dysentery, typhoid fever
Glucose tolerance test (GTT)	Hypoglycemia, diabetes mellitus
Heterophil antibody or "mono" test	Infectious mononucleosis
Lactate dehydrogenase (LD); formerly lactic acid dehydrogenase (LDH)	Myocardial infarction
PKU test (phenylpyruvic acid in urine; phenylalanine in serum)	Phenylketonuria
Prothrombin time (PT), platelet count, bleeding time, fibrinogen, activated partial thromboplastin time (aPTTT), thrombin time (TT)	Anticoagulation therapy or coagulation disorders
Red blood cells, hematocrit, hemoglobin, iron, total iron-binding capacity, reticulocyte count	Anemia
Sickle cell test	Sickle cell trait or sickle cell disease
Sodium (Na) and Potassium (K)	Fluid and electrolyte balance
Sugar (glucose), FBS (fasting blood sugar), 2-h postprandial blood sugar, hemoglobin A_{ic} (glycohemoglobin)	Diabetes mellitus
Total protein, globulin, albumin, albumin/globulin ratio	Cirrhosis, hepatitis, nephrosis, multiple myeloma
Thyroid-stimulating hormone (TSH), triiadothyronine (T_3), thyroxine (T_4)	Thyroid function
Uric acid	Gout
White blood count (total WBC and differential count)	Infections, leukemias, leukopenia

THE CLINICAL LABORATORY IMPROVEMENT AMENDMENTS: REGULATIONS AND REQUIREMENTS

Prompted by press and television reports of deaths resulting from misdiagnosed Pap smears, Congress passed the Clinical Laboratory Improvement Amendments (CLIA) of 1988. The CLIA are intended to regulate all human testing and apply to anyone who performs testing of human specimens for the diagnosis, prevention, or treatment of disease or health problems. This includes physicians who perform the most basic tests to those who operate moderately complex or highly complex POLs. The Health Care Financing Administration (HCFA) and the Centers for Disease Control (CDC) regulate CLIA standards at the federal level; but states can seek to implement their own standards, provided that the state standards are equivalent to the federal standards. Information on whether state standards are in place can be obtained by contacting the state health department.

Table 28-2
COMMON LABORATORY PROFILES

Coagulation Profile
Bleeding time
Activated partial thromboplastin time (aPTT)
Platelet count
Prothrombin time (PT)

Diabetic Management Profile
Glucose
Hemoglobin A$_{ic}$ (glycohemoglobin)

Electrolyte Profile
Carbon dioxide (CO)
Chloride (Cl)
Potassium (K)
Sodium (Na)

General Health Profile
Albumin
Alkaline phosphatase
Aspartate aminotransferase (AST); formerly serum glutamic-oxalacetic transmainase (SGOT)
Bloodurea nitrogen (BUN)
Calcium
Cholesterol
Creatinine
Glucose
Lactic dehydrogenase (LD)
Phosphorus
Potassium
Sodium
Total bilirubin
Total protein
Triglycerides
Uric acid

Kidney Function Profile
Albumin/globulin ratio
BUN
Clearance tests
Creatinine
Total Protein

Lipid Profile
Cholesterol
Triglycerides
Lipoprotein fractions (high-density lipoprotein [HDL], low-density lipoprotein [LDL])

Liver Function Profile
Albumin
Alkaline phosphatase
alanine aminotransferase (AST); formerly serum glutamic-pyruvic transaminase (SGPT)
AST (SGOT)
Bilirubin (direct)
Bilirubin (total)
Cholesterol
Gamma-glutamyl transferase (GGT)
LD
PT
Total protein

Myocardial Infarction Profile
CK
CK isoenzymes (MB fraction)
LD
LD isoenzymes

Prenatal Profile
ABO grouping and Rh typing
Antibody screen
Complete blood count (CBC)
Syphilis
Rubella

The *degree* of applicable federal or state regulation of the POL depends on the complexity of tests performed. Three categories of testing have been established: waiver tests, moderate complexity tests, and high complexity tests. Waiver tests are simple, stable tests that require a minimal degree of judgment and interpretation. Waiver tests also include tests approved by the Food and Drug Administration (FDA) for patient self-testing at home. The following tests are considered waiver tests:

Urine
Dipstick or tablet
Reagent
Urinalysis for:
  Bilirubin
  Glucose

Blood
Erythrocyte
  sedimentation rate
Hb-copper sulfate
  (nonautomated)
Spun microhematocrit

Urine
  Hemoglobin (Hb)
  Ketone
  Leukocytes
  Nitrites
  pH
  Protein
  Specific gravity
  Urobilinogen
  Pregnancy tests (visual
    color comparison
    tests)

Blood
Blood glucose testing
  (using monitoring
  devices cleared by the
  FDA for home use)

Other
Fecal occult blood
Ovulation tests (visual
  color tests for human
  luteinizing hormone)

Moderately complex tests make up approximately 75% of the 10,000 laboratory tests and test methods performed on human specimens in bacteriology, myco-bacteriology, mycology, parasitology, virology, immu-

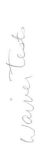

nology, chemistry, hematology, and immunohematology. High complexity tests include the more complex tests performed in each of these disciplines as well as those performed in clinical cytogenetics, histopathology, histocompatibility, and cytology disciplines. HCFA publishes lists of all the moderately complex tests and test methods. If a test is not on a HCFA list, it must be considered high complexity until it can be categorized. The best way to find out if a particular instrument or commercial test kit is on the moderately complex list is to call the manufacturer and ask.

Moderately and highly complex POLs must meet specific standards for personnel training and experience, on-site proficiency testing, and continuing education, QA, QC, and facility inspections. All laboratories, including waiver laboratories in the physician's office, must participate in three proficiency testing events each year and at least one on-site inspection to maintain a certificate of approval to perform the tests and continue receiving Medicare laboratory payments.

QUALITY ASSURANCE

The CLIA requirements include a QA program for all laboratory testing. QA is an ongoing program designed to monitor and evaluate objectively and systematically the quality and appropriateness of patient care, to pursue opportunities to improve patient care, and to resolve identified problems in the laboratory. QA in the laboratory must ensure the safety, reliability, and medical usefulness of each laboratory test performed. The six characteristics of any QA assurance program include the following:

1. Written policies on the standards of patient care and professional behavior
2. A QC program
3. A training and continuing education program
4. An instrument maintenance program
5. Documentation requirements
6. Evaluation methods and frequency

Requirements for a laboratory QA program under CLIA include written policies and procedures for patient preparation; specimen collection, labeling, preservation, and transportation; test methods and methodologies; alternative testing methods; inconsistent results; personnel training; complaints; subsequent investigations; and corrective actions.

QUALITY CONTROL

In the laboratory, QC methods include the following:

1. Running control samples for each test performed
2. Reagent management
3. Instrument calibration
4. Documentation
5. Preventive maintenance of the equipment

Control Sample

A *control sample* is a manufactured sample that resembles a human specimen. The control sample has an exact, known value. Each time a test is performed, a control sample should be run as if it were another patient specimen to ensure that the reagents, temperatures, instruments, and techniques at the time the test is performed are within an acceptable range of accuracy. Control samples also should be run every time a new kit or new lot of reagents is opened to ensure that the materials have not been damaged or altered in shipping or storage.

Some control samples, for example, whole blood, have a list of expected values or ranges of values and are run separately to confirm that the equipment, reagents, and technique can produce a *normal* value or a *normal* range. Others come as sets of normal (negative) and abnormal (positive) control samples. This is a way of testing that the technique, reagents, and equipment can produce an *abnormal* as well as a *normal* test result.

Control samples should be run each day of testing. For *qualitative* tests, a positive and negative control sample should be run; for *quantitative* tests, at least two samples of different concentrations should be run. For tests requiring antigen-antibody determinations, the systems should be evaluated for their detection ability. Staining materials should be checked for reactivity. Culture material should be checked for reactivity, sterility, and ability to support growth. The medical assistant must always adhere to the manufacturer's instructions for control procedures.

Reagents

Reagents are testing substances used to produce chemical reactions. Each resulting chemical reaction helps the physician to detect or measure a change in a body function or to identify the characteristics of a condition or disease.

Each reagent is manufactured with a lot number and an expiration date. Reagent package inserts describe the stability of the reagent, its expected shelf-life, and the storage requirements. Both the lot number and the expiration date must be recorded into a reagent QC log both when it is received and on the date it is opened. The log helps to identify reagents that should be replaced. A reagent must be used before the stated expiration date.

Occasionally, unreliable test results can occur as the result from a defective reagent. In this case, lot numbers help the manufacturer identify a reagent when there is a question as to the integrity of its contents. Defective products should be returned to the manufacturer.

Reagents, solutions, culture media, control samples, and calibration materials should be carefully labeled. The labels should indicate the identity, storage requirements, preparation dates, and expiration dates. Do not use expired reagents, solutions, media, or kits, or interchange different lot numbers of reagents, solutions, or media. Rotate stock so that older materials are used before the newer inventory. Discard expired reagents according to manufacturers' directions.

When pouring liquids from a bottle, tilt the bottle so the label is toward the ceiling so that the liquid does not soil the label. Reagent container covers, tops, and lids should be securely replaced as soon as the reagents have been used.

Calibration

Instruments are usually operated by electrical or battery power or by using a light source. Because laboratory instruments are very sensitive, instrument performance can fluctuate owing to decreased electrical or battery power, changes in the quality of light used, or repeated use. Specimen testing is not reliable unless the equipment works the same with each test. Calibration must be performed regularly to determine the accuracy of the instrument or to ascertain the necessary corrective factors and adjustments to make testing accurate. The medical assistant must completely understand the operation and maintenance of a piece of laboratory equipment before attempting to use it or attempting appropriate instrument calibration and recalibration.

Standards

Instruments are calibrated with a set of *standards,* usually a chemical of exact known values. Unlike control samples, standards, which may or may not be the same as the control samples that resemble human specimens, are run before patients' specimens are tested. Instruments should be calibrated as often as the manufacturer recommends and at any time the value of a control sample fails to fall within an expected range. A complete set of standards should also be run each time a new lot of reagents is opened.

Quality Control Logs

Quality control logs must be updated every time a control sample or standard is run (see the section titled Recordkeeping). The entry should include the date and time, the expected results of the control or standard, whether the expected results were obtained, and any corrective actions taken.

Should a control sample or standard fail, the expiration dates of all reagents should be checked first. If the

expiration date is not the problem, then a control sample should be repeated using reagents with different lot numbers. Instrument malfunction should be investigated next. If neither the reagents or the instrument can be pinpointed as the source of error, the procedural technique should be investigated.

Maintenance guidelines are provided by each manufacturer at the time of purchase. Maintenance may be required daily, weekly, monthly, semiannually, or annually (Fig. 28–1). Document any manufacturer-serviced maintenance and whether it was a scheduled or unscheduled service call. Manufacturers' representatives are available to provide training for office staff, to perform daily or routine maintenance, and to answer questions or troubleshoot new problems by telephone.

Food and Drug Administration–Approved Equipment and Procedures

Quality control requirements under CLIA vary depending on the complexity of the test and on whether the laboratory instruments, kits, and testing methods are FDA-approved or modified from those approved by the FDA. The medical assistant must explicitly follow each manufacturer's directions when using commercially prepared FDA-approved reagents or kit methods for laboratory testing. FDA-approved instrument manuals and package inserts are the best source for determining the QC requirements. Whenever possible, FDA-approved kits and equipment should be used.

When using FDA-approved instruments and kits to perform either waiver tests or moderately complex tests, the role of the medical assistant in laboratory quality control is to:

1. Follow the manufacturer's instructions for specimen collection, labeling, and transportation
2. Perform only tests and methodologies assigned
3. Follow the manufacturer's instructions for the operation of instruments and kits
4. Maintain and use a POL procedure manual
5. Conduct routine maintenance and troubleshooting
6. Perform and document calibration procedures
7. Follow the manufacturer's directions for reagent stability and storage

Date	Cleaning	Repair	Initials
7/7	Microscope Stage, Objective	Changed bulb	MWW
7/20	Microscope High Objective	Cleaned	MWW
7/23	Microscope Eyepiece	Cleaned	MWW

Figure 28–1. Form used to record microscope maintenance.

Date	Instrument	Maintenance	Calibration	Temperature	Reagent	Expiration Date	Control	Expiration Date	Tech.
7/12	Coulter	Cleaned 7/12	7/12	37°C	(2)	8/15	Normal	156 8/15	MAW

Figure 28–2. Example of a quality control daily worksheet.

8. Be knowledgeable of normal test values and factors influencing test results
9. Perform and document QC procedures using control materials on each day of testing
10. Validate patient test results with QC before reporting them
11. Perform and document remedial actions when problems or errors are identified

RECORDKEEPING

The medical assistant must maintain accurate documentation of all laboratory tests performed. In addition to the maintenance log mentioned earlier, four more records make up a complete recordkeeping system. The required records are:

- ❑ The patient's medical record
- ❑ QC daily worksheets
- ❑ Reference laboratory log sheets (specimens sent out to a separate laboratory)
- ❑ Daily workload log sheets

The patient's medical record documents all procedures performed by the medical assistant. Procedures include the collection of the specimen, the tests ordered and performed, and the test results. A charting example is:

June 18, 1993, 10 AM: Venipuncture, right arm for fasting blood sugar (FBS), Hb, and white blood count (WBC). Results: FBS = 145 mg/dL; Hb = 12.8 g; WBC = 9500. (signature)

A QC daily worksheet (Fig. 28–2) helps the medical assistant review reagent and control expiration dates and provides documentary proof that equipment has been properly calibrated.

A reference laboratory log sheet is a record of all laboratory specimens sent to a reference laboratory (Fig. 28–3). This log verifies when and where specimens were sent and also documents turnaround time. Most results are reported within 24 hours.

Finally, the physician may also require maintenance of a daily laboratory work log that indicates the laboratory testing done on site (Fig. 28–4).

REGULATIONS CONCERNING HAZARDOUS AND TOXIC SUBSTANCES

The POL can contain flammable and toxic chemicals, infectious materials, and electrical equipment. The law (OSHA: Access to Information About Hazardous and Toxic Substances Act, 29 CFR 1910.1200) requires employers to make an inventory and list of all hazardous equipment and toxic substances used in the workplace. The Occupational Safety and Health Administra-

Date	Patient's Name	Type of Specimen	Test Ordered	Where Sent	Initials	Results Rec'd	Initials
7/7	Jones, Molly	Serum	Cholesterol	Roche	MWW	7/9	MWW
7/10	Smith, Sue	Serum	CPK	Biomedical	MWW	7/11	MWW
7/12	Jones, John	Serum	Acute Viral Study	State Laboratory	MWW	7/20	MWW

Figure 28–3. Example of a reference laboratory log sheet.

Date	Patient's Name	Test	Results	Control Values Normal	Abnormal	Initials
7/7	Jones, Molly	FBS	195 mg/dl	70 mg/dl	250 mg/dl	MWW
7/10	Smith, Sue	PTT	20.5 mg/dl	11.5 mg/dl	28 mg/dl	MWW
7/12	Johnson, Sally	Pregnancy Test	Positive	Positive	Negative	MWW

Figure 28–4. Example of a daily laboratory work load log.

tion (OSHA) requires each medical facility to have a written *Hazard Communication Program.* As part of the program, employers must post Material Data Safety Sheets (MSDSs) for all hazardous substances and equipment and properly label the containers of all hazardous chemicals (Fig. 28–5). The law specifies that all employees are entitled to information about the hazardous substances in their workplace and are entitled to be trained in the safe use of such materials.

MATERIAL SAFETY DATA SHEETS

Material Safety Data Sheets permit cross-referencing of hazardous materials from inventory sheets to labels. Each MSDS should list the following:

1. Substance stated on the label
2. Chemical and common names of each ingredient
3. Chemical characteristics of each chemical (e.g., vapor pressure or flash point)
4. Physical hazards associated with the substance (e.g., fire or explosion)
5. Potential health hazards and risks, including the signs and symptoms of exposure, and the medical conditions aggravated by exposure
6. Primary routes of entry
7. OSHA exposure limits
8. Whether the ingredients are carcinogens
9. Precautions that should be taken when handling the substance

The information sheet should also list the personal protective equipment (PPE) required (see the Highlights at the end of this chapter), protective measures for repair and maintenance of contaminated containers or equipment, spill and leak cleanup procedures, emergency first aid procedures, and how to contact the manufacturer of the substance or equipment.

The following is a partial list of some typical hazards in the medical office:

❏ Disinfectants—1% phenol, bleach, hydrogen peroxide, isopropyl alcohol, acetone, provodone iodine
❏ Cleaning compounds—ammonia, Lysol, Comet, Windex

❏ Laboratory reagents, pharmaceuticals, vaccines, antiseptics
❏ Office supplies—toner, liquid paper
❏ Equipment—x-ray machine, diathermy, autoclave, laser equipment, electrical equipment

Useful information for writing MSDSs can be gathered from package inserts, instrument manuals, the local fire department, OSHA, and state departments of natural resources. Manufacturers are required to supply MSDSs when requested. MSDSs should be arranged in alphabetical order so that they can be found quickly during an emergency. Before the sheets are filed, they should be photocopied and posted on a bulletin board. All employees should sign that they have read and understood the data.

HAZARD LABELS

Each hazardous substance also must have a hazard label. The label should be a condensed version of the MSDS. Hazard labels can be attached over the original label with a rubber band. The original label must not be removed. If a solution has more than one hazardous chemical, the label must contain all of the ingredients or, at least, those with the worst ratings. Drugs and injectables do not require additional labeling, unless the drug is considered a carcinogen. Large containers, storage boxes, cabinet doors, and the outsides of drawers should be labeled when any hazardous substances are stored in them. Dispensers also must be labeled. Dispensers include soap dispensers, alcohol dispensers, covered disinfectant trays, reagent bottles, or any other container into which hazardous substances are transferred.

If cleaning products are supplied to janitorial personnel, the physician is responsible for providing on-site training of the janitorial staff. It is best to have the cleaning service purchase its own supplies and store the supplies in an area outside the office. The medical facility should provide the janitorial staff with an instruction sheet describing the hazardous chemicals in the office. Janitorial personnel should not touch or come into contact with any medical wastes.

Material Safety Data Sheet

May be used to comply with
OSHA's Hazard Communication Standard,
29 CFR 1910.1200. Standard must be
consulted for specific requirements.

U.S. Department of Labor

Occupational Safety and Health Administration
(Non-Mandatory Form)
Form Approved
OMB No. 1218-0072

IDENTITY *(As Used on Label and List)* Acetone	*Note: Blank spaces are not permitted. If any item is not applicable, or no information is available, the space must be marked to indicate that.*

Section I

Manufacturer's Name	Emergency Telephone Number
Address *(Number, Street, City, State, and ZIP Code)*	Telephone Number for Information
	Date Prepared January 2, 1989
	Signature of Preparer *(optional)*

Section II — Hazardous Ingredients/Identity Information

Hazardous Components (Specific Chemical Identity; Common Name(s))	OSHA PEL	ACGIH TLV	Other Limits Recommended	% *(optional)*
2-Propanone, Ketone propane	TWA 1000ppm	TWA 750ppm		
Dimethyl Ketone				
Acetone				
Note: All of the above in Section II are different chemical names				
for the same material.				

Section III — Physical/Chemical Characteristics

Boiling Point	133°F	Specific Gravity (H$_2$O = 1)	Unk
Vapor Pressure (mm Hg.)	at 77°F 266mm	Melting Point	-169°F
Vapor Density (AIR = 1)	Unk	Evaporation Rate (Butyl Acetate = 1)	Unk

Solubility in Water
miscible

Appearance and Odor
Colorless liquid with a fragrant mint-like odor.

Section IV — Fire and Explosion Hazard Data   Rating: 3

Flash Point (Method Used) 1.4°F	Flammable Limits	LEL 2.6%	UEL 12.8%

Extinguishing Media
see below

Special Fire Fighting Procedures
use CO$_2$; dry chemical; alcohol foam

Unusual Fire and Explosion Hazards
dangerous disaster hazard due to fire and explosion

(Reproduce locally)   OSHA 174, Sept. 1985

Figure 28–5. For each hazardous substance used in the workplace, OSHA requires the employer to fill out and display this form.

Section V — **Reactivity Data**   Rating: 0

Stability	Unstable		Conditions to Avoid
	Stable	X	

Incompatibility (*Materials to Avoid*)
nitric and sulfuric acid; oxidizing materials; acids; chloroform

Hazardous Decomposition or Byproducts
Unk

Hazardous Polymerization	May Occur		Conditions to Avoid
	Will Not Occur	X	

Section VI — **Health Hazard Data**   Rating: 1

Route(s) of Entry: Inhalation? yes   Skin? yes   Ingestion? no
TARGET ORGANS: respiratory system; skin

Health Hazards (*Acute and Chronic*)
Moderately toxic by various routes. A skin and eye irritant. Possible mutagenesis.

Carcinogenicity: NTP? no   IARC Monographs? Unk   OSHA Regulated? yes

Signs and Symptoms of Exposure
Inh: irritating to eyes, nose, and throat

Ing: headaches, dizziness, and dermititis

Medical Conditions
Generally Aggravated by Exposure   Unk

Emergency and First Aid Procedures
Eyes: irrigate immediately   Skin: soap wash immediately

Ing: seek medical attention immediately   Breath: artificial respiration

Section VII — **Precautions for Safe Handling and Use**

Steps to Be Taken in Case Material Is Released or Spilled
use gloves or forceps; ventilate

Waste Disposal Method
See Hazardous Waste Management or consult the manufacturer.

Precautions to Be Taken in Handling and Storing
Use forceps or gloves when handling contaminated gauze or brushes. Keep bottles tightly

closed. Store bottles on flat surfaces. Don't store near an open flame.

Other Precautions
Unk

Section VIII — **Control Measures**

Respiratory Protection (*Specify Type*)
Unk

Ventilation	Local Exhaust well ventilated	Special several air exchanges per hour
	Mechanical (*General*) Unk	Other vent outside if using high concentrations

Protective Gloves rubber gloves	Eye Protection should use in case of splash or spill

Other Protective Clothing or Equipment
Unk

Work/Hygienic Practices   Remove contaminated clothing; may be flammable after exposure. Don't
eat, drink, or smoke in vicinity.

Figure 28-5. Continued.

OCCUPATIONAL EXPOSURE TO BLOODBORNE PATHOGENS

Another aspect of the OSHA Hazard Communication Program is the Occupational Exposure to Bloodborne Pathogens regulation (OSHA 29 CFR 1910.1030). In the same manner as for hazardous chemicals, this law outlines infection control for the protection against occupational exposure to hepatitis B virus (HBV) and the human immunodeficiency virus (HIV).

The law defines infectious materials as semen, vaginal secretions, cerebrospinal fluid, synovial fluid, pleural fluid, pericardial fluid, peritoneal fluid, amniotic fluid, saliva in dental procedures, any body fluid visibly contaminated with blood, and all body fluids in situations where it is difficult or impossible to differentiate between body fluids. It also includes under its definition of infectious materials any unfixed tissue or organ other than intact skin from a human (living or dead) and HIV-containing cell or tissue cultures, organ cultures, and HIV or HBV-containing culture medium or other solutions as well as blood, organs or other tissues from experimental animals infected with HIV or HBV.

Universal precautions are designed to minimize needle sticks and splashing and spraying of blood, to ensure appropriate packaging of specimens with biohazard labeling before shipping to laboratories, and to regulate wastes by either decontamination or labeling before shipping to waste servicing facilities.

The law requires that the orange or orange-red biohazard symbol be affixed to containers of regulated waste, refrigerators and freezers, and other containers that are used to store or transport blood or other potentially infectious materials (Fig. 28–6). Red bags or containers may be used instead of labeling. If the medical office uses universal precautions in its handling of all specimens, labeling is not required within the office. If all linens are handled and laundered with universal precautions, the laundry need not be labeled. Blood that has been tested and found free of HIV and HBV and released for clinical use and regulated waste that has been decontaminated need not be labeled.

STANDARD OPERATING PROCEDURES

The bloodborne standard requires employers to identify, in writing, tasks and procedures as well as job classifications where occupational exposure to blood occurs—without regard to personal protective clothing and equipment. These are called *standard operating procedures* (SOPs).

Medical facilities classify work-related tasks into three categories of potential exposure (Table 28–3):

Category I. Those tasks for which protective equipment must be worn

Category II. An intermediate grouping of tasks that do not require protective equipment but have the potential for unexpectedly or on short notice converting to category I tasks

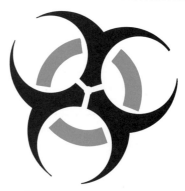

Figure 28–6. The law requires that this orange-red symbol be visibly attached to all waste containers, refrigerators, and other receptacles that contain material defined by law as hazardous because of their potential for exposure to bloodborne or other pathogens.

Category III. Those tasks that do not require any protective equipment

Examples of category I tasks are capillary puncture, phlebotomy, blood testing, culturing, dressing changes, needle biopsies or aspirations, pelvic examinations and procedures, and surgical procedures.

Examples of category II tasks are urinalysis; fecal occult blood; examination of sweat, tears, saliva, or nasal secretions; x-rays; ultrasound; electrocardiogram; and injections (unless injecting blood).

Category II tasks can be performed on the following body fluids, *provided the fluid does not contain visible blood*: feces, sweat, nasal secretions, tears, sputum, urine, vomitus, breast milk, and saliva (except in dentistry).

For all category I and II tasks, SOPs are used to ensure procedural uniformity and safety. SOPs include the name of the procedure, the protective equipment required, disposal methods, sterilization procedures, other procedures necessary to the task, the type of body fluid with which there will or may be contact, and the volume of blood or body fluid likely to be encountered.

Physicians must provide and require employees to use appropriate personal protective equipment (PPE). Employers must clean, repair and replace PPEs whenever necessary. (See Highlights at the end of this chapter for more details.) Gloves must be worn for phlebotomy except in volunteer blood donation centers, where gloves must be made available to employees who want them. The standard also requires a written schedule for cleaning and identifying the method of decontamination to be used for equipment, in addition to instructions for cleaning equipment after it has come into contact with blood or other potentially infectious materials. The standard specifies the methods for disposing of contaminated sharps and handling contaminated laundry. (See also Chapter 17 Highlights.)

Table 28–3

CATEGORIES OF JOBS ACCORDING TO LEVELS OF EXPOSURE TO BLOODBORNE PATHOGENS

Category	Example
I. Normal Tasks Involve Exposure to Blood, Body Fluids, or Tissues All procedures or other job-related tasks that involve an inherent potential for mucous membrane or skin contact with blood, body fluids, or tissues or that carry the potential for spills or splashes of these materials. Use of appropriate protective measures should be required for every employee engaged in category I tasks.	Capillary puncture Blood testing Culturing Dressing changes Needle biopsies or aspirations Pelvic examinations and procedures Surgical procedures Emergency medical care and first aid Contact with saliva during dental procedures
II. Normal Tasks Involve No Exposure to Blood, Body Fluids, or Tissues, but Employment May Require Performing Unplanned Category I Tasks The normal work routine involves no exposure to blood, body fluids, or tissues, but exposure or potential exposure may be required as a condition of employment. Appropriate protective measures should be readily available to every employee engaged in category II tasks.	Urinalysis Fecal occult blood examination Examination of sweat, tears, saliva, or nasal secretions x-Ray procedures Ultrasound procedures Electrocardiographic procedures Injections (unless injecting blood) Procedures involving sputum, vomitus, breast milk, and saliva (except in dentistry)
III. Tasks Involve No Exposure to Blood, Body Fluids, or Tissues; Performing Category I Tasks Is Not a Condition of Employment The normal work routine involves no exposure to blood, body fluids, or tissues (although situations can be imagined or hypothesized under which anyone, anywhere, might encounter potential exposure to body fluids). Persons who perform these duties are not called on as part of their employment to perform or assist in emergency medical care or first aid or to be potentially exposed in some other way. Tasks that involve handling of implements or utensils, use of public or shared bathroom facilities or telephones, and personal contacts such as handshaking are category III tasks.	Administrative, secretarial, and reception procedures with patients Patient interviews Obtaining vital signs Patient assistance before or after examination

Source: Adapted from the Department of Labor/Department of Health and Human Services: Joint Advisory Notice—Protection Against Occupational Exposure to Hepatitis B Virus (HBV) and Human Immunodeficiency Virus (HIV), October 19, 1987.

PERSONNEL TRAINING AND EVALUATION

Annual office training sessions and performance evaluations ensure staff compliance with OSHA standards. On-site training must include the following:

- Exposure control plan
- Recordkeeping
- Protective equipment
- Housekeeping
- Labels, signs, and color-coding
- Work practice controls
- Hepatitis B vaccine
- Response to emergencies involving blood
- How to handle exposure incidents (See Chapter 23 Highlights)

SPECIMEN COLLECTION

Quality control is continued by properly collecting and labeling the specimen. If a specimen is mislabeled or collected in an incorrect container, the results could be invalid. There are five basic steps for properly collecting a specimen:

1. Confirm the identification of the patient.
2. Screen the patient regarding compliance with pretest preparation (fasting, premedication, discontinuing certain medications, etc.).
3. Use good collection techniques.
4. Select the proper collection containers with or without specified preservatives.
5. Label specimens accurately and without delay.

PREPARATION AND COLLECTION

The patient should be asked to state his or her name or to spell his or her last name to confirm patient identification. Next, the patient must be screened to verify that the required preliminary restrictions and requirements have been followed. Dietary restrictions, especially, must be carefully monitored. Some tests require the patient to fast (usually for 6 to 8 hours) before the blood sample is collected. Food intake can affect some tests. If specimens requiring fasting are obtained from nonfasting patients, the results will reflect the meal consumption rather than the patient's true metabolic state.

Specimen collection at specifically timed intervals is important for some tests. For example, timely analysis of cardiac enzymes that are released within 2 to 48 hours after a heart attack can assist the physician in making a diagnosis of myocardial infarction. As another example, glucose tolerance test samples are collected periodically for up to 6 hours to obtain differing blood sugar levels.

When tests for the presence or effects of medication are performed, specimens are collected $\frac{1}{2}$ to 1 hour after a medication is taken for "peak" levels or $\frac{1}{2}$ to 1 hour before the next dose of medication for "trough" levels, that is, when the medication is at the lowest level in the bloodstream.

Many medications alter laboratory test values. Over-the-counter drugs such as aspirin can affect urine tests, blood tests, and thyroid function tests. Starting a patient on antibiotics before culturing an infected area could seriously inhibit the growth of a suspected organism, resulting in a missed diagnosis. Each laboratory has reference tables available that list which drugs can produce increased or decreased values, false-positive values, and false-negative values. Many drug references and medical dictionaries also contain this information.

Correct collection technique is necessary if laboratory results are to reflect the true health status of the patient. Frequently, the causative agent for a communicable disease may be identifiable only if the specimen is free of external contamination from the skin or mucosal surfaces. Sterile equipment and proper skin cleaning procedures and aseptic techniques are necessary to control external contamination.

Selection of appropriate specimen containers is necessary to preserve some specimens before laboratory testing. Often, anticoagulants or preservatives are premeasured and added to containers. Reference laboratories will clearly state the type of specimen, the amount, and any special additives or containers required for the test (Table 28–4).

The specimen must be accurately labeled at the time of collection. Label information should include the following:

1. Patient's full name
2. Date and time of collection
3. Test requested
4. Name of the phlebotomist or the person who received the specimen from the patient

All laboratory request forms for outside reference work must match the information on the specimen label and in the office's reference laboratory log book.

TRANSPORT

Specimens that are tested by an outside laboratory must be transported to the laboratory by the patient, through a daily or on-call pickup service, or through the postal service. Regardless of the delivery system, each laboratory will supply mailing containers, directions for obtaining the specimens (including the amount and storage requirement), and directions for packaging the specimens for transport to the laboratory.

Patient delivery is the fastest method and should be encouraged when results are needed quickly or the specimen can quickly deteriorate. Patient instructions should include the address and phone number of the laboratory and directions to the laboratory.

The mail service is the least desirable method of transport. The postal service cannot guarantee specimen storage requirements such as refrigeration or incubation, and the specimen integrity can be altered before the specimen reaches the laboratory. If a specimen is mailed, it is best to collect the specimen and place it in a mailbox as close as possible to a scheduled pickup time.

Laboratory pickup is the most reliable transport method. Carriers are trained in the proper handling and preservation of specimens and are aware of the universal precautions for handling biomedical packages. Carriers may be scheduled to pick up *morning* specimens and then to return later in the day for *randomly collected* specimens. It is important to take laboratory pickup times into consideration when scheduling patients for specimen collection procedures.

Mailing containers are designed to protect those who must handle the specimen in transport. In general, all specimens are double-packed in crushproof boxes, leakproof bags, or crushproof mailing tubes and identified with a "biomedical" label to protect the handlers from contamination. Most containers also contain packing material to protect both the specimen and the inner specimen container from breakage. The inner specimen containers may be microscope slides packed in a cardboard slide holder, plastic or cardboard cups with lids, or plastic tubes containing a transport medium to keep the specimen from drying. The inner specimen container is considered sterile; the outer container is not.

Each slide, cup, or tube inside the outer mailer must be individually labeled with the patient's name, the type of specimen, and the date and time of collection. To avoid contamination, it is best to label the specimen holders *before* the specimen is placed in the container.

A laboratory requisition form is included in every mailer (Fig. 28–7). It is vital that these forms be completed accurately and completely. The request form must be placed on the outside of bags. The laboratory requisition includes the following:

- Physician's name and address
- Patient's name and address

Text continues on p. 725.

Table 28–4

LABORATORY PROCEDURES FREQUENTLY PERFORMED OR REQUESTED IN THE MEDICAL OFFICE

Test	Purpose	Specimen Required	Preparation Required	Equipment	Test Interferences	Specimen Preservation	Transportation
			Bacteriological Specimens				
Routine throat culture (TC)	To identify specific organisms: (1) Rapid screening Group A step test; (2) culture as confirmation	Collect from nasopharynx on sterile swab; if two swabs used, collect from each tonsillar area with separate swab; obtain prior to initiating antibiotic therapy	None	Culturette (sterile specimen transport container) or sterile cotton or dacron or calcium alginate swabs; tongue blade	Patient on antibiotics, false negative; Contamination of specimen or break of sterile technique, false positive; Delay in processing can cause overgrowth (false positive) or death (false negative) of pathogens	Place swab in Culturette and crush ampule; or process within 2–3 h of collection; include time of culture collection on label and requisition; do not refrigerate; if Gram stain required, second swab should be in Culturette tube with **unbroken** ampule, or prepare two labeled, unstained slides	Swabs in media should be processed within 24 h; transport media is effective for 72 h
Sputum culture	Identify specific micro-organisms in the respiratory tract; Gram stain routinely performed on all sputum	First morning sputum (not saliva) expectorated into a sterile contain (not Culturette); examine to ensure at least 1 mL thick mucus collected; obtain prior to initiating antibiotic therapy	Brush teeth and rinse to flush food particles, oropharyngeal secretions, and upper respiratory flora	Sterile sputum cup and lid	Saliva obtained instead of sputum; Patient on antibiotics, false negative; Contamination of specimen or break of sterile technique, false positive; Delay in processing can cause overgrowth (false positive) or death (false negative) of pathogens	Do not refrigerate	Must be received by lab within 2 h of collection

719

Continued

Table 28–4

LABORATORY PROCEDURES FREQUENTLY PERFORMED OR REQUESTED IN THE MEDICAL OFFICE—*Continued*

Test	Purpose	Specimen Required	Preparation Required	Equipment	Test Interferences	Specimen Preservation	Transportation
Urine culture	Identify specific microorganisms and diagnose and cause of urinary tract infections	Clean-catch, midstream preferred or catheterized urine, if sterile specimen required; obtain prior to initiating antibiotic therapy	Cleanse vulvourethral area; counts more accurate if urine is permitted to remain in the bladder 3 h or more before collection	Sterile urine container, tightly capped; cleansing kit, urine collection kit or pediatric urine collection kit	Patient on antibiotics, false negative. Contamination of specimen or break of sterile technique, false positive. Delay in processing can cause over-growth (false positive) or death (false negative) of pathogens. Patient taking urinary antiseptics or antibiotics	Process immediately or refrigerate; culture must be performed prior to routine tests; record time of collection on label and requisition	Transport immediately or refrigerate
Wound culture	Identify specific microorganisms in wounds	Exudate within the wound in an area with most drainage or pus; lesion without pus may be injected with sterile saline (without preservative) then aspirated; obtain prior to initiating antibiotic therapy	Decontaminate unbroken skin or mucous membranes first with alcohol	Note: most labs request use of an aerobic Culturette system; otherwise use sterile cotton, dacron, or calcium alginate swabs	Patient on antibiotics, false negative. Contamination of specimen or break of sterile technique, false positive. Delay in processing can cause over-growth or death of pathogens, false positive or false negative	Anerobic transfer system: quickly insert swab to within 5mm from bottom of media; break shaft of swab even with lip of tube, tighten cap. Process within 2–3 h of collection or refrigerate; keep genital cultures at room temperature	Swabs in media should be transported immediately after collection; transport media is effective for 72 h
Ova and Parasites (O&P)	Identify parasitic infestations such as pinworm and roundworm	Fresh stool and preserved stool	None	Stool collection kit: dry plastic container; one vial with formalin; one	Stool containing mineral oil. Stool containing barium	Preserved specimen should be sent to the lab immediately after collection	Fresh specimen should be received by the lab within 1 h after collection

Test	Purpose	Collection instructions	Patient preparation	Specimen container	Interfering substances / comments	Handling	Transport
				vial with polyvinyl alcohol		or refrigerated up to 24 h	
Ova and Parasite smear (infants & small children)	Identify parasitic infestations such as pinworm and roundworm	Collect thin smear by inserting moistened swabs, one at a time, 1–1½ inch into the rectum	None	Swabs moistened with water, glass slide		Specimen should be sent to the lab or refrigerated immediately	Transport within 48 h
Occult blood	Detect blood in stool with the chemical guaiac	Three specimens of a thin smear of stool from two different areas of stool and from three separate bowel movements	Medication and diet restrictions 2 days before the 1st specimen is collected	Hemoccult slide testing kit (commercial test cards)	Stool containing mineral oil; Stool containing barium; Foods: false positive; Drugs: false positive; Menses: false positive; Bleeding from other condition (i.e., hemorrhoids): false positive; Vitamin C false positive; Iron: false positive	Room temperature; out of sun light and heat; unpreserved	Within 12 days
Semen	Quantitatively measure semen for fertility studies; post vasectomy sterility confirmation	1.0 mL semen; 2–3 separate specimens collected by masturbation or interruption of intercourse with ejaculation into a specimen container	Collect after 2–3 days abstinence	Clean glass jar	Condoms contain a spermicide that can cause false decreased values; Delay in processing results in decreased values	Keep at body temperature; record time of collection and time of last previous ejaculation	Within ½ h of collection
Phenylketonuria (PKU)	Screening for the amino acid phenylalanin Required by law	Three samples of capillary blood from one puncture site; enough blood to entirely saturate and fill three test circles on treated paper	None	PKU kit; capillary puncture materials	Inadequately filled circles	None	Transport as soon as possible after collection in container provided; observe universal body fluid precautions

Continued

Table 28–4

LABORATORY PROCEDURES FREQUENTLY PERFORMED OR REQUESTED IN THE MEDICAL OFFICE—*Continued*

Test	Purpose	Specimen Required	Preparation Required	Equipment	Test Interferences	Specimen Preservation	Transportation
Wet preparations (India ink)	Identify trichomonas, yeast infections, protozoan infections, or Gardnerella vaginalis	Endocervical or urethral exudate obtained on a swab passed through a speculum or with a vaginal aspirator	No intercourse or douching 24 h prior to collection; for urogenital specimens, do not urinate 1 hr prior to collection	2 swabs: one for microscopic, the other for culture; tube of 0.5 mL sterile saline; Gram stain slides	Menses Intercourse or douching within 24 h	Swab placed in tube of 0.5 mL sterile saline or air dry then heat fix; Gram stain on site; process within 30 minutes; keep at room temperature	Specify to lab that specimen should be divided for fungus culture, KOH prep, mycobacterial culturing, smear, and routine bacteriologic culture, also Gram stain, if sufficient quantity
Vaginal smear; urethral smear in males	Identify micro-organisms (yeast, protozoa, chlamydia, gonorrhea)	Endocervical or urethral exudate obtained on a swab passed through a speculum or a vaginal aspirator	No intercourse or douching 24 h prior to collection; for urogenital specimens, do not urinate 1 hr prior to collection	Anaerobic collection system; sterile cotton or calcium alginate swabs treated with charcoal; frosted glass slides (pre-labeled) and or petri dish	Nontreated swabs are toxic to gonorrhoea; Menses, intercourse, or douching within 24 h	Gram stain on stie (air dry then heat fix); keep at room temperature; wet preps must be processed within 30 min	Transport at room temperature in a cardboard slide holder or anaerobic collection system; specify to lab that specimen should be divided for fungus culture, KOH prep, mycobacterial culture, smear, and routine bacteriologic culture (also Gram stain, if sufficient quantity)
Cytology smear (Pap smear)	Diagnose malignant lesions	Endocervical, cervical, vaginal, oral, nipple, burshings, imprints, scrapes obtained on a spatula, swab, or brush	No intercourse or douching 24 h prior to collection; for urogenital specimens, do not urinate 1 h	Sterile cotton swabs or Ayer spatulas; frosted, labeled glass slides, fixative spray, "Pap" transport bottles	Menses; Air drying results in poor cellular detail	Wet fix in 95% ethyl alcohol fixative for 10 minutes or immediately spray with fixative	Transport immediately or refrigerate until time of transportation

Bacteriologic smear	Identify micro-organisms taken from the throat, mouth, ear, nose, anus, neonate conjunctiva, surface of the skin, or wounds	Exudate or wound drainage	directly or through a speculum Aseptic technique prior to collection	with 95% ethyl alcohol Sterile cotton, dacron, or calcium alginate swabs; frosted, prelabeled glass slides	Air dry then heat fix on site; Gram stain on site	Medications; Contamination of specimen by break in sterile technique (false positive Delay in processing (false positive or negative)	Transport at room temperature in a cardboard slide holder

TYPES OF BLOOD SPECIMENS

Type of Specimen	Purpose of Specimen	Tube Color/Additives	Tube Requirements	Specimen Requirements	Storage Requirements	Anticoagulant Action	Types of Tests
Clotted blood (serum)	Serum determinations in chemistry, serology, and blood banking	Red; when multiple Vacutainer tubes are required use in order: (1) red; (2) lavender; (3) blue; (order washes out thromboplastin released by the blood vessel at the site of penetration; no additives)	No tube inversions necessary	2–20 mL; not affected by volume collected	Best on fresh (within 30 min)	No anticoagulant	Chemistry profiles, drug levels, BUN, creatinine, uric acid, cholesterol, high-density lipoproteins (HDL)
Serum (obtained from separating the clot from clotted blood)	Chemistry studies; Emergency studies	Red/Gray mottled (speckled) Brown mottled	Five inversions Five inversions	2.5–13 mL; not affected by volume collected	Serum must be separated from blood within 30 minutes, then centrifuged. May be kept at room temperature, refrigerated, or frozen; protect from light	Polymer gel and clot activator (inert serum separator gel) physically separates serum	Emergency chemistry and lipid studies Stat serum determinations

Continued

Table 28–4

LABORATORY PROCEDURES FREQUENTLY PERFORMED OR REQUESTED IN THE MEDICAL OFFICE—*Continued*

TYPES OF BLOOD SPECIMENS—*continued*

Type of Specimen	Purpose of Specimen	Tube Color/Additives	Tube Requirements	Specimen Requirements	Storage Requirements	Anticoagulant Action	Types of Tests
Plasma (whole blood that has been centrifuged) or whole blood	Hematology determinations	Lavender; ethylenediaminetetraacetic acid (EDTA) Gray (potassium oxalate and sodium fluoride)	Eight inversions; tube at room tempertaure	3–7 mL; at least ⅔ full (larger tubes with Na₂ powder not affected by volume; prevent hemolysis	Best on fresh (within 30 min); refrigerate at 39°F (4°C) for 2 h; never freeze	EDTA prevents coagulation by binding calcium; preserves the cellular constituents of blood; potassium oxalate is a dry additive that prevents coagulation by removing calcium (calcium alters cell morphology)	Complete blood cell count, erythrocyte sedimentation rate, platelet studies, hemoglobin, hematocrit, blood grouping. VDRL (Venereal Disease Research Laboratory) test for syphilis
Plasma (whole blood that has been centrifuged)	Coagulation studies	Light blue (buffered sodium citrate)	Eight inverstions	1.8–4.5 mL; full draw needed	Certain tests require chilled specimens; follow recommended procedures for collection and transportation	Prevents coagulation by removing calcium	Prothrombin time; partial prothrombin time; erythrocyte sedimentation rate
Plasma (whole blood that has been centrifuged)	Endocrine studies, plasma determinations, electrolyte and blood gas studies	Green (heparin)	Eight inversions	2–10 mL; not affected by volume collected	Must be processed immediately (can prevent coagulation for only 24 h)	Prevents coagulation by inhibiting thrombin formation; the best anticoagulant because it is a normal body constituent, but expensive	Electrolyte panels, blood gases, pH assays
Plasma (whole blood that has been centrifuged)	Blood culture	Yellow (SPS—sodium polyanetholesulfonate)	Eight inversions	4–16 mL; not affected by volume collected	Used for the sterile interior of the tube	Preserves the red blood cell and material for culture	Blood culture, immunocompetency profile, blood banking

	TEST REQUEST SLIP ROUTINE URINALYSIS				DATE _____ TIME _____
	TEST REQUEST SLIP ROUTINE URINALYSIS				

Figure 28–7. An example of a laboratory requisition form. (From Wedding MD and Toenjes SA: Medical Laboratory Procedures. FA Davis, Philadelphia, 1992, p. 91, with permission.)

- Patient's age and gender
- Patient's insurance billing information
- Test ordered
- Type and source of specimen collected
- Date and time of collection
- Any medications taken by the patient
- Physician's clinical diagnosis
- Any special orders, such a "stat" (immediate results required)

CHAIN OF CUSTODY

A chain of custody exists for the preservation and protection of every specimen collected. This is especially important in medicolegal cases or drug testing. A chain of custody form is supplied by the laboratory, and all persons involved in specimen handling must use and verify proper protocols throughout the collection and testing process. The chain of custody ensures that there is no mixup or tampering with a specimen.

The first person responsible in the chain of custody is the person collecting the specimen; this is usually the medical assistant. As the first person handling the specimen, it is the medical assistant's job to do the following:

1. Observe that the specimen is actually collected from the patient.
2. Label the specimen and complete the requisition form.
3. Sign and date the form attesting to use of correct procedure.
4. Have the patient initial or sign the form verifying that the specimen is his or hers.

The original copy of the chain of custody form is sealed in a bag with the specimen. Once the bag is sealed, it may not be reopened. The second copy is attached to the outside of the sealed container and is signed by every person handling the specimen; a third copy is retained in the patient record.

SPECIMEN WASTE

Specimen waste is considered to be biohazardous waste. Every article coming into contact with a human specimen and the specimen itself must be double-bagged in a red bag or tagged with a red biohazard warning label before disposal. The more common hazardous medical waste products in the medical office include blood products, body fluids, tissues, cultures, live and attenuated vaccines, sharps, table paper or gowns with body fluids on them, gloves, disposable specula, swabs, and inoculation loops. Reagents and other chemicals used in specimen handling should be disposed of according to the manufacturers' directions.

Hazardous sharp containers are necessary for needles, syringes with needles, scalpel blades, glass slides and coverslips, broken glass, and lancets. Biohazard containers are necessary for tubes of blood, disposable pipette tips, test tubes, microbiology specimens after testing, used specimen collection swabs, used specimen collection containers, dressings, table paper or gauze soaked with body fluids, and used gloves. (Single-use gloves must not be reused. Heavier utility gloves may be processed for reuse provided that the gloves are intact and undamaged in any way.)

Materials that may be considered nonhazardous and discarded in the normal way include all items that have not been exposed to body fluids, such as gowns, table paper, paper towels, tissues, and paper sheaths of disposable supplies.

The Hazard Communication Program (see above) specifically sets standards for the management of hazards in the workplace and medical waste disposal. Each medical facility will have specific *written* guidelines for waste management, based on state requirements and the local availability of services. Waste management includes, but is not limited to, the use of the following:

- Hazardous labeling
- Biohazard containers
- Biohazard sharps containers
- Autoclaving techniques before disposal

❏ Chemicals approved for disinfection of materials and contamination
❏ Incineration
❏ Licensed waste removal service company

PHLEBOTOMY

Phlebotomy is an invasive procedure in which a sterile needle is inserted into a vein for the purpose of obtaining a large blood sample for diagnostic testing. Another term for this procedure is *venipuncture.* Capillary blood can be used when a blood test requires a small amount of blood. The terms for obtaining blood from the capillaries is *capillary puncture,* or *finger puncture.* The medical assistant may or may not be able to perform venipuncture depending on state laws. Before performing a venipuncture, the medical assistant should contact his or her state medical society.

PATIENT TEACHING CONSIDERATIONS

The medical assistant must establish an environment that encourages the patient to relax. Patients usually view a venipuncture as a traumatic event and are very apprehensive. It is the medical assistant's job in the role of phlebotomist to complete the procedure with a minimal amount of pain or discomfort to the patient. The medical assistant must maintain a professional attitude while simultaneously being sympathetic to the fears and concerns of the patient.

The patient who has a positive attitude toward phlebotomy will need little explanation about the procedure and may, in fact, wish to tell the medical assistant what sites have been successful previously. The medical assistant should heed these suggestions, using a combination of patient-supplied information and knowledgeable judgment in choosing an appropriate site. The patient's positive attitude is usually related to a past venipuncture experience with a skilled technician. This patient will appear relaxed, talkative, and confident. The goal is to help every patient to develop a positive attitude.

The patient who has a negative attitude has probably experienced unpleasant, possibly traumatic events associated with phlebotomy procedures. The patient will appear nervous, apprehensive, and quite ill at ease. The medical assistant must make every effort to perform the phlebotomy rapidly, efficiently, and effectively.

Medical Assistant: Mr. Jones, your doctor would like to have some laboratory work done.

Mr. Jones: Oh, no! No blood tests for me!

Medical Assistant: Your doctor needs these test to aid in your diagnosis. Is there some reason you don't want the test done?

Mr. Jones: The last time they couldn't find a vein and after three times, you know, well, I just fainted. I said "never again."

Medical Assistant: Let's do it with one phlebotomy this time, Mr. Jones. Since you fainted before, please lie down and then you will be more comfortable.

Mr. Jones: Well, uh, one try, understand, but that's all I'll stand for.

The medical assistant should exercise particular caution with any patient who has previously fainted. The patient must lie down for the procedure, and the physician should be present in the office before the phlebotomy is attempted. By identifying the patient's past problem, as in the previous dialogue, the medical assistant was able to reassure the patient that he or she had the professional skills to achieve results with one venipuncture. This type of confident, firm, reassuring professional care may eventually transform negative resistance into a positive attitude toward phlebotomy. The medical assistant must always be aware, however, that the patient has the right to refuse to have the procedure done. If this occurs, notify the physician immediately.

The first-time patient who has never had a phlebotomy is often apprehensive and nervous, but negative attitudes have not yet been formed. When dealing with this patient, it is important to explain the procedure, answer any questions, and perform a skilled venipuncture before anxiety is allowed to build. By answering all questions, the medical assistant reassures the patient. When questions concerning the patient's diagnosis are asked, broad, nonspecific answers should be given. For instance, the medical assistant should say, "The doctor has ordered a blood sugar test," rather than "The doctor has ordered a blood sugar test because he thinks you have diabetes mellitus." It is the medical assistant's responsibility as a phlebotomist to make sure that each first-time phlebotomy patient leaves the office with a positive attitude toward the phlebotomy experience.

Medical Assistant: Mr. Green, your doctor would like you to have some laboratory tests done. Have you ever had a blood test?

Mr. Green: No. Why do I need blood tests? Does he think I have a serious disease?

Medical Assistant: The blood test will just aid in your diagnosis. By obtaining a small sample of blood from your arm, we can gain an overall picture of the functioning of your body.

Mr. Green: What tests are ordered?

Medical Assistant: You are to have a test to see how much sugar is in your blood and one to count your white blood cells.

Mr. Green: How long will this take?

Medical Assistant: I will draw the blood sample now and give your doctor the test results while you are waiting. Now, just have a seat and I will explain everything. I'll tie this tourniquet around your arm and locate your vein. There will be a small pinch, and I'll fill these two tubes. I will apply a bandage, and you may leave after 5 minutes.

VENIPUNCTURE

The process of venipuncture consists of patient preparation, collecting the needed equipment and blood collection tubes, performing the venipuncture, labeling the specimens, and disposing of the equipment properly. The medical assistant must work rapidly and must perform a skilled venipuncture to gain the patient's confidence and to limit discomfort. There are four major factors that can affect the venipuncture procedure: (1) the patient's cooperation, (2) the patient's vein status, (3) the equipment, and (4) the medical assistant's skill level as a phlebotomist.

The medical assistant can use various techniques to encourage patient cooperation but has no control concerning the patient's vein status. Vein condition can be assessed, but it cannot be changed.

The equipment used can influence venipuncture to a great degree. Most facilities use either a nonevacuated blood collection system or an evacuation collection system to obtain blood specimens. The *Vacutainer* (Becton Dickinson & Co., Rutherford, NJ) is an evacuation blood collection system composed of (1) a reusable plastic holder, (2) double-ended, sterile collection needles of different lengths and gauges, and (3) interchangeable Vacutainer tubes, each containing a premeasured evacuated space (Fig. 28–8). The major advantages to the evacuated tube system are that it allows for multiple tubes of blood to be drawn from a single venipuncture and that there is less chance of labeling error or blood sample hemolysis. Both pediatric and adult adapters are available.

The medical assistant's skill level as a phlebotomist exerts the greatest influence on the quality of the veni-

puncture. Venipuncture is a skill, and it is develope and perfected through study and practice. It is the medical assistant's responsibility to master this skill. Remember that various factors affect a venipuncture, and not every attempt will be successful.

No more than three venipuncture attempts should be made on any patient. After two attempts, quietly inform the physician of the situation; usually, the physician will then obtain the specimen. Never be discouraged by an unsuccessful venipuncture. Each phlebotomy presents different circumstances, and a difficult situation should be viewed as a new challenge for the future. (See the detailed description of this procedure at the end of this chapter.)

SPECIMEN TUBES

Each laboratory test requires a specific specimen. Blood obtained by venipuncture may be tested as whole blood or coagulated blood or prepared so that only plasma or serum is used for testing.

Whole blood is collected in a tube containing an *anticoagulant* to prevent the blood from separating and clotting.

Coagulated blood is collected in a plain tube with no additives.

Plasma is obtained by drawing blood into a tube with an anticoagulant and then centrifuging the blood.

Serum is obtained from coagulated blood that has been centrifuged or by using a *serum-separator* tube that contains a clot activator and a gel that physically separates the serum from the cells. During centrifugation, the gel temporarily becomes fluid and moves to the dividing point between the serum and the cells.

To obtain the correct blood components for the requested test, the proper specimen collection tube must be selected. The Vacutainer system uses color-coded rubber stoppers to indicate the presence of or to identify the type of additives contained in the tube (Table

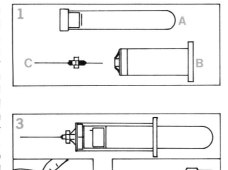
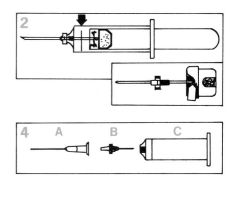

Figure 28–8. The Becton Dickinson Vacutainer system is used in many medical offices. (**1**) DESCRIPTION OF PARTS: (*A*) glass tube with rubber stopper; (*B*) plastic holder with guide line; (*C*) double-pointed needle. ASSEMBLY: (**2**) Thread needle into holder and tighten firmly. Place tube in holder with needle touching stopper. (**3**) Push tube forward until top of stopper meets guide line and then let go. Tube stopper will retract below guide line and should be left in that position. At this stage, the full point of the needle is embedded in the stopper, thus avoiding blood leakage upon venipuncture and preventing premature loss of vacuum. (**4**) ALTERNATE ASSEMBLY METHOD, using (*A*) Luer hub needle; (*B*) Vacutainer adapter; and (*C*) plastic holder. Thread adapter into holder and tighten firmly. Attach Luer needle to adapter, in the way that a needle is attached to a syringe. Place tube in holder with needle touching stopper, then proceed to **3**.

on to Vacutainer tubes, *microcon-
...ble* for small sample volumes and are
.e same manner.

.an one type of blood test is performed,
Vacutainer may be needed. To avoid
...tion of tube additives, the order of
...d collection is important. Each health
care facility should have a policy governing the order of
tubes of blood drawn for laboratory analysis. In general,
the following order applies when drawing blood with
evacuated systems:

1. Draw blood culture specimens first (yellow stopper).
2. Specimens that require no additive next (plain tubes, red, or mottled red and gray stoppers). Some facilities treat clot activators as an additive tube.
3. Tubes needed for coagulation studies (usually sodium citrate or heparin—green or blue stopper). Because blue tubes need to be completely filled, it is best to fill these tubes after at least one other tube of blood has been drawn and the blood is flowing freely.
4. Last, tubes of blood with additives, first with EDTA (ethylenediaminetetraacetic acid) (lavender), then oxilates and fluorides (gray stopper), are drawn.

When blood is added to tubes from a syringe, the following order is usually observed:

1. Coagulation tubes with citrate (blue)
2. EDTA tubes (lavender)
3. Other coagulants (gray, green)
4. Plain tubes (red)

It is recommended, however, that if a green tube containing heparin is used for electrolyte levels and if coagulation studies (blue tubes) or a complete blood count (lavender tube) is also ordered, the order of the tubes for drawing blood should be (1) green, (2) blue, then (3) lavender.

The choice of needle size usually depends on the size of the vein. Most facilities use a 21-gauge needle. For small veins, the 22- to 23-gauge needle is better. The length of the needle (from 1 inch to 1½ inches [2.5 to 3.8 cm]) is usually a matter of individual choice.

SITE SELECTION

The most common site for the venipuncture are the cephalic, median cubital, and median basilic veins in the forearm (Fig. 28–9). The median cubital vein is the easiest to stabilize because of its centralized position and because it bruises less. Choose the cephalic vein next, although the skin over the cephalic may be tougher to penetrate. The cephalic vein does not roll and is as slow to bruise as the median cubital vein, but the blood flows more slowly in the cephalic vein. The median basilic should be a last choice as it tends to roll or move, and the area bruises easily.

Even if the vein can be clearly seen, it should be palpated to make sure of its direction and location. A vein should feel elastic and give under pressure. If a satisfactory vein cannot be found in one arm, examine the other arm. Sometimes veins in one arm are larger than those in the other. Veins are palpated after the tourniquet is applied. Although the tourniquet helps to make the veins more prominent, it should not be left on for longer than 1 minute.

Infrequently, the phlebotomist cannot locate a vein by palpation in either of the patient's arms, or intrave-

Table 28–5

VACUTAINER STOPPER COLOR CODE IN ORDER OF DRAW

Stopper Color	Additive	Specimen Usage
Yellow	SPS (sodium polyanethole sulfonate)	Tests using plasma for culturing
Red	No additive; no anticoagulant	Tests using serum (e.g., most blood chemistries); acquired immunodeficiency syndrome antibody, viral studies, serology tests, blood typing
Red and black mottled top	Silicone (serum separating material)	Tests using serum except blood bank testing
Red Monoject	Gel energizer and microscopic glass particles	Tests using serum except blood bank testing
Blue	Sodium citrate	Coagulation studies
Green	Sodium heparin	Blood chemistries (e.g., electrolytes)
Lavender	EDTA (ethylenediaminetetraacetic acid)	Hematology studies
Gray	Potassium oxalate, sodium fluoride	Blood glucose
Black	Sodium oxalate	Westergren sedimentation rate determinations

Source: Wedding ME and Toenjes SA: Medical Laboratory Procedures. FA Davis, Philadelphia, 1992, p 144, with permission.

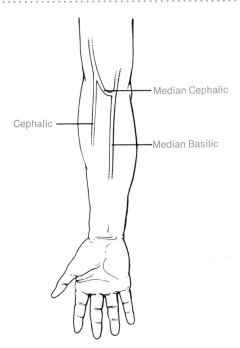

Figure 28-9. Major veins of the arm.

nous (IV) lines prevent the use of the most readily available veins. *Never draw a blood sample from an extremity with an IV.* A tourniquet application could occlude veins, possibly dislodge the IV needle, or cause a clot to be formed in the needle. Also, the IV solution will dilute the blood sample, giving erroneous results.

An alternate method for obtaining venous blood is to use the more visible veins in the back of the hand or ankle. A syringe, rather than a Vacutainer system, is frequently used when drawing blood from these areas because the veins are small and narrow, and the amount of suction can be better controlled when the blood is drawn. Venipuncture performed on the hands, legs, and feet are difficult and potentially dangerous. Only specifically trained phlebotomists should try to obtain blood from these sites. If a site cannot be palpated or blood successfully drawn after two attempts, notify the physician.

SYRINGE METHOD

For patients with small or fragile veins, blood specimens should be obtained by using a needle and syringe. This method is frequently used for children and the elderly. The vacuum in the Vacutainer tube may cause small or fragile veins to temporarily collapse, preventing blood from entering the tube. With a syringe system, the vacuum can be controlled by the medical assistant by the degree of pull exerted on the plunger.

The needle gauge usually used for venipuncture is 20 or 21. The larger the gauge number, the thinner the needle. For patients who have particularly difficult veins, a butterfly infusion set may be the equipment of

choice. A butterfly infusion set is a needle with a butterfly holder and a tube 11¾ inches (30 cm) long that attaches to either a syringe tip or a Vacutainer holder (Fig. 28-10).

WITHDRAWING A BLOOD SAMPLE FOR CULTURING

Normally, blood is sterile; however, in a disease state, microorganisms may have invaded the bloodstream. Blood is cultured in the laboratory. A blood sample is provided under sterile conditions to determine the presence or amount of pathogens present in the blood.

A venipuncture for a blood culture must be collected by special aseptic technique to prevent contamination. Prevention of the growth of external contaminants is necessary if the causative agent for the disease is to be isolated. Generally, appropriate blood culture collection procedure requires that the venipuncture site must be cleansed with alcohol for 2 full minutes followed by a

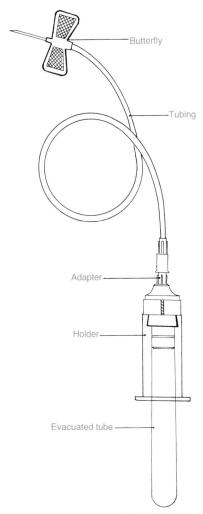

Figure 28-10. For small or fragile veins, the butterfly-winged infusion set with adapter, holder, and evacuated tube allows the phlebotomist to control the rate at which the vacuum in the tube draws blood from the vein.

"painting" of 2% providone iodine. The site must be cleansed in enlarging circles, with care taken never to cross the same area. Begin at the site previously palpated as suitable for a phlebotomy and work outward. The same pattern is followed with the iodine. After the venipuncture, the needle is replaced with a sterile needle, and culture bottles are filled with the blood sample. Some microbiology laboratories use a sterile Vacutainer tube. The microbiology reference laboratory used by the physician will provide exact procedures for their particular facility.

SERUM SEPARATION

The red-stopper Vacutainer tube contains no anticoagulant. A blood specimen collected in this tube will form a clot in approximately 15 to 20 minutes. The clot is a jelly-like mass held together by fibrin. Centrifuge covers must be in place during centrifugation, and the centrifuge should be placed as far from personnel as possible. Spin at the recommended speed for the recommended length of time. The yellow liquid portion in the top of the tube is serum (Fig. 28–11). The clot remains in the bottom of the tube. The serum should be immediately siphoned from the clot with a mechanical suction pipetter or a serum separator and placed in a properly labeled test tube for further diagnostic testing.

Generally, serum is refrigerated or frozen to prevent chemical changes unless it can be tested immediately. Commercially available serum separator tubes provide a silicone barrier material to facilitate the separation of serum.

HEMOLYSIS

Whole blood, plasma, and serum must be handled with care to prevent hemolysis, the most common problem with drawing blood. Hemolyzed blood specimens (cells broken down) produce invalid laboratory results. As the red blood cells are lysed or destroyed, chemical components contained in the cells are released into the serum or plasma, producing a reddish color.

Hemolysis can be caused by trauma at the vein site due to poor venipuncture technique. Collecting and transferring blood to a dirty or wet test tube can hemolyze the red cells. Hemolysis can also be caused by freezing, by prolonged exposure to heat, by too forceful spraying of blood through the needle, or by allowing the sample to sit too long before separating the serum or plasma from the cells.

CAPILLARY PUNCTURE

Because of the risk of contamination by tissue fluid and the inability to repeat the test owing to the small volume of blood obtainable from finger puncture, venipunctures are generally preferred over capillary methods. However, the capillary method is used if the patient has extremely poor veins, or with children and newborns from whom removal of large amounts of blood is not feasible. A note that the sample is capillary blood should always be made on the laboratory slip when the specimen is obtained from a capillary puncture.

The capillary puncture can be made in the ear lobe, finger, toe, or heel. The lateral side of the "cushion" of the palmar aspect of the middle (index) finger is the usual site used for toddlers up through adults (Fig. 28–12). One disadvantage is that this area is quite sensitive. At the end of this chapter, a step-by-step description of the procedure for a capillary puncture on a finger or heel is given.

The heel is the common puncture site for infants. Obtaining a blood specimen from a heel stick follows the general procedure for a capillary finger puncture.

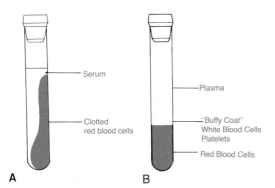

Figure 28–11. (**A**) A sample tube with no anticoagulant; after centrifugation, the coagulated blood has separated into serum and clotted red blood cells. (**B**) A blood sample with anticoagulant added: after centrifugation, the uncoagulated blood has separated into plasma, the buffy coat, and packed red blood cells.

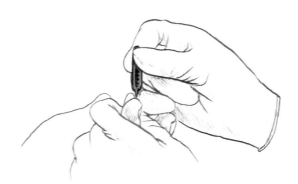

Figure 28–12. To obtain blood by finger puncture, the medical assistant uses a lancet, usually choosing the middle or fourth finger. The lateral tip of the finger is less sensitive than the dorsal tip.

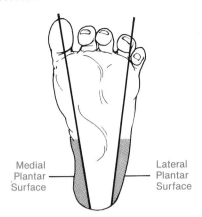

Figure 28–13. Recommended sites for capillary heel puncture of the infant or newborn.

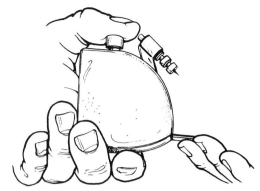

Figure 28–14. The Autolet automatic capillary puncture kit is often used by diabetic patients for self-monitoring of blood glucose.

From a study of heel sticks performed on infants, it is recommended that the medial or lateral portions of the plantar surfaces of the heel be used and that the puncture be no more than 2.4 mm ($\frac{1}{8}$″) in depth to avoid injury or complications. This area is shaded in Figure 28–13. When the infant's heel is punctured, special care must be taken to protect the area from further injury. A previously used puncture site should never be repenetrated. To improve circulation before puncturing, commercially prepared heel warmers can be applied to the infant's foot or the heel may be warmed by wrapping the foot in a warm washcloth or by placing the heel in warm water. If the heel is submerged in water, it must be dried thoroughly before proceeding with the puncture.

AUTOMATIC SAMPLE COLLECTING DEVICES

The use of small volumes of blood for diagnostic testing is also known as a *microtechnique* and is frequently used because laboratories have adopted automated technologies that require minimum amounts of serum for testing. The Autolet kit (Ames Co) and microcontainer tubes (Becton Dickinson & Co.) with flow-directed tips are two devices designed for the collection of blood from capillary finger and heel sites (see also Fig. 30–4).

A lancet is secured in the Autolet, which punctures the skin when the activating button is depressed and then retracts. Diabetic patients frequently use the Autolet system for blood glucose self-monitoring (Fig. 28–14).

The Microtainer System (Becton Dickinson & Co.) also offers a means of collecting capillary blood directly into the container by using a "Flotop" collector.

BASIC LABORATORY EQUIPMENT

To obtain results that are as accurate as possible, the best possible methods and instruments must be used. It is also necessary to use good quality laboratory glassware and plastic ware to collect, transport, and measure specimens. Other important equipment includes centrifuges and microscopes, used to prepare and examine blood, urine, and tissues; and colorimeters and spectrophotometers, used to determine the concentration of substances.

Most glassware can be divided into two categories: containment (noncalibrated) and volumetric (calibrated). Noncalibrated test tubes, reagent bottles, and cuvettes are examples of containment ware. Manual and automatic pipettes are examples of volumetric ware. Because volumetric ware is calibrated, it is more expensive than noncalibrated containment ware.

PIPETTES

A pipette is a cylindrical glass tube for measuring fluids. It is calibrated to deliver or transfer a specified volume from one container to another. Each pipette has at least one calibration mark on it. Pipettes are filled by suction or aspiration devices.

Pipettes also are classified according to whether they deliver (TD—to deliver) or contain (TC—to contain). The TD pipette is filled and allowed to drain into another container by the force of gravity as it is held in a vertical position. When the fluid is drained a drop of fluid remains inside the tip. Since the remaining drop is accounted for in the calibration, the drop should never be "blown" out of the tip.

A TD pipette that is known as a *volumetric* (or *transfer*) pipette. Volumetric pipettes are used for volumes of 1 mL or more. When filled to the calibration mark, the pipette is designed to deliver the amount inscribed on it. For example, a 2-mL pipette, when filled to the calibration mark, will deliver 2 mL of fluid. Volumetric pipettes are used to measure standard solutions, serum, plasma, urine, and some reagents.

Another way to deliver fluids is to use a *graduated* (or *measuring*) pipette. Graduated pipettes are used when great accuracy is not required. Like the syringe, the graduated pipette is used to deliver volumes from 1.0 to 25 mL. Graduated pipettes are commonly used to measure reagents.

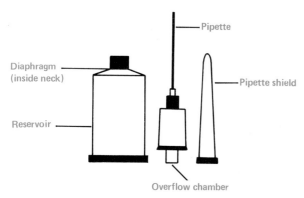

Figure 28-15. The Unopette disposable micropipette system consists of a reservoir containing a diluent, a pipette, and a pipette shield.

The *micropipette* is a TC pipette. It is calibrated to contain a specified amount of liquid but will not necessarily deliver that exact amount. Micropipettes are designed to contain precise amounts of fluid, ranging from 1 to 500 μL (0.001 to 5.0 mL). When using TC pipettes, the medical assistant must make sure that none of the contents remain inside the pipette. Therefore, the specimen is rinsed with a diluting fluid to assure that all the contents will be removed when emptied. To properly use a TC pipette, the receiving container must contain a diluent. A TC pipette should never be used to deliver a specimen into an empty test tube or cuvette.

Capillary pipettes are inexpensive, disposable glass pipettes used for obtaining blood specimens. Blood flows into the pipette by capillary attraction. A capillary pipette is filled to its single calibration mark, and the measured blood is then delivered by positive pressure.

The *Unopette* (Becton Dickinson Co., Rutherford, NJ) is a disposable micropipette used mostly in hematology and blood chemistry testing (Fig. 28-15). A glass capillary tube is fitted into a plastic holder and automatically fills with blood by capillary attraction. The plastic reagent bottle (reservoir) is squeezed while the pipette is inserted into it. On release of pressure, the blood is drawn into the diluent in the reservoir. Intermittent squeezing rinses the contents.

CENTRIFUGE

Centrifuges are used to separate solid material from a liquid with the increased gravitational force created by spinning or rotating motion. Solid materials or suspended particles settle to the bottom of a centrifuge tube because they are heavier than the liquid portion.

Centrifugation is used to recover solid materials suspended in urine. After centrifugation, the solid material at the bottom is called the *sediment* or *precipitate*, and the remaining liquid portion is called the *supernatant.* To prepare urinary sediment for microscopic examination, the supernatant is decanted, and the remaining sediment is examined.

The centrifuge can also be used to separate serum or plasma from cells in blood. If coagulated blood is centrifuged, two layers are formed: the formed elements of blood (cells and platelets) and the plasma. If anticoagulated blood is centrifuged, three layers are formed: the red cells, the *buffy coat* (white blood cells and platelets) and the plasma (see Fig. 28-11).

For separating serum from the clot, the centrifugal force is not critical. Usually a force of at least 1000 g for 10 minutes gives a good separation. When serum separator tubes are used a greater force is needed to displace the gel. Usually a force of 1000 to 1300 g for 10 minutes displaces the gel. Centrifuges revolutions per minute should be checked at least every 3 months.

A smaller, tabletop version of the centrifuge has been specially designed for microhematocrit determinations (Fig. 28-16). This *microhematocrit centrifuge* attains a speed of about 10,000 to 15,000 rpm, usually averaging 12,000 g (force of gravity).

Tubes placed in the centrifuge must always be balanced. The centrifuge cup directly opposite the specimen must contain a tube of equal size and shape with an equal volume of liquid with the same specific gravity of the load (specimen being tested). Usually water may be placed in the balancing load.

Tubes being centrifuged must be capped. Never centrifuge blood without a tube stopper. White bandage tape can be placed around the rim of the centrifuge to provide a visible means of detecting splatter of blood during centrifugation. Capping also prevents evapora-

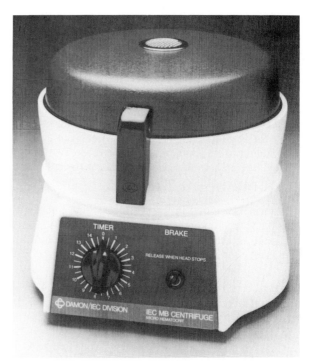

Figure 28-16. There are several types of laboratory centrifuges; this is designed specifically for the microhematocrit procedure. (From Wedding MD and Toenjes SA: Medical Laboratory Procedures. FA Davis, Philadelphia, 1992, p. 230, with permission.)

tion of the sample from occurring. It is best to place the centrifuge in a place that is as far away from personnel as possible. Personnel should not work near a centrifuge while it is in use.

Centrifuge tubes usually are thicker than other test tubes. Some tubes are conical, others have rounded bottoms. Centrifuge tubes are disposable or reusable. Even though the glass is thick and strong, a tube should not be placed into the centrifuge unless a rubber cushion is positioned in the test tube compartment. If some cushions are missing, the centrifuge will not balance properly.

Centrifuge covers prevent laboratory personnel from being exposed to aerosol spray and flying glass, should a tube break in the centrifuge. Do not stop the centrifuge with the hands. "Braking" the centrifuge may cause a resuspension of the sediment and could create dangerous aerosols. Should a tube break, both the cup and the rubber cushion must be decontaminated (see Housekeeping, p. 737) and all glass particles removed wearing utility gloves. Centrifuges must be cleaned, lubricated, and serviced regularly.

SPECTROPHOTOMETER

Many office-based laboratories use the spectrophotometer for quantitatively determining the exact amount of an unknown substance in human specimens. The spectrophotometer is based on principles of colorimetry.

Colorimetry, or photometry, uses color and color variations to determine the concentration of a substance. The use of colorimetry is based on two factors: the color itself and the intensity of the color. Originally, colorimetric procedures used only a visual (naked-eye) comparison of the color of an unknown substance with that of a standard. One application of visual colorimetry still in use is the dry reagent strip tests used in urinalysis. These reagent strips are compared against a color chart with the naked eye. (Instruments now are available to read urine color comparisons electronically.)

Colorimetry instruments work at the invisible level by isolating a narrow wavelength of the color spectrum for measurements. To isolate wavelengths, instruments use filters (filter photometers), prisms (spectrophotometers), or gratings (photoelectric colorimeters). The principle of each instrument is the same, however: the light transmitted by the *standard* solution is compared with the amount of light transmitted by the solution of an unknown specimen.

Specimens measured by spectrophotometry must have color or be capable of being colored. Hemoglobin is an example of a specimen that has measurable color. Glucose, on the other hand, is a colorless substance and first must be colored by the use of certain reagents and reactions. Unknown, colored substances are compared with a similar substance of known strength (the standard), based on the principle that the intensity of color is directly proportionate to the concentration of the substance being tested. Light is passed through a wavelength isolator that allows only one particular portion of the color spectrum to pass through a specimen.

Cuvettes are special test tubes used in photometry. They are made of glass or plastic, and may be round, square, or rectangular. Since the amount of light transmitted by a cuvette must be uniform, cuvettes must be of high quality and calibrated before use.

Depending on the concentration and thus the color of the solution, a certain amount of light is absorbed by the solution, and the remainder is transmitted through the solution (Fig. 28–17). The light that is transmitted through the solution passes on to a measuring device consisting of a photoelectric cell and galvanometer. The measuring device is connected to a viewing device. The viewing scale reports the result in percent of transmittance (some instruments measure absorbance). A concentrated substance transmits less light, and the reading on the viewing scale will be lower than for a dilute (pale) solution. The differences in percent of transmittance is the basis for comparing color intensity in spectrophotometry.

When substances are colored with reagents, the color of the reagents can sometimes alter test results. To eliminate test misinterpretation from any color emitted by the reagents themselves, a *blank solution* is used to make corrections. A blank solution contains the same reagents as the unknown sample and the standard tubes but not the unknown substance being measured. Spectrophotometers and cuvettes must be regularly calibrated using the directions of each specific manufacturer.

THE MICROSCOPE

The microscope is the most frequently used laboratory instrument in the POL. The *microscope* is an optical instrument used to magnify small structures for morphologic study. It is a vital laboratory tool and one that the medical assistant must be able to operate properly. The medical assistant should be familiar with the parts of the microscope and their functions, as well as with proper maintenance (see procedure at end of chapter).

MICROSCOPE COMPONENTS

Figure 28–18 shows the major parts of a *binocular compound microscope*. Table 28–6 summarizes the purposes of the various parts.

Of the three objective lenses of a compound microscope, the most powerful is usually an *oil immersion lens*. An oil immersion lens is designed to be lowered onto a drop of oil placed on the slide to be examined. The oil corrects the tendency of light rays to *defract* (bend) and scatter as they pass through the glass slide (Fig. 28–19).

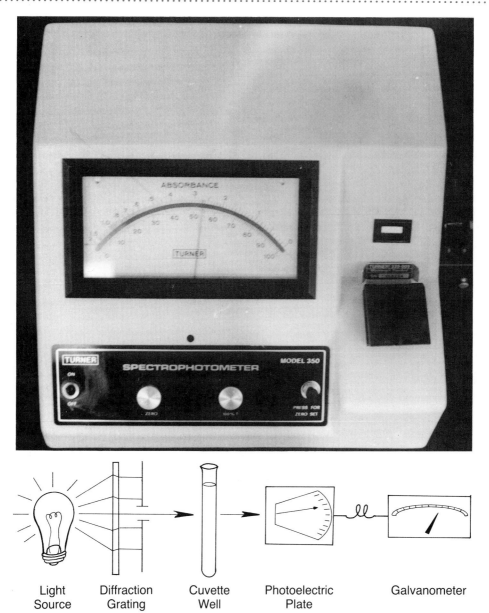

Light   Diffraction   Cuvette   Photoelectric   Galvanometer
Source   Grating   Well   Plate

Figure 28-17. The spectrophotometer *(top)* consists of a light source, monochromator, cuvette, photodetector, and galvanometer. (From Wedding MD and Toenjes SA: *Medical Laboratory Procedures.* FA Davis, Philadelphia, 1992, p. 163, with permission.)

MAGNIFICATION

The total magnifying power of the microscope is the product of the magnification of the objective lens times that of the eyepiece. For example, a low-power dry objective (10×) used with a 10× eyepiece results in a magnification of 100×.

The ability of the microscope to produce a sharp image depends not only on its magnification qualities, but also on the resolving power of the lens. Resolution is the ability of the objective to present details of separate images, making them sharp and clear. The *numerical aperture* (NA) is an index used to indicate the resolving power of the objective. The higher the NA, the greater the resolution.

CARE AND MAINTENANCE

Since the microscope is a delicate instrument, it must be properly maintained to ensure an optimal working condition. The microscope will give many years of service if the following rules are adhered to:

1. Carry the microscope in an upright position by grasping the arm of the instrument with one hand while placing the other hand securely under the base of the instrument for support.
2. Inspect the oculars, objectives, stage, and light source, and clean if necessary.
   a. Rotate the eyepiece and observe if a pattern moves; if so, the eyepiece needs to be cleaned.

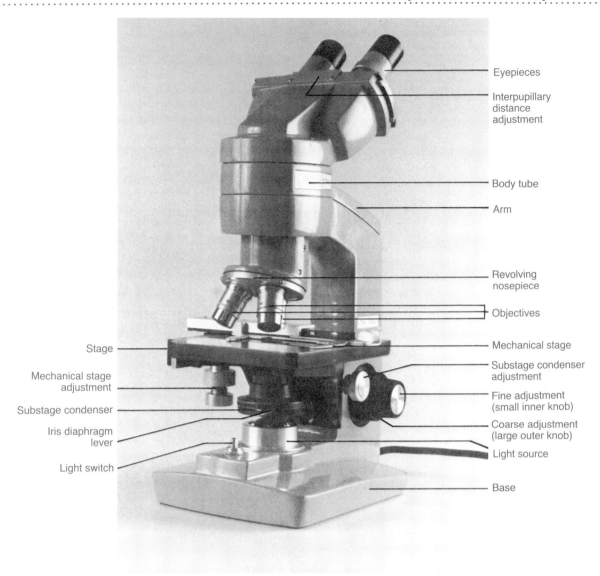

Eyepieces

Interpupillary distance adjustment

Body tube

Arm

Revolving nosepiece

Objectives

Mechanical stage

Substage condenser adjustment

Fine adjustment (small inner knob)

Coarse adjustment (large outer knob)

Light source

Base

Stage

Mechanical stage adjustment

Substage condenser

Iris diaphragm lever

Light switch

Figure 28–18. A binocular compound microscope.

b. Never touch the optical areas. Use only lens paper for cleaning.

c. For a heavy oil film, special lens cleaners or xylene may be used sparingly on lens paper to dissolve the oil. Pay particular attention to the amount of xylene used as too much xylene may loosen the cement holding the lenses in place.

3. Always keep a stock of extra light bulbs available if a rheostat is not used. To change the microscope bulb, follow these steps:

a. Carefully place the microscope on its side and open the cover plate.

b. Using a protective bulb holder, cover the bulb and twist gently, freeing the bulb.

c. Discard the old bulb and place a new one in the protective holder.

d. Properly align the bulb and twist it into place.

The holder will prevent the bulb from shattering under pressure.

e. Close the cover plate and return the microscope to the upright position.

4. Store the microscope as follows:

a. Place the low-power objective as close to the stage as possible.

b. Remove the plug from the electrical outlet and wrap the cord around the base of the microscope.

c. Place a protective cover over the microscope to shield it from dust.

d. Place the covered microscope in a wooden carrying case, if available.

e. Never allow chemicals to touch the microscope.

5. Daily maintenance of the microscope is mandatory. Inspect the equipment. As equipment is inspected or repaired, document both in a log (see Fig. 28–1).

Table 28-6
PARTS OF THE BINOCULAR MICROSCOPE

Part	Purpose
Eyepiece (ocular lens)	The eyepiece is the lens system that is closest to the eye, on which the magnification is printed.
Interpupillary distance adjuster	The binocular compound microscope has two eyepieces that can be adjusted to the width between the individual's eyes by means of the knob found between the oculars.
Body tube	The body tube directs the light path from the light source to the eyepiece.
Arm	The arm is used to carry the microscope with one hand on the arm handle and the other firmly holding the base of the microscope.
Base	The base of the microscope is its foundation or platform.
Revolving nosepiece	The revolving nosepiece holds the objectives and permits their movement for selection.
Objectives	The objectives constitute the lens system found on the nosepiece. There are usually three objectives (low-power dry, high-power dry, and oil immersion), each having the magnification engraved on the barrel.
Stage clip	The stage clip is a movable spring device used to secure a slide to the top of the stage.
Stage	The stage is a movable platform allowing the entire slide to be scanned.
Stage mechanism	The stage mechanism consists of two knobs that control the vertical and horizontal movement of the slide.
Fine adjustment	Fine adjustment provides better resolution by exact focusing with slow movement within a limited range.
Coarse adjustment	Coarse adjustment provides better resolution by approximate focusing within a wide range of movement.
Substage condenser	The substage condenser is a lens system used to increase the light and converge the rays for a sharper focus.
Diaphragm	The diaphragm is an adjustable aperture that controls the intensity of light.
Light source	An in-base illuminator usually serves as the microscope's light source.
Rheostat	Some microscopes have the light source connected to a rheostat, which regulates the intensity of the light.

This log provides a recording that maintenance has taken place.

GENERAL RULES OF SAFETY

Even when precautions are observed, laboratory accidents can occur. Glassware breaks, chemicals spill, and electrical equipment fails. The medical assistant who understands the principles presented in this chapter and Chapter 27 is prepared to react to an accident or emergency instantaneously and to administer first aid immediately.

Establish an appropriate environment for testing. All laboratory facilities and equipment must be kept clean and orderly at all times, with all unnecessary articles properly stored. Follow *written* safety policies and procedures, and use MSDSs. Compliance with the following safety rules should ensure safe laboratory practice:

1. Wear appropriate PPE.
2. Avoid hand-to-mouth contact. No food or drink and no smoking restrictions should be observed.
3. Do not mouth pipette.
4. Do not store caustic material above eye level as there is the potential for spillage when reaching up for the container stored on a shelf.
5. Be sure hands are dry when transferring a reagent bottle from one place to another.
6. Locate a fire extinguisher in the laboratory area. Know how to operate it.
7. Keep a first aid manual and supplies available in the laboratory area.

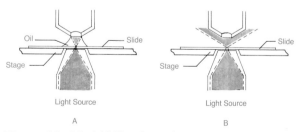

Figure 28-19. (**A**) The drop of oil causes the light rays passing through the slide to be directed into the oil immersion lens. (**B**) Without oil, some light rays are scattered as they emerge from the slide and do not pass into the lens. (From Wedding MD and Toenjes SA: Medical Laboratory Procedures. FA Davis, Philadelphia, 1992, p. 48, with permission.)

8. Avoid inhaling any chemical substances that might cause injury to nasal membranes or lungs. Flammable substances frequently have noxious fumes; be sure such materials are kept away from heat sources and are used only in a well-ventilated room.

9. Never use chipped, broken, or cracked glassware.

HOUSEKEEPING

Follow *written* cleanup policies and procedures for all housekeeping and spills.

1. Wash hands with soap and water before and after working in the laboratory area.

2. Disinfect the work area with 5.25% sodium hypochlorite (bleach) diluted 1:10 with water at the start and end of each day.

3. Clean up spills immediately with 5.25% sodium hypochlorite (bleach) diluted 1:4 with water. (Remember, a wet surface is dangerous.)

4. When infectious materials are spilled, cover the area with paper towels, pour 5.25% sodium hypochlorite (bleach) diluted 1:4 with water liberally over the towels, and allow to stand for 15 minutes. After putting on nonsterile utility gloves, wipe up the spill completely and discard the waste into a biohazard container labeled for infectious waste.

5. Needles have the potential for injuring and infecting the phlebotomist. The intact needle must be disposed of immediately after use. Place all materials capable of skin puncture in a puncture-resistant container available nearby. Never recap, bend, or remove a used needle as there is a possibility of puncturing yourself with the contaminated needle. Containers must be color-coded red, have a lid, and remain upright to keep liquids and sharps inside. If recapping is required for a specific medical procedure, such as blood gas analysis, the needle must be recapped with a mechanical device (tongs or forceps) or a one-handed technique. In the one-handed technique, use the needle itself to "scoop" up the cap, then push the cap and sharp together against a hard surface.

6. When a specimen is known or suspected to be infectious, dispose of the waste by double bagging in red bags or bags labeled with a red biohazard label. Reusable materials coming in contact with potentially infectious specimens must be sterilized by wrapping in a cloth (cotton) wrapper and autoclaving for the recommended period of time *before* sanitizing (cleaning) for reuse. Clean the work area carefully with a disinfectant after the laboratory procedure is completed.

EMERGENCY PRECAUTIONS

Every office laboratory, no matter how small, should have a posted plan for evacuation in the event of a fire or contamination with dangerous fumes. Safety practices should include periodic unannounced fire and safety drills, and safety equipment, such as fire extinguishers, emergency eye washers, and fire blankets should be on hand.

A hazard identification system was developed by the National Fire Protection Association. The system consists of four diamond-shaped symbols that form a larger diamond shape (Fig. 28–20). Each smaller diamond is color-coded to depict a specific type of hazard. The top diamond is red and indicates a flammability hazard. The bottom diamond is white and indicates special hazards, such as radioactivity. The diamond on the left is blue and indicates a possible health hazard, and the diamond on the right is yellow and indicates a reactivity-stability hazard. Inside each diamond is a number from zero to four, with four being extremely hazardous and zero no hazard.

In the case of fire, it is important to know the correct use of the fire extinguisher and alarm systems. It is also important to know which type of extinguisher to use. Red and yellow fire extinguishers use the same color-coded hazard identification system. Whenever possible use the correct type of fire extinguisher to extinguish a fire. Water must never be used in an attempt to put out a fire.

PROTECTION FROM AEROSOLS

Another type of hazard in the POL is the potential health hazard posed by pathogenic organisms in the

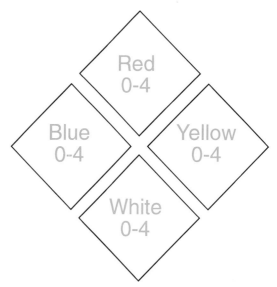

Figure 28–20. Hazard identification sign system developed by the National Fire Protection Association. Each color represents a different type of fire hazard; the number used in each diamond indicates the degree of hazard relative to that type of hazard.

environment. Biohazard aerosols can be found anywhere there are human specimens. Aerosols are generated from spills, splashes, and splatter of blood and body fluids. Several procedures are responsible for aerosol production, especially procedures involving culturing, centrifugation, and the preparation of direct smears. Protective devices and techniques must be used to prevent aerosols from entering the nose, eye, or mouth.

The first line of defense is the use of masks and eye protectors. Some laboratories prefer that their personnel use face shields. Laboratory personnel should wear protective eye gear when transferring blood from a collection syringe into a specimen container, using chemicals, cleaning glassware, and preparing laboratory reagents.

Biosafety cabinets can be used to contain and remove air contaminants through an outside exhaust system, heat, or ultraviolet light. Specially constructed splash shields are used for blood processing. The shield acts as a barrier between the person and the specimen. Laboratory safety boxes are commercially available for use in procedures that might cause splattering. Splash shields and safety boxes should be decontaminated with disinfectants on a regular basis.

A common source of splatter is the blood-collecting tube stopper. Substances can become airborne when the stopper is removed from the tube, a serum sample is poured from one tube to another, or a serum tube is centrifuged. Safety boxes are ideal when removing stoppers from blood samples.

In addition, stoppers should be removed using a disposable 4 × 4 gauze square or special gauze pads with an impermeable plastic coating on one side to reduce contamination of the gloves. When removing a blood tube stopper, always hold the tube away from the body and gently twist the stopper to remove. When not on the container, stoppers should remain wrapped in the gauze and not come into contact with any work surface or tabletop. When centrifuging, the stopper must be firmly attached to the tube. Centrifuge covers should be used and left down until the centrifuge comes to a full stop.

PIPETTING SAFEGUARDS

Pipetting may be done only with a mechanical suction device or aspirator bulbs. Mouth pipetting is never done. One alternative for pipetting is the automatic pipetting device. Automatic pipetters can be set to deliver specific volumes of blood and reagents. The equipment parts are autoclavable and the pipette tips are disposable. The most commonly used automatic system is the Unopette system (see Fig. 28–15). Unopettes already contain the specified amount of reagent, and are entirely disposable after each use.

Some reusable laboratory ware, such as pipettes, cannot be presoaked with bleach, as bleach corrodes stainless steel and coagulates proteins. If laboratory ware cannot be presoaked in bleach or treated with some other procedure, such as autoclaving, a strong detergent such as 3% phenol can be used to decontaminate reusable equipment before autoclaving. Reusable pipettes should be placed in a covered tray containing 3% phenol before being transported to the autoclave room. Phenol can cause caustic burns or contact dermatitis, even on slight exposure. In case of contact, skin should be rinsed with water or alcohol. Instruments soaked in phenol should be rinsed in alcohol before cleaning or autoclaving. Soap, detergents, or cleaning powders are specially manufactured for laboratory equipment. Allowing dirty glassware or plastic ware to soak in a solution of detergent and water prevents debris from drying on the surface and makes the task of cleaning much easier.

RELATED ETHICAL AND LEGAL IMPLICATIONS

A few special legal situations warrant consideration with regard to drug testing. When obtaining a sample for drug testing, the medical assistant should follow procedures exactly. Courts of law require absolute adherence to procedures for collecting, handling, and analyzing specimens and complete and exact documentation of the chain of events.

Skin preparation for a blood alcohol level test must be done with providone-iodine (Betadine) rather than with alcohol, as the alcohol could falsely elevate the blood alcohol level. Many states have statutes that specify exactly how, when, and under what circumstances this testing can be done. The medical assistant should request a copy of the legislation from the state hospital association, the state police, or a state representative.

SUMMARY

The medical assistant who is responsible for laboratory testing must clearly understand the basic concepts of laboratory medicine. This chapter has introduced the medical assistant to the various components of laboratory medicine: QC, specimen collection, venipuncture, capillary puncture, basic laboratory equipment, and safety. The medical assistant should stay current with the rapid technological advances in laboratory medicine and assist in establishing protocols for those tests best suited to the physician's practice.

The key to successful administration of any POL lies first in determining the needs of the individual physician based on his or her diagnostic approach and then deciding which tests and instruments are best suited to the work performed. QC measures also must be performed daily to ensure reproducible laboratory tests and quality of health care delivery.

The medical assistant working in the POL has primary responsibility for properly collecting and accurately testing specimens. The medical assistant should approach office laboratory testing as a challenging opportunity to work with the physician to improve and promote health care.

DISCUSSION QUESTIONS

1. The patient refuses to have a venipuncture and states that she fears needles. What is your response?
2. A venipuncture procedure results in the tube filling slowly and only partially. The needle remains in the patient's arm. What is your response?
3. While performing a venipuncture, you notice that the patient is becoming pale and is perspiring profusely. What is your response?

BIBLIOGRAPHY

Clinical laboratory improvement amendment, 1988. Superintendent of Documents, U.S. Government Printing Office, Washington, DC. Federal Register Stock No. 069-001-00042-4 (Feb 28, 1992).

Henry JB (ed): Clinical Diagnosis and Management by Laboratory Methods, ed 18. WB Saunders Philadelphia, 1991.

Lane K: AIDS Concepts for the Medical Assistant, Part I. American Association of Medical Assistants, Chicago, 1993.

Lane K (ed): Saunder's Manual of Medical Assisting Practice. WB Saunders, Philadelphia, 1992.

Linne J and Ringsrud K: Basic Techniques in Clinical Laboratory Science, ed 3. CV Mosby, St Louis, 1992.

Manual of BBL Products and Laboratory Procedures, ed 6. Becton Dickinson and Company, Cockeysville, Maryland, 1989.

National Fire Protection Association: Hazardous Chemical Data, No. 49. National Fire Protection Association, Boston, MA, 1975.

Occupational exposure to bloodborne pathogens, final rule. 54 Federal Register Stock No. 23042–23139 (Dec 12, 1991).

Occupational exposures to hazardous chemical in laboratories, final rule. 55 Federal Register Stock No. 3327–3335 (Jan 31, 1990).

Occupational safety and health standards. 43 Federal Register (Oct 24; Nov 17, 1978).

Pendergraph G.: Handbook of Phlebotomy, ed 3. Lea & Febiger, Philadelphia, 1992.

Recommendations for prevention of HIV transmission in health-care settings. MMWR 36(Suppl):3s, 1987.

Standards for the tracking and management of medical waste, interim final rule and request for comments. 40 Federal Register 12326 (Mar 24, 1989).

Update, universal precautions for prevention of transmission of human immunodeficiency virus, hepatitis B virus, and other bloodborne pathogens in health-care settings. MMWR 37:377, 1988.

Wedding ME and Toenges SA: Medical Laboratory Procedures. FA Davis, Philadelphia, 1992.

PROCEDURE: Withdraw a venous blood sample using the evacuated blood collecting system or a syringe

OSHA STANDARDS:

Terminal Performance Objective: Obtain a single sample or multiple blood samples for diagnostic testing and prepare the specimen(s) for transport within a reasonable time.

EQUIPMENT: Nonsterile gloves
Tourniquet
70% alcohol preparation pads
Dry gauze pads
Vacutainer brand blood collection system holder or syringe
Color-topped evacuated tubes for the specific tests ordered
Single-sample or multiple-sample needle of the appropriate length and gauge
Band-aid and adhesive tape
Biohazard sharps container
Disposable biohazard container

PROCEDURE	PRINCIPLE
Equipment Preparation	
1. Prepare the equipment, including extra supplies.	1. Equipment readily at hand allows for a quick, efficient, and skillfully performed phlebotomy.
2. Prepare the area by checking the orderliness and cleanliness of the room and appropriate lighting. Don gloves.	2. To reduce the chance of transmitting microorganisms and to provide adequate light.
3. Review the request form for the test(s) ordered.	3. To select the appropriate evacuated tubes and to set up the correct order for drawing the blood samples when more than one tube must be filled.
4. Identify the patient and explain the procedure.	4. The patient needs to understand the procedure to be performed.
5. Recheck the request form.	5. As a second check to verify the procedure ordered and the patient's identity and to ensure that all the equipment has been gathered for the venipuncture.
6. Check for dietary or other restrictions.	6. For fasting specimens, the patient should not have eaten since midnight of the previous day.
7. Reassure the patient.	7. Patients are very nervous and anxious about a venipuncture. They should be reassured that it may be painful but will not take long.
8. Comfortably and safely seat the patient.	8. Patients should arrive about 15 minutes before blood is drawn. A venipuncture chair should be available.
9. Position the arm on a slanting armrest in a straight line from the shoulder to the wrist, with the elbow joint fully extended.	9. A venipuncture chair should be available to position the arm for the best visualization and result from a free-flowing vein.
10. Assemble the tube(s), needle holder, and syringe and needle and place the gauze, Band-aid, and alcohol nearby.	10. From the time the tourniquet is applied, the procedure should not take more than 1 minute. It is essential to have all equipment at hand.
a. Break the seal of the needle by twisting and inspect the needle. Leave the needle loosely covered without contaminating it.	a. The end of the needle point must be free of hooks and have a clear opening.
b. Thread the needle into the Vacutainer holder.	b. If multiple tubes are to be filled, a multisample Vacutainer needle with a rubber sleeve should be used, to prevent blood from seeping into the Vacutainer holder.

PROCEDURE

    c. Place the tube in the holder and on the needle until the rubber stopper reached the holder guideline.

11. Recheck the request form

Patient Preparation

1. Select the site for venipuncture. Observe both arms.

2. Apply the tourniquet around the arm approximately 3 to 4 inches (7.5 to 10 cm) above the vein area to be felt.

3. Hold one end taut, then tuck a portion of the other end under the taut end so as to form a loop.

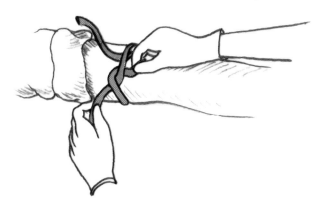

4. Ask the patient to open and close the fist twice. The fist should then remain closed.

5. Palpate the vein with the index finger to make sure the vein feels like an elastic tube and gives under pressure. Palpate and trace the vein several times.

6. Release the tourniquet before cleaning the venipuncture site.

7. Cleanse the site with alcohol in a circular motion working from the inside outward and allow to air dry.

8. Place the patient's arm in a downward position. Remove the cap from the needle.

9. Reapply the tourniquet and grasp the patient's arm 1 to 2 inches (2.5 to 5 cm) below the venipuncture site with your nondominant hand. Pull the skin tight with the thumb.

Performing the Venipuncture

10. Turn the needle so that the bevel is in an upward position and position the tube or syringe below the venipuncture site with the needle at approximately a 15° angle to the arm and in a direct line with the vein.

PRINCIPLE

    c. If inserted past the guideline, the needle will puncture the rubber stopper and break the vacuum seal in the tube.

11. As a third check for tube verification.

1. Avoid areas that have rash, burns, bruises, scars, edematous areas, or blood concentration. Select the vein that looks the fullest.

2. The tourniquet constricts venous blood returning from the arm which causes the veins to distend. If veins are prominent, a tourniquet is not necessary. If possible, select the site without the use of a tourniquet. Even if a vein can be seen, however, it must be palpated.

3. The tourniquet must be tight enough to obstruct venous return, but not so tight as to cut off arterial circulation.

4. The closed fist increases venous stasis (distension) and makes the veins more prominent. Avoid vigorous pumping which could overdistend the veins.

5. To be certain of the vein's location and direction and to palpate that no pulse is present indicating a vein rather than an artery. If a vein cannot be palpated, release the tourniquet and repeat the process on the other arm.

6. The tourniquet should be released after 1 minute because prolonged application of the tourniquet will cause hemoconcentration and patient discomfort. Hemoconcentration is a cause of specimen hemolysis.

7. Alcohol mixed with blood by the needle tip will alter test results. If the vein has to be palpated again, repeat the cleaning procedure.

8. A downward position helps to prevent backflow.

9. Pulling the skin taut will keep the vein from rolling.

10. The downward position and the small angle provide for the most uninterrupted flow and prevent backflow into the vein. Backflow can be a cause of specimen hemolysis. The bevel-up position facilitates skin and vein puncture and provides a better flow.

PROCEDURE

PRINCIPLE

11. Puncture the skin and the vein in a single motion to a depth of 1/2 to 3/4 inch (1.25 to 1.88 cm), following the longitudinal line of the vein. Hold the syringe or assembled Vacutainer system by placing the thumb and forefinger on the barrel or holder and using the other three fingers to support the syringe or rear of the Vacutainer system.

11. The depth depends on the proximity of the vein to the skin. A greater depth or a greater angle could puncture the other side of the vein, resulting in a hematoma and a hemolyzed specimen. A sensation of resistance will be felt followed by ease of penetration as the vein is entered.

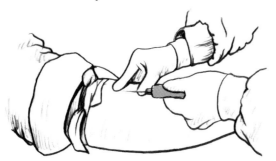

Holding the skin taut helps to anchor the vein.

12. As soon as the needle enters the vein, push the Vacutainer tube into the holder as far as it will go. This is done by grasping the holder flange with the index and third fingers and pushing the tube forward with the thumb. If using a syringe, begin pulling on the plunger, taking care not to pull too rapidly or forcefully. Blood should freely fill the tube or syringe.

12. When the needle punctures the vacuum, blood will flow into the tube. Have spare tubes available in case the vacuum in the first tube has broken. With the syringe technique, too great a suction causes hemolysis and tends to collapse the vein, causing blood flow to cease.

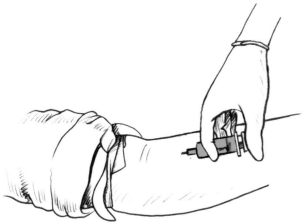

Once the needle is in the vein, push the tube firmly into the holder.

A. Steady the needle holder or syringe barrel so that the needle does not come out of the vein.

B. Allow the tube to fill or aspirate the amount of blood needed into the syringe.

A. Moving the needle out of the vein will interrupt the blood flow and result in a "short draw."

B. The vacuum contained in the tube predetermines the amount of blood drawn. Blood flow into the Vacutainer will cease automatically once the tube is filled. Removal of the Vacutainer tube before complete filling results in air rushing inside the tube, causing hemolysis. Tests involving the use of an anticoagulant are based on a ratio of blood volume to anticoagulant. If an inadequate volume is drawn, this ratio will be affected and yield inaccurate results.

C. If the blood flow is rapid, release the tourniquet and have the patient relax the fist.

C. Too rapid a blood flow could cause hemolysis. Releasing the tourniquet and relaxing the fist decreases the vein distension, thus slowing the flow.

PROCEDURE

13. To take more than one sample, remove the tube as soon as the blood flow stops and insert the next tube in the holder. Adhere to the proper tube order for blood collection. Do not change the position of the needle in the vein.

14. Mix any tubes with additives by inverting gently.

15. Have the patient relax the fist and release the tourniquet by pulling one end.

16. Place sterile gauze over the site and quickly withdraw the needle from the arm. Ask the patient to hold the gauze in place until the bleeding stops or for 3 to 5 minutes. Pay special attention to patients with prolonged bleeding.

Post-Venipuncture Procedures

17. Grasp the Vacutainer holder and press firmly on the bottom of the tube to extract a drop of blood 1 to 2 mm in diameter onto a slide or coverslip.
18. Label tubes with the patient's name, time specimen collected, date, and initials of the collector.
19. Immediately dispose of the needle into a biohazard sharps container.
20. Dispose of gauze and any other blood-soaked equipment in a biohazard container.
21. Remove gloves and dispose of in a biohazard container. Wash hands.
22. Check the patient's arm and apply an adhesive bandage. If the patient continues to bleed apply a pressure dressing with gauze and tape. Tell the patient to leave the bandage on for 15 to 30 minutes.
23. Thank the patient. Have the patient wait 5 minutes before leaving the office. Release the patient only after all signs of bleeding have stopped.
24. Properly process the test tubes for testing or transportation to the reference laboratory.

Problems During Venipuncture

1. If blood does not flow, palpate the vein with the forefinger of the free hand. A slight needle adjustment to the side or in depth should create an adequate blood flow.

PRINCIPLE

13. The shut-off valve in the hub of the needle covers the point and keeps the blood from flowing until the next tube is inserted. The order of the tubes for drawing blood is:
    a. Sterile tubes for culture
    b. Nonadditive tubes
    c. Tubes for coagulation studies
    d. Tubes with additives.
14. Tubes with additives should be mixed immediately. Failure to mix the blood will cause the blood to clot, and the specimen will be inadequate for testing. Hemolysis will occur if the blood is shaken.
15. To decrease physical pressure on the blood flow. The tourniquet must be loosened from the arm before the needle is removed. If the needle is removed first, blood will gush from the puncture site or cause a severe hematoma. The tourniquet should be released as soon as blood flow is established in the last tube to be drawn.
16. Pressure reduces pain and allows time for the blood to clot in order to prevent a hematoma. Keep the arm straight. Bending the elbow may cause a hematoma. Never press on the needle in the arm with the gauze pad while withdrawing the needle.

17. Preparing blood slides has the advantage that the blood does not mix with anticoagulants, which distorts the cells.
18. Never label the tubes before withdrawing the blood.

19. To reduce the chance of accidental puncture or blood spill, splash, or splatter.
20. To reduce the chance of blood contamination.

21. Used gloves are considered hazardous waste.

22. To observe for abnormal coloration or excessive bleeding and to protect the site.

23. This shows appreciation for the patient's cooperation and assures that the patient is stable and no adverse reactions, such as fainting, will result.
24. Maintaining specimens under proper storage conditions assures accurate laboratory test values.

1. Failure of blood to enter the tube necessitates reevaluation of the vein. Adjusting the needle should be performed with extreme care and only for a short duration since it causes patient discomfort.

PROCEDURE

2. If unable to get into a vein, remove the tourniquet, release the tube from the needle, then remove needle and notify the physician.

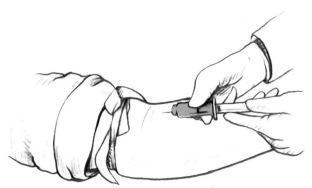

If it is necessary to withdraw the needle from the arm, first remove the Vacutainer tube from the holder.

3. If the venipuncture area begins to swell during blood collection, immediately release the tourniquet, remove the needle, and apply pressure with the gauze.

PRINCIPLE

2. The patient should not be "stuck" more than two times. To minimize patient discomfort, remove tube from holder before removing the needle from the arm.

3. Swelling indicates extravasation of blood in the tissues, which could cause hemolysis and invalid test results, as well as hematoma and injury to the patient.

PROCEDURE: Perform a capillary puncture on a finger or heel

OSHA STANDARDS:

Terminal Performance Objective: Obtain a small volume of capillary blood for diagnostic testing and prepare the specimen(s) for transport within a reasonable time.

EQUIPMENT: Nonsterile gloves
Sterile lancet (tip up to 5 mm [approx. $\frac{1}{4}''$] for adults and
    older children; 2.4 mm ($\frac{1}{8}''$) or less for newborns and
    infants)
70% alcohol preparation pads
Dry gauze pads
Warming towels or basin of warm water
Capillary tubes or microcontainers
Glass slide or coverslips
Biohazard sharps container
Disposable biohazard container

PROCEDURE

Equipment Preparation

1. Prepare the equipment, including extra supplies.

2. Prepare the area by checking the orderliness and cleanliness of the room and appropriate lighting. Don gloves.
3. Identify the patient and explain the procedure.

4. Recheck the request form.

5. Reassure the patient.

6. Comfortably and safely seat the patient.
7. Assemble the equipment quickly.

8. Recheck the request form.

Puncture Technique

9. Select the puncture site. Observe both hands.

10. Warm the puncture site by covering the hand with a warm towel.
11. Cleanse the site with alcohol in a circular motion working from the inside outward and allow to air dry.
12. Grasp the finger with your thumb distal to and well away from the puncture site.
13A. FINGER: Penetrate the pulp of the finger in one continuous motion at a 10° to 20° angle to the longitudinal axis of the phalangeal bone. Penetrate to the depth of the lancet point length.

PRINCIPLE

1. Equipment readily at hand allows for a quick, efficient, and skillfully performed capillary puncture.
2. To reduce the chance of transmitting microorganisms and to provide adequate light.

3. The patient needs to understand the procedure to be performed.
4. As a second check to verify the procedure ordered and the patient's identity and to ensure that all the equipment has been gathered for the capillary puncture.
5. Patients are very nervous and anxious about a finger puncture. They should be reassured that it may be painful but will not take long.
6. Patients should never stand when blood is drawn.
7. Many patients become apprehensive about a capillary puncture.
8. As verification of the procedure ordered.

9. Avoid areas that have callouses, burns, bruises, scars, edematous or cyanotic areas, or blood concentration.
   Select the lateral side of the middle or fourth finger.
10. To increase the blood flow.

11. Alcohol mixed with blood from the needle tip will hemolyze the blood.

12. To keep the finger immobile.

13A. The lancet or Autolet (Ames Co, Elkhart, IN) has a calibrated system so that an excessively deep puncture cannot be made. The pain of a deep puncture is no more than that of a superficial puncture, and a deep puncture establishes better flow of blood.

PROCEDURE

13B. HEEL: Place the forefinger around the ankle, and the thumb over the arch of the foot. Use lancets with a maximum tip length of 2.4 mm ($\frac{1}{8}''$). Puncture in one motion perpendicular to the site on the most medial or most lateral portion of the plantar surface (bottom of the foot). Do not stick an infant's heel more than twice. Immediately place the lancet in a nearby sharps container or on a dry gauze pad, safely out of reach of the patient.

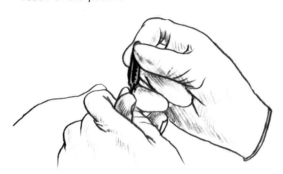

14. After removing the lancet, wipe away the first drop of blood with a sterile gauze.

15. Fill the capillary tube(s) with the free-flowing blood. Gentle pressure may be applied to form a round drop.

16. Collect the specimens by holding a capillary tube to the blood drop or by touching the drop to a glass slide. Adhere to the proper order of collection.

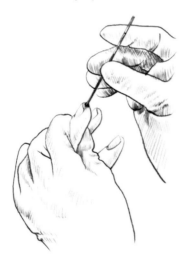

17. Collect the blood rapidly.

18. Place sterile gauze on the puncture site. Ask the patient to hold the gauze in place with gentle pressure until the bleeding stops or for 3 to 5 minutes. Pay special attention to patients whose blood continues to flow after 5 minutes.

19. Label specimen with the patient's name, time specimen collected, date, and initials of the collector, and that the collection was by capillary puncture.

PRINCIPLE

13B. To keep the infant or child immobile. Do not perform skin punctures on the posterior (back) curvature of the heel. The depth of puncture must not exceed 2.4 mm ($\frac{1}{8}''$) in infants, as bone damage and infection is a danger at greater depths.

14. Because the first drop of blood may contain antiseptic and tissue fluid, it is an inadequate blood specimen.

15. Squeezing or vigorously massaging will increase tissue fluid, yielding false laboratory test results.

16. The order for tube filling is:
   a. Hematology specimens
   b. Chemistry specimens
   c. Blood bank specimens

17. Rapid collection is necessary to prevent coagulation, especially when multiple samples are being drawn from the same site.

18. Pressure reduces pain and allows time for the blood to clot in order to prevent a hematoma.

19. Never label blood specimens before withdrawing the blood.

PROCEDURE

20. Immediately dispose of the lancet into a biohazard sharps container (if not done in 13.) by grasping the gauze pad away from the lancet tip and placing the lancet-gauze unit into the container.
21. Dispose of gauze and any other blood-soaked equipment in a biohazard container.
22. Seal one end of each tube and place all the tubes used in a single large test tube for transport to the reference laboratory.
23. Remove gloves and dispose of in a biohazard container. Wash hands.
24. Check the patient's finger.

25. Thank the patient and have the patient wait 5 minutes before leaving the office. Release the patient only after all signs of bleeding have stopped.

PRINCIPLE

20. To reduce the chance of accidental puncture or blood spill, splash, or splatter.

21. To reduce the chance of blood contamination.

22. To avoid loss of any of the tubes or errors in identification.

23. Used gloves are considered hazardous waste.

24. To observe for abnormal coloration or excessive bleeding.
25. This shows appreciation for the patient's cooperation and ensures that the patient is stable and that no adverse reactions, such as fainting, will result.

PROCEDURE: Focus and care for the microscope

OSHA STANDARDS:

Terminal Performance Objective: Focus the microscope on specimens prepared for low-power, high-power, and oil immersion examination, and care for the microscope, to keep it in good condition, within a reasonable time.

EQUIPMENT: Binocular compound microscope
Nonsterile gloves
Prepared microscope slides
Cover glass
Lens paper
Immersion oil
Xylene or other commercial lens cleaner
Towel for work surface
Disposable biohazard container
Biohazard sharps container

PROCEDURE

1. Prepare the equipment.
2. Prepare the area by checking the room for orderliness, cleanliness, and appropriate lighting. Don gloves.

Focusing the Microscope

3. Place the specimen slide on the stage and secure it with the stage clip.
4. Adjust the eyepieces.

5. Turn on the light switch and adjust the light to a comfortable level.

6. Rotate the nosepiece until the low-power dry objective (10X) is directly over the slide.

7. While looking through the eyepiece, close the diaphragm until the light just begins to be reduced.

8. Use the coarse adjustment and move the stage and objective close together. Watch from the side to make sure the objective does not touch the specimen.
9. Look through the eyepiece and, using the fine adjustment, focus a microscopic field on the slide.

10. Further adjust light intensity with the brightness control.
11. Adjust the iris diaphragm by opening it completely, then closing it until the light intensity just begins to be reduced.

PRINCIPLE

1. To reduce the chance of transmitting microorganisms.
2. To reduce the chance of transmitting microorganisms and to provide adequate light.

3. The mechanical stage is the shelf on which the object being observed is placed.
4. The interpupillary distance knob is used to adjust the distance of the eyepieces to the proper width of the individual's eyes. The interpupillary distance is correct when the right and left fields merge into one.
5. The light is directed up through the condenser system and iris diaphragm. Light adjustment is made before focusing.
6. The nosepiece allows for the objective to be changed depending on the magnification needed. The low-power dry objective has the smallest magnification and is used to perform the initial focusing on a wide range.
7. At the start of the adjustment, the condenser should be 1 to 2 mm (less than $\frac{1}{8}$") below the slide and the condenser iris diaphragm all the way open. Light adjustment is helped by raising and lowering the condenser and opening and closing the diaphragm. Closing the diaphragm too much or lowering the condenser too far, although it can increase contrast and depth of focus, will reduce resolution.
8. The coarse adjustment is used to bring the objective down as far as it will go, so that it almost meets but does not touch the specimen.
9. When the object is nearly in focus with the coarse adjustment, it is brought into clear focus with the fine adjustment knob.
10. The background light should be sufficiently white and comfortable to the eyes.
11. The iris diaphragm regulates the field size. As the size of a field is decreased, the resolution increases.

PROCEDURE	PRINCIPLE
12. Rotate the nosepiece to the high-power dry objective (40×).	12. Most microscopes are parfocal, which means the microscope can be first adjusted under low power, then switched to high power without a loss of focus. The nosepiece should be grasped not the objective to prevent damage to the objective.
13. Focus with the fine adjustment.	13. Fine adjustment is used continuously during microscopic examination.
14. Raise the condenser to alter the light refraction and open the diaphragm.	14. When greater magnification is needed, more light is necessary.
15. Rotate the nosepiece until the slide is free of all objectives.	15. To prevent the objectives from being damaged. The oil immersion lens is used to examine blood smears and microorganisms. Because of the short working distance between the slide and objective, wet preparations with coverslips cannot be fitted under the oil immersion objective.
16. Place one drop of oil on the slide area to be examined.	16. Immersion oil provides additional light and directs the light rays to a finer point.
17. Move the oil immersion objective (100×) directly into the drop of oil, while observing from the side. Raise the condenser to its maximum position. Open the iris diaphragm.	17. Side observation prevents damage to the slide or objective should the distance be too little. Partial closing of the iris diaphragm may be necessary.
18. Move the objective side to side.	18. To eliminate any air bubbles.
19. Focus using the fine adjustment.	19. Fine adjustment is used continuously throughout the microscopic examination.
20. Observe the slide.	20. Low-power examination is used for examination of urinary casts; dry high-power examination with coverglass is used for examination of urine sediment, red blood counts and wet preparations; oil immersion examination is used for white blood counts, differential counts, and dry microbe smears.

Clean-Up

21. Rotate the nosepiece until the slide is free from all objectives and turn off the light switch. Release the slide from the spring clip.	21. To ready the microscope for storage.
22. If the slide is not to be kept, discard the slide in a biohazard sharps container.	22. Unless the slide was heat-fixed using a heat block, treat it as potentially infectious. Glass should be placed in a sharps container.
23. Clean the eyepieces and objectives by first blowing away dust and debris with an air syringe or air compressor, then wiping with lens paper.	23. Optical glass is softer than ordinary glass and should never be cleaned with paper tissue or gauze. The oil immersion lens must be wiped completely dry to prevent the oil from seeping inside the lens. If the lens is extremely dirty, xylene or a commercial lens cleaner can be applied to the lens paper. Only a small amount of xylene should be used, as xylene can damage the lens mounting seals. Clean in a circular motion from inside to outside. Do not use plastic with any cleaning agents, as it will be dissovled by the cleaning agent and ruin the lens.
24. Clean the metal parts of the microscope.	24. Neutral soap and water and a soft cloth should be rubbed in a circular motion to remove any dust or debris.
25. Rotate the nosepiece until the low-power dry objective is in place and as close to the stage as possible.	25. This is the proper storage position for the microscope.
26. Unplug the electrical cord and wrap it carefully around the base of the microscope.	26. The cord should not be allowed to dangle. A loose cord could cause the microscope to be pull from the shelf.
27. Cover the microscope with protective covering.	27. Covering protects the microscope from dirt, dust, and lint.
28. Carry the microscope to the storage area with two hands.	28. It should be carried by the arm in one hand and supported under the base with the other hand.
29. Remove gloves and dispose of them in a biohazard container.	29. Used gloves are considered hazardous waste.

HIGHLIGHTS

Personal Protective Equipment Cuts Risk*

Wearing gloves, gowns, masks, and eye protection can significantly reduce health risks for workers exposed to blood and other potentially infectious materials. The new Occupational Safety and Health Administration (OSHA) standard covering bloodborne disease requires employers to provide appropriate personal protective equipment (PPE) and clothing free of charge to employees.

Workers who have direct exposure to blood and other potentially infectious materials on their jobs run the risk of contracting bloodborne infections from hepatitis B virus (HBV), human immunodeficiency virus (HIV), which causes acquired immunodeficiency syndrome (AIDS), and other pathogens. About 8700 health care workers each year are infected with HBV, and 200 die from the infection. Although the risk of contracting AIDS through occupational exposure is much lower, wearing proper PPE can greatly reduce potential exposure to all bloodborne infections.

SELECTING PPE

Personal protective clothing and equipment must be suitable. This means the level of protection must fit the expected exposure. For example, gloves would be sufficient for a laboratory technician who is drawing blood, whereas a pathologist conducting an autopsy would need considerably more protective clothing.

Personal protective equipment may include gloves, gowns, laboratory coats, face shields or masks, eye protection, pocket masks, and other protective gear. The gear must be readily accessible to employees and available in appropriate sizes.

If an employee is expected to have hand contact with blood or other potentially infectious materials or contaminated surfaces, he or she must wear gloves. Single-use gloves cannot be washed or decontaminated for reuse. Utility gloves may be decontaminated if they are not compromised. They should be replaced when they show signs of cracking, peeling, tearing, puncturing, or deteriorating. If employees are allergic to standard gloves, the employer must provide hypoallergenic gloves or similar alternatives.

Routine gloving is not required for phlebotomy in voluntary blood donation centers, although it is necessary for all other phlebotomies. In any case, gloves must be available in voluntary blood donation centers for employees who want to use them. Workers in voluntary blood donation centers must use gloves (1) when they have cuts, scratches, or other breaks in their skin; (2) while they are in training; and (3) when they believe contamination might occur.

---

*Source: US Department of Labor, Occupational Safety and Health Administration.

Employees should wear eye and mouth protection such as goggles and masks, glasses with solid side shields, and masks or chin-length face shields when splashes, sprays, splatters, or droplets of potentially infectious materials pose a hazard through the eyes, nose, or mouth. More extensive coverings such as gowns, aprons, surgical caps and hoods, and shoe covers or boots are needed when gross contamination is expected. This often occurs, for example, during orthopedic surgery or autopsies.

AVOIDING CONTAMINATION

The key is that blood or other infectious materials must not reach an employee's work clothes, street clothes, undergarments, skin, eyes, mouth, or other mucous membranes under normal conditions for the duration of exposure.

Employers must provide the PPE and ensure that their workers wear it. This means that if a laboratory coat is considered PPE, it must be supplied by the employer rather than the employee. The employer also must clean or launder clothing and equipment and repair or replace it as necessary.

Additional protective measures such as using PPE in animal rooms and decontaminating PPE before laundering are essential in facilities that conduct research on HIV or HBV.

EXCEPTION

There is one exception to the requirement for protective gear. An employee may choose, temporarily and briefly, under rare and extraordinary circumstances, to forego the equipment. It must be the employee's professional judgment that using the protective equipment would prevent the delivery of health care or public safety services or would pose an increased hazard to the safety of the worker or coworkers. When one of these excepted situations occurs, employers are to investigate and document the circumstances to determine if there are ways to avoid it in the future. For example, if a firefighters's resuscitation device is damaged, perhaps another type of device should be used or the device should be carried in a different manner. Exceptions must be limited—this is not a blanket exemption.

DECONTAMINATING AND DISPOSING OF PPE

Employees must remove personal protective clothing and equipment before leaving the work area or when the PPE becomes contaminated. If a garment is penetrated, workers must remove it immediately or as soon as feasible. Used protective clothing and equipment must be placed in designated containers for storage, decontamination, or disposal.

Continued

OTHER PROTECTIVE PRACTICES

If an employee's skin or mucous membranes come into contact with blood, he or she is to wash with soap and water and flush eyes with water as soon as feasible. In addition, workers must wash their hands immediately or as soon as feasible after removing protective equipment. If soap and water are not immediately available, employers may provide other handwashing measures such as moist towellettes. Employees still must wash with soap and water as soon as possible.

Employees must refrain from eating, drinking, smoking, applying cosmetics or lip balm, and handling contact lenses in areas where they may be exposed to blood or other potentially infectious materials.

> Results of medical technology procedures are a valuable tool used in the process of determining a diagnosis or course of treatment.
>
> Margaret Watkins

CHAPTER OUTLINE

LEARNING OBJECTIVES

Upon completing this chapter, you will be able to:

1. List the physical properties of urine.
2. List the considerations in collecting and preserving urine specimens.
3. List the normal appearance or values for the physical tests of urine as they appear on a urinalysis reporting form.
4. Identify the chemical tests of urine as they appear on a 10-test reagent strip.
5. Describe at least four types of confirmatory tests and methods for urinalysis quality control.
6. List the reference values for the constituents of normal urine sediment as they appear on a urinalysis reporting form.
7. Identify the types of abnormal cells, casts, crystals, and artifacts that may appear in urine sediment.
8. Give an example of at least one organism and the disease it causes for each of the five types of bacteria.
9. Outline the procedure for collecting and transporting specimens in transport media.
10. List the precautions necessary in collecting bacterial specimens for testing.

Chapter 29

The Physician's Office Laboratory: Part II

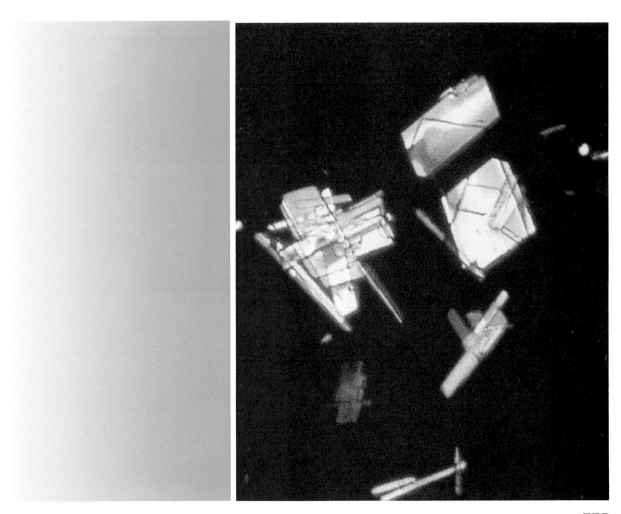

11. Describe the streak plate technique of inoculating media.
12. Describe the principle on which rapid manual non-growth-dependent tests are based.
13. Describe the principles on which stains to differentiate cellular and bacterial morphology are based.

PERFORMANCE OBJECTIVES

Upon completing this chapter, you will be able to:

1. Examine and report the physical properties of urine.
2. Test and report the chemical results in a routine urinalysis.
3. Examine and report the findings in a microscopic examination of urinary sediment.
4. Obtain a throat specimen for transport or for isolation and identification of bacteria by culturing or rapid screening technique.
5. Prepare and stain a bacterial smear for microscopic classification based on the Gram stain reaction.

Glossary

Acid-base balance: maintaining a constant balance between acids and alkaline substances; maintaining a constant pH

Albumin: water-soluble serum or plasma protein responsible for much of the blood's osmotic pressure and for transporting fatty acids, bilirubin, many drugs, and hormones; albumin in the urine indicates malfunction of the kidney

Amorphous: having no shape or definite form

Antibody: protein substance found in the body as the result of antigen stimulation that is specific for the antigen against which it is formed

Antigen: foreign substance that when introduced into the body of a person lacking the antigen results in an immune response and formation of a corresponding antibody

Brownian movement: peculiar random movement of microscopic particles, both organic and inorganic, when suspended in liquid

Dehydration: removal of water from the body when fluid intake is insufficient or the output is excessive

Direct test: examination that specifically detects or directly effects the source being tested

Ehrlich unit: unit for measuring the presence of urobilinogen in the presence of specific chemical; named after Paul Ehrlich, the founder of hematology

Electrolytes: chemical substances which, when dissolved in water, become electrically charged particles (ions) capable of producing electric current; positively charged ions (cations) include sodium, potassium, calcium, and magnesium; negatively charged ions (anions) include chloride, bicarbonate, and phosphate; calcium electrolyte imbalance is often a cause of renal disease.

Flagellum (pl. Flagella): long, mobile, whiplike appendage on a cell used to produce locomotion

Hemolysis: rupture of red blood cells with release of hemoglobin

Homeostasis: ability of the body systems to remain stable while continually adjusting to conditions necessary for survival

Hypha (pl. Hyphae): filaments protruding from a mold

Incubate: to provide ideal conditions, such as temperature, humidity, and nutrients, for growth and development

Indirect test: to look for an associated condition or substance to give evidence through a causal relationship

Lyse: to cause the disintegration of a cell or substance

Macroscopic: visible to the naked eye

Meniscus: curved upper surface of a liquid in a container

Methylene blue: synthetic organic compound used as a stain in bacteriology or as an antibiotic

Normal flora: bacteria normally residing in a nonpathogenic existence on or in a particular area of the body; infection can sometimes result when resident bacteria are accidentally introduced into tissue through trauma, contamination, or inhalation

Occult: not observable to the naked eye, but requires a test to be detected

Postprandial: after a meal

Precipitation: visible result when the solid particles of a substance settle in a solution

Qualitative assay: determining the presence or purity of a substance

Quantitative assay: determining the amount of any particular substance in a mixture
Refractive: ability of light to deviate when passing obliquely from one medium to another of a different density
Supernatant: the clear upper portion of a mixture after it has been centrifuged
Turbid: cloudy

As a continuation of the chapters on the physician's office laboratory, this chapter discusses the first two basic specialty areas of laboratory medicine: urinalysis and bacteriology.

URINALYSIS

Urinalysis, or examination of the urine, provides information concerning the state of health and functioning of many body systems. Routine urinalysis is one of the most commonly performed laboratory tests in the physician's office. More than 100 tests are available to assist the physician in diagnosing diseases of the kidney, urinary tract, urinary bladder, and liver, as well as diseases of the endocrine system and metabolism. Because routine urinalysis involves very little specialized equipment, it is frequently used both in screening and as a diagnostic tool.

Urine is composed of 95% water and 5% waste products, including urea, ammonia, creatinine, uric acid, and electrolytes. Since the primary function of the kidneys is to eliminate excess water and to remove waste products from the blood in the form or urine, the constituents of urine can be used as a prime indicator of kidney function and diseases such as nephritis, renal failure, and kidney malfunction during pregnancy. Urinalysis is also used as a primary tool for diagnosis of lower urinary tract infections, such as cystitis, urethritis, and prostatitis, and bladder conditions. In addition, an abnormal urinalysis is often the first indicator of diabetes and drug overdose or toxicity.

The medical assistant should have a listing of normal urine values available for easy reference so the physician can be alerted immediately when any deviations from the normal ranges are found (Table 29–1). The procedures for physical, chemical, and microscopic examination are described in detail at the end of this chapter.

URINE COLLECTION

Four basic types of urine specimens are used in diagnostic tests: random, first morning, clean-catch, and 24-hour collection. Others include the second-voided specimen, the catheterization specimen, infant collection, and the postprandial collection.

1. *Random specimen.* A freshly voided specimen is collected in a nonsterile container any time during a 24-hour period. This type of specimen is most convenient and most common. It is best for chemical screens and microscopic examinations.

2. *First morning specimen.* A specimen is collected during the first voiding after sleep. This is the preferred specimen type because it is most concentrated and the bladder contents have had a chance to incubate; however, the formed elements may have disintegrated if the urine pH is high, or the specific gravity, low. The specimen container is usually nonsterile. This type of specimen is best for chemical examination of nitrite and protein and for microscopic examination.

3. *Clean-catch specimen.* A specimen is collected midstream in a sterile container after using a special skin cleansing kit (Fig. 29–1). It is frequently used for bacterial studies, particularly urine cultures. (See procedure for obtaining a clean-catch urine specimen in Chapter 21.)

4. *24-hour specimen.* A 24-hour specimen is collected to measure the amount of urine output in a 24-hour period (quantitative assay) or to diagnose a relatively rare disease known as *pheochromocytoma.* Twenty-four hour urine output studies may be helpful in diagnosing renal disease, dehydration, and urinary tract obstructions. The normal adult volume of urine in a 24-hour period is 750 to 2000 mL. Collection of a 24-hour specimen is described in Table 29–2.

5. *Catheterized specimen.* Some patients consistently test positive for bacteria in the urine even after careful cleansing for a clean-catch specimen. A catheterized specimen, obtained under strict sterile conditions, can confirm whether the bacteria is residing in the urinary tract or is a vaginal or skin contaminant. Specimens should be labeled "catheterized." Because catheterization is a difficult procedure, it should be performed by the physician or those who have had specific training in the procedure. Disposable catheterization kits are usually purchased. The kits contain all the equipment needed to set up the sterile field, the catheter, and the collection container.

6. *Infant specimen.* Pediatric urine collection kits are available for collecting urine specimens from infants and small children. The kit contains a bag with an adhesive backing that is designed to fit over the genital area of either sex. The parent or care provider should be instructed to wash and dry the infant's skin, then apply the bag. The urine collected should be removed as soon

Table 29–1
NORMAL URINE VALUES IN ADULTS

Test	Normal Values
Albumin	
Qualitative	Negative
Quantitative	10–100 mg/24 h
Aldosterone	2–23 μg/24 h
Amino acid nitrogen	100–290 mg/24 h
Ammonia	700 mg/24 h
Bence Jones protein	Negative
Bilirubin	Negative
Blood, occult	Negative
Calcium	
Qualitative	Positive 1+ (Sulkowitch method)
Quantitative	30–150 mg/24 h
Chloride	110–250 mEq/24 h
Creatine	Less than 100 mg in 24 h, or less than 6% of creatinine. Pregnancy: up to 12% of creatinine. Children under 1 y: may equal creatinine. Children over 1 y: up to 30% of creatinine.
Creatinine	Females: 0.8–1.7 g/24 h Males: 1–1.9 g/24 h
Estrogens	Females: 4–60 μg/24 h Males: 4–25 μg/24 h
Glucose	
Qualitative	Negative
Quantitative	50–500 mg/24 h
Lead	0.021–0.038 mg/L
pH	4.8–7.8
Phenylpyruvic acid	Negative
Phosphorus	0.9–1.3 g/24 h
Porphobilinogen	Negative
Potassium	25–100 mEq/24 h
Sodium	About 110 mEq/24 h
Specific gravity	1.002–1.030 (single specimen) 1.015–1.025 (24-h specimen)
Uric acid	0.5–1.0 g/24 h
Urobilinogen	
Semiquantitative	Up to 1 Ehrlich unit/2 h
Quantitative	1.0–4.0 mg/24 h
Volume	Adults: 1000–1500 mL/24 h (about 15–21 mL/kg body weight) Children: 3 to 4 times as much as adults per kg body weight

as it is voided and transferred to a sterile specimen cup.

7. *Postprandial specimen.* The postprandial specimen is collected after a meal and is used for glucose testing in the diabetic patient. A 2-hour

postprandial volume collection is sometimes required for urobilinogen testing.

PHYSICAL EXAMINATION OF URINE

The first aspect of urinalysis is the visual examination of the physical characteristics of urine. The appearance, color, volume, and specific gravity of the specimen are observed.

Appearance

The appearance of normal, freshly voided urine is clear and transparent, but the presence of pus, blood, mucus, or bacteria causes turbidity, or cloudiness. Certain foods may cause turbidity, as does allowing the urine to remain at room temperature for an extended period. Refrigerating urine also increases turbidity; therefore, the appearance of the specimen should be recorded as soon as possible. The terms used to record appearance (transparency) are "clear," "slightly cloudy," or "turbid."

Color

The color variations of urine range from very pale yellow (straw) to amber yellow to deep orange, depending on food and fluid intake, medications taken, or the amount of waste products contained in the urine (Table 29–3). Normal urine color is due to the presence of a yellow pigment called *urochrome* and is most often a pale, straw-yellow in color. A very pale color may indicate a dilute urine, whereas a dark color may indicate a concentrated urine. A red color may be due to blood; a greenish shade may indicate *Pseudomonas* organisms; and dark yellow urine is associated with the presence of bile. Food can alter urine color. Beets can turn urine red and asparagus can tinge the urine green. Medicines can also affect the urine color. Iron preparations can turn the urine dark brown or black, vitamin B can turn the urine bright yellow, and methylene blue can turn the urine blue-green. Table 29–3 includes some of the commonly used drugs that can affect urine color.

The color of the specimen should be recorded as light or dark yellow, light or dark red, or orange (or any other abnormal color just described).

Odor

Normal, freshly voided urine has a characteristic odor that is distinct yet not unpleasant. Urine that has been standing for some time develops an ammonia-like odor, which is due to the decomposition of urea by the bacteria in the specimen. Urine in patients with diabetes mellitus may have a fruity odor due to the presence of ketones. Urine in patients with urinary tract infections usually has a foul-smelling odor. In addition to abnormal conditions, urine odors may be altered by food, such as garlic or asparagus.

With a few exceptions, the odor of urine is not considered to be of special clinical significance. The exception to this is the strange, "mousey" odor in an infant's diaper which is an indication of phenylketonuria, a congenital metabolic disease. (Because of the danger of

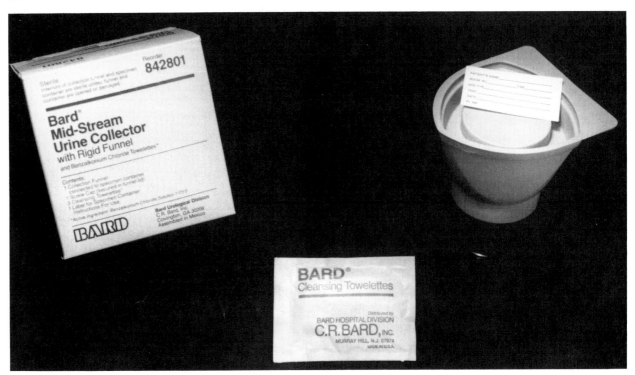

Figure 29–1. A midstream clean-catch urine specimen kit. (From Wedding MD and Toenjes SA: *Medical Laboratory Procedures.* FA Davis, Philadelphia, 1992, p. 69, with permission.)

aerosol contamination, "smelling" a patient's urine is no longer accepted as safe practice.)

Specific Gravity

The kidneys regulate the volume of urine that is produced and the concentration of the substances in urine to maintain balance, or homeostasis, of fluids and electrolytes. Since urine specific gravity indicates the total solute concentration (dissolved solids) of the urine, it measures the kidney's ability to concentrate

urine. An abnormal measurement is one of the first indications of kidney disease.

The specific gravity of water distilled at 68°F (20°C) 1.000. The normal range of specific gravity for urine is between 1.003 and 1.030, depending on the fluid intake of the individual, but is usually between 1.010 and 1.025. Specific gravity is highest in the first morning specimen, in which it is usually greater than 1.020. Specific gravity may be increased in dehydration, adrenal insufficiency, hepatic disease, congestive heart fail-

Table 29–2

PATIENT TEACHING FOR COLLECTION OF A 24-HOUR URINE SPECIMEN

1. Instruct the patient to obtain the collection container from the reference or hospital laboratory that will be doing the test.
2. Have the patient void and *discard* the first urine specimen and note the time. This initial voiding begins the 24-h collection period.
3. The patient collects all urine samples during the next 24 h in a nonsterile container.
4. Instruct the patient to purposely void to close out the collection period exactly 24 h after the test was initiated. *Include* this last specimen as part of the 24-h collection.
5. It is important to further instruct the patient to transport the collected specimen to the laboratory without delay. Most 24-h specimens require a preservative, and some require refrigeration during the collection period. All special collection requirements will be designated by the reference laboratory. Initial specimen time may need to be adjusted in order to facilitate transportation. In other words, the patient should not begin and end the testing period at bedtime or any other time the laboratory is not open for receiving the specimen.
   Example: The patient voids at 6:30 AM and discards the urine. The patient collects urine for the next 24 h, and includes the voiding at 6 AM the following day. The urine specimen is refrigerated until 8 AM, when the patient takes the specimen to the laboratory.

Table 29–3

ABNORMALITIES IN URINE CHARACTERISTICS ASSOCIATED WITH PATHOLOGY

Color

	Possible Source	Possible Pathologic Cause
Yellow-brown	Bilirubin	Excessive destruction of red blood cells Obstruction of the bile duct Diminished function of liver cells
Orange-yellow	Urobilin, bilirubin	Excessive destruction of red blood cells Diminished function of liver cells
Dark red	Porphyrin products	Disturbance in porphyrin metabolism, which produces precursors necessary for heme synthesis
	Red blood cells	Hemorrhage in urinary structures Menstrual contamination
	Hemoglobin	Lysed erythrocytes Excess free hemoglobin in plasma
Red-brown	Myoglobin Red blood cells Hemoglobin	Excessive destruction of skeletal or cardiac muscle See above See above
Clear red	Hemoglobin Porphyrin	See above See above
Cloudy red	Red blood cells	See above
Green	Biliverdin	Oxidation of bilirubin

Odor

Ammonia	Splitting of urea molecule by bacteria	Urinary tract infection; "stale" urine
Sweet/fruity	Acetone and acetoacetic acid (ketone)	Fat metabolism due to starvation, diabetes mellitus, etc.
Putrid/foul	Decomposition of leukocytes; bacterial growth	Leukocytes associated with urinary tract infection
"Mousey"	Phenylketonuria	Congenital metabolic disease

Source: Adapted from Wedding ME and Toenjes SA: Medical Laboratory Procedures. FA Davis, Philadelphia, 1992, p 81.

ure, or the presence of glucose and protein in the urine. A decrease is usually associated with overhydration, diabetes insipidus, or chronic renal diseases where the kidney has lost its ability to concentrate the urine.

There are four types of equipment that can be used to measure specific gravity: (1) the urinometer (a glass cylinder with a floating device called a *hydrometer*), (2) the refractometer, (3) the colorimetric method using a reagent stick, and (4) the falling drop method.

A *urinometer* is a bulb filled with mercury attached to a stem on which is engraved a scale graduated from 1.000 to 1.040. The tester puts the urinometer in a cylindrical container that is three-fourths filled with a well-mixed urine sample, giving the stem a gentle spin to ensure that the urinometer is floating freely (Fig. 29–2). The specific gravity of the urine determines how deeply the float sinks into the sample. The tester reads the specific gravity by noting the point on the scale at which the top surface of the sample touches the stem. For an accurate reading, the tester must keep his or her eye level with the bottom of the sample's *meniscus.* The meniscus is the slight curve in a column of liquid caused by the tendency of the liquid to adhere to the sides of a container (Fig. 29–3).

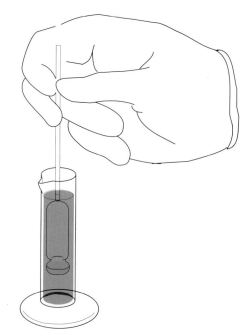

Figure 29–2. Give the urinometer a gentle spin to ensure that it is free floating.

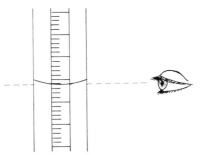

Figure 29–3. Read the scale at the lowest point of the meniscus, with the eye level with the meniscus. (From Wedding MD and Toenjes SA: *Medical Laboratory Procedures.* FA Davis, Philadelphia, 1992, p. 82, with permission.)

Check the urinometer daily for accuracy by reading it in a sample of distilled water at room temperature. The specific gravity of the sample is 1.000; if the reading is more or less than 1.000, replace the urinometer.

Certain precautions must be taken in reading specific gravity. Surface bubbles should be avoided, and the hydrometer should not be allowed to touch the sides or bottom of the cylinder, as this will result in an inaccurate reading. If the quantity of urine is not sufficient to fill the urinometer three-fourths full (approximately 20 to 25 mL of urine), the test should not be attempted but is reported as "QNS" (quantity not sufficient).

The hydrometer and cylinder should be cleaned at the end of the day by presoaking them in 5% bleach, then washing with a laboratory detergent and rinsing with water. Never allow dirty glassware to dry out. Between specimens, rinse the equipment with water and dry the stem. Urine samples can be flushed down the sink with copious amount of running water.

A *refractometer* is an optical instrument that measures specific gravity with a single drop of well-mixed urine. Light is refracted (refractive index) in proportion to the dissolved solids present. The result is determined by reading the scale through the eyepiece (Fig. 29–4). The refractometer has two advantages over the urinometer: It requires only one drop of urine for specific gravity readings, and in most cases, it compensates for temperature variations. The refractometer must be calibrated daily with distilled water and two standard solutions with a known specific gravity. The water tests its ability to measure a normal value; the standards, its ability to accurately measure abnormal values.

The *colorimetric reagent strip* method of measuring specific gravity, by the Ames Specific Gravity Reagent Strip method (Ames Co. Elkhart, IN), uses color reactions on commercially prepared reagent paper. It is the newest method of estimating specific gravity. The chemical reactions between the urine and the reagents impregnated on the strip pad result in color changes that are interpreted at timed intervals according to the manufacturer's instructions.

The *falling drop* method is a procedure performed with the Ames Clinitek Auto 2000 analyzer (Ames Co.),

and is more accurate than refractometry and hydrometers. The equipment is designed to measure the time required for a precisely measured specimen drop to fall a defined distance. A drop of urine is dispensed into a column of oil by a pipette, and the falling time is measured electronically and computed in specific gravity units. The system comes equipped with a waste disposal system that allows the urine to drain into a liquid waste container without losing any of the oily fluid through which the urine falls.

CHEMICAL EXAMINATION USING REAGENT STRIPS

Urine reagent strips (dipsticks) are used for detecting the presence of, and sometimes the amount of, specific substances contained in the urine. Some dipsticks test for single substances, whereas many are designed to test for groups of substances. The Ames Co for example, markets the Multistix-10 SG (10 tests plus specific gravity) reagent strip that tests for glucose, blood, pH, protein, ketone bodies, urobilinogen, bilirubin, leukocytes, nitrite, and specific gravity. Two other examples are the Urostix strip (tests for glucose and protein) and the Multistix 2 strip (tests for leukocytes and nitrite). Comparable reagent strips (except for measuring specific gravity) are available from Boehringer Mannheim Diagnostics Co (Biodynamics/BMC, Indianapolis, IN) as Chemstrip 9, Chemstrip GP, and Chemstrip LN strips, respectively. Which brand or type of reagent strip is best suited to the practice is determined by the

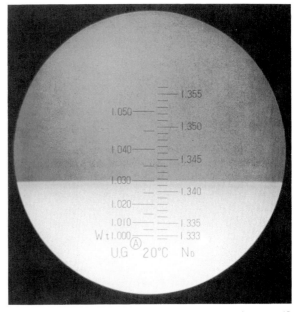

Figure 29–4. The refractometer measures the specific gravity of urine by the way light waves are bent (refracted) as they pass through a single drop of well-mixed urine sample. The tester holds the rectrometer toward a light source and looks into the eyepiece. The line between light and dark indicates the specific gravity. In this example, the reading is 1.030.

types of equipment and urine screening most often performed.

CONFIRMATORY TESTS

Confirmatory testing is used to substantiate that a test result is correct. It is used in chemical testing of urine when there is doubt about either a positive or negative result on a dipstick. When dipstick results are positive, confirmatory testing may further quantify or qualitatively differentiate the first result. Sometimes, a positive or negative result seems illogical in view of other test results or the patient's symptoms. Confirmatory testing in these cases can check an expected positive or negative result that was *not* obtained. Confirmatory testing is performed by:

1. Repeating the same test on the same specimen
2. Repeating the same test on a new specimen
3. Using a different test on the same specimen
4. Testing another component of urine or another system (e.g., blood), or collecting more information from the patient

The following sections list the substances that may be measured using the Ames Multistix 10 SG Reagent Strip for urinalysis and includes the confirmatory tests for each substance, when applicable.

Leukocytes

The leukocyte esterase test detects the presence of a significant number of white blood cells in the urine and is an indication of *bacteriuria* or a urinary tract infection. Reagent strips work by detecting the presence of leukocyte esterase, which is released from white blood cells in the urine and indicates an infection. Whereas the nitrite test (see next section) is a direct test for infection, leukocyte detection is an indirect test. When bacteria are present, white blood cells assist the body in fighting the infection and then break down into pus (*pyuria*), which is detected as a by-product of the inflammatory process.

A specimen preservative should never be used, as it will slightly inhibit the leukocyte esterase reaction. Values are recorded as negative, trace, 1+ (small amount), 2+ (moderate amount), or 3+ (large amount). The intensity of the color is proportionate to the number of white blood cells in the urine and, therefore, the intensity of the infection. In infection, a positive result on the nitrite test and a high pH correlates with a positive result on the leukocyte strip test. Positive results are confirmed by microscopic examination for white blood cells and bacteria and bacterial culture. When the result of the leukocyte strip test is positive, the medical assistant should carefully look for bacteria on microscopic examination. In many cases where there are two positive strip test results for infection, the physician may forego the microscopic examination and confirm directly with a culture.

Nitrites

Certain nitrates are found in all urines as a result of protein metabolism. Bacteria, however, contain enzymes that reduce nitrates to nitrites; thus, a positive nitrite test result indicates bacteriuria. Common organisms that infect the urinary tract include *Escherichia coli* (usually from the intestines), *Klebsiella, Enterobacter, Proteus, Staphylococcus,* and *Pseudomonas.*

Some patients have a condition known as *asymptomatic bacteriuria.* Since this condition can cause severe kidney damage even though the patient experiences no symptoms, many physicians routinely screen high-risk patients. High-risk groups include pregnant women, school-age children (especially girls), diabetics, the elderly, and patients with a history of chronic urinary tract infections.

A clean-catch sample in a sterile container immediately closed with a sterile cap is preferred; however, a positive nitrite test on any random specimen always indicates bacteriuria. A specimen preservative should never be used, as it would produce false-negative culture results. The first morning specimen is the specimen of choice, but urine that has incubated in the bladder for at least 4 hours should be adequate.

Values are recorded as negative or positive. Any coloration of the pad is considered a positive result. The Multistix 10 SG is most often used, but other test strips with seven or more tests may be used. Microscopic examination and a urine culture are the confirmatory testing methods. Bacteriuria is considered significant if microscopic findings show the presence of moderate to high counts of bacteria on three separate urine specimens. Low counts on a single specimen are probably due to specimen contamination during collection.

Urobilinogen

Urobilinogen is a compound formed by the reduction of bilirubin. Small amounts may normally be present in the urine, but increased amounts are associated with liver disease or conditions where there is excessive destruction of red blood cells. These conditions include hemolytic anemia, cirrhosis, hepatitis, hepatic jaundice, and congestive heart failure.

Urinary urobilinogen may also be decreased or absent as a result of partial or complete obstruction of the bile ducts or during antibiotic therapy, when there is destruction of the normal intestinal flora needed to convert bilirubin to urobilinogen.

Values are recorded as normal (0.2 or 1 Ehrlich unit/dL urine) or positive (2, 4, or 8 Ehrlich units/dL urine). The Multistix 10 SG or other multiple testing strip is used. Testing must be performed on freshly voided urine. The preferred sample should be collected over a 2-hour period in the early afternoon when urinary urobilinogen is the highest for the day. The strip is read exactly 60 seconds after the strip is removed from the urine.

The test will not detect a decrease or absence of urobilinogen. A more thorough diagnosis can be obtained from comparing urine urobilinogen results to urine bilirubin results. Confirmatory tests include the serum urobilinogen test or a 24-hour urobilinogen test.

Protein

Trace quantities of protein may be found in most urines. The majority of normal proteins are globulins and albumin, but other proteins that may be present include hemoglobin, fibrinogen, and Bence Jones protein (present in some cancers). *Proteinuria* refers to an increased amount of protein in the urine and is one of the most important indicators of renal disease or lower urinary tract inflammation or degeneration. Benign proteinuria may be found in the urine of patients with fever or emotional stress, after heavy exercise or exposure to extreme heat or cold, during pregnancy, and in newborns.

Values are recorded as negative, trace, 1+, 2+, 3+, and 4+. Albustix and most multiple reagent strips can be used. Highly alkaline urines may give false-positives results. Microscopic examination of a positive strip test is important to confirm the type of renal disorder. Other confirmatory tests include the precipitation test using the sulfosalicylic acid method or the acetic acid test (Table 29–4).

pH

While the lungs regulate metabolism by the excretion of carbon dioxide, the kidneys regulate the excretion of nonvolatile acids produced as by-products of metabolism. These two processes regulate the body's acid-base balance. The acidity of urine is due mainly to salts, primarily sodium, potassium, calcium, and ammonium salts. Urine usually becomes increasingly more acid as the amount of sodium retained by the body increases.

pH values are recorded using the Multistix 10 SG as ranging from 5.0 to 8.5. For exact determinations and confirmation, a pH meter is used.

The normal freshly voided urine is acid with a pH of about 6.0, with the normal range varying from 4.5 to slightly higher than 8.0. A pH below 7.0 indicates an acid urine, and above 7.0, an alkaline urine. An acid urine is expected in patients on high protein diets and certain medications and in patients with acidosis or uncontrolled diabetes mellitus. An alkaline urine is expected in patients on diets high in vegetables and dairy products or on certain medications and in patients with renal disease and urinary tract infections.

pH determination must be done on fresh urine as urine becomes alkaline on standing. If urine must be stored before pH testing, it must be stored in the refrigerator. Knowledge of the urine pH is necessary for interpreting other strip test results and for proper microscopic reporting of crystals found in urine (see Crystals, p. 767).

Blood

Hematuria is the presence of red blood cells in the urine. *Hemoglobinuria* is the presence of free hemoglobin in the urine, which is usually caused by the rupture of red blood cells as they pass through the kidneys and urinary tract. Because the strip tests are now so sensitive to occult blood (hemolyzed blood), differentiating small amounts of hemoglobin from red blood cells is no longer clinically significant. Most urines containing red blood cells also contain hemolyzed occult blood.

Blood in the urine usually indicates bleeding in the urinary tact due to renal disorders, infectious diseases, tumors, or trauma. It may also indicate a transfusion reaction, poisoning, hemolytic anemia, or traumatic muscle injury, and it can be found in patients with severe burns.

Most reagent strips with four or more testing areas can be used to test for urine occult blood. Values are recorded as negative, nonhemolyzed trace, nonhemolyzed moderate, hemolyzed trace 1+ (small amount), 2+ (moderate amount), or 3+ (large amount). The color of the strip is compared the color chart 50 seconds after the strip is dipped into the urine. Confirmatory testing is performed with microscopic examination.

Specific Gravity

See Physical Examination of Urine section.

Ketones

Ketone bodies are the waste products of fat metabolism. Whenever there is inadequate intake, metabolism, or absorption of carbohydrates, the body metabolizes fatty acids instead to meet the body's energy requirements. Since diabetes mellitus is a disorder of glucose metabolism, *ketonuria* is almost always present in uncontrolled diabetes mellitus. Ketonuria is also present in other conditions associated with restricted carbohydrate intake, such as fever, anorexia, digestive disturbances, fasting, starvation, excessive vomiting or diarrhea, or after anesthesia. Popular diets that severely restrict carbohydrate intake should be regularly monitored for ketones.

Values are recorded as negative, trace, small amount, moderate amount, or large amount. The strip tests used are the Ketostix, Keto-Diastix, or most multiple strips with five or more test areas. Testing with Acetest tablets (Ames Co) is the test used for confirmation (see Table 29–4).

Bilirubin

Bilirubinuria is the presence of bilirubin in the urine. Bilirubinuria is associated with obstructive jaundice, hepatitis, and cirrhosis. Bilirubin is a normal by-product of hemoglobin breakdown, which is usually processed by the liver into bile and excreted by the intestines. Normally, bilirubin is present in urine in such low amounts that it is not detected during routine testing. The presence of bilirubin in urine is often the first sign of liver dysfunction or biliary tract disease.

Values are recorded as negative, 1+ (small amount), 2+ (moderate amount), or 3+ (large amount). Usually the Multistix 10 SG is used. The test is read 30 seconds

Table 29–4
URINE CONFIRMATION TESTING PROCEDURES*

Protein: Sulfosalicylic acid (precipitation; other tests include quantitative 24-h sulfosalicylic turbidity test, precipitation tests with a photometer, and acetic acid test for Bence Jones Protein)

Equipment: Centrifuge, centrifuge tube, test tube, gloves

Reaction: 1. Urine is centrifuged and mixed with sulfosalicylic acid.

2. Turbidity is estimated and compared and interpreted as follows:

Negative—no turbidity

Trace—perceptible turbidity

1+—distinct turbidity

2+—turbidity with granulation but no flocculation

3+—turbidity with granulation and flocculation

4+—clumps of precipitated protein or solid precipitate

Into test tube add:

3 mL centrifuged urine

3 mL 3% sulfosalicylic acid (3 g dissolved in 100 mL water)

Read: After 10 min

Note: The strip method is sensitive to albumin but less sensitive to globulins; therefore, a negative (−) strip test result may still produce a positive (+) precipitation or other confirmatory test result.

Ketones: Acetest reagent tablets

Equipment: White paper, dropper, gloves

Reaction: 1. The paper absorbs the urine.

2. If ketones are present, the solution changes color and is read at a timed interval.

Place on paper:

Urine Sample	Serum/Plasma Specimen	Whole Blood Specimen
1 tablet	1 tablet	1 tablet
1 drop urine	1 drop serum or plasma	1 drop whole blood
Compare to chart in 30 sec	Compare to chart in 2 min	Remove blood and compare to chart in 10 min

Note: If urine is not completely adsorbed into the tablet in 30 sec, the tablet most likely has been contaminated with moisture and may give a false reading.

Bilirubin: Ictotest reagent tablets (replaces older oxidation tests)

Equipment: Test mat, dropper, gloves

Reaction: 1. If bilirubin is present, the urine will be absorbed onto the mat surface.

2. The testing is interpreted by color changes within 1 minute.

Add to test mat: 10 drops urine

Place over moistened area: 1 tablet

Flow over tablet: 2 drops water

Read: Compare to color chart in 60 sec

Glucose: Clinitest reagent tablets (Cooper reduction test, Benedict's test)

Equipment: Small test tube, test tube holder, dropper, gloves

Reaction: 1. The tablet dissolves and produces CO_2 and heat.

2. If glucose is present, the solution changes color from blue to orange.

5-Drop Test	2-Drop Test
Add: 10 drops water	10 drops water
5 drops urine	2 drops urine
1 Clinitest tablet	1 Clinitest tablet
Read: Compare to color chart	Compare to 2-drop chart

Note: Sugars other than glucose present will not react with the dipstick method, therefore, a positive Clinitest may be a false-positive value for glucose.

Negative (−) Diastix and Clinistix results and a positive (+) Clinitest result may indicate presence of lactose, galactose, fructose, or pentose, or other nonglucose substances.

Positive (+) Diastix and Clinistix results and a negative (−) Clinitest result may be due to too small glucose levels (> 0.1% [100 mg/dL] but < 0.25% [250 mg/dL]).

---

*Using Ames Co. (Elkhart, IN) products.

after the strip has been dipped in the urine. Testing with Ictotest tablets (Ames Co) is the test for confirmation (see Table 29–4).

Bilirubin is unstable on standing or if exposed to light. If left to stand, it disappears from urine, so testing should be performed right away. Universal precautions should always be taken owing to the possibility of hepatitis if bilirubin results are positive.

Glucose

Glucose is not normally present in urine and, if found in large amounts with a marked increase in urine volume, can be indicative of diabetes. Some causes of *glycosuria* are benign, such as in emotional stress, after eating a heavy meal, or after ingesting large amounts of ascorbic (vitamin C).

The Plastix, Keto-Diastix, and Clinistix strip tests specifically test for glucose in the urine (glycosuria). The strips are not sensitive to other urine sugars that may be present. Values are both quantitative and qualitative and are recorded as negative, trace, 1+, 2+, 3+, and 4+. Testing with Clinitest tablets is the test used for confirmation (see Table 29–4). Confirmation is, however, qualitative only; that is, the test can detect the presence of sugar but not the amount of sugar in the urine.

Other sugars that may be detected in urine include lactose, galactose, fructose, and pentose. The sugar lactose may be present temporarily in lactating women or in children and adults who are deficient in intestinal lactase. Fructose is sometimes present in patients with hepatic disorders, and pentosuria can be present in patients who are on certain drug therapies or with hereditary conditions. Pentosuria is usually a benign condition.

Children who are deficient in an enzyme necessary for converting galactose into glucose develop a life-threatening condition called *galactosemia.* Many pediatricians routinely screen infants for galactosemia using both the Clinistix and the Clinitest methods.

A negative Clinistix and a positive Clinitest result usually indicates the presence of a sugar other than glucose or other nonglucose substances. Because the Clinitest will detect any sugar and some other substances present in urine, it can also produce false-positive results.

Phenylpyruvic Acid

Phenylketonuria is a disease of infants caused by the hereditary absence of an enzyme needed to convert phenylalanine (found in milk and other foods) to tyrosine. As phenylalanine accumulates in the body, phenylpyruvic acid is produced and, if production of this acid is left unchecked, will result in brain damage and severe mental retardation. By the age of 4 weeks, phenylpyruvic acid begins to appear in the urine. PKU testing is *required* on all infants. When detected early and treated with a diet low in phenylalanine, the disease process can be prevented.

Testing is done with the Phenistix test strip. The strip is dipped in fresh urine or pressed against a wet diaper and read after exactly 30 seconds. Values are read as negative, 1+, 2+ or 3+. Color changes that may interfere with test results are produced if the urine is contaminated with salicylates or phenothiazine derivatives, in the presence of high concentrations of bilirubin, or in very alkaline urines.

AUTOMATED CHEMISTRY SCREENING AND CONTROLS

Visual interpretation of the subtle color changes that can occur on the reagent strip has been a major drawback of their use. Many people have difficulty matching the color on the strips with the charts. The commercial availability of automatic reagent strip readers, such as the Ames Clinitek, is eliminating human error in visual interpretation and standardizing chemical testing.

The Clinitek 100 Urine Chemistry Analyzer (Ames Co.) is a semiautomatic, bench-top instrument that is designed for the small- to moderate-sized office performing urinalysis screens (Fig. 29–5). It is designed to read Ames Multistix 10 SG, Multistix 9, and Uristix 4 reagent strips. A strip is immersed in urine, placed on the feed-load table and automatically drawn into the instrument for analysis. Specimen results appear on a screen and are printed through a built-in printer. The instrument also can be linked to an office host computer. The Clinitek 100 also calibrates itself when it is turned on and before each specimen is read.

Another quality control measure that can be used is urine control samples. These are artificial urine samples that have specific values for each component being tested. Values are printed on the control package insert and are given in ranges that are considered acceptable. If the reagent strip values being tested fall within this acceptable range, the reagents are performing adequately and the test was performed correctly. A negative control sample and a positive control sample should be run on reagent strips each day. Controls should also be performed when a new bottle of reagents is opened, and whenever results are doubtful. A patient's urine that is known to be negative can be used as a negative

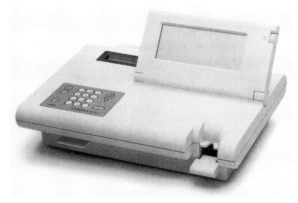

Figure 29–5. The Clinitek 100 Urine Chemistry Analyzer. (Courtesy Miles, Inc., Elkhart, IN)

control sample, as can distilled water. Positive control samples should not be borderline. Control samples may be purchased in liquid form or as a powdered dry reagent strip, such as the Ames Chek-Strip Urinalysis Control Strip. Control results should be recorded in a quality control log each time they are performed (Fig. 29–6).

When unexpected control results occur, the results may be due to an interfering substance in the urine or a technical error. If the instrument is suspected, the manufacturer's operating manual should be consulted. One backup control method is to test the sample with reagent tablets. If control results are still out of the normal range, the reagent manufacturer should be contacted. Ames provides a urinalysis problem identification and resolution checklist for use in control testing (Fig. 29–7).

Inaccurate tests can result from outdated or improperly stored reagent strips. The caps must be kept on the reagent strip bottles at all times to prevent moisture in the air from deteriorating the strips. Manufacturers' instructions should be followed exactly because the procedures and the reagents specified vary. The lot

number and expiration dates of the reagent strips, as well as results from quality control tests, must be recorded daily to ensure accuracy.

Accuracy is a must because results from the chemical examination of urine alerts the medical assistant to what substances should be found during the microscopic examination of urine. For instance, a positive blood (hemoglobin) specimen alerts the medical assistant to look for the presence of intact red blood cells on microscopic examination. With a specimen that tests positively for protein, the medical assistant must look for microscopic evidence of bacteria, white blood cells, and casts.

MICROSCOPIC EXAMINATION OF URINARY SEDIMENT

Microscopic examination identifies cells and other elements that cannot be identified or quantified by chemical reaction strips or can help to confirm a positive or negative strip test result. With the improved sensitivity of chemical strip testing and in view of the importance placed on cost containment by the govern-

URINALYSIS DAILY QUALITY CONTROL CHART

Reagent Strip Name_____

Control Name_____

Date	Control		Reagent Strip		LEU	Nitrite	pH	Protein	Glucose	Ketone	Urobili.	Bili.	Blood	SG	Tech	Comments
	Lot #	Exp. date	Lot #	Exp. Date												

Figure 29–6. Results of the daily quality control tests must be recorded in the appropriate log. (Courtesy Miles, Inc., Elkhart, IN)

CLERICAL ERRORS

Yes   No

- Were sample identification numbers assigned to the correct specimens?

- Were any letters or numbers omitted or transposed while being copied onto the Urinalysis Report—Running Log, Urinalysis Daily Quality Control Chart, Urinalysis Lab Result Slip, or the Maintenance, Repair, and Problem Resolution Record?

- Were results entered for the correct control sample level?

- Were results entered for the correct test?

REAGENT ERRORS
(Refer to the package insert and/or written procedure to check these issues.)

- Were control specimens reconstituted and mixed properly?

- Were control specimens and reagents at the right temperature?

- Were reagents, controls, or calibrator within their expiration dates when used?

PROCEDURAL ERRORS
(Refer to the instrument operating manual and/or written procedure to check these issues.)

- Was the appropriate reagent strip used?

- Should the specimen have been diluted?

PREVIOUS RECORDS
Reviewing past problems—and then solutions—often helps solve existing problems. Refer to the Maintenance, Repair, and Problem Resolution Record and the Urinalysis Daily Quality Control Chart for a record of previous problems that have caused results to fall outside of acceptable control value limits.

Figure 29–7. *Medical assistants who run daily quality control tests can use a checklist, like this, to investigate incorrect or unexpected control readings. (Courtesy Miles, Inc., Elkhart, IN)*

ment and the insurance industry, the need for microscopic examination as a routine procedure or as an appropriate confirmatory test for certain conditions is declining. Strip tests are usually considered reliable for detection of white blood cells and bacteria and have nearly eliminated the need to examine urine sediment for red blood cells. However, microscopic examination is still the only method available for the detection and identification of casts.

When used as confirmatory testing, microscopic results must be compared to the results of chemistry tests. Contradictory or illogical findings must be further investigated before reporting the results. It should be noted that the results of chemistry tests are considered very reliable, whereas the microscopic examination of urinary sediment can be very inaccurate because of the many variables in the techniques of collection and preparation of the specimen and the subjectivity of the person viewing the specimen. Procedures for examining urine microscopically should be standardized whenever possible to ensure the most reliable testing possible.

Urinary sediment is obtained by centrifuging 10 to 15 mL of a well-mixed, freshly obtained urine specimen at a standard speed and time, usually 2000 rpm for 5 minutes. This forces the solid particles to the bottom of the test tube. All but 1 mL of the liquid portion, known as the *supernatant,* is poured off. The remaining urine and sediment are resuspended, and 1 drop is placed on a microscope slide with a coverslip.

Several stains are available to color the constituents of urine sediment, especially the cellular elements, either free or embedded in casts. The most common,

all-purpose stain used is a crystal violet and safranin mixture known as the *Sternheimer-Malbin stain.* It is commercially available as Sedistain (Clay-Adams, division of Becton Dickinson & Co, Parsippany, NJ) and KOVA stain (ICL Scientific, Fountain Valley, CA). Complete descriptions of the various elements when stained are completely described in each company's literature. Other stains are as follows:

1. *Acetic acid.* Useful for differentiating white blood cells from red blood cells.
2. *Methylene blue.* Used to visualize bacteria.
3. *Sudan dyes or oil red O.* Useful for differentiating triglycerides from cholesterol droplets and for visualizing fat globules, either free or in casts.
4. *Gram's stain.* Useful for differentiating gram-negative and gram-positive bacteria. The Gram-staining procedure is described at the end of this chapter.

It is recommended that both a stained and unstained specimen be examined as some elements, such as crystals, are more easily identified *without* stain. Stain can also obscure some important findings, especially in alkaline urine.

The slide specimen is first scanned for casts using the microscope's low-power objective with a low light. The high-power dry objective is then used for identifying cells, the types of casts, and any other elements present, such as crystals, bacteria, or parasites. Normally, the urine sediment may contain a few white blood cells and epithelial cells, occasional crystals, and rarely one or two red blood cells per field. Five to 10 high-power fields (HPFs) are observed, and for each element, the field counts are averaged and recorded. This system for reporting is listed under the procedure for examining microscopic urine at the end of this chapter.

Red Blood Cells

Red blood cells are always significant when found in the urinary sediment, except in the cases when the specimen has been obtained by catheterization, after the passage of a stone, or in menstruating females. Red blood cells indicate urinary tract injury or disease or systemic hemorrhagic diseases such as hemophilia. They appear as refracting, nongranular, non-nucleated small cells with a pale greenish-blue sheen (Fig. 29–8). In dilute urine, the red blood cells may be swollen and rounded; in concentrated urine, they may appear crenated and shrunken. Red blood cells rapidly lyse in alkaline or dilute urine; for this reason, the specimen must be absolutely fresh. After lysing, red blood cells appear as faint, colorless shells and are reported as "ghost" or "shadow" cells. A 2% acetic acid solution lyses red blood cells and is an excellent test for differentiating red blood cells from yeast cells or oil droplets.

Red blood cells should be recorded as the average number per HPF after 5 to 10 fields are observed. Less than one to two red blood cells per HPF is considered normal. More than three red blood cells per HPF is

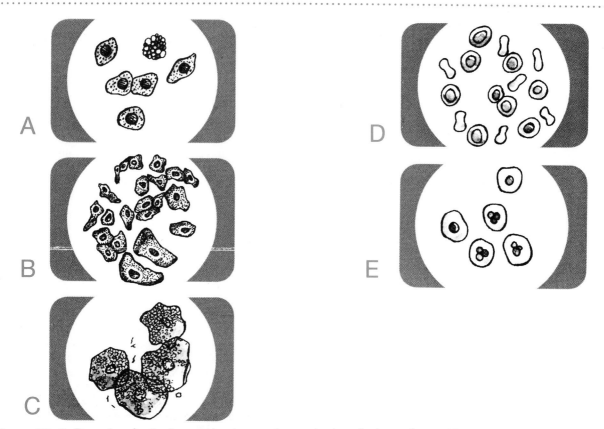

Figure 29–8. Examples of cells observed in microscopic examination of urine sediment. (**A**) Renal tubular epithelial cells; (**B**) transitional epithelial cells; (**C**) squamous epithelial cells; (**D**) red blood cells (RBCs); (**E**) white blood cells (WBCs). Adapted from Ames Atlas of Urinary Sediment. Miles, Inc., Elkhart, IN)

considered abnormal. The red blood cells counted in each field are totaled and divided by the number of fields examined to obtain the average number of red blood cells per HPF. The red blood cell average is reported as the numerical range in which it falls, for example: "red blood cells, 5 to 10 per HPF." The ranges are as follows:

0	10 to 20
0 to 1	20 to 30
1 to 2	30 to 40
2 to 5	40 to 50
5 to 10	More than 50

White Blood Cells

White blood cells in urine signify infection somewhere in the urinary tract or kidney disease. Leukocytes are approximately two times larger than red blood cells. Segmented neutrophils appear round, granular, and nucleated (see Fig. 29–8). Some neutrophils are so large that their cytoplasmic granules show Brownian movement. These large white blood cells are called "glitter" cells. White blood cells often appear in large clumps.

White blood cells in each field are totaled and recorded as the average number per HPF after 5 to 10 fields are observed. More than five white blood cells per HPF is considered significant; less than five signals a possible contamination of the specimen during collection. The white blood cell average is reported as the numerical range in which it falls, for example: "white blood cells, 5 to 10 per HPF." The ranges are listed in the previous section on red blood cells.

Epithelial Cells

Normally, a few squamous epithelial cells are found in the urine and appear as large, flat, cells with prominent nuclei and large cytoplasm (see Fig. 29–8). These normal-appearing cells arise from the urethra and the vagina. The presence of large numbers of renal epithelial cells or transitional epithelial cells is abnormal (see Fig. 29–8). Renal tubular epithelial cells originate in the kidney. They are round with a large nucleus and slightly larger than white blood cells. They are difficult to identify and often confused with white blood cells. Transitional epithelial cells tend to be pear-shaped. Bladder epithelial cells are larger than renal epithelial cells and may appear as flat, cuboidal, or columnar. Rarely seen are oval fat bodies, which are special renal epithelial cells that have undergone fat degeneration. They contain refractive fat droplets within the cell. (See also fatty casts, below.)

Normal squamous epithelial cells are reported as few, moderate, or many per HPF. Abnormal epithelial cells are examined under high power (×40) magnification, and counts in each field are totaled and recorded as the average number per HPF after 5 to 10 fields are observed. The cell average is reported as the numerical range in which it falls, for example: "renal tubular epithelial cells, one to two per HPF." The ranges are listed in the section on red blood cells.

Casts

A cast is a positive copy (mold) of a particular spot of blockage in the lumen of a kidney tubule. It can be compared to a sculptured biopsy of the kidney. The classic shape is molded from the shape of the tubule lumen: it is definitively outlined as a cylindrical structure with even parallel sides and two rounded ends.

Since casts are, in essence, a gelatinous substance, they may also capture any material that may be present in the tubule such as cells or cellular debris. Empty casts are called *hyaline casts;* casts full of cells or other material are named according to the type of material contained in them (Fig. 29–9). Once the cast is formed, it is sloughed into the urine. Table 29–5 summarizes the most common kinds of urinary casts.

Certain conditions must exist before a cast can develop in the renal tubules. The urine must be acid with high salt concentrations; urine output must be lower than normal; and protein must be present in the urine. Because of these conditions, most urines that contain casts show some cloudiness and test positive for protein on chemical testing.

There is a direct correlation between the presence of protein and casts in urine sediment. In the presence of the conditions just listed, it is the protein that becomes concentrated and precipitated by the low pH condition and eventually changes to a mucoprotein matrix that forms the cast.

Simple hyaline casts are translucent albuminoid casts that are empty or contain only a small amount of debris. The refractive index of the hyaline cast is nearly the same as that of flat glass. It is extremely difficult to see. In small numbers (less than two per HPF) they may not be clinically important. Hyaline casts are further classified according to their inclusions as *hyaline cellular, hyaline granular,* and *hyaline fatty* casts.

Casts are formed in the presence of serious renal disease, and their presence in urinary sediment is very significant. They almost always indicate damage to the kidney. For proper viewing, the microscope should have a very low light, the condenser should be down, and the diaphragm should be closed, because casts, particularly hyaline casts, tend to be transparent.

Casts tend to migrate to the edges of the coverslip. The edges of the coverslip should be observed first, and the average *number* of casts per low-power field (LPF) should be reported after 5 to 10 fields have been counted. The ranges are listed in the previous section on red blood cells. Casts are then specifically *identified* under high-power examination.

Unfortunately with the microscopic examination of urine, the easiest-to-see objects are often the most insignificant findings and, conversely, the most significant findings are also the most difficult to see. Casts are probably the single most significant finding in urine yet the hardest to find and identify. Serious abnormalities in urine usually do not stand alone, however. Often the nature of the other urinary constituents can best alert the medical assistant to look for a specific finding in the urine sediment or to confirm a tentative finding.

Eventually the beginning medical assistant learns not only to identify the constituents of urinary sediment but also to correlate multiple urinalysis findings and the certain patterns they follow. The beginning medical assistant, however, should not make independent judgments about casts; rather all cast identifications should be verified by the physician.

Crystals

Crystals and amorphous salts are compounds often found during a routine urinalysis. The type and amount of crystals vary depending on the pH of urine (Fig. 29–10). Their presence does not indicate abnormality and usually is not addressed unless the patient is re-

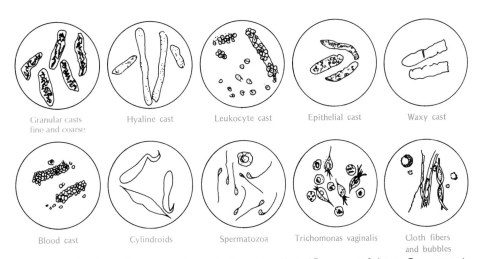

Granular casts fine and coarse   Hyaline cast   Leukocyte cast   Epithelial cast   Waxy cast

Blood cast   Cylindroids   Spermatozoa   Trichomonas vaginalis   Cloth fibers and bubbles

Figure 29–9. Casts and other microscopic elements found in urine. (Courtesy of Ames Company, Inc., Elkhart, IN)

Table 29-5
SUMMARY OF URINE CASTS

Type	Origin	Clinical Significance
Hyaline	Tubular secretion of Tamm-Horsfall protein that aggregates into fibrils	Glomerulonephritis Pyelonephritis Chronic renal diseae Congestive heart failure Stress and exercise 0-2/LPF normal
Red blood cell	Red blood cells enmeshed in or attached to Tamm-Horsfall protein matrix	Glomerulonephritis Strenuous exercise
White blood cell	White blood cells enmeshed in or attached to Tamm-Horsfall protein matrix	Pyelonephritis
Epithelial cell	Tubular cells remaining attached to Tamm-Horsfall protein fibrils	Renal tubular damage
Granular	Disintegration of white cell casts Bacteria Urates Tubular cell lysosomes Protein aggregates	Stasis of urine flow Urinary tact infection Stress and exercise
Waxy	Hyaline casts	Stasis of urine flow
Fatty	Renal tubular cells Oval fat bodies	Nephrotic syndrome
Broad casts	Formation in collecting ducts	Extreme stasis of urine flow

ceiving specific drugs (e.g., sulfonamides) or if there is a problem with protein synthesis. In normal urine, crystals form as the urine cools.

Normal crystals are reported as few, moderate, or many per HPF. Abnormal crystals are estimated by observing a minimum of five microscopic fields and reporting the average number per HPF of the five fields observed. Estimation of the microscopic field can be done by dividing the field into four sections, counting the number in one section, and multiplying by four.

Bacteria

Normal urine does not contain bacteria. Most bacteria found in the urine are bacilli (rod-shaped) or cocci (round-shaped) bacteria. Rods are fairly easy to identify, but cocci may be confused with crystals and more difficult to detect. The finding of 20 or more bacteria per HPF may indicate urinary tract infection. The presence of a few bacteria combined with a positive or negative nitrite test result and a negative leukocyte esterase test result usually indicates a collection contamination or it may represent the beginnings of a urinary tract infection that cannot be confirmed without further testing. Any bacteria present combined with both positive nitrite and leukocyte esterase test results indicate infection, usually in the lower urinary tract. Bacteria is examined under high-power magnification and reported as few, moderate, or many.

Yeast

Yeast are refractive, flat, oval bodies that vary in size and have buds. They are often confused with red blood cells. Yeast cells are often a vaginal contaminant. Found in great numbers, yeast with hyphae may indicate a vaginal infection. Yeast may also be seen in diabetes, pregnancy, and obesity. Yeast are examined under high-power magnification and reported as few, moderate, or many.

Parasites

Parasites are usually a contaminant. The most common parasite seen is *Trichomonas vaginalis* (see Fig. 29-9). *Trichomonas* is a flagellate protozoan that should be reported only when the flagellates are motile. Inactive *Trichomonas* organisms can easily be confused with leukocytes. *T. vaginalis* can be present in male (urethritis) and female (vaginitis) patients. In urines from female patients, *T. vaginalis* are associated with increased vaginal epithelial cells, leukocytes, and bacteria. Parasites are examined under high-power magnification and reported as few, moderate, or many.

Mucous Threads

Mucous threads are found in normal urine but increased amounts usually indicate urinary tract inflammation. Mucous threads are examined under low-power magnification and reported as "present."

Spermatozoa

Spermatozoa may be present in female urine after sexual intercourse and usually is not reported (see Fig. 29-9). A few spermatozoa in male urine are normal, but abnormal amounts are significant and should be reported. Sperm is examined under high-power magnification and reported as "present."

CRYSTALS FOUND IN ACID URINE (X400)

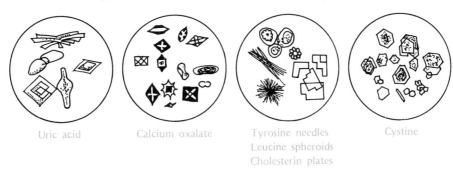

Uric acid   Calcium oxalate   Tyrosine needles
Leucine spheroids
Cholesterin plates   Cystine

CRYSTALS FOUND IN ALKALINE URINE (X400)

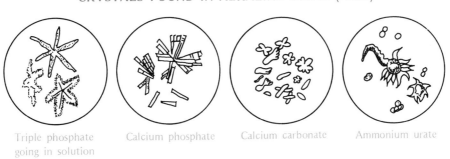

Triple phosphate
going in solution   Calcium phosphate   Calcium carbonate   Ammonium urate

SULFA CRYSTALS

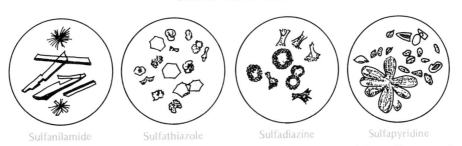

Sulfanilamide   Sulfathiazole   Sulfadiazine   Sulfapyridine

Figure 29–10. Crystals found in microscopic examination of urine. (Courtesy of Ames Company, Inc., Elkhart, IN)

Other Contaminants

Contaminants are often present in urine and can be confused with pathologic cells or crystals. Talcum powder and glove starch often resemble calcium crystals or fat bodies. Scratches on the glass slide or coverslip, wood fibers from spatulas, hairs, bubbles, or material fibers may be mistaken for casts or cells (see Fig. 29–9). Oil droplets from dirty equipment may be mistaken as red blood cells. These contaminants are often frustrating to the student when first examining urine. One good rule to remember, however, is: if the object is easily viewed, it most likely is a contaminant and not significant.

Recording Urinalysis Results

With the new CLIA standards, the physician's office laboratory must keep records of the number and types of tests performed. These records provide a backup to patient charts and documentation of a quality assurance and quality control program. As each urinalysis is performed, a laboratory result form (Fig. 29–11) and a running log of all urinalysis performed (Fig. 29–12) must be completed. The laboratory result form is filed in the patient's chart. The running log is filed with the laboratory records. The running log can be particularly helpful for troubleshooting out-of-control range values. Running logs also can show trends in biased reporting or in the reliability of a reagent for a particular component being tested.

Pregnancy Tests

Pregnancy tests are based on the presence or absence in urine or serum of a hormone called *human chorionic gonadotropin (hCG)*. The hormone hCG is produced by

LAB RESULT SLIP

PATIENT _____

DATE _____   TIME _____

LEUKOCYTES	NEGATIVE ☐	TRACE ☐	SMALL + ☐	MODERATE ++ ☐	LARGE +++ ☐
NITRITE	NEGATIVE ☐	POSITIVE ☐	POSITIVE ☐	(Any degree of uniform pink color is positive)	
UROBILINOGEN	NORMAL 0.2 ☐	NORMAL 1 ☐	mg/dL 2 ☐	4 ☐	8 ☐ (1 mg = approx. 1 EU)
PROTEIN	NEGATIVE ☐	TRACE ☐	mg/dL 30 + ☐	100 ++ ☐	300 +++ ☐ 2000 or more ++++ ☐
pH	5.0 ☐	6.0 ☐	6.5 ☐	7.0 ☐	7.5 ☐ 8.0 ☐ 8.5 ☐
BLOOD	NEGATIVE ☐	NON-HEMOLYZED TRACE ☐	HEMOLYZED TRACE ☐	SMALL + ☐	MODERATE ++ ☐ LARGE +++ ☐
SPECIFIC GRAVITY	1.000 ☐	1.005 ☐	1.010 ☐	1.015 ☐	1.020 ☐ 1.025 ☐ 1.030 ☐
KETONE	NEGATIVE ☐	TRACE mg/dL 5 ☐	SMALL 15 ☐	MODERATE 40 ☐	LARGE 80 ☐ LARGE 160 ☐
BILIRUBIN	NEGATIVE ☐	SMALL + ☐	MODERATE ++ ☐	LARGE +++ ☐	
GLUCOSE	NEGATIVE ☐	g/dL (%) mg/dL ☐	1/10 (tr.) 100 ☐	1/4 250 ☐	1/2 500 ☐ 1 1000 ☐ 2 or more 2000 or more ☐

MICROSCOPIC

WBC _____ /HPF   EPITHELIAL CELLS _____ /HPF   COMMENTS _____

RBC _____ /HPF   TYPE _____   _____

CASTS _____ /LPF   TRICHOMONAS _____   _____

TYPE _____   BACTERIA _____   _____

CRYSTALS _____   OTHER _____   _____

YEAST _____   COLOR _____   _____

CLARITY _____   TESTED BY: _____

BLOOD GLUCOSE RESULTS

_____ mg/dL

Figure 29–11. Federal regulations require the completion of a laboratory result slip for each test performed. (Courtesy Ames Company, Inc., Elkhart IN)

the placenta about 7 to 10 days after fertilization. In normal pregnancies, hCG levels continue to rise during the first trimester, then peak and decrease during the second and third trimesters. Levels of hCG are much lower in abnormal or ectopic pregnancies; hCG may also be produced by other conditions, such as tumors, hydatidiform moles, chorionic carcinoma, and testicular tumors. These conditions may produce false-positive results in pregnancy testing.

Traditional agglutination inhibition tests are relatively insensitive and subject to false reactions. Newer enzyme immunoassay color-change tests have a high level of sensitivity, and many types of kits are available that offer ease of performance. (Chapter 30 discusses these types of tests more fully.)

The first morning urine specimen with a specific gravity of at least 1.015 should be used for laboratory testing because it is more concentrated. Testing should be on very fresh urine. Specimens that contain blood or

protein are likely to give false-positive results. Drugs can also cause false-positive results. False-negative results may occur if the urine is too diluted or it is too early in the pregnancy for a positive result to register.

The stage of pregnancy determines the concentration of hCG. Owing to variations in hCG concentrations in specimens, positive and negative control samples must be run with each test to ensure accurate readings. Most manufacturers include positive and negative control samples with their kits. Sources of error include failure to add reagents properly, inadequate washing, improper storage of reagents, and interfering substances as mentioned above.

BACTERIOLOGY

Bacteriology is the study of microorganisms. Medical bacteriology deals primarily with pathogenic (disease

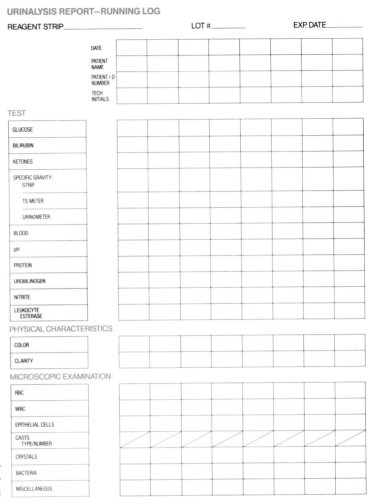

Figure 29–12. Federal regulations also require that a running log of all uranalyses performed be kept. (Courtesy Ames Company, Inc., Elkhart, IN)

producing) organisms. Most bacteriology laboratory specimens are obtained and the tests run in hospitals or reference laboratories. These facilities employ microbiologist or pathologists to read and interpret test results.

This section provides a general overview of bacterial culture, isolation, and sensitivity techniques, and the macroscopic and microscopic identification of bacteria. The medical assistant will gain a general knowledge of the basic steps in studying bacterial cultures, even though the technical procedures are often done at reference laboratories. Although it is beyond the scope of this text to discuss every pathogen, the medical assistant will find bacteriology reference texts to be a valuable tool for interpretating the significance of individual pathogens found in patients' cultures.

The collection of urine, blood, and throat cultures is often performed by the medical assistant in the physician's office. The physician may also request the medical assistant's aid in the collection of material from the nose, eye, or ear, or from wounds and other body openings, such as the vagina.

Bacteriology testing includes the preparation of cultures, wet preparations, and potassium hydroxide (KOH) preparations, direct smears, Gram staining, and direct non-growth-dependent screening tests for strep throat and mononucleosis. Table 29–6 lists the sources and specimen collection methods of commonly cultured organisms.

Since the presence of a pathogenic organism is suspected in all microbiologic testing, the medical assistant must follow the general safety rules of the laboratory for self-protection and to prevent the spread of infection. Good handwashing technique and the wearing of gloves are mandatory. Face masks or face shields are also recommended any time there is the danger of aerosol contamination. In cases of contamination with bacterial specimens, soiled containers and surfaces must be soaked with commercial disinfectants of the correct concentration and for the time required by the manufacturer.

CLASSIFICATION AND IDENTIFICATION OF BACTERIA

The classification of microorganisms is based on their *morphology* (form and structure) and the metabolic and chemical characteristics of the individual microorganisms. Bacteria represent a family of microorganisms.

Table 29–6
COMMONLY CULTURED BACTERIA

Source	Method	Organism
Blood	Blood culture tube containing transport medium and an anticoagulant. Collected by venipuncture at two separate sites to rule out collection contamination. Puncture sites and the vacutainer tops should be cleaned with providone-iodine.	*Bacteriodes, Brucella, Clostridium, Histoplasma, Listeria, Vibrio, Salmonella Staphylococcus, Streptococcus, Pseudomonas, Pasteurella, Mycoplasma Neisseria,* Pneumococci.
Ear	Culture swab placed in the ear canal.	*Staphylococcus, Streptococcus, Pneumococcus, Pseudomonas, Proteus Candida, Haemophilus*
Eye	Culture swab placed at the site of infection or into the pus	*Streptococcus, Staphylococcus, Pneumococcus, Neisseria, Pseudomonas Haemophilus, Cornebacterium.*
Feces	Stool specimen collected in early morning or with a rectal swab.	*Salmonella, Shigella, Proteus, Pseudomonas*
Sputum	Sterile sputum collection container. The patient must obtain a sputum specimen by coughing deeply when getting up in the morning.	*Diplococcus pneumoniae, Streptococcus, Staphylococcus, Mycobacterium, Haemophilus, Klebsiella, Neisseria.*
Throat and nasopharynx	Culturette swab touched to the site of inflammation and/or pus at the back of the throat.	Streptococci (group A), Staphylococcus, Pneumococcus, Candida, Bordetella, Haemophilus.
Urine	First morning voided midstream clean-catch specimen in sterile container. Refrigerate if transportation is delayed.	*Escherichia coli, Klebsiella, Enterobacter, Serratia, Proteus, Pseudomonas, Streptococcus, Staphylococcus, Candida, Neisseria.*
Wounds	Culture swab placed into the pus.	*Staphylococcus,* enterococci, *Streptococcus, Clostridium, Bacteroides, Pseudomonas, Proteus, E. coli.*

Bacteria generally have two names. The first name designates the genus and is capitalized. It usually indicates general structure and the shape of the organism or is derived from its discoverer's name. For example, the first name of *Diplococcus pneumoniae* refers to spherical bacteria occurring in pairs, and the second name refers to the disease produced. Table 29–7 summarizes various classes of microorganism and their associated diseases.

The morphologic classification of bacteria consists of five categories: (1) cocci, (2) bacilli, (3) vibrios, (4) spirillae, and (5) spirochetes (Fig. 29–13). A sixth classification, *mycoplasma,* is a genus of gram-negative bacteria that lack cell walls and cannot be morphologically classified.

Cocci are spherical bacteria that vary according to their patterns of arrangement. Diplococci occur in pairs. Pneumonia (*D. pneumoniae*), gonorrhea (*Neisseria gonorrhoeae,* or gonococcus), and meningitis (*Neisseria meningitidis,* or meningococcus) are three diseases caused by pathogenic diplococci. (**Note:** meningitis may also be caused by *Staphylococcus pneumoniae* [pneumococcus] and *Haemophilus influenzae.*)

Staphylococci appear in irregular, grapelike clusters. Staphylococci are constantly present on the skin and in the upper respiratory tract. One of the pathogenic species, *S. aureus,* is the causative agent of food poisoning, boils, abscesses, acne, osteomyelitis, and another type of pneumonia.

Streptococci appear in chains. Streptococci organisms can be further classified by whether or not they are capable of hemolyzing red blood cells and into three groupings as follows:

1. *Streptococcus pyogens.* Also called β-hemolytic streptococci. β-hemolytic types produce a clear zone of hemolysis immediately around the colony on blood agar. The most virulent streptococci are the beta type.

   In addition to classifying streptococci by its characteristic hemolysis, streptococci can be classified according to its cellular carbohydrate content, called the *Lancefield groups A through H and K through T.* The organism in primary infections is usually group A, which primarily invades the body through the throat. The group A β-hemolytic pyogens group contains the more serious pathogenic organisms causing streptococcal sore throat ("strep throat"), scarlet fever, rheumatic fever, puer-

Table 29–7
Table 29–7
TYPES OF MICROORGANISMS AND THEIR ASSOCIATED DISEASES

Classification	Subclassification	Microorganism	Diseases
		Bacteria	
Bacilli	Gram-positive	*Clostridium botulinum*	Botulism (food poisoning)
		Clostridium perfringens	Gas gangrene
		Clostridium tetani	Tetanus (lockjaw)
		Cornybacterium diphtheria	Diphtheria, diplcoccal pneumonia
		Norcardia asteroides	Lung and brain lesions
	Gram-negative	*Bacteroides* species	General infections, abscesses, endocarditis
		Bordetellea pertussis	Whooping cough
		Enterobacter aerogenes	Some urinary tract infections (UTIs), other systemic infections
		Escherichia coli	Some UTIs, systemic infections, and normal intestinal flora
		Gardnerella vaginalis	Nonspecific vaginitis
		Haemophylus ducreyi	Chancroid
		Haemophilus influenzae	Meningitis
		Klebsiella pneumoniae	Pneumonia, UTI, osteomyelitis, superinfections
		Legionella pneumophilia	Legionnaire's disease
		Leptothrix buccalis	Vincent's disease
		Proteus species	UTI
		Pseudomonas aeruginosa	UTI, upper respiratory infection (URI), skin and systemic infections
		Salmonella species	Typhoid fever, gatroenteritis, bacteremia
		Serratia marcenscens	Systemic superinfections in immunocompromised patients
		Shigella species	Gastroenteritis
	Acid-fast	*Mycobacterium leprae*	Leprosy
		Mycobacterium tuberculosis	Tuberculosis
Cocci	Gram-positive staphylococci	*Staphylococcus aureus*	Food Poisoning, abscesses, boils, toxic shock, surgical wounds, pneumonia, otitis, bacteremia, endocarditis, osteomyelitis, normal skin flora
	Gram-positive Streptococci	*Streptococcus faecalis*	Endocarditis, peritonitis, bacteremia, normal intestinal flora (enterococcus)
		Streptococcus pneumoniae (also called *Diplococcus pneumoniae*)	Pneumonia, meningitis, otitis, endocarditis
		Streptococcus pyogens (group A β-hemolytic type)	URI, otitis, scarlet fever, strep throat, rheumatic fever, glomerulonephritis
		Streptococcus viridins (α-hemolytic type)	Endocarditis, bacteremia, normal respiratory tract flora

Continued

<u>Table 29–7</u>
TYPES OF MICROORGANISMS AND THEIR ASSOCIATED DISEASES — *Continued*

Classification	Subclassification	Microorganism	Diseases
	Gram-negative diplococci	*Neisseria gonorrhoeae*	Gonorrhea (vaginitis, urethritis, salpingitis, endocarditis, arthritis)
		Neisseria meningitidis	Meningitis, bacteremia
Spirillum	—	*Vibrio cholerae*	Cholera
Spirochetes	—	*Borrelia burgdorferi*	Lyme disease
		Treponema pallidum	Syphilis
		Treponema pertenue	Yaws
Mycoplasm	Gram-negative	*Ureaplasma urealyticum*	Nonspecific urethritis
Chlamydia			
—	—	*Chlamydia psittaci*	Psittacosis (Parrot fever)
		Chlamydia trachomatis	Sexually transmitted diseases (STDs): conjunctivitis, lymphogranuloma venereum, nongonococcus urethritis, genital infection
Rickettsiae			
—	—	*Rickettsiae* species	Rocky Mountain spotted fever, typhus, Q fever, trench fever
Fungi			
Yeast	—	*Candida albicans*	Candidiasis (skin infection, thrush, vaginitis, jock itch, panonychia)
		Coccidioides immitis	Coccidioidomycosis
		Histoplasma capsulatum	Histoplasmosis
Molds	—	*Aspergillus* species	Systemic fungal infections, skin and bone lesions
		Dermatophytes (*Tinea* species)	Ringworm, jock itch, athlete's foot, barber's itch
Viruses			
Arthropodborne	—	Arboviruses	Yellow fever, equine encephalitis
Enteric	—	Enteroviruses	Polio (infantile paralysis)
Exanthem	Herpesviruses	Herpes simplex virus type I	Cold sores, fever blisters, herpes labialis
		Herpes simplex virus type II	Genital herpes
		Varicella-zoster virus	Chickenpox, shingles
	—	Paramyxoviruses	Rubeola
Persistent	—	Cytomegaloviruses	Cytomegalovirus infections
		Hepatitis A virus	Hepatitis A
		Hepatitis B virus	Hepatitis B
		Hepatitis C virus	Hepatitic C (non-A, non-B hepatitis)
		Papovaviruses	Warts
		Retroviruses	Leukemia, lymphoma, AIDS

Continued

Table 29-7

TYPES OF MICROORGANISMS AND THEIR ASSOCIATED DISEASES—*Continued*

Classification	Subclassification	Microorganism	Diseases
Neurotropic	—	Rabies viruses	Rabies (hydrophobia)
Respiratory	—	Adenovirus Herpes-like Epstein-Barr virus Myxoviruses Rhinoviruses	Viral pneumonia Infectious mononucleosis Influenza, croup, mumps (paromyxovirus) Common cold (over 100 rhinoviruses and some other species can cause the common cold)
Protozoa			
Amoeba	—	*Entamoeba histolytica* *Giardia lamblia* *Plasmodium* species	Amebiasis Giardiasis Malaria
Flagellates	—	*Trichomonas vaginalis*	Trichomoniasis (STD)
Helminths			
Roundworms	—	*Enterobius vermicularis*	Pinworm
Tapeworms	—	Various organisms	Tapeworms (from beef, pork, or fish)
Flukes	—	*Schistosoma* species	Schistosomiasis (blood flukes), swimmer's itch (skin infection)
Insects	Mites	*Sarcoptes scabiei*	Scabies
	Lice	*Pediculus* species	Pediculosis (head and body lice, genital lice [crabs])

peral fever, glomerulonephritis, endocarditis, and other acute conditions.

2. *Streptococcus viridans.* α-Hemolytic parasitic forms occur as normal flora in the upper respiratory tract. α-Type streptococci produce a smaller greenish discoloration immediately surrounding the colony on blood agar due to incomplete hemolysis of the blood agar.
3. *Streptococcus enterococcus.* α-Hemolytic parasitic forms that occur as normal flora in the digestive tract.

Bacilli are straight, cylindrical rods. Examples of diseases caused by bacilli include tuberculosis (tubercle bacillus), dysentery (*Shigella*), whooping cough (*Bordetella pertussis*), food poisoning (*Clostridium botulinum,* or botulism), gas gangrene (*Clostridium perfringens*), gastroenteritis (*Clostridium difficile*), and tetanus (*Clostridium tetani*).

Vibrios are curved or sickle-shaped bacteria. The pathogen *Vibrio cholerae* is the causative organism of cholera. *Spirilla* are spiral, nonmotile rods. *Spirillum minus* is a species that causes rat-bite fever in humans. Spirochetes are spiral, motile bacteria. Syphilis is caused by the spirochete *Treponema pallidum.*

SPECIMEN COLLECTION

Great care must be taken to prevent contamination when specimens are collected and prepared. Aseptic technique is used in collecting and preparing all specimens for microbiologic studies to ensure accurate laboratory results. All containers and instruments must be sterile.

Most cultures are obtained using a sterile swab, which is a round wooden stick with a Dacron, rayon, or calcium alginate applicator at one end. (Cotton swabs are not used for bacteriologic specimen collection.) The swab is then placed in a transport media for shipment to a laboratory, or used on site to make a direct smear for immediate examination or to inoculate a culture plate for growing the organisms.

The Culturette Collection and Transport System, manufactured by Becton Dickinson & Co (Rutherford, NJ), is a self-contained culturing packet system that readily adapts to most office specimen collections from the throat, nose, eye, ear, rectum, wound, and urogenital sites (Fig. 29–14). The Culturette has a sterile, disposable plastic tube containing a soft rayon applicator swab and a sealed ampule of holding (transport) medium. The holding medium is the transport sub-

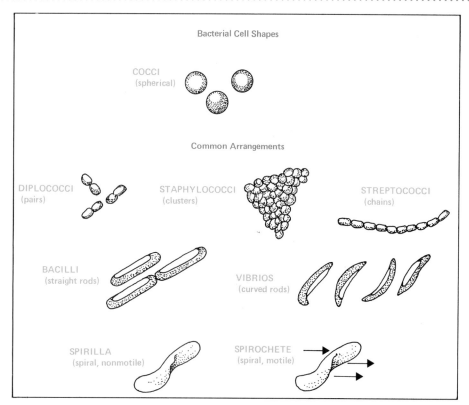

Figure 29-13. Bacteria are classified according to their shapes.

stance and prevents drying and deterioration of the specimen.

The plastic tube is removed from the sterile envelope, and the applicator swab is used to collect the specimen. Caution must be used to avoid contamination from the surrounding skin or mucosa. The swab is placed back into the plastic tube and immediately recapped, and the ampule of holding medium is crushed. This system permits culture storage for up to 72 hours at room temperature. The plastic tube is placed in its envelope. The specimen must be labeled with the patient's name, date and time, specimen source, test(s) ordered, physician's name, and any special instructions. The specimen is then mailed to or picked up by a reference laboratory. The culture specimen must be quickly transported so that the microorganisms are vital when they reach the laboratory. Biohazard warnings are required when transporting hazardous biologic material to a reference laboratory.

There is also a commercially available two-swab Culturette II Collection and Transport System that allows the medical assistant to obtain two separate specimens from a single infected area. This is useful particularly when performing a group A streptococcal screen or a Gram stain on site. The second swabbed specimen can be transported to the reference laboratory for culturing.

A culture specimen should be collected before initiating antibiotic therapy to provide a baseline reference. If the patient is already taking antibiotic medication, the laboratory receiving the specimen must be informed. The test requisition accompanying the culture should indicate the name of the antibiotic being taken by the patient. (See the description of this procedure at the end of this chapter).

CULTURE MEDIA

A culture is the propagation of living organisms in a special *medium* (plural *media;* a substance that is conducive to the growth of the organism). Microorganisms grow on the prepared media in *colonies,* which are discrete groupings of single types of organisms. The type of organism growing in a colony may or may not be identifiable by the colony characteristics alone.

A variety of culture media are available for transporting specimens or for growing cultures at the time of collection (Table 29-8). Culture media may be liquid, semisolid, or solid. Liquid media are called media *broth.* A broth can be solidified in a tube or on a plate (Petri dish) by adding agar, a seaweed extract.

Media either inhibit or encourage the growth of certain pathogens and are classified as differential, enrichment, or supportive. Media is selective or nonselective. Selective media supports the growth of specific bacteria while inhibiting the growth of other organisms. Nonselective media supports the growth of almost all bacteria. The most common nonselective media used in the physician's office are sheep blood and tryptic soy broth (TSB, also called *blood agar*), used for throat cultures, and eosin-methylene blue (EMB), used with blood agar for urine cultures.

Some microorganisms cannot survive in oxygen; they are said to be *anaerobic.* Anaerobic organisms require a high concentration of carbon dioxide for growth and

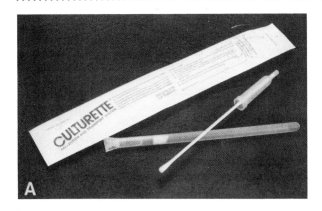

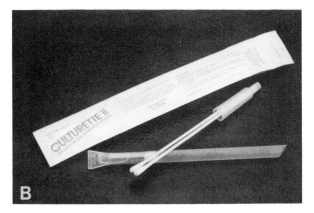

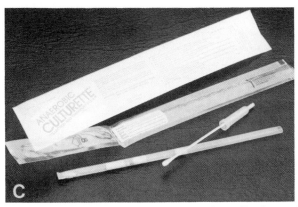

Figure 29–14. *Self-contained systems for collection and transport of specimens. (**A**) Single swab aerobic specimen package. (**B**) Double-swap aerobic specimen package. (**C**) Single swab anaerobic specimen package. (Courtesy Becton Dickinson & Company, Rutherford, NJ)*

must be transported in media that generates carbon dioxide and in a carbon dioxide gas-generating container.

The type of media stocked in the physician's office laboratory depends on the practice and the needs of the physician. Media containers (plates or tubes) must not be opened before plating, or they will not be sterile. Culture plates are stored in the refrigerator upside down to prevent condensation from falling on the agar.

CULTURING EQUIPMENT

Special equipment is needed to culture specimens in the physician's office laboratory. In addition to culture media, inoculating loops and needles are used to transfer microorganism colonies to new culture plates or glass slides for microscopic examination. Disposable loops and needles may be purchased for single use. Reusable loops of platinum or nicrome wire that fit into loop holders are also available. The loops are sterilized by incinerating before and after each transfer of material.

A bunsen or alcohol burner is used to sterilize the loop. Introducing a wet inoculating loop into a hot flame can cause a splattering of live bacteria into the air. The laboratorian must be careful to prevent this type of aerosol contamination. Wear gloves and a face protector. When flaming the loop, first introduce the loop into the bottom colorless portion of the flame for a few seconds, then carefully raise the loop to the hotter, blue area of the flame (Fig. 29–15). Keep the wire in the flame until it begins to glow red. Remove the loop and allow it to cool for a few seconds before transferring material. If the loop is hot, it could kill the organisms and interfere with accurate test results.

Some states prohibit the use of Bunsen and alcohol burners. Specialized incinerators that sterilize loops and needles by infrared heat are available. Organic material is incinerated deep within a ceramic funnel tube to prevent infectious splatter or cross-contamination. Complete sterilization takes only 5 to 7 seconds at a sterilizing temperature of 1600°F (871°C).

Another piece of equipment required for growing cultures is an incubator. For the physician's office laboratory, small incubators that maintain culture plates at or near 99°F (37°C) are available. A pilot light should be included to ensure that the power is on. Cultures are usually incubated for 24 hours.

BACTERIAL CULTURES

Primary culture growths are performed to identify which disease-producing bacteria are present in infection. Culture results can also be used to diagnose or rule out the cause of a fever of unknown origin, to determine the source of an epidemic, or to test for the complete resolution of an infection after treatment.

Most throat specimens are taken for the detection of group A β-hemolytic streptococci. The specimen can be cultured on sheep blood media or screened using one of the commercial rapid direct tests, which tests by extracting the streptococcus antigen and its recognition antibody (see below, and also Chapter 30).

Either selective or nonselective media is used. When grown in sheep blood agar, the specimen is transferred to the culture material by rolling the swab on the agar, then *streaking* the plate with a loop. In the streak plate method, the loop gently spreads the inoculum (specimen) in a pattern (Fig. 29–16) designed to dilute the inoculum by dragging less and less of the material over the medium with each pass. The loop is incinerated

Table 29–8
COMMONLY USED CULTURE MEDIA

Medium	Used to Isolate
Blood agar (BA)	Many organisms; generic medium
Chocolate agar (Choc)	*Neisseria; Haemophilus*
Phenylethyl alchohol agar (PEA)	Gram-positive organisms
MacConkey agar (Mac)	*Enterobacter* species; *Escherichia coli*
Thioglycollate broth (Thio broth)	Anaerobic microorganisms
Thayer-Martin agar	*Neisseria*
Eosin-methylene blue (EMB)	*Escherichia coli* in urine
Group A-selective streptococci agar	Group A streptococci in throat specimens

between each quadrant to avoid contamination from the previous pass.

The primary culture plate is inverted and incubated in a culture incubator. This allows moisture to collect on the plate lid instead of the agar. Excess moisture would interfere with colony growth. The primary culture is incubated for 24 hours under a controlled incubation temperature of 99°F (37°C).

After incubation, the organisms may be identified macroscopically by their characteristic colony growth.

For example, β-hemolytic streptococci produce zones of clear hemolysis around each colony, whereas α-streptococci colonies are surrounded by a green discoloration which is due to incomplete hemolysis of the sheep blood.

In addition to hemolysis detection, most bacteria grow in colonies that are specific in size, texture, color, and shape. For example, many gram-positive organisms present in urine have a specific appearance on EMB media. EMB promotes the growth of gram-negative organisms and inhibits that of gram-positive organisms. EMB also contains both eosin and methylene dyes. Acids produced by *Escherichia coli* organisms (normal flora in the intestines) and other gram-negative organisms react with the eosin, giving a metallic sheen to the media, while the methylene blue inhibits the growth of gram-positive organisms and gives gram-negative

Figure 29–15. Sterilize inoculating loops and needles in the flame of a Bunsen burner before and after each transfer of material. In order to avoid spattering live bacteria, (*A*) first insert the loop into the colorless cone in the center of the flame, which is cooler than the outer, blue portion. Any live bacteria are heat dried without splattering. (*B*) Then move the needle or loop into the hotter blue portion of the flame and hold it there until all the wire glows red. Allow the loop to cool before transferring specimen. (From Wedding MD and Toenjes SA: Medical Laboratory Procedures. FA Davis, Philadelphia, 1992, p. 359, with permission.)

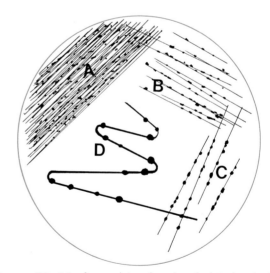

Figure 29–16. Agar plate showing isolated colonies. (*A*) First quadrant shows the growth of many microorganisms, with no isolated colonies. (*B*) Second quadrant shows thinning of microorganisms. (*C*) Third quadrant has a few isolated colonies. (*D*) Fourth quadrant has several isolated colonies. (From Wedding MD and Toenjes SA: Medical Laboratory Procedures. FA Davis, Philadelphia, 1992, p. 360, with permission.)

colonies a purple center. The result is a distinctive growth of colonies with a purple metallic sheen.

Even though the experienced physician or laboratory technician can tentatively diagnose an organism by macroscopic examination of the colonies present on the culture plate, the final diagnosis must be confirmed by isolating the organism in a pure culture or by examining it under the microscope.

CULTURE ISOLATION

The medical assistant should have general information about the procedure used to isolate and identify bacteria, even though this is usually done by the reference laboratory. The medical assistant needs to be able to understand and interpret information in laboratory culture reports. A *pure culture* is used for the following reasons:

1. To confirm or differentiate the contents of a primary culture by placing specific colonies in various selective media
2. To perform a special streaking technique for determining a colony count (the number of organisms present in infection)
3. To determine the susceptibility of a pathogen to antibiotics by sensitivity testing

This secondary culture is made by selecting one isolated pathogenic-appearing colony from the primary culture plate. The laboratory worker picks up a small inoculum of the first incubated specimen (one colony) and streaks it onto other Petri dishes containing media specific for the suspected specimen source and the test being performed.

The *streak plate* method promotes the isolation of pathogens by separating and thinning even further the organisms in the first isolated colony. The transference of the colony and streaking of the agar plate is done with an inoculating wire loop. The key in applying any method is to obtain isolated colonies of pathogens from normal flora on the primary culture.

As with a primary culture, isolation cultures are incubated at 99°F (37°C), allowing a *pure culture* to grow. The result should be a pure culture, meaning it only contains a single type of organism.

Although most organisms show a characteristic colony growth and expert clinicians can identify an organism by the macroscopic appearance of the colony, further identification of the organism is confirmed by using the pure culture to prepare special stains and by performing various biochemical tests. By observing the morphology and chemical characteristics present under the microscope, laboratory personnel can definitively identify the organism.

Control cultures should be used to test the quality of materials and techniques. Control cultures are available to check the accuracy and precision of testing procedures and of personnel who report gram-positive, gram-negative, anaerobic, and fungal strains.

SENSITIVITY TESTING

Once the organism has been isolated and identified, it is necessary to determine which antibiotic will have the greatest therapeutic effect. Sensitivity testing determines the susceptibility of an organism to specific antibiotics. The disk method is used routinely by most medical laboratories. A pure culture is used for sensitivity testing to be sure that only one type of organism will react with the antibiotic disks. A pure culture is placed on a Petri dish containing Mueller-Hinton agar. Antibiotic disks are placed on the agar, and the Petri dish is incubated overnight at 99°F (37°C). The size of the zone of growth inhibition, which is an area of clear medium around the disk where the organisms did not grow in the presence of a particular antibiotic, is measured to determine the degree of sensitivity of the organism to each particular antibiotic disk. The zone of most inhibition denotes the antibiotic to which the organism is most susceptible. The absence of a zone of inhibition means that the organism grew up to the antibiotic and is resistant to it (Fig. 29–17).

Automated susceptibility testing equipment, such as the Becton Dickinson & Co. Sensi-Disc System, uses automated dispensing techniques to identify the most effective antibiotic (Fig. 29–18). For this equipment to be cost-effective, large volumes of susceptibility tests must be done daily; for this reason, they are used mostly by hospitals and reference laboratories. After the most effective antibiotic is identified, the patient is started on drug therapy.

GROUP A STREPTOCOCCAL SCREEN

Instead of traditional manual growth bacteriology tests, many office laboratories use newer and faster, direct, non-growth-dependent, manual testing proce-

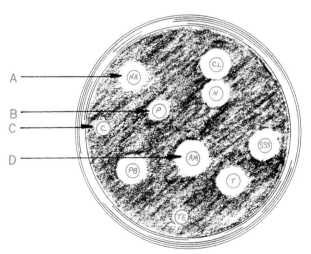

Figure 29–17. Antibiotic sensitivity (susceptibility) test. (*A*) Moderately sensitive. (*B*) Moderately sensitive. (*C*) Resistant. (*D*) Highly sensitive. (From Wedding MD and Toenjes SA: *Medical Laboratory Procedures.* FA Davis, Philadelphia, 1992, p. 398, with permission.)

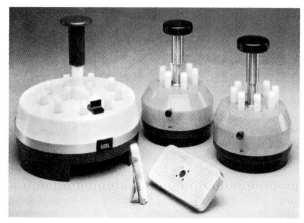

Figure 29–18. *Self-delivering dispenser system for antibiotic and antimicrobial sensitivity discs. (Courtesy Becton Dickinson & Company, Rutherford, NJ)*

dures. One type of rapid manual screening is the group A streptococcal screen. This is a frequently requested test in pediatric practices because children are especially susceptible to sore throats caused by group A β-hemolytic streptococci.

Most rapid screening tests are based on serologic detection using latex agglutination or enzyme immunoassay color-change tests (see Chapter 30). Enzyme tests are easier to interpret because a positive reaction is indicated by a visible color change. Compared with the 24 to 48 hours needed to obtain the result of a throat culture, these tests can be quickly run while the patient waits in the office. Antibiotic therapy can be initiated quickly if needed.

Several commercial kits are available. The kits are self-contained and include a self-contained testing station with a testing device, reagents, collection and dispensing tubes, and a procedural chart. The kits should be stored at room temperature. If group A streptococci are present in the specimen, a colored geometric shape (for example, a pink triangle) appears on the test device. The appearance of a second shape of a specified color (e.g., a pink circle) serves as an automatic control check that confirms proper execution of the test and the use of good reagents. If the test is performed incorrectly or the reagents are inactive, nothing will appear in the testing area.

WET PREPARATIONS AND POTASSIUM HYDROXIDE PREPARATIONS

A direct *wet saline mount* is prepared by placing a small inoculum on a clean dry glass slide. Wet preparations are usually used to detect simple vaginal infections, specifically trichomoniasis (caused by *Trichomonas vaginalis*). In addition to the saline preparation, potassium hydroxide (KOH) can be used as the wetting agent to diagnose moniliasis and bacterial vaginitis caused by the *Gardnerella* organism (*G. vaginalis*). For both males and females, the diagnosis is usually made

by observing the mobile organisms mounted on the slide from freshly voided urine, prostatic secretions, or vaginal fluids.

The specimen is rolled onto the slide with the collection swab. If the specimen is too thick, a drop of saline or water may be mixed on the slide with the specimen. A coverslip is then placed on the slide, and the organisms observed immediately under the microscope. The smear may be observed directly or with the aid of special stains used to enhance the morphologic characteristics of the organism. Preparations should be examined within 30 minutes of collection. All slides should be labeled first to avoid contact with the organisms.

SMEAR PREPARATIONS

A smear is a bacterial specimen that is placed on a glass slide, then dried, heat fixed, and stained. A direct smear is taken from the body with a collection swab (Fig. 29–19). A culture (indirect) smear is taken from a culture plate by transferring one colony (cluster of organisms) to the glass slide with an inoculating loop (Fig. 29–20). The material is applied thinly to aid in visualization under the microscope. Since most bacteria are colorless under the microscope, red and purple stains are applied to the specimen to aid viewing. The most commonly used staining technique is the Gram stain.

GRAM STAINING

The medical assistant must have a general knowledge of the principles involved in the Gram-staining technique. The Gram stain differentiates, or separates, bacteria into two groups: gram-positive and gram-negative. The purpose of any staining technique is to color the organism so its cell structure can be identified and studied. Although the actual principles involved in Gram staining are not fully understood, it is believed that an acid substance (magnesium ribonucleic acid) is present in all gram-positive organisms. This acid causes the Gram stain to adhere to and color the structures of

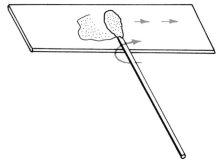

Figure 29–19. *Preparing a bacterial smear from a clinical specimen collected with a sterile swab (direct smear). (From Wedding MD and Toenjes SA: Medical Laboratory Procedures. FA Davis, Philadelphia, 1992, p. 372, with permission.)*

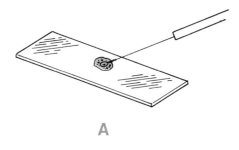

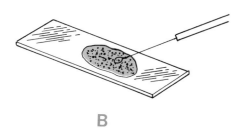

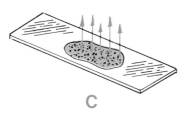

Figure 29–20. Preparing a bacterial smear from a culture plate (indirect smear). (**A**) Place two or three loopfuls of inoculum on a glass slide. (**B**) Spread the inoculum over a large area of the slide with the inoculation loop. (**C**) Allow the slide to air dry. (From Wedding MD and Toenjes SA: Medical Laboratory Procedures. FA Davis, Philadelphia, 1992, p. 371, with permission.)

specific organisms purple. If the color cannot be removed by an alcohol-acetone solution, the organism is identified as gram-positive. If the color is able to be removed by this solution, the organism is classified as gram-negative. (See Table 29–7 for a partial list of organisms defined by these Gram stain characteristics.)

A counterstain, safranin, is then used to stain the gram-negative organisms red.

Four basic steps are involved in gram staining: (1) smear preparation, (2) staining with crystal violet and iodine Gram's stain, (3) decolorization with alcohol-acetone solution, and (4) counterstaining with safranin. Gram-positive organisms appear deep purple; gram-negative organisms stain red. The procedure for performing a Gram stain is given at the end of this chapter.

Gram-Staining Precautions

Gram-positive bacteria may appear as gram-negative because of such factors as temperature, incubation time, age of the culture, and autolysis. The timing element of the Gram stain is critical and may change owing to the age of the reagents and individual techniques. Because many Gram stains may be misinterpreted, preliminary Gram stain results must be followed with culture and isolation techniques for macroscopic colony identification and confirmation.

SUMMARY

The type and amount of testing performed in the physician's office laboratory depends on the individual physician's diagnostic approach. Screening kits available today are less complicated and costly than those of the past. Nevertheless, the time, labor, and materials required for quality control can often offset the costs of these newer advances. Quality control measures must be performed daily to ensure reproducible laboratory tests and the quality of health care delivery. Quality control capabilities and CLIA restrictions play a part in deciding which tests and instruments are best suited and most cost-effective for a particular office laboratory.

The medical assistant who is responsible for specimen collection and office laboratory testing must clearly understand the basic concepts of laboratory medicine. This chapter has introduced the medical assistant to the various components of the routine urinalysis and basic bacteriologic tests. The medical assistant should stay current with the rapid technological advances in laboratory medicine and assist in establishing protocols for those tests performed in the physician's office laboratory. The medical assistant should also approach office laboratory testing as a challenging opportunity to work with the physician to improve and promote health care.

DISCUSSION QUESTIONS

1. During a patient's visit, you obtain a urine specimen and complete the test. Before leaving, the patient asks you what the results of the test are. What is your response?
2. In the examining room, you ask the patient to provide a midstream clean-catch urine sample. The patient insists that she cannot urinate at the moment and offers you a urine specimen that she had collected at home before coming to the office. What is your response?
3. After the patient hands you her midstream clean-catch urine sample, she asks you if you will be able to tell if she is pregnant. (The physician requested collection to assist in confirming or denying cystitis.) What is your response?

BIBLIOGRAPHY

Haber MH: A Primer of Microscopic Urinalysis. ICL Scientific, Fountain Valley, CA, 1978.

Hopp J, Rogers E: AIDS and the Allied Health Professions. FA Davis, Philadelphia, 1989.

Lane K (ed): Saunders Manual of Medical Assisting Practice. WB Saunders, Philadelphia, 1993.

Linne J, Ringsrud K: Basic Techniques in Clinical Laboratory Science, ed 3. St. Louis, Mosby Year Book, 1992.

Modern Urine Chemistry. Ames Division, Miles Laboratory, Elkhart, IN, 1991.

Physician's Office Laboratory Guidelines, Tentative Guidelines. National Committee for Clinical Laboratory Standards, Villanova, PA, 1989; 9(4) POL 1-T, 9(5) POL 2-T.

Sacher R: Widman's Clinical Interpretation of Laboratory Tests, ed 10. FA Davis, Philadelphia, 1990.

Schweitzer SS, Schumann JL, Schuman GB: Quality assurance guidelines for the urinalysis laboratory. J Med Technology 3:11, 1986.

Strasinger S: Urinalysis and Body Fluids, ed 2. FA Davis, Philadelphia, 1989.

Urinalysis Today, Boehringer Mannheim Diagnostics, Indianapolis, 1987.

PROCEDURE: Perform a physical examination of urine

OSHA STANDARDS:

Terminal Performance Objective: Examine and report the physical properties of urine.

EQUIPMENT: Universal precautions barriers, as necessary*
Nonsterile gloves
Disposable urine cup or container
Transfer pipette or eye dropper
Urinometer
Lens paper
Gauze and tissues
Towel for work surface
Detergent
Biohazard container

PROCEDURE

Color and Clarity

1. Mix the urine by gently swirling it in the test cylinder.
2. Label a standard-sized centrifuge tube.
3. Pour the specimen into the centrifuge tube and assess the color.
4. Assess the clarity.

Specific Gravity

Urinometer method:

1. Fill the urinometer cylinder two-thirds to two-fourths full with distilled water and check that the specific gravity is 1.000.
2. Fill the urinometer cylinder two-thirds to three-fourths full with urine.
3. If 20 to 25 mL of urine is not available label the test QNS (quantity not sufficient).
4. Float and spin the hydrometer in the urine.

5. While the float is slowly revolving, read the scale at eye level where it meets the lower curve of the urine meniscus.
6. Obtain a duplicate reading by repeating the procedure.
7. Dispose of the urine down a sewage drain and clean the urinometer with cold water and a mild detergent.
8. Remove gloves and dispose of them in a biohazard container.

Refractometer method:

1. Place a drop of distilled water on the refractometer prism and ensure that the reading is 1.000. Wipe off the distilled water with lens paper.
2. Using a Wintrobe pipette or an eye dropper, place a drop of urine on the refractometer prism.

PRINCIPLE

1. Substances in urine settle on standing.
2. Labeling first avoids contact with the specimen.
3. To record as straw, yellow, amber orange, red, blue-green, or brown, etc.
4. To record as clear, slightly cloudy, cloudy, very cloudy, or foamy, etc.

1. As a quality control check. If the hydrometer does not read 1.000, the room temperature may be the cause or a new hydrometer may be necessary.
2. To make the urinometer float, 20 to 25 mL of urine is necessary.
3. If the quantity of urine is not sufficient, an accurate specific gravity cannot be obtained by this method.
4. To keep the hydrometer from touching the sides of the cylinder.
5. Always read the meniscus at eye level on a flat surface. If the urine is too cloudy to read the meniscus, measure at the top of the urine and add 0.002 to the reading.
6. Two readings provide a quality control check. Record the reading to the nearest one thousandth (0.001).
7. Urine is a biohazardous body fluid. Dried urine salts on the equipment will affect the accuracy of future tests.
8. Gloves should remain on during the cleanup process. Used gloves are considered hazardous waste.

1. To calibrate the refractometer as a quality control. The boundary line should fall at 1.000, or the refractometer must be recalibrated by adjusting the calibration screw.
2. The prism will be used to measure the refractive index of the fluid.

---

*Because urine is not considered likely to transmit human immunodeficiency virus (HIV), urine examination is generally considered a category II task. However, gloves should be worn when handling all wet preparations. If any specimen is suspected of containing blood, the task is considered a category I task and gloves are required.

PROCEDURE

3. Point the instrument toward the light.
4. Rotate the eyepiece until the calibrated scale is in view and read the scale where the light and dark portion meet.
5. Clean the prism with lens paper.

PRINCIPLE

3. The light is refracted along the prism.
4. The denser a liquid, the less refractive the passage of light through the liquid.
5. To prevent scratching the glass.

PROCEDURE: Perform a chemical examination of urine

OSHA STANDARDS:

Terminal performance Objective: Test and report the chemical results in a routine urinalysis.

EQUIPMENT: Universal precautions barriers, as necessary*
Nonsterile gloves
Disposable urine cup or container
Reagent dipsticks
Stopwatch
Gauze and tissues
Towel for work surface
Detergent
Biohazard container

PROCEDURE

1. If the sample has been refrigerated, allow the sample to warm to room temperature.
2. Check the reagent container for the expiration date.

3. Take one strip out of the container and immediately close the container lid.
4. Compare the dry patches to the negative color blocks on the chart of the container.
5. Mix the urine by gently swirling.

6. Dip the reagent strip briefly into the urine and note the time on the stopwatch.
7. With a sharp tap, shake off excessive urine.

8. Hold the strip horizontally next to the corresponding color blocks and read each test at the appropriate time on the stopwatch as follows:
   At 30 seconds: glucose, bilirubin, phenylketonuria (Phenistix)
   At 40 seconds: ketone bodies
   At 45 seconds: specific gravity
   At 50 seconds: blood
   At 60 seconds: pH, protein, blood urobilinogen, and nitrite
   At 2 minutes: leukocytes
9. Record each result on the proper laboratory form as each test time occurs.
10. Dispose of the urine down a sewage drain and clean the test tube with cold water and a mild detergent.
11. Dispose of the reagent strip in a biohazard container.

12. Remove gloves and dispose of them in a biohazard container.

PRINCIPLE

1. The reagent patches are temperature-sensitive. Cold urine may produce false-negative results.
2. Reagent reactivity is altered by age, moisture, and chemical reactions
3. To prevent the strips from being exposed to environmental moisture, light, or heat.
4. To check for discolored patches that could produce false readings.
5. If settling occurs, certain elements may not be detected.
6. To moisten all the reagent patches but not leave the pads saturating for more than 1 second.
7. To keep excess urine from leaking from one pad to another.
8. Timing is critical in measuring the reactivity of each test. Any color changes that occur after 2 minutes should be considered invalid and not recorded.

9. To avoid forgetting readings as you move to the next timed test.
10. Urine is a biohazardous body fluid. Dried urine salts on the equipment will affect the accuracy of future tests.
11. Contaminated reagent strips are considered biohazardous waste.
12. Gloves should remain on during the cleanup process. Used gloves are considered hazardous waste.

---

*Because urine is not considered likely to transmit HIV, urine examination is considered a category II task. However, gloves should be worn when handling any wet preparation. If any specimen is suspected of containing blood, the task is considered a category I task and gloves are required.

PROCEDURE: Perform a microscopic examination of urine

OSHA STANDARDS:

Terminal Performance Objective: Examine and report the findings of a microscopic examination of urinary sediment.

EQUIPMENT:
Universal precautions barriers, as necessary
Centrifuge
Microscope
Nonsterile gloves
Disposable urine cup or container
Two centrifuge tubes
Transfer pipette or eye dropper
Sediment stain
Lens paper
Microscope slides and coverslips
Gauze and tissues
Towel for work surface
Detergent
Biohazard container
Biohazard sharps container

PROCEDURE

1. Label a clean microscope slide.
2. Gently mix the urine.
3. Pour 10 mL of well-mixed urine in a prelabeled centrifuge tube and place the tube in the urine centrifuge.
4. Pour 10 mL of water in a similar tube and place it in the centrifuge opposite the urine sample.
5. Secure the lid and centrifuge for the time and speed recommended by the manufacturer.
6. After the centrifuge has come to a full stop, remove the tube of urine.
7. Pour off the clear liquid at the top of the tube into a sewage drain.
8. Hold the tube upright and tap the bottom of the tube with the fingertips.
9. To stain, add 2 drops of stain to 1 drop of urine sediment, and mix by flicking the tube with the fingers.
10. Transfer 1 drop of urine to the microscope slide with a transfer pipette. Place a coverslip over the drop.
11. Focus under LPF and reduce the light.
12. Focus on an area of the slide edge, using the coarse adjustment, until the edge appears as a sharp, distinct line; then scan the entire coverslip for abnormal findings.
13. Examine five LPFs and count and classify (if possible) the types of casts, if any, and note mucus, if present.

14. For each type of cast, add the number of casts counted in each of the five LPFs. Divide that total by five to get the average. Record the total counted, the average, and the appropriate reporting range. For instance, an average of 5 red blood cells is reported as 5 to 10.

PRINCIPLE

1. Labeling first avoids contact with the specimen.
2. To resuspend any settled elements.
3. Reference values are based on a specific concentration of urine.
4. Centrifuges must be balanced.
5. Timing varies according to the speed and size of the centrifuge.
6. Stopping the rotations with the hand throws the sediment back into the liquid portion of the urine.
7. Only the heavier sediment at the bottom is viewed microscopically.
8. To resuspend the sediment in the remaining liquid.
9. Urine sediment is usually examined unstained, but staining may be helpful to the beginning microscopist.
10. This prepares a wet mount specimen for examination under the microscope.
11. Mucus and casts may be missed under bright light.
12. Casts tend to migrate to the edges of the coverslip.

13. Examine all four corners and the center of the coverslip. If nothing is viewed in any one of the five fields, record the field as zero.
14. REPORTING RANGES:

Normal (two per LPF)	Abnormal (three per LPF)
0 to 1	2 to 5
1 to 2	5 to 10
	10 to 20
	20 to 30
	30 to 40
	40 to 50
	More than 50

PROCEDURE	**PRINCIPLE**

PROCEDURE

15. Switch to the high-power objective and focus with the fine adjustment. Increase the intensity of the light source.

16. In five HPFs, count each of the following elements: red blood cells, white blood cells (red-blue nucleus with red cytoplasm, or unstained), and casts, including red blood cell casts, hemoglobin casts, hyaline casts, finely granular casts, and coarsely granular waxy casts.

    Add the number of each element counted in each of the five HPFs. Divide that total by five to get the average. Record that average in the appropriate reporting range. For each element, record the total counted, the average, and the reporting range.

17. Using the high-power lens, examine five fields and count, total, and average the number of round, transitional, and squamous epithelial cells. Record the total, average, and recording range for each type of epithelial cell.

18. Examine five HPFs and count, total, average, and record the number of crystals; rod-shaped bacteria; cocci-type bacteria; and miscellaneous elements, such as spermatozoa or parasites.

19. Dispose of the urine down a sewage drain and clean the test tube with cold water and a mild detergent.

20. Dispose of the slide and cover glass in a biohazard sharps container.

21. Remove gloves and dispose of them in a biohazard container.

PRINCIPLE

15. High-power magnification is necessary to see and count the smaller elements.

16. REPORTING RANGES:

Normal (two per HPF)	Abnormal (three per HPF)
0 to 1	2 to 5
1 to 2	5 to 10
	10 to 20
	20 to 30
	30 to 40
	40 to 50
	More than 50

17. RECORDING RANGES:

    0 = 0
    0 to 3 = occasional
    3 to 6 = few
    6 to 12 = moderate
    More than 12 = many
    For example, an average of four squamous epithelial cells would be recorded as "few."

18. REPORTING RANGES:

    Not seen in every field = occasional
    Cover less than one fourth of the field = moderate
    Cover entire field = many

19. Urine is a biohazardous body fluid. Dried urine salts on the equipment will affect the accuracy of future tests.

20. Urine is considered a biohazardous waste. Glass is considered a sharps containment material.

21. Gloves should remain on during the cleanup process. Used gloves are considered hazardous waste.

PROCEDURE: Obtain a throat specimen using the Culturette
System

OSHA STANDARDS:

Terminal Performance Objective: Obtain a throat specimen for transport or for isolation and identification of bacteria by culturing or rapid screening technique.

EQUIPMENT: Culturette or Culturette II Collection package
Sterile tongue depressor
Nonsterile gloves
Biohazard container

PROCEDURE

1. Don gloves. Explain the procedure to the patient. Peel the plastic tube from the envelope and pull the sterile swab out of the tube by holding the cap.
2. Depress the tongue with a sterile tongue depressor and firmly rotate the sterile swab directly on the back of the throat.

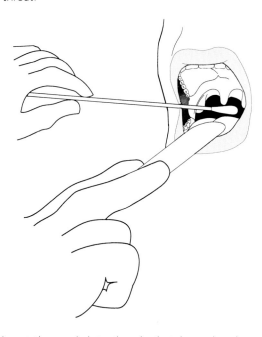

3. Insert the swab into the plastic tube and replace the cap.
4. Crush the ampule of holding medium.

5. Place the plastic tube in the envelope and staple the ends securely.
6. Complete the laboratory request form.

7. Remove gloves and dispose of them in a biohazard container. Wash hands.
8. Arrange for immediate transport of the culture or for a rapid screening test.

PRINCIPLE

1. Do not contaminate the sterile swab or touch the swab to any of the surfaces of the package.

2. Care must be taken to avoid contamination from the teeth, gums, tongue, or cheeks. Rotation of the swab on the infected area obtains a good specimen. White patches of exudate in the tonsillar area usually indicate the presence of streptococcal organisms.

3. Immediately placing the swab in the plastic tube prevents contamination.
4. The ampule contains 0.5 mL of modified Stuart's transport medium to prevent drying or deterioration of the specimen.
5. To prevent the plastic tube from falling out of the envelope during transport.
6. The form must be filled out with the patient's name, date, specimen, source, probable diagnosis, laboratory test requested, and a list of any medication that the patient is receiving.
7. Used gloves are considered hazardous waste.

8. Streptococcal organisms can survive on dry swabs for 2 to 3 hours. In a holding media, the organisms can survive for 24 to 48 hours if refrigerated.

PROCEDURE: Perform a gram stain*

OSHA STANDARDS:

Terminal Performance Objective: Prepare and stain a bacterial smear for microscopic classification based on the Gram stain reaction.

EQUIPMENT:
Universal precautions barriers, as necessary
Nonsterile gloves
3 inches × 1 inch (7.5 × 2.5 cm) microscope slides
Sterile cotton swabs or inoculating loop and saline
Patient specimen or bacterial culture
Wax pen
Diamond tip pen
Gauze and tissues
Forceps
Bunsen or alcohol burner
Gram stain reagents
    Crystal violet
    Gram's iodine
    Acetone alcohol
    Safranin
Staining rack and basin
Water in a squeeze bottle
Stopwatch
Bibulous blotting paper
Lens paper
Microscope
Immersion oil
Xylene
Towel for work surface
Biohazard container
Biohazard sharps container

PROCEDURE

Making the Direct Smear

1. Label a clean microscope slide with a diamond tip pen.

2. Obtain a swabbed specimen from the infected site on the patient.

3. Hold the slide between the thumb and index finger of your nondominant hand. Starting ½ inch (1.25 cm) from the thumb, roll the swab along the lower half of the slide's length, stopping ½ inch (1.25 cm) from the index finger. Make sure that the swab is always touching the slide as it rolls along.

PRINCIPLE

1. Labeling first avoids contact with the specimen. The marks made by the diamond tip will not wash off.

2. A direct smear is made from a swab of the infected area. If the same swab will be used to inoculate culture medium, inoculate the medium first. Once the swab has touched the slide, it must be considered contaminated.

3. The ½-inch (1.25 cm) allowance prevents contamination of the gloves. Keeping the swab in constant contact ensures that as much as possible of the inoculate is deposited on the slide.

---

*Illustrations in this procedure are adapted from Wedding ME and Toenjes SA: Medical Laboratory Procedures. FA Davis, Philadelphia, 1992, p 383, with permission.

PROCEDURE

4. Turn the slide 180°, so that the smeared half of the slide is at the top, and roll the swab along the untreated bottom half of the slide. Roll from index finger to thumb, leaving a ½ inch (1.25 cm) space at either end of the slide.

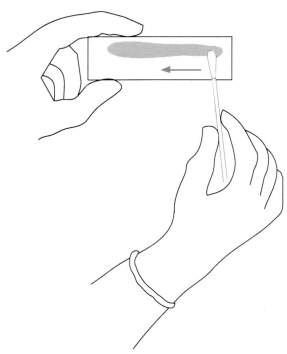

After rolling the swab along the bottom half of the slide, rotate the slide 180° and roll the swab in the opposite direction on the unsmeared half, which is now on the bottom.

5. Allow the slide to air dry for 20 to 30 minutes.

6. Discard the swab in a biohazard container.
7. Remove gloves and dispose of them in a biohazard container.

Making a Culture Smear

1. Label a clean microscope slide with a diamond tip pen.

2. Select the colony to be lifted from the culture plate and label the colony by circling the area on the back of the plate with a wax pencil.
3. Number the circled area, then label the slide area to be used with the same number using a diamond-tip pen. If multiple smears are to be made, number each smear site at the same time.

4. Incinerate the loop before and after each transfer of material.

5. Put a small drop of saline solution on the slide with a loop.
6. Touch only the top of the colony chosen with the loop and transfer the specimen to the slide.
7. Spread the specimen in a circular motion from the center outward. The smear should be about the same diameter as a dime.

PRINCIPLE

4. Thin smears are best for microscopic examination. This two-step smear method allows the maximal transfer of microorganisms from swab to slide.

5. Waving the slide would distort the distribution of organisms; heating would distort the cells.
6. Microorganisms are considered hazardous waste.
7. Used gloves are considered hazardous waste.

1. Labeling first avoids contact with the specimen. The marks made by the diamond tip pen will not wash off.
2. To ensure accurate identification of the colony being examined under the microscope.

3. If multiple smears are made on one slide, each smear can be matched to its corresponding colony on the culture plate. All sites are numbered in advance to avoid touching the slide once the microorganisms are applied.

4. The loop must be sterilized before and after touching any materials or colonies and at the end of the procedure.

5. Liquid is need to emulsify the colony growth.

6. The colony is a very concentrated area of microorganism growth. Not much of the colony is needed.

7. To ensure an even distribution of the organisms.

PROCEDURE

8. Repeat the procedure for any other colonies chosen.

9. Allow the slide to air dry for 20 to 30 minutes.

10. Replace the culture plate in the incubator until the examination is complete.

11. Remove gloves and dispose of them in a biohazard container.

Fixing the Smear

1. Grasp the slide with forceps or hold the slide at its ends between the thumb and forefinger.
2. Hold the slide with the specimen up and pass the slide through a Bunsen or alcohol flame so that the flame travels the length of the slide.
3. Pass through the flame in 1 to 2 seconds. Repeat this step three to four times.

4. Touch the back of the slide to ensure that the slide is warm.

5. Allow the slide to cool.

Staining the Smear

1. Place the slide on the staining rack, smear side up.

2. Flood the slide with crystal violet and let stand for 30 seconds.

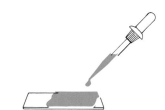

Flood the slide with crystal violet.

3. Use forceps to hold the slide at about a 45-degree angle and wash the stain off with a strong stream of water from the squeeze bottle.

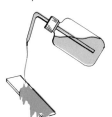

Wash the violet off with water.

PRINCIPLE

8. Up to three colonies can be examined. Be sure to keep each smear site ½ inch from any other site.
9. Waving the slide would distort the distribution of organisms; heating would distort the cells.
10. The culture plate must be carefully handled until the physician gives the order to have it disposed of in a biohazard container.
11. Used gloves are considered hazardous waste.

1. To prevent being burned as the slide is brought down until the flame hits it close to the fingers.
2. After a smear is dried, it must be fixed; otherwise it will wash off during the staining procedure.

3. The object of fixing is to gel slightly the protoplasm of the cells so that they adhere to the slide. Even this small amount of heat distorts the cells by shrinkage.
4. Apply only enough heat to ensure the slide is warm, not hot. Excess heat will distort the organisms and destroy the specimen.
5. A warm slide would prevent proper staining.

1. The staining rack is designed to collect the staining fluids. **Note:** Unless the slide was heat-fixed, treat it as potentially infectious.
2. Crystal violet is the primary stain, staining all material purple.

3. To stop the staining process and wash the crystal violet from the slide.

PROCEDURE

4. Put the slide on the rack and flood the slide with Gram's iodine. Let stand for 60 seconds.

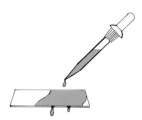

Flood the slide with Gram's iodine.

5. Use forceps to hold the slide at about a 45° angle and wash the stain off with a strong stream of water from the squeeze bottle.

6. Use forceps to hold the slide at about a 90° angle and flood the slide with alcohol. Let the alcohol run down the slide until the violet stain no longer discolors the alcohol running off the slide (about 10 seconds).

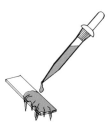

Flood the slide with alcohol, keeping up the flow of alcohol until the violet stain no longer flows from the slide.

7. Wash the slide with water and replace it on the staining rack.

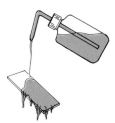

Stop the decolorizing effect of alcohol by washing it with water.

8. Flood the slide with safranin and let it stand for 60 seconds.

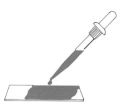

Flood the side with safranin, which stains the decolorized, gram-negative organisms red.

PRINCIPLE

4. Gram's iodine is the mordant stain that combines with crystal violet to set the purple stain in organisms that are gram-positive. The stain in these organisms now will not wash away.

5. To stop the staining process and wash the Gram iodine from the slide.

6. The alcohol acts as a decolorizer that washes away the purple stain from the gram-negative organisms.

7. To stop the decolorizing process and wash the alcohol from the slide.

8. Safranin is the counterstain that will stain the decolorized, or gram-negative, cells a red color.

PROCEDURE

9. Wash the slide with water and wipe dry the back of the slide with an alcohol tissue.

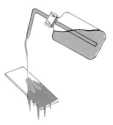

Wash the slide with water one last time.

10. Blot the slide dry or allow it to air dry in a vertical position.

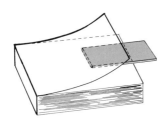

Blot the slide with bibulous paper.

11. Discard the blotter tissue in a biohazard container.
12. Discard the used stains down a sewage drain with plenty of running tap water.
13. Remove gloves and dispose of them in a biohazard container.

Examining Gram-stained Smears

1. Focus the area to be examined under the low-power objective.

2. Place a drop of immersion oil on the slide area to be examined.
3. Focus using the oil-immersion objective with the condenser up and the diaphragm open.
4. Observe that the cells and background look pink or red.
5. Examine the slide, looking for Gram's reaction and cell morphology of any bacteria present, also noting the presence of any white blood cells, yeast, or epithelial cells. Look for and report groupings.
6. Save the smear for review by the physician.

7. Remove the oil from the slide by blotting it with lens paper and xylene.
8. If the slide is not to be kept, discard the slide in a biohazard sharps container.

9. Remove gloves and dispose of them in a biohazard container.

PRINCIPLE

9. To stop the staining process and wash the safranin excess from the slide. Stain on the back of the slide would make microscopic visualization difficult.

10. Wiping could rub off the stains.

11. Microorganisms are considered hazardous waste.
12. The stains have been contaminated with living bacteria.
13. Used gloves are considered hazardous waste.

1. To bring the specimen into view using the coarse adjustment. The microscope can be focused on the line made by the wax pencil.
2. Bacteria can be identified only using the oil-immersion objective.
3. To clear the image using the fine adjustment knob and adding light as needed.
4. If the predominant color is purple, the slide was not decolorized enough.
5. Do not identify bacteria by genus and species name based on smear observation alone. For a positive diagnosis, the organisms must be cultured and examined by the physician or trained laboratory personnel.
6. The physician or a trained laboratory person will identify the organism by genus and species, depending on the smear, the bacterial growth on the media, and the patient's clinical signs and symptoms.
7. Xylene is an oil solvent.

8. Unless the slide was heat-fixed using a heat block, treat it as potentially infectious. Glass should be placed in a sharps container.
9. Used gloves are considered hazardous waste.

CHAPTER OUTLINE

LEARNING OBJECTIVES

Upon completing this chapter, you will be able to:

1. Identify the composition of blood and list its three cellular elements.
2. Delineate the parameters of a complete blood count.
3. Identify two types of automated cell counting systems generally used in hematology.
4. Discuss the principles of serology testing as applied to antigen-antibody reactions.
5. List and describe at least three general methods for most assays in clinical chemistry.

Chapter 30

*T*he Physician's Office Laboratory: Part III

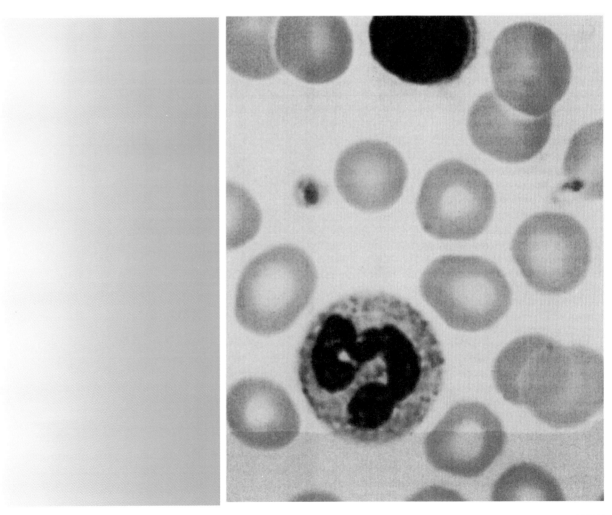

6. Describe the various processes used in the different types of rapid manual serology test kits.
7. List the specimen collection and storage requirements for each hematology and blood chemistry test listed in this chapter and for blood glucose testing.

PERFORMANCE OBJECTIVES

Upon completing this chapter, you will be able to:

1. Determine the hematocrit by comparing the amount of packed red blood cells with the total blood volume.
2. Determine the concentration of cyanmethemoglobin in grams per deciliter (100 mL) of blood.
3. Determine the number of white blood cells in thousands per microliter (1 μL) of blood.
4. Determine the number of red blood cells in thousands per microliter (1 μL) of blood.
5. Determine what percentage of the total leukocyte count each type of white blood cell represents, evaluate the morphology of RBCs, and estimate the number of platelets per microliter of blood.

DACUM EDUCATIONAL COMPONENTS

1. Apply procedures of aseptic technique and infection control (4.1).
2. Use quality control (4.9).
3. Collect and process specimens (4.10).
4. Screen and follow up patient test results (4.12).
5. Document accurately (5.1).
6. Operate and maintain facilities and equipment safely (6.2).

Glossary

Agglutination: clumping together of cells
Antibody: substance produced in response to a specific antigen
Antigen: foreign substance whose presence in the body stimulates the body's immune response
Batch-test analyzer: instrument designed for one type of test to be performed on a group of specimens
Coagulation: process by which blood clots
Enzyme: complex protein capable of inducing a chemical change and speeding up chemical reactions without itself being structurally changed
Erythropoiesis: development of erythrocytes
Hemagglutination: clumping together of red blood cells
Hematopoiesis: production and development of the cellular element of blood
Leukopoiesis: development of leukocytes
Packed cell volume: volume of packed red blood cells compared by percentage to the total blood volume (hematocrit)
pH: measurement of the acidity or alkalinity of a solution
Partial prothrombin time (PTT): screening test for coagulation disorders used to monitor heparin therapy
Polymorphonuclear (PMN) cell: granular leukocyte that has a segmented nucleus; a neutrophil
Prothrombin time (PT): screening test for coagulation disorders used to monitor anticoagulant (coumarin) therapy
Qualitative test: relating to quality, the clinical analysis for the presence or absence of a substance
Quantitative test: relating to quantity, the clinical analysis for the specific amount of a substance
Standard solution: solution containing a known value
Thrombopoiesis: development and production of platelets
Wright's stain: eosin and methylene blue stain used for differential counts

This laboratory chapter discusses the basic specialty areas of hematology, serology, and clinical chemistry.

Hematology is the study and testing of blood cell components and some of their constituents. These tests represent the most commonly performed procedures in routine blood testing. Most procedures are performed on anticoagulated venous blood or capillary whole blood specimens.

Clinical chemistry is perhaps the most complicated division of laboratory testing, an area of study that is constantly changing and growing. *Clinical chemistry* is the quantitative analysis of glucose, electrolytes, nonprotein nitrogen compounds, bilirubin, and enzymes; it also includes drug testing. Most of these tests are performed on serum or plasma.

Serology is a division of immunology that detects and measures specific antibodies that develop in the blood serum as a result of antigen-antibody reactions. Some antigen-antibody reactions may be detected in other body fluids, such as the urine or bacterial smears; therefore, a discussion of a few of these tests is included in Chapter 28 rather than here. Serology techniques are used to test for syphilis, streptococcal infections, rubella infections, infectious mononucleosis, rheumatoid conditions, and pregnancy.

COMPOSITION OF BLOOD

Blood is composed of two major parts: the cellular, or formed elements, and the plasma (Fig. 30–1).

The plasma consists of water, blood proteins, salts, and immune substances necessary for the body's protection. As the fluid portion of the blood, plasma also contains the substances that it transports — specifically, blood gases, food nutrients, hormones, and waste products. Plasma is composed of approximately 90% water and 10% solid matter.

The largest group of substances circulating in the plasma are the plasma proteins: serum albumin, globulins, fibrinogen, and prothrombin. Serum albumin regulates plasma volume and water balance between the blood and tissues, and gives viscosity to the blood, which in turn regulates blood pressure. Serum globulins are important to antibody formation — the reaction of blood to toxins formed by bacteria and other foreign proteins — and to the functioning of the immune system. Fibrinogen and prothrombin are essential for blood clotting.

The plasma carries sodium, chloride, potassium, calcium, phosphate, bicarbonate, and magnesium, which are the electrolytes that maintain the fluid and acid-base balance of the body. Nutrients carried by the plasma include glucose, amino acids, and lipids. Amino acids are the building blocks for all proteins found in the body. Waste products circulating in the plasma and carried to the organs of excretion consist of urea, uric acid, lactic acid, and creatinine. Respiratory gases include carbon dioxide and oxygen. Hormones, antibodies, enzymes, and vitamins regulate and control the overall functions of the body.

When the formed cells and the blood-clotting proteins (fibrinogen and prothrombin) are separated from the plasma, a yellowish fluid remains which is called *serum.* When a blood sample is allowed to stand, serum can be separated. This occurs because the chemical substances essential for blood clotting interact and separate in the plasma to form a clot.

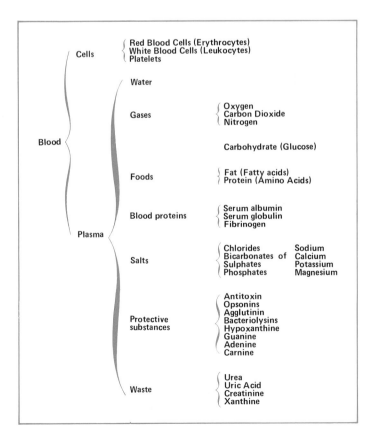

Figure 30–1. The constituents of human blood.

The cellular elements are divided into red blood cells, white blood cells, and platelets (thrombocytes). A discussion of each of these constituents of blood follows.

RED BLOOD CELLS

Most of the cells in the blood are red blood cells. There are approximately 5 million red blood cells in a speck of blood about the size of the head of a pin. Red blood cells are responsible for the exchange of oxygen in the body and the maintenance of the acid-base balance.

During erythropoiesis, red blood cells are formed in the bone marrow. The erythrocyte develops from a rubriblast into a metarubricyte, then into a reticulocyte, and finally into an erythrocyte (Fig. 30–2).

The hemoglobin (Hb) in red blood cells is responsible for the transport of the body's oxygen, carbon dioxide, and other body wastes. Hb is made from *heme,* an iron-containing substance, and *globin,* a protein.

WHITE BLOOD CELLS

There are five types of white blood cells: neutrophils, eosinophils, basophils, lymphocytes, and monocytes. Neutrophils, basophils, and eosinophils are called *granulocytes.* Granulocytes phagocytize (engulf and digest) bacteria, detoxify blood of foreign substances, and play a vital role in the mechanisms required for the resolution of inflammation. The *nongranular* leukocytes are the lymphocytes and monocytes. Lymphocytes function primarily in antibody production, and monocytes play a different type of role in phagocytizing bacteria. The following morphologic descriptions of the various white blood cells are divided into the granulocytic and nongranulocytic types.

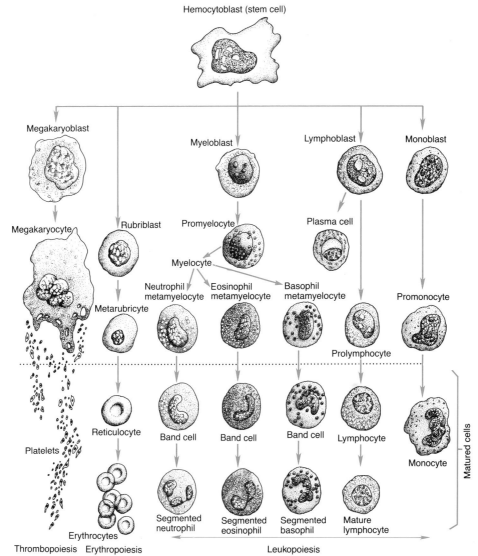

Figure 30–2. Hematopoiesis—the maturation of blood cells. (From Gylys B and Wedding ME: *Medical Terminology: A Systems Approach,* ed 2. FA Davis, Philadelphia, 1978, p. 175, with permission.)

Granulocytic White Blood Cells

Granulocytic development involves the progression of the white blood cell from myeloblast to promyelocyte to myelocyte to metamyelocyte to band cells (see Fig. 30–2). At this point, the granular cells can develop into one of the following types of matured white blood cells:

1. *Neutrophils* function in phagocytosis by killing bacteria. They also release pyrogens which cause fever. Neutrophils may be elevated by physical or emotional stress, acute infections with suppuration, trauma, ketoacidosis, and myelocytic leukemia. Neutrophils may be decreased in aplastic anemia, chemotherapy, dietary deficiency, and severe bacterial infection, especially in the elderly.
2. *Basophils* release chemicals that assist the body in coping with allergies and exaggerated immune responses such as anaphylaxis.
3. *Eosinophils* function in the phagocytosis of antigen-antibody complexes and the killing of parasites. Eosinophil counts are increased in parasitic infections, allergic reactions, eczema, autoimmune diseases, and leukemia. Eosinophils may be decreased in patients with increased adrenocorticosteroid production.

Nongranular White Blood Cells

The formation and development of nongranular white blood cells involves the progression from the immature blast stage through the intermediate stages (prolymphocyte, promonocyte) to the matured circulating lymphocyte and monocyte (see Fig. 30–2).

1. *Lymphocytes* are classified into two groups: B lymphocytes, which produce specific antibodies against viruses, bacteria, and other proteins; and T lymphocytes, which regulate the immune response by such functions as delaying allergic reactions and graft or transplant rejection (Fig. 30–3). T lymphocytes may be helper cells that enhance the activity of other leukocytes, or suppressor cells that suppress the immune (antibody) response and destroy infected cells. Lymphocytes may be elevated in chronic bacterial infection, viral infection, infectious mononucleosis, lymphocytic leukemia, and multiple myeloma. Lymphocytes may be decreased in sepsis and in immunodeficiency diseases, such as AIDS; in leukemia; and in patients taking chemotherapeutic drugs.
2. *Monocytes* function in phagocytosis by ingesting microorganisms and removing cell debris.

PLATELETS

Platelets, or thrombocytes, are disk-shaped, nonnucleated structures that form the smallest of the formed elements in blood. They are formed in the red bone marrow by fragmentation or megakaryocytes (see Fig. 30–2) and average about 250,000 per μL of blood. Platelets assist in blood coagulation and clotting. Platelets function either to accelerate the coagulation process in fibrin-fibrinogen reactions or to form the jelly-like substance that is the clot. Platelets tend to adhere to uneven or damaged surfaces. When a blood vessel is damaged, platelets form and adhere to the break, forming a plug in the vessel wall and eventually sealing off the leak.

Abnormally high platelet counts occur in the presence of malignancy, splenectomy, asphyxiation, polycythemia vera, and acute infections. Low platelet counts result from thrombocytopenia purpura, pernicious ane-

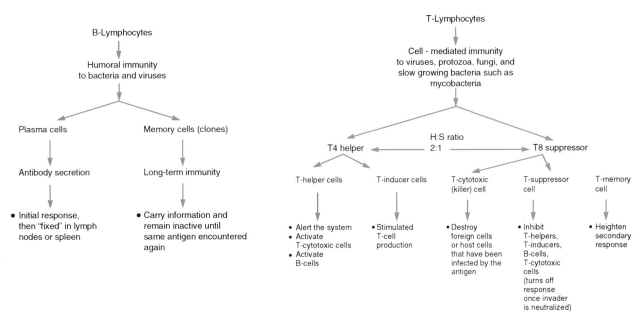

Figure 30–3. Both kinds of lymphocyte have important functions in the immune response.

mia, allergic conditions; during cancer chemotherapy; and on taking certain drugs.

HEMATOLOGY

The entire range of human diseases can be examined in hematology. Often, hematology testing by itself can lead to a diagnosis; in other cases, it can be a major contributor to a final diagnosis. Abnormal blood composition can indicate specific hematologic disease conditions or can denote hematologic changes secondary to the malfunction of any of the body's systems.

Most hematology specimens are obtained by venipuncture or capillary puncture. Because venipuncture and capillary puncture are convenient procedures to perform, blood tests are a frequently ordered diagnostic aid. The medical assistant student should review the techniques for venipuncture, capillary puncture, specimen handling, and the approaches to the patient in general before performing any of the tests presented in this chapter (see Chapter 28).

A *complete blood count* (CBC) is the number of blood cells (red blood cells, white blood cells, and platelets) in a given sample of blood, usually expressed as the number of cells in a microliter (μL) of blood. Each blood component can be counted separately, but collectively they comprise the complete blood count, as follows:

1. Red blood cell count (RBC) and morphology
2. White blood cell count (WBC) and differential count
3. Platelet estimate
5. Hb determination
5. Hematocrit (Hct)
6. Mean corpuscular volume (MCV)
7. Mean corpuscular hemoglobin concentration (MCHC)

A *differential* WBC determines the number and percentage of each type of white blood cell contained in a blood specimen. A CBC with differential count is one of the most common hematology tests performed on the blood.

The medical assistant should have a listing of normal hematology reference values and common hematology abbreviations available for each referencing (Tables 30–1 and 30–2). The physician must be alerted immediately to any deviations from the normal range. Normal value ranges can differ slightly depending on the testing methods used. When using normal values, it is important to know not only what test was performed but also what method was used.

BLOOD COLLECTION

Blood is collected by standard venipuncture technique. (See Chapter 28.) Most hematologic tests are performed on whole blood. Five to seven milliliters of blood is collected in a lavender-top Vacutainer tube

Table 30–1

NORMAL ADULT HEMATOLOGY VALUES

Hematocrit	Men: 40–54% Women: 38%–47%
Hemoglobin	Men: 13.5–18.0 g/d Women: 12.0–16.0 g/d
Red blood cells per microliter	Men: 4.6–6.2 × 10⁶/μL Women: 4.2–5.4 × 10⁶/μL
White blood cells	4.5–11.0 × 10³/μL
Differential count, adult (%)	Neutrophils 52–64 Eosinophils 1–4 Monocytes 2–6 Basophils 0–1 Lymphocytes 25–35
Mean corpuscular volume	80–96 fl
Mean corpuscular hemoglobin	27–31 pg
Mean corpuscular hemoglobin concentration	32%–36%
Platelets	150,000–400,000/μL
Erythrocyte sedimentation rate, Modified Westergren method, in millimeter per hour	Men below age 50: 1–15 Men above age 50: 1–20 Women below age 50: 1–20 Women above age 50: 1–30
Reticulocytes	0.5%–1.5%

treated with ethylenediaminetetracetic acid (EDTA) or a capillary specimen may be obtained for some individual tests by using an Autolet and the Microtainer or Unopette systems (all by Becton Dickinson & Co, Rutherford, NJ).

Microtainers are special capillary blood collectors for simplified, single-tube capillary punctures. These tubes are ready for use in the centrifuge and eliminate the problem of clogged capillary tubes. Microtainers are available as plain tubes, tubes with EDTA preservatives, or serum-separator tubes (Fig. 30–4).

THE UNOPETTE SYSTEM

If undiluted blood were examined, the cells would be too numerous to count accurately, the blood would clot, and the red blood cells would break down. The blood sample, therefore, is first diluted with a suitable solution in a blood-diluting pipette. Older methods included the use of reusable glass pipettes, such as the Thoma red blood cell and white blood cell pipettes. These reusable glass pipettes consist of a calibrated stem for aspirating blood and diluting fluid, an enlarged bulb with a mixing bead where the blood sample is mixed with the diluting fluid, and a short stem to which rubber tubing and a mouthpiece or an aspirating bulb is attached.

Table 30–2

COMMON HEMATOLOGY ABBREVIATIONS

Abbreviation	Meaning
Band	a band-shaped immature granulocyte
Baso	basophil
Coag	coagulation
CBC	complete blood count (usually includes Hb, Hct, WBC, RBC, MCV, MCH, MCHC)
Diff	differential leukocyte count of peripheral blood
EDTA	ethylenediaminetetraacetic acid (a common blood anticoagulant)
Eos	eosinophilic leukocyte
ESR	erythrocyte sedimentation rate
Hgb, Hb	hemoglobin
Hct	hematocrit or packed cell volume
LE	lupus erythematosus
Leukocyte	white blood cell
Lymph	a type of leukocyte
MCH	mean corpuscular hemoglobin
MCHC	mean corpuscular hemoglobin concentration
MCV	mean corpuscular volume
MONO	monocyte
MPV	mean platelet volume
PLT	platelet
PMN (polys)	polymorphonuclear leukocyte (neutrophil)
PT	prothrombin time
PTT	partial thromboplastin time
RBC	red blood count
Segs	segmented polymorphonuclear neutrophil leukocyte (polys)
Retic	reticulocyte
Stab	a band
WBC	white blood (leukocyte) count

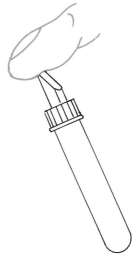

Figure 30–4. Peripheral blood sample collected in a micro blood collection tube; the tube is ready for transport or centrifugation. (From Wedding ME and Toenjes SA: Medical Laboratory Procedures. F A Davis, Philadelphia, 1992, p. 205, with permission.)

The Centers for Disease Control (CDC) universal precautions, however, have banned the method of mouth pipetting, and automatic pipetting systems or the disposable blood-diluting units, such as the Unopette System (see Fig. 28–15), are replacing the Thoma pipetting technique. Automatic pipetters and Unopettes automatically draw the correct amount of sample without mouth pipetting.

Unopettes are also designed for the preparation of micro blood specimens. As with other Unopette types, this is a single-use, self-contained collection and diluting unit with a reservoir containing a premeasured amount of diluting fluid (Fig. 30–5). Different Unopettes are available for counting red blood cells, white blood cells, and platelets, and for performing hemoglobin testing. They are available for automatic and man-

ual cell counting. Each type of Unopette contains its own specific diluting fluid or reagent for directions.

Red blood cells are destroyed by solutions not isotonic (having equal osmotic pressure) to blood plasma. If the red blood cell is placed in a solution more dilute than plasma (such as water), the red blood cell swells and bursts. If the red blood cell is placed in a solution more concentrated than plasma, the cell loses water and shrivels (crenate). For this reason, the diluting fluid for red blood cells is a physiologic saline solution, which will keep the red cells from breaking down during testing. Red blood cell Unopettes contain 1.99 mL of 0.85% saline solution in a 10-mL pipette for a 1 : 200 dilution. White blood cell Unopettes, on the other hand, contain 1.98 mL of 3% acetic acid in a 20-mL pipette (1 : 100 dilution) or 0.475 mL of 3% acetic acid in a 25-mL pipette (1 : 20 dilution). Acetic acid (or 0.1 normal hydrochloric acid) destroys red blood cells while preserving white blood cells. To perform a WBC and platelet count on a single blood sample, a 20-mL pipette containing 1.98 mL of 1% ammonium oxalate is used.

Unopettes have the advantage over older blood-diluting pipettes in that they eliminate the need for mouth pipetting, storage of diluting chemicals, and cleaning. They also provide standardized procedures for collection, pipetting, and dilution. Disposable tests have premeasured, prefilled reagent reservoirs that provide accurate dilutions with minimal handling.

See the procedure at the end of this chapter for a step-by-step description of this process.

HEMATOCRIT DETERMINATION

The Hct, or packed cell volume (PCV), is the percentage, after a sample has been centrifuged, of packed red blood cells as compared with the total blood volume.

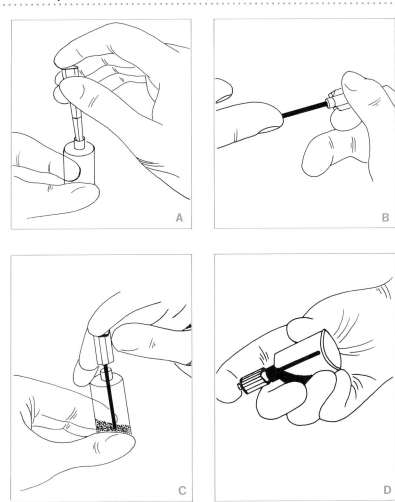

Figure 30–5. The Unopette system allows blood collection and the mixing of the sample with a premeasured diluting fluid. (**A**) Use the shield of the capillary pipette to puncture the diaphragm of the reservoir. (**B**) Fill the capillary with peripheral blood from a finger stick. (**C**) After gently squeezing the reservoir to force out some air (do not expel any liquid), insert the pipette into the reservoir, while covering the opening at the overflow end of the pipette with your index finger. When the pipette is securely inserted in the reservoir, stop squeezing and take your finger off the overflow end of the pipette; the blood will flow into the reservoir. Then squeeze and release the reservoir several times to rinse the bore of the pipette, taking care not to expel any liquid. (**D**) Cover the opening of the pipette overflow chamber with your index finger and gently invert the unit several times in order to thoroughly mix sample with diluent. (From Wedding ME and Toenjes SA: Medical Laboratory Procedures. FA Davis, Philadelphia, 1992, p. 256, with permission.)

There is a direct relationship between the hemoglobin concentration of a blood sample (see p. 803) and its Hct value. The Hct value should be approximately three times the hemoglobin reading, plus or minus two. For example, if the hemoglobin reading were 15 g, the hematocrit value should be 45%, with a range of 43% to 47%.

Anticoagulated blood is spun in a centrifuge to find the hematocrit value. Venous blood is drawn into a lavender EDTA tube, then transferred to a capillary tube for centrifugation. When anticoagulated venous blood is first collected in an EDTA Vacutainer tube, plain blue-tip microhematocrit capillary tubes are used.

Capillary blood may be used for the micromethod, or microhematocrit. To run a microhematocrit, the laboratorian fills two special red-tip capillary hematocrit tubes with blood directly from the puncture site. Two tubes are always run, to provide a backup test and to balance the centrifuge. The inner surface of the red-tipped tube is coated with ammonium heparin as an anticoagulant.

Seal the microhematocrit tube with capillary tube sealant (Fig. 30–6). After sealing, the two samples are centrifuged for 3 to 5 minutes at high speed in a micro-hematocrit centrifuge. The centrifuged sample will be layered: packed red blood cells will be at the bottom then, moving upward, the buffy coat layer and the plasma layer on top (Fig. 30–7). The reading of the volume of packed red blood cells is accomplished by lining up the layers on various scale markings as directed on hematocrit reader cards. Two types of micro-hematocrit readers are available; circular and columnar (Fig. 30–8).

Blood collected for a microhematocrit should be fresh, anticoagulated, and unhemolyzed. Duplicate tests should agree within 2%. Sources of error include poor venipuncture technique, such as leaving on the tourniquet too long, puncturing the vein more than twice, or otherwise hemolyzing the specimen during blood collection; inadequate skin puncture; too little or too much mixing with the anticoagulant in the EDTA tube; overfilling or underfilling the capillary tube; or failing to seal the tube with a tight clean plug. Hemolysis colors the plasma layer pink to red and must be reported with the results.

See the procedure at the end of this chapter for a step-by-step description of this process.

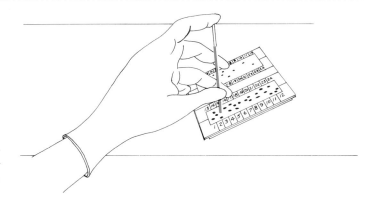

Figure 30–6. Sealing the capillary tube with sealing clay. (From Wedding ME and Toenjes SA: Medical Laboratory Procedures. FA Davis, Philadelphia, 1992, p. 229, with permission.)

ERYTHROCYTE SEDIMENTATION RATE

The erythrocyte sedimentation rate (ESR) is the distance that red blood cells settle out in a column of *anticoagulated, noncentrifuged* blood during a 1-hour period. As the blood sits, the red blood cells settle and separate from the plasma. An elevated ESR is an indicator of increased plasma proteins and inflammatory conditions. It is used in adults to monitor rheumatoid arthritis and in pediatric patients to indicate acute infections.

Three basic methods are used for determining the ESR: the Wintrobe, Westergren, and zeta sedimentation rate (ZSR). All use anticoagulated blood specimens.

The specimen is collected in a lavender (EDTA) tube. The Wintrobe method uses a special Wintrobe sedimentation tube and transfer pipette. With the pipette, the tube is filled with blood to the O-mm mark, and the tube is placed in a vertical rack (Fig. 30–9) for exactly 60 minutes. The erythroycte column is read in millimeters per hour. The measurement is taken by reading the number at the point where the RBC meniscus crosses the scale (Fig. 30–10).

Quality control measures using known specimens are not available. *Parallel testing* is recommended. In parallel testing, a specimen is divided in half, and two separate facilities perform the analysis.

Sources of error when performing an ESR include an incorrect ratio of anticoagulant to blood; samples older than 2 hours at room temperature or 6 hours in refrigeration, or samples not at room temperature when the test is performed; bubbles in the tube; equipment not level; or damaged tubes or equipment.

HEMOGLOBIN DETERMINATION

Hemoglobin tests measure the concentration of Hb in the blood. Hb is recorded in grams (g) per 100 mL of blood. Normal values for men are approximately 13 to 18 g/100 mL; for women 12 to 16 g/mL. The Hg determination test is used to screen the severity of anemia and to monitor the patient's response to anemia treatment.

Hemoglobin testing can be performed on either venous or capillary whole blood specimens. Venous blood is drawn into tubes containing an anticoagulant, preferably EDTA (lavender tube). Blood that is drawn for Hb study in an EDTA tube can be stored at room temperature for up to 1 week.

There are many methods for Hb determination. The Sahli, Tallequest, and Dare methods are based on the visual matching of sample colors with a standard. This visual color comparison is not reliable because it is difficult for the eye to accurately estimate color intensity.

The cyanmethemoglobin method is more reliable and uses a photoelectric colorimetric procedure. Red blood cells are hemolyzed and the released Hb reacts with potassium ferricyanide and potassium cyanide (Drabkins' solution) to produce cyanmethemoglobin which gives a measurable bright cherry-red color to the blood. A photometer measures color differences. The spectrophotometer is the apparatus used for determining the quantity of coloring matter in a solution by measuring the transmitted light by means of a color spectrum. Most hematology analyzers are designed for either capillary or venous specimens. Some systems use reader

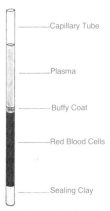

Capillary Tube

Plasma

Buffy Coat

Red Blood Cells

Sealing Clay

Figure 30–7. Diagram of a microhematocrit tube after centrifugation. (From Wedding ME and Toenjes SA: Medical Laboratory Procedures. FA Davis, Philadelphia, 1992, p. 228, with permission.)

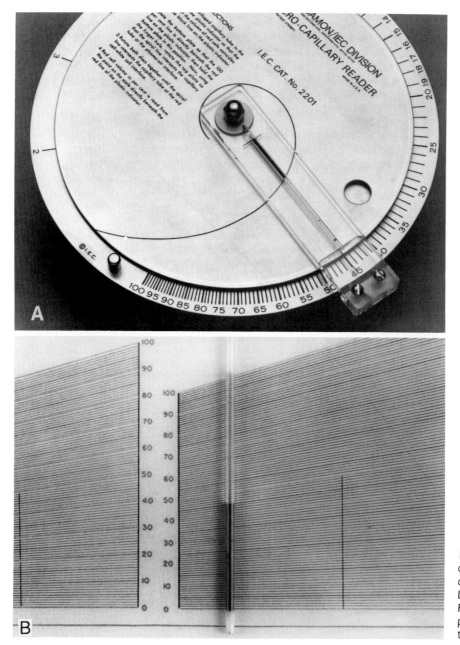

Figure 30–8. (**A**) Circular microhematocrit reader. (From Wedding ME and Toenjes SA: Medical Laboratory Procedures. FA Davis, Philadelphia, 1992, p. 231, with permission.) (**B**) Columnar hematocrit reader.

cards similar to the hematocrit reader card. Others provide results in a display panel. The operation of, quality control measures, types of testing pipettes and tubes, and diagnostic wall charts for comparisons vary with each manufacturer.

Methods using manufacturer-supplied pipettes or the Unopette System should be used because cyanmethemoglobin is a poison, and consequently it is dangerous to pipette by mouth. With the Unopette System, diluents of cyanmethemoglobin are already aliquotted (divided into small portions) and manual pipetting is not required (see Fig. 30–5).

Deviations in Hb concentrations closely parallel those for the RBC and the Hct. Hb concentrations are increased in polycythemia vera, severe burns, chronic obstructive pulmonary disease, and congestive heart failure. Hb is decreased in anemia, hyperthyroidism, cirrhosis, severe hemorrhage, Hodgkin's disease, leukemia, hemolytic conditions, and during pregnancy. Hb levels are very high at birth, decrease throughout childhood, and increase again during adolescence until adult levels are reached.

Increased levels of bilirubin in the blood increase the Hb level. Certain drugs and high levels of lipids can also alter Hb test results.

THE HEMACYTOMETER

The *hemacytometer* is a special slide consisting of a counting chamber of uniform depth that is covered by a

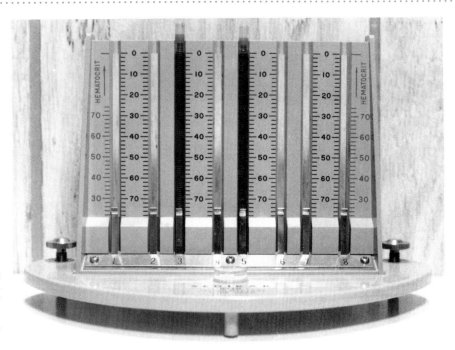

Figure 30–9. Wintrobe tubes in sedimentation rack. (From Wedding ME and Toenjes SA: Medical Laboratory Procedures. FA Davis, Philadelphia, 1992, p. 217, with permission.)

ruled over glass; the region under each ruled square contains a known volume of anticoagulated blood. It is used in manual microscopic methods for expressing the white blood cells, red blood cells, and platelets in 1 μL of anticoagulated blood. The physician's office laboratory employs the hemacytometer primarily for counting white blood cells, although it can readily be used for counting red blood cells, platelets, sperm, or any other type of cell count.

Most frequently used hematocytometer is the Neubauer type (Fig. 30–11). The glass slide is divided into two separate chambers. Each chamber has a total ruled area measuring 3 mm by 3 mm (9 mm²). This area is subdivided into nine squares measuring 1 mm by 1 mm (Fig. 30–11).

The four corner squares are subdivided into 16 squares measuring 0.25 mm by 0.25 mm. White blood counts are performed viewing these four corner squares using the 10× objective lens.

The middle square is subdivided into 25 squares measuring 0.2 mm by 0.2 mm. These 25 squares are subdivided into 16 squares measuring 0.05 mm by 0.05 mm, which makes a total of 400 tiny squares in the middle counting area. Eighty of the tiny squares, or the four corner squares and the central square, are used for red cell counting using the 40× objective lens.

Pattern for Counting Cells

To prevent individual cells from being counted twice, cells on the upper and left borders of a counting area are included, but those on the lower and right borders are not (Fig. 30–12). This method is used for *all* particles being counted by means of a manual counting chamber.

There should be an even distribution of cells in the various counting areas. Poor cell distribution may be due to one or more of the following:

1. Inadequate mixing of the sample at collection
2. Incorrect pipetting
3. Inadequate mixing of the reservoir before filling the hemacytometer
4. Dirty coverslip or hemacytometer
5. Overfilling the counting chamber
6. Underfilling the counting chamber
7. Trapped air bubbles under the coverslip
8. Drying of the solution caused by taking too long to count the cells
9. Bumping or tilting the hemacytometer while focusing with the microscope

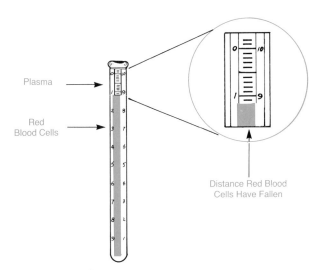

Figure 30–10. After 60 minutes, sedimentation of erythrocytes in Wintrobe tube; inset shows an ESR of 12 mm/hr. (From Wedding ME and Toenjes SA: Medical Laboratory Procedures. FA Davis, Philadelphia, 1992, p. 217, with permission.)

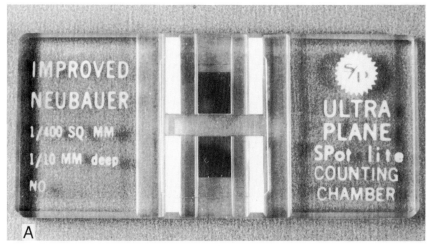

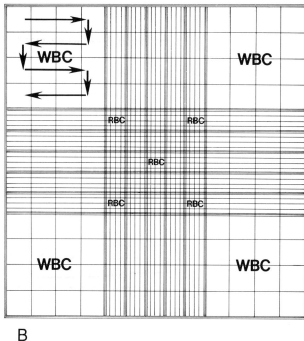

B

Figure 30–11. (**A**) A Neubauer-type, double chamber hematocytometer with cover glass. (From Wedding MD and Toenjes SA: Medical Laboratory Procedures. FA Davis, Philadelphia, 1992, p. 257, with permission.) (**B**) Each chamber of the hematocytometer is etched with rules that divide it into 9 squares, 1 mm per side; the 1-mm squares are further subdivided by etched rules.

10. Errors in counting cells
11. Transcription errors
12. Using counting areas or dilutions other than those prescribed without changing calculation factors

RED BLOOD CELL COUNT

The RBC approximates the number of circulating red cells in the body. The normal number of red blood cells remains fairly constant: between 4 and 5 million/μL of blood in women, and between 4 to 6 million/μL in men. Patients with an RBC below 10% of the normal values are considered anemic. Causes of anemia include bleeding, red blood cell destruction, dietary deficiency, genetic disorders, drug ingestion, bone marrow disease, chronic illness, and diseases of blood-associated organs, such as the spleen or liver.

Red blood cell production may be increased in high altitudes where the body requires greater oxygen-carrying ability; in diseases that interfere with the flow of blood and its transport of oxygen (e.g., congenital heart disease); in severe dehydration; and in polycythemia vera, a neoplastic condition of unknown origin.

Counting and Calculating RBCs

Since red blood cells and white blood cells appear in dense concentrations in the blood, blood specimens must be diluted to be counted microscopically. Red blood cells are counted under the 40X microscope objective. As the cells are counted, a hand counter is used to tally the totals. Figure 30–12 is an enlargement of the central red blood cell counting area. This area measures 0.04 mm² and is one of the five areas used for red cell counts. Red blood cells appear as small round dots and are best seen with a low light. The refraction of light enables the viewer to distinguish between a cell and debris such as dust or stain sediment. The move-

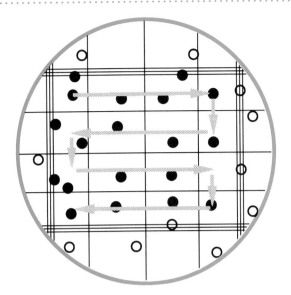

● Cells to be counted
○ Cells not to be counted

Figure 30–12. *When counting cells in a hematocy-tometer, use the zigzag pattern shown here.*

ment of the microscopic field during the actual counting is from the left to right, down to the next row, then right to left, and down again, until all cells in the counting area have been included. (See the end-of-chapter procedure for a description of this process.)

To calculate a RBC, the tester counts five squares in each chamber of the hemacytometer. The difference between any two squares in each set of five squares counted should not be more than 15 cells. The total of the five squares over the first chamber is multiplied by 10,000, then the total in the second chamber is multiplied by 10,000. Duplicate counts (chamber counts) should be within 300,000 cells of one another.

The two chamber counts are averaged and reported as the number of red blood cells per microliter (**Note:** Cell counts were formally reported as the number per cubic millimeter [mm³]. However, the liter has been adopted as the standard for blood counting, and cubic millimeter is expressed in its liter equivalent the microliter) For example:

	Hemacytometer Side One		Hemacytometer Side Two
Square 1	90	Square 1	95
2	85	2	80
3	85	3	80
4	90	4	90
5	95	5	90
Total	445	Total	440
	×10,000		×10,000
	4,450,000		4,400,000

Average of the two sides:
$$4,425,000 = 4.425 \text{ red blood cells}/\mu L$$

Round off to nearest 100 cells:
$$= 4.4 \text{ red blood cells}/\mu L$$

WHITE BLOOD CELL COUNT

The WBC approximates the number of circulating white cells. The normal number of white blood cells is 4,500 to 11,000 cells/μL of blood in both men and women. The WBC normally fluctuates during the day, especially after food intake. The chief function of white blood cells is to protect the body against microorganisms that cause disease. White blood cells are classified into two groups: granular (basophils, eosinophils, neutrophils) and nongranular (lymphocytes and monocytes). See the procedure at the end of this chapter for a detailed description of obtaining a WBC count.

Counting and Calculating White Blood Cells

As with red blood cells, white blood cells must be diluted to be counted microscopically. Using the hemacytometer, white blood cells are counted under the 10× microscope objective. White blood cells are colorless, nucleated cells. White blood cells are far less numerous than red blood cells; however, they are much larger than red blood cells.

Calculations for the WBC are determined by counting four large squares over both chambers of the hemacytometer (see Fig. 30–11). White blood cells are counted in the same manner as red blood cells, as is shown by the arrows in the upper left corner of Figure 30–11. The movement of the microscopic field during the actual counting is from the left to right, down to the next row, then right to left, and down again, until all cells in the counting area have been included. The difference between any two squares in the set of five squares counted should not be more than 10 cells.

The total of the four squares in one chamber is multiplied by 50, then the total in the second chamber is multiplied by 50. Duplicate counts (chamber counts) should be within 1000 cells of one another; for WBCs below 5000, the duplicate count should be within ± 10% of one another.

The two chamber counts are averaged and reported as the number of white blood cells per microliter. (**Note:** Cell counts were formerly reported as the number per cubic millimeter [mm³]. However, the liter has been adopted as the standard for blood counting, and cubic millimeter is expressed in its liter equivalent the microliter.) For example:

	Hemacytometer Side One		Hemacytometer Side Two
Square 1	50	Square 1	50
2	55	2	45
3	45	3	45
4	50	4	50
Total	200	Total	190
×	50	×	50
	10,000		9,500

Average of the two sides: 9,750 WBC/μL

Table 30–3 lists the comparisons between a manual WBC and RBC.

MICROSCOPIC EXAMINATION OF THE PERIPHERAL BLOOD SMEAR

The microscopic examination of peripheral blood is another routine hematology procedure. It involves the preparation, staining, and examination of a dried film of fresh capillary blood or anticoagulated venous blood on a glass slide. The blood smear (blood film) is the only permanent record of the human blood specimen. It can be reexamined at a later time or used in research. The blood smear contains more information about the patient's blood than any other single test, and it is vitally important that it be properly prepared (see the procedures at the end of this chapter for a detailed description of this process).

The blood smear is used for the following examinations:

1. To study the morphology of white blood cells, red blood cells, and platelets
2. To perform a differential WBC
3. To verify Hb and Hct determinations and the RBC
4. To estimate the WBC, platelet count, and RBC

Once the hemacytometer blood cell counts are completed, the medical assistant should closely examine the peripheral blood smear, first under the 10X objective then under the oil-immersion objective. A well-made smear is essential. Usually 2 slides are prepared. Only *very* fresh blood or EDTA blood collected within 2 hours should be used.

The smear is first scanned under 10X for overall quality and an estimation of the WBC and RBC. This provides a check on the WBC and RBC obtained by the hemacytometer method.

A quality slide is vital. If the initial scan reveals a smear that is too thick, too thin, or otherwise defective, the examination must end and a new slide examined or prepared. The slide is scanned from the thick end to the thin, feathered area. The ideal counting area is the area where there is no clumping or rouleaux formation and red blood cells lie side by side without touching or overlapping. The margins and the feathered edges are also examined, as immature or abnormal cells tend to congregate near feathered edges and the side of the slide.

White Blood Cell Estimation

Using the 10X eyepiece and the 10X objective (100X magnification), the laboratorian scans five fields for white blood cells. At this magnification, 20 to 30 white blood cells per low-power field (LPF) is approximately equivalent to a 5000 white blood cell/μL count: 40 to 60 cells is equivalent to a 10,000 white blood cells/μL. In general, five white blood cells per LPF is equal to a count of 1000 white blood cells. The number of white blood cells in five LPFs are counted and the results averaged to *estimate* the WBC.

Red Blood Cell Morphology

The medical assistant may be responsible for reporting the red cell morphology. Red blood cells may appear in the specimen in varying stages of development or in abnormal shapes or sizes. The normal, mature red blood cell is a biconcave disk with no nuclei and, when stained, it appears to be pale pink. Table 30–4 lists terms related to abnormal red cell morphology. Figure 30–13 illustrates the types of abnormal red blood cell morphology.

When the optimal counting area is viewed under the

Table 30–3

DIFFERENCES BETWEEN WHITE BLOOD CELL AND RED BLOOD CELL MANUAL CELL COUNTS

	RBC	WBC
Pipette used	RBC (red bead)	WBC (white bead)
Dilution range	1:100–1:1000	1:10 to 1:100
Outstanding marks	0.5, 1.0, 101.0	0.5, 1.0, 11.0
Diluent	Hayem's solution (mercury chloride and sodium sulfate)	2% acetic acid
Blood is drawn to "x" mark	0.5 mL	0.5 mL
Diluent is drawn to "x" mark	101 mL	11 mL
Dilution	1:200	1:20
Ruled area counted	Five red blood cell areas	Four white blood cell areas
Microscope power used	High power	Low power
Calculations	Red blood cells/μL = count $\times$ 10 (depth factor) $\times$ 5 (area factor) $\times$ 200 (dilution factor). Red blood cells/μL = count $\times$ 10,000	WBC/μL = count $\times$ 10 (depth factor) $\times$ ¼ (area factor) $\times$ 20 (dilution factor). WBC/μL = count $\times$ 50
Normal range	Men: 4.5–6.0 million/μL Women: 4.3–5.5 million/μL	5,000 to 10,000/μL

<u>Table 30–4</u>
TERMINOLOGY OF RED BLOOD CELL MORPHOLOGY

Anisechromia	Variation in color.
Anisocytosis	Variation in cell size.
Basophilic stippling	Fine blue granules found in red blood cells, possibly diagnostic of lead poisoning.
Crenated cells	Cells with a scalloped or notched appearance, due to shrinkage.
Howell-Jolly bodies	Small nuclear fragments in the red blood cells which stain deep blue.
Hyperchromia	A condition in which cells have increased hemoglobin.
Hypochromia	A condition in which cells have decreased hemoglobin.
Inclusion bodies	Particles, such as secretory granules and crystals, in the cytoplasm of a cell. Not found in normal red blood cells.
Macrocyte	An abnormally large cell (10–12 μm in diameter).
Megalocyte	An exceptionally large cell (12–25 μm in diameter).
Microcyte	An abnormally small cell (5 μm or less in diameter).
Nucleated red blood cells	The number of red blood cells containing a nucleus seen in a count of 100 white blood cells.
Ovalocytes	Oval-shaped cells, also called elliptocytes.
Poikilocytosis	Variation in cell shape.
Polychromasia	A condition in which stained cells show bluish shades with tinges of pink.
Reticulocytes	Immature red blood cells showing a blue reticulum when stained with methylene blue (appear as polychromasia on Wright stained smear).
Rouleaux	Red blood cells having the appearance of stacked coins.
Schistocytes	Fragmented cells, also called helmet cells.
Sickle cells	Crescent-shaped cells occurring in hereditary anemias.
Spherocytes	Small, round, completely spherical cells.
Target cells	Abnormally thin red blood cells with a dark center and a surrounding ring of hemoglobin, occurring in anemia and jaundice.

oil-immersion objective normal (normocytic) red blood cells appear 7 to 8 μm in diameter, consistent in size, and round in shape; when stained, they have a pink color with a paler central area. Red blood cells in 10 fields are evaluated. Any variations is size, shape, color, and intercellular structure should be recorded.

Although most counts will reveal mature cells, immature cells may be circulated into the peripheral blood in various disease states or conditions. On the smear, immature red blood cells can be differentiated from mature cells because they appear in the peripheral blood as *nucleated* red blood cells. These immature, nucleated cells must be reported separately.

Nucleated red blood cells (normoblasts) are not destroyed by acetic acid diluting fluids and will be mistakenly counted as white blood cells in the hemacytometer. If nucleated red blood cells are observed, they are counted during the WBC and reported separately in number per 100 white blood cells. In this case, the hemacytometer WBC must also be corrected with the following formula:

$$\text{Correct WBC} = \frac{\text{Incorrect WBC} \times 100}{100 + \text{Number of nucleated red blood cells per white blood cells}}$$

Sources of error in examining blood cells on a peripheral smear include using blood that has been stored too long or time delays during the slide preparation; poor quality or unclean slides; lack of correct speed, angle, and pressure on the spreader slide; high humidity in the laboratory or not allowing slides to dry; outdated or deteriorated reagents; improper timing or use of reagents; examination of cells in wrong areas of the smear; and misidentification of cells.

Platelet Estimation

Under 10X power, the slide should be scanned for any clumps which may indicate an increased platelet count. Then under the oil-immersion field, an estimation of the number of platelets should be performed next. Although platelet studies should be performed by trained laboratory technicians, a platelet *estimation* can be performed on a stained smear. Platelets are observed for any abnormalities and their appearance in adequate numbers. Normal values for platelets may be placed at 150,00 to 400,000/μL or approximately one platelet to each 17 to 70 red blood cells. Platelets vary from 2 to 5 μm in diameter and stain as light blue, small irregularly-shaped bodies with a dark nucleus. It is important to remember that this type of count is an estimation only and therefore reported as *increased, decreased*, or *normal*. Five to 25 platelets per oil-immersion field is considered within normal range and is equivalent to the normal platelet count range. The average number of platelets seen in 10 to 15 fields is reported. Errors in the platelet count include a false decrease due to the presence of clots in the blood collection tube.

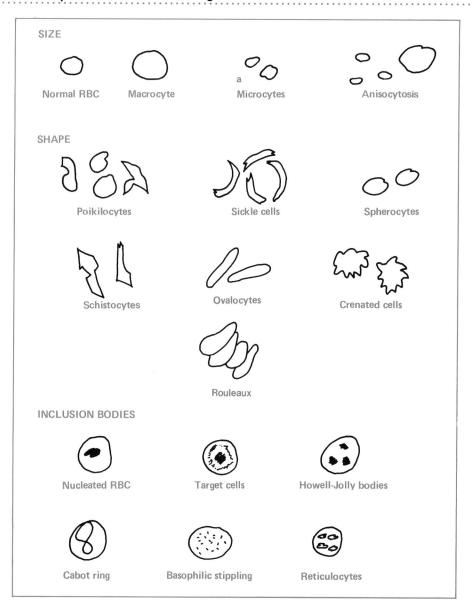

SIZE

○ Normal RBC   ○ Macrocyte   ᵃ Microcytes   Anisocytosis

SHAPE

Poikilocytes   Sickle cells   Spherocytes

Schistocytes   Ovalocytes   Crenated cells

Rouleaux

INCLUSION BODIES

Nucleated RBC   Target cells   Howell-Jolly bodies

Cabot ring   Basophilic stippling   Reticulocytes

Figure 30-13. Examples of abnormal RBC morphology.

White Blood Cell Differential Count

Finally, with the oil-immersion objective focused over the area of optimal counting, the percentage distribution of each type of white blood cell is calculated after identifying 100 *consecutive* white blood cells. A special counting pattern is used (Fig. 30-14). Starting at the feathered end *of the optimal area*, count the cells moving from the bottom margin upward until the top margin is reached. Move the visual field toward the thicker end (1 to 2 fields), and beginning at the top margin, count downward to the bottom margin. Continue the pattern, counting from margin to margin, then moving once again toward the thick end of the slide until 100 cells are counted.

The cells are counted with the aid of a mechanical counter that provides a separate key for recording each type of white blood cells counted and maintains a run-ning total. The counter automatically rings when 100 cells have been recorded. The following types of blood cells may be seen. Their appearances, as described, are the result of staining with *Wright's stain*.

1. *Neutrophils.* Neutrophils (segmented or band) average about 12 μm in diameter, and when stained, they have a pale pink granulated cyto-plasm and a dark purple segmented nucleus, usually having three to five lobes connected by strands of chromatin. If the nucleus is unseg-mented, the cell is known as a *band* or *stab cell* and is an immature neutrophil. The most nu-merous of the white blood cells, the percentage of segmented neutrophils in the normal white blood cell, is 52 to 64%; the percentage of bands is 3%. Segmented and band neutrophils are re-ported separately. An increased WBC usually

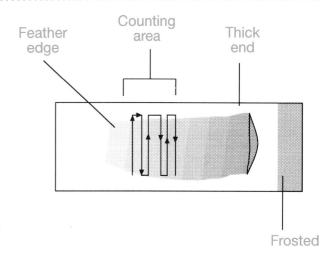

Feather edge   Counting area   Thick end

Figure 30–14. Counting pattern for the WBC differential.

Frosted

results from an increase in neutrophils. *Neutrophia* is usually accompanied by a "shift to the left," which means an increase in the number of immature cells.

2. *Basophils.* Basophils average about 12 μm in diameter, and when stained, they have dark blue-black granules in the cytoplasm and a purple nucleus, which is usually indented. The percentage of basophils in the normal white blood cell is 0% to 1%.

3. *Eosinophils.* Eosinophils average about 13 μm in diameter, and when stained, they appear with bright orange granules in the cytoplasm and a purple nucleus, usually with two lobes. The percent of eosinophils in the normal blood count is 1% to 4%.

4. *Lymphocytes.* Lymphocytes may be small or large, and their sizes range from 7 to 20 μm in diameter. They have a dark purple nucleus filling almost the entire cell with a faint blue cytoplasm. The percentage of lymphocytes in the normal white blood cell is 25% to 35%. Small leukocytes may be confused with red blood cells; therefore, the staining reaction is the way to distinguish between the two (blue versus red or pink stain).

5. *Monocytes.* Monocytes are the largest of the normal leukocytes, ranging between 13 and 25 μm in diameter. They are identifiable by their largeness. They appear with a gray-blue cytoplasm and a kidney-shaped nucleus. The percentage of monocytes in the normal white blood cell is 2% to 6%.

If any of the following conditions are encountered during the WBC differential 100-cell count, 200 cells should be counted and reported: (1) more than 5 eosinophils, (2) more than 2 basophils, (3) more than 10 monocytes, (4) less than 15 or greater than 40 lymphocytes in an otherwise normal adult WBC, or (5) if the lymphocyte percentage is greater than the neutrophil percentage (except in children). The percentage of each cell type per 200 cells is recorded, with a notation indicating that a 200-cell count was performed. If the WBC count is less than 1000 white blood cells/μL, only 50 cells are counted.

Personnel not having special hematologic training should easily be able to identify normal cells, but should seek the physician's assistance when a questionable or abnormal cell is observed, because it is often difficult to classify each white blood cell observed. No white blood cells should be skipped. Figure 30–15 identifies some abnormal white blood cells. Table 30–5 provides a list of terms used to describe abnormal blood cell morphology.

AUTOMATED CELL COUNTING

The medical assistant should be familiar with the basic types of automation used in hematology. In addition to the equipment mentioned earlier, some physicians may use a white blood cell and red blood cell counter to decrease the time involved in processing individual tests if a large volume of tests are handled in the office.

There are basically two types of cell counting systems:

1. The optical system counts particles appearing as light on a dark-field illumination, which is converted to an electrical impulse by a photomultiplier.

2. The electrical system counts particles that are suspended in an electrolyte solution by measuring the resistance of the particles. For example, red blood cells and white blood cells are poor conductors of electricity. When they pass through an opening that measures voltage, there will be a drop in voltage represented by each cell. The most commonly used type of electrical system is the *Coulter counter.* It provides results for all CBC parameters. The WBC, RBC, and MCV count are performed electrically, and the Hb is done colorimetrically. Mean corpuscular hemoglobin (MCH) and MCHC are then derived for the other readings.

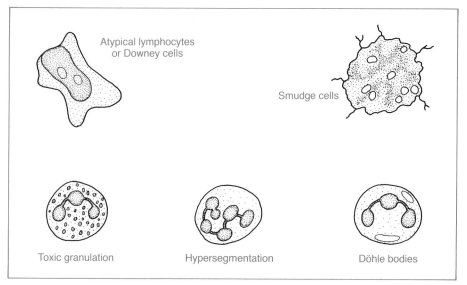

Figure 30–15. Examples of abnormal WBC morphology.

The medical assistant should be prepared to undertake special training in the operation and maintenance of sophisticated laboratory instruments.

The medical assistant should be familiar with a Coulter Model S and the newer Coulter Model S Plus (Coulter Diagnostics, Hialeah, FL) processing cards since most reference laboratories will report patient results in this format (Fig. 30–16). The medical assistant should be able to rapidly visualize the card format when entering laboratory results reported by telephone.

OTHER HEMATOLOGIC TESTS

Other hematologic studies include red blood indices, reticulocyte counts, eosinophil counts, red blood cell osmotic fragility tests, sickle cell screening tests, and tests for coagulation and hemostasis. A brief introduction to red blood cell indices and coagulation studies are given below.

Red Cell Indices

Red cell indices are mathematical calculations derived from the RBC and from hemoglobin and hematocrit determinations. Many medical offices do not report MCV, MCH, and MCHC values. Red blood cell indices are used primarily to differentiate the types of anemia and represent an average value that must be correlated with the blood smear findings. The medical assistant will find these mathematic calculations to be very useful in studying red blood cell morphology. A low MCH, for example, would alert the medical assistant to look for the presence of hypochromic red blood cells.

Mean corpuscular volume is the average volume of individual red blood cells. The normal range is 80 to 95 cubic microns per cell.

$$MCV = \frac{Hct \times 10}{RBC \text{ in millions per microliter}}$$

Table 30–5

TERMINOLOGY OF WHITE BLOOD CELL MORPHOLOGY

Döhle bodies	Round or oval, small clear light blue staining areas found in neutrophilic cytoplasm, usually present in infections, severe burns, chemical toxicity, and pregnancy; often seen in combination with toxic granulation.
Downey cells	Oval or kidney-shaped lymphocytes with heavy clumps of stained chromatin, seen in infectious mononucleosis and viral infections; also called reactive lymphocyte, atypical lymphocyte, or reticular lymphocyte.
Hypersegmentation	Neutrophils that contain five or more lobes in their nuclei, characteristics of vitamin B_{12} and folic acid deficiency (pernicious anemia)
Smudge cells	Damaged white cells with frayed nuclei and no cytoplasm, and not counted as part of the white blood cell differential if a few are observed (normal). Increased numbers are associated with the leukemias and are reported.
Toxic granulation	Basophils that stain deeply or blue-black, enlarged granules found in the cytoplasm of neutrophils and associated with acute bacterial infections, drug toxicity, and severe burns.

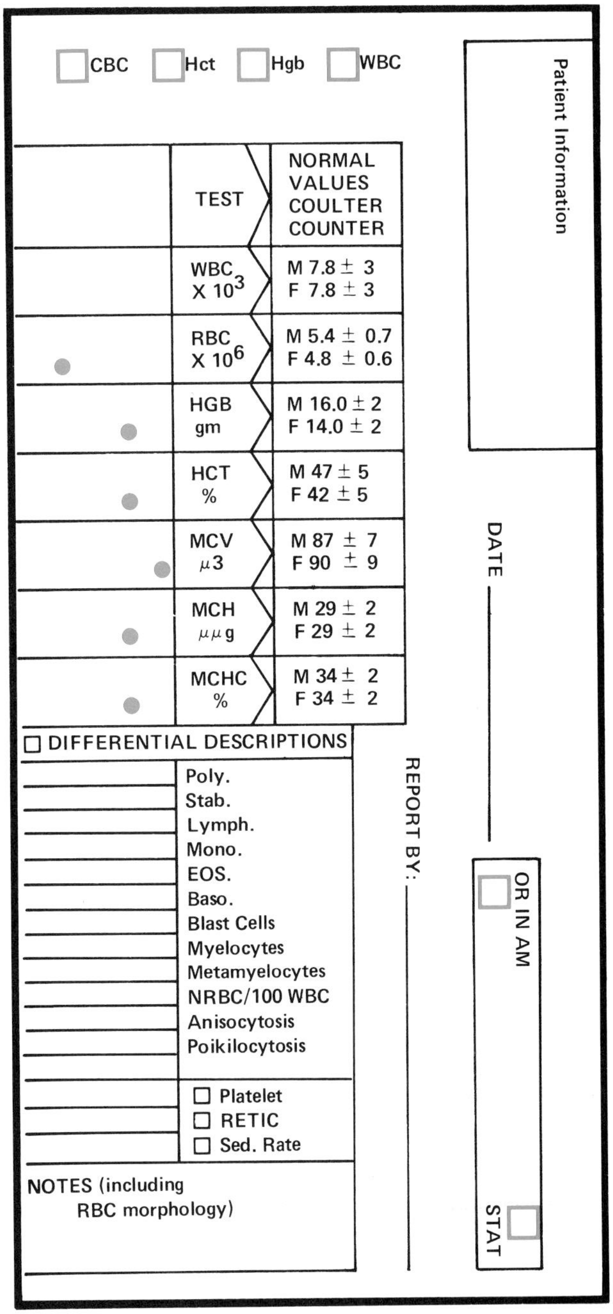

	TEST	NORMAL VALUES COULTER COUNTER
	WBC X 10³	M 7.8 ± 3 F 7.8 ± 3
●	RBC X 10⁶	M 5.4 ± 0.7 F 4.8 ± 0.6
●	HGB gm	M 16.0 ± 2 F 14.0 ± 2
●	HCT %	M 47 ± 5 F 42 ± 5
●	MCV μ3	M 87 ± 7 F 90 ± 9
●	MCH μμg	M 29 ± 2 F 29 ± 2
●	MCHC %	M 34 ± 2 F 34 ± 2

☐ DIFFERENTIAL DESCRIPTIONS

Poly.
Stab.
Lymph.
Mono.
EOS.
Baso.
Blast Cells
Myelocytes
Metamyelocytes
NRBC/100 WBC
Anisocytosis
Poikilocytosis

☐ Platelet
☐ RETIC
☐ Sed. Rate

NOTES (including RBC morphology)

☐ CBC ☐ Hct ☐ Hgb ☐ WBC

Patient Information

DATE _____

REPORT BY: _____

☐ OR IN AM

☐ STAT

Figure 30–16. Standard Coulter Model S processing card.

Mean corpuscular hemoglobin is the Hb content of the average red blood cell. The normal range is 27 to 34 picograms (micromicrograms) per cell.

$$MCH = \frac{Hb \times 10}{RBC \; in \; millions \; per \; microliter}$$

Mean corpuscular hemoglobin concentration is the average Hb concentration per 100 mL of packed red blood cells expressed as a percentage. The normal range is 31% to 36%.

$$MCHC = \frac{Hb}{Hct} \times 100 = \%$$

Coagulation Studies

The medical assistant employed in the office of a cardiologist may routinely perform coagulation tests, such as the prothrombin time (PT) and the partial thrombinplastin time (PTT). A chart of normal values should be available for reference (Table 30–6).

The physician uses the PT monitor anticoagulant (coumarin) therapy to adjust drug dosage accordingly. An extended prothrombin test time may indicate hemorrhaging, and a low test time may suggest thrombosis. Therefore, accurate quality control measures are vital. The PTT is used to monitor heparin therapy. Both tests are frequently ordered as a routine test before surgery to identify any abnormal bleeding problems.

Table 30-6
NORMAL COAGULATION VALUES IN ADULTS

Bleeding time	
Ivy	1-6 min
Template	3-6 min
Fibrinogen	150-450 mg/dL
Partial thromboplastin time	60-85 sec
Partial thromboplastin time, activated	35-40 sec or within 5 sec of control test
Plasminogen	10-20 mg/dL
Platelets	150,000-450,000/μL
Prothrombin time	11-13 sec or within 2 sec of control test
Thrombin clotting time	10-15 sec or within 1.3 times as long as control test

Because of the difficulty in interpretating the classic manual "tilt" tube method, most offices now use automated analyzers for coagulation studies that determine results by electrodes of photometric techniques. Available coagulation test systems are Fibrometer (BBL Microbiolgy Systems, Cockeysville, MD), Du 500 (Boehringer Mannheim Diagnostics, BMC/Bio-Dynamics, Indianapolis, IN), and Coag-a-mate 150 and 2001 (General Diagnostics, Elk Grove, IL).

CLINICAL CHEMISTRY

Clinical chemistry is the quantitative analysis of the chemicals contained in blood or other body fluids, such as urine, spinal fluid, and synovial fluid. The test values are compared with known normal values (Table 30-7). Deviations from this normal range may indicate a disease state or a dietary deficiency. Because the results of so many clinical chemistry tests are used by the physician to diagnose and treat patient illnesses, the medical assistant must know the type of specimen required for each test and make certain that it is collected, prepared, and preserved properly. As in other types of laboratory testing, the medical assistant is specially trained to perform chemistry tests, must master the basic principles of use and care of the laboratory equipment, proper preparation of reagents, recognition of problems when they arise, quality assurance protocol for performing procedures, and correct reporting of results.

General methods for most assays in clinical chemistry involve the use of spectrophotometry, photometry, and immunoassays involving enzymes as markers or tags. Strict adherence to quality control procedures as listed by the manufacturers of the testing products is necessary. Table 30-8 provides the commonly used clinical chemistry abbreviations.

Manual techniques for analysis—such as the preparation of solutions by tedious weighing of dry volumes, mixing reagents, pipetting diluents, observing chemical reactions, and interpreting results by visual methods—

represent the classical methodology for diagnostic procedures. While the medical assistant is encouraged to develop an understanding of chemical reactions through the classical study of clinical chemistry, it must be understood that these time-consuming activities are not practical.

Table 30-7
NORMAL BLOOD CHEMISTRY VALUES FOR ADULTS

Substance	Normal Values
Acetone	0.3-2.0 mg/dL
Albumin	3.5-5.0 g/dL
Alanine aminotransferase, formerly serum glutamic-pyruvic transaminase	6-53 U/mL 4-36 U/L
Ammonia	45-50 μg/dL
Amylase	80-150 U/dL
Ascorbic acid	0.6-2.0 mg/dL
Aspartate aminotransferase, formerly serum glutamic-oxaloacetic transaminase	12-36 U/mL
Bilirubin (total/direct)	0.8/0.2 mg/dL
Calcium	4.25-5.25 mEq/L 8.5-10.5 mg/dL
Chloride	98-106 mEq/L
Copper	Men: 70-140 μg/dL Women: 80-155 μg/dL
Creatine kinase	Men: 55-170 U/L Women: 30-135 U/L
Creatinine	0.6-1.2 mg/dL
Fibrinogen	200-400 mg/dL
Globulins	2.3-3.5 g/dL
Glucose	70-110 mg/dL
Iron	56-183 μg/dL
Lactate dehydrogenase	100-190 U/L
Lipase	0.1-1.0 U/mL
Lipids (total)	450-1000 mg/dL
Magnesium	1.4-2.2 mEq/L 1.7-2.7 mg/dL
Nitrogen (nonprotein nitrogen)	25-40 mg/dL 5-25 mg/dL
pH (blood urea nitrogen)	Arterial: 7.37-7.42 Venous: 7.34-7.39
Phosphatase, acid	2.2-10.5 U/L
Phosphatase, alkaline	20-90 U/L
Phospholipids	150-380 mg/dL
Phosphorus, inorganic	2.6-4.8 mg/dL
Potassium	3.5-5.3 mmol/L
Sodium	135-148 mmol/L
Uric acid	Men: 3.0-7.0 mg/dL Women: 2.0-6.0 mg/dL

Table 30-8
COMMONLY USED CLINICAL CHEMISTRY ABBREVIATIONS

Abbreviation	Meaning
Ab	Antibody
ACTH	Adrenocorticotropic hormone
A/G	Albumin/globulin ratio
Ag	Antigen
Alb	Albumin
Alc	Alcohol
Alk	Alkaline
ALT	Alanine aminotransferase, formerly serum glutamic-pyruvic transminase
AST	Aspartate aminotransferase, formerly serum glutamic-oxaloacetic transaminase
BJP	Bence Jones protein
BUN	Blood urea nitrogen
Ca	Calcium
CEA	Carinocembryonic antigen
CK	Creatine kinase
FBS	Fasting blood sugar
GA	Gastric analysis
G6PD	Glucose-6-phosphate
GTT	Glucose tolerance test
5-HIAA	5-Hydroxyindole acetic acid
ICD	Isocitric dehydrogenase
IgE	Immunoglobulin E
17KS	17-Ketosteroids
LAP	Leucine aminopeptidase
LD	Lactate dehydrogenase
PKU	Phenylketonuria
Sp Gr	Specific gravity
T_3	Triiodothyronine
T_4	Tetraiodothyronine (thyroxine)
TBG	Thyroxine-binding globulin
TIBC	Total iron-binding capacity
TSH	Thyroid-stimulating hormone

CHEMISTRY PROFILES

Specimens are frequently sent to reference laboratories where large analyzers provide highly reliable results and volume testing at a relatively low cost. These autoanalyzers are particularly useful for profile testing (multiple tests run on a single specimen), and many physicians order profiles as a general health screen.

The blood chemistry profile usually evaluates several of the 12 body systems by including one or more of the following tests: glucose, blood urea nitrogen, uric acid, calcium, total bilirubin, albumin, total protein, inorganic phosphorus, cholesterol, alkaline phosphatase, lactic dehydrogenase, and glutamic-oxaloacetic transaminase. The profile should provide the physician with a good overview of the health of the patient.

Specific profiles are used to perform multiple tests that can assist the physician in diagnosing conditions within in single system. Some commonly run profiles include the renal, liver, lipid, and cardiac profiles.

SPECIMEN COLLECTION

The medical assistant is responsible for collecting the specimen and for its transportation to a reference laboratory. Chemical tests are performed on whole blood, plasma, or serum. Most tests are done on plasma or serum processed from whole blood obtained by venipuncture. Occasionally microsamples are collected using special microcontainer tubes or capillary tubes. If plasma is used, the specimen must be drawn in a Vacutainer containing an anticoagulant. After centrifugation, whole blood treated with an anticoagulant separates into plasma, buffy coat, and packed red blood cells. The plasma is then drawn off the sample.

Serum is plasma with the fibrinogen removed, which is accomplished by coagulating blood. To obtain coagulated blood, the medical assistant draws blood into a plain Vacutainer tube, containing no anticoagulant, and allowed to sit for at least 15 to 20 minutes at room temperature. Allowing this time minimizes hemolysis and results in a greater volume of serum for testing. If the specimen is allowed to sit too long, however, glycolysis can occur and alter the test results. Speckled-top Vacutainer tubes may be used to separate the serum from the cells. After sitting, the tube is centrifuged and the supernatant serum is removed. Universal precautions must be strictly adhered to (see Chapter 28).

Ideally, all chemistry tests should be performed within 1 hour of collection. The specimen should be carefully observed for color changes. If the serum appears red, the specimen has hemolyzed and is unfit for testing.

Jaundiced serum or plasma appears either brownish-yellow or bright yellow. This abnormal coloring will interfere with photometric results and should be reported immediately. Extreme caution must be taken in handling the specimen as jaundiced serum is a good indication of hepatitis.

When high levels of lipids are present in the serum, the appearance is that of a milky white. As with any coloring of serum, the presence of these particles will interfere with photometric testing.

Glucose specimens can be preserved with sodium fluoride, if the testing cannot be performed on fresh blood. Specimens that cannot be tested immediately must be refrigerated to retard bacterial growth and glycolysis. Refrigerated specimens must be brought to room temperature before testing.

OFFICE LABORATORY ANALYZERS

Less costly than in the past, several types of automated chemistry analyzers are feasible for the office. Most chemistry tests are run with a photometer (light source). Some photometers accept only one brand of reagent, whereas others accept a variety of brands. All analyzers come equipped with the manufacturer's operating instructions and directions for daily calibration.

An analyzer may be semiautomated or fully automated. Semiautomated analyzers require the operator to mix reagents, prepare the specimen, select the machine wavelength, and calculate the readings. Fully automated analyzers need only minimal handling of the specimen by the operator or are self-calibrating. Many fully automated analyzers also run controls automatically.

While the variety of analyzers is diverse, there are some general principles that should be understood by the medical assistant. There are three basic types of analyzer: (1) single test, (2) batch test, and (3) automated random access.

Single-test analyzers test samples one at a time. This method adapts well to low-volume testing, but the actual cost per test may be high. Batch testing enables one type of test to be performed on a number of specimens. This method is highly suited to reference laboratories, where, for example, they are able to batch 100 specimens together at the same time, for example, for a glucose test. Automated random access analyzers have the capability to readily switch from a single test mode to the batch test mode for testing numerous patient samples. This type of analyzer is more expensive but highly efficient if the volume of testing is great.

Kits are purchased with reagents. Control samples should be run with every test or test batch to ensure that the reagents are good and technique is correct (see Chapter 28). One drawback to chemistry equipment is that, because of rapid technological advances, equipment is often obsolete within 5 years. Frequently, however, manufacturers will update or upgrade equipment.

ROUTINE CLINICAL TESTING IN THE PHYSICIAN'S OFFICE LABORATORY

The role of clinical chemistry in the physician's office laboratory (POL) has generally been limited to tests such as glucose or blood urea nitrogen. These are screening methods using chemically impregnated reagent strips (dipsticks) and are performed in a manner similar to the chemical analysis of urine. For example, the Dextrostix (Ames, Elkhart, IN), a reagent strip that measures blood glucose levels from a finger puncture, continues to be a frequently ordered test in physicians offices. The medical assistant has the responsibility for patient education as well as testing. When Dextrostix is used by the diabetic patient for self-monitoring of blood glucose levels, the medical assistant must provide special instruction in the use and interpretation of this test.

Increasingly, the medical assistant is being challenged to acquire specific training for the operation of semiautomated and automated blood chemistry analyzers in the POL. The medical assistant's rapidly changing role in the laboratory is best illustrated in the field of clinical chemistry, and the medical assistant is encouraged to stay abreast of the technical advances that provide newer chemistry techniques for on-site testing. The medical assistant must also stay abreast of the test-site regulations for training and testing imposed by the 1988 CLIA standards (see Chapter 28).

GLUCOSE TESTING

One of the most commonly performed chemistry tests is the blood glucose determination. Blood glucose tests are performed for the diagnosis and control of diabetes mellitus. The most common method to quantitatively measure blood glucose is colorimetry, either visually or by photometry. Both the nonautomated and the automated methods are being performed routinely in the POL and by diabetics in the control and self-management of their disease.

SPECIMEN COLLECTION

Glucose specimens must be collected at specific times. Blood may be collected from patients in a fasting state, from patients 2 hours after the patient has consumed a high-glucose meal or drink (postprandial), or during a glucose tolerance test (GTT). A random sample is of no value in glucose determination.

A fasting blood specimen is drawn in the morning before breakfast. The patient should be instructed not to eat or drink before the test (including coffee) and not to take caffeine or any other medication. An early specimen collection also assumes that there have been no emotional disturbances that could release glucose into the blood.

The 2-hour postprandial collection is timed to measure the "stress" placed on the body after a defined glucose load, in the form of a high carbohydrate drink or meal, is given to the patient. Blood is collected 2 hours after breakfast or lunch. The 2-hour specimen provides a more complete picture of the patient's diabetic condition.

Glucose determinations can be performed on whole blood, plasma, or serum, but plasma and serum, free of hemolysis, is the preferred specimen. There are many substances in whole blood, particularly the enzymes in red blood cells, that affect the stability of glucose in the blood. If whole blood is allowed to stand at room temperature in a test tube, the red blood cells will destroy glucose (glycolysis) at an average rate of 5% per hour.

Specimens for glucose determination should be transported to the laboratory as soon as possible. Adequate centrifugation is necessary to produce plasma free of both red blood cells and white blood cells. In unhemolyzed, cell-free plasma, the glucose concentration is stable for up to 8 hours at room temperature and up to 72 hours under refrigeration.

Blood should be centrifuged and separated from the clot and cells as soon as possible or within 30 minutes, unless a specific additive (such as fluoride) is used. Sodium fluoride is one anticoagulant that preserves glucose by tying up calcium (thus preventing clotting) and inhibiting enzymes production of the enzymes that destroy glucose.

If the blood must be stored for several hours, fluoride-oxalate is the anticoagulant mixture of choice. When enzyme immunoassay methods of testing are used, fluoride anticoagulant should not be used, as the enzymes used in the test kit could be inhibited by the fluoride. For enzyme immunoassay methods, use serum separator gel tubes and process the specimen within 30 minutes.

GLUCOSE TOLERANCE TEST

Patients with diabetes may have normal fasting blood glucose levels, but they may be unable to produce a sufficient amount of insulin when needed to metabolize normal loads of carbohydrates. In these cases, blood glucose levels rise to abnormally high levels and remain high for a long period of time. The GTT is performed to measure the patient's overall ability to respond appropriately to a heavy load of glucose. It is usually a confirmatory test on patients who have a glucose concentration in excess of 105 mg/dL but it can also be done to determine hypoglycemia (low glucose levels) (Table 30–9).

The test begins with the patient in the fasting state. Blood is collected as the baseline control. Glucose is then administered and blood samples are obtained at intervals of 30, 60, 120, and 180 minutes. Urine specimens may also be tested coinciding with the blood sampling.

GLUCOSE REAGENT STRIPS

Although plasma and serum samples tend to be more specific for glucose, whole blood provides the advantage of measuring glucose directly from capillary blood with a glucose reagent strip. Capillary blood specimens are especially convenient for testing infants, in mass screening programs, and for in-home monitoring by the patient. Patient self-monitoring with a reagent strip allows the patient to know his or her blood glucose level at the time of the test. Urine glucose testing can only estimate what the glucose levels have been in the hours before the urine was tested.

When blood glucose is tested with a reagent strip, the color changes on the reactive pad are visually compared with a color chart or measured by electronic reflectance meter, such as the Glucometer Blood Glucose Meter (Ames) is used. Important factors in blood glucose testing include using the correct amount of capillary blood, waiting the correct time allowed for the reaction, correct washing and wiping of the strips, and calibration of the reflectance meter. Control tests are available. There are three control levels: low range, normal range, and high range.

Patient glucometer systems are easy to use. Systems such as the Glucometer II (Ames) System (Fig. 30–17) consist of an electronic glucometer, reagent strips, reagent control strips, an automatic lancing device, and a recordkeeping log. Most glucometers have a built-in timing device, so a stopwatch is not necessary. The only other material needed is absorbent tissue.

The Glucometer II with Memory (Ames) can store measurements until the patient is able to record the information in a log or diary. Records should include the times and results of blood glucose measurement, the amount and types of food eaten, exercise, medication time and dosage, and special events, such as stressful situations or illness. When the patient uses a diary, he or she can see patterns in blood glucose levels that may indicate adjustments to the diabetes management program (Fig. 30–18).

The Glucometer M Blood Glucose Meter hooks up to a computer or printer in the physician's office to analyze patterns of blood glucose control. This system is particularly valuable for patients with diabetes that is characterized by unexplained oscillation between hypoglycemia and diabetic ketoacidosis and therefore difficult to control. This condition is referred to a "brittle" diabetes.

PATIENT SELF-TESTING FOR GLUCOSE

This procedure is followed by patients using the Ames Glucometer II Blood Glucose Meter:

1. Turn on the meter by pressing the ON/OFF button. Check that the number on the meter display matches the Program Number on the

Table 30–9

GLUCOSE TOLERANCE TEST RESULTS

| | Normal Range | | Fasting Specimen | 2-Hour Specimen |
	Serum/Plasma	Whole Blood		
Nondiabetic				
Adult	70–105 mg/dL	65–95 mg/dL	<105 mg/dL	<120 mg/dL
Child	60–100 mg/dL	30–80 mg/dL		
Impaired glucose tolerance			115–140 mg/dL	>200 mg/dL (on one occasion)
Diabetes mellitus			>140 mg/dL (on two occasions)	>200 mg/dL (on two occasions)

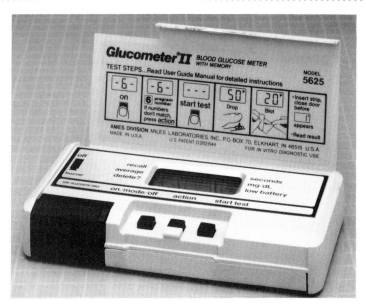

Figure 30-17. The glucometer, which uses a photometer to read a reagent strip, allows for quick, accurate blood glucose readings. (Courtesy of Ames Co., a division of Miles, Inc.)

R/NPH

Date	BLOOD GLUCOSE					KETONE TESTS Time	Result	MEDICATION (eg Insulin) Time	Type/Amount	COMMENTS
7/22 Time	6:30 A			7:30 PM				6:30	5/7	Did not sleep well
7/22 Result	110			180						
7/23 Time	6:30 A	11:15	4:00 P	6:00				6:45 / 12:00	5/15 / 6/–	Tired
7/23 Result	150 A	180	160	277				7:00	4/2	
7/24 Time	6:30 A	11:30	8:45 P	11:30				7:00 / 1:15 / 8:00	5/15 / 61 / 9/3	
7/24 Result	125	160	195	296						
7/25 Time	7:00 A	2:00	4:30	11:30 P				7:05 / 12:00 / 8:10	6/15 / 8/ / 6/3	
7/25 Result	220	195	180	273						
7/26 Time	7:00 A	11:45	8:30	11:30				7:05 / 12:00	5/15 / 7/ / 4/6	
7/26 Result	110	150	289	161						
7/27 Time	12:45 A	7:30 A	8:30 P	11:30				8:00 / 1:30 / 8:00	5/15 / 7/ / 6/	
7/27 Result	55	87	180	161						
7/28 Time	2 AM	2:00 PM	9:15	12:00 A				7:05 / 2:30 / 9:30	5/15 / 7/ / 4/6	Hypo episode @ 6:00 p.m.
7/28 Result	178	96	298	324						

Figure 30-18. An example of a log kept by a patient with diabetes. (Courtesy of Ames Co., a division of Miles, Inc.)

bottle of Glucostix Reagent Strips being used. If it does not match, press the PROGRAM button repeatedly until the number matches.

2. Wash hands with soap and warm water. Rinse and dry thoroughly. Remove a Glucostix strip from the bottle and tightly replace the cap. Fold tissue in half, then in quarters. Obtain a large drop of blood from the outer edges of a fingertip using the Glucolet (Ames).

3. Press the meter START button. When the "beep" first sounds, apply blood to the Glucostix strip, completely covering the two yellow reagent pads.

4. When the warning "beeps" sound at 22 and 21 seconds, be prepared to blot the strip using the folded tissue. When the number 20 appears on the display and a longer "beep" sounds, blot the test pads as follows:

❏ Place a reacted strip, pad side up, on the tissue.
❏ Fold tissue over the pads and firmly press it against the pads for 1 to 2 seconds.
❏ Move the strip to a clean area and blot again.

5. Immediately after blotting, open the test door and insert the strip with the test pads facing the test window and close the door. This last step must be done before the meter display reaches one (in the countdown). Record the glucose value that appears in the display window.

This procedure is followed by patients using Ames Glucostix Reagent Strips for Visual Color Matching:

1. Wash hands with soap and warm water. Rinse and dry thoroughly. Remove a Glucostix strip from the bottle and tightly replace the cap. Fold tissue in half, then in quarters. Obtain a large drop of blood from the outer edges of a fingertip using the Glucolet.

2. Apply blood to the Glucostix strip, completely covering the two yellow test pads. Begin timing immediately. Be prepared for step 3 in 30 seconds.

3. At exactly 30 seconds, blot the test pads as follows:

❏ Place a reacted strip, pad side up, on the tissue.
❏ Fold tissue over the pads and firmly press it against the pads for 1 to 2 seconds.
❏ Move the strip to a clean area and blot again.

4. Continue timing for 90 seconds more (120 seconds total). Now read the glucose value by comparing the test pads with the color chart on the label of the Glucostix Reagent Strip bottle:

❏ If the green pad on the strip is darker than the 110-mg/dL color block, compare the

orange pad to the closest matching orange block and record the glucose result.
❏ When comparing either the green or orange test pad, if the color is between two color blocks, estimate the glucose result.

A newer Ames system is the Glucometer 3 Diabetes Care System for use with Glucofilm Test Strips. The meter is smaller and simpler to use and the Glucofilm has a smaller test area to cover than the Glucostix. Ames maintains a center for diabetes education and has available publications and films for patients with diabetes.

CHOLESTEROL

Now recognized as a more prevalent problem than in the past, abnormalities of lipid metabolism are clearly one focus of routine screening for general health status and mass public screening.

Cholesterol is a steroid alcohol substance found in all animal fats and oils. It is a precursor of bile acids and steroid hormones and is found in considerable concentration in nerve tissue, adrenal glands, and the skin. Most serum cholesterol is synthesized by the body, but it is also obtained from the diet (dietary cholesterol). *Serum cholesterol* may exist free in the blood but most is combined with acids in the form of cholesterol esters.

The major *plasma lipids* are serum cholesterol and the triglycerides. Plasma lipids cannot circulate freely in the blood. Instead they attach themselves to blood proteins and are transported as *lipoproteins*. Triglyceride and cholesterol make up the major lipoproteins that are called *chylomicrons*. The cholesterol lipoproteins are classified as follows:

1. Very low density lipoproteins (VLDL)—produced by the liver and intestines from lipids stored after a meal. It is the main source of plasma low-density lipoprotein (LDL).

2. Low-density lipoproteins—produced by the metabolism of VLDL. LDL carries most of the plasma cholesterol (60% to 75%). Elevated LDL is associated with coronary artery disease.

3. High-density lipoproteins (HDL)—produced by the liver and intestines from lipids stored after a meal. HDL is *inversely* associated with cardiovascular risk. It is a protector against the harmful effects of the LDL and VLDL. HDL removes excess cholesterol from the tissues and the body. It normally accounts for 20% to 25% of the total plasma cholesterol. Although it is believed that HDL levels may be genetically controlled, they are also positively associated with exercise and the low intake of alcohol and inversely associated with smoking and certain contraceptives.

In contrast to cholesterol, it is not clear whether or not elevated serum triglycerides are an *independent* risk factor; however, in combination with elevated cholesterol levels, triglycerides are now considered important in the development of heart disease. The triglycerides are the major lipids transported through the blood and are also called simple lipids (true fat, neutral fat).

Serum lipid studies include the testing for total lipids, cholesterol, triglycerides, and the cholesterol lipoproteins. The formula used for the relationship of these lipids is:

$$\text{Cholesterol} = \frac{\text{Triglycerides}}{5} + \text{HDL} + \text{LDL} + \text{VLDL}$$

Abnormal levels of blood lipids usually are a result of metabolic disorders that may be due to hereditary causes, endocrine disorders, specific organ diseases, or external causes, such as diet. More than the value of any single lipid test, most physicians view the relationship of all the lipid values to one another (ratios) as the key to diagnosing diseases related to lipid metabolism.

SEROLOGY

Traditionally, serology was a branch of laboratory medicine restricted to reference and hospital laboratories. Originally, serology was the study of the in vitro reactions of immune sera. *Immune sera* is the serum obtained from an immunized individual, containing specific antibody or antibodies. These studies included precipitin, agglutination, and complement fixation reactions. Currently the term is used to refer to a broader use of serologic tests to measure the body's immune responses by detecting antibodies in the serum or by detecting special enzymes produced from an increased white blood cell production during infection. Serology tests can be used to evaluate the immunization status of an individual or an exposure to specific pathogenic microorganisms. Serology tests are also available to detect the presence of drugs, hormones, and vitamin levels in the body.

Serology is the study of the immune system's antigen-antibody reactions. The immune response is the body's ability to recognize the presence of a foreign agent and to produce a defense mechanism against it. The foreign agent is called an *antigen*. The *antibody* is the body's defense mechanism. Antibodies are produced when antigens are detected in the blood. Antibodies are specific for inactivating one particular matching antigen.

The same antigen-antibody reaction produced in the body can produce a visible or measurable result in the laboratory. Testing a patient's serum with a known antigen (reagent) can reveal the presence of a corresponding antigen. Testing is done on serum, urine, or other body fluids. Table 30–10 list abbreviations associated with serology.

TYPES OF ANTIGEN–ANTIBODY REACTIONS

In the body, the ability of an antibody to bind with or stick to an antigen allows it to destroy the antigen in a

Table 30–10

COMMONLY USED SEROLOGY ABBREVIATIONS

Abbreviation	Meaning
ASO	Antistreptolysin-O titer
CRP	C-reactive protein
CSF	Cerebrospinal fluid
FA	Fluorescent antibody; febrile antigens
FTA	Fluorescent treponemal antibody
hCG	Human chorionic gonadotropin
LE test	Rapid slide test method for systemic lupus erythematosus
Mono-Spot	Test for mononucleosis
RA test	Rapid slide test for rheumatoid arthritis
RF	Rheumatoid factor
RIA	Radioimmunoassay
rpm	Revolutions per minute
RPR	Rapid plasma reagin
SLE	Systemic lupus erythematosus
TB	Tuberculin
VD	Venereal disease
VDRL	Venereal Disease Research Laboratory

number of ways. Laboratory tests are based on the same reactions that occur in the body (Fig. 30–19).

One antigen-antibody reaction is *agglutination* (clumping). Agglutination occurs when bacterial antigens are forced to clump together by the action of a specific antibody. Agglutination may occur in other body fluids. *Hemagglutination,* for instance, is the clumping of red blood cells when they are mixed with the blood cells of another type. Platelets also agglutinate in the presence of different platelet types. This type of agglutination is the basis of laboratory platelet typing. Agglutination only occurs if the antigen is in the form of particles, such as bacteria, red blood cells, white blood cells, latex particles, or any substance appearing cloudy when suspended in saline. Commercial reagents for slide agglutination tests contain artificial carriers, such as latex particles, treated with red blood cells or bacterial cells that can carry antigen on their surface. The artificially introduced antigens bind with antibodies produced by the host during the test.

Antibodies also "fix" or activate *complement.* Complement fixation is a complex series of events occurring when a united antigen-antibody becomes bound (fixed, fixation) with a series of enzymatic proteins. When complement fixation occurs, the cell membrane (usually a bacteria) ruptures, resulting in a leakage of its substances into the body fluids. The destructive rupturing of the cell membrane is termed *lysis.*

Opsonization occurs when an antibody combines with an antigen and makes the antigen susceptible (sensitizes) to phagocytosis by leukocytes. Another defense reaction is *antitoxin production.* In the body,

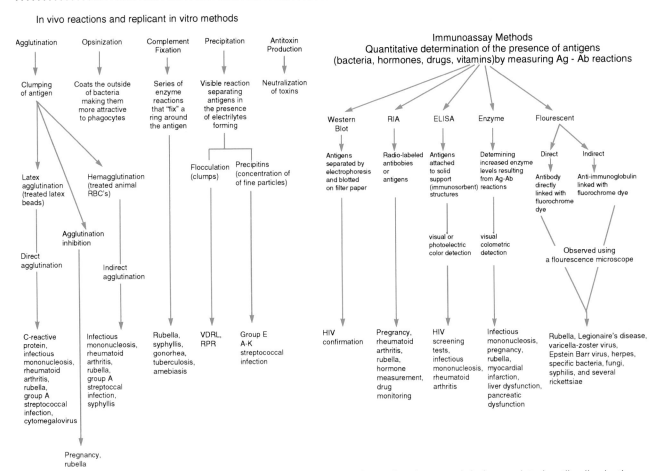

In vivo reactions and replicant in vitro methods

Figure 30–19. Many serologic procedures are based on the reactions of antigens and their associated antibodies in the blood.

certain bacteria release toxins. It is the toxins from toxin-producing bacteria that produce disease rather than the bacteria themselves. Antitoxins are special antibodies that are produced in the body in response to bacterial toxins. Antitoxin go to work to specifically destroy bacterial toxins.

Immunoassay is a term relating to any of several methods that measure antibody-antigen interactions. The detection of these interactions confirms the presence of antigens (hormones, drugs, vitamins, bacteria) in the body. *Radioimmunoassay (RIA)* involves a process where antibodies or antigens are tagged with radioisotopes. RIA is an extremely sensitive testing method that can detect a minute amount of antigen-antibody reaction. RIA methods require blood specimens, expensive laboratory equipment, and specialized personnel. It is rarely used for screening or pregnancy testing. Most reference laboratories use RIA techniques. Patients' blood samples are drawn in the office by venipuncture and sent to the reference laboratory. Each reference laboratory provides special instruction for collection and transportation of laboratory specimens.

Other types of immunoassay include *enzyme-linked immunosorbent assay (ELISA)*, which uses an enzyme-labeled antigen or antibody (immunoreactant) and

an antibody or antigen bound to an insoluble support (immunosorbent) substance which absorbs the antigens; and *fluorescent antibody immunoassay*, in which antibodies coat antigens with a fluorochrome dye that cannot be washed away. The dyed substances can then be seen under the fluorescent microscope. Enzyme immunoassay measures the enzymes released from injured tissues and white blood cells into the blood when tissue is damaged by the presence of antigens. Thus, detecting increased serum enzyme levels can aid in the diagnosis of infection. Reference laboratories perform ELISA tests to confirm the presence of HIV antibodies. Many other enzyme immunoassay kits are quick and easy to use in the office laboratory.

RAPID MANUAL SEROLOGY TESTS KITS

Rapid manual serology screening test kits are available to test for infectious diseases, such as strep throat, syphilis, herpes, hepatitis, rubella or infectious mononucleosis; for autoimmune diseases, such as rheumatoid arthritis; and for pregnancy. (Pregnancy testing is covered in the Urinalysis section of Chapter 29.)

Many commercial tests that have been long used in the POL are slide or tube tests based on the inhibition of latex particle agglutination. Currently, these types of tests have expanded to include hemagglutinin inhibition tests, latex particle inhibition tests, direct latex particle agglutination tests, and enzyme immunoassay tests. These tests are easy to perform, and many of them are manufactured for in-home use. The effectiveness of these tests depends on following the manufacturer's directions, using good reagents, good specimen collection technique, and proper storage. Table 30–11 summarizes the guidelines for interpreting the more commonly used serologic tests.

RAPID SLIDE TEST FOR INFECTIOUS MONONUCLEOSIS

Infectious mononucleosis is caused by the Epstein-Barr virus. Patients infected with the Epstein-Barr virus produce heterophil antibodies. The heterophil antibody is detectable on the rapid slide test.

The most common slide test for infectious mononucleosis is based on a latex agglutination reaction (see Fig. 30–19). The test can detect the presence of antibodies with a reagent made up of mononucleosis antigen attached to latex particles. The reagent agglutinates in the presence of heterophil antibodies. If agglutination occurs, the test is positive; if no agglutination occurs, the test is negative.

Serum is the usual specimen, although plasma can be used. The presence of hemolysis in the specimen makes the blood unfit for testing. At least 0.5 mL of serum is necessary for the test. The blood is centrifuged and the serum removed. The slide test is then performed according to the manufacturer's instructions.

A false-negative result can occur if the testing is done too early. A detectable level of heterophil antibody usually does not occur until 2 weeks after the onset of symptoms. Certain leukemias, rheumatoid arthritis, viral hepatitis, cytomegalovirus infections, and myocardial infarction may produce a false-positive result.

GROUP A STREP SCREEN

As an alternative to traditional manual growth microbiology tests (culturing), the group A streptococcal screen is a frequently requested test in pediatric practices because children are especially susceptible to sore throats caused by group A β-streptococci. Most group A streptococcal screens are based on serologic detection using latex agglutination or enzyme immunoassay color-change tests. Enzyme tests are easier to interpret because a positive reaction is indicated by a visible color change. Compared with the 24 to 48 hours needed for a throat culture result, the test can be quickly run while the patient waits in the office, and antibiotic therapy can be quickly initiated.

Because the group A streptococcal screen is performed on a throat specimen, the group A streptococcal screen is described in the Bacteriology section of Chapter 29.

SUMMARY

The medical assistant has the responsibility for properly collecting specimens and accurate testing. The medical assistant should approach office laboratory testing as a challenging opportunity to work with the physician to improve and promote health care.

Table 30–11

GUIDELINES FOR INTERPRETING SEROLOGIC TEST RESULTS

Test	Result	Observation
Hemagglutination inhibition	Positive	No agglutination.
	Negative	Agglutination in the second stage of the test.
Latex particle agglutination inhibition	Positive	A colored symbol becomes visible.
	Negative	No color symbol appears.
	Quality control (QC)	A separate, QC, color symbol should appear with both negative and positive results. If the control symbol does not appear, the test is considered uninterpretable.
Latex particle agglutination	Positive	Agglutination occurs.
	Negative	No agglutination occurs.
	QC	Both positive and negative controls are run with every test.
Enzyme immunoassay	Positive	A colored symbol appears.
	Negative	No colored symbol appears.
	QC	A separate, QC, color symbol should appear with both negative and positive results. If the control symbol does not appear, the test is considered uninterpretable.

DISCUSSION QUESTIONS

1. When performing a specimen collection, the specimen spills. What is your immediate response?
2. Discuss the importance of safeguarding the transport of microbiological specimens.
3. How would you describe the purpose of a complete blood count to the patient?

BIBLIOGRAPHY

Finegold S and Baron E: Bailey and Scott's Diagnostic Microbiology, ed 7. CV Mosby, St. Louis, 1986.
Lifshitz M and DeCresce R: An overview of equipment for the physician's office laboratory. Laboratory Medicine 17(6):337, 1986.
Sacher A and McPherson A: Widmann's Clinical Interpretation of Laboratory Tests, ed 10. FA Davis Co, Philadelphia, 1991.

PROCEDURE: Perform a hematocrit determination using the Unopette System and the microhematocrit method

OSHA STANDARDS:

Terminal Performance Objective: Determine the hematocrit by comparing the amount of packed red blood cells with the total blood volume within a reasonable time.

EQUIPMENT: Universal precautions barriers, as necessary
Nonsterile gloves
Microhematocrit (high speed) centrifuge with timer
Microhematocrit reader
Microhematocrit capillary tubes, heparinized (if used with free-flowing blood from a capillary puncture site)
Microhematocrit capillary tubes, plain (if used with 5 to 7 mL Vacutainer tube with ethylenediaminetetraacetic acid–treated [EDTA] blood)
Capillary tube sealing compound
Adhesive tape
Two wooden sticks
Gauze
Towel for work surface
5% bleach and towels
Two disposable biohazard bags
Sharps collector

PROCEDURE

Obtaining the Specimen

1. Holding the capillary tube at a 10° angle, touch the tip directly to a free-flowing capillary puncture site or a Vacutainer tube with a well-mixed EDTA coagulant (lavender stopper) and fresh blood sample. Fill the capillary tube two-thirds full (one-half to three-fourths full).
2. If blood from a Vacutainer tube is used, first rim the inside of the tube with two wooden applicator sticks.

3. Use a plain capillary tube for blood withdrawn from a Vacutainer tube with EDTA; for free-flowing blood from a skin puncture, use heparinized capillary tubes.
4. If air enters the capillary tube, expel the blood past the bubble and refill.
5. Remove the tube from the blood and allow the blood in the tube to flow an additional 1.3 inches (0.5 cm) toward the clean end of the tube.
6. Remove any blood from the outside of the tube with clean gauze, without touching blood inside the pipette.
7. Hold the tube near the clean end that is to be inserted into sealing clay and insert at a 90° angle. Rotate the tube to fill with the clay and prevent any blood from seeping out the ends during the process.
8. Fill and seal a second capillary tube.

9. Fill and seal two tubes with a control sample.
10. Tape the patient tubes and control tubes to a sheet of paper.

PRINCIPLE

1. Blood must be fresh and free-flowing or well-mixed to avoid clots. Blood samples begin to clot and the cells begin to break down from the time it is collected. Clotting blood will produce falsely high values.

2. Clotted blood will give a falsely high result. Rimming is accomplished by running the applicator sticks around the rim of the tube.
3. Blood must be anticoagulated, unclotted, and unhemolyzed.

4. Air displaces the blood, causing the tube to be underfilled.
5. This clears the end of the tube of blood for sealing with clay. Blood mixed with the sealing clay could splatter during centrifugation.
6. Blood on the outside of the tube will enter the reservoir and add more blood to the solution, thus elevating the count.
7. Holding near the end prevents breaking the tube, which could cause an injury with blood. If tubes are not sealed properly, more red blood cells than plasma will be lost, resulting in false-low results.
8. The second tube will be used as a balance in the centrifuge and will provide a check for accuracy.
9. Two samples are required for centrifugal balance.
10. To properly identify the specimens and the control samples.

PROCEDURE

11. Place white tape on the inside of the microhematocrit centrifuge.

12. Place the two patient tubes into two grooves of the centrifuge head with the sealed end facing outward and record the groove numbers for the two samples.

13. Place the two control tubes on the opposite side of the centrifuge head with the sealed end facing outward and record the groove numbers.

14. Carefully lower and secure the inner lid, then lower the outer lid and seal.

15. Centrifuge for 3 to 5 minutes at 10,000 rpm.

16. Allow the centrifuge to stop on its own.

17. Line up the bottom of the packed red cell column (just above the clay sealer) with zero on the microhematocrit reader. Turn the reader until the top of the plasma is at the 100 mark. The hematocrit is read at the line between the packed red cells and the buffy coat.

18. Read the results as a percentage on the hematocrit reader within 10 minutes.

19. The two patient samples should be within ± 0.02 (2%) of one another. The two control samples should be within the manufacturer's specified range.

20. Average the two readings if they are within 2% of each other. Report the results as a decimal fraction. For example, a 40% result is reported as 0.45.

PRINCIPLE

11. If blood leakage occurs, the tape will show a band of blood. If leakage occurs, the centrifuge must be cleaned with a solution of 5–10% household bleach.

12. With the sealed end to the outside, blood will be prevented from spinning out during centrifugation.

13. During high speed rotation, the material in the centrifuge head must be in balance.

14. The inner lid could break the capillary tubes.

15. The time is needed to force the red blood cells to become packed on the bottom of the tube. Inadequate time will give falsely high results.

16. Stopping the rotations with the hand throws cells back into the plasma and invalidates the results.

17. The buffy coat is a gray-white layer of white cells and platelets, and the area should not be included on the measurement. The reading represents the percentage of the total volume of blood occupied by the red blood cells.

18. The horizontal position of the tubes will allow the cells to start traveling back into the plasma.

19. Duplicate testing and control samples provide quality assurance.

20. Proper documentation is an important part of quality assurance.

PROCEDURE: Perform a white blood cell count using the Unopette System and the Neubauer ruled hemacytometer*

OSHA STANDARDS:

Terminal Performance Objective: Determine the number of white blood cells in thousands per microliter (1 μL) of blood within a reasonable time.

EQUIPMENT: *For Diluting:*
Universal precautions
  barriers, as necessary
Nonsterile gloves
Unopette unit
  25-μL pipette
  Pipette shield
  Prefilled reagent reservoir
    (3% acetic acid to make 1:20 solution when 25 μL of
    blood is added)
5 to 7 mL EDTA anticoagulated blood or free-flowing
  blood from a capillary puncture
Whole blood control sample of known value
Test tube rack
Two wooden sticks
Gauze
Towel for work surface

For Counting:
Microscope
Neubauer ruled hemacytometer
Coverslip, plane on both sides within 0.002 mm
Hand tally
Lens paper
70% alcohol
Covered petri dish with moist filter paper
Interval timer
5% bleach and towels
Biohazard disposal bags
Biohazard sharps collector

PROCEDURE

Preparation

1. Perform a manual white blood count (WBC) on a whole blood control of known value.
2. Gather enough materials to perform a duplicate WBC.

PRINCIPLE

1. To conduct a quality control test of the equipment and performance of the technician.
2. White blood cells should be counted in duplicate (pipetted in duplicate and each pipette counted on two sides of a hemacytometer, giving four counting areas) by the beginning student until accuracy is attained. The more experienced student and practicing medical assistant need only duplicate low counts or counts of critical importance.

---

*Illustrations in this procedure from Wedding ME and Toemjes SA: Medical Laboratory Procedures. FA Davis, Philadelphia, 1992, p 258, with permission.)

PROCEDURE

Filling a Unopette

1. Puncture the test reservoir diaphragm with the pipette shield to form a hole large enough to allow the pipette to freely enter the system.
2. Holding the pipette (capillary tube) horizontally, touch the tip directly to a free-flowing capillary puncture site or Vacutainer tube with a well-mixed EDTA coagulant (lavender stopper) and blood *not more than 24 hours old.*
3. If blood from a Vacutainer tube is used, first rim the inside of the tube with two wooden applicator sticks.

4. Remove any blood from the outside of the pipette with clean gauze, without touching the tip of the pipette.
5. Squeeze the sides of the reservoir, cover the pipette overflow chamber with the index finger, and securely seat the pipette into the reservoir neck with a twisting motion.
6. Release pressure on the reservoir, then remove the finger from the overflow chamber.
7. Squeeze the reservoir three times to rinse the pipette, without expelling the reservoir contents through the top of the overflow chamber.
8. Place the index finger over the overflow chamber and gently invert several times.
9. Let the sample stand for 10 minutes.
10. If the sample is to sit for longer than 10 minutes, reverse the position of the pipette and cover it with the pipette shield.

Charging (Filling) the Hemacytometer

1. Clean and dry the hemacytometer and coverslip with 70% alcohol and lens paper.
2. Check the surface of the hemacytometer and coverslip for scratches.
3. Align the cover slip over the ruled chamber.

4. Mix the sample well, then convert the Unopette assembly by withdrawing the pipette from the solution and reseating it in the reverse position.

PRINCIPLE

1. Too small a hole can result in the lose of a portion of the sample when the pipette is inserted into the reservoir.
2. Well-mixed blood must be inverted eight times to suspend the cells. Blood samples begin to clot and the cells begin to break down from the time blood is collected. The filling will stop by itself when the pipette is full.
3. Clotted blood will give a falsely high result. Rimming is accomplished by running the applicator sticks around the rim of the tube.
4. Blood on the outside will enter the reservoir, adding more blood to the solution and elevating the count.

5. Squeezing the reservoir will create a vacuum that will draw the sample into the reservoir.

6. This allows the blood to flow into the diluting fluid.

7. To ensure that all of the blood sample is delivered into the reservoir.

8. To thoroughly mix the sample with the diluting fluid.

9. To hemolyze the red cells.
10. To prevent evaporation. The sample is stable for *3 hours.* If the sample is allowed to sit, mix it again to suspend the cells before performing the actual count.

1. Dirt, fingerprints, and grease interfere with blood cell distribution.
2. Scratches will interfere with blood cell distribution and visualization.
3. The coverslip must not be moved after the chamber is filled.
4. Shaking the Unopette and reservoir is an important factor in obtaining good distribution of cells and accurate cell counts.

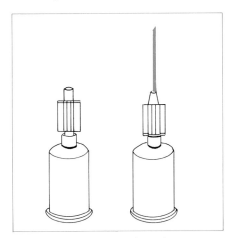

Convert the Unopette reservoir to dropper assembly.

PROCEDURE

5. Invert the reservoir and gently squeeze out 3 or 4 drops onto a gauze square.

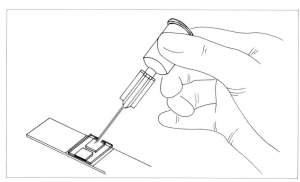

Charge the hematocytometer by gently squeezing the reservoir bottle.

6. Touch the tip of the pipette to the edge of the cover-slip in the loading area at a 40° angle.

7. Fill the chamber by controlling the flow with the finger on the pipette or by squeezing the reservoir sides until 1 drop of blood is drawn rapidly under the coverslip by capillarity, and the ruled area is full but not overfull.

8. Do not move the coverslip. If blood spills into the dividing moats or is unevenly distributed, recharging with a new sample is necessary.

9. Fill both sides of the hemacytometer.

10. Allow the chamber to sit for 1 minute covered in a Petri dish lined with moist filter paper.

11. Keeping the hemacytometer horizontal and without touching the coverslip, place it on the lowered micro-scope stage.

12. Center one of the ruled areas over the condenser and using the low-power objective.

13. Reduce the light intensity by adjusting the diaphragm and slightly lowering the condenser.

14. Turn the coarse adjustment slowly until the ruled area comes into focus; then use the fine adjustment to bring the area into perfect focus and adjust the light if necessary.

PRINCIPLE

5. Discarding the first 3 to 4 drops clears any blood standing in the pipette and is an important factor in obtaining good distribution of cells.

6. The chamber fills by capillary attraction. If the pipette tip is not touching the edge of the coverslip, the chamber will not fill properly.

7. Any unevenness or slowness in filling affects the cell distribution. Only 1 drop can be used — 2 or more partial drops is unsatisfactory.

8. Excess blood could raise the coverslip and change the depth factor of the sample, which would result in inaccurate results.

9. Two separate counts are performed with each charging.

10. Sitting allows the cells to settle to a single plane. Moisture prevents evaporation. Evaporation contracts the sample and elevates the cell count.

11. The hemacytometer is too thick for a raised stage. Raise the stage carefully.

12. Unstained cells require reduced light for counting.

13. To adjust the light so that the field is evenly illuminated and easy to view. Raise the stage carefully.

14. Careful movement is necessary so as not to damage the coverslip. If the objective touches the coverslip, the cell distribution is altered and the hemacytometer must be recharged.

Counting White Blood Cells in the Neubauer Hemacytometer

1. Using the 10X objective, focus on the ruled area and scan the entire ruled area.

2. Move the chamber to center the upper left white blood cell square in the microscopic field and focus using the coarse adjustment and mechanical stage simultaneously.

3. Count the white blood cells that touch the top and left hand boundaries of each of the 16 smaller squares by depressing the hand tally once for each cell seen.

4. Start at the top row, far left, move visually from left to right across the top row, drop down to the second row and move right to left, then drop down to the third row and visually move left to right.

1. To check that the cells are evenly distributed.

2. To avoid miscounting cells or counting cells twice, a specific winding pattern is used to scan and count the cells.

3. Cells touching the right hand and bottom boundaries are not counted to avoid counting cells twice or missing cells altogether.

4. To avoid counting cells twice or missing cells altogether.

PROCEDURE

5. Record the number tallied on the 16 squares and return the counter to zero.

6. Count the cells in the large white blood cell squares 2, 3, and 4 and record the number tallied in each of these areas.

7. Count the white blood cells on the second side of the chamber in the same manner.

8. Total the four white blood cell squares and multiply the result by 50 on each side.

9. Compare the totals from each side.

10. Average the totals from the two sides and round off to the nearest 100 cells.

11. Record the results.

12. Perform a second count as necessary (see Preparation, above).

13. Disinfect the hemacytometer and cover slip in 5% bleach solution for 10 minutes, rinse with tap water, and dry with lens paper.

14. Dispose of the Unopette System and contaminated materials in a biohazard container and sharps collector.

PRINCIPLE

5. Each of the four large counting areas are tallied separately.

6. The totals should agree within 10 cells of each other. If the count does not agree within 10 cells, the hemacytometer should be cleaned and refilled, and the procedure repeated.

7. Two counts provide a check on the accuracy of the prepared specimen.

8. To obtain the total number of white blood cells per microliter of blood.

9. The totals should agree within 1000 cells.

10. Only one total can be reported.

13. Bleach is the acceptable disinfectant for equipment coming into contact with blood.

14. To prevent transmitting microorganisms or patient access to blood.

PROCEDURE: Perform a red blood count using the Unopette
System and the Neubauer ruled hemacytometer

OSHA STANDARDS: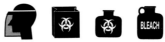

Terminal Performance Objective: Determine the number of red blood cells in millions per microliter ($1\ \mu L$) of blood within a reasonable time.

EQUIPMENT: *For Diluting:*
Universal precautions barriers, as necessary
Nonsterile gloves
Unopette unit
   $25\text{-}\mu L$ pipette
   pipette shield
   prefilled reagent reservoir (Hayem normal saline $1:200$
      solution when $25\ \mu L$ of blood is added)
5 to 7 mL EDTA anticoagulated
   blood or free-flowing blood from a capillary puncture
Whole blood control of known value
Test tube rack
Two wooden sticks
Gauze
Towel for work surface

For Counting:
Microscope
Neubauer ruled hemacytometer
Coverslip, plane on both sides within 0.002 mm
Hand tally
Lens paper
70% alcohol
Covered Petri dish with moist filter paper
Interval timer
5% bleach and towels
Biohazard disposal bags
Biohazard sharps collector

PROCEDURE

Preparation

1. Perform a manual red blood count (RBC) on a whole blood control of known value.
2. Gather enough materials to perform a duplicate RBC.

Filling a Unopette

(See preceding WBC procedure).

Charging (Filling) the Hemacytometer

(See preceding WBC procedure.)

Counting Red Blood Cells in the Neubauer Hemacytometer

1. Using the 10× objective, focus on the central ruled area and scan the entire area.

PRINCIPLE

1. To conduct a quality control test of the equipment and the technician's performance.
2. Because the RBC is one of the least accurate manual procedures performed in the laboratory, every sample should be pipetted in duplicate, and each pipette is charged on two sides of the hemacytometer, giving four counting areas in all.

1. To check that the cells are evenly distributed.

PROCEDURE

2. Move the chamber to center the central ruled square in the microscopic field and switch to 40X power; adjust the light and focus.
3. Count the red blood cells that touch the top and left-hand boundaries of each of the 16 squares by depressing the hand tally once for each cell seen.
4. Start at the top row, far left, move visually from left to right across the top row, drop down to the second row and move right to left, then drop down to the third row and visually move left to right.
5. Record the number tallied on the 16 squares and return the counter to zero.
6. Count the cells in the corner squares 2, 3, 4, and 5 and record the number tallied in each of these areas.

7. Count the red blood cells on the second side of the chamber in the same manner.
8. Total the five red blood cell squares and multiply the results on each side by 10,000.
9. Compare the totals from each side.
10. Average the two side totals and round off to the nearest 100 cells.
11. Record the results.
12. Disinfect the hemacytometer and coverslip in 5% bleach solution for 10 minutes, rinse with tap water, and dry with lens paper.
13. Dispose of the Unopette System and contaminated materials in biohazard bag and sharps collector.

PRINCIPLE

2. The central counting area is counted before the four corner areas.

3. Cells touching the right-hand and bottom boundaries are not counted to avoid counting cells twice or missing cells altogether.
4. To avoid counting cells twice or missing cells altogether.

5. Each of the five large counting areas are tallied separately.
6. The totals agree within 20 cells of each other. If the count does not agree within 20 cells, the hemacytometer should be cleaned and refilled, and the procedure repeated.
7. Two counts provide a check on the accuracy of the prepared specimen.
8. To obtain the total number of red blood cells per microliter of blood.
9. The total should agree within 300,000 cells.
10. Only one total count per microliter of blood is reported.

12. Bleach is the acceptable disinfectant for equipment coming into contact with blood.

13. To prevent transmitting microorganisms or patient access to blood material and to prepare the room for the next blood test.

PROCEDURE: Perform an examination of a peripheral blood smear

OSHA STANDARDS:

Terminal Performance Objective: Determine what percentage of the total WBC each type of white blood cell represents, evaluate the morphology of red blood cells, and estimate the number of platelets per microliter of blood.

EQUIPMENT: *For Staining:*
Universal precautions barriers, as necessary
Nonsterile gloves
Clean glass slides with frosted ends
Transfer pipette or capillary tubes
Wright's stain
Buffer
Distilled water
Forceps and staining rack
5 to 7 mL EDTA anticoagulated blood or free-flowing
    blood from a capillary puncture
Whole blood control of known value
Drying rack
Stopwatch
Two wooden sticks
Gauze
Towel for work surface
Biohazard disposal bags
Biohazard sharps collector

For Counting:
Microscope
Immersion oil
Lens paper
Hand tally
Differential counter
Ethanol
Calculator

PROCEDURE

Preparing the Smear

1. Holding the pipette (capillary tube) horizontally, touch the tip directly to a free-flowing capillary puncture site or Vacutainer tube with a well-mixed EDTA coagulant (lavender stopper) and blood *not more than 1 hour old.*
2. If blood from a Vacutainer tube is used, first rim the inside of the tube with two wooden applicator sticks.

3. Remove any blood from the outside of the pipette with clean gauze, without touching the tip of the pipette.
4. Place the slide on a flat surface with the frosted end on the side of the dominant hand.

PRINCIPLE

1. Well-mixed blood must be inverted eight times to suspend the cells. Blood samples begin to clot and the cells begin to break down from the time blood is collected. The filling will stop by itself when the pipette is full.
2. Clotted blood will give a falsely high result. Rimming is accomplished by running the applicator sticks around the rim of the tube.
3. Blood on the outside will enter the reservoir and add more blood to the solution and elevate the count.

4. The smear will be made with the dominant hand in a direction away from the frosted end.

PROCEDURE

PRINCIPLE

5. Place 1 small drop of blood on the slide approximately ¾ inch (1.9 cm) from the nonfrosted end in the center of the slide.

5. Smears should be thin to stain satisfactorily, to eliminate cell overlapping, and to prevent white blood cells from being too small to view.

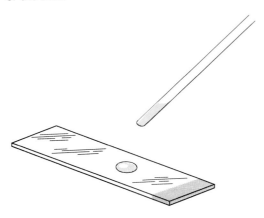

6. Place a second slide (called the spreader slide) in front of the drop of blood at a 30° to 45° until it touches the blood. The drop will quickly spread along the edge of the spreader slide, because of capillary action. Allow the blood to spread only three fourths along the spreader edge.

6. If blood spreads to the far edges of the slide, the white blood cells at the side margins cannot be seen under the microscope. White blood cells tend to migrate to the edges.

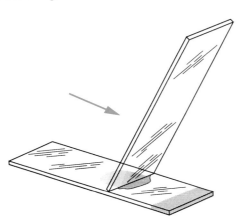

7. Quickly push the spreader forward in one movement while maintaining the same angle and keeping the spreader in contact with the first slide.

7. A smooth motion prevents ridges from occurring in the smear. Pushing too rapidly produces a short, thick smear; too slowly, a long thin smear. The smear should be at least 1½ inches (3.8 cm) long, smooth, and have margins on all sides.

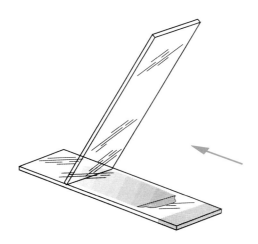

PROCEDURE

8. Finish the motion by raising the spreader in a smooth, low arc to produce a "feathered" edge.

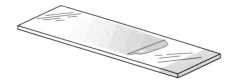

9. Prepare a second smear in the same manner.
10. Allow the smears to air-dry 15 minutes. Gently wave the slide in a horizontal position, then stand the slides with the thick end down until dried.

11. Label the slides with the patient's name and the date.

Staining the Smear

1. Place the smear on a staining rack blood side up with the thin end of the smear away from you.
2. Flood the smear with Wright's stain and leave on for 2 to 3 minutes.
3. Add one to one and one-half times buffer drop by drop onto the Wright's stain.
4. Blow gently along the length of the slide and let stand for the time recommended by the manufacturer (usually 10 minutes).
5. Rinse thoroughly with distilled water and drain water from the slide.
6. Wipe the back of the smear with gauze and air-dry in a vertical position with the thickest part down.
7. Examine the smear under 10X power to check the stain quality and blood cell distribution. If the red blood cells appear too red and the nuclei of the white blood cells too pale or colorless, the stain is too acidic. If the red blood cells appear blue, the stain is to alkaline. If the smear is of poor quality, repeat the process, adjusting the time of the staining procedure.
   Neutrophils — pale pink with dark purple nucleus
   Basophilic granules — stain deep blue to black with purple nucleus
   Eosinophils — stain orange with a purple nucleus
   Lymphocytes — stain pale blue with a dark purple nucleus
   Monocytes — stain gray-blue
   Platelets — stain lilac with multicolor central granules

Examining the Smear

1. Move the smear to view an area where at least 50% of the red blood cells touch or are slightly overlapping under 10X, then focus under 40X with the fine adjustment knob and increased light.
2. Count the number of white blood cells in 10 fields, average, and multiply the average by 2000.

PRINCIPLE

8. The slight lifting movement at the end produces a smear having gradation from thick at the beginning to very thin at the end. The central half of the smear should be of a thickness that allows the red blood cells to touch each other but not overlap. The red blood cells will be in the thin end studied and must not touch each other.

9. It is good practice to make two smears for each test.
10. Air drying accelerates the process. If the thick end is up, blood could run down onto the thin end and ruin the smear. The smear should be stained as soon as possible but can sit for a maximum of 24 hours.
11. To provide a means of identification.

1. The tray will catch the overflow from the staining solution.
2. The Wright's stain is an eosin (acid dye) and methylene blue (alkaline) stain.
3. The timing will vary according to the specific technique.
4. To mix the stain and buffer until a green metallic sheen appears.
5. To remove the metallic sheen that has formed on top of the stain.
6. The quicker it dries, the less cell shrinkage. The smear should have a lavender-pink color.
7. The red blood cells should be evenly stained a light buff color and free of precipitated stain. The red cells should be evenly distributed without streaks. There should be at least 10X power fields in which the red cells are lying side by side but not touching. The white blood cells should be stained so that there is a prominent distinction between their nuclei and cytoplasm. The white blood cells should be evenly distributed and not clumped along the edges. There should be not more than five times the number of white cells at the feathered edge than at the examination area. The platelets should not be clumped at the feathered end or at the edges of the smear.

1. To check that the distribution of white blood cells is without clumps in some spots and sparse in others.

2. To estimate the number of white blood cells. The count should be within 20% of the WBC obtained in the hemacytometer. A larger count may be ordered if the white count is elevated.

PROCEDURE

3. Begin counting near the top of the smear, moving the field of view down, then to the right and back up in an "S" pattern over the area to be counted.

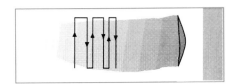

4. Move the smear to an area where the red cells are side by side but not overlapping (thin end of smear).
5. Move the 40× objective aside and add a drop of oil immersion to the slide, then lock the 100× objective in place.
6. Evaluate the red blood cells in 10 fields. Report any variations in size, shape, or color.

7. If nucleated erythrocytes are seen, count them separately while performing the white blood cell differential count and report them in number per 100 white blood cells.
8. Estimate the platelets by counting 10 fields, average the field count and multiply the average by 15,000.

9. Perform a white blood cell differential count following a winding pattern from the top of the smear downward.
10. As each white blood cell comes into view, record it on the differential counter by depressing the appropriate key for each type of cell, until 100 cells have been counted.
11. Record the number of cells for each category and verify that the total equals 100.

PRINCIPLE

3. To avoid duplication.

4. Cells that overlap are too difficult to count.
5. The differentiation of cells can be performed only when details are visualized under oil-immersion power.
6. The red blood cells should be uniform in size, shape, and color and free of excess stain. The central pallor of the cell should occupy approximately 30% to 40% of the cell.
7. Any abnormalities should be reported. Nucleated erythrocytes or immature red cells may be indicative of bone marrow dysfunction.

8. The normal platelet count is 150,000 to 400,000/μL. Report the estimate as normal, decreased, or increased. The average field count should be 10 to 20 platelets per field. Platelets are one fourth to one third the size of red cells and have a fuzzy periphery.
9. To avoid duplication.

10. One hundred cells are counted so that each differential count can be counted as a percentage of 100.

11. The differential report shows whether individual types of white cells are increased or decreased, which in turn can help the physician in arriving at a more specific diagnosis.

> Obtaining a quality electrocardiogram requires a skillful combination of art and science.
>
> Anonymous

CHAPTER OUTLINE

LEARNING OBJECTIVES

Upon completing this chapter, you will be able to:

1. Define the terminology related to electrocardiography (ECG).
2. Describe the structure and function of the heart, and relate function to electrical activity.
3. Identify the components of the ECG cardiac cycle.
4. Describe the basic functions of the ECG.
5. List the twelve ECG leads, and identify the sensor placement for each lead.
6. Describe the preparation of a patient for an ECG procedure.
7. Describe the procedure for obtaining an accurate ECG.
8. Discuss the procedures for eliminating artifacts.
9. Discuss the international marking system.
10. Explain the procedure for mounting an ECG.

Chapter 31

*E*lectrocardiography

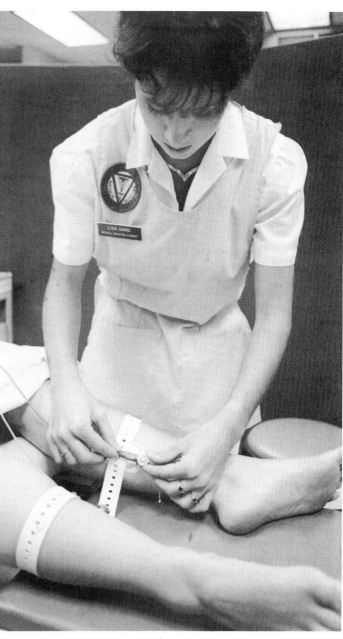

PERFORMANCE OBJECTIVES

Upon completing this chapter, you will be able to:

1. Instruct and position the patient, correctly position all electrodes and leads, and operate the electrocardiograph (ECG) machine.
2. Mount the ECG tracing in a way that will make it easy to read and ensure its preservation in the patient's file.

DACUM EDUCATIONAL COMPONENTS

1. Run an electrocardiogram and record the results for 12 leads and the rhythm strip (4.11–G).
2. Maintain and operate the electrocardiograph (6.2–E).

Glossary

Arrhythmia: alteration in cardiac rate, rhythm, or conduction

Artifact: extraneous voltages that interfere with recording the electrocardiographic (ECG) cycle on the graph paper

Cardiac cycle: period from the beginning of one beat or contraction of the heart to the beginning of the next succeeding beat including systole (contraction) and diastole (relaxation) of the atria and ventricles

Electrocardiogram: recording of the electrical impulses associated with cardiac contraction and relaxation; the two functions recorded include the amount of voltage generated by the heart and the time required for the voltage to travel through the heart

Sensors: originally called electrodes. Made of conductive metal (nickel-silver), they are attached to the limbs and chest and serve as receiving antennas to detect voltage from the skin and feed it into the ECG instrument (using the term "electrodes" may cause the patient to think of electricity, thereby inducing fear)

An electrocardiogram, abbreviated EKG or ECG, usually is included as part of a patient's routine physical examination to establish a baseline ECG for future reference and to detect the presence of heart abnormalities. Even though it is a simple procedure to perform, often the tracings are not accurate or of good quality.

The information presented in this chapter will assist the medical assistant in efficiently performing the ECG procedure. However, only practicing the art and science of ECG can ensure the task is performed accurately and with confidence and expertise. It is vital for the medical assistant to acquire the knowledge and skills essential for performing an accurate ECG.

CARDIAC ANATOMY AND PHYSIOLOGY

The heart is a hollow muscular organ that pumps blood throughout the body. The muscle tissue composing the heart walls is called the *myocardium.* When stimulated, cardiac muscle contracts. Through this contraction process, or pumping action, the heart circulates blood through the body, carrying the oxygen d nutrients needed by the tissues and removing the te by-products of metabolism.

Each side of the heart contains two hollow chambers. The upper chambers are referred to as *atria* and the lower chambers as *ventricles.* The right and left sides of the heart are separated by a partition, or *septum.* Valves separate the atria from the ventricles. The *tricuspid valve* is between the right atria and ventricle; and the *bicuspid,* or *mitral, valve* is located between the left atria and ventricle. The valves prevent the backflow of blood. Valves are hinged flaps that permit blood to flow in only one direction. When the ventricle contracts, it forces blood against the valve, thus pushing it closed. As the ventricle contraction empties the blood from the chamber, the mechanical pressure against the valve decreases and the valve reopens to let blood from the atrium again fill the ventricle. This process repeats itself with each ventricle contraction.

Figure 31–1 shows the way that blood flows through the heart and lungs. Blood being returned from the body to the heart contains little oxygen but has a high carbon dioxide content. This oxygen-poor or -depleted blood enters the right atria by way of the superior and inferior vena cava. The blood is pumped from the right atria through the tricuspid valve into the right ventricle. Right ventricle contraction forces the blood through the pulmonary valve into the pulmonary artery, which provides passage to the lungs. Capillary

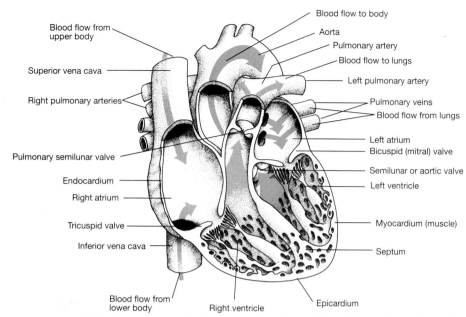

Figure 31–1. Anatomy of the heart; arrows indicate the direction of blood flow. (From Gylys BA and Wedding ME: *Medical Terminology: A Systems Approach*, ed 2. F. A. Davis, Philadelphia, 1988, p. 149, with permission.)

action in the lungs removes the carbon dioxide and replaces it with oxygen. This oxygen-rich blood returns to the left atrium by way of the pulmonary veins. (Note that this is one of the two instances in which oxygenated blood is transported by veins and oxygen-depleted blood by arteries. The other instance occurs in umbilical arteries and veins.) The blood next flows from the left atrium through the bicuspid valve into the left ventricle. Contraction of the left ventricle forces the blood through the aortic valve into the aorta and into the body's systemic circulation. The blood again gives up its oxygen and begins to collect carbon dioxide. It returns to the vena cava and is transported back to the right atrium, where the cycle is repeated.

CONDUCTION SYSTEM

Cardiac muscle differs from skeletal muscle in that it is able to contract rhythmically and conduct impulses. Although the heart contains many autonomic nervous system nerve fibers that can alter the beat of the heart, the heart muscle does not require *any* nerve supply to function. The heart can be removed from the body and continue to beat because of its self-contained pacemaker system. Specifically, this intrinsic or pacemaker system functions because of specialized cells located within the muscle tissue. These special cells conduct an electrical impulse that initiates the muscle contraction.

The transmission of this impulse follows a specific pathway. Contraction of heart muscle results from the stimulus initiated by the sinoatrial node (SA or pacemaker). The unique facet of the SA node is that it initiates activity without being stimulated by a nerve impulse. (Figure 31–2 shows the impulse transmission pathway.) This mass of specialized tissue is located in

the right atrial wall near the opening of the superior vena cava. The SA node has an intrinsic rhythm that acts as the pacemaker in initiating a cardiac muscle contraction, or a heartbeat. The SA node merges with the surrounding cardiac muscle, and as a result, the impulse for muscle contraction spreads throughout the atrium. This wave of excitation passes through the atrial muscle to the junction of the ventricles, where the atrioventricular (AV) node or junction is located. The AV node is stimulated and passes the stimulation on to the bundle of His, which acts as the relay station for continuing the stimulation on to the Purkinje fibers. The bundle of His relay performs a vital function in that it does not let the impulse proceed to the ventricles until the atrium has completed its contraction. The

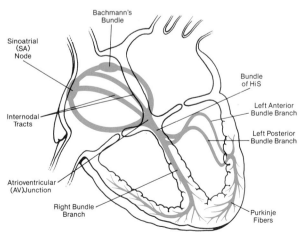

Figure 31–2. The conduction system of the heart.

Purkinje fibers are intertwined with the cardiac muscle fibers of the ventricles, and when the wave of excitement reaches the ventricles, they respond by contracting to eject blood into the pulmonary and systemic circulation.

This conduction mechanism appears as the peaks and valleys inscribed on the paper when a patient has an ECG performed. These peaks and valleys, or deflections, were named P, Q, R, S, and T waves (Fig. 31–3). These letters were arbitrarily chosen because they were not being used for anything else in medicine at the time the waves were named.

The P wave represents transmission of the stimulus of the atria. The QRS complex represents ventricular transmission of the stimulus of the ventricles followed by ventricular recovery, which is represented by the T wave. The time required for the impulse to travel from the SA node to the AV junction is represented on the ECG tracing by the PR interval. The PR interval in an adult varies from 0.12 to 0.20 of a second. It is measured from the beginning of the P wave to the beginning of the Q or R wave in the QRS complex. The QT interval represents ventricular stimulation and recovery and is measured from the beginning of the Q wave to the end of the T wave. The amount of time required for the QT interval varies with heart rate, sex, and age. The ST segment is between the end of the QRS complex (ventricular contraction) and the beginning of the T wave (ventricular recovery). The ST segment is normally isoelectric (straight baseline). Finally, there may be a U wave that appears after the T wave. Its presence may be due to slow recovery of the Purkinje fibers or due to low serum potassium. Table 31–1 summarizes the electrical stimuli, mechanical actions, and graphic representations of the ECG.

ELECTROCARDIOGRAPHIC COMPONENTS

To better understand what is represented by the ECG tracing, the medical assistant must understand the ECG

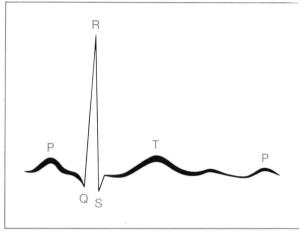

Figure 31–3. Normal ECG inflections. (From Gylys BA and Wedding ME: Medical Terminology: A Systems Approach, ed 2. FA Davis, Philadelphia, 1988, p. 152, with permission.)

components and the rate of paper movement through the machine. The procedure for obtaining an ECG is given on p. 872.

RECORDING PAPER

The ECG paper consists of two layers (Fig. 31–4). The bottom layer is black or pink paper, and the top layer is a grid of horizontal and vertical lines. The paper is both heat and pressure sensitive. The horizontal and vertical lines of the grid show heart rate and length of conduction period. The horizontal lines measure the voltage of the electrical impulse and the vertical lines measure time (Fig. 31–5).

CONTROL PANEL

The location of the control knobs and buttons on the machine varies with each model, but all machines generally have the following features (Fig. 31–6):

Table 31–1

ELECTRICAL STIMULI, HEART ACTIONS, AND THEIR RELATED ELECTROCARDIOGRAPHIC FORMS

Electrical		Mechanical		Graphic
I. Atrial transmission				
A. Sinoatrial node	→	Atrial contraction	→	P wave
B. Delay of impulse	→	Blood enters ventricle	→	PR Interval
II. Atrial recovery				
Ventricular transmission				
A. Atrioventricular node				
B. Bundle of His				
C. Bundle branches	→	Ventricles contract	→	QRS complex
D. Purkinje fibers	→	Blood leaves ventricle	→	ST segment
E. Silence				
III. Ventricular recovery				
A. Charges inside and outside the cell reverse due to active transport mechanisms	→	Rest	→	T wave

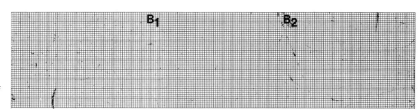

Figure 31–4. ECG paper. (Courtesy of Burdick Corporation.)

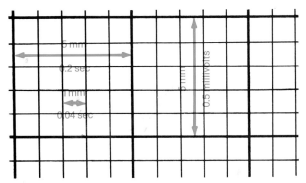

Figure 31–5. The grid of horizontal and vertical lines on the ECG paper measure voltage and time.

1. *Indicator light.* A red pilot light that indicates when the power is on.
2. *Power switch.* When the machine power cable is plugged in, the main switch turns the ECG on or off.
3. *STD control.* By international agreement, all ECG tracings should be standardized. This control adjusts the voltage (height) of the standardization mark. When this button is depressed,

the stylus should move upward 10 small squares (Fig. 31–7).

4. *Stylus heat.* This control adjusts the temperature of the stylus, which results in a heavier (higher temperature) or lighter (lower temperature) line.
5. *Stylus position.* This control adjusts the stylus position so it is centered on the graph paper.
6. *Record switch.* A speed selector runs the paper at 25 or 50 mm per second. The speed selector is usually set at 25 mm per second (2.5 cm [1 inch]) for adults and may be 50 mm per second for infants and small children or adults with tachycardia. *Speed selection is changed only at the direction of the physician.*
7. *Marker.* A code marker identifies each of the 12 leads on the ECG paper. The newer machines may not have this control because it is built into the lead selector and codes automatically.
8. *Sensitivity.* This control adjusts the voltage (height) of the standardization mark. This control is normally set on 1. If the height of the tracing is so high that the upward and downward deflections do not fit on the graph paper, the sensitivity control should be set on $\frac{1}{2}$. On the other hand, if the complexes are so small that

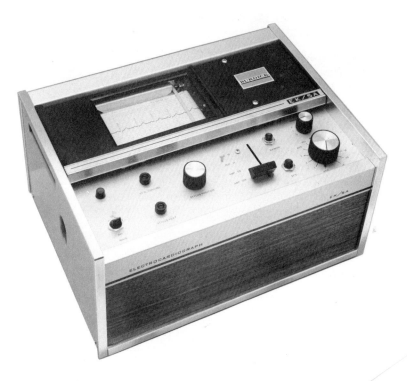

Figure 31–6. ECG control panel. (Courtesy Burdick Corporation.)

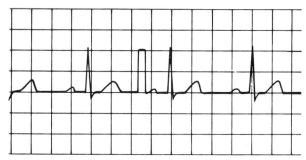

Figure 31–7. This pattern verifies that the ECG tracing has been standardized.

they are barely discernible, the control is set on 2. If it is necessary to adjust sensitivity, the selection number should be clearly marked on the tracing to inform the physician of the change, and the standardization button should be depressed at the beginning of the change.

9. *Lead Selector.* A lead selector dial marked SRD, I, II, III, aVR, aVL, aVF, V_1, V_2, V_3, V_4, V_5, V_6 indicates the lead currently being recorded.

SENSORS

Sensors are small metal plates, made of conductive metal, that are attached to the patient's limbs with stretchable rubber straps (Fig. 31–8). Another type of sensor, Welsh sensors, adheres to the skin surface by suction. Sensors detect electrical voltage on the skin surface, and the ECG machine translates the impulses into a recording (ECG tracing).

Before the sensors are attached to the patient, an electrolyte-saturated pad or electrode paste or cream must be applied to the sensor plate to ensure conduction of the impulses from the skin to the machine. The conductive paste is necessary because the skin is a poor conductor of electricity. After attaching the sensors, cables are attached which are affixed to the ECG machine.

LEADS

The ECG consists of 12 leads that are obtained by placing the sensors at specific locations on the body. There are four stationary sensors and one movable chest sensor (some ECG machines have six separate chest sensors). The four stationary sensors are attached to:

RA: right arm

LA: left arm

RL: right leg (the ground, or reference, sensor that simply serves as an electrical reference point; helps to stabilize the tracing)

left leg

chest

By using various combinations of sensors, the electrical activity of the heart can be recorded from different angles. The lead selector switch automatically designates different sensor combinations to view the heart's electrical activity from 12 different angles. The heart's electrical activity, which is detected by the sensors, is transmitted through the ECG machine, amplified, and then recorded on the paper. Figure 31–9 illustrates standard lead placement.

Leads I, II, and III are called the *standard,* or *bipolar, leads* because each lead uses two limbs for recording the electrical force of the heart. Placement consists of three points in a triangle and is called *Einthoven's triangle.* These leads allow a frontal visualization of the heart's electrical activity from side to side.

An additional lead is added for the augmented ECG recording. Augmented leads are *unipolar,* recording midpoint positions between the limbs. These include leads aVR, aVL, and aVF, which allow visualization from a frontal view top to bottom.

Leads V_1 through V_6 are known as the *precordial,* or *chest, leads.* The chest sensor placements are as follows (Fig. 31–10):

V_1: fourth intercostal space at the right of the sternum (right sternal border)

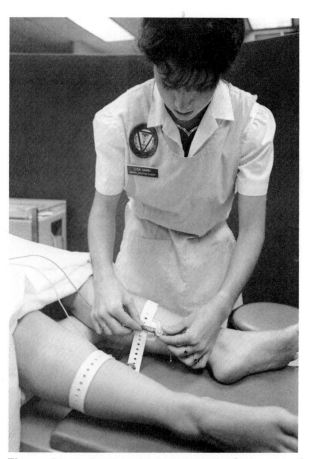

Figure 31–8. Position the sensor on the fleshy part of the leg with the lead connector pointing at the foot.

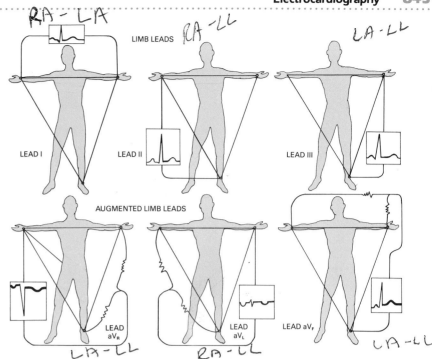

Figure 31–9. Electrocardiogram leads. (From Thomas CL [ed]: Taber's Cyclopedic Medical Dictionary, ed 17. F. A. Davis, Philadelphia, 1993, p. 614, with permission.)

V_2: fourth intercostal space at the left of the sternum (left sternal border)

V_3: midway between V_2 and V_4

V_4: fifth intercostal space, left midclavicular line

V_5: same level as V_4 at the left anterior axillary line

V_6: same level as V_5 at the left midaxillary line

These six chest leads are also unipolar, recording electrical activity of the heart in six areas of the chest wall and an area within the heart itself. The chest leads allow a horizontal visualization of the myocardium's electrical activity (from the front to the back). Unlike the standard leads, in which sensor placement on the limbs is somewhat arbitrary, chest sensors require precise placement in order for the ECG to be accurate and reliable.

After all 12 leads have been recorded, the physician examines the entire ECG strip and compares it with known standards to determine if abnormalities exist in the heart's electrical conduction system.

ARTIFACTS

Artifacts are ECG tracings that are created because of poor conduction, patient movement, electrical interference, and other sources of interference. They are outside (or external) phenomena attributable to improper technique or mechanical problems. An artifact is *not* a recording of cardiac electrical activity. The most common artifacts are caused by muscle movement, wandering baseline, and alternating current interference. The

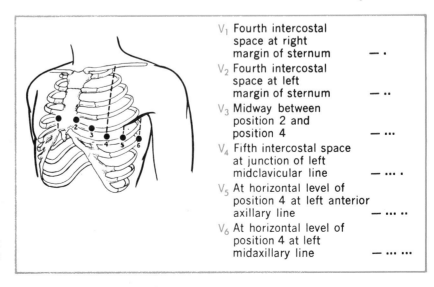

Figure 31–10. Sensor placement for recording chest leads V_1 through V_6. (Courtesy Burdick Corporation.)

V_1 Fourth intercostal space at right margin of sternum — ·

V_2 Fourth intercostal space at left margin of sternum — ··

V_3 Midway between position 2 and position 4 — ···

V_4 Fifth intercostal space at junction of left midclavicular line — ···· ·

V_5 At horizontal level of position 4 at left anterior axillary line — ···· ··

V_6 At horizontal level of position 4 at left midaxillary line — ···· ···

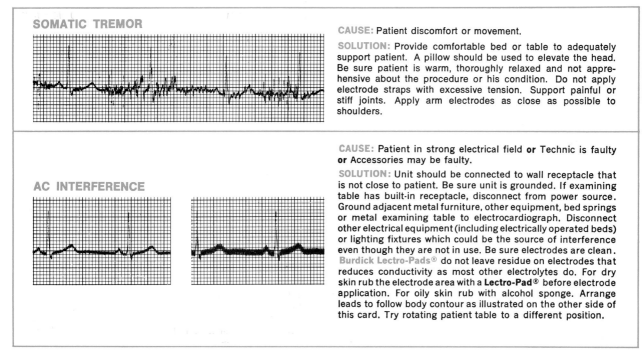

SOMATIC TREMOR

CAUSE: Patient discomfort or movement.

SOLUTION: Provide comfortable bed or table to adequately support patient. A pillow should be used to elevate the head. Be sure patient is warm, thoroughly relaxed and not apprehensive about the procedure or his condition. Do not apply electrode straps with excessive tension. Support painful or stiff joints. Apply arm electrodes as close as possible to shoulders.

CAUSE: Patient in strong electrical field **or** Technic is faulty **or** Accessories may be faulty.

AC INTERFERENCE

SOLUTION: Unit should be connected to wall receptacle that is not close to patient. Be sure unit is grounded. If examining table has built-in receptacle, disconnect from power source. Ground adjacent metal furniture, other equipment, bed springs or metal examining table to electrocardiograph. Disconnect other electrical equipment (including electrically operated beds) or lighting fixtures which could be the source of interference even though they are not in use. Be sure electrodes are clean. Burdick Lectro-Pads® do not leave residue on electrodes that reduces conductivity as most other electrolytes do. For dry skin rub the electrode area with a **Lectro-Pad**® before electrode application. For oily skin rub with alcohol sponge. Arrange leads to follow body contour as illustrated on the other side of this card. Try rotating patient table to a different position.

Figure 31–11. Common artifacts and their solutions. (Courtesy Burdick Corporation.)

medical assistant must be able to identify and eliminate artifacts because they interfere with obtaining an accurate recording of the cardiac cycle. Figure 31–11 shows two commonly occurring artifacts.

Artifacts created by voluntary patient movement or by involuntary muscle tremors are characterized by a fuzzy, irregular tracing baseline. Before starting the ECG, instruct the patient about the need to remain motionless in order to obtain an accurate tracing that is free of artifacts.

Patient reassurance may be all that is required to resolve or decrease anxiety and to eliminate the cause of artifact. ECG tracings detect and translate muscle tension as artifact. Frequently, these artifacts can be eliminated by placing a pillow under the patient's head and knees and having the patient place his or her hands with palms up under the buttocks. When obtaining an ECG on a patient with a nervous system disorder such as Parkinson's disease, for example, the tracing will need to be interrupted and then resumed as necessary to accommodate the patient's involuntary movement.

Wandering baseline, or baseline artifacts (Fig. 31–12), are mechanical in nature. The application or condi-

tion of the sensors may be faulty. Electrolyte solution that has not been evenly applied can cause interference. Likewise, body creams and cosmetics previously applied to the skin may cause disruptive electrical conduction. Both sensors and skin must be dry before electrode attachment.

Alternating current artifacts are usually caused by power demand overloads. Nearby electrical equipment may be competing for the available voltage resource. Improper grounding or dangling lead wires can also cause electrical interference.

The source of interference can usually be identified by (1) recording leads I, II, and III; and (2) examining the recording to determine which two leads have the most interference.

Lead Interference Source

Leads I and II	Patient's right arm
Leads I and III	Patient's left arm
Leads II and III	Patient's left leg

If the medical assistant is unable to identify or eliminate the artifact(s), the ECG recording is discontinued

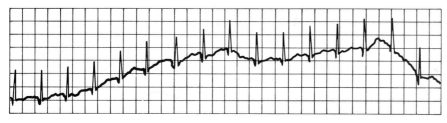

Figure 31–12. An example of the artifact known as wandering baseline.

and the physician notified. Provide the physician with a sample of the artifact and identify the lead so that further investigation can be done.

MOUNTING THE ECG

Mounting procedures depend on the physician's preference and the method and materials being used. Stock mounting forms can be purchased, or they can be specifically designed by office staff. The procedure for mounting ECGs is explained on p. 849.

STRESS TESTING

In some specialty offices, particularly cardiology, stress ECGs are performed. During the stress (exercise) ECG, the patient is monitored while exercising on a treadmill, stairs, or bicycle to increase oxygen demand of the heart muscle. This test provides an evaluation of the functional performance and capacity of the heart, lungs, and blood vessels. The stress ECG is done similarly to the resting ECG except the skin surfaces are prepared differently for the placement of the sensors. Excess hair is shaved, and the skin is prepared with alcohol to degrease or defat the skin.

During the test, the patient is observed closely for any signs or symptoms of cardiac decompensation. Blood pressure recordings and ECG are monitored throughout the test. A common phenomenon is that the patient has a normal, or negative, ECG and an abnormal stress ECG.

A stress test is *never* to be conducted unless a physician is in attendance because of the potential for sudden development of a life-threatening crisis. The medical assistant should be alert for and prepared to handle cardiac or respiratory arrest, transient ischemic attack, or fainting. Emergency resuscitation equipment and drugs should be readily available, preferably in the testing room during the procedure.

HOLTER MONITOR

The Holter monitor provides another unique method for recording cardiac electrical activity. The small recorder, about 3 inches by 6 inches, records on a magnetic tape cassette and is worn like a shoulder purse or attached to a belt.

The patient proceeds about his or her normal daily activities while cardiac response to these usual activities is recorded. The recorder is attached to the patient by sensors and lead wires that are miniature versions of the ones used when running an ECG. The sensors are adhesive backed and disposable. Patients are instructed not to shower or swim while being monitored because of the potential for electrode detachment.

Many physicians have their patients keep a diary while wearing the Holter monitor. The patients are asked to write down all of their activities for the 24-hour period and any symptoms experienced. When the patient experiences symptoms, he or she should press the event marker on the Holter monitor recorder. Each time the button is pressed, it makes a mark on the ECG recording so the physician can correlate the interpretation of the Holter ECG with the diary notes of activities and symptoms.

THE MEDICAL ASSISTANT'S ROLE IN ELECTROCARDIOGRAPHY

The ECG is a graphic display of the electrical activity of the heart that is measured and compared with known values. A physician is trained to interpret the ECG and to determine the presence, type, location, and severity of the abnormalities. The patient's progress can be monitored by periodic ECG comparisons. Remember that each ECG is used in different ways. It not only detects or verifies any current problems, but will also be used in comparison with previous or future ECGs to identify any changes that have occurred.

As with any other diagnostic tool, the ECG tracing is useful only if the recording accurately depicts cardiac activity. To accomplish this, the medical assistant must have an understanding of normal cardiac function and its relationship to the graphic ECG printout. The machine must be properly set up and the patient adequately prepared to obtain an accurate graphic representation of the patient's cardiac activity. The medical assistant must be able to recognize electrical interference, determine its origin, and then make the needed corrections or adjustments.

PATIENT TEACHING CONSIDERATIONS

The first and most important step in ECG recording is the patient preparation. Patients who have never had an ECG may be afraid that the procedure will be painful or that electricity will enter their bodies during the procedure. Patients who have had previous ECGs may be anxious about what the results might indicate.

Explaining the step-by-step procedure clearly can eliminate or decrease the stress the patient is experiencing. A relaxed patient can eliminate or significantly reduce tremor artifacts. The pre-ECG education should include the following:

1. Clothing will need to be removed from the chest and extremities (shirt, blouse, bra, hose, socks, and so forth).
2. A blanket or drape will cover the area to avoid undue exposure and provide warmth.
3. Pillows can be placed under the head and knees if necessary for comfort.
4. There should be no movement or talking during the procedure because it interferes with the recording.
5. Ask the patient if there are any questions or if further clarification is needed.

SUMMARY

Modern technology has made available computerized ECG machines. Depending on the type of practice and the frequency of use, this type of machine may be more appropriate for a particular office practice. Operating computerized ECG machines requires the same understanding of the concepts presented in this chapter.

The ECG is a valuable diagnostic tool and one that is indispensable in the diagnosis and treatment of heart disease. The ECG procedure requires precise skill and knowledge. The medical assistant who is competent in performing this procedure will be a valuable asset to the medical office practice.

DISCUSSION QUESTIONS

What would the medical assistant's response be in the following situations?

1. The patient expresses fear of the procedure.
2. The patient is moving about during the procedure.
3. After the procedure, the patient inquires if the ECG findings are normal.
4. Before the procedure, the patient asks what the ECG will show.
5. You have stopped the machine to correct an artifact. When you restart the machine, you notice that the patient appears apprehensive. You conclude that you must have looked perplexed while correcting the artifact.
6. Mrs. Jones has a coughing episode during the procedure.
7. An artifact appears. The patient has been motionless and quiet.
8. The patient is obese. You are not certain that you have correctly placed the leads.
9. The patient's relative wants to remain in the room with the patient during the procedure.
10. The stylus is not marking the cardiac cycle.

BIBLIOGRAPHY

Memmler RL and Wood DK: The Human Body in Health and Disease. JB Lippincott, Philadelphia, 1987.
Thaler MS: The Only EKG Book You'll Ever Need. JB Lippincott, Philadelphia, 1988.

PROCEDURE: Obtain an accurate electrocardiographic tracing

OSHA STANDARDS: III

Terminal Performance Objective: Instruct and position the patient, correctly position all electrodes and leads, and operate the electrocardiograph (ECG) machine to obtain an accurate, artifact-free reading.

EQUIPMENT:
ECG machine and paper
Treatment table
Pillows
Disposable razor
Paper towels
Alcohol wipe
Patient drapes
Four limb electrodes (strap, bulb, or disposable)
Electrolyte gel or paste, according to the electrode manufacturer's instructions
Chest electrode and strap, if necessary
Felt tip marking pen
Ballpoint pen

PROCEDURE	PRINCIPLE
1. Wash hands.	1. To prevent cross-contamination and infection.
2. Identify the patient. Explain the procedure and instruct the patient to lie still, breathe normally, and refrain from talking.	2. To reduce patient anxiety and avoid artifacts.
3. Ask the patient to disrobe to the waist. Assist the patient onto the treatment table. Position the patient on the table, placing pillows under head and knees as needed for patient comfort. Drape the patient so that the arms and lower legs are exposed.	3. The ECG requires skin-to-electrode contact for proper reading. Ensuring patient comfort helps to reduce tremor artifacts.
4. Check the ECG's cord and three-prong plug. Plug the cord into a properly grounded outlet.	4. To avoid AC interference, which could distort the ECG tracing.
5. Turn the machine on to warm up the stylus.	5. The ECG graph paper is heat-sensitive.
6. Mark the 6 electrode placement spots on the patient's chest; where necessary, shave excessive hair.	6. The felt tip marks can be removed with an alcohol wipe. Chest hair between electrode and skin will interfere with the recording.
7. Apply electropads or electrogel to the sensors.	7. Electropads or electrolyte gel enhance conduction of the impulses from the skin to the sensor.
8. Place the sensors on the arms and legs and on the fleshy parts of the extremities distal to the wrists and ankles. Place each sensor so the lead connector points toward the patient's head. a. With *regular sensors*, secure by wrapping the rubber strap around the limb until a hole in the strap meets the sensor hook. Stretch the strap one hole tighter, then fasten. b. With *bulb suction sensors*, rub a little electrogel over the sensor location spot on the patient's body. Compress the bulb to create suction, press the sensor to the spot, and release the bulb. c. With *disposable electrodes*, peel off the protective adhesive backing and press the electrode firmly into place. Each disposable electrode contains electrogel.	8. Putting the electrode over a bony prominence increases the chance of artifacts.
9. Attach leads to the sensors.	9. Accuracy of placement is essential for obtaining an accurate tracing.
10. When all sensors are connected, double-check for accurate placement.	10. Accuracy of placement is essential for obtaining an accurate tracing.

PROCEDURE

11. Turn the lead selector switch to "standardize" (STD).

12. Set the record switch to RUN 25.
13. Make sure sensitivity is set at 1.
14. Depress the STD and note if the standard is 10-mm high. If not, make the necessary adjustments. The physician may call for standardization between complexes in each lead or in specified leads. *Follow agency or physician preference.*

15. Center the stylus. Run leads I, II, III, aVR, aVL, and aVF. Run 5- to 10-inch (12.5 to 25 cm) strips for each lead. Correct any artifacts. If any unusual complexes (not caused by interference) appear, run a strip that records the entire incident.

16. If the ECG instrument does not automatically mark each lead, code the beginning of the tracing for each lead, using the code below:

Lead	Code
I	.
II	..
III	...
aVR	-
aVL	--
aVF	---
V_1	-.
V_2	-..
V_3	-...
V_4	-... .
V_5	-... ..
V_6	-... ...

17. Place the chest sensor on each of the marked spots and record the six chest leads. Turn the machine off between recordings, while moving the sensor. Twist the chest sensor each time it is moved.

18. Turn off the machine.
19. Remove all sensors and clean the patient's skin with a clean moistened cloth to remove the electrolyte solution. Use an alcohol soaked sponge to clean the marker off the patient's chest. Clean the straps as needed.

20. Coil all lead wires and the power cord and put them in their storage positions.
21. Write the patient's name, age, sex, height and weight, the date, and a list of the patient's medications on the recording. Be careful to avoid scratches. Roll the strip; never fold it.

PRINCIPLE

11. To verify that the accuracy of the recording of the impulse voltage.
12. To begin recording.
13. To provide a standard for amplitude.
14. This ensures an accurate tracing.

15. Centering the stylus ensures an accurate tracing.

16. Without the marking code, physicians would find it difficult to know which leads were recorded and it would be most difficult to mount the tracing.

17. Turning the machine off between recordings prevents the stylus from thrashing when the sensor is moved. Twisting the sensor releases electrolyte gel, which ensures good impulse conduction.

18. This completes the procedure.
19. Cleaning the skin is necessary to remove the residual electrogel.

20. To ready the equipment for its next use.

21. To ensure proper patient identification. Folding the strip could cause unwanted marks; such marks and scratches could obscure the tracings. The strip is now ready for mounting.

PROCEDURE: Mount the electrocardiographic tracing

OSHA STANDARDS:

Terminal Performance Objective: Mount the ECG tracing in a way that will make it easy to read and ensure its preservation in the patient's file.

EQUIPMENT: ECG strip
Ruler
ECG mount
Scissors
Pen

PROCEDURE

1. Gather equipment together on a flat, uncluttered work surface.
2. Label the mount with all the required information: patient's name, age, sex, height and weight, the date, and a list of the patient's medications.
3. Unroll the ECG and locate lead I. Locate the standardization mark for that lead. Determine the physician or facility preference as to where to place the standardization tracing. Use ruler to find out the length of lead I and its associated standard and cut the required length of mount.
4. Open mount slot by sliding ruler into the lead I slot. Remove ruler while holding strip securely. Slide strip into the slot. If using self-stick mounts, remove the protective paper strip, carefully position the ECG strip, and press to attach. Remove ruler from slot; fold ¼ inch (0.0625 cm) of the ECG paper over the ruler edge and tear.
5. Repeat step 4 for all leads. Make sure that the correct lead is mounted in each designated mounting section.
6. Review the entire mount. It should be neat without extraneous scratch marks; it should have at least one standardization tracing (depending on the preference of the physician or facility). Check for:

   ❏ Straight baseline
   ❏ Good contact
   ❏ No apparent somatic tremor
   ❏ Correct standardization
   ❏ Leads marked properly
   ❏ Proper patient identification and other pertinent information

7. Put away all supplies. File the mounted ECG in the proper place.

PRINCIPLE

1. To save time and unnecessary steps and to avoid making extraneous marks on the ECG tracing.
2. To avoid confusion as to the identity of the tracing.

3. Some physicians or facilities prefer the standard at the beginning of the ECG leads; others like the standards placed between complexes.

4. The ruler makes it easier to slide the ECG strip into the slot, which may be tight. Self-stick mounts can become loose if not securely attached to the mount sheet.

5. Always double-check work for accuracy.

6. To ensure an accurate, neatly mounted ECG.

7. Neatness ensures that supplies will be readily available for the next mounting. Consistent filing prevents loss of strips.

HIGHLIGHTS
Limitations of the Electrocardiogram

Electrocardiography (ECG) is used to diagnose an evolving heart attack (myocardial infarction), identify arrhythmias, and determine the effects of hypertension or other disorders. When included as part of a routine examination, the ECG will provide information on the heart's status. The ECG in routine examination cannot predict a heart attack. It can only serve as a reference point (baseline) to compare changes in the heart over time or after disease. It is particularly useful in measuring heart damage caused by a heart attack since an ECG performed during the routine examination would provide a representation of the heart before the attack.

If an ECG cannot predict a heart attack, then you may wonder about the value of the stress test. The stress test, also called an exercise tolerance test, is usually ordered to assess the presence and severity of coronary heart disease when the baseline ECG is normal. The patient exercises on a treadmill or stationary bicycle while connected to a 12-lead ECG monitor. Since the graded exercise puts increasing demands on the heart, if cardiac oxygen exceeds consumption, electrocardiographic changes and symptoms such as chest pain and shortness of breath will occur. False readings may occur, but are rare.

The ECG, then, should be regarded as an important diagnostic tool. However, the health professional should help patients to understand both the role of the ECG and its limitations. Unfortunately, a normal baseline ECG is not a guarantee against the occurrence of a heart attack or other cardiac disorder.

*D*iagnostic Imaging

> **A** picture is worth a thousand words.
>
> Chinese proverb

LEARNING OBJECTIVES

Upon completing this chapter, you will be able to:

1. Define the terms related to diagnostic imaging.
2. Describe the clinical uses of specific imaging procedures.
3. Describe the advantages of and necessary precautions related to each of the imaging techniques discussed in this chapter.
4. Describe the patient preparation needed for specified diagnostic procedures.
5. List radiation and safety precautions to be observed in the medical office.

PERFORMANCE OBJECTIVES

Upon completing this chapter, you will be able to:

1. Assist the physician or radiographer in obtaining radiographs of acceptable quality with minimal exposure and patient discomfort.

Chapter 32

*D*iagnostic Imaging

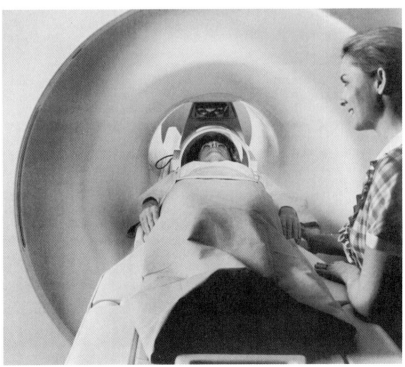

DACUM EDUCATIONAL COMPONENTS

1. Receive incoming telephone calls regarding x-ray reports (2.8B).
2. Observe guidelines for scheduling imaging study appointments for patient services outside the office setting (4.7E).
3. Instruct patients in preparation for radiographic examination (4.7D).
4. Apply principles of radiation safety if assisting with radiographic procedures, wear dosimetry badge, and protect the patient from undue exposure (4.7E).

Glossary

Cassette: lightproof container that holds x-ray film and serves to intensify the image

Contrast medium (plural **media):** a radiopaque substance used in radiography to permit visualization of internal structures

Enhancement: to increase image contrast or detail with the use of chemical agents or special imaging methods

Film: photosensitive material capable of producing a transmission image. (See *radiograph*)

Invasive procedure: procedure in which the body cavity is entered, either by tube, needle, scalpel, or ionizing radiation

Ionizing radiation: radiation that causes ionization in the tissues that absorb it

Isotope: one of two or more varieties of an element that vary only in mass; the chemical properties of isotopes of a single element are nearly identical. Many isotopes are radioactive

Pixels: picture elements of a computed tomography scan; cross-sectional area of the patient

Radiograph: film after exposure to radiation that has been processed to bear a stable, visible image

Radionuclide: material whose unstable atoms give off electromagnetic radiation

Radiopaque: a substance that can obstruct x-ray passage, resulting in white or light areas on x-ray film

Roentgenogram: older term for radiograph, named for the discoverer of x-rays

Scan: an image produced on film by a sweeping beam of radiation

Scintillation camera: camera used in special diagnostic procedures that photographs emissions that come from radioactive substances; it is also known as a gamma camera, because the emissions are gamma rays

Tracer: a radioactive isotope added to a material that is then introduced into the body; the isotope "tags" the material, so that its course through the body can be traced

Uptake: absorption of nutrients or chemicals (including those containing radioactive tracers) by the body's tissues

x-Ray: high-energy electromagnetic wave capable of penetrating most solid matter

---

Today, diagnostic imaging consists of various x-ray techniques, such as radiographs using dyes, specifically controlled radiation, radioactive isotopes, and non-radiographic, noninvasive imaging. Diagnostic imaging has changed drastically in recent years; the term now covers, in addition to traditional radiography and fluoroscopy, the use of computers, image-intensifying screens, high-speed film processing, radiographic enlargement through closed-circuit television, radio waves, magnetism, and sound waves.

Hospital radiology divisions are divided into many departments: x-ray, angiography, computed tomography (CT), magnetic resonance imaging (MRI), and ultrasound. In recent years, the increase in methods of viewing human tissues has been paralleled by the spread of independently owned, outpatient imaging centers. These private facilities are capable of performing most noninvasive imaging procedures by appointment and on referral from a physician. If covered by insurance, patients also may schedule routine annual or biannual procedures, such as mammograms, on their own.

Diagnostic imaging consist of five distinct areas:

1. *Diagnostic radiology.* Skeletal, screen-film radiography; fluoroscopy; and mammography
2. *CT.* Computerized analysis of the varying absorption by body tissues of a high-energy, pinpoint radiographic beam to produce a precise, reconstructed image of a selected plane (slice) of the body
3. *Nuclear medicine.* Use of radionuclides injected or inhaled in the body to aid in diagnosis
4. *MRI.* Use of electromagnetic energy to produce image information about body tissues
5. *Ultrasound.* Production of images of body structures from the reflection of sound waves.

CONVENTIONAL X-RAY MACHINE

Until recently, most x-ray machines in physician's offices were comparatively simple, manual models designed exclusively for chest x-rays. In recent years, however, fully automatic equipment has become available. Figure 32–1 shows a standard machine that can be used for various types of x-rays.

The x-ray machine has four basic parts: (1) table, (2) x-ray tube, (3) control panel, and (4) high-voltage generator. The table is usually adjustable, so that the patient can be placed in various positions at various angles to the x-ray beam. The x-ray tube, above the table, produces and transmits the x-radiation, and the control panel operates and controls x-ray emissions. The machine is placed behind a specially constructed lead-lined wall that shields the operator from exposure to the radiation.

Most states require all x-ray equipment, including tabletop machines used in physician's offices, to be operated by licensed radiographers. Medical assistants can be called on to assist in radiographic procedures, and of course, the medical assistant must be able to instruct patients in and prepare them for such procedures. Therefore, the medical assistant must understand the principles behind radiographic procedures.

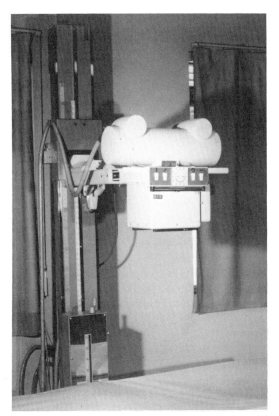

Figure 32–1. A standard medical office x-ray machine.

PROCESSING RADIOGRAPHIC FILM

X-ray film is developed in the darkroom, which is designed to eliminate all natural light. The only acceptable light in a darkroom is a specially designed, low-wattage darkroom bulb. Figure 32–2 illustrates the steps involved in x-ray film processing. Proper preparation, use, and processing and storage of the film are essential for obtaining high-quality and permanently fixed (stable) radiographs.

The manual processing cycle takes about 1 hour. In recent years, automated processors have been developed that mechanically process and dry ready-to-read radiographs in as little as 90 seconds. Automatic processing systems require expensive processors, special chemicals, and compatible films, but they can greatly increase the efficiency and capacity of an x-ray facility.

CONVENTIONAL SCREEN-FILM RADIOGRAPHY

In general, most x-rays are of specific bones or the chest. The limb or body part in question is placed between the tube and the film. The tube generates the wave of electromagnetic energy called the *x-ray* and directs it toward the film. The film is coated with a material that is sensitive to the energy of the x-ray. When the film is processed, the resulting image, known as a *radiograph*, is a record of the x-ray energy that struck the film. Areas that received no x-ray energy are black, and areas that received maximal energy are white, with variations in energy resulting in varying shades of gray.

As the x-ray passes through the specified body part, the radiation passes freely through softer, less dense tissue, such as muscle. Such areas show up dark on the radiograph. Denser tissue, such as bone, permits less radiation to pass through and strike the film. Such areas show up light on the radiograph. Radiography, therefore, uses the varying tissue densities to produce varying shades of black to white on the processed film.

SPECIAL IMAGING METHODS

CONTRAST MEDIA STUDIES

The variances in the black-to-white gradations recorded on x-ray film can be enhanced by the use of a contrast media. The most commonly used contrast media are barium sulfate powder for studies of the gastrointestinal tract and an iodine compound used for vessel studies (arteries, veins), urinary system studies, myelograms, and other areas. Bone x-ray does not require use of contrast media.

Contrast media is a radiopaque substance that creates increased density of the area being studied. The increased density clearly delineates the boundaries or function of the specific area for more complete and accurate visualization.

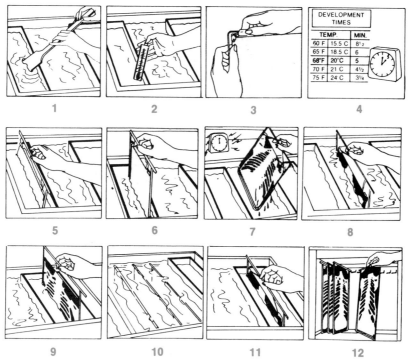

Figure 32-2. Steps in x-ray film processing. (**1**) Stir developer and fixer solutions to equalize their temperature. (Use a separate paddle for each to avoid contamination.) (**2**) Check the temperature of the solutions with an accurate thermometer. Adjust to 68°F (20°C) if possible. (**3**) Attach the film carefully to a hanger of the proper size. (Attach at lower corners first.) Avoid finger marks, scratches, or bending. (**4**) Set the timer for the desired period of development, based on the temperature of the developer. Consult the chart on the back of the timer for the correct temperature and time. (**5**) Immerse the film completely, smoothly, and without pause to avoid streaking, then start the timer. (**6**) Raise and lower the hanger several times to bathe the film surfaces thoroughly, repeating this once each minute. (**7**) When the alarm rings, lift out the hanger quickly, then drain the film for a moment into the space between the tanks. (**8**) Place the film in an acid rinse bath or under running water. Agitate the hanger vigorously, and rinse for 2 seconds. If a water rinse is used, lift the film and drain well. If an acid bath is used, plunge the film immediately into the fixer. (**9**) Immerse the film and agitate the hanger vigorously. Most films are fixed a 60-70°F (15.5-20°C) for 4-10 minutes in Kodak x-ray Fixer, or for 2-4 minutes in Kodak Rapid Fixer. (**10**) Place the film in a tank of running water with ample space between hangers. Length of time will vary according to the type of film used. (**11**) If facilities permit, use a final rinse of Kodak Photo-Flo solution to speed drying time and prevent water marks. Immerse the film for about 30 seconds and drain for several seconds. (**12**) Place the film in a dryer, or on a rack in a current of air. Keep films well separated. When dry, remove films from their hangers and trim the corners to remove top marks. Insert each film in an identifying envelope. (Drawings courtesy of the Radiography Market Division, Eastman Kodak Company.)

The most commonly ordered contrast media studies are intravenous pyelogram (IVP), barium enema, and upper gastrointestinal (GI) examinations. Table 32-1 outlines the applications, procedures, and patient preparations for these and other contrast media studies.

Patient preparation required before the specific examination varies greatly from facility to facility. The medical assistant is responsible for obtaining and maintaining an office supply of preexamination patient instruction sheets from the radiology facilities used by the physician. Instruction sheets must be available to provide the patient with proper instructions specific to the radiologist's directions. See Table 32-2 for sample pre-x-ray examination instructions for several contrast media tests.

Figures 32-3 and 32-4 are examples of an upper GI examination and an IVP film.

FLUOROSCOPY

Fluoroscopy allows for visualization of organs in motion. The advantage of fluoroscopy is that it provides a method of visualizing activity in real time. Structures, processes, and functions can be observed as they occur. The contrast medium can be viewed as it moves through the structure, organ, or system during activity. The images are projected onto a television screen via a closed-circuit television system.

CINEFLUOROGRAPHY

Cinefluorography is an x-ray motion-picture study that records the movement of an organ. The method is used most often for coronary arteriography. Coronary arteriography uses image intensifiers, which make the

Table 32–1

CONTRAST MEDIA STUDIES

Test	Area Studied	Procedure Information	Patient Preparation	Exam Time
Sialography	Salivary gland duct	1. Patient sucks on lemon wedge to open duct. 2. Catheter inserted into duct and contrast medium.	None	1–2 h
Hysterosal-pingography	Uterus and uterine tubes	1. Procedure is very uncomfortable, but premedication for relaxation is given.	None	1–2 h
Voiding cystourethrography	Bladder and urethra	1. Catheter is inserted into the bladder and dye is instilled. 2. Catheter is removed and x-rays are taken during voiding.	None	1–2 h
Intravenous pyelogram (IVP)	Renal pelvis, ureters, and bladder	1. Dye is injected IV. 2. x-Rays are taken at intervals as kidneys excrete the dye.	1. Laxative is taken the night before examination. 2. Eat light evening meal. 3. Fast after evening meal.	1½ h
Retrograde pyelogram	Ureters, bladder, and urethra	1. Dye is inserted via cytoscope and uretoscope. 2. x-Rays are taken of the urinary tract.	Same as for IVP.	1½ h
IV cholangiography	Bile ducts	1. Dye is inserted via IV.	1. Laxative is taken the night before. 2. Eat light evening meal. 3. Fast after midnight.	2–3 h
Cholecystogram	Gallbladder	1. Oral contrast media is taken the evening before exam. 2. Some require 2-d preparation.	1. Low-fat diet evening meal. 2. Take oral contrast media at 8 PM evening before. 3. Fast after midnight. 4. Laxative is sometimes ordered.	15 min
Upper gastrointestinal series	Esophagus, stomach, and sometimes small bowel	1. Patient drinks barium sulfate solutions.	Fast after midnight.	5–6 h if small bowel film is requested
Barium enema (single- or double-contrast study)	Colon and sometimes ileum	1. Single-contrast: barium is instilled into the colon. Double-contrast:	1. Instruct patient to expect some discomfort during both bowel	1–2 h

Continued

Table 32–1
CONTRAST MEDIA STUDIES—*Continued*

Test	Area Studied	Procedure Information	Patient Preparation	Exam Time
		when barium is evacuated, air is forced into the colon.	preparation and procedure. 2. Frequent side-to-side turning is required during examination. 3. Hand pressure is often applied to lower abdomen. 4. Low-residue diet for 2 d before examination. 5. Hydration and laxative preparation. 6. Enemas may be ordered. 7. Use rectal suppositories morning of examination. 8. Clear-liquid breakfast day of examination.	

Table 32–2
SAMPLE PATIENT PREPARATION INSTRUCTIONS FOR X-RAY EXAMINATION

Upper Gastrointestinal Series

1. Please do not eat, drink, or chew gum after midnight before your appointment.
2. Laxatives and enemas are not required.

Colon Exam (Barium Enema)

1. Please report to the x-Ray Office to pick up a bowel preparation kit to be used the day before the examination as directed.
2. Where time permits, maintain a low-residue diet (eliminate roughage, such as lettuce, celery, etc.) for 2 days before the examination.

Gallbladder Examination

Please report to x-Ray Office for gallbladder capsules.
First Day
1. Do not eat fried or fatty foods, eggs, butter, cream, or any dairy products. You may have toast, jelly (no butter), fruit, jello, tea, black coffee, water, and soups. Cooked foods may be baked or boiled.
2. At 7 PM (after the evening meal), take the first packet of capsules, one at a time, with water.
Second Day
1. Remain on low-fat diet as outlined above.
2. At 7 PM take the second packet of capsules, as above.
3. After taking the capsules, DO NOT eat or drink anything until your examination is finished.

Intravenous Urogram

1. Please drink 10 oz of citrate of magnesia at 3 PM the day before the examination.
2. Eat a light supper.
3. No food or liquids in the morning before the examination.

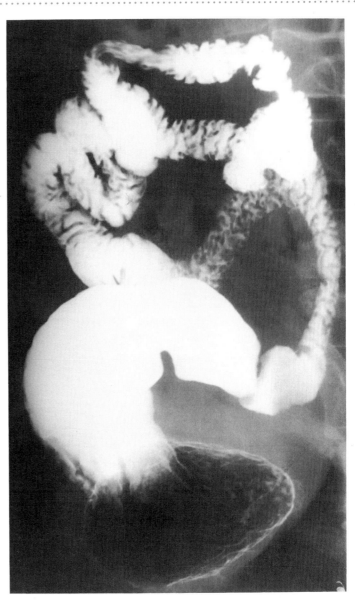

Figure 32–3. A radiograph of the upper gastrointestinal tract following barium ingestion. (Courtesy of Michael Ramer, MD, from Judd E: Nursing Care of the Adult. F. A. Davis, Philadelphia, 1983, p. 192, with permission.)

image many times brighter, and radiographic enlargement techniques to magnify the small vessels. The method also allows for camera spot filming, which produces permanent, still radiographs of selected phases of the examination.

MAMMOGRAPHY

Mammography is the radiologic study of the breast used in the diagnosis of cancer. The most common form is film-screen mammography; three other forms are thermography, diaphanography, and ultrasonography (ultrasound).

Patient preparation for mammography consists of informing the patient that she will be standing for the entire procedure, which requires about 5 minutes, and explaining the procedure. Each breast is individually compressed by the machine. Breast compression is a necessary element of this examination. This compression may be slightly uncomfortable, but the mammography is not painful for the patient. However, patients with pendulous breasts may experience some increased discomfort from the physical compression.

Imaging centers request that the patient apply no perfume, deodorant, or powder the morning of the examination. The medical assistant will need to obtain complete patient instructions from the facility performing the test and arrange for time to discuss these with the patient.

The medical assistant should also provide patient education about the screening guidelines for mammography. The general rule is a woman should have a baseline mammogram between ages 35 and 40. Since one third of the women with breast cancer are between the ages of 45 and 50, it is recommended that women in this age range have a mammogram every 1–2 years,

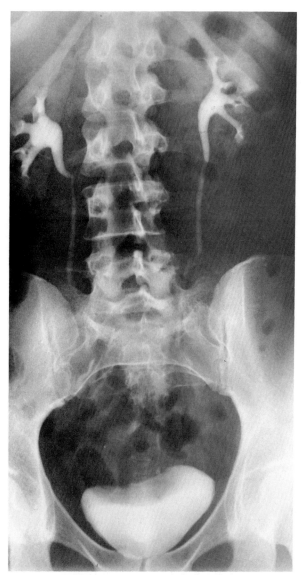

Figure 32–4. Intravenous pylogram. (Courtesy of Michael Ramer, MD, from Judd E: Nursing Care of the Adult. F. A. Davis, Philadelphia, 1983, p. 589, with permission.)

unless identified as a member of a risk group. After age 50, it is recommended that a woman have an annual mammogram.

Diaphanography is a relatively new form of imaging using light. It is not commonly used but is an excellent diagnostic tool for breast examination. A high-intensity light is directed through the breast or soft tissue to produce images on a screen. This process is called *transillumination*. The imaging equipment is highly specialized. The advantage of diaphanography is that no ionizing radiation is used. Preparation for diaphanography examination is essentially the same as for mammography.

TOMOGRAPHY

Tomography, or body-section radiography, provides visualization of an organ or body area in cross-section, or "slices." Tomography differs greatly from traditional radiography, which can only view the target organ, along with the structures above and below it, as a whole. Tomography provides an image of any selected plane (slice) through the body. This gives physicians the ability to visualize extremely small tissue differences. For instance, a series of tomographic scans can differentiate white matter from gray matter in the brain. Tomography is also useful in cases where the patient's condition makes more conventional imaging methods impossible or not useful.

In conventional linear tomography, the plane of the image recorded is always parallel to the long axis of the body. *Axial transverse tomography* allows visualization of structures at right angles (transverse) to the long axis.

Computed Tomography

Computed tomography (CT) combines radiographic images of the same organ or body area from many different angles to produce three-dimensional visualizations of tissues or structures (Fig. 32–5). This procedure has revolutionized radiography by making it possible to "see" deep into the body without invasive procedures.

The technology behind CT continues to change and grow rapidly. By combining CT with the materials and methods of nuclear medicine and nuclear MRI, researchers and manufacturers are finding ever newer, more precise ways of visualizing tissues, organs, and other structures.

Patient Instruction for Tomography Procedures

For the medical assistant, patient preparation includes reassuring patients about the procedure (CT machines are large and complicated) and explaining the necessity of lying still for the duration of the procedure. Some of these examinations can take from 45 to 90 minutes, although some of the newer scanners take less time.

Some tomography or CT procedures require the injection of contrast agents, for instance, for the accurate definition of tumor borders. In these cases, the medical assistant must ask the patient about allergies and any previous adverse reaction to such agents. Although tomography and CT are noninvasive techniques that can be done on an outpatient basis, the patient must sign a consent form at the time of the examination. The medical assistant should also explain to the patient that there can be no metallic objects, skin staples, and metallic prostheses in the path of the x-rays.

Table 32–3 is a sample patient information sheet for CT scanning procedures.

Diagnostic Uses of Tomography and CT

Tomography and CT scanning are useful for:

Assessment of aneurysms in the aorta and heart
Clinical evaluation of the liver and biliary system

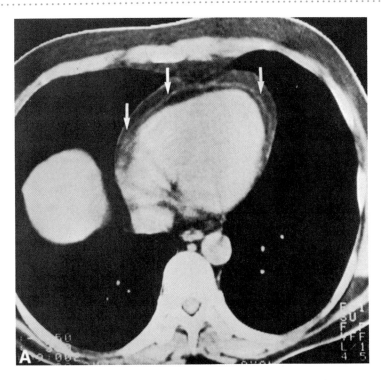

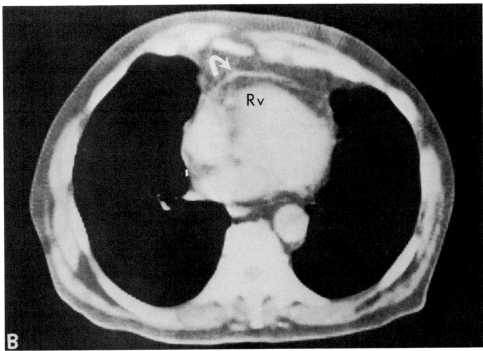

Figure 32–5. Two CT scans of the chest, showing the heart enclosed within its pericardium (indicated by the arrows in [**A**]. Rv, right ventricle. (From Kotler MN and Steiner RM: Cardiac Imaging: New Technologies and Clinical Applications. F. A. Davis, Philadelphia, 1986, p. 412, with permission.)

Evaluation of renal and pulmonary tumors

Diagnosing abdominal conditions

Guiding catheter placement when draining abscesses

Diagnosing brain tumors and trauma and evaluating brain swelling

Evaluating spinal disorders, including herniated disks

Guiding biopsy procedures

Detecting cancer in some breasts that are difficult to examine by mammography

Table 32–3

SAMPLE PATIENT INFORMATION SHEET FOR COMPUTED TOMOGRAPHY SCANNING PROCEDURES

Length of Exams: CT Scans, on the average, are approximately 1 h long. However, your scan may take longer depending upon how many views the radiologist must take to determine this diagnosis.

CT preps:

CT HEAD: NO FOOD 4 h before; NO LIQUIDS 2 h before examination.
CT CHEST: NO FOOD 4 h before; NO LIQUIDS 2 h before examination.
CT ABD OR CT PELVIS: You must pick up a preparation kit and special instructions for your examination at least the day before the examination.
CT SPINE: NO PREPARATION
CT BONE DENSITOMETRY: NO PREPARATION

YOUR PHYSICIAN HAS ASKED US TO PERFORM A CT (COMPUTED TOMOGRAPHY) SCAN ON EITHER YOU OR YOUR FAMILY MEMBER. MANY QUESTIONS ARISE WITH REGARDS TO THIS EXAMINATION, AND HOPEFULLY MOST OF THEM WILL BE ANSWERED WITH THIS INFORMATION SHEET. IF YOU HAVE ADDITIONAL QUESTIONS, PLEASE CALL, OR THE DAY OF THE EXAMINATION YOU COULD TALK WITH THE TECHNOLOGIST OR RADIOLOGIST.

Questions	Answers
1. HOW LONG DOES THE EXAMINATION TAKE?	The amount of time required for your examination is dependent on the area being scanned, and the amount of information needed to determine a diagnosis. Usually, for most examinations, 45–60 min is adequate, though examinations of multiple areas can range beyond 90 min.
2. WILL THERE BE ANY SIDE EFFECTS?	No. Since this is strictly a diagnostic examination and not a treatment, you will feel no "after effects" of the CT scan.
3. DO I NEED TO HAVE AN INJECTION SHOT?	For most CT examinations (except CT spine), an intravenous injection into the arm or back of the hand is required. This injection is performed by the radiologist and will cause only minimal discomfort. The contrast material injected is essential in helping the radiologist determine normal from abnormal areas.
4. WHY DO I HAVE TO FAST BEFORE A CT BRAIN SCAN?	If you have a very full stomach, you may experience a mild nausea after receiving the intravenous injection of contrast material. If you fast for 4 h with no food and 1 h with no liquids before examination, you should not experience any discomfort.
5. FOR CT ABD AND/OR PELVIS: WHY DO I HAVE TO DRINK A PREPARATION?	The gastrografin preparation which you are required to drink for a CT scan of the ABD/pelvis is designed to outline your intestines and colon, and therefore aids the radiologist in distinguishing normal from abnormal structures. This preparation is not designed to produce a laxative effect and should not provide any discomfort. It is very important that you pick up your gastrografin preparation in time to begin drinking the night before your examination date (some preparations are longer than others depending on the area to be scanned). The scheduling coordinator or CT technologist can help you with any questions you may have regarding this preparation.
6. WHEN WILL MY PHYSICIAN GET THE RESULTS?	The written report is usually available within 24 h of the examination. A typed report is sent to each of your physicians, and the original films of your examination may be furnished to your physician on request.

ULTRASOUND

Ultrasound is the process of recording the deflection of high-frequency sound waves directed at an organ or into tissue. During an ultrasound procedure, the operator moves a device called the *transducer* over the skin above the area to be examined. Special ultrasound gel, applied to the skin, enhances the transmission of the sound waves. The transducer both emits the sound waves and receives their echoes as they bounce back from underlying tissues and structures. The ultrasound machine records the echoes as a series of dots that together make up a composite "picture" of the tissue through which the waves travel and return. The picture, an image on a television monitor, is what is referred to as a "real-time image"; this means that what the monitor shows is what lies underneath the transducer at that moment.

Ultrasound is painless and noninvasive. It is useful in imaging low-density soft tissues (Fig. 32–6) without the use of radiation. Such tissues include organs, fluids, muscles, and abnormal masses, such as tumors or cysts. Ultrasound is well-suited to distinguishing solid tumors that may be malignant or premalignant from benign growths, such as cysts (which are encapsulated and usually harmless), sacs containing a liquid or semi-solid substance. The technique can also help in detecting hidden lesions. Other uses of ultrasound include:

Measuring the velocity of blood flow through vessels

Visualization of the abdomen, brain, heart and blood vessels, and biliary tract

Clinical evaluation of aneurysms, urogenital problems, infertility problems, and breast lesions

Routine prenatal visualization of the fetus and placenta

Table 32–4 lists other ultrasound applications and summarizes patient preparation.

MAGNETIC RESONANCE IMAGING

Magnetic resonance imaging (MRI) is a diagnostic procedure that uses a magnetic field (rather than ionizing radiation) to produce images of structures and tissues of the body. MRI combines the advantages of CT scanning with ultrasound by using nonionizing radiation and providing tomography on any plane. The process yields high-resolution images without any risk to the patient.

In MRI, the patient's head or body is placed in a strong magnetic field. One of the effects of such a field is that all the hydrogen protons within the field (including those within the patient) become aligned with the

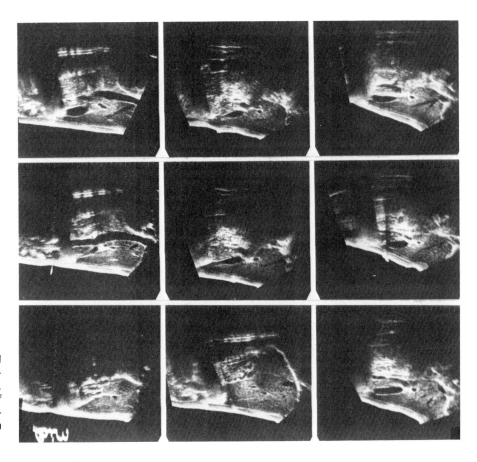

Figure 32–6. Ultrasound study of the abdomen. (Courtesy of Michael Ramer, MD, from Judd E: Nursing Care of the Adult. F. A. Davis, Philadelphia, 1983, p. 435, with permission.)

Table 32–4
ULTRASOUND APPLICATIONS AND PREPARATION

Procedure	Visualizes	Patient Preparation	Procedure Time
Cardiac ultrasound	Internal cardiac structures	1. Test is done lying down. 2. Will need to assume and hold various positions. 3. Transducer is held to chest using moderate pressure.	1½ h
Pelvic ultrasound	Masses and fluid accumulations	1. Laxative taken day before examination. 2. Drink 3–4 glasses of water 1 h before examination. 3. Do not void for 1 h before examination	1–2 h
Abdominal ultrasound	Abdominal organs and organ blood vessels	1. Laxative taken day before examination. 2. No food or fluid for 8 h before test.	½–1 h

direction of the field. The MRI machine then emits a pulse of radiofrequency energy that "flips" the hydrogen protons into a higher energy state. When the radiopulse ends, the hydrogen protons "relax," and the energy they emit produces signals that the MRI machine records and translates into anatomic images.

Magnetic resonance imaging is especially effective in imaging tissues with high fat and water content, the kind of tissues that are not visualized with other radiologic techniques. Magnetic resonance imaging is very sensitive to the differences in the chemical makeup of various kinds of tissue. This capability helps physicians identify and tell the difference between normal and cancerous tissue, for instance, or between atherosclerotic tissue and blood clots. Magnetic resonance imaging is also useful in visualizing heart valves, the brain, spine, and joints.

Patient preparation for MRI requires screening for internal metal, such as a pacemaker or bone pins. If internal metal is present, notify the physician immediately. This is most important as the magnetic force is so strong it can remove metal from the patient. Patients should be instructed that they will be placed into a long, narrow tube of about 22 inches (56 cm) in diameter for the test (Fig. 32–7) and that they will hear a loud knocking noise during the examination. Patients susceptible to claustrophobia or unable to lie still for a long period may need sedation. Assure patients that the radiologists and technologists will be attentive and in attendance during the entire time that they are inside the tube. Examination time varies from 45 minutes to 2 hours depending on the extent of the examination. Table 32–5 provides instructions for both the medical assistant and the patient requiring MRI.

NUCLEAR MEDICINE

Nuclear medicine is the use of unsealed radioactive materials (radionuclides) and special equipment to help diagnose and treat various diseases and the results of injury.

Nuclear medicine professionals administer radionuclides orally, parenterally, or through intracavitary routes. The radioactive material they introduce into the patient's body is designed to travel to and be localized in the organ to be imaged. The technicians then use specialized equipment and material to produce images from the gamma rays (photons) emitted by the radionuclides. The production of the image may take place immediately or up to several days after the radionuclide is introduced, depending on the type of study being done. Such procedures usually result in much lower doses of radiation than other radiographic techniques. Another advantage of nuclear medicine diagnostic techniques is that they can be used with patients whose allergic reactions to contrast media make them poor candidates for other radiographic procedures.

When the radionuclide concentrates in the target organ, the radioactivity it emits will cluster there as well. The radiographers use special probes, scintillation cameras, and computers to translate the radioactivity into light flashes. The light flashes, in addition to forming an image on a television monitor, strike and expose photographic film. The resulting image is called a *scan* (Fig. 32–8). A nuclear medicine physician interprets the resulting radiographs and dictates a report which is sent to the referring physician or attached to the patient's hospital record. Table 32–6 explains the patient preparation requirements for a nuclear medicine examination.

INPATIENT IMAGING PROCEDURES

Patients are admitted to hospitals for invasive radiology procedures and, when the patient's condition warrants, subsequent treatment. Invasive procedures involve the introduction of catheters, wires, or other

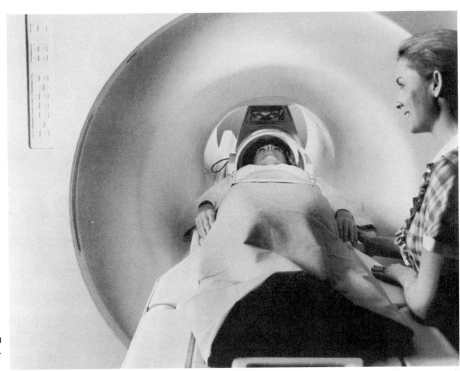

Figure 32-7. Technician with a patient about to proceed with MRI.

<u>Table 32-5</u>
MAGNETIC RESONANCE IMAGING SCHEDULING AND SCREENING PROCEDURE

Schedule: Call the MRI Department to schedule the patient.
The TIME and DATE will be set up when possible.

Screening: The patient must pass the basic screening in order to be scheduled. The questions are as follows:
1. Pacemaker?
2. Brain or aneurysm clips?
3. Brain or heart surgery; what and when?
4. Shunts or heart valves; type?
5. Any other surgery; what and when?
6. Shrapnel or metal fragments; what and when?

Some questions and answers about your examination are listed below:

1. HOW LONG DOES THE EXAMINATION TAKE?	MRI examinations take about 60–90 min. The radiologist will tailor the examination to your clinical history, so the individual examination may be shorter or longer.
2. WILL THERE BE ANY SIDE EFFECTS?	No, you will feel no "after effects."
3. DO I NEED TO GET AN INJECTION OR DRINK A PREPARATION?	No injection or drinking of oral preparations is routinely required. We request that the patient refrain from caffeine for 4 h before examination and also refrain from wearing eye makeup on the day of examination.
4. DO I NEED TO FAST BEFORE AN MRI EXAMINATION?	No, you may eat your normal meals with the exception of MRI of the pelvis, which requires no solid food 6 h before examination and no liquids 4 h before examination. YOU MAY TAKE YOUR PRESCRIPTION MEDICATIONS.
5. WHEN WILL MY PHYSICIAN GET THE RESULTS?	The preliminary report is available on request within 24 h of the examination. A typed report is sent to each of your physicians, and the original films of your examination may be furnished to your physician upon request.

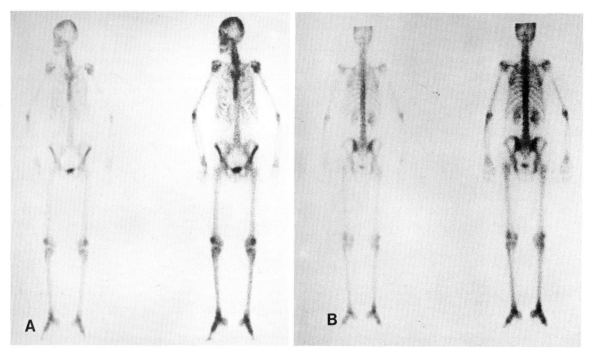

Figure 32–8. Radionuclide bone scan film. (**A**) Anterior; (**B**) posterior. (Courtesy of Michael Ramer, MD, from Judd E: *Nursing Care of the Adult.* F. A. Davis, Philadelphia, 1983, p. 189, with permission.)

foreign objects into vessels and organs. They require strict asepsis and local or general anesthesia and have the potential for causing life-threatening complications. After the procedure, the patient requires close and frequent monitoring, which can only be done in the hospital.

Vascular procedures, called *angiography,* study blood and lymph vessels after a contrast media is injected directly into the vessel. Angiography studies include carotid, coronary, renal, abdominal or cerebral vessels, phlebography (ascertain blood clot[s] location), or lymphography. Figure 32–9 is an aortic angiogram study.

Other inpatient radiology invasive procedures, called

Table 32–6
NUCLEAR MEDICINE EXAMINATION PREPARATION REQUIREMENTS

Nuclear Medicine examinations require an intravenous injection and the examination is performed at various time intervals after the injection.

Bone scan	15 min for the injection. 2–3 h after the injection, scan will be done, taking about 1 h. Between the injection and the scan, patient must drink a quart of liquid. Patient may eat a normal diet.
Liver/spleen Lung	No diet restrictions. Approximately 1 h.
Renal	No diet restrictions. Approximately 2 h.
Gastrointestinal bleed	NO LAXATIVES 4 DAYS BEFORE EXAMINATION. Approximately 2 h and possibly to return after several hours.
Hepatobiliary	NO FOOD OR DRINK 8 HOURS BEFORE EXAMINATION. Approximately 3 h day 1 and possibly asked to return at a later hour or even the following day, depending on information needed.
Galium 67 Cisternogram	Each has specific instructions provided at the time of scheduling. Each takes several time intervals for about 1 wk to complete examination.
III in leukocyte	Special study to be arranged at the time of scheduling. Various time intervals over a 2-d period.
Thyroid studies	DAY 1 LIQUID DIET. Special instructions given at time of scheduling. Usually takes 2 visits and at least 1 h.

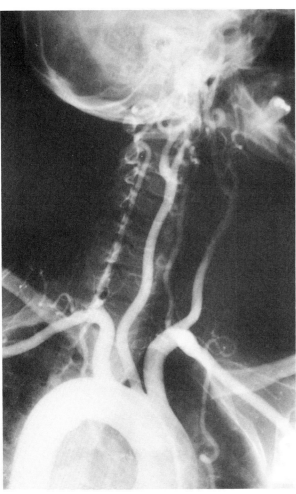

Figure 32–9. An aortic angiogram. (Courtesy of Michael Ramer, MD, from Judd E: Nursing Care of the Adult. F. A. Davis, Philadelphia, 1983, p. 330, with permission.)

interventional, are used in conjunction with surgical procedures to restore normal function. These procedures use needles, coils, and other specialized devices, in conjunction with fluoroscopy and cinefluorography to visually direct the insertion, use, and location of these devices and to document the procedure process and results. Table 32–7 lists other restorative radiology interventional procedures.

Although the medical assistant is not expected to provide patient education and pretest instruction for invasive radiology procedures, he or she is responsible for scheduling the patient for a particular procedure and understanding the general procedure process. The medical assistant should encourage patients to ask questions so they can feel comfortable about the procedure. A detailed description of the radiology procedure is provided at the end of this chapter.

Patient preparation is provided by the physician or radiologist performing the examination. The medical assistant should inquire if any patient pretest instructions are needed when scheduling the test.

RADIATION THERAPY

Radiation therapy is used in the treatment of cancer. Radiation is capable of killing cells by destroying the cell nucleus and preventing cell reproduction.

There are two major forms of radiation therapy: teletherapy and brachytherapy. The specific treatment chosen provides optimum results for the patient.

Teletherapy permits deeper penetration and is used primarily for deep tumors. It spares damage to superficial tissues, and untoward effects are minimal. This type of radiation therapy is done on an outpatient basis.

Brachytherapy uses local, temporary, radioactive implants. It is used to treat localized cancers where the implant can be placed close to the cancer or directly into the cancerous tissue. Special safety precautions are necessary to protect both patient and staff from radiation exposure.

Table 32–7

RADIOLOGIC RESTORATIVE INTERVENTIONAL PROCEDURES

Procedure	Process	Purpose
Percutaneous transluminal angioplasty	Catheter is inserted into major blood vessels. "Umbrella" tip is opened and catheter is pulled along vessel, removing any obstructions.	Increase vessel lumen diameter previously occluded by atherosclerosis. Improve blood flow.
Transcatheter embolization	Substance injected via catheter to occlude blood vessel.	Stop localized bleeding.
Percutaneous nephrolithotomy	Small cannula is inserted through flank into renal pelvis or ureter.	Remove renal stone.
Transcatheter endarterectomy	Arterial angioplasty.	Removes atherosclerotic plaques from arteries.
Thrombolytic therapy	After locating blockage with x-ray, catheter is inserted and thrombolytic drugs injected to break down clot.	Restore blood flow.

Some major side effects of radiation therapy are extremely uncomfortable to the patient, but most of these are reversible. Patients should be encouraged to discuss possible palliative measures with their oncologist to minimize their distress and discomfort. Side effects include nausea and vomiting, epilation (hair loss), ulceration of mucous membranes, weakness, and malaise. Radiation therapy can also produce localized areas of tissue burn or may damage organs in the path of the treatment. Radiation oncologists discuss these side effects with their patients before treatment is initiated. Patients should be informed to immediately report any additional symptoms noted.

STANDARDIZED POSITIONING TERMINOLOGY

To provide adequate patient education and to prepare the patient for unusual, uncomfortable, or prolonged angulated or oblique positions, the medical assistant must understand radiographic positions and projections.

Radiographic positioning refers to specific patient body positions, as follows:

1. *Supine.* Lying flat on the back

2. *Prone.* Lying on the stomach with the face downward
3. *Recumbent.* Lying in any position
4. *Trendelenburg.* Lying on a table angled with the patient's head lower than the feet
5. *Oblique.* Various angled positions (standing or lying)

Radiographic projection refers to the portion of the body the x-ray beam enters first. Projection should not be confused with patient positioning. Figure 32–10 illustrates some of the radiographic projections.

1. *Anteroposterior.* The central ray (beam) enters anterior and exits posterior.
2. *Posteroanterior.* The beam enters posterior and exits anterior.
3. *Oblique.* The beam enters at an oblique point and exits at the opposite oblique point.
4. *Lateral.* The beam crossed the side plane of the patient either through the left or right side.

RADIATION SAFETY AND PROTECTION

Protection and safety of both patients and personnel are of primary concern when x-rays are taken. The

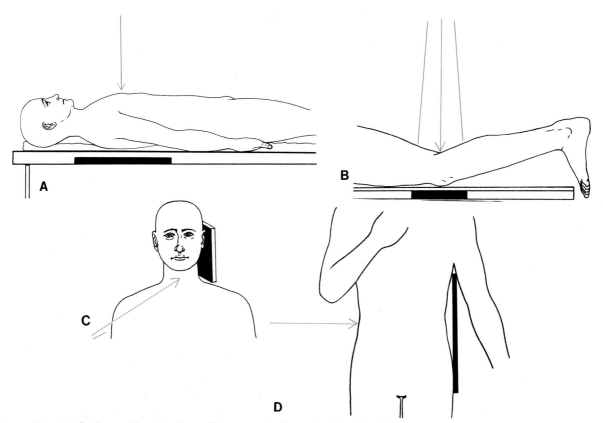

Figure 32–10. Radiographic projections. The arrows indicate the direction of the x-ray; the black bar represents the x-ray film. (**A**) AP chest, patient recumbent. (**B**) PA knee, patient prone. (**C**) Oblique cervical spine (top view). (**D**) Lateral lumbar spine, patient recumbent (top view). (From Drafke MW: Trauma and Mobile Radiography. F. A. Davis, Philadelphia, 1990, pp. 160, 212, 156, 174, with permission.)

long-term effects of radiation exposure can result in genetic defects in offspring or radiation malignant disease. Very high doses of radiation can cause short-term erythema (redness of skin), burns, and epilation (loss of hair by the roots). Cumulative radiation exposure of technologists and physicians must be carefully monitored according to the National Council on Radiation Protection and Measurement. Patients whose x-ray exposure is not monitored may be at risk for long-term effects. Safety precautions must be observed at all time, as follows:

1. Film badges that detect and record the amount of radiation received must be worn by the operator of the machine and by assistants participating in the procedure. These badges are regularly evaluated by specially qualified personnel.
2. The equipment must be kept in good working order and checked routinely to detect any radiation leakage in the machinery that would be dangerous to both patient and operator.
3. Always follow the "10-day rule" which consists of scheduling elective abdominal x-rays on females of child-bearing age (10 to 50 years old) during the 10 days after their last menstrual period. This eliminates the possibility of performing an abdominal x-ray on a patient who is unaware of her pregnancy. Elective procedures are those that are nontrauma and nonemergency x-rays.
4. Always question female patients about the possibility of pregnancy. Never schedule an x-ray for a pregnant woman until the radiologist has approved the examination.
5. Always question the patient about the number and type of x-rays received in the past and the possibility of exposure to radiation in the home, school, or workplace.
6. Provide a lead apron or barrier for the patient.
7. The technician should use a lead barrier.

Information about safety regulations is available from state and local health departments as well as the following agencies:

Bureau of Radiological Health
Rockville, MD 20857

American College of Radiology
20 North Wacker Drive
Chicago, IL 60606

The National Council on Radiation Protection and Management
7910 Woodmont Avenue
Washington, DC 20014

National Bureau of Standards
Washington, DC 20234

THE ROLE OF THE MEDICAL ASSISTANT IN DIAGNOSTIC IMAGING

Patients are routinely scheduled for skeletal x-rays and diagnostic x-ray procedures at radiology centers and hospital radiology departments. The medical assistant's role in making arrangements for these radiologic procedures is as follows:

1. Schedule the appointment for the patient.
2. Instruct the patient in pre-examination preparations.
3. Educate the patient concerning the procedure.

Thorough patient education can result in greater patient cooperation during the examination and possibly reduce exposure to radiation.

Many physicians have x-ray equipment in the office. The physician or radiology technician will operate the office x-ray machine while the medical assistant is responsible for assisting the patient and team members with the procedure.

OFFICE RADIOGRAPHS

In some states, the medical assistant can be trained for limited operation of x-ray equipment in the medical office. x-Ray procedures are usually performed in conjunction with the physical examination or diagnostic examinations. More commonly, the assistant may be expected to assist the physician or x-ray technician when radiographic procedures are performed in the office.

PATIENT TEACHING CONSIDERATIONS

To adequately prepare the patient for a diagnostic imaging procedure, the medical assistant is responsible for providing information to correspond with the patient's ability and willingness to comprehend the procedure, knowledge of body functions, and familiarity with the procedure. The goal of the patient education process is to assist the patient in alleviating fear and anxiety and achieving a feeling of comfort about the procedure. The medical assistant should use the following guidelines when conducting adult patient education before procedures to be performed in diagnostic imaging centers or hospital imaging departments.

1. Avoid the use of complex medical terms when possible. Use proper terminology, but explain it fully.
2. Outline the procedure briefly and clearly.
3. Provide information about frequently asked questions, such as:
   a. length of the examination
   b. side effects (patient sensations)
   c. injections, catheterizations, or other uncomfortable procedures
   d. pretest requirements or restrictions

    e. when test results will be available
    f. costs and insurance coverage
    g. location, time, and date of the scheduled procedure
4. Encourage patients to ask questions.
5. Provide brochures or other written materials that discuss the procedures.
6. Remember that each imaging facility has its own patient preparation requirements. The medical assistant must ensure that the correct facility's instructions are given to the patient.
7. Reinforce the physician's rationale for the test.
8. Request feedback from the patient to verify information accuracy and understanding.

The preceding guidelines should also be used when explaining procedures to pediatric patients and their parents. Calm, properly prepared parents will not transfer feelings of fear and anxiety to the child. Ask the parents' advice when determining the type and amount of information to be given to the child. It is important to remember the following:

1. Patience, honesty and empathy will make the medical assistant more effective.
2. Explain the procedure to the parent first.
3. Explain parental rights to assist with and stay with the child during a procedure.
4. Explain the advantages and disadvantages of parental assisting.
5. If the patient is under 3 years of age, technicians may or may not request parental or adult assistance, depending on the facility's policy and the procedure.
6. Providing a pacifier or bottle may ease the procedure for an infant or toddler.
7. Prepare the parent for the child's immobilization.

Tables 32–8 and 32–9 provide samples of pediatric pretest preparations required for contrast media studies.

Patients often ask questions about safe levels of radiation. The medical assistant should research health effects of common radiology examinations in order to address these concerns. An excellent reference source on this subject is Gofman JW and O'Connor E: x-Rays, Health Effects of Common Exams. Sierra Club Books, San Francisco, 1985.

LEGAL AND ETHICAL IMPLICATIONS

The medical assistant must be aware of state laws designating the specific individuals who may perform diagnostic imaging procedures. Regulations vary depending on whether or not procedures are invasive, and on whether or not they are connected with radiation, either ionizing or nonionizing. Many states, such as California, have regulations and certification requirements for all persons who use x-ray equipment. The

---

Table 32–8

SAMPLE PEDIATRIC PREPARATION FOR A BARIUM ENEMA

0–3 y
1. Nothing by mouth for 3 h before the examination.
2. No solid foods on the day of the examination.
3. No milk.

3–6 y
1. Light, low-residue supper.
2. No solid foods on the day of the examination.
3. Nothing by mouth for 4 h before the examination.
4. One-half rectal suppository (laxative) ordered 3 h before the examination. If the result is poor, give the pediatric enema ordered.

6–11 y
1. Light, low-residue supper.
2. Nothing by mouth after midnight.
3. One rectal suppository (laxative) ordered early on the evening prior to the examination and another one on the day of the examination, 3 h before the study. If the result is poor, give the pediatric enema ordered.

Table 32–9

SAMPLE PEDIATRIC PREPARATION FOR AN INTRAVENOUS PYELOGRAM

0–2 y
1. Nothing by mouth for 3 h before the examination.
2. No solid foods on the day of the examination.

2–6 y
1. Nothing by mouth for 4 h before the examination.
2. No solid foods on the day of the examination.
3. One-half rectal suppository (laxative) ordered in the early evening before the examination. Repeat the same dosage very early in the morning of the examination. If this second dosage does not result in a fairly large bowel movement, an enema is recommended.

6–11 y
1. Nothing by mouth after midnight unless the examination is scheduled for the afternoon.
2. No solid foods on the day of the examination.
3. One rectal suppository (laxative) ordered in the early evening before the examination. Repeat the same dosage very early in the morning of the examination. If this second dosage does not result in a fairly large bowel movement, use the pediatric enema ordered.

11–14 y
1. Drink 5 oz (½ bottle) of citrate of magnesia at 3 PM the day before the examination.
2. For your evening meal, you may have only <u>clear liquids</u>.
3. No food or liquids after midnight.
4. No food or liquids in the morning before the examination.

medical assistant must be sure to practice within the framework of individual state regulations.

Imaging is an important diagnostic tool. The patient must be informed about each procedure and the preparation necessary for and side effects of all scheduled radiographic examinations. Any procedure that is invasive requires that an informed, written consent be obtained from the patient. This consent is obtained by the facility doing the procedure.

SUMMARY

The medical assistant must have a basic understanding of imaging technology to properly explain the procedure to the patient and to provide physician assistance.

This chapter has provided an overview of the relationship of diagnostic imaging to medical office practice. Certainly not all diagnostic procedures have been discussed. Information regarding additional studies in the specialty areas of medicine can be obtained through local medical centers and radiology departments. Touring a department of radiology and nuclear medicine may be a possibility in your area and could be arranged through your instructor.

An expert in the area could be invited as a guest speaker so that questions may be asked, the newest procedures explained, and information updated.

Most important, the medical assistant should be aware that radiology, like other fields of medicine, is a dynamic field. Even though the medical assistant's responsibilities are limited, it is essential that he or she be knowledgeable about changing technology and its impact on patient care.

DISCUSSION QUESTIONS

1. The patient asks you what the x-ray shows during a chest x-ray in the physician's office. How would you respond?
2. The patient tells you that he has read that x-rays are harmful, and is not sure that he wants to have the x-ray ordered by the physician performed. How would you respond?
3. Many radiologists are opposed to medical assistants taking x-rays. How would you explain the medical assistant's role in this process in the physician's office?

BIBLIOGRAPHY

Ballinger PW: Merrill's Atlas of Radiographic Positions and Radiologic Procedures, ed 7. CV Mosby, St Louis, 1990.
Chabner DE: Language of Medicine, ed 4. WB Saunders, Philadelphia, 1991.
Gofman JW and O'Connor E: x-Rays, Health Effects of Common Exams. Sierra Club Books, San Francisco, 1985.
Gurley LT et al: Introduction to Radiologic Technology, ed 3. Mosby Multi-Media, St Louis, 1992.
Meschan I and Ott DJ: Introduction to Diagnostic Imaging. WB Saunders, Philadelphia, 1984.
Thomas CL (ed): Taber's Cyclopedic Medical Dictionary, ed 17. FA Davis, Philadelphia, 1992.

PROCEDURE: Assist with office radiology

OSHA STANDARDS:

Terminal Performance Objective: Assist the physician or radiographer in obtaining radiographs of acceptable quality, with minimal exposure and patient discomfort.

EQUIPMENT: Examination order
X-ray machine and x-ray film cassette
X-ray shield
Patient drape
Patient lead apron

PROCEDURE

1. Identify the patient. Determine that the patient has complied with any instructions to prepare for the procedure.
2. Review with the patient the steps involved in the procedure and the rationale behind the procedure.
3. Instruct the patient to remove clothing as needed according to the physician's or facility's policy (e.g., for a chest x-ray, the patient may be required to remove shirt and undershirt or blouse and bra) and don the robe. Allow the patient the necessary privacy by leaving the room.
4. Make sure that the patient has removed all metal objects from the area to be examined.
5. Position the patient according to the x-ray view ordered; drape the patient and apply the patient shield appropriately.

6. Instruct the patient about the need to remain still and to hold their breath when requested.
7. Leave the room or place yourself behind a lead shield during the x-ray exposure.
8. After the examination, wait until the operator releases the patient.
9. Return the patient to the physician's office for consultation.

PRINCIPLE

1. Noncompliance with procedure preparations will result in false readings or cancellation of the examination.
2. To allay patient fear and encourage patient cooperation.
3. In some cases, clothing may interfere with proper positioning or reduce the image quality.

4. Metal objects will show up on the film and interfere with clear visualization of the target area.
5. Proper positioning ensures good image quality. Appropriate draping is necessary to protect patient privacy and to promote patient comfort. The abdominal x-ray shield protects reproductive organs.
6. Movement, even that associated with respiration, will blur the image and necessitate a retake.
7. To minimize radiation dosage.

8. If the image is unclear, the procedure may have to be repeated.
9. To provide immediate feedback and to reduce patient anxiety.

HIGHLIGHTS

Exposure to X-Rays

Thirty years ago, in most states, mobile x-ray units were driven into neighborhood communities for the purpose of making available x-ray screening for tuberculosis. About as many years ago, x-rays were also used as a treatment for enlarged tonsils and adenoids. The dosage of these x-rays was large and unsafe by contemporary standards. Today, medical scientists have established correlations between the use of high-dosage x-rays and the development of cancer, birth defects, cataracts, and other disorders, and they warn against high dosages and the unwarranted use of x-ray examination. In the McCall's July 1984 issue, an article concerning the safety of x-rays quoted Dr. Eve Bargmann, a physician and researcher with the Public Citizens Health Research Group, as stating that approximately 30% of x-rays taken were unnecessary. The American College of Radiology is also concerned with the number of unnecessary x-ray examinations conducted. In addition, Dr. Reynold Brown, former chairman of the US Commission on Public Health and Radiation Protection and professor of radiology at the University of California, San Francisco, echoes this concern and maintains that "there are many conditions in clinical situations where x-rays are simply not necessary." The sharing of these findings with the patient population, while necessary, oftentimes is misconstrued by articles appearing in the media, and has unfortunately led to much confusion, fear, and the potential for overreaction.

Health professionals, in order to provide accurate information, to educate patients, and to respond to their concerns regarding the use and safety of x-ray examinations, should be aware of the current guidelines for x-ray examinations established by the American College of Radiology. While those listed below are current, health professionals should keep abreast of new developments regarding the understanding of the risks associated with x-ray examinations.

The contemporary view of the role of x-ray examination is that patient exposure to all x-ray radiation (not ultrasound waves) should be minimized. In addition, patients are being instructed to:

1. Ask why an x-ray is necessary and whether the risks can be justified
2. Question the need for annual company or preemployment x-rays, especially if the patient's physician has records on file
3. Avoid mobile x-ray examinations (they tend to be higher exposure)
4. Avoid fluoroscopy (higher exposure) when regular x-rays could be substituted
5. Question x-ray safeguards: regular inspection and licensure

6. Avoid dental x-rays performed by using wide- rather than narrow-beamed plastic cones: narrow cones enable the long, lead-lined cylinders to radiate more precisely and less dangerously (be aware that the American Dental Association and the National Conference of Dental Radiology have condemned the use of x-rays solely for insurance purposes to prove that dental procedures were performed as reported on insurance claims)
7. Wear lead aprons or shields on vital organs not being x-rayed
8. Cooperate with x-ray technicians in remaining still and thereby avoid blurred images (caused by moving or breathing), which would necessitate a retake
9. Understand that x-rays are, in many instances, absolutely essential for determining an accurate diagnosis
10. Keep a family record of x-ray examinations (the Federal Drug Administration supplies x-ray record cards free of charge: x-Rays, Bureau of Radiological Health, HFX-28, Rockville, MD 20857)
11. Be cognizant that the American Cancer Society recommends that women without symptoms of breast disease follow this schedule for mammography:
    a. Obtain a baseline mammogram between the ages of 35 and 40
    b. Between the ages of 40 and 49 — frequency recommended is at the discretion of the patient and physician (usually every 2 years)
    c. After 50 — annually
    Note that breast x-rays are indicated at any age when masses, lumps, or persistent nipple discharge occurs

Finally, health practitioners should advise patients that today's x-ray equipment and procedures are greatly improved and that a much lower-dosage radiation is used than in the past. A combination of newly developed sensitive x-ray film and intensifying screen is now in use throughout the United States. The American College of Radiology further cautions: "Many consumers have exaggerated fears about medical radiation and refuse x-ray examinations that are truly needed. For the individual, avoiding a needed x-ray can be far riskier than the radiation involved in the exam. We believe that informed consumers make better patients . . . patients who communicate effectively with physicians and who play a constructive role in x-ray protection."

APPENDICES

1. Punctuation Patterns in Medical Correspondence
2. Symbols Used in Medical Writing
3. Commonly Used Medical Abbreviations
4. Medical Prefixes and Suffixes
5. Some Medical Terms and Their Latin or Greek Equivalents
6. Latin and Roman Numerals
7. Insurance Vocabulary
8. Medical Law Vocabulary
9. Medical Ethics Vocabulary
10. Universal Precautions

Punctuation Patterns in Medical Correspondence*

	Open	**Mixed**	**Difference**
Dateline	January 28, 1982	January 28, 1982	No difference. The comma is retained in both styles between day and year.
Inside address	Mr. John Wilkes 2970 East Lake Road Fairview, Pennsylvania	Mr. John Wilkes 2970 East Lake Road Fairview, Pennsylvania	No difference. No punctuation is used at the ends of lines in either style.
Salutation	Dear Mr. Wilkes	Dear Mr. Wilkes:	No punctuation is used after the salutation in the open style; a colon or comma is used in the mixed style.
Complimentary close	Sincerely	Sincerely,	No punctuation is used in the open style; a comma is always used in the mixed style.
Signature block line	Joseph Caruso	Joseph Caruso	No difference

*Both open and mixed punctuation patterns are acceptable in office correspondence, provided that consistency is maintained throughout. Open punctuation is preferred for letters typed in block form.

Symbols Used in Medical Writing

♍	Minim	—	Minus; deficiency; alkaline reaction; negative
℈	Scruple	±	Plus or minus; either positive or negative; indefinite
ʒ	Dram		
fʒ	Fluidram	#	Number; following a number, pounds
℥	Ounce	÷	Divided by
f℥	Fluidounce	×	Multiplied by; magnification
O	Pint	/	Divided by
℔	Pound	=	Equal to
℞	Recipe (Latin take)	≈	Approximately equal to
M	Misce (Latin mix)	>	Greater than; from which is derived
$\overline{aa}$	Of each	<	Less than; derived from
A, Å	angström	≮	Not less than
C-1, C-2, etc.	Complement	≯	Not greater than
c, c̄	cum (Latin with)	≦	Equal to or less than
Δ	Change; heat	≧	Equal to or greater than
E_0	Electroaffinity	≠	Not equal to
F_1	First filial generation	√	Root; square root, radical
F_2	Second filial generation	$\sqrt[2]{}$	Square root
mμ	Millimicron, nanometer	$\sqrt[3]{}$	Cube root
μg	Microgram	∞	Infinity
mEq	Milliequivalent	:	Ratio; "is to"
mg	Milligram	::	Equality between ratios, "as"
mg%	Milligrams percent; milligrams per 100 mL	∴	Therefore
QO_2	Oxygen consumption	°	Degree
m-	Meta-	%	Percent
o-	Ortho-	π	3.1416 — ratio of circumference of a circle to its diameter
p-	Para-		
p̄	After	□, ♂	Male
PO_2	Partial pressure of oxygen	O, ♀	Female
PCO_2	Partial pressure of carbon dioxide	⇌	Reversible reaction
s̄	Without	n	Subscripted n indicates that number of molecules can vary from 2 to greater
s̄s̄, ss	(Latin semis). One half		
μm	Micrometer	↑	Increase
μ	Micron (former term for micrometer)	↓	Decrease
μμ	Micromicron		
+	Plus; excess; acid reaction; positive		

Source: From Thomas CL (ed): Taber's Cyclopedic Medical Dictionary, ed 17. FA Davis, Philadelphia, 1993, p 2351.

APPENDIX 3

Commonly Used Medical Abbreviations

Abbreviation	Latin (unless indicated)	English definition
ad	Ad	To; up to
ad lib.	Ad libitum	Freely; at pleasure
ALT		Alanine aminotransferase (formerly SGPT)
AQ	Aqua	Water
AST		Aspartate aminotransferase (formerly SGOT)
AV		Atrioventricular
av.	(French)	Avoirdupois
		Average
B.P.		British Pharmacopeia
BUN		Blood urea nitrogen
C		Calorie (kilocalorie)
		Celsius
		Centigrade
C	Congius	Gallon
ca.	Circa	About
CBC		Complete blood count
cc.	(French)	Cubic centimeter
CDC		Centers for Disease Control
cg	(French)	Centigram
cm	(French)	Centimeter
comp.	Compositus	Compound
CNS		Central nervous system
cong.	Congius	Gallon
CSF		Cerebrospinal fluid
CV		Cardiovascular
d	Dexter	Right
	Dies	Day (24 h)
/d		Per day
D&C		Dilatation and curettage
DPT		Diphtheria-pertussis-tetanus
dr.	Drachma	Dram
ECG		Electrocardiogram
ECT		Electroconvulsive therapy

Continued

Abbreviation	Latin (unless indicated)	English definition
EEG		Electroencephalogram
elix.	(Arabic)	Elixir
EMG		Electromyogram
emp.	Emplastrum	A plaster
ENT		Ear, nose, and throat
ESR		Erythrocyte sedimentation rate
F	(proper name)	Fahrenheit
f		Female
FDA		Food and Drug Administration
FEV		Forced expiratory volume
Fld	Fluidus	Fluid
fl. dr.	Fluidrachma	Fluidram
fl. oz.	Fluidus uncia	Fluidounce
FSH		Follicle-stimulating hormone
GI		Gastrointestinal
Gm; gm	Gramme (French)	Gram
Gr	Granum	Grain
Gtt, gtt	Guttae	Drops
h.	Hora	Hour
hgb		Hemoglobin
I.M.		Intramuscular
inf.	Infusum	Infusion
inhal.	Inhalatio	Inhalation
inj.	Injectio	Injection
instill.		Instillation
IQ		Intelligence quotient
I.U.		International unit
IUD		Intrauterine device
I.V.		Intravenously
kg	(French)	Kilogram
l	Litre (French)	Liter
lab.		Laboratory
lb.	Libra	Pound
LD$_{50}$		Lethal dose, median
liq.	Liquor	Liquid; fluid
m		Male
	(French)	Meter
	Minimum	Minim
MED		Minimum effective dose
mEq		Milliequivalent
mg		Milligram
mL		Milliliter
mM		Millimole
mm	(French)	Millimeter
mol. wt.		Molecular weight
mph		Miles per hour
MPN		Most probable number
µEq		Microequivalent
µg		Microgram
no.	Numerus	Number
NPN		Nonprotein nitrogen
O	Octarius	Pint
OC		Oral contraceptive

Continued

Abbreviation	Latin (unless indicated)	English definition
O.D.	Oculus dexter	Right eye
O.L.	Oculus laevus	Left eye
O.S.	Oculus sinister	Left eye
oz.	Unica	Ounce
paren.		Parenterally
PBI		Protein-bound iodine
pH		Hydrogen ion concentration
ppm		Parts per million
pt	Pinte (French)	Pint
qt	Quartina	Quart
rad		Radiation absorbed dose
s	Sans	Without
$\bar{s}$	Sine	Without
S	Signa	Mark
s.c.	Sub cutis	Subcutaneously
s.cut.		Subcutaneously
SGOT		Serum glutamic oxaloacetic transaminase (see AST)
SGPT		Serum glutamic pyruvic transaminase (see ALT)
sp. gr.	Gravitus	Specific gravity
spt.	Spiritus	Spirit
s.q.		Subcutaneously
stat.	Statim	Immediately
syr.	Syrupus	Syrup
top.		Topically
tr., tinct.	Tinctura	Tincture
UHF		Ultrahigh frequency
ung.	Unguentum	Ointment
UV		Ultraviolet
vin.	Vinum	Wine
Vo_2		Maximum oxygen consumption
vol.%		Volume per cent
WBC		White blood count
Wt.	Wiht (Old English)	Weight
w/v.		Weight in volume
x		Multiplied by

Source: From Thomas CL (ed): Taber's Cyclopedic Medical Dictionary, ed 17. FA Davis, Philadelphia, 1993, p 2352.

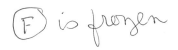
Ⓕ is frozen

Medical Prefixes and Suffixes

a, an-: Negative

a-, ab-, abs-: Away from

ad-, -ad: Toward

-aemia: Blood

aer-: Air

-aesthesia: Sensation

-algesia, -algia: Suffering; pain

algi-: Pain

all-: Other

amb-: Both; on both sides

amph-: Around; on both sides

ana-, an-: Up

angio-: Relating to blood or lymph vessels

ante-: Before

anti-: Against

apo-: From; opposed

-ase: Enzyme

aut-, auto-: Self

bi-, bis-: Twice; double

brachy-: Short

brady-: Slow

cac-, caco-: Bad; evil

cat-, cata-, cath-: Down

-cele: A tumor; a cyst; a hernia

cent-: Hundred

cephal-: Relating to a head

chrom-, chromo-: Color

-cide: Causing death

circum-: Around

co-, com-, con-: Together

contra-: Against

cyst-, -cyst: Bag; bladder

-cyte: Cell

dacry-: Tears

dactyl-: Fingers

de-: From; not

deca-: Ten

deci-: Tenth

demi-: Half

dent-: Relating to the teeth

derma-: Skin

di-: Double; apart from

dia-: Through; between; asunder

dipla-, diplo-: Double

dis-: Negative; double; apart; absence of

-dynia: Pain

dys-: Difficult; bad

ec-, ecto-: Out; on the outside

-ectomy: Cutting out

ef-, es-, ex-, exo-: Out

-emesis: Vomiting

-emia: Blood

en-: In; into

endo-: Within

entero-: Relating to the intestine

ento-: Within

epi-: Upon; above

-esthesia: Sensation

eu-: Well

ex-, exo-: Out

extra-: On the outside; beyond

fore-: Before; in front of

-form: Form

-fuge: To drive away

galact-, galacto-: Milk

gaster-, gastro-: The stomach; the belly

-gene, -genesis, -genetic, -genic: Production; origin, formation

glosso-: Relating to the tongue

-gog, -gogue: To make flow

-gram: Tracing; mark

-graphy: Writing; record

hem-, hemato-: Relating to the blood

hemi-: Half

hepa-, hepar-, hepato-: Liver

hetero-: Other; indicating dissimilarity

holo-: All

homo-, homeo-: Same; similar

Continued

hydra-, hydro-: Relating to water

hyp-, hyph-, hypo-: Under

hyper-: Over; above; beyond

hypo-: Under

-iasis: Condition, pathologic state

idio-: Peculiar to the individual or organ

ileo-: Relating to the ileum

in-: In; into; not

infra-: Beneath

inter-: Between

intra-, intro-: Within

-ism: Condition; theory

iso-: Equal

-itis: Inflammation

-ize: To treat by special method

juxta-: Near

karyo-: Nucleus; nut

kata-, kath-: Down

kera-: Horn; indicates hardness

kinesi-: Movement

-kinesis-: Motion

lact-: Milk

laparo-: Loin; relating to the loin or abdomen

laryng-, laryngo-: The larynx

latero-: Side

lepto-: Small; soft

leuko-: White

-lite, -lith: Stone; calculus

lith-: Stone

-logia, -logy: Science of; study of

-lysis: Setting free; disintegration

macro-: Large; long; big

mal-: Bad; poor; evil

med-, medi-: Middle

mega-, megal-: Large; great

-megalia, -megaly: Large, great, extreme

melan-, melano-: Black

mes-, meso-: Middle

meta-: Beyond; over; between, change, or transposition

-meter: Measure

metra-, metro-: Uterus

micro-: small

mio-: Less; smaller

mono-: Single

multi-: Many

my-, myo-: Muscle

myel-, myelo-: Marrow

myxa-, myxo-: Mucus

neo-: New

nephr-, nephra-, nephro-: Kidney

neu-, neuro-: Nerve

niter-, nitro-: Nitrogen

non-, not-: No

nucleo-: Nucleus

ob-: Against

oculo-: Eye

-ode, oid: Form; shape; resemblance

odont-: Tooth

oligo-: Few

-oma: A tumor

omo-: Shoulder

o-: Egg; ovum

oophoron-: Ovary

opisth-: Backward

orchid-: Testicle

ortho-: Straight; normal

os-: Mouth; bone

-osis-: Condition; disease; intensive

oste-, osteo-: Bone

-ostomosis, -ostomy: To furnish with a mouth or an outlet

-otomy: Cutting

oxy-: Sharp; acid

pachy-: Thick

pan-: All; entire

para-: Alongside of

path-, -path, -pathy: Disease; suffering

-penia: Lack

per-: Excessive; through

peri-: Around

phobia: Fear

-phylaxis: Protection

-plasm: To mold

-plastic: Molded; indicates restoration of lost or badly formed features

-plegia: Stroke

plur-: More

pneu-: Relating to the air or lungs

poly-: Much; many

post-: After

pre-: Before

pro-: Before; in behalf of

proto-: First

pseud-, pseudo-: False

psych-: The soul; the mind

py-, pyo-: Pus

re-: Back; again

retro-: Backward

-rhage, -rhagia: Hemorrhage; flow

-rhaphy: A suturing or stitching

-rhea: To flow; indicates discharge

sacchar-: Sugar

sacro-: Sacrum

salping-, salpingo-: A tube; relating to a fallopian tube

sarco-: Flesh

sclero-: Hard; relating to the sclera

-sclerosis: Dryness; hardness

-scopy: Sight

semi-: Half

-stomosis, -stomy: Artificial mouth or outlet

sub-: Under

Continued

super-, supra-: Above

syn-: With; together

tele-: Distant; far

tetra-: Four

thio-: Sulfur

thyro-: Thyroid gland

-tomy: Cutting

trans-: Across

tri-: Three

-trophic: Relating to nourishment

tropho-: Relating to nutrition

uni-: One

-uria: Relating to the urine

urino-, uro-: Relating to the urine or urinary organs

vaso-: A vessel

venter-, ventro-: The abdomen

xanth-: Yellow

Source: From Thomas CL (ed): Taber's Cyclopedic Medical Dictionary, ed 17. FA Davis, Philadelphia, 1993, p 2360.

Some Medical Terms and Their Latin or Greek Equivalents

Medical Words

Acid: Acidum
Ague: Febris
And: Et
Arm: Brachium. Gr., brachion
Artery: Arteria
Attachment: Adhesio
Back: Tergum; dorsum
Backbone: Spina
Backward: Retro
Bath: Balneum
Beef: Bubula
Belly: Venter; abdomen
Bend: Flexus
Bile: Bilis. Gr., chole
Bladder: Vesica
Bleed: Fluere
Blind: Obscurus
Blister: Pustulo; vesicatorium
Bloat: Tumeo
Blood: Sanguis. Gr., haima
Blood vessel: Vena
Body: Corpus. Gr., soma
Boiling up: Effervescens
Bone: Os. Gr., osteon.
Bony: Osseus
Bowels: Intestina; viscera
Bowlegged: Valgus
Brain: Cerebrum. Gr., enkephalos
Breach: Ruptura
Breast: Mamma. Gr., mastos
Breath: Halitus
Bubble: Pustula
Bulb: Bulbus
Buttock: Clunis. Gr., gloutos
Calcareous: Calci similis

Canal: Canalis
Cartilage: Cartilago. Gr., chondros
Catarrh: Coryza
Cavity: Caverna
Change: Mutatio
Chest: Thorax. Gr., thorax
Chin: Mentum. Gr., geneion
Choke: Strangulo
Clavicle: Clavicula
Confinement: Puerperium
Congestion: Conglobatio
Consumption: Phthisis, pulmonaria
Convulsion: Convulsio
Cord: Corda
Corn: Callus; clavus
Cornea: Cornu. Gr., keras
Costive: Astrictus
Cough: Tussio
Countenance: Vultus
Cramp: Spasmus
Crisis: Dies crisimus
Cup: Poculum
Cure: Sano
Curvature: Curvatura
Cuticle: Cuticula
Daily: Diurnus
Dandruff: Furfures capitas
Day: Dies
Dead: Mortuus; defunctus
Deadly: Lethalis
Deafness: Surditas
Decompose: Dissolvo
Dental: Dentalis
Depression: Depressio
Digestive: Digestorius; pepticus

Dilute: Dilutus
Discharge: Eluvies; effluens
Disease: Morbus
Dorsal: Dorsalis
Dose: Potio
Dram: Drachma
Drink: Bibo; potis
Dropsy: Hydrops; opis
Drug: Medicamentum
Duct: Ductus
Dysentery: Dysenteria
Ear: Auris, Gr., ous
Eat: Edo. Gr., phagos
Egg: Ovum
Elbow: Cubitum. Gr., ankon
Embryo: Partus immaturus
Emission: Emissio
Entrails: Viscera
Epidemic: Epidemus
Epilepsy: Morbus comitalis; epilepsia
Epileptic: Epilepticus
Erection: Erectio
Erotic: Amatorius
Eunuch: Eunuchus
Every: Omnis
Excrement: Excrementum
Excretion: Excrementum; excretio
Exhalation: Exhalatio
Exhale: Exhalo
Expel: Expello
Expire: Expiro
External: Externus
Extract: Extractum
Eye: Oculus. Gr., ophthalmos
Eyeball: Pupula
Eyebrow: Supercilium
Eyelid: Palpebra
Eyetooth: Dens caninus
Face: Facies
Faculty: Facultas
Faint: Collabor
Fat: Adeps. Gr., lipos
Feature: Lineomentum
Febrile: Febriculosus
Fecundity: Fecunditas
Feel: Tactus
Fever: Febris
Film: Membranula
Filter: Percolo
Finger: Digitus. Gr., daktylos
Fistula: Fistula putris
Fit: Accessus
Flesh: Carnis. Gr., sarx
Fluid: Fluidus

Food: Cibus
Foot: Pes, pedis. Gr., pous.
Forearm: Brachium
Forehead: Frons
Freckle: Lentigo
Gall: Bilis
Gangrene: Gangraena
Gargle: Gargarizo
Gland: Glandula
Gleet: Ichor
Gout: Morbus articularis; (in feet) podagra
Grain: Granum
Gravel: Calculus
Grinder tooth: Dens maxillaris
Gullet: Gula
Gum: Gingiva
Gut: Intestinum
Hair: Capillus. Gr., thrix
Half: Dimidius
Hand: Manus. Gr., cheir
Harelip: Labrum fissum
Haunch: Clunis
Head: Caput. Gr., kephale
Heal: Sano
Healer: Medicus
Healing: Salutaris
Health: Sanitas
Healthful: Salutaris; saluber
Healthy: Sanus
Hear: Audio
Hearing: Auditio; (sense of) auditus
Heart: Cor. Gr., kardia
Heartburn: Redundatio stomachi
Heat: Calor
Hectic: Hecticus
Heel: Calx, talus
Hirsute: Hirsutus
Homeopathic: Homeopathicus
Hysterics: Hysteria
Illness: Morbus
Incisor: Dens acutus
Infant: Infans; puerilis
Infect: Inficio
Infectious: Contagiosus
Infirm: Infirmus; debilis
Inflammation: Inflammatio; (of lungs) inflammatio pulmonaria
Injection: Injectio
Insane: Insanus
Intellect: Intellectus
Intercourse: Congressus
Internal: Intestinus
Intestine: Intestinum. Gr., enteron
Itch: Scabies

Continued

Itching: Pruritus
Jaw: Maxilla
Joint: Artus. Gr., arthron
Jugular vein: Vena jugularis
Kidney: Ren. Gr., nephros
Knee: Genu. Gr., gonu
Kneepan: Patella
Knuckle: Condylus
Labor: Partus
Labyrinth: Labyrinthus
Lacerate: Lacero
Larynx: Guttur
Lateral: Lateralis
Leech: Sanguisuga
Leg: Tibia
Leprosy: Leprosus
Ligament: Ligamentum. Gr., syndesmos
Ligature: Ligatura
Limb: Membrum
Lime: Calx
Listen: Ausculto
Liver: Jecur. Gr., hepar
Livid: Lividus
Loin: Lumbus. Gr., lapara
Looseness: Laxitas
Lotion: Lotio
Lukewarm: Tepidus
Lung: Pulmo. Gr., pneumon
Lymph: Lympha
Mad: Insanus
Malady: Morbus
Male: Masculinus
Malignant: Malignus
Maternity: Conditio matris
Medicated: Medicatus
Medicine: (Remedy) Medicamentum
Milk: Lac
Mind: Animus
Mix: Misceo
Mixture: Mistura
Moist: Humidus
Molar: Dens molaris
Month: Mensis
Monthly: Menstruus
Morbid: Morbidus
Mouth: Os. Gr., stoma
Mucous: Mucosus
Muscle: Musculus. Gr., mys.
Mustard: Sinapis
Nail: Unguis
Navel: Umbilicus. Gr., omphalos
Neck: Cervix; collum. Gr., trachelos
Nerve: Nervus. Gr., neuron
Nipple: Papilla

no, none: Nullus
Normal: Normalis
Nose: Nasus. Gr., rhis
Nostril: Naris
Not: Non
Nourish: Nutrio
Nourishment: Alimentus
Now: Nunc
Nudity: Nudatio
Nurse: Nutrix
Obesity: Obesitas
Ocular: Ocularis
Oculist: Ocularis medicus
Oil: Oleum
Ointment: Unguentum
Operator: Manus curatio
Opiate: Medicamentum somnificum
Optics: Optice
Orifice: Foramen
Pain: Dolor
Palate: Palatum
Palm: Palma
Parasite: Parasitus
Part: Pars
Patient: Patiens
Pectoral: Pectoralis
Pedal: Pedale
Phlegm: Pituita
Pill: Pilus
Pimple: Pustula
Plaster: Emplastrum
Poison: Venenum
Poultice: Cataplasma
Powder: Pulvis
Pregnant: Gravida
Prepare: Paro
Prescribe: Praescribo
Prescription: Praescriptum
Puberty: Pubertas
Pubic bone: Os pubis. Gr., pecten
Pulverize: Pulvero
Pupil: Pupilla
Purgative: Purgativus
Putrid: Putridus
Quinsy: Cynanche; angina
Rash: Exanthema
Recover: Convalesco
Recumbent: Recumbens
Recur: Recurro
Redness: Rubor
Remedy: Remedium
Respiration: Respiratio
Rheum: Fluxio
Rib: Costa

Continued

Rigid: Rigidus
Ringing: Tinnitus
Rupture: Hernia
Saliva: Sputum
Sallow: Salix
Salt: Sal
Salve: Unguentum
Sane: Sanus
Scab: Scabies
Scalp: Pericranium
Scaly: Squamosus
Scar: Cicatrix
Sciatica: Ischias
Scruple: Scrupulum
Seed: Semen
Senile: Senilis
Serum: Sanguinis pars equosa
Sheath: Vagina
Shin: Tibia
Shock: Concussio; (of electricity) ictus electricus
Short: Brevis
Shoulder: Humerus. Gr., omos
Shoulder blade: Scapula
Shudder: Tremor
Sick: Aegrotus
Side: Latus
Sinew: Nervus
Skeleton: Gr., skeleton
Skin: Cutis. Gr., derma
Skull: Cranium. Gr., kranion
Sleep: Somnus
Smallpox: Variola
Smell: Odoratus
Soap: Sapo
Socket: Cavum
Soft: Mollis
Solid: Solidus
Solution: Dilutum
Soporific: Soporus
Sore: Ulcus
Spasm: Spasmus
Spinal: Dorsalis; spinalis
Spine: Spina
Spirit: Spiritus
Spittle: Sputum
Spleen: Lien
Spoon: Cochleare
Sprain: Luxatio
Stomach: Stomachus. Gr., gaster
Stone: Calculus
Stricture: Strictura
Sugar: Saccharum
Suture: Sutura
Swallow: Glutio

Sweat: Sudor. Gr., hidros
Symptom: Symptoma
System: Systema
Tail: Cauda:
Take: Sumo
Tapeworm: Taenia
Taste: Gustatus
Tear: Lacrima
Teeth: Dentes
Tendon: Tendo. Gr., tenon
Testicle: Testis. Gr., orchis
Thigh: Femur
Throat: Fauces. Gr., pharynx
Throb: Palpito
Thumb: Pollex
Tongue: Lingua. Gr., glossa
Tonsil: Tonsilla
Tooth: Dens. Gr., odous
Troche: Trochiscus
Tube: Tuba
Twin: Geminus
Twitching: Subsultus
Ulcer: Ulcus
Unless: Nisi
Urine: Urina
Uterine: Uterinus
Vaccine: Vaccinum
Vagina: Vagina. Gr., kolpos
Valve: Valvula
Vein: Vena. Gr., phleps
Vertebra: Vertebra. Gr., spondylos
Vessel: Vas
Wash: Lavo
Water: Aqua
Wax: Cera
Waxed dressing: Ceratum
Weary: Lassus
Wet: Humidus
Windpipe: Arteria aspera
Wine: Vinum
Woman: Femina
Womb: Uterus. Gr., hystera
Worm: Vermis
Wound: Vulnus
Wrist: Carpus. Gr., karpos
Yolk: Luteum

Colors

Black: Niger; nigra, nigrum
Blue: Caeruleus; cyaneus; lividus
Brown: Fulvus
Crimson: Coccum; coccineus
Gray: Cinereus
Green: Viridis

Continued

Lemon: Citreum
Pink: Rosaceus
Purple: Purpura; purpureus
Red: Ruber
Scarlet: Coccineus
Violet: Violaceus
White: Albus
Yellow: Flavus; luteus; croceus.

Qualities

Bitter: Acerbus
Chill: Friguscolum
Cold: Frigidus
Dry: Aridus
Dull: Stupidus; hebes
Faintness: Languor
Fat: Obesus; pinguis
Heat: Calor; ardor; fervor
Heavy: Gravis; ponderosus
Hot: Calidus; fervens; candens
Light: Levis
Liquid: Liquidus
Moist: Humidus; uvidus
Sharp: Acutus
Short: Brevis
Sour: Acidus
Sweet: Dulcis
Tall: Longus; celsus; procerus
Thick: Densus
Thin: Tenius; macer
Warm: Calidus
Warmth: Calor:
Weary: Lassus; languidus; fatigatus
Wet: Humidus

Metals

Copper: Cuprum; cuprinus
Gold: Aurum; aureus
Iron: Ferrum; ferreus
Silver: Argentum; argenteus
Tin: Stannum; plumbum album

Time

Afternoon: Post meridiem
Age: Aetas; maturas; adultas; impubis
Autumn: Autumnus
Birth: Partus; natales
Breakfast: Prandium
Child: Infans; puer; filius
Daily: Diurnus
Date: Status dies
Dawn: Prima lux
Day: Dies
Death: Mors
Dinner: Cena
Evening: Vesper
Hour: Hora
Infant: Infans
Maturity: Maturitas; aetas matura
Meal: Epula
Midnight: Media nox
Midsummer: Media aestas
Moment: Punctum
Month: Mens
Monthly: Menstruus
Morning: Matutinum
Night: Nox
Noon: Meridies
Old: Antiquus
Puberty: Pubertas
Second: Secundum
Spring: Ver; veris
Summer: Aestas
Sunrise: Solis ortus
Sunset: Solis occasus
Supper: Cena
Time: Tempus
Winter: Hiems, hiemis
Year: Annus
Young: Parvus; infans
Youth: Adolescentia

Source: From Thomas CL (ed): Taber's Cyclopedic Medical Dictionary, ed 17. FA Davis, Philadelphia, 1993, p 2362.

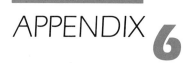

Latin and Roman Numerals

	Latin Numerals			Roman Numerals*	
Cardinal		**Ordinal**			
1	Unus	1st	Primus	1	I
2	Duo	2nd	Secundus	2	II
3	Tres	3rd	Tertius	3	III
4	Quattuor	4th	Quartus	4	IV
5	Quinque	5th	Quintus	5	V
6	Sex	6th	Sextus	6	VI
7	Septem	7th	Septimus	7	VII
8	Octō	8th	Octāvus	8	VIII
9	Novem	9th	Nōnus	9	IX
10	Decem	10th	Decimus	10	X
11	Undecim	11th	Ūndecimus	11	XI
12	Duodecim	12th	Duodecimus	12	XII
13	Tredecim	13th	Tertius decimus	15	XV
14	Quattuordecim	14th	Quartus decimus	20	XX
15	Quīndecim	15th	Quīntus decimus	30	XXX
16	Sēdecim	16th	Septus decimus	40	XL
17	Septendecim	17th	Septimus decimus	50	L
18	Duodēvīgintī	18th	Duodēvīcēsimus	60	LX
19	Ūndēvīgintī	19th	Ūndēvīcēsimus	70	LXX
20	Vīgintī	20th	Vīcēsimus	80	LXXX
21	Vīgintī ūnus; ūnus et vīgintī	21st	Vīcēsimus primus; prīmus et vīcēsimus	90	XC
22	Vīgintī duo; duo et vīgintī	22nd	Vīcēsimus secundus; duo et vīcēsimus	100	C
28	Duodētrīgintā	28th	Duodētrīcēsimus	500	D
29	Ūndētrīgintā	29th	Ūndētrīcēsimus	1000	M
30	Trīgintā	30th	Trīcēsimus	2000	MM
40	Quadrāgintā	40th	Quadrāgēsimus	5000	V̄
50	Quīnquāgintā	50th	Quīnquāgēsimus	10,000	X̄
60	Sexāgintā	60th	Sexāgēsimus	100,000	C̄
70	Septuāgintā	70th	Septuāgēsimus	1,000,000	M̄
80	Octōgintā	80th	Octōgēsimus		
90	Nōnāgintā	90th	Nōnāgēsimus		
100	Centum	100th	Centēsimus		

Continued

	Latin Numerals			Roman Numerals*
Cardinal		*Ordinal*		
101	Centum ūnus; centum et ūnus	101st	Centēsimus prīmus; centēsimus et prīmus	
102	Centum duo; centum et duo	102nd	Centēsimus secundus; centēsimus et secundus	
200	Ducentī	200th	Ducentēsimus	
300	Trecentī	300th	Trecentēsimus	
400	Quadringentī	400th	Quadringentēsimus	
500	Quīngentī	500th	Quīngentēsimus	
600	Sēscentī; sexcenti	600th	Sēscentēsimus	
700	Septingentī	700th	Septingentēsimus	
800	Octingentī	800th	Octingentēsimus	
900	Nōngentī	900th	Nōngentēsimus	
1,000	mīlle	1,000th	Mīllēsimus	
2,000	Duo mīllia	2,000th	Bis mīllēsimus	
10,000	Decem mīllia	10,000th	Decies mīllēsimus	
100,000	Centum mīllia	100,000th	Centiēs mīllēsimus	

*A line over a letter increases its value 1000 times.

Source: From Thomas CL (ed): Taber's Cyclopedic Medical Dictionary, ed 17. FA Davis, Philadelphia, 1993, p 2366.

Insurance Vocabulary

Assignment of insurance benefits: Authorization granted to the insurance company by an insured individual to pay policy benefits to another individual.

Attending physician: The physician ultimately in charge or the overseer of the patient's care.

Authorization to release information: Signed permission given by the patient, authorizing the physician to release privileged information.

Benefits: Services provided under the insurance agreement.

Carrier: The agent designated by the policy holder to process claims. The carrier can be a commercial company or a federal agency, such as Medicare.

Certification of eligibility: Written verification of the policy holder's entitlement to benefits.

Claimant: The individual making a formal request to receive payment or benefits as mandated by the insurance policy.

Claim form: A written statement listing services rendered, usually signed by both the physician and the patient. Payment is made on the basis of the information specified on the form.

Claim payments: Payments made by the insurance company, under terms of the agreement, to the insured (the patient) as reimbursement or the physician for services rendered.

Coinsurance: Payment for services shared by the insurance company and the insured.

Coverage: Benefits forthcoming to the insured, stated in the insurance plan.

Effective date: The date on which coverage can be granted and the contractual agreement is binding.

Eligibility rules: Specific criteria, stated in the insurance plan, indicating when benefits may be granted, to whom, and for how long.

Eligible members: Individuals in a family or group plan who qualify, by reason of their relationship, for benefits stated in the plan.

Exclusions (exceptions): Circumstances specified by the policy for which there is no coverage.

Expiration date: The date on which coverage can no longer be granted; termination of the contract (see "termination date").

Explanation of benefits: The statement that accompanies benefit payment, describing in detail how the amount of payment was calculated.

Extended care: Health care provided by a facility other than a hospital that specializes in long-term care.

Fee (or benefit) schedule: The policy statement listing specified amounts to be paid for specified services.

Group plan: An insurance policy providing coverage to several individuals who share premium costs. Companies may share premium costs as well.

Income limit: (1) The maximum income an individual can earn and still be eligible for insurance benefits. (2) The maximum amount of income protection to which the insurance company will agree in the contract.

Indemnity allowance (or schedule): The fee amount to be paid by the insurance plan. Coverage differences less than the physician's fee are the patient's responsibility.

Individual insurance plan: An insurance policy purchased by an individual who accepts full responsibility for premium payment.

Inpatient: The hospital patient receiving room and board.

Insuring clauses: Statements in the policy that specify the terms and conditions of coverage and benefits.

Manual of procedures: The insurance company's instructions for interpreting its plans and processing the related forms.

Maximum benefit: The dollar amount of benefits that the insurance company will pay for processed claims in any year.

Outpatient: A patient receiving hospital treatment without room and board.

Participating physician: A physician member of a group or organization providing health care, such as Blue Shield.

Preexisting condition: An abnormal physical or mental condition existing prior to the date on which the policy becomes effective.

Primary physician: The physician who first cares for the patient.

Physician's profile: The physician's statement of the patient's general health status following a comprehensive physical examination.

Referring physician: The physician who recommends another physician to the patient. The term may also be used of the physician who authorized the patient's hospital admission.

Release of information: A form signed by the patient, granting permission to the physician to release medical information to the insurance company.

Retroactive: Made effective to an earlier date.

Rider: An amendment to an original policy statement that increases, decreases, or excludes certain aspects of coverage.

Schedule of allowances: A list of specified amounts to be paid by the insurance company for medical services.

Subscriber: The insured representing the family unit in the insurance agreement.

Termination date: The date on which insurance protection and coverage cease (see "expiration date").

Time limit: The time in which a claim must be filed so that the patient can receive benefits.

Usual and customary fees: Normal or average charges or fees for services rendered.

APPENDIX 8

Medical Law Vocabulary

Assault: An expressed threat to do bodily harm.

Battery: Body contact that is unauthorized.

Board of Medical Examiners: The licensure board of the American Medical Association, which is responsible for suspending or revoking a physician's license to practice medicine.

Breach: A violation of law, promise, or duty.

"Captain of the ship" doctrine: The legal doctrine holding that a physician is in complete charge of individuals present and those providing assistance during and until the conclusion of an operative procedure.

Committee: The guardian of a mentally incompetent individual.

Consent: The agreement, authorization, or permission that allows the physician to act on the patient's body.

Consent implied in action: Permission given nonverbally but evidenced in the patient's activity, such as the patient's keeping an appointment for x-ray testing.

Consent implied in emergency: Permission given nonverbally but evidenced in the urgency of the patient's condition when the patient cannot clearly respond. Consent is implied for life-saving measures. It is deemed reasonable that an individual would give permission for any procedure required to save his or her life.

Consent implied in law: Consent implied in emergency and consent of parent or guardian are also termed consent implied in law because legal statutes govern their use.

Consent of parent or guardian: Written permission given by the parent or guardian to the physician so as to act on the body of the patient.

Criminal offense: An act for which there is no legal support, such as the practice of medicine by an unlicensed person.

Damages: The approximated money equivalent for a detriment or damage sustained by the plaintiff.

Defamation: Written or oral statements or representations that attack the character of an individual, resulting in an unfavorable impression or unjust actions.

Defendant: The individual being prosecuted or sued.

Direct liability: Responsibility of the physician for willful or negligent acts performed during the rendering of services.

Discreet disclosure: The principle that allows the physician to not disclose all information relating to the patient's condition as long as no form of consent is elicited.

Dying declaration: Statements made by an individual approaching death that are witnessed and can be used in a court action.

Emancipated minor: A person who is not of legal age but is married and therefore has legal rights and responsibilities.

Endorsement: The acceptance by some states of the National Board of Medical Examiners certification in lieu of a state licensure examination for the practice of medicine.

Excess damages: Damages that exceed the amount covered by the insurance policy.

Express consent: Written permission, authorization, or agreement given by a relative of the deceased for the performance of an autopsy on the deceased.

Expert witness: A professional (physician) who testifies against another professional (physician) in the legal determination of negligence or malpractice.

Fee splitting: An arrangement in which a physician-specialist charges the patient a fee and then returns a portion of the fee to the referring physician. This act may result in the suspension or revocation of the physician's license to practice medicine.

Fraud: Deceit or misrepresentation used to obtain unfair advantage.

"Good Samaritan" statute: The statute that protects the physician from legal action for the treatment of an accident victim requiring emergency care.

Implied (oral) contract: The contractual agreement that pertains to the physician-patient relationship and usually begins when the patient first visits the medical office and the physician touches the patient for the purpose of examination.

Informed consent: Agreement, authorization, or permission that, to be legally valid, requires the physician to share information in the following five areas before a procedure can be performed:

1. The nature of the illness and why it needs treatment

894

2. The nature of the proposed treatment, the details of the procedure, and who will perform the procedure
3. The risks or consequences and their probability of occurrence
4. Alternative treatment methods and the reasons for their appropriateness or inappropriateness related to this illness
5. Reasonable expectations for recovery and chances of failure

Insanity: Mental incompetence precluding legal responsibility for one's actions. An individual must be declared insane by a court of law.

Law of contracts: The legal framework for unwritten agreements between two parties, as between physician and patient. To be binding, such agreements must satisfy four requisites:

1. Manifestation and assent. The individual must request the services of the physician, and the physician must accept the responsibility to render care
2. The legal subject matter of the agreement must bear on the relationship between physician and patient
3. The patient and physician must be of legal age and sound mental capacity
4. Consideration must exist. This term refers to the assumption that the patient will pay for the services rendered

Liable: Legally responsible for one's actions.

Liability suit: A legal action taken when one individual (the plaintiff) seeks damages from another (the defendant). The plaintiff assumes a breach of the defendant's legal obligation.

Licensed physician: A physician who has passed a state licensure examination and has been determined to be competent to practice medicine.

Majority: The age at which full civil rights are granted.

Malfeasance claim: A malpractice claim charging that the physician treated the patient wrongfully. An example would be the surgical removal of a healthy organ.

Malpractice: Dereliction of professional skill through carelessness, ignorance, or intent, resulting in undesirable consequences of the treatment rendered. Malpractice claims fall into one of three categories: malfeasance, misfeasance, and nonfeasance.

Medical practice acts: Legal statutes that govern the practice of medicine.

Minority: The age at which full civil rights cannot be granted and during which the parent or guardian has the right of jurisdiction.

Misfeasance claim: A malpractice claim involving the wrongful manner of an act, as when a physician is alleged to have performed a procedure incorrectly, although the procedure itself was rightful.

Moral turpitude: Acts or actions of an immoral or shameful nature.

Nonfeasance claim: A malpractice claim charging the physician with failure to act in accordance with duty or necessity.

Plaintiff: The individual seeking legal resolution (damages) and initiating legal action (suit).

Professional fee: Payment due from the patient for professional services. Medical fees are determined by geographic averages and the fee schedule recommendations of the American Medical Association.

Professional liability insurance: Insurance available to health professionals for protection from monetary loss from legal action.

Proximate cause: For negligence to be proved and liability charged, the injury to the patient cannot have occurred without the physician's action, thus establishing the proximate, or direct, cause.

Reciprocity: The granting of licensure without medical examination in one state to a physician who has successfully passed the medical board examination in another state in which the requirements meet or surpass those in the state granting reciprocity.

Registration fee: The fee paid periodically to the Board of Medical Examiners to maintain the licensure to practice.

Reregistration: Periodic payment of the registration fee.

Res ipsa loquitur: (Latin, "The thing speaks for itself.") A doctrine applied to malpractice cases to assist in the determination of negligence. There are several requirements for the application of *res ipsa loquitur.*

1. The consequences of treatment must be out of the ordinary; that is, not within the normal range of expectations. It must be proved that "the thing speaks for itself" and occurred solely as a result of the physician's negligence
2. The physician must be directly or vicariously liable for the action
3. The patient must be free of any contribution to the consequences through his or her own actions

Respondeat superior: (Latin, "Let the master answer.") *Respondeat superior* places responsibility on the physician for the liability of employees. The physician is ultimately responsible for the wrongful acts of others, be they junior partners, office staff members, or those assisting in surgery.

Standards of care: The qualifications of the physician who serves as expert witness. The expert witness must occupy a position in which the quality of care (techniques and procedures) is expected as that maintained by the defendant.

Statute: A legal doctrine set forth by a legislative body to govern specific acts.

Statute of fraud: The doctrine bearing on the failure of the patient or the patient's agent to pay the physician's fee when agreement had been assumed.

Statute of limitations: A statute restricting the time in which a claim may be prosecuted. For instance, in some states, legal action cannot be initiated for treatment received when 3 years have lapsed from the time of treatment.

Suit: The act of seeking legal resolution in the form of damages in a court of law.

Tort: Any wrongful act (not involving breach of contract) for which civil or legal action can be initiated.

Vicarious liability: The physician's responsibility for the wrongful acts committed by others, as in employees or persons whom the physician supervises.

Medical Ethics Vocabulary

Amniocentesis: Withdrawal of a sample of amniotic fluid from the uterine cavity through a needle inserted into the abdomen.

Artificial insemination: The introduction of seminal fluid from a donor into the female reproductive organs.

Atopogenics: Highly controversial studies in biologic engineering for such purposes as the development of "genetically superior" offspring.

Cloning: Experiments in biologic engineering concerned with genetic duplication of individual organisms through asexual reproduction, as by cellular stimulation.

Code of medical ethics: Guidelines for the moral conduct of physicians.

Confidentiality: The responsibility of all health professionals to safeguard the privacy of patient records, files, and discussions.

Eugenics: The applied science of genetics that deals with efforts to improve the hereditary qualities of a species.

Euthanasia: The "merciful killing" of another human being, usually deemed to be terminally ill, and often at the patient's own request.

Genotype: The aggregate of genes that constitutes the individual's biologic heredity.

Hippocratic Oath: The oath concerning ethical professional behavior taken by physicians and attributed to the Greek physician, Hippocrates (460?–377? BC).

Medical ethics: The application of a moral code of behavior to medical practice.

Morality: The evaluation of human conduct in terms of the inherent rightness and wrongness of human actions.

Phenotype: The appearance, structure, and functional state of the body at a given moment in time. (Phenotype depend on genotype.)

Psychoanalysis: The technique, originated by Sigmund Freud, that explores and interprets past experiences to enable the patient to make personality adjustments. A specially trained psychoanalyst leads the patient through the course of treatment.

Psychosurgery: Surgical intervention for the purposes of altering behavior.

Psychotherapy: Therapeutic intervention, such as group and individual counseling, for the purpose of altering behavior.

Spontaneous abortion: The natural termination of a pregnancy; miscarriage.

Sterilization: Procedure by which an individual is made incapable of reproduction, such as castration, vasectomy, or salpingectomy (surgical removal of the fallopian tube).

Therapeutic abortion: The termination of a pregnancy for specific medical reasons.

Tubal ligation: The surgical tying or binding of the fallopian tubes as a contraceptive measure.

Vasectomy: The surgical removal of the ductus deferens (the excretory duct of the testis) or a portion of it as a contraceptive measure.

Universal Precautions

PART 1: GUIDELINES FOR
PREVENTION OF TRANSMISSION OF
HUMAN IMMUNODEFICIENCY VIRUS
AND HEPATITIS B VIRUS TO
HEALTH-CARE AND PUBLIC-SAFETY
WORKERS

In 1985, the Centers for Disease Control (CDC) developed the strategy of "universal blood and body fluid precautions" to address concerns regarding transmission of human immunodeficiency virus (HIV) in the health-care setting. The concept, how referred to simply as "universal precautions," stresses that *all patients should be assumed to be infectious for HIV and other blood-borne pathogens.* In the hospital and other health-care settings, universal precautions should be followed when workers are exposed to blood, certain other body fluids (amniotic, pericardial, peritoneal, pleural, synovial, and cerebrospinal fluids, semen, and vaginal secretions), or any body fluid visibly contaminated with blood. Because HIV and HBV transmission have not been documented from exposure to feces, nasal secretions, sputum, sweat, tears, urine, and vomitus, universal precautions do not apply to these fluids, or to saliva, except in the dental setting, where saliva is likely to be contaminated with blood.

For the purpose of this document, human "exposure" is defined as contact with blood, or other body fluids to which universal precautions apply, through percutaneous inoculation or contact with an open wound, nonintact skin, or mucous membrane during the performance of normal job duties.

The unpredictable and emergent nature of exposures encountered by emergency and public-safety workers may make differentiation between hazardous and nonhazardous body fluids very difficult and often impossible. Therefore, *when emergency medical and public-safety workers encounter body fluids under uncontrolled, emergency circumstances in which differentiation between fluid types is difficult or impossible, they should treat all body fluids as potentially hazardous.*

DISINFECTION, DECONTAMINATION, AND DISPOSAL

1. *Needle and sharps disposal.* All workers should take precautions to prevent injuries caused by needles, scalpel blades, and other sharp instruments or devices during procedures; when cleaning used instruments; during disposal of used needles; and when handling sharp instruments after procedures. To prevent needle-stick injuries, needles should not be recapped, purposely bent or broken by hand, removed from disposable syringes, or otherwise manipulated by hand. After they are used, disposable syringes and needles, scalpel blades, and other sharp items should be placed in puncture-resistant containers for disposal; the puncture-resistant containers should be located as close as practical to the use area (e.g., in the ambulance or, if sharps are carried to the scene of victim assistance from the ambulance, a small puncture-resistant container should be carried to the scene). Reusable needles should be left on the syringe body and should be placed in a puncture-resistant container for transport to the reprocessing area.
2. *Hand washing.* Hands and other skin surfaces should be washed immediately and thoroughly if contaminated with blood, other body fluids to which universal precautions apply, or potentially contaminated articles. Hands should always be washed after gloves are removed, even if the gloves appear to be intact. Hand

Source: Adapted from Thomas CL (ed): Taber's Cyclopedic Medical Dictionary, ed 17. FA Davis, Philadelphia, 1993, p. 2392, with permission. Adapted from Centers for Disease Control: Guidelines for prevention of transmission of human immunodeficiency virus and hepatitis B virus to health-care and public-safety workers. MMWR 38 (S-6), 1989. Recommendations for preventing transmission of human immunodeficiency virus and hepatitis B virus to patients during exposure-prone invasive procedures. MMWR CDC Surveill Summ 40 (R-8), 1991.

washing should be completed using appropriate facilities, such as utility or restroom sinks. Waterless antiseptic hand cleanser should be provided on responding units to use when hand-washing facilities are not available. When hand-washing facilities are available, wash hands with warm water and soap. When hand-washing facilities are not available, use a waterless antiseptic hand cleanser. The manufacturer's recommendations for the product should be followed.

3. *Cleaning, disinfecting, and sterilizing.* The following table presents the methods and applications for cleaning, disinfecting, and sterilizing equipment and surfaces in the prehospital setting. These methods also apply to housekeeping and other cleaning tasks.

REPROCESSING METHODS FOR EQUIPMENT*

Sterilization	Destroys:	All forms of microbial life, including high numbers of bacterial spores.
	Methods:	Steam under pressure (autoclave), gas (ethylene oxide), dry heat, or immersion in EPA-approved chemical "sterilant" for prolonged period of time, eg, 6–10 hours or according to manufacturers' instructions. Liquid chemical "sterilants" should be used only on instruments that are impossible to sterilize or disinfect with heat.
	Use:	Instruments or devices that penetrate skin or contact normally sterile areas of the body, eg, scalpels, needles, etc. Disposable invasive equipment eliminates the need to reprocess these items. When indicated, however, arrangements should be made with a health-care facility for reprocessing of reusable invasive instruments.
High-Level Disinfection	Destroys:	All forms of microbial life except high numbers of bacterial spores.
	Methods:	Hot water pasteurization (80°–100°C, 30 min) or exposure to an EPA-registered "sterilant" chemical as above, except for a short exposure time (10–45 min or as directed by manufacturer).
	Use:	Reusable instruments or devices that come into contact with mucous membranes (eg, laryngoscope blades, endotracheal tubes, etc.).
Intermediate-Level Disinfection	Destroys:	*Mycobacterium tuberculosis*, vegetative bacteria, most viruses, and most fungi, but does not kill bacterial spores.
	Methods:	EPA-registered "hospital disinfectant" chemical germicides that have a label claim for tuberculocidal activity; commercially available hard-surface germicides or solutions containing at least 500 ppm free available chlorine (a 1:100 dilution of common household bleach—approximately ¼ cup bleach per gallon of tap water).
	Use:	Surfaces that come into contact only with intact skin, e.g., stethoscopes, blood pressure cuffs, splints, and have been visibly contaminated with blood or bloody body fluids. Surfaces must be precleaned of visible material before the germicidal chemical is applied for disinfection.
Low-Level Disinfection	Destroys:	Most bacteria, some viruses, some fungi, but not *Mycobacterium tuberculosis* or bacterial spores.
	Methods:	EPA-registered "hospital disinfectants" (no label claim for tuberculosis activity).
	Use:	These agents are excellent cleaners and can be used for routine housekeeping or removal of soil in the absence of visible blood contamination.
Environmental Disinfection		Environmental surfaces that have become soiled should be cleaned and disinfected using any cleaner or disinfectant agent intended for environmental use. Such surfaces include floors, woodwork, ambulance seats, countertops, etc.

EPA—Environmental Protection Agency.

*To ensure effectiveness of any sterilization or disinfection process, equipment and instruments must first be thoroughly cleaned of all visible soil.

4. *Cleaning and decontaminating spills of blood.* All spills of blood and blood-contaminated fluids should be promptly cleaned up using an EPA-approved germicide or a 1:100 solution of household bleach in the following manner *while wearing gloves.* Visible material should first be removed with disposable towels or other appropriate means that ensure against direct contact with blood. If splashing is anticipated, protective eyewear should be worn along with an impervious gown or apron. The area should then be decontaminated with an appropriate germicide. Hands should be washed following removal of gloves. Soiled cleaning equipment should be cleaned and decontaminated or placed in an appropriate con-

tainer and disposed of according to agency policy. Plastic bags should be available for removal of contaminated items from the site of the spill.

Shoes and boots can become contaminated with blood. Where there is massive blood contamination on floors, disposable impervious shoe coverings should be used. Protective gloves should be worn to remove contaminated shoe coverings. The coverings and gloves should be disposed of in plastic bags.

5. *Laundry.* Although soiled linen may be contaminated with pathogenic microorganisms, the risk of actual disease transmission is negligible. Rather than rigid procedures and specifications, hygienic storage and processing of clean and soiled linen are recommended. Soiled linen should be handled as little as possible and with minimum agitation to prevent gross microbial contamination of the air and of persons handling the linen. All soiled linen should be bagged at the location where it was used. Linen soiled with blood should be placed and transported in bags that prevent leakage. Normal laundry cycles should be used according to the washer and detergent manufacturer's recommendations.

6. *Decontamination and laundering of protective clothing.* Protective work clothing contaminated with blood or other body fluids to which universal precautions apply should be placed and transported in bags or containers that prevent leakage. Personnel involved in bagging, transport, and laundering contaminated clothing should wear gloves.

7. *Infective waste.* The selection of procedures for disposal of infective waste is determined by the relative risk of disease transmission and application of local regulations, which vary widely. In all cases, local regulations should be consulted prior to disposal procedures and then followed. Infective waste in general should be incinerated or decontaminated before disposal in a sanitary landfill. Bulk blood, suctioned fluids, excretions, and secretions may be carefully poured down a drain connected to a sanitary sewer, where permitted. Sanitary sewers may also be used to dispose of other infectious wastes capable of being ground and flushed into the sewer, where permitted. Sharp items should be placed in puncture-proof containers and other blood-contaminated items should be placed in leak-proof plastic bags for transport to an appropriate disposal location.

Prior to the removal of protective equipment, personnel remaining on the scene after the patient has been cared for should carefully search for and remove contaminated materials. Debris should be disposed of as noted above.

FIRE AND EMERGENCY MEDICAL SERVICES

Fire and emergency medical service personnel deliver medical care in the prehospital setting. The following guidelines are intended to assist these personnel in making decisions concerning use of personal protective equipment and resuscitation equipment, as well as for decontamination, disinfection, and disposal procedures.

1. *Gloves.* Disposable gloves should be a standard component of emergency response equipment. All personnel should put them on before initiating any emergency patient care tasks involving exposure to blood or other body fluids to which universal precautions apply. Extra pairs should always be available. Considerations in the choice of disposable gloves include dexterity, durability, fit, and the task being performed. Thus, there is no single type or thickness of glove appropriate for protection in all situations. For situations where large amounts of blood are likely to be encountered, it is important that gloves fit tightly at the wrist to prevent contamination of hands around the cuff. For multiple trauma victims, gloves should be changed between patient contacts, if the emergency situation allows.

While wearing gloves, avoid handling personal items, such as combs and pens, that could become soiled or contaminated. Gloves that have become contaminated with blood or other body fluids to which universal precautions apply should be removed as soon as possible, taking care to avoid skin contact with the exterior surface. Contaminated gloves should be placed and transported in bags that prevent leakage and should be disposed of or, if reusable, cleaned and disinfected properly.

2. *Masks, eyewear, and gowns.* Masks, eyewear, and gowns should be kept in all emergency vehicles that respond to medical emergencies or victim rescues. These protective barriers should be used in accordance with the level of exposure encountered. Minor lacerations or small amounts of blood do not merit the same extent of barrier use as required for exsanguinating victims or massive arterial bleeding. Management of the patient who is not bleeding, and who has no bloody body fluids present, should not routinely require use of barrier precautions. Masks and eyewear (e.g., safety glasses) should be worn together, or a face shield should be used by all personnel before splashes of blood or other body fluids to which universal precautions apply are likely to occur. Gowns or aprons should be worn to protect clothing from splashes with blood. If large splashes or quantities of blood are present or anticipated, impervious gowns or aprons should be worn. An extra

change of work clothing should be available at all times.

3. *Resuscitation equipment.* No transmission of HBV or HIV infection during mouth-to-mouth resuscitation has been documented. However, because of the risk of salivary transmission of other infectious diseases (e.g., herpes simplex and *Neisseria meningitidis* infection) and the theoretical risk of HIV and HBV transmission during artificial ventilation of trauma victims, disposable airway equipment or resuscitation bags should be used. Disposable resuscitation equipment and devices should be used once and disposed of, or if reusable, thoroughly cleaned and disinfected after each use according to the manufacturer's recommendations.

Mechanical respiratory assist devices (e.g., bag-valve-masks, oxygen demand valve resuscitators) should be available on all emergency vehicles and to all personnel who may respond to medical emergencies or victim rescues.

Pocket mouth-to-mouth resuscitation masks designed to isolate emergency response personnel (e.g., double lumen systems) from contact with victims' blood and blood-contaminated saliva, respiratory secretions, and vomitus should be provided to all personnel who provide or potentially provide emergency treatment.

OTHER CONSIDERATIONS

1. *Handling deceased persons and body removal.* For any personnel who may have to touch or remove a body, the response should be the same as for situations requiring cardiopulmonary resuscitation or first aid: wear gloves and cover all cuts and abrasions to create a barrier and carefully wash all exposed areas after any contact with blood. The precautions to be used with blood and deceased persons should also be used when handling amputated limbs, hands, or other body parts. Such procedures should be followed after contact with *any* blood, regardless of whether the person is known or suspected to be infected with HIV or HBV.

2. *Autopsies.* Personnel should wear protective masks and eyewear (or face shields), laboratory coats, gloves, and waterproof aprons when performing or attending all autopsies. All autopsy material should be considered infectious for both HIV and HBV. Onlookers who risk exposure to blood splashes should be similarly protected. Instruments and surfaces contaminated during postmortem procedures should be decontaminated with an appropriate chemical germicide.

3. *Forensic laboratories.* Blood from *all* individuals should be considered infective. To supplement other worksite precautions, the following precautions are recommended for workers in forensic laboratories.
   a. All specimens of blood should be put in a well-constructed, appropriately labeled container with a secure lid to prevent leaking during transport. Care should be taken when collecting each specimen to avoid contaminating the outside of the container and of the laboratory form accompanying the specimen.
   b. All persons processing blood specimens should wear gloves. Masks and protective eyewear or face shield should be worn if mucous-membrane contact with blood is anticipated (e.g., removing tops from vacuum tubes). Hands should be washed after specimen processing.
   c. For routine procedures, such as histologic and pathologic studies or microbiologic culturing, a biologic safety cabinet is not necessary. However, biologic safety cabinets (Class I or II) should be used whenever procedures have a high potential for generating droplets. These include activities such as blending, sonicating, and vigorous mixing.
   d. Mechanical pipetting devices should be used for manipulating all liquids in the laboratory. Mouth pipetting must not be done.
   e. Use of needles and syringes should be limited to situations in which there is no alternative, and the recommendations for preventing injuries with needles should be followed.
   f. Laboratory work surfaces should be cleaned of visible materials and then decontaminated with an appropriate chemical germicide after a spill of blood, semen, or blood-contaminated body fluid and when work activities are completed.
   g. Contaminated materials used in laboratory tests should be decontaminated before reprocessing or be placed in bags and disposed of in accordance with institutional and local regulatory policies for disposal of infective waste.
   h. Scientific equipment that has been contaminated with blood should be cleaned and then decontaminated before being repaired in the laboratory or transported to the manufacturer.
   i. All persons should wash their hands after completing laboratory activities and should remove protective clothing before leaving the laboratory.
   j. Area posting of warning signs should be considered to remind employees of continuing hazard of infectious disease transmission in the laboratory setting.

PART 2: RECOMMENDATIONS FOR PREVENTING TRANSMISSION OF HUMAN IMMUNODEFICIENCY VIRUS AND HEPATITIS B VIRUS TO PATIENTS DURING EXPOSURE-PRONE INVASIVE PROCEDURES

INFECTION CONTROL PRACTICES

Previous recommendations have specified that infection-control programs should incorporate universal precautions (i.e., appropriate use of hand washing, protective barriers, and care in the use and disposal of needles and other sharp instruments) and should maintain these precautions rigorously in all health-care settings. Proper application of these principles minimizes the risk of transmission of HIV or HBV from patient to health-care worker, health-care worker to patient, or patient to patient.

As part of standard infection control practice, instruments and other reusable equipment used in performing invasive procedures should be appropriately disinfected and sterilized as follows:

1. Equipment and devices that enter the patient's vascular system or other normally sterile areas of the body should be sterilized before being used for each patient.
2. Equipment and devices that touch intact mucous membranes but do not penetrate the patient's body surfaces should be sterilized when possible, or under high-level disinfection if they cannot be sterilized before being used for each patient.
3. Equipment and devices that do not touch the patient or that touch only intact skin need be cleaned only with a detergent or as indicated by the manufacturer.

Compliance with universal precautions and recommendations for disinfection and sterilization should be scrupulously monitored in all health-care settings. Training of health-care workers in proper infection control technique should begin in professional and vocational schools and continue as an ongoing process. Institutions should provide all health-care workers with appropriate in-service education regarding infection control and safety and should establish procedures for monitoring compliance with infection control policies.

All health-care workers who might be exposed to blood in an occupational setting should receive hepatitis B vaccine, preferably during their period of professional training and before any occupational exposures can occur.

EXPOSURE-PRONE PROCEDURES

Despite adherence to universal precautions, certain invasive surgical and dental procedures have been implicated in the transmission of HBV from infected health-care workers to patients, and should be considered exposure-prone. Reported examples include certain oral, cardiothoracic, colorectal, and obstetric-gynecologic procedures.

Certain other invasive procedures should be considered exposure-prone. In a prospective study CDC conducted in four hospitals, one or more precutaneous injuries occurred among surgical personnel during 96 (6.9%) of 1382 operative procedures on the general surgery, gynecology, orthopedic, cardiac, and trauma services. Percutaneous exposure of the patient to the health-care worker's blood may have occurred when the sharp object causing the injury recontacted the pa-

tient's open wound in 28 (32%) of the 88 observed injuries to surgeons.

Characteristics of exposure-prone procedures include digital palpation of a needle tip in a body cavity, or the simultaneous presence of the health-care worker's fingers and a needle or other sharp instrument or object in a poorly visualized or highly confined anatomic site. Exposure-prone procedures present a recognized risk of percutaneous injury to the health-care worker, and — if such injury occurs — the health-care worker's blood is likely to contact the patient's body cavity, subcutaneous tissues, and mucous membranes.

Experience with HBV indicates that invasive procedures that do not have the above characteristics pose substantially lower risk, if any, of transmission of HIV and other blood-borne pathogens from an infected health-care worker to patients.

RECOMMENDATIONS

Investigations of HIV and HBV transmission from health-care workers to patients indicate that, when health-care workers adhere to recommended infection control procedures, the risk for transmitting HBV from an infected health-care worker to a patient is small, and the risk for transmitting HIV is likely to be even smaller. However, the likelihood of exposure of the patient to a health-care worker's blood is greater for certain procedures designated as exposure-prone. To minimize the risk of HIV or HBV transmission, the following measures are recommended:

1. All health-care workers should adhere to universal precautions, including the appropriate use of hand washing, protective barriers, and care in the use and disposal of needles and other sharp instruments. Health-care workers who have exudative lesions or weeping dermatitis should refrain from all direct patient care and from handling patient-care equipment and devices used in performing invasive procedures until the condition resolves. Health-care workers should also comply with current guidelines for disinfection and sterilization of reusable devices used in invasive procedures.
2. Currently available data provide no basis for recommendations to restrict the practice of health-care workers infected with HIV or HBV who perform invasive procedures not identified as exposure prone, provided the infected health-care workers practice recommended surgical or dental techniques and comply with universal precautions and current recommendations for sterilization or disinfection.
3. Exposure-prone procedures should be identified by medical, surgical, and dental organizations and institutions at which they are performed.
4. Health-care workers who perform exposure-prone procedures should know their HIV antibody status. Health-care workers who perform exposure-prone procedures and who do not

have serologic evidence of immunity to HBV from vaccination or from previous infection should know their Hepatitis B surface antigen (HbsAg) status and, if that is positive, should also know their Hepatitis Be surface antigen (HBeAg) status.

5. Health-care workers who are infected with HIV or HBV (and are HBe Ag positive) should not perform exposure-prone procedures unless they have sought counsel from an expert review panel and been advised under what circumstances, if any, they may continue to perform these procedures. Such circumstances should include notifying prospective patients of the health-care worker's seropositivity before the procedure.

The review panel should include experts who represent a balanced perspective. Such experts might include all of the following: (1) the health-care worker's personal physician, (2) an infectious disease specialist with expertise in the epidemiology of HIV and HBV transmission, (3) a health-professional with expertise in the procedures performed by the health-care worker, and (4) state or local public health officials. If the health-care worker's practice is institutionally based, the expert review panel might also include a member of the infection-control committee, preferably a hospital epidemiologist. Health-care workers who perform exposure-prone procedures outside the hospital or institution should seek advice from appropriate state and local public health officials regarding the review process. Panels must recognize the importance of confidentiality and the privacy rights of infected health-care workers.

6. Mandatory testing of health-care workers for HIV antibody, HBsAg, or HBeAg is not recommended. The current assessment of the risk that infected health-care workers will transmit HIV or HBV to patients during exposure-prone procedures does not support the diversion of resources that would be required to implement mandatory testing programs. Compliance by health-care workers with recommendations can be increased through education, training, and appropriate confidentiality safeguards.

CHAPTER OUTLINE

THE RESUME

PRODUCING THE FINAL RESUME
    Resume Length
    Typing the Resume
    Reproduction and Paper Quality
    Quantity

THE RESUME WITH COVER LETTER AND
    REFERENCE LIST

ENTERING THE JOB MARKET

THE INTERVIEW
    Professional Traits
    Questions to Anticipate
    Questions to Ask of the Interviewer

SUMMARY

BIBLIOGRAPHY

HIGHLIGHTS
    And the Winner Is . . .

LEARNING OBJECTIVES

Upon completing this chapter, you will be able to:

1. List and describe the parts of a resume.
2. Explain the purpose of the interview.
3. List at least three characteristics the interviewee ideally would display during the interview.
4. Describe the purpose and method of the postinterview follow-up.
5. Construct a resume.
6. Simulate the externship and employment interviews.

DACUM EDUCATIONAL COMPONENTS

1. Project a positive attitude (1.1A–E).
2. Show initiative and responsibility in past experience and education (1.8A–E).
3. Promote the profession by projecting the concept of the professional medical assistant (1.9C).

Afterword

Entry into Professional Employment

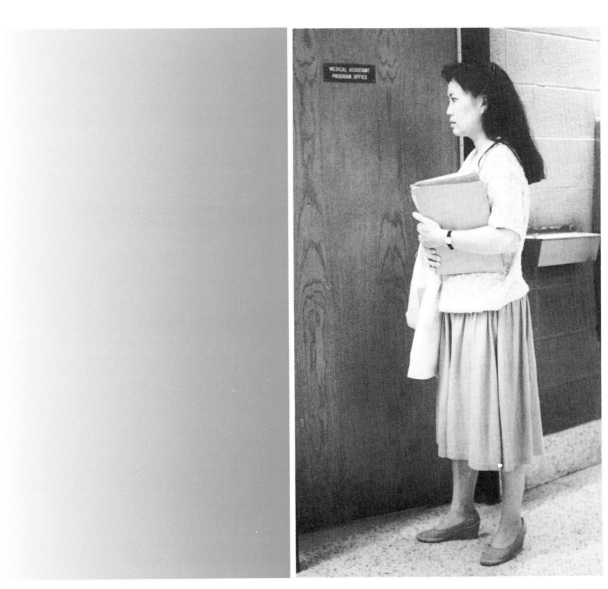

The final step in becoming a professional medical assistant is the task of finding appropriate and satisfactory employment after graduation. This process is a continuing aspect of professional development both for new graduates and for working medical assistants who are seeking to upgrade their positions. Therefore, this chapter provides information that will be useful to the medical assistant attempting to secure professional employment. In an effort to personalize the job-seeking process, we have deviated from the traditional third-person discussion characteristic of other chapters and have entered into dialogue with the student by using first- and second-person pronouns when appropriate.

Many students, and for that matter, many employed professionals, make the mistake of presuming that their educational training or their experiences represent an automatic calling card. They assume that potential employers will immediately recognize their competence and seek them out and hire them. Nothing could be farther from the truth. For those of us who are not movie stars or superathletes, the process of obtaining employment is not glamorous or ego supporting. We must, in effect, sell ourselves.

Unfortunately, most of us do not have formal training in sales and marketing. It is this fact that often leads to frustration and underutilization of medical assistants and other professionals. We simply fail to do a good job of marketing ourselves to prospective employers or we fail to recognize potential opportunities. Before seeking employment, we must orient ourselves to the concept of marketing and then choose, plan, and prepare the marketing tools that can be used to help us achieve our goal.

THE RESUME

The resume is a marketing tool of primary importance. It is to the job seeker what the brochure or catalog is to the salesperson. A salesperson must have up-to-date information about the product, and the information must be attractively presented. Likewise, the job seeker must have an attractive and effective resume. Remember that many inadequate products have been successfully marketed by individuals who were using "flashy three-colored brochures," whereas some of the best products ever developed have gone unnoticed because of poor advertising. It is also true that some very competent people have not been able to secure employment because of poor resumes.

A proper resume must be impeccable. It must be attractive, absolutely error-free, and inoffensive in its language and style. The major objective in designing a resume is to open doors to obtain an interview. Once an interview is obtained, personality and interpersonal skills will determine the outcome. First, however, our focus is to create the best possible resume that is compatible with our objective.

Many of the most essential aspects of resume construction are controversial. One reference source on resume design suggests that "no competent resume can

be without a particular feature," whereas another expert says "under no circumstances should you ever. . . ." While there are many alternatives available, the resume model discussed and illustrated here contains some aspects that are commonly desirable. A sample resume is depicted in Figure A–1 and contains the following primary sections:

1. *Name.* Begin with your name and be sure that your name stands out (is not overwhelmed by the address). The name should be italicized or written in all caps.
2. *Education.* Recent graduates should list their educational experiences next, beginning with the most recent schooling. It may be advisable for older persons to omit references to their high school and to begin with the employment section, placing the education section third (this places emphasis on the older person's best and most recent professional experiences).
3. *Employment.* Prospective employers are interested in seeing evidence of a work ethic. This means that it is useful to list the widest possible array of job experiences. For each job, list the firm, the job title, and an explanation of primary duties, responsibilities, and special accomplishments.
4. *Honors and Organizations.* As evidence of both breadth and accomplishment, it is useful to include a list of not only the organizations that you have participated in (be sure to mention offices held) but also the special honors that you have earned: academic, athletic, and service. These are indicative of potential for success.
5. *Interests and Activities.* Employers are interested in well-rounded individuals who will be able to bring fresh ideas into the office and relate well to a broad array of patients. For this reason, it almost always is useful to develop a comprehensive list of hobbies and interests.
6. *References.* We are advising persons against including a list of actual references with the resume. Since it is common within the course of a job search to learn that a particular reference person is not doing a good job of representing the applicant, or that for a particular opening a different reference would be better, we have found that it is best to list the names of the references on a separate sheet that can be given to the potential employer on request. On the actual one-page resume, simply state that "references will be furnished on request." This makes it more likely that the resume, itself, will be useful for a variety of situations.
7. *Statement of Professional Objectives.* There appears to be consensus that statements of objectives are better addressed in the cover letter. The rationale for this placement is that objectives may be contingent on the opportunities

Résumé

MARY ANN NISHIMURA
529 Shenley Drive
Erie, PA 16505
814 455-0724

Education

1985–87	Gannon University; Erie, Pa.
	Associate Degree in Medical Assisting, Academic minors in Management and in English. Vice President of the Student Medical Assisting Club, Member of Delta Chi Sorority, and two year participant on the intercollegiate Women's Soccer Club. Quality Point Average 3.40.
1982–84	Strong Vincent High School; Erie, Pa.

Employment

9/87 to present	Work-Study Aid, Gannon University; Erie, Pa.
	Various part time secretarial and administrative duties in offices of the University—
6/87–9/87	Clerk/Typist, Shotz Beer Co.; Erie, Pa.
	Served as one of three persons in the office secretarial pool. Had complete responsibility for various reports and the weekly newsletter—
9/86–6/87	Sales Clerk, Bentleys Dept. Store; Erie, Pa.
	Worked as part-time salesperson and had customer service and advertising duties—

Honors & Organizations	American Association of Medical Assistants, Pa. Academy of Science, Big Brothers and Sisters of Erie, Dean's List (Gannon U.) 1986 & 1987, Who's Who Among College Women: 1987, Honor Student (Strong Vincent H.S.) 1984 and 1985.
Interests & Activities	Tennis, Jogging, Coin Collecting, Classical Music, and Antiques.
References	Will be furnished upon request.

Figure A–1. A sample resume.

presented. Therefore, a more generic approach is preferred.

PRODUCING THE FINAL RESUME

The resume, like all other writing projects, is refined through a process of drafts culminating in a final perfect product. This final draft must be an attractive and professional representation of the individual seeking employment. Although graduation may be some time away, it is useful to begin thinking about resume design and perhaps to begin writing a resume for current use. The practice of writing a resume will alert the student to the areas needing particular attention in planning and perfecting the resume. Grammatical errors, word usage, and writing style are among the items that must

receive critical attention. Errors will obviously act as a significant roadblock to employment.

RESUME LENGTH

Many employment counselors recommend that younger persons or those just entering the job market should present one-page resumes. The experienced individual may need to expand the resume. In these instances, a maximum of two pages is advisable. It is also accepted practice to reproduce the resume "back to back" so that one sheet of paper is still all that is required.

Regardless of the length, the page or pages should be completely filled. A partially filled page gives the employer the impression that an applicant has too few accomplishments. One should get the impression from a resume page that the candidate had to struggle to get all of the accomplishments or experiences on the page. This creates a psychological expectation that the candidate is "even better" than the resume description.

TYPING THE RESUME

The particular style of type and the issue of whether or not a resume should be word-processed is not as important as quality. The work should not be flamboyant in style or type. It should be clear, easy to read, and perfect with regard to spelling, layout, and grammar. Many job applicants are finding that a word processor makes it both easier to achieve this level of aesthetic quality and to make changes from draft to draft.

REPRODUCTION AND PAPER QUALITY

If it is possible, the final copies should be professionally printed. The paper should be of the highest quality available and of a tasteful but distinctive weave. Although the use of colored paper for resumes is controversial, its use is becoming more widespread and acceptable. Many job applicants have had success with the use of a conservative color such as pale green, off-white, or beige. Remember that the point of a resume is to make you "stand out" from other candidates and to ensure that you obtain an interview. Paper quality and color may help to achieve this end.

QUANTITY

As you try to decide how many resumes to produce, remember that you will be using these to market yourself for some time and that you may be sending the completed resume to a large number of potential employers. The more resumes you distribute, the greater your potential market.

THE RESUME WITH COVER LETTER AND REFERENCE LIST

The rationale for choosing the generic resume with cover letter and reference list approach is based on the need for flexibility and efficiency. The generic resume contains only the basic information about the job applicant described previously. A carefully designed cover letter specifically addresses the job in question and includes an appropriate statement of your professional objectives. A separate list of references is developed for each particular job application.

The cover letter provides the opportunity to individualize the resume presentation. The cover letter may be a response to a specific advertisement or an inquiry into a potential opening. When the availability of the position is known, the cover letter should reflect this and should mention how you learned of the opening. Before writing the cover letter, try to learn as much as possible about the position and the potential employer. A telephone call to the potential employer's office to speak to an individual who can provide information regarding the nature and characteristics of the position will help to direct the choice and style of the content. It is also useful during this preliminary phone call to inquire about references. Ask if it would be appropriate to include references or letters of reference when mailing or presenting the resume. Once armed with this information, create a cover letter to accompany the resume which speaks specifically to your own suitability for the position and how your own professional objectives might be satisfied by employment. This can be a powerful method of stating professional objectives in lieu of using the more traditional format that lists the objectives on the resume. The letter should be brief (one page), include the date when you would be available to begin employment, and personalized using the potential employer's name and title. The neatness and general aesthetics of the cover letter and reference list are just as important as those aspects in the resume itself. A sample cover letter is included in Figure A–2.

Depending on the information regarding references obtained during the preliminary telephone conversation, references will be listed, included as reference letters, or furnished on request. When a list of references is preferred, it can be placed on a single 8½ by 11 sheet of paper with the heading "Professional References." Include for each reference a complete address, business name and title, and telephone number to facilitate the employer's contact with the individuals listed. A sample of a reference list is included in Figure A–3.

The individuals who are included in your list should be asked in advance for their permission to serve as references. If an individual seems to be reluctant, it is best to omit him or her from the list and include only those persons who are interested and willing.

The strategy of using one basic or generic resume and designing special cover letters and lists of references for each position represents a substantial advantage over a single mass-produced product. It allows for personalization and adaptation to a number of different circumstances.

The objective for designing the "promotional" material according to these guidelines is to obtain an interview. Marketing considerations, however, do not end once the interview is scheduled. The information that follows will alert you to the interviewer's concerns and the methods of assessment that he or she will display during the interview. In addition, you will be alerted to using the interview process as a tool for conducting your own evaluation of your suitability regarding the nature and characteristics of the position. However, before the interview process can be discussed, certain other considerations regarding marketing strategy must be mentioned. When the resume, cover letter, and reference list are developed, you must next determine where and how you will distribute them. In effect, you are now ready to enter the professional medical assisting job market.

M. P. Johnson, M.D.
10 Golfview Road
West Palm Beach, Florida 33401

Dear Dr. Johnson:

The placement office at the University of South Florida has announced an opening for a medical administrative office assistant in the offices of Anesthesiology Associates. In this regard I have enclosed my résumé for your consideration.

I will be graduating on May 27th and will be available for full-time employment anytime thereafter. May I see you at your convenience for an interview? You may reach me at the telephone number given on my résumé.

Thank you for your kind consideration.

Sincerely,

Sally M. Brown

Figure A-2. *A sample cover letter.*

ENTERING THE JOB MARKET

While preparing the resume, you reviewed your qualifications and most likely began to imagine yourself in a particular employment setting. In assessing your education and experience, you were able to recognize certain employment parameters, both personal and professional. For instance, if you have earned an associate's degree in medical assisting, you will most likely not be interested in becoming a unit secretary in a medical center that lists a high school diploma as the sole prerequisite. In addition, you may have determined that you are not willing to relocate. Conducting a personal inventory such as this will influence how and where you will direct your efforts in obtaining employment. You must also determine the types of practices or employment settings for which you are best suited and which capture your interest. Following one or more of these steps will help you to formulate a strategy for seeking employment that is compatible with your own needs and interests:

1. Visit the placement office at your school. Ask about job opportunities in the particular fields and geographic areas of your choice.
2. Contact by phone or in writing the officers of the associations of medical office professionals in specific areas and inquire about the opportunities available. Likewise, contact medical organizations, which often serve as placement referral services for physicians in their areas.
3. Contact medical centers and agencies (e.g., hospitals, health maintenance organizations, and medical specialty clinics) to inform them of your interests and availability and to learn of potential openings. Consult the Yellow Pages of the telephone book, the chamber of commerce, and the state employment service to identify health care organizations in your area.
4. Review classified listings in the newspaper.
5. Utilize the services of a professional employment service but be cautious about signing any agreement that requires you to pay a high percentage of your prospective salary or a large down payment for their services.
6. Ask for—and listen to—the advice of medical assistants working in your particular area of interest.

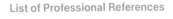

List of Professional References

1. Academic

Professor Philip Morley
Department of Secretarial Science
Milwaukee Junior College
Milwaukee, Wisconsin 53208
814-452-1110

2. Employment

Arnold Shotz, II
Managing Director
Shotz Beer Company
Milwaukee, Wisconsin 53207
814-481-8231

3. Character

Fr. Peter Black
Our Lady of Victory R.C. Church
212 Lilly Lane
Milwaukee, Wisconsin 53230
814-481-5061

Figure A-3. *A sample reference list.*

These suggestions will enable you to survey the market for the type and number of employment opportunities. You can then decide on the method of initial approach: contact by phone or in writing. Once the resume is received by the potential employer, a phone call to solicit an interview is appropriate. It is the interview that will ultimately determine the outcome of your pursuit of a particular position.

THE INTERVIEW

Because the interview is the most important phase of acquiring employment, the preparation, the content of the interview, and the follow-up must be accomplished appropriately.

Much of the time and effort spent on preparing for the interview will be focused on creating a particular image. Personal image is created not only by appearance (clothing and grooming) but by projected attitudes as well. Deciding how you will conduct yourself is as important as determining what to wear. The discussion that follows will alert you to what attitudes and personal characteristics are most often desirable. However, there are also certain modes of appearance acceptable in medical office settings. Those listed here are most common.

Wearing attention-getting colors or styles of clothing is not acceptable. Dark or neutral and well-fitting business attire is usually more appropriate. In choosing clothing for the interview, remember that your desire is to have the interviewer's attention focus on what you know rather than how you look. Avoid jeans and revealing clothing. Wear a clean, pressed, and comfortable outfit. Accessories should be subtle and be coordinated with the outfit. Hair and nails should be well groomed. Try on your chosen outfit in advance to test its comfort and appropriateness. Likewise, rehearse responses to anticipated questions. Adequate preparation will help you to be more confident during the interview.

The following guidelines will assist you in making a positive impression on the interviewer:

1. Arrive unescorted for the interview 10 to 15 minutes in advance of the appointed time. This practice demonstrates independence and dependability.
2. Introduce yourself to the secretary to demonstrate that you can take charge of the situation and use your own initiative.
3. When approached by the interviewer, introduce yourself and shake hands if you are comfortable doing so.
4. Listen attentively. Display eye contact.
5. Answer questions directly and honestly. Avoid one word answers except when appropriate. Ask for clarification when necessary.
6. Ask the interviewer questions related to the position.
7. When the interview is completed, thank the interviewer and acknowledge the secretary as you leave. Write a follow-up letter thanking the interviewer for the opportunity to discuss the position and include any pertinent information you may have forgotten during the interview.
8. Phone the interviewer when the appropriate amount of time has lapsed to learn the outcome if you have not been notified. You will ask the interviewer during the interview when you might expect to know his or her decision.

PROFESSIONAL TRAITS

The following professional traits are commonly preferred by interviewers:

1. *Confidence.* Confidence is displayed through eye contact, responding without hesitation, and asking pertinent questions.
2. *Assertiveness.* It is desirable and acceptable for the interviewee to ask the interviewer questions concerning the position.
3. *Interpersonal Communication Skills.* The skills discussed in Chapter 3 can be applied appropriately to the interview situation. Enthusiasm, interest, warmth, and confidence in your own educational and experiential preparedness are most often viewed as desirable characteristics.

QUESTIONS TO ANTICIPATE

The interviewer will most likely be interested in the manner in which you respond as well as in the specific content of your responses. It will be helpful to you in preparing for the interview to anticipate the types of questions that may be asked. Among the types of questions frequently asked on the interview are those listed below:

1. What are you seeking from this position?
2. Why did you choose the medical assisting profession?
3. What would you like to be doing 5 years from now?
4. What are your strengths? Weaknesses?
5. What administrative and clinical duties can you perform?

Some questions that might be asked are illegal, and you can decline to respond. These are related to:

1. Birthplace
2. Citizenship
3. Religion
4. Maiden name
5. Marital status
6. Children
7. Age
8. Height
9. Weight
10. Place of employment of your spouse or relatives

QUESTIONS TO ASK OF THE INTERVIEWER

After the interviewer has finished questioning the applicant, he or she usually invites the applicant's questions related to the opening being discussed. Because the period of questioning may distract you from remembering the questions you may want to ask, bringing a written list of general questions with you to the interview is recommended. You may wish to include the following questions:

1. Why has the position become available?
2. If not previously discussed, ask what administrative and clinical duties you would be expected to perform?
3. How will your performance be evaluated?
4. What are the opportunities for advancement?
5. What are the particulars: fringe benefits, vacation policy, work schedule, and salary.

After the interview, analyze your own performance and the information you received about the opening. Think positively about the interview, viewing it as a learning experience and practice session. Rate the potential for job satisfaction that the opening represents. Table A–1 is an example of a chart that can help in evaluating the attractiveness of the position. To construct such a chart, each factor to be considered is listed in the first column. Each factor is then rated on a 10-point scale (1 equals least important; 10 equals most important). For example, vacation and schedule are recorded as very importance (10) in the sample chart. The next step is to list each job offer in a separate column and to rate each factor separately on the same 10-point scale. For example, Drs. Smith and Green had excellent educational reimbursement plans, whereas Drs. Jones and Brown had none. Each factor rating is now multiplied by the general importance of that factor. Dr. Smith's salary offer is rated as 6 on a 10-point scale. This is multiplied by 9, the general importance of salary, to yield 54. On adding all of the totals in a column, you will find the value of a particular job offer to you. This process enables you to be thoughtful in making the employment decision and helps you to carefully prepare your response to offers.

All offers require a courteous response in writing that includes a thank you and, when nonoffensive, an explanation regarding your inability to accept the position. An affirmative response may be expressed in writing or by telephone.

SUMMARY

Seeking professional employment requires a thoughtful strategy and perseverance. The first posi-

Table A–1
JOB SELECTION CHART

Decision Factor	Importance	Job Offers			
		Dr. Smith	Dr. Jones	Dr. Brown	Dr. Green
Salary	9	6 (54)	2 (18)	8 (72)	1 (9)
Medical insurance	5	1 (5)	2 (10)	2 (10)	0 (0)
Dental insurance	4	0 (0)	0 (0)	0 (0)	5 (20)
Education plan	8	10 (80)	0 (0)	0 (0)	10 (80)
Uniforms	3	0 (0)	10 (30)	5 (15)	0 (0)
Sick Pay	2	0 (0)	0 (0)	5 (10)	5 (10)
Vacation	10	6 (60)	7 (70)	3 (30)	1 (10)
Pension	4	0 (0)	0 (0)	5 (50)	3 (15)
Office atmosphere	9	9 (81)	8 (72)	7 (63)	3 (27)
Schedule	10	5 (50)	5 (50)	6 (60)	2 (20)
Reputation	8	8 (64)	7 (56)	4 (32)	10 (80)
Total		394	306	312	259

tion begins your work history as a professional medical assistant and will have an impact on all future employment decisions. Energy and enthusiasm displayed in the first position, as well as clear goal setting, will help to make the first position satisfying and will open the door for greater opportunities.

BIBLIOGRAPHY

Balasa DA: Results of the 1991 AAMA Employment Survey. Professional Medical Assistant. XXIV:6, 1991.
Brown KW: How Employers Look At Job Applicants. Business Education Forum, January 1985, pp 5–6.
Drafke MW: Becoming a Professional in Health Care. FA Davis, Philadelphia, 1994.
Green D: Career second strategies. The Professional Medical Assistant XVIII:3, 1985.
Teel MR: Marketing yourself. The Professional Medical Assistant XX:2, 1987.

HIGHLIGHTS
And the Winner Is . . .

In applying for positions in medical assisting, you will be competing with other qualified medical assistants. Which of you will win the position? While there are many obvious factors that influence the interviewer's selection, a not-so-obvious factor is your own self-knowledge and your own determination of the characteristics of a desirable position.

Critical self-assessment is an essential prelude to obtaining job satisfaction. Self-assessment necessitates the evaluation of your own strengths and weaknesses. There are several ways of participating in self-evaluation assessment. A tool that can be used for this purpose is the Myers-Briggs Personality Test, which can help you determine what general work-related areas hold your greatest interest. Equipped with this information, you can set your own goals. Where do I want to be in 3 years, in 5, and 10, and what do I want to be doing? What types of positions and work settings would be most helpful in aiding me to achieve my goals? While these goals will remain flexible, they do provide some direction.

Another helpful tool in getting to know yourself and setting goals is "informational interviewing." Talking to other professionals working in the field and in situations that you regard as desirable can be help-ful in providing the perspective of reality — of real life experience. To be most productive, these "interviews" should provide you with the opportunity to ask questions and to check your own understanding of the profession and its opportunities. Be careful to select individuals who express enthusiasm and are willing to explain the benefits related to their careers but are also willing to share their own frustrations.

Know what you want and what you need to get there, and then set your sights on realistic goals. The employment opportunities today for medical assistants are boundless. The United States Department of Labor projects that the need for medical assistants will increase by 62 percent and that 207,000 medical assistants will be needed to fill the demands in 1995 (US News and World Report, December, 1985). The projection represents an 80,000 increase in the number of jobs from 1985 to 1995. Most assuredly, you will be enabled to attain your goals by becoming a highly qualified medical assistant who keeps current through continuing education programs, who maintains a vigil over the profession, and who is deeply concerned about health care issues and their impact on the profession.

And the winner is . . . YOU.

Index

A *t* following a page number indicates a table; an *f* indicates a figure.